Operative Techniques in Vascular Surgery

Second Edition

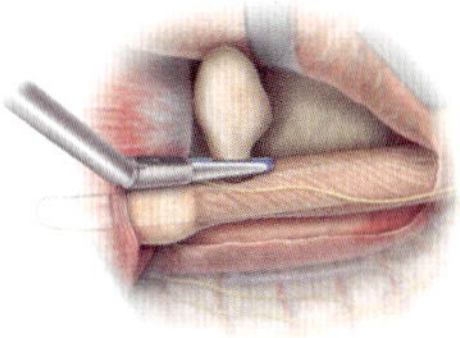
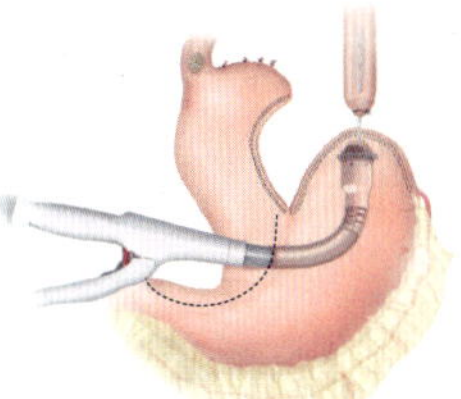
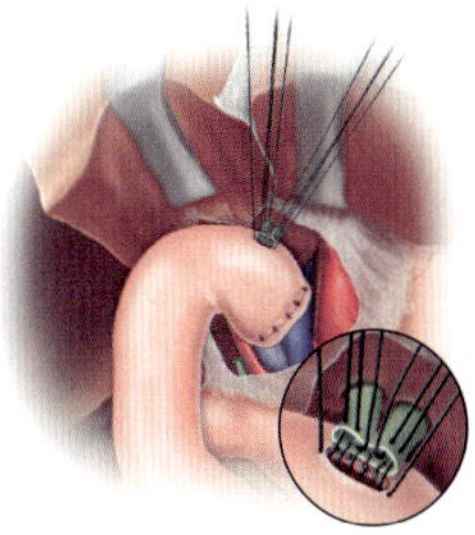
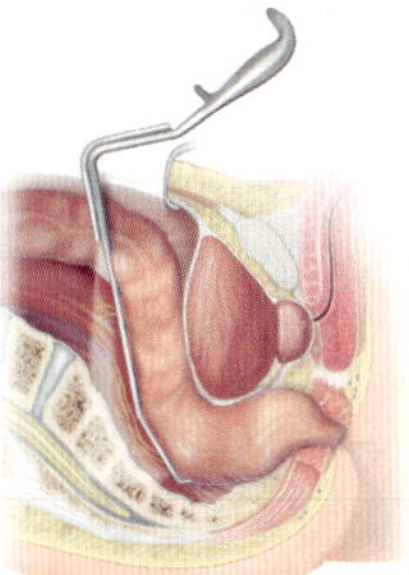
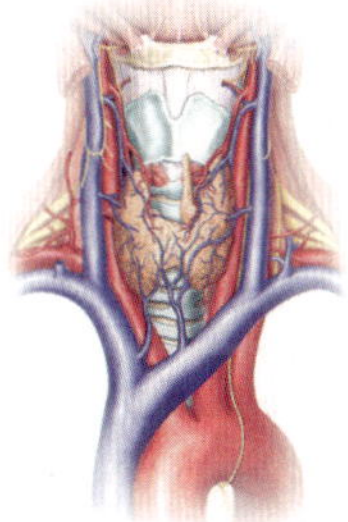
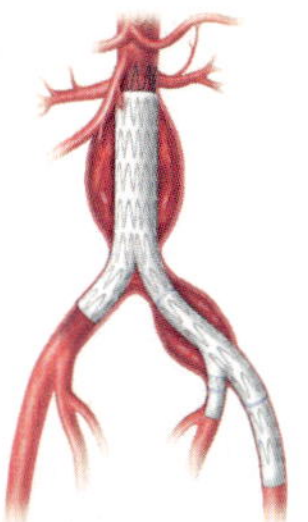
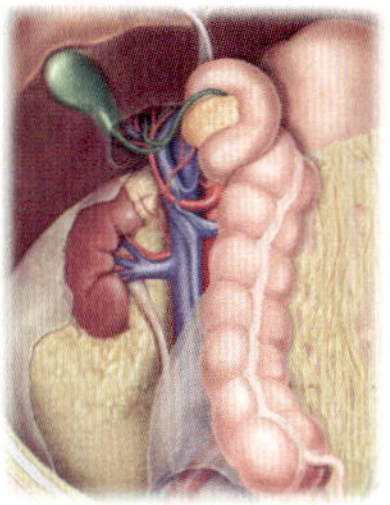

OPERATIVE TECHNIQUES IN VASCULAR SURGERY

Second Edition

Mary T. Hawn, MD, MPH
EDITOR-IN-CHIEF

Emile Holman Professor and Chair
Department of Surgery
Stanford University School of Medicine
Stanford, California

EDITOR
Kellie R. Brown, MD
Tenured Professor of Surgery
Division of Vascular and Endovascular Surgery
The Medical College of Wisconsin
Milwaukee, Wisconsin

Illustrations by: Body Scientific International, LLC

Wolters Kluwer

Philadelphia • Baltimore • New York • London
Buenos Aires • Hong Kong • Sydney • Tokyo

Senior Acquisitions Editor: Keith Donnellan
Senior Development Editor: Ashley Fischer
Development Editor: Barton Dudlick
Editorial Coordinator: Erin E. Hernandez
Marketing Manager: Kirsten Watrud
Production Project Manager: Bridgett Dougherty
Manager, Graphic Arts & Design: Stephen Druding
Manufacturing Coordinator: Lisa Bowling
Prepress Vendor: TNQ Technologies

9 8 7 6 5 4 3 2 1

Printed in Mexico.

Library of Congress Cataloging-in-Publication Data

ISBN-13: 978-1-9751-7664-8

Cataloging in Publication data available on request from publisher.

shop.lww.com

QUADM0323

Contributing Authors

Steven D. Abramowitz, MD, RPVI
Assistant Professor of Surgery
Chair, Department of Vascular Surgery
Georgetown University School of Medicine
Washington, DC

Georges E. Al-Khoury, MD
Assistant Professor of Surgery
Division of Vascular Surgery
University of Pittsburgh Medical Center
Pittsburgh, Pennsylvania

Olamide Alabi, MD, FACS
Assistant Professor of Surgery
Division of Vascular Surgery and Endovascular Therapy
Department of Surgery
Emory University School of Medicine
Atlanta, Georgia

Adham N. Abou Ali, MD
Division of Vascular Surgery
Department of Surgery
University of Pittsburgh Medical Center
Pittsburgh, Pennsylvania

Shipra Arya, MD, SM
Associate Professor of Surgery
Division of Vascular Surgery
Department of Surgery
Stanford University School of Medicine
Stanford, California
Section Chief, Vascular Surgery
VA Palo Alto Health Care System
Palo Alto, California

Bernadette Aulivola, MD, MS, RVT, RPVI
Professor
Department of Surgery
Loyola University Stritch School of Medicine
Director, Division of Vascular Surgery and Endovascular Therapy
Department of Surgery
Loyola University Medical Center
Maywood, Illinois

Kellie R. Brown, MD
Tenured Professor of Surgery
Division of Vascular and Endovascular Surgery
The Medical College of Wisconsin
Milwaukee, Wisconsin

Christopher Burke, MD
Assistant Professor of Cardiac Surgery
Department of Cardiac Surgery
University of Washington
Seattle, Washington

Ruth L. Bush, MD, JD, MPH, FACS
Associate Dean for Medical Education
Professor
University of Houston College of Medicine
Houston, Texas
Vascular Surgeon
Department of Surgery
Central Texas VA Healthcare System
Temple, Texas

Rabih A. Chaer, MD, MSc
Professor of Surgery
Department of Surgery
University of Pittsburgh Medical Center
Pittsburgh, Pennsylvania

Venita Chandra, MD, FACS
Clinical Associate Professor of Surgery
Division of Vascular Surgery
Department of Surgery
Stanford University School of Medicine
Stanford, California

Mark F. Conrad, MD, MMsc
Associate Professor of Surgery
Department of Surgery
Harvard Medical School
Boston, Massachusetts
Chief, Vascular and Endovascular Surgery
Department of Surgery
St. Elizabeth's Hospital
Brighton, Massachusetts

Esmaeel Reza Dadashzadeh, MD, MS
Vascular Surgery Fellow
Department of Vascular Surgery
Washington University School of Medicine
Saint Louis, Missouri

Ronald L. Dalman, MD
Walter Clifford Chidester and Elsa Rooney Chidester Professor of Surgery
Department of Surgery
Stanford University School of Medicine
Stanford Healthcare
Stanford, California

Elizabeth Dauer, MD
Associate Professor of Surgery
Department of Surgery
Lewis Katz School of Medicine at Temple University
Temple University Hospital
Philadelphia, Pennsylvania

Brian G. DeRubertis, MD
Assistant Professor
Chief, Division of Vascular and Endovascular Surgery
Department of Surgery
Weill Cornell Medicine
New York, New York

Peter DeVito, Jr., MD
Division of Vascular Surgery and Endovascular Surgery
Department of Surgery
University of Arizona Health Sciences
Tucson, Arizona

Kathryn Lambeth DiLosa, MD, MPH
Division of Vascular Surgery
Department of Surgery
University of California Davis School of Medicine
Sacramento, California

Shernaz S. Dossabhoy, MD, MBA
Division of Vascular Surgery
Department of Surgery
Stanford University School of Medicine
Stanford, California

Adam Joseph Doyle, MD
Associate Professor of Surgery
Associate Program Director Vascular Surgery Integrated Residency Program
Medical Director Noninvasive Vascular Laboratory
Department of Surgery
University of Rochester School of Medicine and Dentistry
Vascular Surgeon
Department of Surgery
University of Rochester Medical Center
Rochester, New York

Anahita Dua, MD, MSc, MBA
Assistant Professor
Division of Vascular Surgery
Department of Surgery
Harvard Medical School
Vascular Surgeon
Massachusetts General Hospital
Boston, Massachusetts

Audra A. Duncan, MD, FACS, FRCSC
Professor
Department of Surgery
Western University
Chair/Chief, Division of Vascular Surgery
London Health Sciences Centre
London, Ontario, Canada

David T. Efron, MD
Professor of Surgery
Department of Surgery
University of Maryland School of Medicine
Medical Director and Chief of Trauma
R. Adams Cowley Shock Trauma Center
Baltimore, Maryland

Javairiah Fatima, MD, FACS, RPVI, DFSVS
Associate Professor of Surgery
Georgetown University School of Medicine
Co-Director of Complex Aortic Center
Department of Vascular Surgery
MedStar Heart and Vascular Institute
Washington Hospital Center
Washington, DC

Arash Fereydooni, MD, MS, MHS
Department of Vascular Surgery
Stanford University School of Medicine
Stanford, California

Paula Ferrada, MD, FACS, FCCM, MASE
Professor of Medical Education
University of Virginia
Division and System Chief, Trauma and Acute Care Surgery
Inova Healthcare System
Falls Church, Virginia

Julie Ann Freischlag, MD
CEO, Atrium Health Wake Forest Baptist
Dean, Wake Forest University School of Medicine
CAO, Atrium Enterprise
Department of Vascular and Endovascular Surgery
Wake Forest University School of Medicine
Winston-Salem, North Carolina

Elizabeth Leigh George, MD, MSc
Division of Vascular Surgery
Department of Surgery
Stanford University School of Medicine
Stanford, California

Ashley R. Gutwein, MD
Assistant Professor of Surgery
Department of Vascular Surgery
Indiana University School of Medicine
Indianapolis, Indiana

Melike N. Harfouche, MD
Assistant Professor
Department of Surgery
University of Maryland School of Medicine
Attending Surgeon
R. Adams Cowley Shock Trauma Center
University of Maryland Medical Center
Baltimore, Maryland

E. John Harris, Jr., MD
Professor
Division of Vascular Surgery
Department of Surgery
Stanford University School of Medicine
Stanford Healthcare
Stanford, California

Joseph Patrick Hart, MD, MHL, FACS
Associate Professor of Surgery and Radiology
Division of Vascular and Endovascular Surgery
Department of Surgery
The Medical College of Wisconsin
Froedtert Hospital
Milwaukee, Wisconsin

Stephen Heisler, DPM, MHSA
Podiatrist
Department of Surgery
University of North Carolina School of Medicine
Chapel Hill, North Carolina

Thomas S. Huber, MD, PhD
Edward R. Woodward Professor and Chief
Division of Vascular Surgery
Department of Surgery
University of Florida College of Medicine
Gainesville, Florida

Misty D. Humphries, MD, MAS, RPVI, FSVS, FACS
Associate Professor of Surgery
Department of Surgery
University of California Davis School of Medicine
Sacramento, California

Jeffrey Jim, MD, MPHS
Chair, Vascular and Endovascular Surgery
Minneapolis Heart Institute
Abbott Northwestern Hospital
Minneapolis, Minnesota

Erika R. Ketteler, MD, MA
Associate Professor
Department of Surgery
University of New Mexico School of Medicine
Chief, Vascular Surgery
Albuquerque VA Medical Center
Albuquerque, New Mexico

Sharon C. Kiang, MD
Chief, Vascular and Endovascular Surgery
Chair, Institutional Review Board
Medical Director, Non-Invasive Vascular Laboratory
Associate Professor of Surgery
Department of General Surgery
Division of Vascular and Endovascular Surgery
Loma Linda Veterans Healthcare System
Loma Linda, California

Young Kim, MD, MS
Vascular Surgery Clinical Fellow
Division of Vascular and Endovascular Surgery
Massachusetts General Hospital
Harvard Medical School
Boston, Massachusetts

Dean Edward Klinger, MD, FACS
Professor of Surgery
Department of Surgery
The Medical College of Wisconsin
Milwaukee, Wisconsin

Matthew P. Kochuba, MD
Assistant Professor of Surgery
Department of Surgery
University of Florida College of Medicine
Jacksonville, Florida

Lindsey Marie Korepta, MD, RPVI
Assistant Professor of Surgery
Division of Vascular and Endovascular Surgery
Department of Surgery
Loyola University Stritch School of Medicine
Loyola University Medical Center
Maywood, Illinois

Rosemary A. Kozar, MD, PhD
Professor of Surgery
Department of Surgery
University of Maryland School of Medicine
Co-Director, Shock Trauma Anesthesia Research (STAR) Center
Shock Trauma Department
Baltimore, Maryland

Ashley Nicole Krepline, MD
Department of Surgery
The Medical College of Wisconsin
Milwaukee, Wisconsin

Nathan W. Kugler, MD
Assistant Professor
Division of Vascular Surgery
Department of Surgery
The Medical College of Wisconsin
Froedtert Memorial Lutheran Hospital
Milwaukee, Wisconsin

Gregory J. Landry, MD
Professor and Chief, Vascular Surgery
Department of Surgery
Oregon Health & Science University
Portland, Oregon

Cheong Jun Lee, MD
Associate Professor
Department of Surgery
University of Chicago
Chicago, Illinois
Division Chief, Vascular Surgery
Department of Surgery
NorthShore University HealthSystem
Evanston, Illinois

Jason T. Lee, MD
Professor
Department of Surgery
Stanford University School of Medicine
Chief, Division of Vascular Surgery
Department of Surgery
Stanford Healthcare
Stanford, California

Meryl Simon Logan, MD
Adjunct Assistant Professor
Department of Surgery
Texas A&M University College of Medicine
Vascular Surgeon
Department of Surgery
Central Texas Veterans Health Care System
Temple, Texas

Diletta Loschi, MD
Contract Lecturer
Medical Assistant
Department of Cardiothoracic Surgery
Vita-Salute University
San Raffaele Scientific Institute
Milan, Italy

Gregory A. Magee, MD, MSc, FACS, FSVS
Assistant Professor of Surgery
Division of Vascular Surgery and Endovascular Therapy
Department of Surgery
Keck School of Medicine of the University of Southern California
Los Angeles, California

Robyn A. Macsata, MD†

Germano Melissano, MD
Professor, Chair of Vascular Surgery
Department of Vascular Surgery
Vita-Salute San Raffaele University
Milan, Italy

Matthew W. Mell, MD, MS
Professor and Chief, Division of Vascular Surgery
Department of Surgery
University of California Davis School of Medicine
Sacramento, California

Joseph P. Minei, MD, MBA
Professor and Executive Vice Chair
Department of Surgery
UT Southwestern Medical Center
Surgeon-in-Chief
Parkland Health and Hospital System
Dallas, Texas

Erica L. Mitchell, MD, MEd
Professor and Interim Chief, Vascular and Endovascular Surgery
Department of Surgery
University of Tennessee Health & Science Center
Medical Director, Vascular & Endovascular Surgery
Elvis Presley Trauma Center
Regional One Health
Memphis, Tennessee

Mark D. Morasch, MD, FACS, RPVI
Chief, Vascular and Endovascular Surgery
Vascular Specialists at St. Mark's
St. Mark's Hospital
Salt Lake City, Utah

Courtney M. Morgan, MD
Assistant Professor of Surgery
Department of Vascular Surgery
University of Wisconsin School of Medicine and Public Health
University of Wisconsin Hospital Clinics
Madison, Wisconsin

Raghu L. Motaganahalli, MD, FRCS, FACS
Professor
Division of Vascular Surgery
Department of Surgery
Indiana University School of Medicine
Indianapolis, Indiana

Michael J. Nabozny, MD
Assistant Professor
Department of Surgery
University of Rochester School of Medicine and Dentistry
Rochester, New York

Robin B. Osofsky, MD
Department of Surgery
University of New Mexico School of Medicine
University of New Mexico Health Sciences Center
Albuquerque, New Mexico

Caroline Park, MD, MPH, FACS
Assistant Professor
Department of Surgery
University of Texas Southwestern Medical Center
Dallas, Texas

Abhijit S. Pathak, MD, FACS, FCCM
Professor of Surgery
Department of Surgery
Lewis Katz School of Medicine at Temple University
Philadelphia, Pennsylvania

Laura B. Pride, MMSc, PA-C
Medical College of Georgia
Athens, Georgia

Benjamin Pomy, MD
Department of Surgery
George Washington University Hospital
Washington, DC

Alyssa Jaesun Pyun, MD
Department of Surgery
Keck School of Medicine of the University of Southern California
Los Angeles, California

John E. Rectenwald, MD, MS
Professor of Surgery
Division of Vascular Surgery
Department of Surgery
University of Wisconsin School of Medicine and Public Health
Madison, Wisconsin

Jennifer E. Reid, MD, MS
Fellow
Department of Surgery
University of California, San Francisco
San Francisco, California

Kyle B. Reynolds, MD, RPVI
Assistant Professor of Surgery
Site Chief, MedStar Montgomery Medical Center
Department of Vascular Surgery
Georgetown University School of Medicine
Washington, DC

Enrico Rinaldi, MD
Chair, Department of Vascular Surgery
Vita-Salute San Raffaele University
San Raffaele Scientific Institute
Milan, Italy

†deceased

Lisbi del Valle RivasRamirez, MD
Assistant Professor
Department of Surgery
Johns Hopkins University
Baltimore, Maryland
Trauma and Acute Care Surgeon
Department of Surgery
Suburban Hospital
Bethesda, Maryland

Matthew John Rossi, MD
Department of Vascular Surgery
MedStar Washington Hospital Center
Washington, DC

Peter J. Rossi, MD
Professor and Chief, Division of Vascular and Endovascular Surgery
Department of Surgery
The Medical College of Wisconsin
Milwaukee, Wisconsin

Vincent Lopez Rowe, MD
Professor of Surgery
Department of Surgery
Keck School of Medicine of the University of Southern California
Los Angeles, California

Salvatore T. Scali, MD
Professor of Surgery
Division of Vascular and Endovascular Surgery
Department of Surgery
University of Florida College of Medicine
Staff Surgeon
Division of Vascular and Endovascular Surgery
Department of Surgery
University of Florida Health Shands Hospital
Gainesville, Florida

Oonagh H. Scallan, MD
Western University
London, Ontario, Canada

Malachi G. Sheahan, MD
Claude C. Craighead, Jr. Professor and Chair
Division of Vascular and Endovascular Surgery
Louisiana State University Health Sciences Center
New Orleans, Louisiana

Benjamin W. Starnes, MD, FACS, DFVS
Professor and Chief, Division of Vascular Surgery
Department of Surgery
University of Washington
Harborview Medical Center
Seattle, Washington

Nicole A. Stassen, MD, FACS, FCCM
Professor of Surgery
Department of Surgery
University of Rochester School of Medicine and Dentistry
Rochester, New York

Deborah M. Stein, MD, MPH
Professor
Department of Surgery
University of Maryland School of Medicine
Director of Critical Care Services
R. Adams Cowley Shock Trauma Center
University of Maryland Medical Center
Baltimore, Maryland

Kelly M. Sutter, MD
Fellow
Department of Trauma & Surgical Critical Care
MedStar Washington Hospital Center
Washington, DC

Kathryn Marie Swanson, MD
Department of Surgery
Louisiana State University Health Sciences Center
New Orleans, Louisiana

Matthew P. Sweet, MD, MS
Associate Professor
Division of Vascular Surgery
Department of Surgery
University of Washington
University of Washington Medical Center
Seattle, Washington

Robert W. Thompson, MD
Professor of Surgery
Director, Center for Thoracic Outlet Syndrome
Section of Vascular Surgery
Department of Surgery
Washington University School of Medicine
Attending Surgeon
Department of Surgery
Barnes-Jewish Hospital
Saint Louis, Missouri

Christine T. Trankiem, MD, FACS
Associate Professor
Georgetown University School of Medicine
Chief, Trauma and Acute Care Surgery
Department of Surgery
MedStar Washington Hospital Center
Washington, DC

Gabriela Velazquez-Ramirez, MD, FACS
Associate Professor
Department of Vascular and Endovascular Surgery
Wake Forest University School of Medicine
Winston-Salem, North Carolina

Michael A. Vella, MD, MBA
Assistant Professor
Department of Surgery
University of Rochester School of Medicine and Dentistry
Rochester, New York

Harold Davis Waller, MD
Department of Surgery
Massachusetts General Hospital
Boston, Massachusetts

Fred Arthur Weaver, MD, MMM
Professor
Department of Surgery
Keck School of Medicine of the University of Southern California
Chief, Division of Vascular Surgery and Endovascular Therapy
Department of Surgery
Keck Hospital of USC
Los Angeles, California

Lauren N. West-Livingston, MD, PhD, MSL
Division of Vascular and Endovascular Surgery
Department of Surgery
Duke University School of Medicine
Durham, North Carolina

Edward Y. Woo, MD
Professor of Surgery
Georgetown University School of Medicine
President
MedStar Medical Group
Washington, DC

Jacob C. Wood, MD
Assistant Professor
Department of Surgery
University of North Carolina School of Medicine
Chapel Hill, North Carolina

Brian K. Yorkgitis, DO, FACS
Associate Professor of Surgery
Department of Surgery
University of Florida College of Medicine
Jacksonville, Florida

Mohamed A. Zayed, MD, PhD
Associate Professor with Tenure
Department of Surgery, Radiology, Molecular Cell
Department of Biology & Biomedical Engineering
Department of Surgery, Section of Vascular Surgery
Washington University School of Medicine
Department of Surgery
Barnes-Jewish Hospital
Saint Louis, Missouri

Jeanette Zhang, MD
Assistant Professor of Surgery
Department of Surgery
University of Florida College of Medicine
Jacksonville, Florida

Wei Zhou, MD
Professor and Chief, Vascular Surgery
Department of Surgery
University of Arizona
Banner-University Medical Center
Tucson, Arizona

Series Preface

Operative interventions are complex, technically demanding, and rapidly evolving. *Operative Techniques in Surgery* seeks to provide highly visual step-by-step instructions to perform these complex tasks. The series is organized anatomically with volumes covering foregut surgery, hepato-pancreato-biliary surgery, and colorectal surgery. Breast and endocrine surgery as well as other topics related to surgical oncology are included in a separate volume. Modern approaches to vascular surgery are covered in a standalone volume. We also have a first edition standalone volume dedicated to trauma surgery. Additionally, many chapters are augmented by video clips dynamically demonstrating the critical steps of the procedure throughout the series.

The series editors are renowned surgeons with expertise in their respective fields. Each is a leader in the discipline of surgery, each recognized for superb surgical judgment and outstanding operative skill. Breast surgery, endocrine procedures, and surgical oncology topics were edited by Dr. Michael S. Sabel of the University of Michigan. Thoracic and upper gastrointestinal surgery topics were edited by Dr. Aurora D. Pryor of Donald and Barbara Zucker School of Medicine at Hofstra/Northwell, with Dr. Steven J. Hughes of the University of Florida directing the section on hepato-pancreatico-biliary surgery. Dr. Daniel Albo of University of Texas Rio Grande directed the section dedicated to colorectal surgery. Dr. Kellie R. Brown of Medical College of Wisconsin edited topics related to vascular surgery, including both open and endovascular approaches. New this year, we have added a section on Trauma and Critical Surgery, led by Dr. Amy J. Goldberg of Temple University.

In turn, the series editors recruited contributors that are world-renowned; the resulting volumes have a distinctly international flavor. Surgery is a visual discipline. *Operative Techniques in Surgery* is lavishly illustrated with a compelling combination of line art and intraoperative photography. The illustrated material provides a uniform style emphasizing clarity and strong, clean lines. Intraoperative photographs are taken from the perspective of the operating surgeon so that operations might be visualized as they would be performed.

The accompanying text is intentionally sparse, with a focus on crucial operative details and important aspects of postoperative management and potential complications. The series is designed for surgeons at all levels of practice, from surgical residents to advanced practice fellows to surgeons of wide experience.

Operative Techniques in Surgery would be possible only at Wolters Kluwer, an organization of unique vision, organization, and talent of Brian Brown, executive editor, Keith Donnellan, senior acquisition editor, and Ashley Fischer, senior development editor.

I am deeply indebted to Dr. Michael W. Mulholland, a master surgeon and leader and the editor in chief of the first series for *Operative Techniques in Surgery*. Without his leadership, this project would not have been successful. I am grateful to our new and returning series editors for their vision on how to make the second edition even more impactful. Curating and editing a major surgical techniques textbook during a worldwide pandemic has not been seamless, yet the outcome is masterful.

Mary T. Hawn, MD, MPH

Preface

As part of the *Operative techniques in Surgery* series, *Operative Techniques in Vascular Surgery* was created as a unique and comprehensive resource for residents, fellows, and practicing vascular surgeons alike. The authors of this text were chosen not only for their clinical expertise, but also their abilities as surgeon-educators. In designing this text, we have presented open, endovascular, and hybrid approaches to clinical problems; and have broken each procedure down into the necessary steps for success. The chapters are presented in outline form, for clarity and efficiency. In addition, the Pearls and Pitfalls section addresses the common areas for difficulty and discusses how to address those issues when they arise. Each chapter is filled with photographs and artwork to fully illustrate the text, allowing the reader to fully comprehend the techniques described.

A text such as this does not complete itself, and special thanks is due to the series editor, Dr. Mary Hawn, and the editorial and project management staff at Wolters Kluwer including Ashley Fischer and Keith Donnellan. On behalf of the authors, editors, and editorial staff, it is our hope that this text will be an invaluable reference for vascular surgeons at all levels.

Kellie R. Brown, MD

Contents

Video Contents List

SECTION I: Cerebrovascular Arterial Surgery/ Intervention

Chapter 1 Arch and Great Vessel Revascularization and Reconstruction

Matthew P. Sweet and Christopher Burke

DEFINITION

- The aortic arch is defined as the segment from the proximal end of the innominate artery ostium through the distal end of the left subclavian ostium (Ishimura Zones 1-3). This segment is a dynamic and complex anatomic structure: with compliance that augments coronary blood flow during diastole; a high degree of curvature as the aorta takes a 180° turn from an ascending to descending direction; and critical branch vessels. Rarely occurring in isolation, aneurysms of the arch are often extensions of aneurysms present in the ascending or descending thoracic aorta. The proximal and mid-arch is best approached surgically via a median sternotomy while the more distal arch is often best approached via a high posterolateral left thoracotomy. Given these anatomic and physiologic factors, surgical intervention on the arch necessitates a specific set of techniques.
- This chapter will focus on the management of aortic arch aneurysm and will attempt to combine the approaches utilized by both cardiac and vascular surgeons, each of whom bring discrete tools to approach these lesions. Leading aortic centers of excellence are moving toward multidisciplinary team-based approach with both cardiac and vascular surgeons and in varying circumstances interventional cardiologists, anesthesiologists, geneticists, and other team members to engage in care of these patients. This multidisciplinary approach facilitates individualization of the surgical approach without regard to which specialty drives the operation, integrates open and endovascular tools, improves comprehensive assessment and risk factor modification, and importantly helps anticipate future needs of the patient so that the operative approach may facilitate future care. Institutional infrastructure required to safely care for these patients includes fixed angiographic imaging, cardiac anesthesia, cardiac intensive care, and endovascular inventory.

PATHOPHYSIOLOGY

- Aortic arch aneurysms can occur from a variety of causes, most commonly atherosclerotic degeneration and degeneration of residual aortic dissection after prior ascending aortic repair for a type A dissection (DeBakey 1).
- Patients with genetic aortopathy (eg, Marfan syndrome) are an important group as they require disease-specific treatment. Genetic aortopathies run a wide spectrum of severity, and familial aortopathies without specifically identified genetic abnormality have worse outcomes than patients without family history.[1] Awareness of a potential genetic cause for aortic pathology can significantly affect treatment decisions and should be a routine component of patient evaluation.
- Less frequent etiologies include inflammatory (eg, giant cell arteritis), traumatic pseudoaneurysm (iatrogenic or traumatic), mycotic infectious aneurysm, and saccular aneurysms associated with penetrating atherosclerotic ulcers.

PATIENT HISTORY AND PHYSICAL FINDINGS

- As with any surgical practice, patient assessment begins with a thorough history and physical examination. History should include any prior chest or neck surgery or radiation, concomitant coronary or peripheral vascular disease, aortic insufficiency, smoking history, chronic obstructive pulmonary disease (COPD), and a thorough family history of aneurysm, dissection, or unexplained sudden death.
- Beyond the routine history and physical examination, we place particular importance on two factors: physiologic fitness and anatomic fitness.

Physiologic Fitness

- Physiologic assessment is a composite assessment of patient age, activity level, medical comorbid illness, and frailty. A young, active patient with few comorbidities who is not frail is more likely to tolerate an open operation and benefit from its long-term effectiveness and durability. Conversely, an older patient with more comorbidities and/or frailty may benefit from a less invasive approach and accept a less well-defined long-term effectiveness. Although age, in and of itself, is a poor metric of wellness, it is often used as a surrogate for anticipated remaining life expectancy, which is a critical concept when determining whether to proceed with prophylactic aneurysm repair. That said, octogenarians are clearly considered higher risk for open repair in general and except in very selected cases would typically be offered endovascular or hybrid repair.
- In terms of medical illness, specific attention needs to be paid to coronary artery disease, heart failure, heart valvular function, renal disease, liver disease, and pulmonary function. Concomitant coronary or valvular heart disease may require treatment at the time of open arch intervention or prior to endovascular therapy. Advanced nonischemic cardiomyopathy and severe COPD are conditions that would portend poor outcome from an open operation, particularly if cardiopulmonary bypass (CPB) is utilized.

- Frailty is different from medical comorbid illness. It is a multifactorial clinical syndrome associated with loss of metabolic reserve, physical capability, cognitive ability, and the ability to withstand physiologic stress. We use the Clinical Frailty Scale (CFS).[2] Open repair is generally considered problematic when the CFS is >4. This constellation of age, comorbid illness, and frailty can be used to classify patients as being at standard, increased, or prohibitive risk for both endovascular and open repair.

Anatomic Fitness

- To assess operative risk, one must understand the anatomic suitability of endovascular treatment and the technical feasibility of open repair.
- Each endovascular device has specific anatomic constraints as outlined in their instructions for use (IFU). Deviation from IFU is associated with a high risk of treatment failure. Similar to physiologic assessment, anatomic fitness can be assessed as standard, increased, or prohibitive risk. Features putting a patient at increased risk include calcific atherosclerosis of the arch vessels, small/diseased iliac access vessels, or significant aortic tortuosity. Prohibitive risk features include severe mural atheroma at the arch vessel ostia (aka "shaggy aorta"), absence of a suitable landing zone, or a dominant intercostal artery (artery of Adamkiewicz) where endovascular coverage might confer a very high risk of spinal cord injury. Furthermore, a patient with multiple moderate risk factors might, collectively, be considered prohibitive risk.
- Analogous anatomic risk factors influence the patient's suitability for open repair. Prior sternotomy with high-risk reentry anatomy, coronary bypass grafts, calcified aorta, and other factors may alter the patient's overall suitability for an open operation.
- To assess anatomic suitability, a computed tomography (CT) angiogram with 3D reconstruction on a workstation (eg, TeraRecon, 3mensio, or other) is essential.

IMAGING AND OTHER DIAGNOSTIC STUDIES

Imaging

- Contrast-enhanced fine-cut CT with arterial phase imaging (CTA) is the most important diagnostic test and is essential for any patient being considered for arch operation. ECG gated CTA is an useful tool when assessing the arch as it improves clarity by capturing images in the same phase of the cardiac cycle. Contrast is essential to assess for vessel patency, the presence of mural atheroma, dissection, wall thickening, and device sizing.
- The standard of care is to utilize a 3D workstation to evaluate the CT images. Two-dimensional imaging can be misleading as device sizing is based on the orthogonal plane (the plane that is perpendicular to the centerline of the aorta.)
- Moving from cranial to caudal, specific anatomic assessments for an endovascular approach include the following:
  - Arch branch vessels: patency, atherosclerotic disease, dissection, and aberrant anatomy (hemi-bovine trunk, left vertebral origin from the arch, etc.). For arch branch devices, one must also know the diameter, length, and quality of the innominate, left common carotid, and/or left subclavian arteries to determine if they will serve as suitable landing zones.
  - Aortic landing zones: defined as a segment of healthy, parallel aortic tissue with a <10% change in diameter or surgical graft without a sharp kink. One needs to assess diameter, presence of atherosclerosis, dissection, and atheroma. One also needs to assess the distance from the leading edge of the stent graft to the aortic valve. If the deployment needs to occur low in Zone 0, then the wire might need to cross the aortic valve to accommodate the nosecone.
  - Gantry angles: views with the fluoroscopy machine to optimize visualization of the arch and target vessels.
  - Aortic arch shape: a steep "gothic" arch may complicate stent graft delivery.
  - Distal aortic disease: occlusive disease, dissection, atheroma burden, or tortuosity that might complicate stent graft delivery to the arch.
  - Iliofemoral arterial access: Suitability of access for appropriately sized sheath (based on device sizing).
- Specific to an open operation:
  - Evaluation of the aortic root and valve for concomitant pathology.
  - Space between the posterior table of the sternum and the aorta, to determine the safety of redo sternotomy.
  - Anterior-posterior orientation of the arch, to assess the accessibility of the left subclavian artery (LSA) and distal sewing cuff.
  - Presence of aberrant arch vessel anatomy.
  - Presence of prior coronary bypass grafts, valvular operation, or other prior cardiac intervention.
  - Location of healthy, nondissected arterial cannulation site.

Other Diagnostic Studies

- Magnetic resonance imaging is useful as a screening tool, but the detail is insufficient for operative planning.
- Carotid duplex ultrasound can be helpful in the setting of concomitant cerebrovascular occlusive disease or prior stroke.
- Transthoracic echocardiogram is routinely ordered. It is required in patients with any clinical history of congestive heart failure, genetic aortopathies, or disease of the aortic root.
- Pulmonary function testing is not routinely obtained, but it is indicated in patients with a heavy smoking history or known COPD in whom an open approach is being considered.
- For patients being considered for open repair, a preoperative left heart catheterization is needed to assess for concomitant coronary artery disease requiring revascularization.

SURGICAL MANAGEMENT

- There are two general approaches to treatment of aortic arch aneurysmal disease, open and endovascular. Combinations of these techniques are termed "hybrid repairs."
- Open repair replaces the diseased aortic segment with a fabric surgical graft (typically Dacron). Open repair requires suitable exposure, use of CPB and often deep hypothermic circulatory arrest (DHCA), control of blood flow to the heart, brain, and viscera, and tissue adequate to sew to.
- Endovascular repair serves to reline the diseased aortic segment. The stent graft seals at either end in healthy aortic tissue or prior surgical graft, serving as a bridge across the diseased aorta. Just as with a bridge across a river with

foundations laid in a sand bar, a stent graft landed into diseased tissue may look good at completion of the procedure but will have poor durability. The depressurization of the aneurysm takes away the risk of rupture and often leads to aortic "remodeling" around the stent graft. This basic conceptual framework is essential as endovascular repair cannot be successful without adequate healthy tissue or graft to land the device within, where the device can both seal and fixate. In evaluating a patient with arch pathology, understanding their treatment options is entirely dependent on a comprehensive and quantitative assessment of their aortic anatomy.

This chapter will describe three options for aortic arch aneurysm repair, progressing from the most to the least invasive.

OPEN ARCH REPLACEMENT (WITH OR WITHOUT FROZEN ELEPHANT TRUNK AKA "FET")

- Meticulous preoperative planning and patient selection is critical to successful open aortic arch replacement. In general, these procedures are performed via a median sternotomy with the use of CPB and various DHCA techniques. Fundamentally, operative strategy is divided into the following aspects:
  - Assessment of reentry into the mediastinum, in the case of a reoperative median sternotomy (need for peripheral cannulation, cooling prior to reentry, need for left ventricular (LV) venting if significant aortic insufficiency is present, etc.).
  - CPB cannulation strategy.
  - Proximal and distal aortic extent of operation.
  - Cerebral protection strategy and temperature management (antegrade vs retrograde cerebral perfusion, or hypothermia only).
- The importance of thorough preoperative CTA evaluation of the aorta cannot be overemphasized. This is especially true in the reoperative setting. Cross-sectional imaging shows the position of critical structures to the posterior table of the sternum (innominate vein, right ventricle, aorta, bypass grafts, etc.). In the case of an aortic aneurysm that is in close proximity to the sternum, this can lead to a lethal situation if the aneurysm is injured on reentry. This is especially true if significant aortic insufficiency is present, as efforts to place on CPB and cool will result in LV distension if/when ventricular fibrillation occurs. In this circumstance, peripheral CPB cannulation is often performed. Lidocaine is given and the patient slowly cooled prior to sternotomy. Depending on risk, a LV vent can be placed directly by utilizing a small left anterior thoracotomy.
- The next critical aspect of preoperative planning is CPB strategy. Effective CPB facilitates a bloodless surgical field and allows cooling for DHCA and aortic arch reconstruction. Certain CPB strategies also allow convenient antegrade cerebral protection (ACP) during DHCA. The most commonly used strategy in this regard is right axillary artery cannulation. By placing clamps on the innominate and left common carotid artery (LCCA) during DHCA, ACP can be given via the right axillary artery to perfuse the brain during arch replacement (**FIGURE 1**). Other arterial cannulation options for CPB include central aortic, femoral, and various much less commonly used sites (eg, left axillary artery, innominate artery, etc.).
- The surgeon must have a clear, defined plan for the proximal and distal aortic extent of the operation. Proximal extent varies from aortic root replacement to supracoronary graft anastomosis. This decision rests on whether root pathology is present. Regarding aneurysmal disease, in general any aortic root with a maximum diameter in the sinus segment of greater than 4.5 cm warrants root replacement. This can be accomplished with associated aortic valve replacement (AVR) (Bentall procedure) or with a valve sparing root replacement (David or Yacoub procedure). In rare cases of asymmetric root aneurysms or sinus of Valsalva aneurysms, selective sinus replacement is possible, most commonly performed in the noncoronary sinus.
- The distal extent of the aortic operation is driven by the pathology being treated. Options include a hemiarch (**FIGURE 2**), which involves resection of the lesser curvature of the aorta and a single aortic anastomosis performed under circulatory arrest, or a variety of more extensive transverse arch operations including several hybrid strategies (**FIGURE 2**). A repair extended to Zone 2 can be performed with a thoracic endovascular aortic repair (TEVAR) stent graft deployed distally across the distal arch and into the descending aorta. The stent graft is then incorporated into the distal surgical anastomosis. This operation is a called a "frozen elephant trunk" as it fixates the TEVAR device and creates a strong platform from which to extend the repair distally in the aorta at a subsequent operation. Recently, due to the emergence of single-side branch aortic arch TEVAR, enthusiasm has increased for a Zone 2 arch replacement concept with creation of a TEVAR landing zone followed by interval endovascular therapy of Zone 3 or the

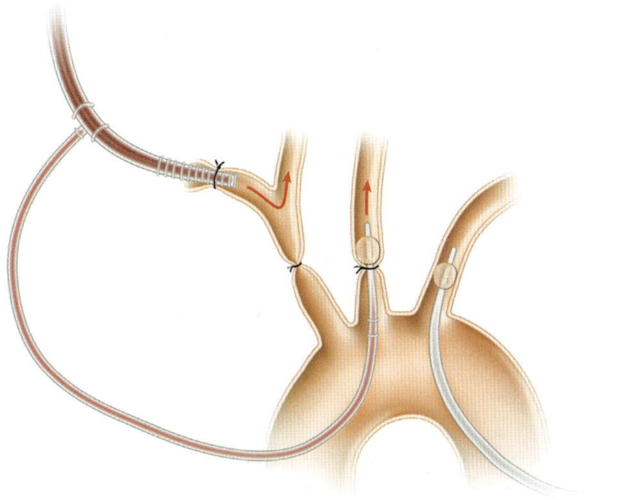

FIGURE 1 • Antegrade cerebral perfusion via axillary cannulation and left common carotid artery (LCA) and left subclavian artery (LSA) cannulation.

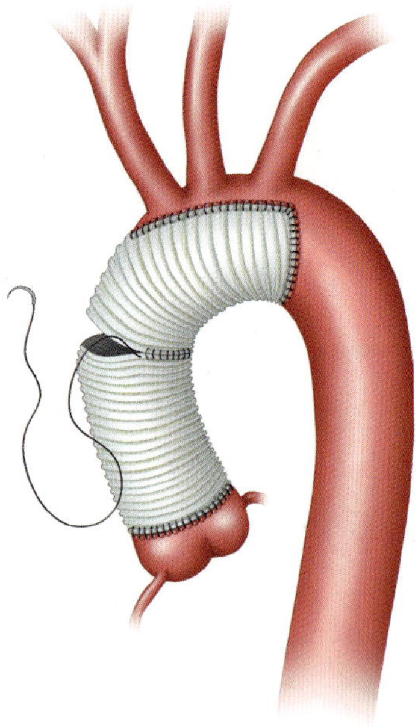

FIGURE 2 ● Ascending aorta and hemiarch reconstruction.

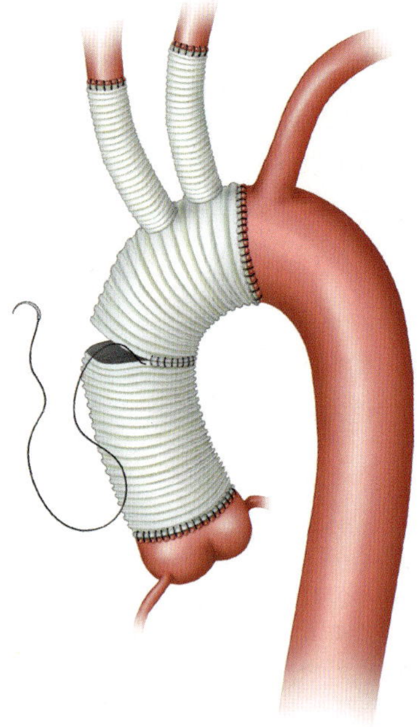

FIGURE 3 ● Ascending aorta and Zone 2 arch reconstruction.

arch as well as DTA (**FIGURE 3**).[3] This allows the surgeon a relatively straightforward arch operation with limited DHCA times.

- Cerebral protection strategies and temperature management are intimately associated. In general, the single most important cerebral protection strategy performed during open arch surgery is hypothermia. Temperature management most commonly varies from moderate hypothermia (MHCA, 22-28 °C) to DHCA (18-22 °C). However, most surgeons in contemporary practice will include cerebral perfusion techniques to supplement hypothermia. These include the antegrade (ACP, via the arterial system) and retrograde (RCP, infused through the venous system, most often the SVC) strategies. Advantages of ACP are the ability to provide nutritive blood flow to the cerebral circulation during periods of circulatory arrest. This also facilitates performance of arch operations at MHCA especially if straightforward repair is being pursued. As mentioned previously, right axillary artery cannulation provides a convenient strategy and is an excellent choice during arch reconstruction. Another option is to use balloon tipped cannulas down the carotid arteries. ACP strategies can be given unilaterally or bilaterally, although no difference in neurologic outcome has been shown between the two techniques. An exception would be when a precipitous fall in left-sided cerebral head saturations during right-sided unilateral ACP, which should mandate addition of LCCA ACP. Retrograde cerebral perfusion involves infusing cold blood into the SVC during periods of DHCA. RCP techniques are commonly used, though not necessarily limited, to straightforward arch reconstructions (hemiarch) and performed at deep hypothermic conditions. Advantages to this technique include the ability to "uniformly" keep the brain cool during circulatory arrest and may provide an "anti-embolic" flushing function as well. No significant difference has been shown in outcomes between ACP and RCP techniques, though there may be some evidence of lower rates of cerebral embolic events during hemiarch with RCP as compared to ACP.[4]
- Left carotid-subclavian (CS) revascularization: The left SCA can be approached in several ways. For complete arch replacement, routine revascularization is indicated to mitigate the risk of perioperative stroke. We generally perform transposition of the LSA to the LCCA in a staged fashion from a supraclavicular approach.[5] Staging the operation simplifies the open arch operation and is of particular importance when the LSA ostium is located more posteriorly, there is a separate origin of the left vertebral from the arch (seen in 5% of cases), or there has been prior open surgical intervention of the distal arch. The transposition also serves as a "stress test" for those patients of uncertain fitness for open repair. If a patient does not tolerate a transposition well, they are unlikely to withstand the stress of an open arch with DHCA and CPB. If the LSA ostium is located anteriorly in the chest making it more easily accessible during sternotomy, the patient has had prior left neck surgery/radiation, the case is urgent, or the logistics of a staged approach are otherwise problematic we tend to do the operation concomitantly with the arch (**FIGURE 4**).

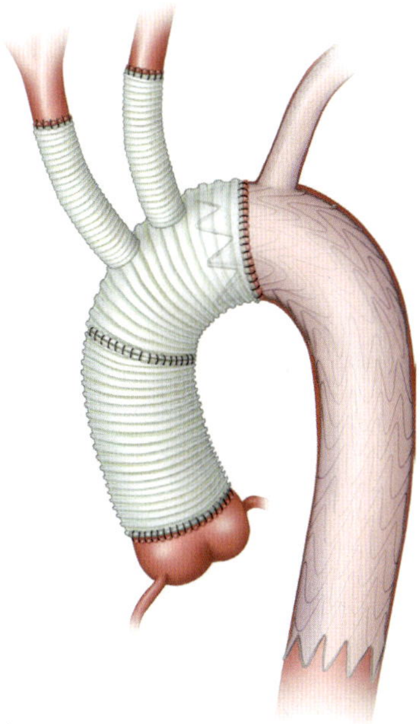

FIGURE 4 • Ascending aorta and Zone 2 arch reconstruction with Zone 2 gore thoracic branched endograft.

HYBRID ARCH DEBRANCHING

- Hybrid arch debranching was an approach that was developed for patients with a healthy ascending aorta and distal arch disease in whom total arch repair was considered to be too stressful. Via median sternotomy, a side-biting clamp is used to control the ascending aorta, from which a 10-mm Dacron graft is sewn on a steep upgoing bevel. This graft is then taken to the innominate artery. An 8-mm Dacron graft is sewn at a 90° angle from the more distal aspect of the 10-mm graft and taken to the LCCA. Following this debranching, a TEVAR procedure is done landing the proximal end of the stent graft in the distal ascending aorta (**FIGURES 5-7**). Several factors have led to a reduction in the use of this approach. First, the majority of patients with arch aneurysms have concomitant abnormalities of the ascending aorta, thereby necessitating a more extensive open operation. Among patients with a healthy ascending aorta or prior graft who are deemed high risk for open arch replacement, the advent of totally branched arch stent grafts has created a far less stressful, safe, and effective treatment option that obviates the need for sternotomy. The third reason is that as multidisciplinary teams have evolved, this operation has fallen out of favor. The appeal of the hybrid operation was that it could be done without CPB, but experience has shown that most patients are well treated with either a definitive arch operation or a branched stent graft, with the exception being the rare patients with severe arch vessel occlusive disease and otherwise healthy ascending aortic tissue.

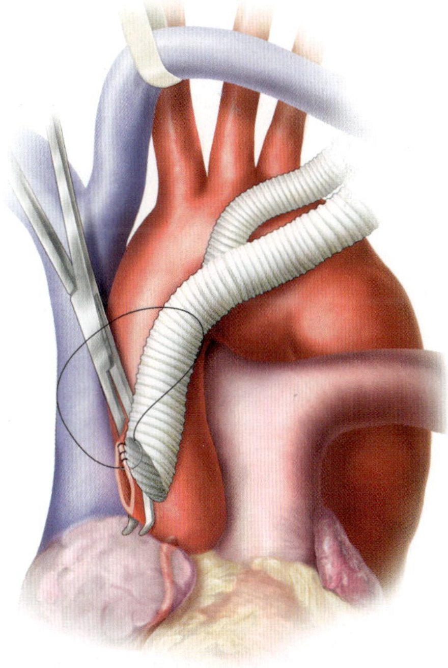

FIGURE 5 • An aortic side-biting clamp is placed on the right anterolateral side (convexity) of the ascending aorta, as low as possible. The proximal end of the larger (10 or 12 mm) graft is beveled and sewn end-to-side to the ascending aorta with a running 3-0 or 4-0 polypropylene suture.

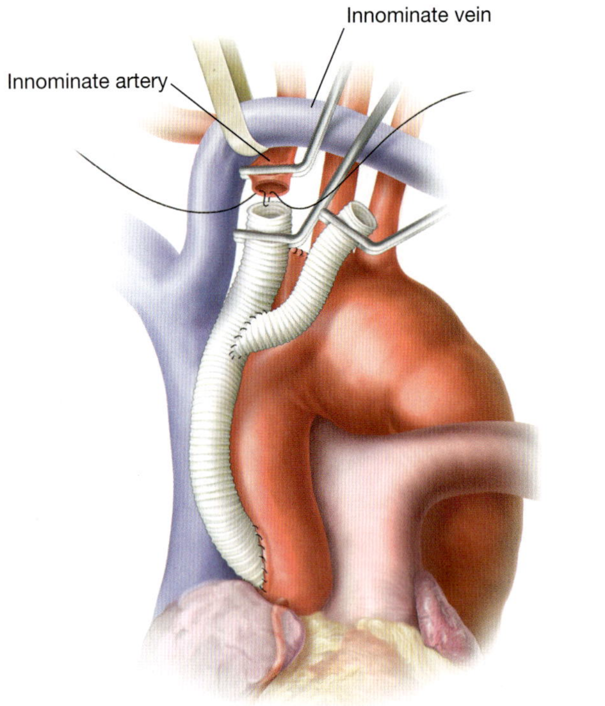

FIGURE 6 • The innominate artery is transected, and the proximal end is oversewn 4-0 polypropylene. The distal large end of the Y-graft is then tunneled underneath the innominate vein and sewn end-to-end to the innominate artery with running 5-0 polypropylene.

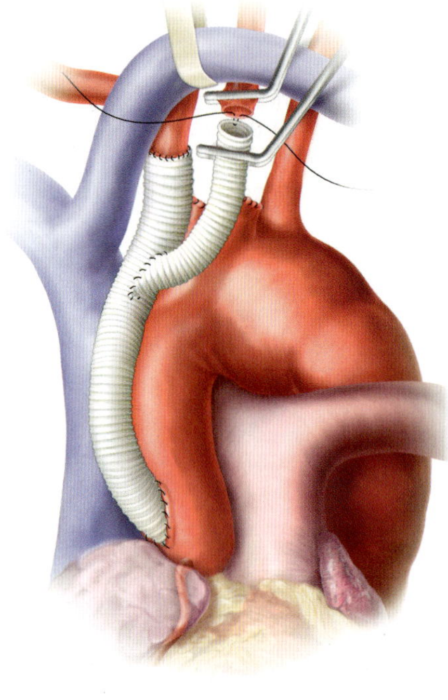

FIGURE 7 • The left common carotid artery is transected, and the proximal end of the carotid artery is oversewn with 4-0 polypropylene. The distal smaller end of the Y-graft is tunneled underneath the innominate vein and sewn end-to-end to the carotid artery with running 5-0 polypropylene.

TOTAL ENDOVASCULAR ARCH REPAIR

- Currently, there are no FDA-approved commercially available arch stent grafts in the United States. Several devices are in use outside the United States and trials for multiple devices are ongoing in the United States. Device design is primarily a function of device curvature to accommodate the arch and Zone 0 landing zone, delivery control, as well as branch and branching stent design. Given the consistency of arch anatomy, standard branch position(s) can accommodate most patients, obviating the need for customization.[6]
- Endovascular treatment of the arch requires several anatomic features:
  - suitable iliofemoral access or the ability to use a surgical iliac conduit
  - a healthy proximal landing zone in Zone 0, with either nondilated tissue or a prior surgical graft
  - distal landing zone in Zones 3 to 5 (or a surgical plan for a staged endovascular repair of the arch and thoracoabdominal aneurysm, which is beyond the scope of this chapter)
  - a thoracic stent graft with one or more side branches
  - patent and nondiseased great vessels to serve as a suitable distal landing zone
  - a strategy for cervical debranching

Access and Landing Zones

- First-generation arch graft technology requires large delivery systems as the branch adds significant material to the device. Current investigational devices run in the 22 to 26F range. It is possible that those sizes will come down as lower profile systems come forward.
- The proximal landing zone is one of the biggest limitations for endovascular arch repair. As described earlier, most patients with arch aneurysms have diseased ascending aorta. Ascending aorta diameters >38 mm is associated with significant increase in adverse events as the landing zone is ecstatic and intrinsically unhealthy. Prior surgical repair of the ascending aorta, as is typical for patients with postdissection arch aneurysms, can provide an excellent landing zone. The primary difficulty with ascending grafts is if they are kinked, leaving a short segment of parallel graft or when they are so short and/or distant from the innominate origin that the stent graft cannot reach the surgical graft when appropriately positioned adjacent to the arch vessels.
- The distal landing zone can be more flexible than the proximal. A grossly aneurysmal descending thoracic aorta will not provide seal, but separate surgical management of the distal aorta can be carried distal to the arch device.

Branched Arch Device

- There are two configurations for arch TEVAR devices: branches and fenestrations.
- A branched device utilizes a manufactured gate or cuff built into the main body of the device. The branching stent then has a 15 to 20 mm length of graft-to-graft interface with the main aortic stent graft, providing a stable and secure connection.
- Fenestrations are simply holes in the graft which can be manufactured with sewn reinforcement, or created using a technique of in situ fenestration with laser perforation and balloon dilation of a hole in the graft.
- There are two problems with the use of fenestrations in the aortic arch.
    - First, fenestrations must be located exactly to align with the target vessel, as malalignment will result in "shuttering" and failure of branch stent placement or excessive torquing on the interface between the branching stent and the aortic stent. Fenestrations for renal targets work well as there is usually a high degree of device rotational control in the abdominal aorta. That rotational control is gone when the device reaches the arch, so trying to align targets in the arch can require multiple attempts to withdraw and advance the device to rotate it in the more distal aorta. These manipulations are a risk factor for stroke and often are ineffective.
    - Secondly, fenestrations provide a very short length of interface between the branching stent and the main body, and as such, they provide a less stable interface. In the setting of in situ fenestration in particular, the repeated movement of the aorta during the cardiac cycle puts a significant stress on the device-to-device interface which likely cause tears in the TEVAR device with uncertain medium- to long-term durability.
- Given these limitations, all commercial arch devices under development in the United States use variations of a branched construct. Branched devices accommodate imperfect rotational alignment and create robust and durable interface between the aortic stent and the bridging stent.

Cervical Revascularization

- Cervical revascularization has been done using a myriad of surgical strategies.
- Our approach is to do a right common carotid to left common carotid bypass with 8-mm Dacron graft in a retropharyngeal tunnel with a concomitant left common carotid to left subclavian end-to-end transposition (**FIGURE 8**).
    - The patient is placed supine with a shoulder roll and their head at the very top of the OR table. The endotracheal tube and associated monitors are taken over the patient's nose/forehead and padded carefully.
    - On the left, a curved supraclavicular incision is taken from the midline for about 10 to 12 cm. Subplatysmal flaps are elevated. The heads of the sternocleidomastoid muscle are separated. The omohyoid is divided. The carotid sheath is then incised longitudinally. Care must be taken to watch for the vagus nerve which sits anterior in the carotid sheath in about 10% of cases. The vein and nerve are retracted laterally and the carotid artery medially. Lymphatic tissues are ligated with silk ligatures, carrying the dissection down to the medial border of the anterior scalene muscle, best identified by palpation as a firm/full structure in the midlateral base of the wound. The entire operation should be done lateral to the strap muscles. It can be difficult to palpate the subclavian artery, as the arch pulsation is transmitted throughout the wound, so I find that following the medial border of the anterior scalene is the best landmark to follow. The left vertebral vein will usually be the last structure to sit on the LSA, again this is ligated with silk ties. Generous use of silk ties is recommended to avoid lymph leak from what may be smaller lymphatic tributaries. The dissection is then taken down on the LSA to ensure exposure proximal to the vertebral ostium.
    - On the right, a 6-cm symmetrical incision is made centered over the anterior border of the sternocleidomastoid muscle, leaving a 1 to 2 cm of intact skin just right of midline of the neck. A similar dissection is performed, but it is necessary to control just a few centimeters of the right common carotid artery (CCA) so a far more limited dissection is required.
    - Once both dissections are complete, the retropharyngeal tunnel is created. To do so, create a small incision on the investing fascia overlying the anterior aspect of the cervical vertebrae. Use finger dissection from both sides, pushing hard against the anterior spinal ligament, to move across the retropharyngeal space. This tunnel is only 2 to 3 cm in length. During this dissection, it is imperative to stay as posterior as possible. One cannot damage the anterior spinal ligament with finger dissection, but you can injury the esophagus/pharynx if the dissection deviates anteriorly.
    - An 8-mm rifampin-soaked nonreinforced Dacron graft is then passed through the tunnel. Heparin is administered. The right CCA is then clamped and the proximal anastomosis created in an end-to-side fashion to the posteromedial aspect of the vessel. Once this is flushed/back-bled, flow is restored to the right CCA and the graft is clamped in the right neck.
    - The distal anastomosis is then created to the mid-left CCA in a symmetrical fashion.
    - Once this is complete, the LSA is ligated proximal to the origin of the left vertebral artery.
    - The LCCA is similarly ligated at the base of the wound.
    - The LCCA and LSA vessels are then anastomosed in an end-to-end fashion.
- This approach definitively deals with the proximal LCCA and LSA and avoids any risk of a stump syndrome. This reconstruction keeps the length of the bypass short and provides a clean and definitive reconstruction.
- This reconstruction is not suitable for a patient with a prior CABG and a left internal mammary artery (LIMA) bypass. In that case, the graft is taken end to side from the right CCA to end to side to the LSA and the LCCA is reimplanted end to side to the graft with ligation of the proximal LCCA. The proximal LSA is then coil embolized after the cervical revascularization is complete (**FIGURE 8**).
- A spectrum of approaches have been used for cervical revascularization, each with advantages and disadvantages.
    - Some surgeons use a ministernotomy and do the bypass in the anterior mediastinum. This minimizes the risk of

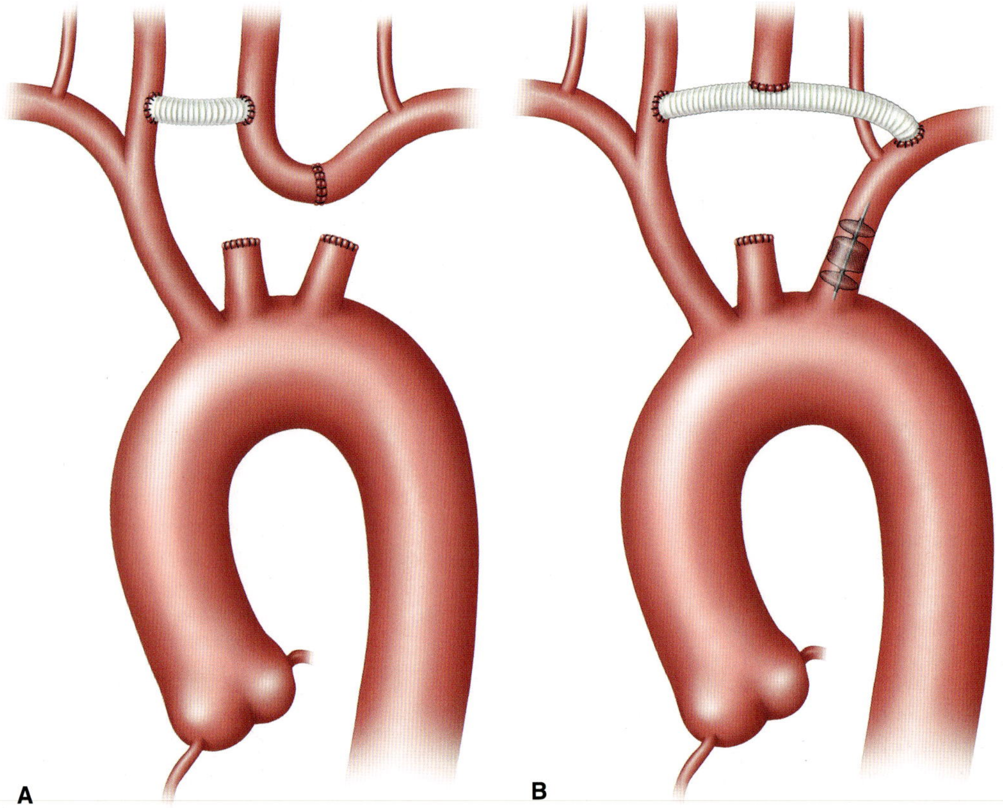

FIGURE 8 • **A,** Right to left carotid-carotid bypass with left carotid-subclavian transposition. The carotid-carotid bypass with a retropharyngeal tunnel minimizes the length of prosthetic graft and definitively deals with the left carotid and subclavian stumps. This does require a deeper neck dissection on the left to control the proximal subclavian and is not appropriate for patients with prior LIMA bypass. **B,** Right carotid to left subclavian bypass with reimplantation of the left carotid. This approach allows for *continued* flow in the LIMA, so is appropriate for patients with a prior CABG and patent LIMA graft. This operation also avoids deep exposure of the left neck but requires endovascular occlusion of the left subclavian ostium during the endovascular portion of the operation.

cranial nerve injury and creates a "near-anatomical" reconstruction, but one primary advantage of endovascular repair is to avoid sternotomy altogether, and this approach is unnecessarily invasive.

- Axillary to axillary collar bypass is a preferred approach by some centers in Japan. This is advocated as it has no risk of cranial nerve injury. Long subcutaneous extra-anatomic bypasses, however, have increased risk of thrombosis and infection in other anatomic locations. There are no data to inform that risk in this setting, but these are potentially catastrophic disadvantages to this approach.
- The retropharyngeal bypass has the advantages of a very short prosthetic bypass that is well protected from the surface within healthy vascularized tissue. Although some authors have expressed concern about dysphagia from a retropharyngeal bypass, this does not happen with nonreinforced Dacron, which will simply ovalize to fit the space. There are anecdotal reports of ringed PTFE used in the retropharyngeal space causing postoperative dysphagia which can be seriously problematic, although other surgeons have advocated for use of this bypass material.

CHALLENGES TO ENDOVASCULAR REPAIR

Stroke

- Stroke remains the greatest concern for total endovascular repair of the arch. Clinical trials have strict inclusion/exclusion criteria and may not reflect the "real-world" risk of this devastating complication. Factors of greatest concern include arch atheroma, diseased arch vessels, aorta-iliac tortuosity, and patients with prior stroke. There is no effective way to mitigate the stroke risk from atheroma at this time. Good case planning should minimize the device manipulation in the arch, but severe tortuosity can be troublesome. In that situation, using a 65-cm DrySeal Sheath (WL Gore) to try to straighten out the iliac and distal aortic tortuosity can help. Generous device flushing, including CO_2 flushing, will also reduce the number of MRI detected cerebral ischemic events.[7]

Aortic Valve

- An AVR is a major difficulty. A bioprosthetic valve can be more difficult to obtain wire access across. A mechanical AVR is essentially a strong contraindication as wire/catheter manipulation in the ascending/root can damage the valve with immediate unfixable aortic insufficiency.

Coronary Arteries

- Current first-generation arch branched endografts are designed to land in the distal 30% to 60% of the ascending aorta. In some cases, such as a patient with prior CABG or a prior short ascending interposition graft, the arch graft may extend in close proximity to a coronary ostium. In this case, it is helpful to consult with interventional cardiology and consider prewiring the coronaries.

Spinal Cord Injury

- Spinal cord injury due to coverage of thoracic intercostal arteries occurs in 2% to 3% of patients requiring treatment of the arch. The incidence rises with increased coverage of the descending thoracic aorta. Prevention is directed at maintaining higher systemic perfusion pressure and treatment uses the same plus lumbar drains to relieve pressure on the injured cord.

PEARLS AND PITFALLS

Endovascular repair

- A written step-by-step operative plan should be shared with team members ahead of the operation. This case plan facilitates each step by outlining the needed devices/wires/catheters/balloons and gantry views. This keeps the surgeon on track without distraction/skipping any steps, serves to remind the team of concerning aspects of the case, and helps the OR team prepare for each step in advance.
- Review the case plan with each operator knowing their role ahead of time. As deployment often requires several operators, it's essential that all team members are coordinated and understand the deployment sequence and their responsibilities during the case.
- Minimize wire/catheter/device manipulation in the arch. Accept "good enough" alignment of the device with the arch vessel rather than worry about "perfect" alignment.
- Cross the aortic valve with an atraumatic floppy wire and exchange for a dedicated intraventricular wire used for transcatheter AVR (eg, Safari wire).
- The device nosecone will often cross the aortic valve, which can cause temporary aortic insufficiency; therefore, the deployment process needs to occur smoothly and expeditiously. Communication with the anesthesia team is essential.
- Generous flushing of all devices/catheters to remove air is critical. Consider CO_2 flushing.
- Post-deployment trans-esophageal echocardiogram (TEE) can help ensure that the ascending aorta and aortic valve are functioning properly.
- Keep track of the length of time the large sheaths are in the femoral arteries. If the case proceeds slowly, these sheaths can be occlusive and cause pelvic and/or limb ischemia with devastating complications.

POSTOPERATIVE CARE

The care of open patients is beyond the scope of this chapter. A contemporary aortic center of excellence will have a dedicated cardiovascular intensive care unit experienced in the care of patients with both open and endovascular repair. Established protocols for neurologic monitoring for stroke and postoperative spinal cord injury in the setting of more extensive aortic coverage should be used to avoid variation in practice.

SUMMARY

- Five steps to proper arch aneurysm repair:
  1. Proper patient selection
  2. Proper case planning, device sizing, and team preparation
  3. Proper technical conduct of the operation
  4. Proper postoperative care, with the ability to recognize complications and "rescue" patients when complications occur
  5. Proper long-term follow-up surveillance and reintervention
- Attention is often focused on step 3, but successful patient treatment requires each of these steps.

REFERENCES

1. Shalhub S, Rah JY, Campbell R, Sweet MP, Quiroga E, Starnes BW. Characterization of syndromic, nonsyndromic familial, and sporadic type B aortic dissection. *J Vasc Surg*. 2021;73:1906-1914.
2. Rockwood K, Song X, MacKnight C, et al. A global clinical measure of fitness and frailty in elderly people. *CMAJ*. 2005;173:489-495.
3. Desai ND, Hoedt A, Wang G, et al. Simplifying aortic arch surgery: open zone 2 arch with single branched thoracic endovascular aortic repair completion. *Ann Cardiothorac Surg*. 2018;7:351-356.
4. Leshnower BG, Rangaraju S, Allen JW, Stringer AY, Gleason TG, Chen EP. Deep hypothermia with retrograde cerebral perfusion versus moderate hypothermia with antegrade cerebral perfusion for arch surgery. *Ann Thorac Surg*. 2019;107(4):1104-1110.
5. Morasch MD. Technique for subclavian to carotid transposition, tips, and tricks. *J Vasc Surg*. 2009;49:251-254.
6. Bosse C, Kolbel T, Mougin J, Kratzberg J, Fabre D, Haulon S. Off-the-shelf multibranched endograft for total endovascular repair of the aortic arch. *J Vasc Surg*. 2020;72:80-811.
7. Charbonneau P, Kolbel T, Rohlffs F, et al. On behalf of STEP collaborators. Silent brain infarction after endovascular arch procedures: preliminary results from the STEP registry. *Eur J Vasc Endovasc Surg*. 2021;61:239-245.

Chapter 2

Extrathoracic Revascularization (Carotid–Carotid, Carotid–Subclavian Bypass and Transposition)

Kyle B. Reynolds, Edward Y. Woo, and Steven D. Abramowitz

DEFINITION

- Extrathoracic revascularization of the proximal great vessels, including carotid–subclavian and carotid–carotid bypass, is characterized by arterial bypass outside of the chest cavity. Initially described for treatment of cerebrovascular and upper extremity occlusive disease, these procedures are also now employed to create a proximal seal zone for the endovascular treatment of thoracic aortic disease by "debranching" the aortic arch.
- Carotid–subclavian bypass is accomplished by creating a conduit between the mid-common carotid artery and the ipsilateral subclavian artery.
- Subclavian artery transposition divides the subclavian artery proximal to the vertebral artery origin and transposes the vessel onto the ipsilateral common carotid artery. It is an alternative means to revascularize the subclavian artery without the use of prosthetic conduit.[1]
- Carotid–carotid bypass provides flow from one common carotid artery to the contralateral common carotid artery.
- Carotid–carotid bypass performed in a right-to-left manner and in conjunction with carotid–subclavian bypass preserves the blood flow to the left brain while allowing for proximal extension of a thoracic endovascular aortic repair (TEVAR) to the distal margin of the innominate artery.

PATIENT HISTORY AND PHYSICAL FINDINGS

- The patient history should be focused on the identification of underlying cerebrovascular disease. A focused review of systems seeks to identify the presence of symptomatic cerebrovascular lesions. The medical history should be reviewed for prior head, neck or carotid surgery, as well as an external beam radiation to the head, neck, or upper chest region. A history of coronary revascularization, specifically with the use of the left internal mammary artery as the inflow, should also be identified due to the impact surgical revascularization may have on coronary flow.
- The physical examination should be focused on the detection of inflow segment atherosclerotic disease. Bilateral upper extremity blood pressures should be obtained; a difference of greater than 15 mm Hg indicates the potential presence of preexisting occlusive disease. Likewise, the presence of carotid bruits, delayed carotid upstrokes, or abnormal upper extremity pulses suggests arterial occlusive disease that should be delineated prior to extrathoracic reconstruction.
- Special attention should be directed toward a baseline examination of the cranial nerves and vocal cord function, particularly in patients with prior cervical surgical procedures. Indirect laryngoscopy should be performed preoperatively in patients with hoarseness or in whom a preexisting vocal cord or cranial nerve deficit had been noted.
- Neck mobility and the presence of cervical spinal disease should be assessed, as neck extension and rotation are required for adequate operative exposure. Patients with significant neck immobility may be poorly suited for these procedures.

IMAGING AND OTHER DIAGNOSTIC STUDIES

- Carotid duplex scanning should be used to identify carotid artery stenosis prior to bypass procedures. Failure to identify and address stenoses at the carotid bifurcation may lead to postoperative steal phenomenon resulting in neurologic sequelae. Manipulation of a diseased carotid artery may also increase the risk of intraoperative stroke. In these circumstances, concomitant or staged carotid intervention may be warranted.
- Computed tomographic (CT) angiography of the aortic arch and extracranial carotid arteries provides the anatomic detail necessary to plan for safe carotid–subclavian bypass, subclavian artery transposition, or carotid–carotid bypass. This study is complementary to duplex scanning, as it provides an anatomic, rather than hemodynamic, assessment of the vessels. For example, CT is helpful in visualizing the distortion caused by a large arch aneurysm to the course of the subclavian artery in relationship to the clavicle. This also allows for the preoperative identification of any aberrant anatomy.

SURGICAL MANAGEMENT

Preoperative Planning

- Neuromonitoring is a useful adjunct to ensure adequacy of cerebral perfusion via contralateral cerebral circulation via collaterals while the ipsilateral common carotid artery is clamped. Numerous modalities exist for neuromonitoring, such as electroencephalography, transcranial Doppler, cerebral oximetry, and somatosensory evoked potentials. Stump pressure measurement has also been shown to be effective in predicting adequate cerebral blood flow. A temporary shunt may be routinely placed prophylactically to maintain ipsilateral blood flow or selectively placed when monitoring indicates cerebral perfusion is inadequate after clamping. Inadequate collateral flow is infrequently encountered, as during these procedures only the common carotid is occluded allowing for retrograde flow from the external carotid artery.
- Invasive continuous arterial pressure monitoring should be routinely employed, with care to place the line relative to

the laterality of the procedure. Typically, the arterial line is placed in the contralateral limb or in a femoral artery.

Positioning

- The patient is positioned supine with the head rotated away from the operative side. A roll or pneumatic pillow is placed below the shoulders to allow for neck extension. Careful attention must be paid to achieve maximum neck extension while still supporting the occiput. The bed may be placed in a semi-Fowler position (supine with back of bed up at 30°) to reduce venous pressure and minimize bleeding.
- For carotid–carotid bypass, the head is positioned midline to facilitate bilateral dissection.

CAROTID–SUBCLAVIAN BYPASS

Exposure of the Subclavian Artery

- An incision is made from the lateral aspect of the clavicular head of the sternocleidomastoid (SCM) muscle laterally across the supraclavicular fossa. This is further developed through the subcutaneous tissue and platysma with electrocautery. If the external jugular vein is encountered, it should be ligated and divided.
- The clavicular head of the SCM may be divided to allow for adequate medial exposure. Up to one-half of the sternal head of the SCM may be divided if needed, but this is rarely necessary. The scalene fat pad is visualized and divided. It is preferable to divide and dissect the fat pad near its inferior and medial border so that most of the fat pad can be preserved and reclosed to cover the reconstruction. Care must be taken to identify and preserve the phrenic nerve as it courses over the anterior scalene muscle deep to the fat pad. The thoracic duct is easily identified. It should be ligated in the field of dissection to prevent significant morbidity from a postoperative lymphatic leak that can occur if unintentional injury occurs during dissection or retraction.
- Once the fat pad has been mobilized and the phrenic nerve identified and protected, the anterior scalene muscle is divided to reveal the subclavian artery (**FIGURE 1**). It is best to divide the muscle slowly and in layers to prevent injury to the underlying vessel. The subclavian artery is dissected circumferentially and controlled with vessel loops. Care must be taken when manipulating this vessel, as the subclavian artery is significantly more fragile and prone to injury than lower extremity arteries of comparable diameter (eg, femoral or popliteal). Depending on the method of reconstruction and location of the planned anastomosis, the thyrocervical trunk, inferior mammary, and vertebral arteries may need to be individually controlled (**FIGURE 2**).

Exposure of Carotid Artery

- In the medial aspect of the wound, the lateral border of the internal jugular vein is identified and dissected. The vein is then retracted posteriorly, and the carotid sheath is entered from the posterolateral margin. Care must be taken to identify the vagus nerve, as its usual posterior position places it immediately in the field of dissection as the sheath is opened from this approach.

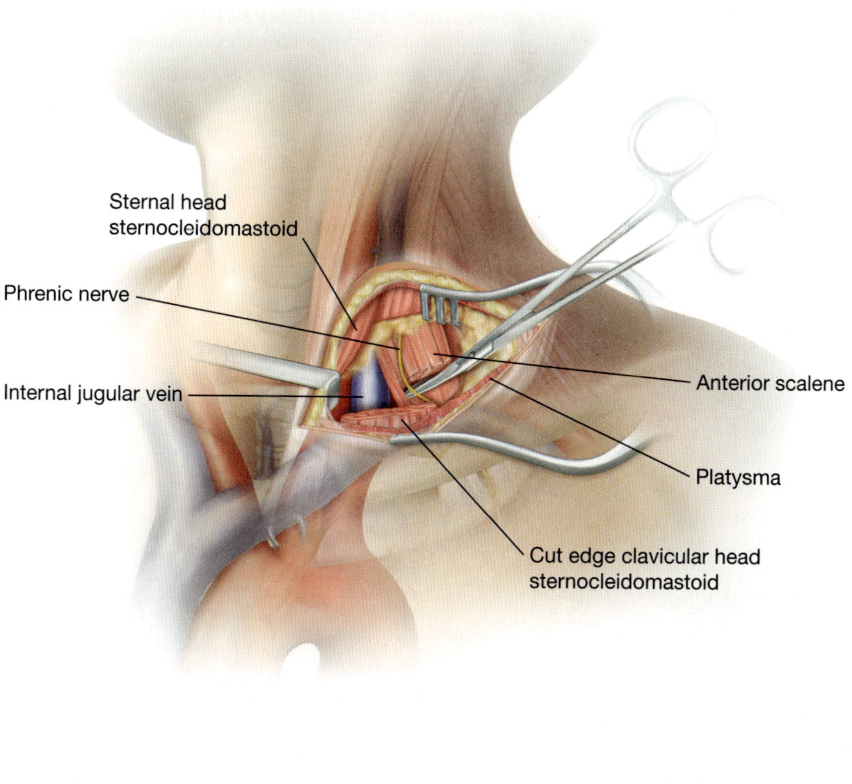

FIGURE 1 • The skin incision is placed in the supraclavicular fossa over the clavicular head of the sternocleidomastoid muscle. The subclavian artery lies directly beneath the anterior scalene muscle. Care must be taken to identify and preserve the phrenic nerve when dividing the anterior scalene muscle.

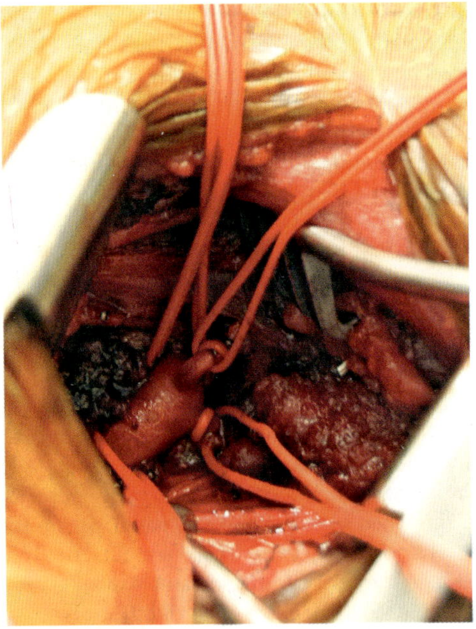

FIGURE 2 • The subclavian artery and its branches are circumferentially dissected and controlled with vessel loops.

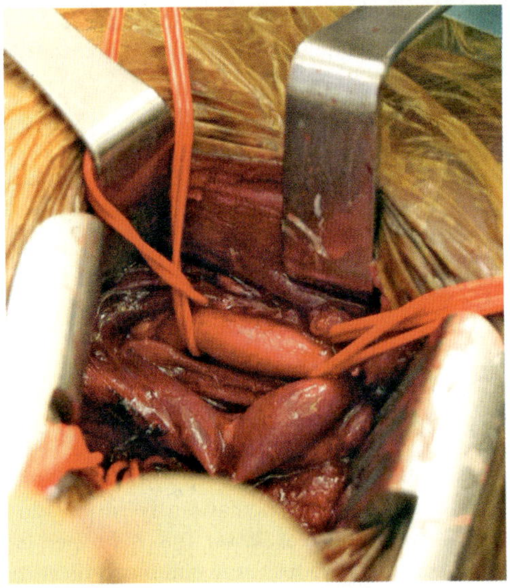

FIGURE 3 • The carotid artery is dissected circumferentially after entering the carotid sheath from its posterior lateral margin. The internal jugular vein can be seen retracted out of the way. The vagus nerve is running parallel to the artery between it and the nerve.

- The common carotid artery is dissected circumferentially (**FIGURE 3**). Only 5 cm of artery needs to be isolated to allow for surgical control and to perform the anastomosis. The dissection should remain proximal to the carotid bulb, thus minimizing the risk of cerebral embolization and injury to more distal nerves.

Bypass

- Dacron or polytetrafluoroethylene (PTFE) grafts can be used as conduits for extrathoracic bypass with no difference in outcomes such as patency or infection.[2] Autogenous vein grafts should be avoided, however, as their long-term patency is inferior to prosthetic in this location.[3]
- Prior to arterial clamping, systemic anticoagulation is achieved with intravenous heparin administration. The activated clotting time should be monitored and additional heparin administered throughout the procedure to maintain adequate anticoagulation.
- The subclavian anastomosis is performed first. Arterial control (vessel loops or clamps) is obtained and the vessel is opened with a longitudinal arteriotomy. The anastomosis should be fashioned in the position most favorable to the anatomic course of the planned graft. The graft is beveled and trimmed so that the graft lies at an approximately 60° angle to the artery. A running Prolene suture is used to perform the anastomosis with completion of the back wall first. Once the anastomosis is complete, the graft is clamped, and flow restored to the arm after flushing the inflow and outflow segments through the graft to remove any potential embolic debris. The graft should also be flushed with heparinized saline and clamped near the anastomosis to avoid thrombosis within the stagnant blood column contained within the graft. If repairs are needed for hemostasis, control is restored and pledgeted sutures are used to avoid injury to the fragile artery.
- The graft is tunneled in a retrojugular fashion. It is then tailored to the appropriate length to prevent redundancy and kinking. If beveling, the heel of the anastomosis should lie proximally on the carotid artery. As the common carotid artery is clamped, special attention should be paid to the patients' mean arterial pressure or systolic blood pressure as well as to any neuromonitoring being used. Shunt placement would be performed during this stage of the procedure. A longitudinal arteriotomy is performed and the proximal anastomosis completed with running Prolene suture, again starting with the back wall (**FIGURES 4** and **5**).
- The final sequence of clamp removal is important to prevent embolism to the brain. Proximal subclavian artery control is again obtained, and the clamp is removed from the graft. The proximal carotid clamp is then removed to allow "flushing" down the arm rather than to the brain. After a few cardiac cycles, the distal carotid clamp is also removed. The proximal subclavian artery clamp is then released.
- When performed in anticipation of thoracic aortic stent grafting, the subclavian artery must be ligated proximal to the origin of the vertebral artery. This can involve dissection deep into the mediastinum, which may be associated with significant morbidity and potentially catastrophic bleeding. Alternatively, the proximal subclavian artery can be occluded via placement of an intra-arterial occlusion device (eg, Amplatzer plug), by endovascular access to the carotid–subclavian bypass or after subsequent stent graft placement via a left radial or brachial artery percutaneous approach.[4]

Closure

- If a pneumatic pillow was used to provide exposure, it is deflated prior to wound closure in order to reduce neck extension and assist in closing the incision without tension from extension.

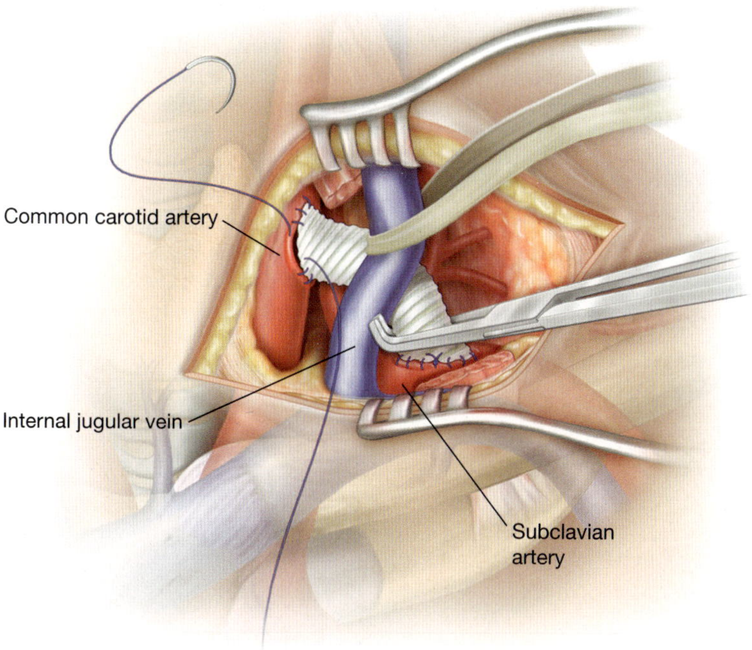

FIGURE 4 • After completing the distal anastomosis, the graft and the subclavian artery are all controlled and the proximal anastomosis is performed in a running fashion. The graft can be tunneled superficial or deep to the internal jugular vein depending on patient anatomy and surgeon preference.

- A closed suction drain may be left in the deep wound and brought out through a separate stab incision, depending on surgeon preference.
- In order to provide coverage for the graft, the scalene fat pad is returned to its anatomic location and sutured in place. The SCM is reapproximated with running absorbable sutures.
- The platysma and subcutaneous tissues are closed in separate layers in a running fashion and the skin is reapproximated with a running dermal suture.

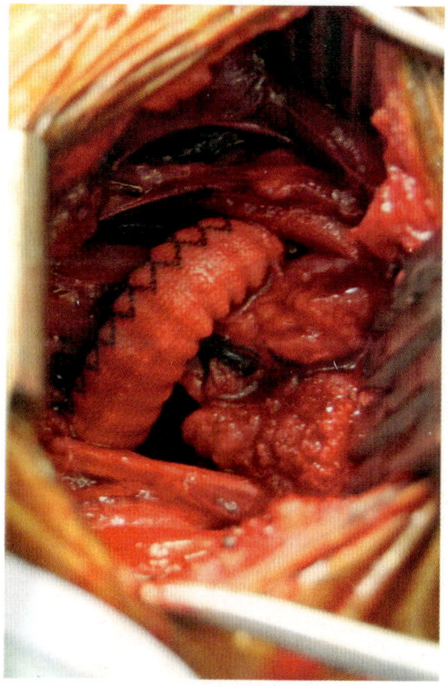

FIGURE 5 • The completed bypass graft can course anterior or posterior to the internal jugular vein. The phrenic nerve is seen in the lower field.

SUBCLAVIAN ARTERY TRANSPOSITION

Exposure

- The subclavian artery is exposed as previously described. The dissection must be carried proximal to the vertebral artery and enough artery must be exposed proximally to allow sufficient length for the anastomosis as well as control of the proximal stump. This can be difficult as an aortic aneurysm can occupy a significant portion of the mediastinum limiting vessel manipulation.
- The carotid artery is exposed in the same manner as described in the previous section.

Division of the Subclavian Artery

- Systemic heparin is administered, and maximum arterial length is obtained by advancing a Cooley clamp as deeply as possible into the mediastinum along the subclavian artery. A distal atraumatic clamp is then applied, typically in the mid-subclavian artery, with the more proximal branches individually controlled with vessel loops. There must be adequate distance between the proximal clamp and the vertebral artery to allow for proximal control, transposition, and anastomosis. Prior to transection, stay sutures, such as pledgeted 5-0 Prolene sutures, are placed on each side of the proximal artery to ensure that if clamp control is lost for any reason, the open, bleeding artery does not retract into the mediastinum (**FIGURE 6**).

- The proximal subclavian artery is then oversewn. Hemostasis is confirmed by slowly releasing clamp control while maintaining traction on the stay sutures. Once hemostasis is ensured, the stay sutures are divided, and the proximal subclavian artery is allowed to retract into the mediastinum.

Carotid–Subclavian Anastomosis

- The subclavian artery, having been freed circumferentially, is then mobilized toward the carotid artery. It may be tunneled either anterior or posterior to the internal jugular vein depending on the length of the mobilized artery. The carotid artery is then clamped proximally and distally and the anastomosis performed in the standard running fashion. Prior control of the subclavian artery is maintained (**FIGURE 7**). As the anastomosis is completed, the unclamping sequence should be repeated as described in the preceding section to prevent inadvertent air or particulate embolization to the brain.

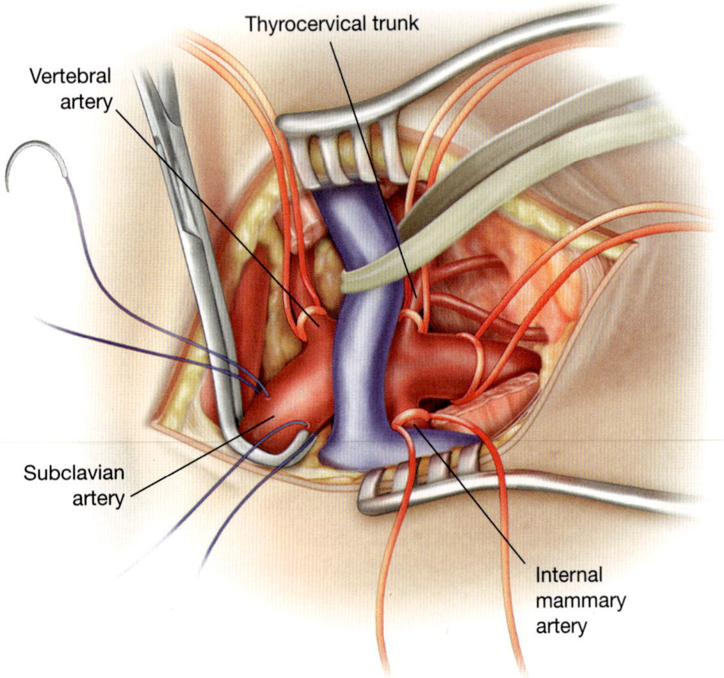

FIGURE 6 • The subclavian artery and its branches are controlled individually with vessel loops and clamps. A Cooley clamp is used proximally on the subclavian artery. Stay sutures of 5-0 Prolene are placed in both ends of the subclavian artery proximal to the transection line.

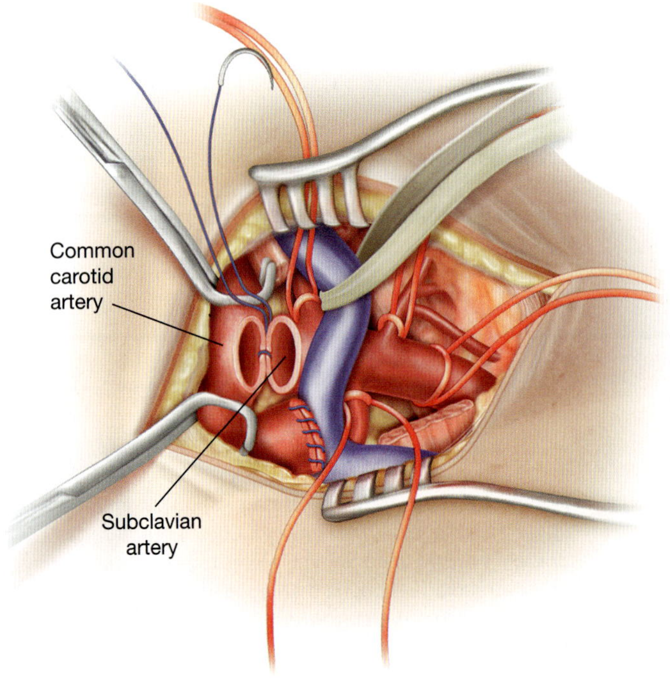

FIGURE 7 • The subclavian artery is mobilized so that it may reach to the carotid artery and the end-to-side anastomosis is performed in the standard running fashion, starting along the back wall. The thyrocervical trunk may be divided if necessary to facilitate mobilization.

Closure

- As described in the section on carotid–subclavian bypass, the wound is closed in multiple layers. A closed suction drain may also be used.

CAROTID–CAROTID BYPASS

Exposure of the Bilateral Carotid Arteries

- Incisions are made over the anterior border of the SCM at the base of the neck bilaterally. The subcutaneous tissues and platysma are then divided and the anterior border of the SCM identified.
- The SCM is mobilized laterally by carrying the dissection down toward the internal jugular vein; this exposes the carotid sheath. Any bridging veins encountered can be divided. Dissection should not extend above the level of the facial vein, as this marks the carotid bifurcation. This limits the risk of injury to adjacent structures and stroke when exposing or manipulating the carotid bifurcation. To obtain sufficient proximal exposure, the omohyoid muscle may need to be divided bilaterally.
- The carotid sheath is entered sharply on its anterior surface. The vagus nerve must be identified within the carotid sheath and protected as the common carotid artery is exposed and controlled.

Graft Tunneling and Anastomosis

- Once the bilateral common carotid arteries are sufficiently exposed and controlled, the appropriate graft tunnel can be created. Tunneling is achieved via blunt finger dissection from both sides of the neck to avoid injuries to these critical structures. The graft may be tunneled either between the trachea and esophagus or behind the esophagus, depending on surgeon preference (**FIGURE 8**). We preferentially create a retroesophageal tunnel, dissecting just anterior to the prevertebral fascia. Placement of an orogastric or nasogastric tube prior to creation of the dissection plane can be helpful for identifying the esophagus.
- Once the tunnel has been developed, the graft is passed and patient systemically anticoagulated with intravenous heparin administration.
- The anastomoses are performed in the standard running fashion; either one may be performed first. Careful attention must be paid to neuromonitoring as the carotid artery is clamped.
- Once the first anastomosis is complete, the graft is clamped and carotid artery flow restored on that side. Prior to removing the distal carotid artery clamp, the distal artery can be back-bled and the proximal artery flushed out the open graft. As with the subclavian artery, the graft should be flushed with heparinized saline and clamped close to the anastomosis to avoid a long stagnant column of blood within the prosthetic graft.

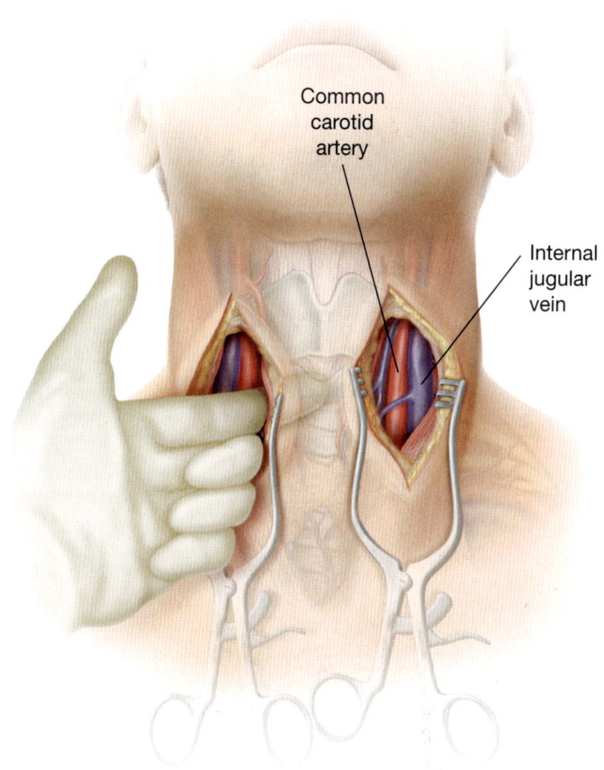

FIGURE 8 • After isolating both common carotid arteries, a retropharyngeal tunnel is fashioned using blunt finger dissection. The placement of a nasogastric or orogastric tube allows for easy identification and protection of the esophagus.

- The contralateral anastomosis is then performed in the same fashion (**FIGURE 9**). The graft should be flushed with heparinized saline and the graft, proximal carotid artery, and distal carotid artery should be vigorously flushed prior to completion.

Closure

- Hemostasis is obtained. The neck wounds are closed in layers, first taking care to reapproximate the SCM in its anatomic position with interrupted absorbable sutures.
- A closed suction drain may be left in each surgical bed.
- The platysma and subcutaneous tissues are closed with running absorbable sutures and the skin reapproximated with a running deep dermal suture.

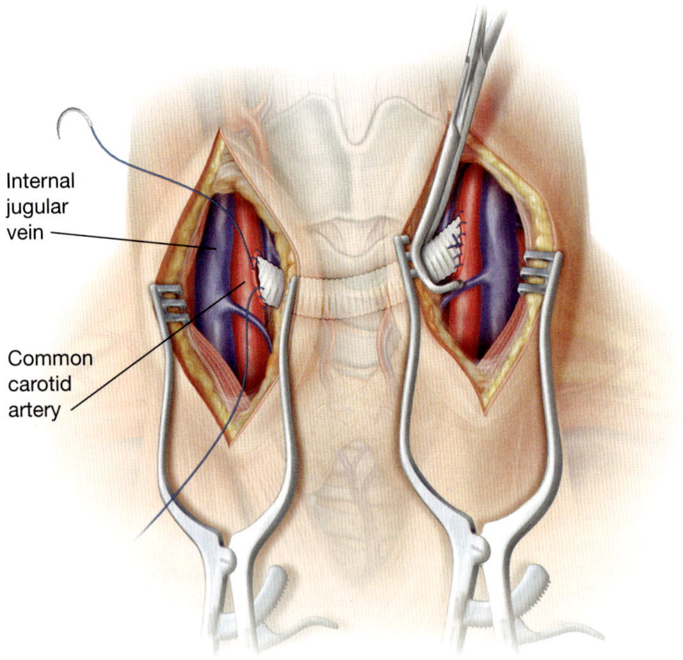

FIGURE 9 • The distal anastomosis is performed in the standard running fashion starting with the back wall. Prior to completing the anastomosis, the carotid arteries and graft should be back-bled and flushed with heparinized saline.

PEARLS AND PITFALLS

Positioning	■ When inflating the pneumatic pillow or placing a shoulder roll, care must be taken to ensure that the occiput is adequately supported. Failure to adequately support the head may result in cervical spine and neurologic injuries.
Thoracic duct	■ Great care must be taken to avoid injuring the thoracic duct when exposing the subclavian artery. All lymphatic tissue encountered should be ligated before being divided as the ensuing lymphatic leak can be quite troublesome for the patient and the surgeon.
Subclavian artery control	■ The subclavian artery can be controlled either with vessel loops or with atraumatic vascular clamps, depending on which helps to better deliver the artery into the wound without undue tension.
Subclavian artery anastomosis	■ In comparison to other peripheral arteries, the subclavian artery is fragile and exceedingly friable, requiring careful handling. Bleeding may best be controlled with pledgeted sutures.
Tunneling	■ The prosthetic graft in a carotid-to-carotid bypass is typically retrojugular. Tunneling in a carotid-to-subclavian bypass is typically posterior to the internal jugular.
Proximal subclavian control during transposition	■ The use of stay sutures on the proximal subclavian artery in subclavian artery transposition is crucial. Once the stay suture on the proximal end of the artery is released, the artery may retract deep into the mediastinum. Uncontrolled bleeding may lead to fatal complications. As such, the proximal oversewn subclavian artery must be hemostatic prior to release of the stay sutures.
Common carotid artery exposure	■ It is neither necessary nor advisable to expose or manipulate the carotid bifurcation in performing these bypasses unless a concomitant CEA is necessary, or the bifurcation is situated unusually low in the neck. These procedures are performed on the common carotid artery, and exposing the bifurcation only increases the risk of cranial nerve injury and stroke.
Closure	■ The pneumatic pillow should be deflated prior to closure to assist in bringing the tissue together without tension.

POSTOPERATIVE CARE

- Careful attention should be paid to both systolic and mean arterial blood pressure in the postoperative period. Invasive arterial monitoring is usually maintained for the first 24 hours. When carotid–subclavian bypass or subclavian artery transposition is performed, blood pressure should be monitored in the contralateral arm.
- Neurologic status and distal pulses should be followed closely in the postoperative period. Any pulse changes need to be rigorously investigated as they may indicate the presence of either graft occlusion or distal embolization.
- When carotid–subclavian bypass is performed as a debranching procedure prior to thoracic aortic stent grafting and the proximal subclavian artery is not ligated, the timing of the endovascular procedure is important. In these patients who tend not to have concomitant occlusive disease, there is competitive flow via the native circulation, putting the newly placed graft at risk of thrombosis. In the absence of complications or other mitigating circumstances, the endovascular aortic procedure should be performed within 3 to 5 days of the debranching bypass.
- Patients should be placed on aspirin therapy and followed at regular intervals with duplex ultrasonography.

OUTCOMES

- A review of the American College of Surgeons National Surgical Quality Improvement Program (ACS-NSQIP) database from 2005 to 2010 demonstrates that extrathoracic revascularization carries a 3.5% risk of stroke and 3.3% risk of death in the immediate perioperative period.[5] Over this time period, 918 procedures were performed, with 10% of them as part of a staged approach to thoracic aortic stent grafting.
- A recent review focusing on outcomes of carotid–subclavian bypass performed in the setting of TEVAR from 2005 to 2016 showed a primary patency of 97% at 5 years.[6]
- Carotid–subclavian bypass has excellent durability. In a series of 284 consecutive patients, Takach and colleagues[2] reported 5-, 10-, and 15-year primary patency rates of 94%, 88%, and 86%, respectively. These results have subsequently been replicated by other large, multiple-decade series.[7] Subclavian artery transposition has similarly outstanding long-term patency, with rates as high as 99% reported at 5 years.[7,8]
- Symptom-free survival following revascularization is likewise excellent, with long-term results approaching 88% to 99% at 5 years.[7,8]

COMPLICATIONS

- The thoracic duct lies at the medial aspect of the field of dissection when dissecting in the supraclavicular fossa. This can be easily injured and remain undetected during the course of the operation. Continued or milky drainage is a clear sign of duct injury. The oral administration of cream can be used to promote chyle flow, and if a leak is present, it will promptly increase drain output. When this occurs, a closed suction drain should be left in place, the patient kept fasting, and parenteral nutrition instituted. With conservative management, some of these injuries may close without further intervention. The complete management of this complication is beyond the scope of this text; however, it should be mentioned that re-exploration of the wound in the early period is relatively straightforward and may represent the best way to resolve the problem. Late re-exploration can be fraught with difficulty finding the leak as the tissue becomes fixed. A muscle flap may then be needed to close the space. The main concern with a persistent leak is the potential for graft infection. Unfortunately, early wound re-exploration significantly increases the risk of prosthetic graft infection.
- The vagus, phrenic, and recurrent laryngeal nerves, as well as the brachial plexus, can all be injured as a result of carotid and subclavian artery exposure. Most injuries are due to traction rather than transection, and conservative therapy will generally resolve symptoms over the course of months to a year. In the case of a staged bilateral subclavian revascularization, it is important to ensure that any vagus or phrenic nerve injury has resolved prior to contralateral intervention, as bilateral injuries can lead to tracheal obstruction and acute respiratory failure.
- Although uncommon, significant bleeding from the wound should mandate immediate re-exploration. More commonly, minor wound hematomas may develop that can be observed. Judgment regarding the need for re-exploration of a neck hematoma is similar to that required during any other neck procedure.
- Infection of the wound can be devastating if prosthetic is involved. Local cellulitis should be treated aggressively with early institution of antibiotics in order to prevent deeper infection. Upon removal of the drain, it is important that the drain site does not continue to leak, as continued leakage may act as an entry point for bacterial contamination. Simple suture closure should resolve this. Prosthetic graft infection necessitates graft removal, which is extremely difficult and beyond the scope of this chapter.
- Although uncommon, stroke is a complication of any carotid procedure. Taking the precautions outlined previously in this chapter should minimize these risks.

REFERENCES

1. Morasch MD. Technique for subclavian to carotid transposition, tips, and tricks. *J Vasc Surg*. 2009;49(1):251-254.
2. Takach TJ, Duncan JM, Livesay JJ, et al. Contemporary relevancy of carotid-subclavian bypass defined by an experience spanning five decades. *Ann Vasc Surg*. 2011;25(7):895-901.
3. Ziomek S, Quiñones-Baldrich WJ, Busuttil RW, et al. The superiority of synthetic arterial grafts over autologous veins in carotid-subclavian bypass. *J Vasc Surg*. 1986;3(1):140-145.
4. Woo EY, Bavaria JE, Pochettino A, et al. Techniques for preserving vertebral artery perfusion during thoracic aortic stent grafting requiring aortic arch landing. *Vasc Endovasc Surg*. 2006;40(5):367-373.
5. Madenci AL, Ozaki CK, Belkin M, et al. Carotid-subclavian bypass and subclavian-carotid transposition in the thoracic endovascular aortic repair era. *J Vasc Surg*. 2013;57(5):1275-1282.
6. Voigt SL, Bishawi M, Ranney D, et al. Outcomes of carotid-subclavian bypass performed in the setting of thoracic endovascular aortic repair. *J Vasc Surg*. 2019;69(3):701-709.
7. Cinà CS, Safar HA, Laganà A, et al. Subclavian carotid transposition and bypass grafting: consecutive cohort study and systematic review. *J Vasc Surg*. 2002;35(3):422-429.
8. Berguer R, Morasch MD, Kline RA, et al. Cervical reconstruction of the supra-aortic trunks: a 16-year experience. *J Vasc Surg*. 1999;29(2):239-246; discussion 246-248.

Chapter 3

Carotid Surgery: Interposition/ Endarterectomy (Including Eversion)/Ligation

Peter DeVito Jr. and Wei Zhou

DEFINITION

- Annually, approximatively 795,000 people experience a new or a recurrent stroke.[1]
- In 2019, stroke was the 5th leading cause of death, accounting for 37 out of 100,000 deaths.[2]
- Pivotal studies have shown the efficacy of carotid endarterectomy (CEA) for stroke prevention in both symptomatic and asymptomatic patients with internal carotid artery (ICA) stenosis vs medical therapy alone.[3,4]
- More recently, there are questions regarding the benefit of intervention on asymptomatic patients primarily due to changes in more modern medical management. However, studies still demonstrate a benefit of intervention in low-risk patients with the high grade stenosis.[5,6]
- CEA is defined as the surgical excision of atherosclerotic lesions of the intima and tunica media of the carotid artery.
- On rare occasions, ICA ligation and/or interposition bypass may be indicated for stroke prevention.

PATIENT HISTORY AND PHYSICAL FINDINGS

- In the United States, most CEA procedures are performed on asymptomatic patients. Symptoms of cerebroembolic disease originating from the carotid bifurcation, when present, may include dysarthria, dysphasia, aphasia, hemiparesis, hemisensory deficit, or amaurosis fugax. Symptoms that resolve within 24 hours are defined as transient ischemic attacks regardless of severity; symptoms that persist past the first day constitute a stroke.
- For patients at risk for cerebroembolic disease, a thorough vascular history is obtained including modifiable risk factors such as smoking, hyperlipidemia, hypertension, and diabetes management. Prior to surgery, antiplatelet therapy is initiated and continued indefinitely following intervention. Blood pressure control at or below 140 mm Hg systolic and 90 mm Hg diastolic is the single most important medical intervention to reduce stroke risk.[7] Sufficient β-blockade to stabilize resting heart rate at 60 to 80 bpm is also instituted prior to surgery to limit perioperative myocardial oxygen demand unless contraindicated.[8]
- Cervical auscultation is performed in both the supraclavicular and mandibular regions. Bruits appreciated at the mandibular angle usually indicate ICA or bifurcation disease. More proximal bruits may indicate common carotid artery (CCA) disease or radiating heart sounds.
- A full neurologic assessment including mental status, speech, facial symmetry, and extremity strength must be obtained and documented prior to surgery.

IMAGING AND OTHER DIAGNOSTIC STUDIES

- All patients exhibiting symptoms of carotid territory ischemia need appropriate vascular imaging studies. Screening is not recommended to detect asymptomatic disease in the general population; patients with atherosclerotic risk factors (age > 65, coronary artery disease, peripheral occlusive disease, tobacco use, hypercholesterolemia)[9] or those with a bruit on physical examination should be evaluated when clinical circumstances warrant.
- Carotid duplex ultrasound provides a reliable and accurate noninvasive tool to identify predicted stenosis and is the initial diagnostic study of choice. Peak systolic velocity (PSV) higher than 125 cm per second predicts angiographic stenosis more than 50% and higher than 230 cm per second predicts more than 70% stenosis. However, a combination of PSV, end diastolic velocity, and the PSV ratio of ICA to CCA is more accurate in estimating significant carotid stenosis. In general, end diastolic velocity higher than 100 cm per second correlates to more than 80% carotid stenosis.
- When duplex imaging is not definitive, as is the case in the setting of extensive carotid bifurcation calcification, additional cross-sectional imaging (computed tomography angiography or magnetic resonance angiography) may be necessary to quantify the degree of stenosis. When accurate velocity information is obtainable, duplex imaging provides the most accurate and physiologically relevant estimates of percent diameter reduction.

SURGICAL MANAGEMENT

Indications

Endarterectomy

- The Society for Vascular Surgery recommends that neurologically symptomatic patients with greater than 50% stenosis or asymptomatic patients with greater than 70% stenosis should be offered CEA to reduce risk of recurrent or initial stroke, respectively.[9]
- Surgical endarterectomy is the procedure of choice for good-risk surgical patients with normal cervical anatomy.[9] For selected high-risk patients, such as those with a tracheal stoma, previously radiated neck, prior cranial nerve injury, or for lesions proximal to the clavicle or distal to the C2 vertebral body endovascular interventions can be considered.[9] These include transcatheter angioplasty and stenting, generally from a transfemoral approach, and TCAR (transcarotid artery revascularization), placement of a stent via open exposure of the proximal CCA.
- Indications and technical guidelines for carotid angioplasty/stenting and TCAR procedures are covered in Chapter 4.

Carotid Artery Interposition Bypass

- Reconstruction for extensive bifurcation disease, injury to the bifurcation during endarterectomy, or aggressive restenosis following previous intervention (endarterectomy or stent placement) is best accomplished by carotid resection and interposition grafting. Other indications include the following:
  - Significant diffuse CCA and ICA disease
  - Radiation-induced stenosis or other forms of arteritis involving long arterial segments
  - Aneurysms (degenerative or traumatic) and invasive carotid body tumors.

Ligation

- Ligation and resection of the proximal ICA may be indicated in the setting of carotid stump syndrome, when persistent distal embolization from the "cul-de-sac" of the occluded ICA into the external carotid artery (ECA) circulation and ultimately into the cerebral circulation via reversed flow in the ophthalmic artery.

Preoperative Planning

- Similar overall outcomes are achieved with general anesthesia or regional anesthesia.
- The use of a shunt during CEA is dependent on operator preference. Most surgeons either shunt selectively or use a shunt for all cases. Surgeons should develop the methods they feel most comfortable with to optimize outcome. Objective measures used in selective shunting include stump pressure measurement, electroencephalographic monitoring, and transcranial Doppler assessment. Data supporting use of these adjuvants are inconsistent, and strategy used should be based on surgeon comfort and local expertise.
- Optimal neck extension is obtained by placing a towel or gel roll behind the scapula. The head is rotated contralateral to the operative side. In patients with limited neck movement or prior cervical fusions, it is critical to carefully pad and support the neck to prevent hyperextension injury. The chin, angle of the mandible, lower earlobe, and sternal angle are prepped and preliminarily draped within the operative field. The bed itself can be flexed with the head in relative extension to aid in positioning (**FIGURE 1**).

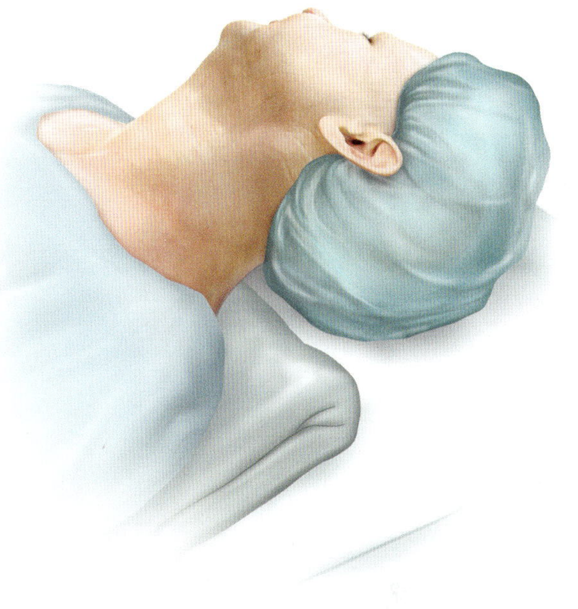

FIGURE 1 • Recommended patient position for a carotid endarterectomy procedure.

- Arterial blood pressure monitoring is necessary for optimal anesthetic management. If endarterectomy is performed with regional anesthesia, an audible squeeze device is placed in the patient's contralateral hand for indirect neurologic monitoring. Preoperative antibiotics are administered routinely.
- Aspirin therapy is initiated well in advance of surgery and continued throughout the perioperative period. Evidence suggests that statin therapy initiated preoperatively reduces postoperative neurologic events and mortality.[10]

CAROTID ENDARTERECTOMY—PATCH ANGIOPLASTY

Incision

- The skin incision is optimally placed along the anterior border of the sternocleidomastoid muscle. This should be curved posterolaterally near the angle of the mandible to avoid dissection into the parotid gland.
- Alternatively, a more transverse incision can be made at the level of the carotid bifurcation. Although providing an improved cosmetic result, exposure of the distal ICA may be compromised with this approach (**FIGURE 2**).

Carotid Exposure and Control

- As the incision is extended through the platysma muscle, the anterior border of the sternocleidomastoid muscle is visualized and retracted posterolaterally. The greater auricular nerve should be identified and protected at the superior extent of the incision.
- Following fascial incision, the facial vein is identified and securely ligated. This vein usually transverses the CCA near the bifurcation. Failure to adequately secure this vein may lead to bleeding and airway compromise during postoperative cough spells or Valsalva maneuvers.
- Within the carotid sheath, the vagus nerve usually extends posterior to, and parallel with, the artery and vein. However, this position relative to the other contents of the carotid sheath may vary, and the vagus should always be identified and protected in the course of the dissection. An anterior vagus nerve can be found in as many as 5% of patients.[11] The ansa cervicalis nerve is commonly much smaller than the vagus and runs anterior to the carotid bifurcation. When completely isolated, the proximal ansa arises from the ipsilateral hypoglossal (XII) cranial nerve. The ansa cervicalis can be divided to improve exposure if

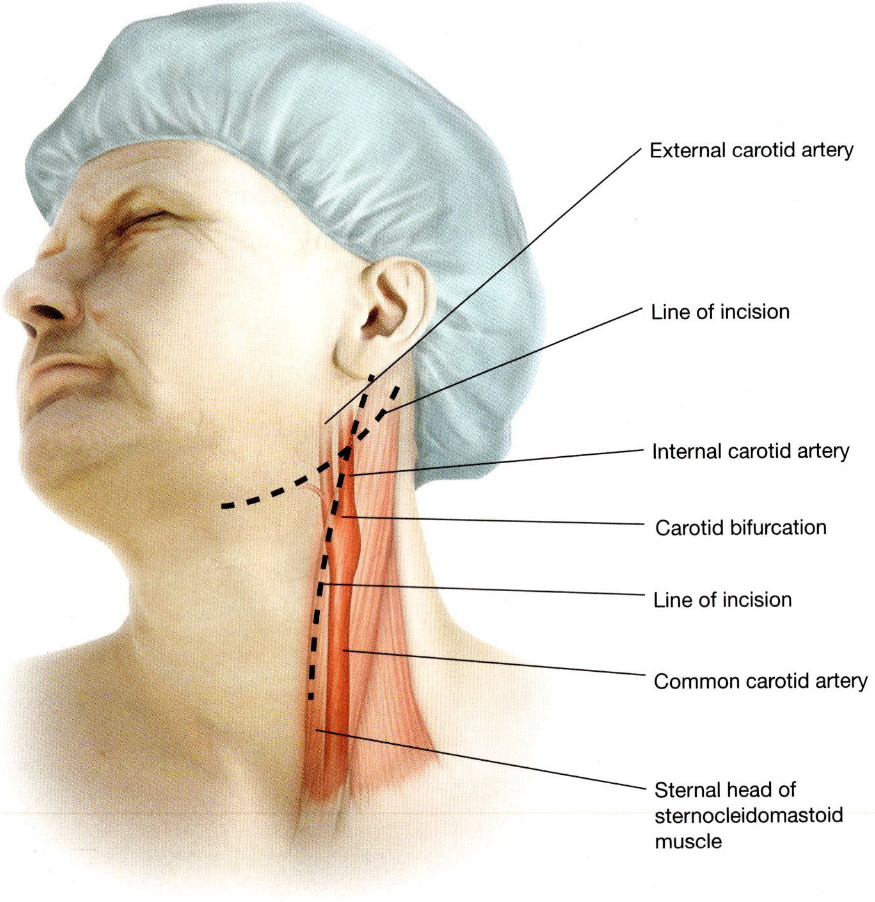

FIGURE 2 • The incision along the anterior border of sternocleidomastoid muscle is the most commonly used incision for a carotid endarterectomy procedure. A transverse incision along a skin crease in the vicinity of the carotid bifurcation is an alternative incision for a better cosmetic result.

necessary or mobilized sufficiently to be gently retracted out of the operative field.

- The CCA is circumferentially dissected from surrounding structures in sufficient length to provide adequate exposure for proximal clamping and control. Passing silastic loops around the CCA can provide temporary control if needed.
- Following common carotid exposure, the dissection is extended cranially and posteriorly along the posterolateral border of the ICA. Development of the dissection plane posterolaterally along the proximal ICA minimizes the risk of hypoglossal nerve injury. This dissection is also performed with minimal displacement and instrumentation of the ICA to reduce intraoperative embolization risk (**FIGURE 3**).
- To complete the necessary exposure, the ECA is dissected and mobilized to at least the level of the superior thyroidal artery. The superior laryngeal nerve may also be encountered posterior to the carotid bifurcation in this area.
- Following dissection, and prior to clamp placement, sufficient unfractionated heparin is administered intravenously to obtain an activated clotting time of more than 200 seconds. With normal circulation times, this is usually accomplished within 2 or 3 minutes of injection.
- Clamping of ICA is performed first, followed by clamping of the external and common carotid arteries. This sequence is followed to minimize embolization risk associated with clamping. When necessary, measurement of ICA stump pressure is obtained at this juncture by cannulation of the carotid bifurcation and selective removal of the internal carotid clamp. The CCA is optimally ultimately controlled by placement of an appropriately sized, atraumatic vascular clamp such as a Gregory profunda clamp, engaged to the minimal force necessary for control.

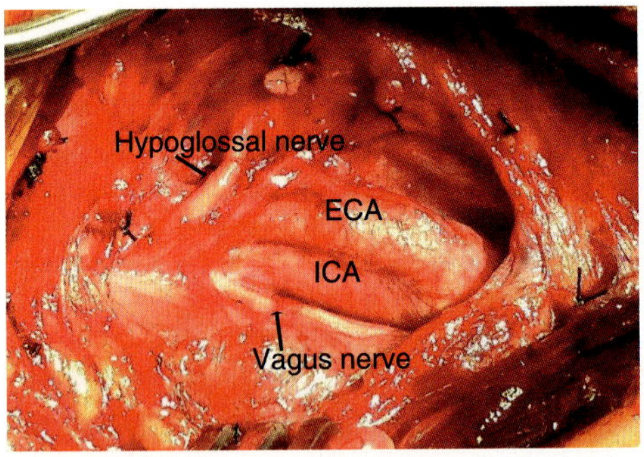

FIGURE 3 • Exposure of carotid bifurcation. Vagus nerve and hypoglossal nerve are the most commonly encountered nerves during carotid dissection. ECA, external carotid artery; ICA, internal carotid artery.

Conventional Endarterectomy

- The arteriotomy is initiated in a soft, uninvolved proximal segment of the CCA and extended cephalad with Potts scissors. It should be positioned on the anterior-lateral surface of the ICA to avoid the flow divider (**FIGURE 4A**).

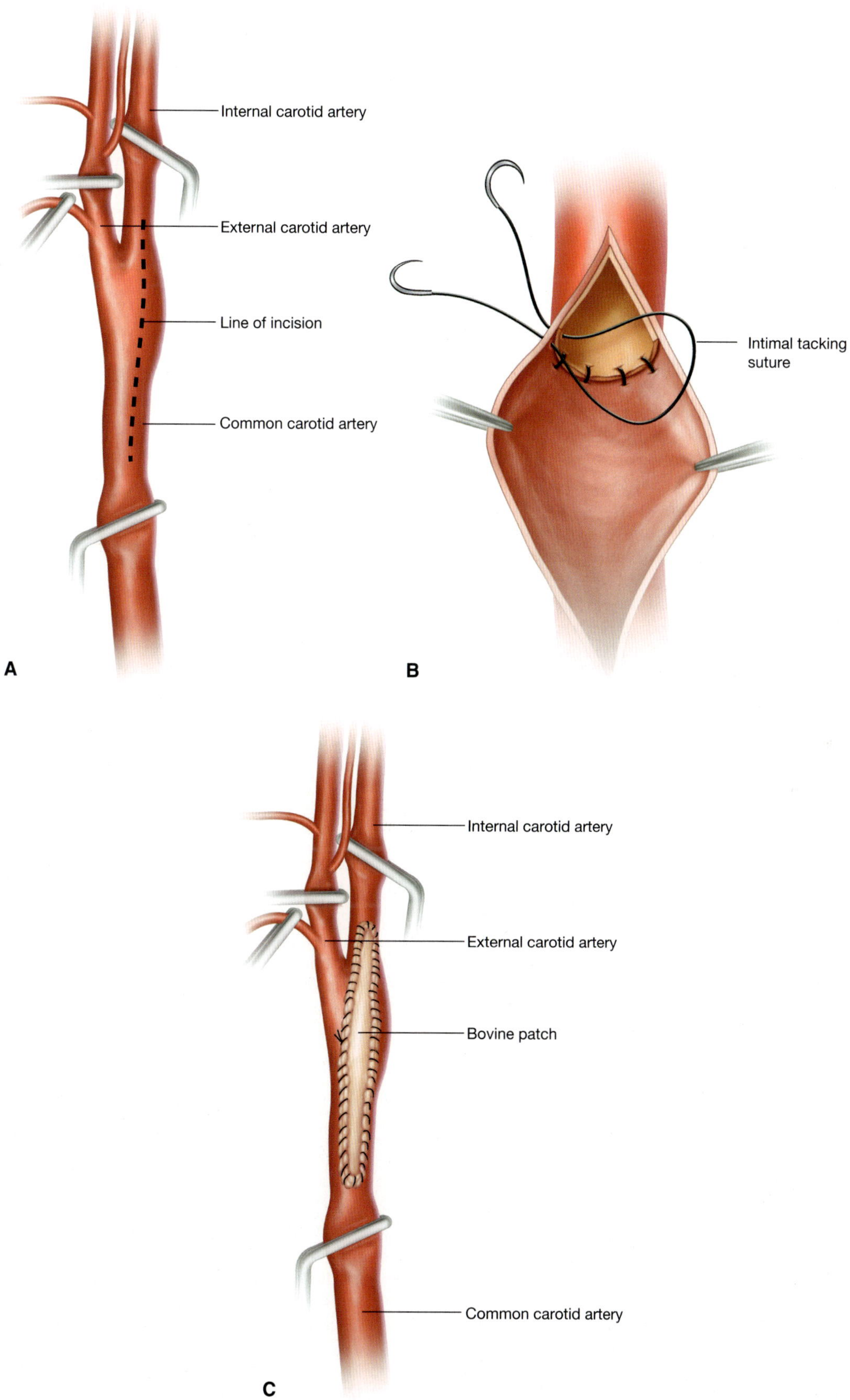

FIGURE 4 • Arteriotomy is extended from the anterior surface of common carotid artery to the anterior surface of internal carotid artery distal to the lesion **(A)**. Intimal flap is tacked down to ensure smooth distal endpoint **(B)**. Arteriotomy is closed with a patch **(C)**.

- When an indwelling shunt is used, the distal tapered end is carefully inserted into the ICA under direct vision. There are multiple shunts available for the purpose including Sundt, Javid, Argyle, Pruitt-Inahara, Brener, and Furui. Each is utilized primarily based on operator preference and familiarity.
- We prefer the Pruitt-Inahara shunt, which has pilot balloons at both ends to maintain shunt position and hemostasis. Once the distal end is inserted, the distal balloon is inflated with less than 1 mL of air until the "pop-off" balloon inflates on the pilot tube. Familiarity with this shunt prior to insertion is essential; if the inflation override cuff covers the "pop-off" balloon on the pilot tube, overinflation may injure or rupture the distal ICA. Following distal ICA cannulation and balloon inflation, the shunt is back-bled to confirm luminal placement and decant air. With the shunt actively back-bleeding, the proximal end is inserted into the CCA followed by proximal clamp removal into the unobstructed lumen. The proximal pilot tube is inflated with the provided syringe until the cuff is palpable in the CCA, after which a prepositioned Rumel tourniquet is gently cinched around the artery. When performed quickly, with concurrent digital control of the CCA following clamp removal and prior to shunt insertion, minimal bleeding ensues. When saline is applied to the shunt tubing, pulsatile flow is appreciable with handheld Doppler insonation.
- At the site of maximal atherosclerotic disease in the CCA, a Penfield dissector or Freer elevator is employed to identify and develop the appropriate endarterectomy plane within the medial layer. When the correct plane is identified, the plaque is easily and rapidly elevated from the underlying adventitia. In areas containing intraplaque hemorrhage, inflammation may increase adherence of the plaque to the adventitia, and care should be taken not to extend the dissection plane into the adventitia itself.
- At the distal extent of the plaque, sufficient exposure should be present to create a defined endpoint, allowing placement of tacking sutures if necessary, ensuring that no further potentially mobile plaque remains. It is essential to "feather" the plaque at the distal endpoint to minimize risk for distal dissection or thrombus accumulation. If the plaque extends past the point where feathering is feasible, a distal endpoint should be determined and created sharply with scissors or a no. 15 blade (**FIGURE 4B**). Tacking sutures, placed circumferentially, can control distal plaque at the transection site. Care should be taken to place the minimal number of sutures necessary to prevent dissection or consider extending the arteriotomy and endarterectomy to identify a more suitable termination site. Successful suture placement requires circumferential dissection and optimal visualization.
- Once the distal endpoint is determined, residual plaque is removed from the ECA by eversion into the CCA and circumferential dissection and traction. Sufficient back-bleeding is performed to remove any luminal debris within the ECA.
- Direct visualization of the endarterectomy bed following plaque removal commonly identifies loosely attached residual medial elements. These are best removed with fine forceps under magnification. Complete removal is facilitated by continuous irrigation to identify mobile medial elements. Integrity of the distal and proximal endpoints is also verified using this technique.

Patch Placement

- An appropriately sized bovine pericardial or prosthetic patch is selected and trimmed as necessary for closure-assisted angioplasty. Both bovine pericardial and prosthetic patches have chirality considerations; one surface is preferred for luminal apposition. Please consult the accompanying instructions for use prior to implantation.
- An autogenous vein patch can be utilized in select cases concerning for infection or in repeat operation with concerns regarding thrombogenicity of the patch.
- Closure is secured with running 6-0 polypropylene suture initiated at the cephalad extent of the arteriotomy and continued proximally along the long axis of the patch.
- After 90% or more of the circumference of the patch is secured, flushing is accomplished by sequential clamp removal and luminal irrigation with heparinized saline. Closure is then completed prior to restoration of flow.
- The declamping sequence is of critical importance. The CCA is released first, followed by the ECA clamp. After several cardiac cycles have ensued, the distal ICA is released (**FIGURE 4C**).
- It is essential to perform a completion assessment prior to closure. We perform intraoperative completion duplex imaging of the endarterectomy site as well as the proximal and distal carotid arteries, with purpose-designed, miniaturized 7 MHz probes. Completion duplex scanning is quick, efficient, highly reproducible, and effective at identifying significant residual luminal defects.[12] Detailed description of the characteristics of significant luminal defects identified by completion ultrasonography is beyond the scope of this chapter. Alternatively, intraoperative insonation can be performed; however, it is not possible through extruded polytetrafluoroethylene (ePTFE) patches. Furthermore, a completion angiogram can also be considered.

Closure

- Following adequate duplex imaging and endpoint determination, anticoagulation may be reversed with protamine sulfate. Some practitioners are reluctant to reverse anticoagulation due to uncertainty regarding thrombogenicity at the endarterectomy site; however, this is unfounded in literature.[13] In our experience, technical issues at the endarterectomy site are most predictive of postoperative neurologic events, and these are efficiently identified and corrected with completion ultrasonography.
- Following reversal, the entire wound is inspected for venous or arterial bleeding. The entirety of the patch angioplasty suture line is reinspected for periodicity of suture placement and potential leaks. Reinforcing sutures are applied liberally as needed to ensure hemostasis, but with experience and even suture spacing, the need for additional sutures should be rare. Bleeding lymph nodes should be sutured and removed from the operative field. Once hemostasis is achieved, the platysma is reapproximated with running absorbable suture followed by skin closure. We usually also perform a Valsalva maneuver to identify occult venous injuries that may not be apparent with positive pressure ventilation prior to closure.

CAROTID ENDARTERECTOMY—EVERSION ENDARTERECTOMY

- The incision, dissection, and control of the carotid artery for eversion endarterectomy are identical to that for CEA with patch angioplasty.
- Once distal and proximal clamps are placed on the carotid artery, an oblique or circumferential incision is made at the junction of the bulbous portion of the ICA and CCA (**FIGURE 5A**).
- The ICA adventitia is grasped with fine forceps and everted away, as gentle traction is placed on the plaque within the artery. This maneuver is extended distally until the feathered endpoint identifies itself. Tacking sutures are not possible using this approach, which can be a deterrent to adoption by surgeons trained with conventional endarterectomy.
- Common and external carotid plaque is subsequently removed by the Penfield dissector or Freer elevator as indicated. The proximal CCA arteriotomy may be extended as possible to ensure complete removal (**FIGURE 5B**).

Anastomosis

- The ICA is reverted and anastomosed end-to-end to the proximal CCA (**FIGURE 5C**).
- If redundant residual ICA is present following plaque removal, the ICA spatulation is extended, as is the CCA arteriotomy, and the two ends are further advanced over each other prior to closure. Alternatively, a portion of the redundant ICA may also be excised. This can prove ideal in circumstances with a kinked ICA.

Closure

- Completion imaging and closure of the incision is identical to that for standard endarterectomy.

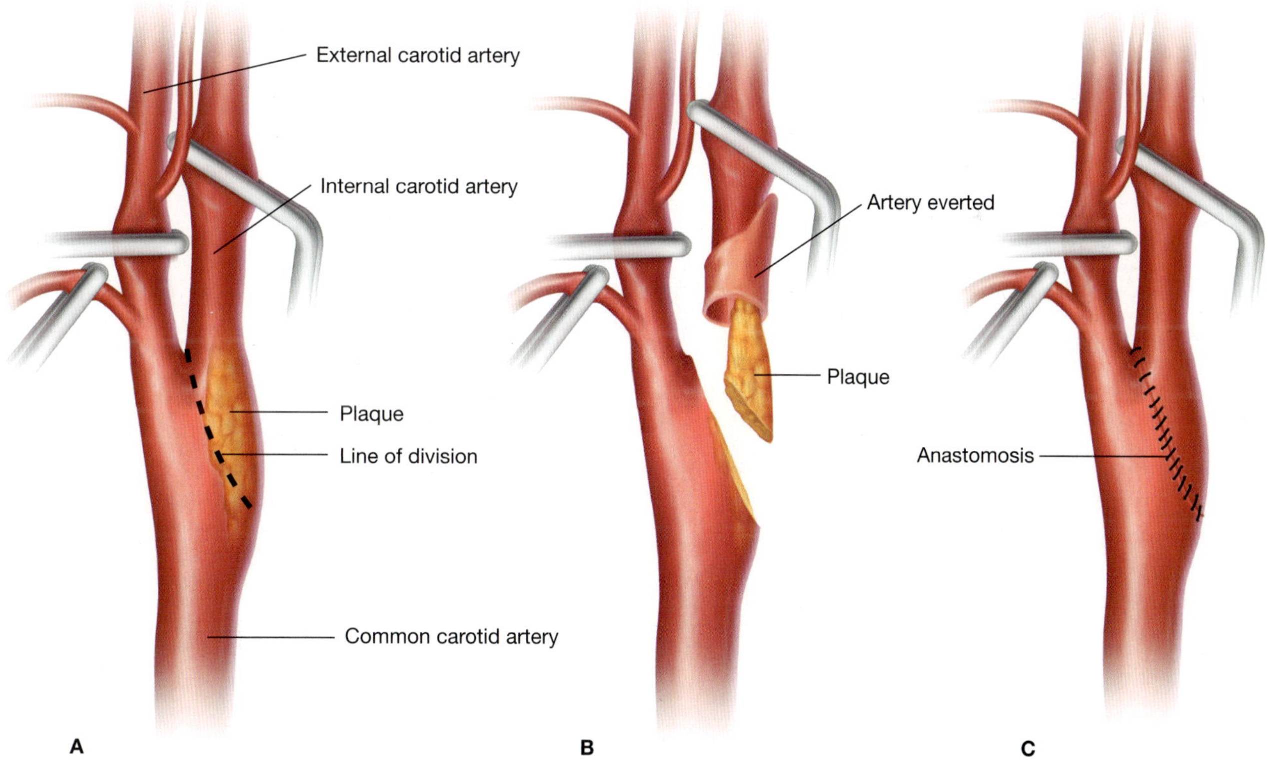

FIGURE 5 • Carotid eversion endarterectomy. The internal carotid artery (ICA) is divided from the common carotid artery (CCA) in an oblique line **(A)**. The divided ICA is everted on itself until the plaque endpoint is encountered and the plaque is removed from the ICA **(B)**. Following endarterectomy, the ICA is reverted and reattached to the CCA **(C)**.

TECHNIQUES

CAROTID ARTERY INTERPOSITION BYPASS

Incision, Dissection, and Control of the Carotid Artery

- The incision, dissection, and control of the carotid artery are identical for a carotid artery interposition bypass as it is for a CEA.
- Although reversed autogenous vein is the preferred conduit when available, ePTFE provides a suitable alternative when necessary.[14]

Anastomosis

- The diseased segment of the carotid artery is resected. Commonly, the ECA is oversewn as well.
- End-to-end anastomoses are performed in standard fashion. Typically, the proximal anastomosis is completed first. Upon completion, a clamp is placed on the bypass and the CCA clamp is removed to test the integrity of the anastomosis.
- Prior to completion of the distal anastomosis, flushing maneuvers are done to evacuate particular matter or residual air (**FIGURE 6**).
- Completion duplex imaging is suggested for this approach as well.

Closure

- Completion imaging and closure of the incision is identical to that for standard CEA.

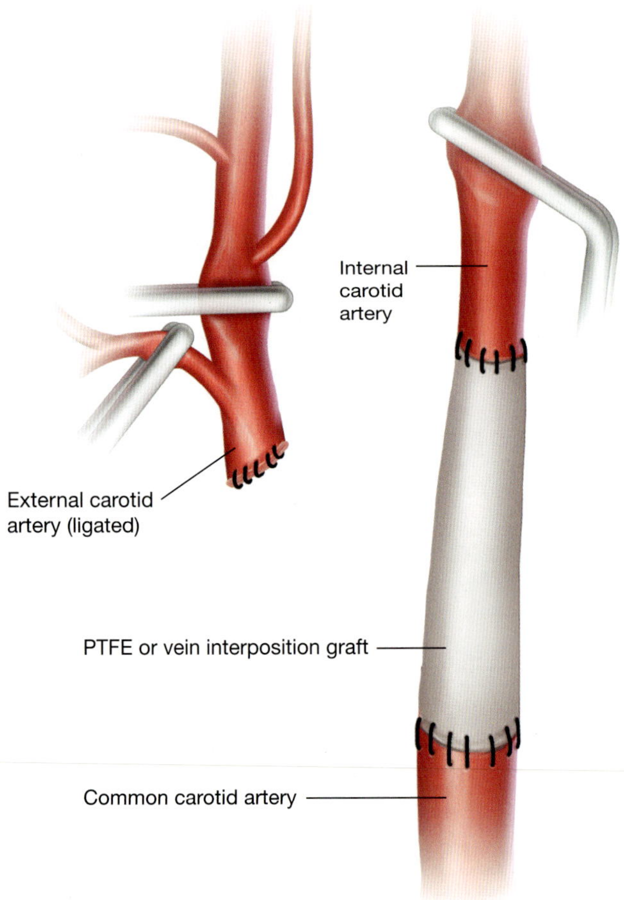

FIGURE 6 • Carotid interposition graft. Following resection of the diseased segment, a prosthetic graft or a segment of reversed greater saphenous vein is used to bridge the common carotid artery and internal carotid artery in an end-to-end fashion.

CAROTID ARTERY LIGATION (CAROTID STUMP SYNDROME)

Incision, Dissection, and Control of the Carotid Artery

- The incision, dissection, and control of the carotid artery are identical in this procedure as it is for CEA.

Endarterectomy

- The technique is similar to that for standard ICA endarterectomy, the difference being the arteriotomy being carried out on the distal CCA into the ECA (**FIGURE 7A**).
- The thrombosed ICA is resected, ideally in line with the common and external carotid arteriotomies. Closure is accomplished via patch angioplasty (**FIGURE 7B** and **C**).

Closure

- The completion imaging and closure is identical to that for standard endarterectomy.

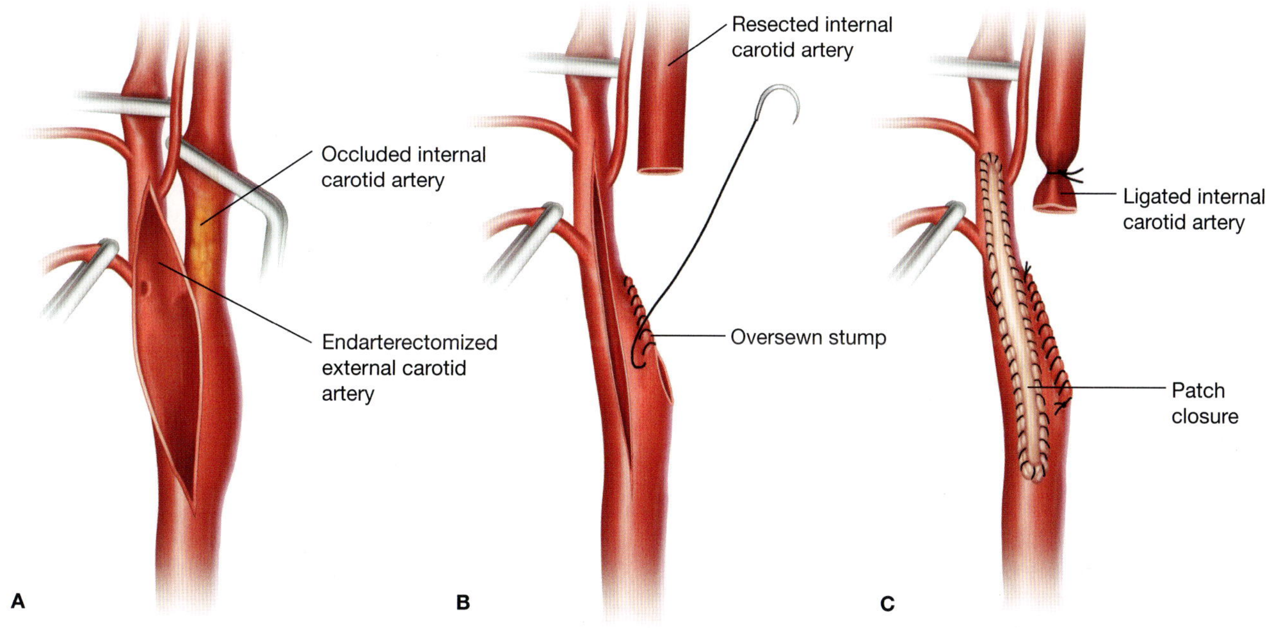

FIGURE 7 • Carotid ligation. The occluded internal carotid artery (ICA) is amputated and removed **(A)**, and the ICA stump is oversewn **(B)**. The plaque in the common carotid artery and external carotid artery is removed, and the arteriotomy is closed with a patch **(C)**.

PEARLS AND PITFALLS

Incision	■ On-table duplex scanning optimizes incision placement, particularly for transverse exposure to localize the bifurcation.
Identifying the vagus nerve and hypoglossal nerve	■ Vagus nerve is located posterolateral to the carotid artery, within the carotid sheath and between carotid artery and internal jugular vein. Hypoglossal nerve typically crosses ICA anteroinferiorly to posterosuperiorly. Following the ansa cervicalis will lead to the hypoglossal nerve.
Clamping	■ A "robin blue" hue is often seen in the distal ICA, which signifies a soft area for safe clamp placement.
Shunting	■ Be prepared in all cases for potential shunt placement. This should be flushed and prepared on the back table prior to performing the arteriotomy.
Conventional endarterectomy	■ Lavage the arterial lumen with heparinized saline to identify and remove luminal debris.
Eversion endarterectomy	■ Use caution in patients with high bifurcation (difficulty visualizing and securing distal endpoint), those who require a shunt, or those with a small ICA. These procedures are best suited for patients with redundant ICAs.
Interposition bypass	■ Use the anastomotic suture line to tack down distal residual plaque as necessary to prevent antegrade dissection.
Ensuring technical perfection	■ A completion imaging study, an on-table angiogram, a carotid duplex, or doppler insonation, must be performed prior to skin closure.
Closure	■ If a closed suction drain is placed, it should be removed on postoperative day 1.

POSTOPERATIVE CARE

- Patients should be placed on continuous monitoring to assess for blood pressure lability. Patients generally are discharged on postoperative day 1.
- A postoperative duplex should be obtained at initial postoperative visit to assess the reconstruction, provide a new baseline for long-term surveillance, and monitor wound healing and plaque incorporation. Serial ultrasounds should be obtained to identify and manage restenosis, which most commonly occurs in the first 2 years following endarterectomy.

OUTCOMES

- The North American Symptomatic Carotid Endarterectomy Trial (NASCET) demonstrated the 30-day CEA stroke and death rate of 5.5% for symptomatic patients. For symptomatic patients with moderate (50%-69%) stenosis, reduced 5-year stroke rate from 22.2% with BMT (best medical therapy) to 15.7% with BMT and CEA.[3]
- The Asymptomatic Carotid Atherosclerosis Study (ACAS) demonstrated a combined 30-day CEA stroke and death rate of 2.3%. For asymptomatic patients with >60% stenosis, reduced 5-year stroke rate from 11% with BMT to 5.1% with BMT and CEA.[4]
- In 2010, the Carotid Revascularization Endarterectomy vs Stenting Trial (CREST) demonstrated the 30-day stroke, death, or rate of myocardial infarction (MI) to be 5.4% in symptomatic patients and 3.6% in asymptomatic patients, and the 30-day death and stroke rates were found to be 3.2% in symptomatic patients and 1.4% in asymptomatic patients undergoing CEA. In the periprocedural period, there is a lower rate of stroke with CEA vs stenting (2.3% vs 4.1%) but a higher rate of MI (2.3% vs 1.1%). Mortality rates are similar.[15]

COMPLICATIONS

- Cervical hematoma
- Hemodynamic instability
- Cerebral hyperperfusion syndrome manifested by severe headache
- Cranial nerve palsy
- Stroke/MI
- Thrombosis (early)
- Recurrent stenosis (late)

REFERENCES

1. Virani SS, Alonso A, Benjamin EJ, et al. Heart disease and stroke statistics—2020 update: a report from the American Heart Association. *Circulation*. 2020;141(9):e139-e596.
2. Kochanek KD, Xu JQ, Arias E. *Mortality in the United States, 2019. NCHS Data Brief, No 395*. National Center for Health Statistics; 2020.
3. North American Symptomatic Carotid Endarterectomy Trial Collaborators. Beneficial effect of carotid endarterectomy in symptomatic patients with high-grade carotid stenosis. *N Engl J Med*. 1991;325:445-453.
4. Walker MD, Marler JR, Goldstein M. Endarterectomy for asymptomatic carotid artery stenosis. Executive committee for the asymptomatic carotid Atherosclerosis study. *JAMA*. 1995;273:1421-1428.
5. Goessens BMB, Visseren FLJ, Kappelle LJ, Algra A, Van Der Graaf Y. Asymptomatic carotid artery stenosis and the risk of new vascular events in patients with manifest arterial disease: the SMART study. *Stroke*. 2007;38(5):1470-1475. doi:10.1161/STROKEAHA.106.477091
6. Howard DPJ, Gaziano L, Rothwell PM. Risk of stroke in relation to degree of asymptomatic carotid stenosis: a population-based cohort study, systematic review, and meta-analysis. *Lancet Neurol*. 2021;20(3):193-202. doi:10.1016/S1474-4422(20)30484-1
7. Brott TG, Halperin JL, Abbara S, et al. 2011 ASA/ACCF/AHA/AANN/AANS/ACR/ASNR/CNS/SAIP/SCAI/SIR/SNIS/SVM/SVS guideline on the management of patients with extracranial carotid and vertebral artery disease: executive summary. A report of the American college of cardiology foundation/American heart association task force on practice guidelines, and the American stroke association, American association of neuroscience nurses, American association of neurological surgeons, American college of radiology, American society of neuroradiology, congress of neurological surgeons, society of Atherosclerosis imaging and prevention, society for cardiovascular angiography and interventions, society of interventional radiology, society of NeuroInterventional surgery, society for vascular medicine, and society for vascular surgery. *Circulation*. 2011;124(4):489-532.
8. American College of Cardiology Foundation/American Heart Association Task Force on Practice Guidelines, American Society of Echocardiography, American Society of Nuclear Cardiology, et al. 2009 ACCF/AHA focused update on perioperative beta blockade incorporated into the ACC/AHA 2007 guidelines on perioperative cardiovascular evaluation and care for noncardiac surgery. *J Am Coll Cardiol*. 2009;54:e13-e118.
9. AbuRahma AF, Avgerinos ED, Chang RW, et al. Society for vascular surgery clinical practice guidelines for management of extracranial cerebrovascular disease. *J Vasc Surg*. 2021;75(1S):4S-22S.
10. Mcgirt MJ, Perler BA, Brooke BS, et al. 3-Hydroxy-3-methylglutaryl coenzyme A reductase inhibitors reduce the risk of perioperative stroke and mortality after carotid endarterectomy. *J Vasc Surg*. 2005;42:829-835.
11. Kawahara I, Shiozaki E, Soejima K, et al. Unusual course of the vagus nerve passing anterior to the internal carotid artery during carotid endarterectomy. *Surg Neurol Int*. 2021;12:278.
12. Ascher E, Markevich N, Kallakuri S, Schutzer RW, Hingorani AP. Intraoperative carotid artery duplex scanning in a modern series of 650 consecutive primary endarterectomy procedures. *J Vasc Surg*. 2004;39(2):416-420. doi:10.1016/j.jvs.2003.09.019
13. Newhall KA, Saunders EC, Larson RJ. Use of protamine for anticoagulation during Carotid Endarterectomy: a meta-analysis. *J Vasc Surg*. 2016;63(6):1662-1663. doi:10.1016/j.jvs.2016.04.017
14. Dorafshar AH, Reil TD, Ahn SS, et al. Interposition grafts for difficult carotid artery reconstruction: a 17-year experience. *Ann Vasc Surg*. 2008;22(1):63-69.
15. Mantese VA, Timaran CH, Chiu D, et al. The Carotid Revascularization Endarterectomy versus Stenting Trial (CREST): stenting versus carotid endarterectomy for carotid disease. *Stroke*. 2010;41(suppl 10):S31-S34.

Chapter 4

Transcarotid Artery Revascularization (TCAR)

Jeffrey Jim

DEFINITION

- Endovascular treatment of carotid artery stenosis was first described in 1997. Carotid angioplasty and stenting (CAS) is typically done through percutaneous access at the common femoral artery. Transfemoral CAS is considered an alternative to traditional carotid endarterectomy (CEA) due to the less invasive nature of this procedure. However, the available clinical evidence has demonstrated this technique to be associated with an increased rate of perioperative neurologic events.[1] As such, CAS is typically reserved for patients considered to be at high risk for complications during a CEA.
- Transcarotid artery revascularization (TCAR) combines open surgical principles with less invasive endovascular techniques. Direct surgical exposure of the common carotid artery (CCA) allows stent delivery to the carotid bifurcation lesion while neuroprotection is provided by creating a reversal of flow through the internal carotid artery (ICA). This technique was first described in small cases series. In 2015, the publication of the results of the ROADSTER clinical trial using the ENROUTE Transcarotid Neuroprotection System (NPS) demonstrated the clinical efficacy of this technique in successfully treating carotid artery stenosis.[2]

PATIENT HISTORY AND PHYSICAL FINDINGS

- A thorough history should be obtained from the patient prior to any intervention. The presence and duration of lateralizing neurologic symptoms (eg, amaurosis fugax, facial droop, slurred speech, paresthesia/paralysis of any extremity) should be elicited. Any underlying cardiovascular risk factors (eg, hypertension, diabetes, smoking history) should be documented and an evaluation of the patient's current medications (including antiplatelet agents, anticoagulation, and statin therapy) should be recorded. A thorough physical examination should be performed with careful attention to any residual neurologic deficits. The presence of a carotid bruit or heart murmur is noted. The presence of prior surgical scars (especially head and neck) as well as effects of radiation therapy should also be documented.

IMAGING AND OTHER DIAGNOSTIC STUDIES

- The presence of carotid artery stenosis is first evaluated using duplex ultrasonography. This diagnostic study has been shown to be reliable in determining the presence of underlying carotid plaque as well as associated level of stenosis. However, the presence of significant calcification as well as vessel tortuosity may limit reliability.
- Catheter-based diagnostic angiography is considered the "gold standard" in determining carotid artery stenosis. However, this is an invasive procedure with associated risks of periprocedural complications. With continued advance in noninvasive axial imaging, patient evaluation with computed tomographic angiography (CTA) or magnetic resonance angiography (MRA) has largely supplanted the need for catheter angiography. In our practice, a CTA of the head and neck is performed with images starting at the aortic arch at the chest and proceed cranially to include the intracranial circulation. This will allow evaluation of the aortic arch, disease at the carotid bifurcation, as well as the presence of intracranial disease (**FIGURE 1**).

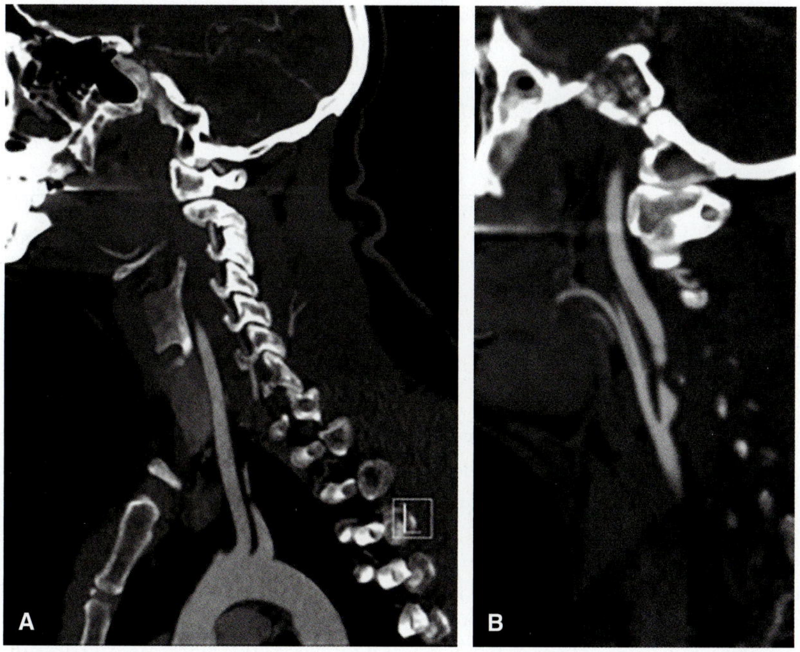

FIGURE 1 • Computed tomographic angiography showing the arterial anatomy. **A,** Sagittal reconstruction demonstrates the aortic arch. **B,** Sagittal reconstruction showing a severe left internal carotid artery stenosis.

SURGICAL MANAGEMENT

- The indication for carotid revascularization depends primarily on the presence of underlying neurologic symptoms as well as the degree of stenosis in the corresponding carotid artery.[3] It is generally accepted that for patients with symptomatic carotid disease, intervention is warranted if the stenosis is between 70% and 99% in severity. Treatment is offered to appropriate patients without prohibitive periprocedural risks. The anticipated periprocedural stroke/death risk must be <6%. The choice to intervene on a patient with severe carotid stenosis without associated neurologic symptoms is less clear. Data from the clinical trials in the 1990s suggest benefit of surgical revascularization in asymptomatic patients with >60% stenosis. However, with advances in medical care (eg, statin medications) and overall decreasing stroke rates in the general population, most physicians typically reserve intervention now for people with much more severe disease. In our practice, we reserve intervention to asymptomatic patients only if they are otherwise healthy with a minimum life expectancy of 3 to 5 years and the presence of a severe >80% stenosis. The anticipated periprocedural stroke/death risk should be well below the recommended 3% standard.

Preoperative Planning

- The instructions for use for TCAR NPS include several anatomic requirements. The patient's anatomy must adhere to three requirements:
  1. ≥5 cm distance between arterial access site to the proximal aspect of lesion
  2. ≥6 mm CCA diameter
  3. CCA free of significant disease (eg, calcification/thrombus) at access site and occlusive site
- While measurements can be obtained through analysis of the CTA, more appropriate measurements may be obtained by performing an ultrasound while the patient is in the surgical position (neck extended and turned). Furthermore, the carotid lesion should be free of acute mobile thrombus or significant calcification that precludes stent placement.[4]
- All patients undergoing TCAR must be on dual antiplatelet therapy (DAPT) prior to the procedure. The most common DAPT regimen includes daily doses of aspirin (81-325 mg) and clopidogrel (75 mg). In cases of urgent intervention, a loading dose may be administered at minimum 4 hours prior to the procedure. Alternative P2Y12 inhibitors (eg, ticagrelor or prasugrel) may also be utilized in place of clopidogrel. Due to the prevalence of clopidogrel resistance in the general population, platelet function testing should be performed if available. It should be noted that systemic anticoagulation (eg, warfarin or direct oral anticoagulants) are not substitutes for DAPT for TCAR. The patient should also be on statin therapy prior to the procedure.
- While fixed fluoroscopic imaging in a hybrid operating room is preferred, the procedure can also be performed in a standard operating room with a mobile fluoroscopy C-arm unit.

TECHNIQUES

ANESTHESIA CONSIDERATIONS

- A TCAR procedure can be done under either general or local anesthesia with moderate sedation. The choice of anesthesia should be determined jointly by the proceduralist, patient, and the anesthesia team. Intraoperative neuromonitoring can be utilized at the physician's discretion but is not considered as mandatory.
- The patient should have a radial arterial line to allow for continuous hemodynamic monitoring during the entire procedure. During the procedure, the patient will be administered a bolus dose (100 U/kg) of heparin to achieve systemic anticoagulation. This is typically given immediately after the surgical incision is made. The target activated clotting time (ACT) is >250 and additional heparin is administered as necessary. The patient should also be given glycopyrrolate (0.2-0.4 mg) to try to mitigate bradycardia/hypotension during balloon angioplasty. During the period of CCA occlusion to establish reversal of flow, the systolic blood pressure should be maintained between 140 to 160 mm Hg and heart rate above 70 beats per minute. The anesthesia team should be ready with necessary vasoactive agents (eg, phenylephrine drip) to maintain the desired hemodynamic parameters during the procedure.

PERCUTANEOUS FEMORAL VENOUS SHEATH PLACEMENT

- It is preferred to obtain venous access in the common femoral vein contralateral to the carotid lesion. This is done using standard ultrasound guidance with a micropuncture system.
- Once the micropuncture sheath is placed into the vein, the NPS 8 French venous sheath should be inserted over an access wire. The sheath is secured to the patient's skin using a 2-0 silk suture.

COMMON CAROTID EXPOSURE

- The patient is positioned similar to a standard carotid endarterectomy. The head should be tilted away from the side of the lesion and a shoulder roll can be placed underneath the patient to elevate the neck and chest. We typically perform a repeat ultrasound to identify the anatomic landmarks (**FIGURE 2**).
- We clearly delineate the two heads of the sternocleidomastoid (SCM) as well as the clavicle. The location of the CCA is identified with ultrasound, with careful attention to the depth of the vessel at the base of the neck and its relation to the internal jugular vein (IJV) (**FIGURE 3**).
- A short transverse skin incision (typically between 2 and 4 cm) is made about a fingerbreadth above the clavicle and

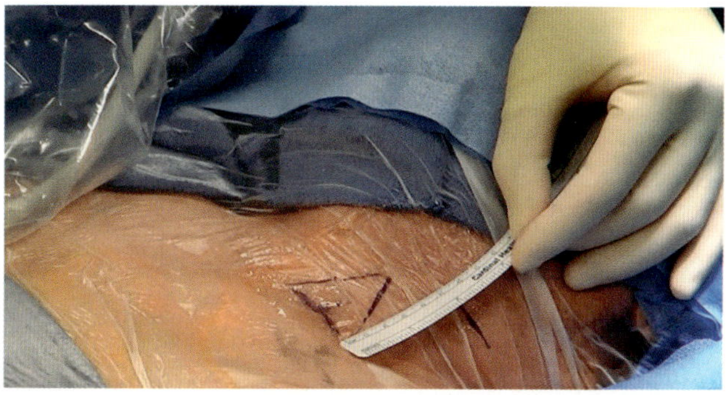

FIGURE 2 • Intraoperative photograph demonstrating preoperative skin marking. The marked triangle is bordered by the clavicle and sternal and clavicular heads of the sternocleidomastoid muscle. A ruler is utilized to confirm adequate distance between the common carotid artery access site and the carotid lesion to be treated.

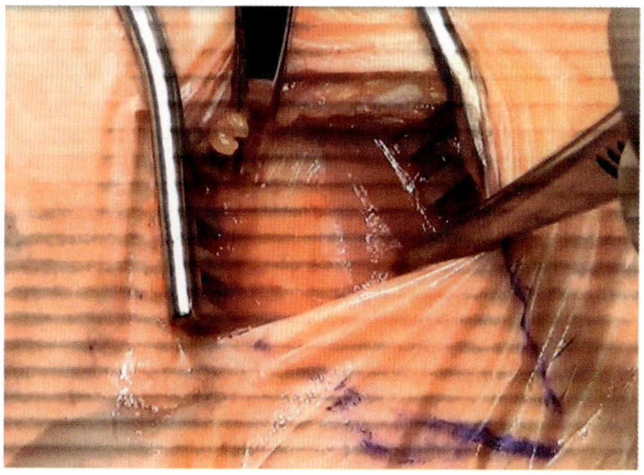

FIGURE 4 • Intraoperative photograph demonstrating the avascular plane between the two heads of the sternocleidomastoid muscle.

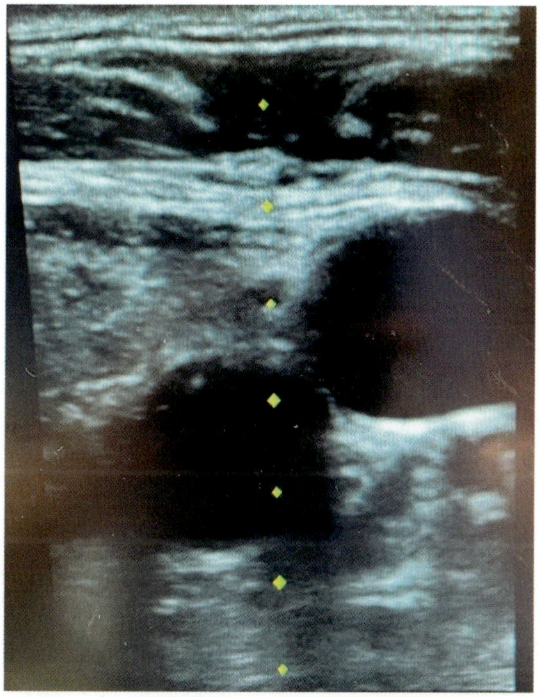

FIGURE 3 • Ultrasound of the base of the neck demonstrating the location of the common carotid artery (bottom left) in relation to the internal jugular vein (upper right). The two heads of the sternocleidomastoid muscle are also identified and the avascular plane is centered at the top of the image.

centered between the two heads of the SCM. Subcutaneous dissection allows identification of the platysma, which is divided utilizing electrocautery. Subplatysmal planes are then developed superiorly and inferiorly. Gentle blunt dissection is utilized to identify the avascular plane between the two heads of the SCM and a self-retaining retractor is placed (**FIGURE 4**).

- There often is a large venous branch coming off medially from the IJV, which may be divided between ties. The proximal CCA is identified and dissected using sharp dissection. The vagus nerve, which usually courses posterior to the CCA, is identified and preserved. The proximal CCA is encircled using a silastic loop close to the clavicle to ensure adequate distance away from the lesion. It is our practice to utilize a 16-gauge vessel loop for retraction and occlusion during the procedure. Alternatively, an umbilical tape can be used for retraction and a surgical clamp for vessel occlusion. The anterior surface of the CCA is dissected clean. A "U-stitch" is then placed and left in place at the intended arterial access puncture site utilizing a 5-0 Prolene suture.

COMMON CAROTID ARTERIAL SHEATH PLACEMENT

- Prior to arterial access, we perform fluoroscopy to ensure that the surgical field is clear of radiopaque materials that may obstruct visualization. Using an ENHANCE Transcarotid Access kit, we puncture the CCA at the site of the U-stitch stitch placement. A key to success is maintaining stability of the CCA during arterial access. This can be done by apply slight caudal retraction of the vessel with retraction of the vessel loop while avoiding CCA occlusion. Once there is adequate blood return from the access needle, the microwire is inserted into the CCA for between 3 and 5 cm using the markings on the wire. The microsheath is then inserted over the wire into the CCA lumen between 2 and 3 cm. With the microsheath in place, an angiogram is performed to delineate the location of the carotid bifurcation.

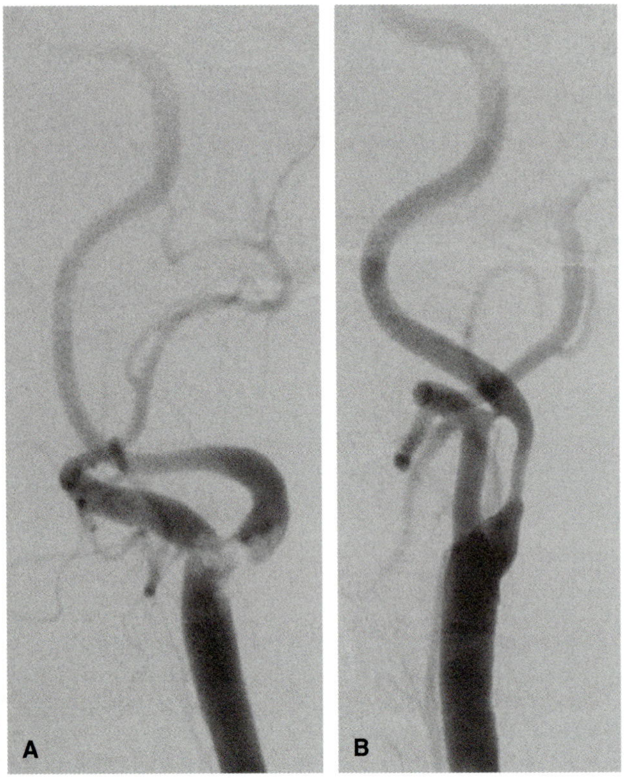

FIGURE 5 • Carotid bifurcation anatomy and arterial sheath insertion technique. **A,** "Stop short" technique is utilized in the presence of disease involving the distal common carotid artery. **B,** "Engage EC" is utilized when the external carotid artery is free of disease and can accommodate wire insertion.

"Stop short" Technique

- In patients with distal CCA involvement or a diseased external carotid artery (ECA), we employ the "stop short" technique to place the arterial sheath (**FIGURE 5A**).
- After the initial angiogram, the provided 0.035″ stiff wire is inserted into the CCA under fluoroscopic guidance. Care should be taken to ensure that the wire does not engage the carotid lesion during sheath insertion. With clear verbal communication between the operators, the microsheath is removed and the arterial sheath is then placed into the CCA by the operator while the assistant maintains caudal retraction of the CCA. The arterial sheath is placed into the CCA until the footplate is placed directly onto the outer wall of the CCA.

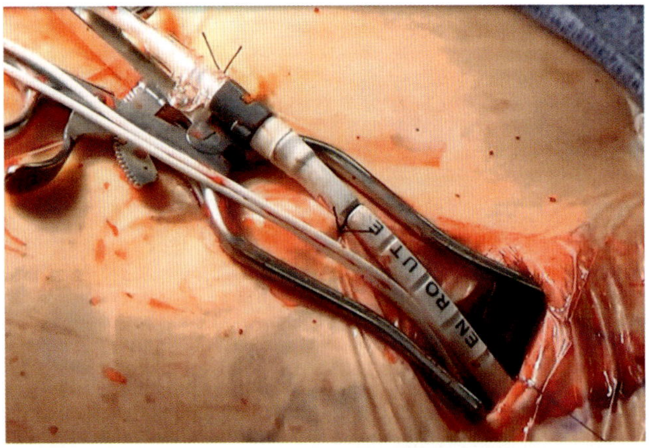

FIGURE 6 • Intraoperative photograph demonstrating the arterial sheath in place after insertion in the common carotid artery. The silastic vessel loop is in place for later vessel occlusion to establish flow reversal. The sheath is secured to the patient at two locations (shaft of sheath and islet of sheath) with sutures.

- The retraction on the CCA is relaxed and the arterial sheath is then secured in place utilizing 2 separate 2-0 silk sutures (**FIGURE 6**). One is placed around the body of the sheath at the base of the neck and the other is placed at the islet of the arterial sheath. The dilator and wire are then removed, leaving the distal 2.5 cm tip of the arterial sheath in the CCA lumen. The NPS flow controller is first connected to the arterial sheath. After appropriate flushing maneuvers to deair the flow controller, the sheath is then connected to the venous sheath and flow between the sheaths is initiated. A "saline bolus test" is performed by infusing heparinized saline into the venous sheath and visualizing the clearance of saline by the patient's blood in the tubing.

"Engage external carotid" Technique

- In patients with a healthy ECA, we employ the "engage EC (external carotid)" technique to place the arterial sheath (**FIGURE 5B**). After the initial angiogram, the microwire is inserted back into the microsheath and the ECA is carefully selected with the wire under fluoroscopy. The microsheath along with the dilator is then inserted into the ECA. The provided 0.035″ stiff wire is then inserted into the ECA. The arterial sheath is then placed into the CCA as above in the "stop short" technique.

ANGIOGRAM AND "TCAR TIMEOUT"

- It is important to point out that there remains antegrade flow through the CCA to the brain during this portion of the procedure. As such, there is no cerebral protection until the CCA is occluded during the angioplasty and stent portion of the procedure. Angiography is performed to further assess the arterial anatomy. This requires a minimum of two angiograms in orthogonal views to identify any possible access site complications (eg, dissection) and to confirm proper positioning of the arterial sheath tip. The images should also clearly delineate the flow channel through the lesion as well as the petrous portion of the ICA (typically represented by a 90° turn of the distal carotid as it enters the skull) (**FIGURE 7A**).
- Once the desired images are obtained, the positions of the patient and image intensifier are locked. The tip of the intervention 0.014″ wire is then shaped as necessary to help facilitate crossing the carotid stenosis. The tip of the wire is inserted into the sheath with care to not engage the lesion with the wire. The predilation angioplasty balloon is then inserted over the wire into the arterial sheath. The balloon should be sized to the nominal ICA diameter. In our practice,

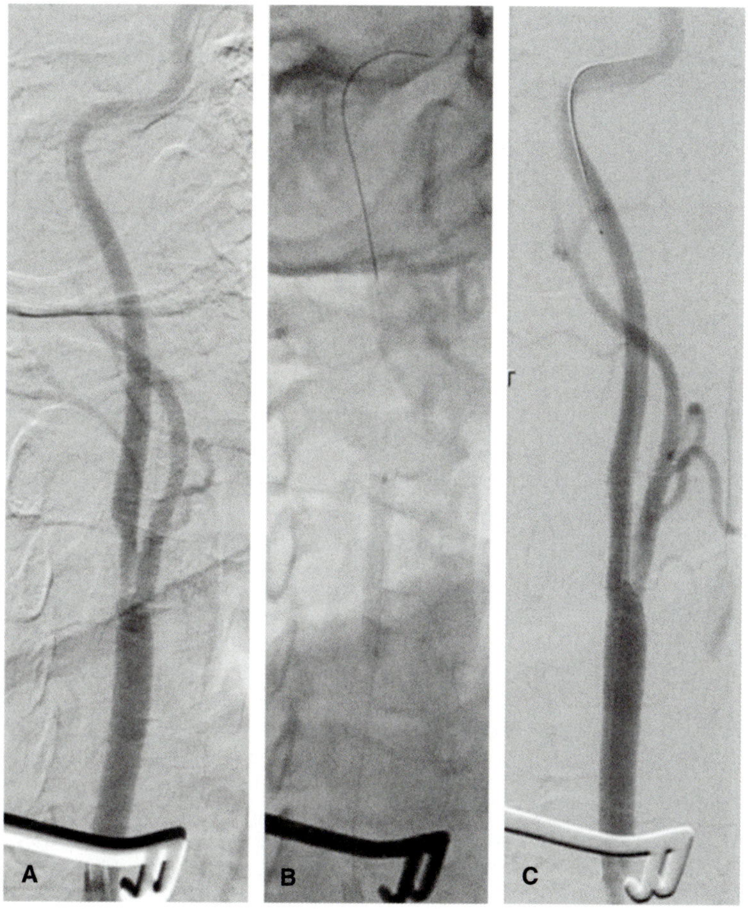

FIGURE 7 • Intraoperative angiograms. **A,** Preintervention angiogram demonstrating carotid stenosis at proximal internal carotid artery. **B,** Balloon angioplasty while under neuroprotection with reversal of flow. **C,** Completion angiogram after stent placement.

we routinely use a 5.5 × 30 mm angioplasty balloon. Once the wire and balloon are in place, a "TCAR timeout" is then performed. This is a second surgical pause (in addition to the standard preincision surgical timeout) to confirm all members of the surgical and anesthesia teams are ready for CCA occlusion. The anesthesia team should confirm adequate blood pressure, appropriate ACT level, and premedication to prevent bradycardia/hypotension during carotid angioplasty. The surgical team should confirm the proper positioning of the wire and balloon in the arterial sheath. The carotid stent should be open, prepped, and ready for use. The stent is typically sized to be 1 to 2 mm greater than the size of the carotid bulb. In our practice, we routinely use 40-mm long stents.

CAROTID ANGIOPLASTY AND STENT PLACEMENT

- After the "TCAR timeout," the common carotid artery is occluded. This can be done by tightening the double looped vessel loop or by placing a surgical clamp. A repeat "saline bolus test" is performed to monitor the rate of saline clearance. Once adequate flow is ensured, the 0.014″ wire is passed through the carotid lesion and the distal tip of the wire is placed at the petrous portion of the ICA. The angioplasty balloon is then placed at the desired location and a predilatation is then performed (**FIGURE 7B**).
- Even though appropriate premedication has been administered, anesthesia personnel should be alert and ready to treat (with atropine administration) any potential bradycardia and hypotension that arise. The balloon is removed, and the stent is then placed at the desired location and subsequently deployed. The degree of residual stenosis can be ascertained with plain fluoroscopic analysis of the stent architecture in orthogonal views (**FIGURE 8**). Postdilatation of the lesion may be performed as necessary, but we typically tolerate a residual stenosis of <30%. After waiting for 2 to 3 minutes of additional flow reversal after the last manipulation, completion angiograms are performed in at least two orthogonal views (**FIGURE 7C**). This is done to ensure adequate flow through the ICA. The wire is then removed and antegrade flow through the CCA is restored by releasing the occlusion (loosening vessel loop or removing clamp).

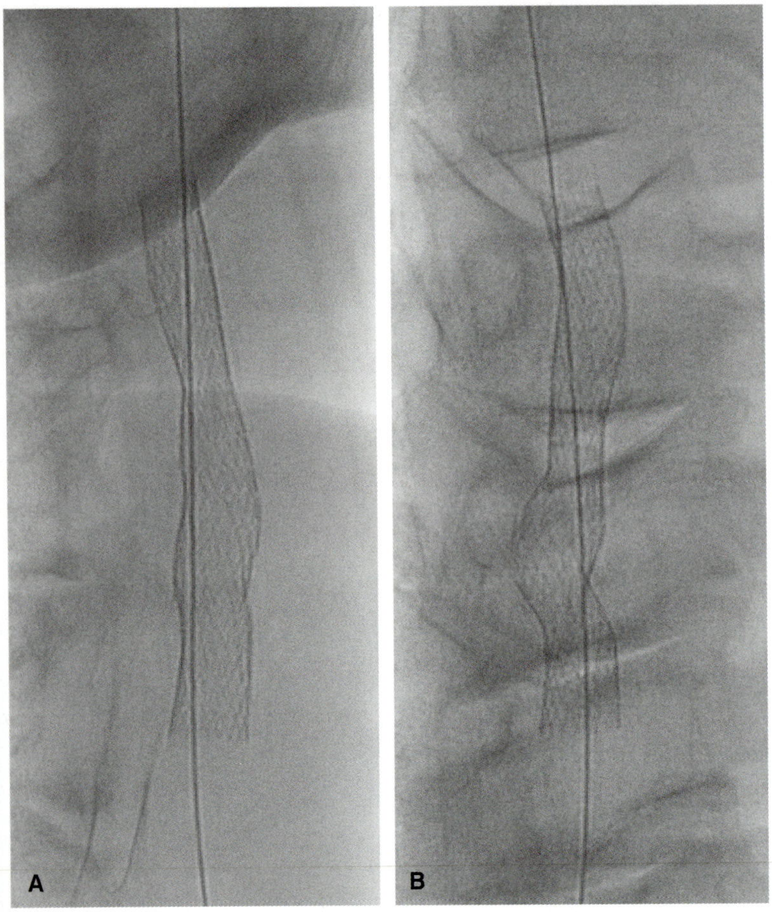

FIGURE 8 • **A** and **B,** Intraoperative plain fluoroscopic images in orthogonal views to demonstrate no significant stenosis based on stent architecture.

NPS REMOVAL AND COMPLETION OF PROCEDURE

- To conclude the procedure, the flow controller is disconnected from the arterial sheath and blood returned to the patient's circulation through the venous sheath. The flow controller is then disconnected from the venous sheath. The filter within the flow controller can be removed and examined to evaluate for the presence of debris (**FIGURE 9**).
- The venous sheath is flushed with heparinized saline and attention is directed back to the neck. The silk sutures securing the arterial sheath are cut. The arterial sheath is removed and the arteriotomy repaired by tying off the previously placed 5-0 Prolene suture. Protamine (typically 40 mg) is routinely administered at this time. After ensuring adequate hemostasis, the platysma is reapproximated utilizing a 3-0 Vicryl suture. The skin is then reapproximated utilizing a subcuticular suture followed by Dermabond. The femoral sheath is removed and manual pressure is utilized for hemostasis.

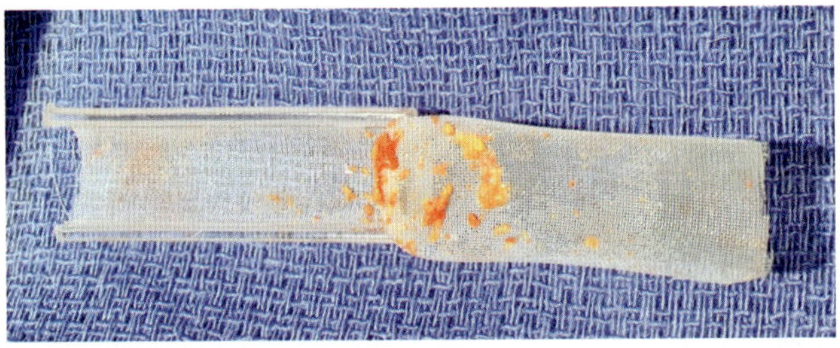

FIGURE 9 • Filter after a TCAR procedure showing the presence of atherosclerotic debris.

PEARL AND PITFALLS

Access site dissection	■ Maintain constant verbal communication between proceduralist and assistant during procedure. ■ Provide slight caudal retraction of CCA to provide stability during needle access. ■ Wire insertion should be gentle and avoid the use of force. ■ Utilize "engage EC" maneuver (if anatomy permits) to provide more wire access/stability during arterial sheath insertion. ■ Careful interrogation of access site with angiography.
Neck hematoma	■ Utilize preoperative ultrasound to identify location of two heads of SCM and depth of CCA. ■ Identify avascular plane during dissection and utilize gentle blunt dissection to identify CCA. ■ Routinely administer protamine after removal of arterial sheath and closure of CCA arteriotomy.
Calcification/ thrombus	■ Obtain high-quality thin cuts (<1 mm) CTA of the head and neck. ■ Carefully perform duplex ultrasound to examine proximal CCA for arterial access/occlusion. ■ Do not perform TCAR in patients with intraluminal thrombus. ■ Avoid stent placement in patients with circumferential (>50%) or thick (>3 mm) calcific burden.
Hypotension	■ Encourage adequate hydration on the night prior to procedure. ■ Hold selected antihypertensive medications day of surgery (continue beta blockers). ■ Appropriate premedication with glycopyrrolate prior to TCAR timeout. ■ Have vasoactive agents prepared and ready for infusion during the procedure. ■ Encourage early ambulation in the postprocedure period.

POSTOPERATIVE CARE

- A neurologic evaluation is performed at the completion of the procedure. The patient should have close neurologic as well as hemodynamic monitoring during the postprocedure period.
- The arterial line is typically left in for a minimum of 4 to 6 hours to determine the need of vasoactive agents. The systolic blood pressure is kept between 100 to 140 mm Hg (20% above baseline). Due to the stent exerting pressure on the carotid bulb, the presence of hypotension after stent placement is more frequent than with CEA. This can be treated with intravenous vasoactive agents (eg, phenylephrine infusion) or with oral medications (eg, pseudoephedrine).
- The patient should remain on bedrest for 1-2 hours due to the presence of the femoral venous puncture. The groin puncture site as well as the surgical wound at the neck will need to be monitored for bleeding/hematoma. Upon discharge, the patient should be maintained on DAPT and statin therapy for a minimum of 1 month. A carotid duplex is obtained at the 1 month follow-up visit to establish a new baseline for long-term monitoring.

OUTCOMES/COMPLICATIONS

- The ROADSTER trial is the first multicenter prospective clinical trial evaluating TCAR using the NPS system.[2] The study enrolled 141 pivotal phase patients between 2012 and 2014 with either symptomatic >50% or asymptomatic >70% stenosis considered to be at "high risk" for complications from CEA. In the pivotal cohort, the all-stroke rate was 1.4% (2 of 141), stroke/death was 2.8% (4 of 141), and stroke/death/MI was 3.5% (5 of 141). These data subsequently led to Food and Drug Administration approval in the United States in 2015.
- The ROADSTER 2 trial is a prospective multicenter postapproval registry for patients undergoing TCAR between 2015 and 2019.[5] The study enrolled 692 "high risk" patients with symptomatic stenosis >50% or asymptomatic stenosis >80% at 43 sites. As 60 cases had major study protocol violations, this left 632 patients (per protocol [PP] population) adhering to the FDA-approved protocol. The technical success occurred in 99.7% of all cases. The primary end point of procedural success (technical success plus the absence of stroke, MI, or death within the 30-day postoperative period) was 97.9% in the PP population. In the PP population, there were strokes in four patients (0.6%), death in one patient (0.2%), and MI in six patients (0.9%) leading to a composite 30-day stroke/death rate of 0.8% and stroke/death/MI rate of 1.7%. In the 60 patients with protocol violations, 11 were for not adhering to the inclusion/exclusion criteria of the study. The remaining 49 patients either did not start or discontinued their DAPT and statin. In this group of 60 patients, there were 11 additional stroke and two additional deaths, emphasizing the detrimental effect of medication noncompliance with the TCAR procedure.
- Data from >95% of TCAR procedures are entered into the TCAR Surveillance Project (TSP), a database created to allow for an evaluation of "real-world" TCAR outcomes compared to CEA.[6] Using data from the TSP and comparing outcomes between 1182 TCAR and 10,797 CEA patients, TCAR patients were older, more likely to be symptomatic, and had more medical comorbidities. On unadjusted analysis, TCAR had similar rates of in-hospital stroke/death (1.6% vs 1.4%) and stroke/death/MI (2.5% vs 1.9%) compared with CEA. There was no difference in the rates of stroke (1.4% vs 1.2%), in-hospital death (0.3% vs 0.3%), 30-day death (0.9% vs 0.4%), or MI (1.1% vs 0.6%). However, TCAR procedures were 33 minutes shorter than CEA and TCAR patients were less likely to incur cranial nerve injuries (CNI) (0.6% vs 1.8%) and less likely to have a postoperative length of stay >1 day (27% vs 30%). On adjusted analysis, there was no difference in terms of stroke/death, stroke/death/MI, or the individual outcomes.
- In an analysis of 86,027 patients that underwent carotid revascularization from over 400 centers in North America between 2015 and 2019, it was shown that the number of centers performing both TCAR and CEA increased from 15

to 247, a more than 16-fold increase.[7] The proportion of all carotid procedures that were TCAR increased from 0.7% to 17.0%, a 24-fold increase. In addition to increased adoption, the study also demonstrated that availability of TCAR at a hospital was associated with a decrease in the likelihood of perioperative major adverse cardiovascular events (MACE). Centers that adopted TCAR had a 10% decrease in the likelihood of MACE at 12 months after TCAR adoption vs if those centers had continued to perform CEA alone.

REFERENCES

1. Brott TG, Hobson RWII, Howard G, et al. Stenting versus endarterectomy for treatment of carotid artery stenosis. *N Engl J Med.* 2010;363:11-23.
2. Kwolek CJ, Jaff MR, Leal JI, et al. Results of the ROADSTER multicenter trial of transcarotid stenting with dynamic flow reversal. *J Vasc Surg.* 2015;62:1227-1235.
3. AbuRahma AF, Avgerinos ED, Chang RW, et al. Society for Vascular Surgery clinical practice guidelines for management of extracranial cerebrovascular disease. *J Vasc Surg.* 2022;75:4S-22S.
4. Kokkosis AA, MacDonald S, Jim J, et al. Assessing the suitability of the carotid bifurcation for stenting: anatomic and morphologic considerations. *J Vasc Surg.* 2021;74:2087-2095.
5. Kashyap VS, Schneider PA, Foteh M, et al. Early outcomes in the ROADSTER 2 study of transcarotid artery revascularization in patients with significant carotid artery disease. *Stroke.* 2020;51:2620-2629.
6. Schermerhorn ML, Liang P, Dakour-Aridi H, et al. In-hospital outcomes of transcarotid artery revascularization and carotid endarterectomy in the Society for Vascular Surgery Vascular Quality Initiative. *J Vasc Surg.* 2020;71:87-95.
7. Columbo JA, Martinez-Camblor P, O'Malley J, et al. Association of adoption of transcarotid artery revascularization with center-level perioperative outcomes. *JAMA Netw Open.* 2021;4:e2037885.

Chapter 5

Carotid Surgery: Distal Exposure and Control Techniques and Complication Management

Cheong Jun Lee

DEFINITION

- The carotid artery typically bifurcates at the level of the C3-C4 cervical spine. Distal internal carotid artery (ICA) exposure for control is required in high carotid bifurcations and lesions that extend to the C1-C2 level. Access to the distal ICA is impeded by the mastoid process and the angle of the mandible and furthermore by its intimate relationship to the hypoglossal and glossopharyngeal nerves. As such, exposure of the vessel cephalad to C3 poses technical challenges that may increase the perioperative risk of stroke and cranial nerve injury.
- To better ascertain the risk of distal ICA exposure, Vang et al subdivided the artery into three anatomic zones based on lesion extent and its relationship to the vertebral body[1]: the proximal segment of the ICA to the level of C3 body is designated Zone 1; Zone 2 extends from the C2 vertebral body but remains below C1; and Zone 3 is the segment of ICA above the C2 vertebral body (**FIGURE 1**).
- Ideally, the need for distal access in carotid surgery should be anticipated preoperatively with appropriate imaging. Familiarity of the anatomy and various exposure techniques are necessary for safe distal carotid control. The optimal level of distal control and which control techniques are employed depends strongly on the underlying pathology as aneurysmal conditions often require higher exposure compared to atherosclerotic disease.[2]

PATIENT HISTORY AND PHYSICAL FINDINGS

- As with any medical therapy, the clinician must first clearly define the goals of treatment and the indication for intervention, as well as thoroughly review the operative risk with the patient.
- An evidence-based approach to the treatment of atherosclerotic carotid disease has been reviewed previously; however, optimal medical therapy must be instituted prior to intervention (eg, antiplatelet agent, statin, appropriate antihypertensive agents).[3-5]
- Patients with hostile neck anatomy, such as those with history of high-dose neck radiation or severe systemic comorbidities contraindicating general or cervical block anesthesia, should be offered carotid angioplasty and carotid stenting (CAS) as an alternative procedure.
- Patients with prior contralateral carotid revascularization procedures should have laryngeal, hypoglossal, and glossopharyngeal nerve function documented prior to ipsilateral dissection and exposure. When evidence of prior injury to CN IX, X, or XII is evident, CAS should be considered as an alternative. If CAS is not feasible under these circumstances, the potential need for tracheostomy to manage postoperative airway obstruction should be reviewed with the patient.

IMAGING AND OTHER DIAGNOSTIC STUDIES

- Although duplex scanning provides accurate and reproducible assessment of the presence and severity of carotid stenosis, precise anatomic detail required for surgical planning is better obtained from computed tomographic angiography (CTA) or magnetic resonance arteriography (MRA). Localization of the carotid bifurcation in regard to cervical landmarks, as well as the distal extent of ICA disease, is best assessed by high-resolution CTA or MRA.
- CTA and MRA have enabled highly accurate characterization of plaque morphology, which may provide useful guidance regarding risk of distal embolization or intimal fractures leading to dissection during operative manipulation.

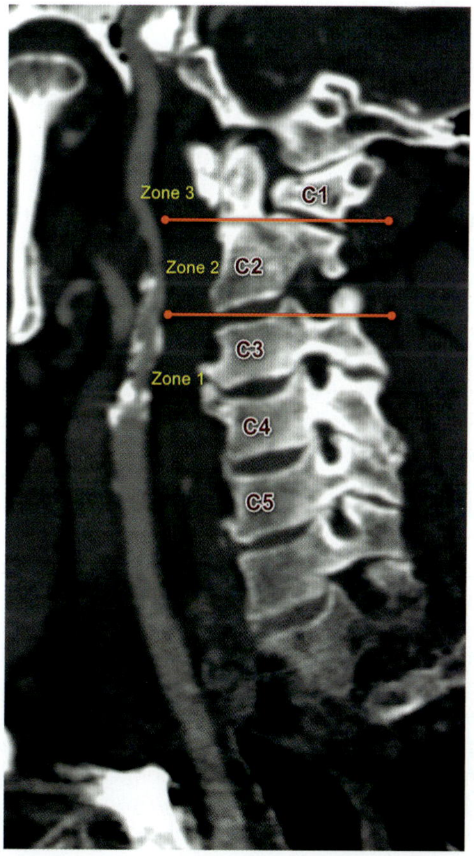

FIGURE 1 • The carotid artery can be divided into three zones respective to the cervical spine. A critical atherosclerotic plaque extending to Zone 1 is pictured in this reformatted computed tomography scan. Lesions that extend Zone 2 and above are deemed high and will require additional surgical maneuvers for exposure and control.

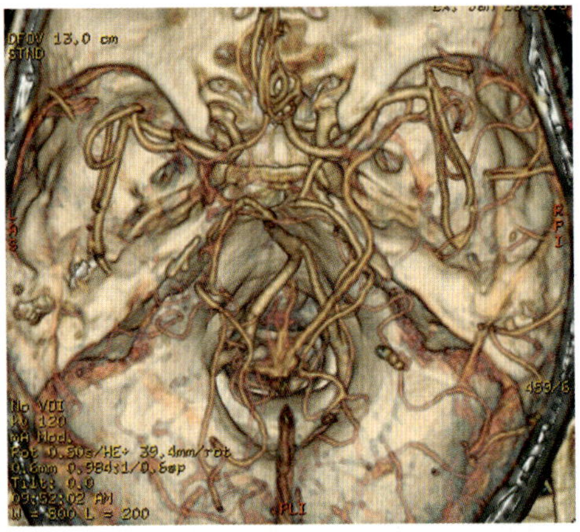

FIGURE 2 • Rendered computed tomographic angiography demonstrating incompetency of the circle of Willis.

- CTA and MRA also provide essential information regarding potential collateral arterial flow through the circle of Willis and the need for adjuvant maneuvers such as shunt placement during carotid revascularization (**FIGURE 2**).

SURGICAL MANAGEMENT

Preoperative Planning for Distal Cervical Carotid Exposure

- "Forewarned is forearmed."
- The degree of difficulty in distal carotid exposure is exacerbated in patients who have a short neck or high carotid bifurcation. As mentioned, for atherosclerotic disease specifically, CAS should be considered when lesion extent is high. However, in select patients with severe ICA tortuosity or heavy calcification, CAS will not be a good option. In these circumstances, CEA remains a safe and viable treatment modality. Nevertheless, being prepared for a challenging endpoint during CEA by having endovascular rescue options readily available is prudent.
- Knowledge of patient-specific cervical spine anatomy and potential patient tolerance for variable neck positioning is important. If neck flexion or extension is not feasible, more invasive maneuvers such as nasotracheal intubation or mandibular subluxation may be required as simple cephalad extension of the cervical incision may not offer significant distal exposure or maneuverability of key anatomic structures.
- Nasotracheal intubation and a chin-up position is an effective method to allow exposure of the distal ICA. Weiss et al. as well as others have described this method allowing operators to obtain as much as 2.5 cm of more distal exposure.[6,7] When recognized as necessary, specifying nasotracheal, rather than orotracheal, intubation for general endotracheal anesthesia is a simple and practical maneuver to improve exposure. Nasotracheal intubation allows the mouth to stay closed during surgery, providing more room between the ramus of the mandible and mastoid process for distal dissection.
- Temporomandibular subluxation may further advantage carotid exposure cephalad to the C2 cervical spine.[8] This technique is more invasive in that it requires subluxation of the ipsilateral mandibular condyle, performed via intraoral wiring. Mandibular subluxation with the addition of mandibular osteotomy and resection of the mastoid process are alternate strategies to obtain additional exposure from the infratemporal ICA to the skull base. Subluxation is distinguished from dislocation, which is more injurious and can potentiate long-term temporomandibular joint pain syndromes. The technique requires craniomaxillofacial surgery or otolaryngology colleagues for assistance. Though rarely utilized in atherosclerotic carotid disease management, anticipation of its application is realized in high extension of carotid body tumors and ICA aneurysms.
- Once the procedure is underway, however, neither nasotracheal intubation nor mandibular subluxation strategies can be used and other exposure methods will need to be considered.

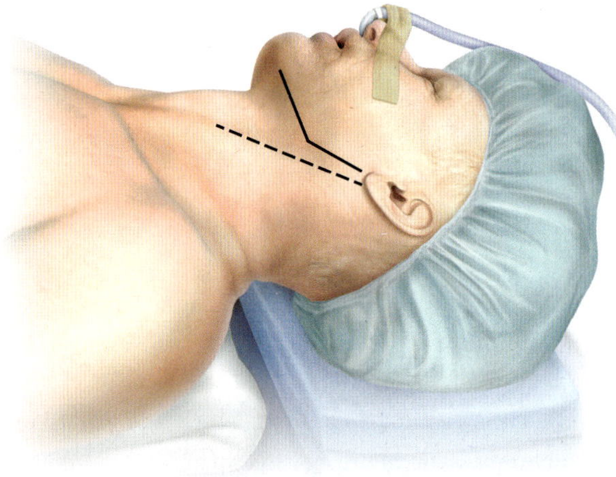

FIGURE 3 • Nasotracheal intubation facilitates exposures of the distal internal carotid artery by opening the angle between the mastoid process and the mandible (*black lines*).

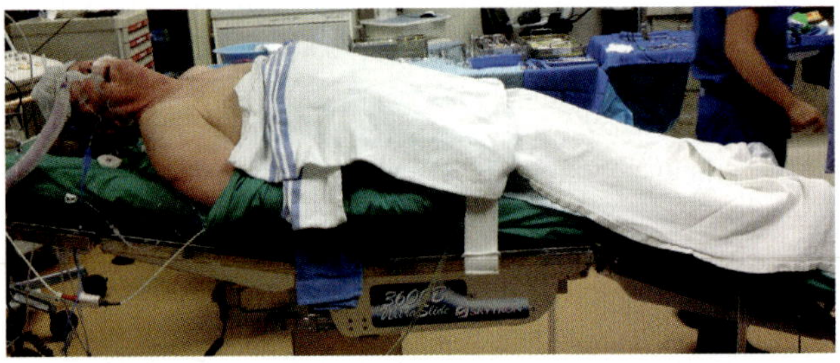

FIGURE 4 • Patient in the "beach chair" position.

Positioning

- The patient is positioned supine, with the head extended and rotated away from the operative site. Shoulder rolls and appropriate padding are placed to stabilize the neck and optimize extension. The nasotracheal tube is secured over the head (**FIGURE 3**).
- Arms are tucked to the patient's side to allow the operator and the assistant to maneuver and stand comfortably. This position also facilitates C-arm positioning when needed.
- The patient is placed in the "beach chair" position to limit venous hypertension (**FIGURE 4**).

ANTERIOR APPROACH TO THE DISTAL INTERNAL CAROTID ARTERY

Incision

- A longitudinal incision along the anterior margin of the sternocleidomastoid muscle (SCM), rather than a transverse cervical incision is recommended for optimal distal ICA access (**FIGURE 5**).

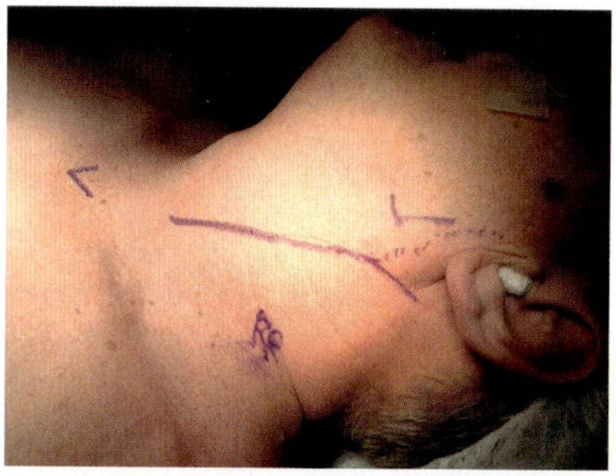

FIGURE 5 • Anatomic landmarks for carotid exposures include the mastoid process, the angle of the mandible, and the sternal notch. Skin incision for carotid exposures is placed anterior to the sternocleidomastoid muscle (*solid line*). If distal exposure is anticipated, the incision can be carried in front of the ear (*dotted line*).

- The incision can be extended anterior to the ear for distal exposure if needed but may require mobilization of the parotid gland in later stages of the dissection when lesion extent is significant.
- At the upper edge of the platysma and SCM, attention must be paid to the great auricular nerve. This nerve exits at the lateral border of the SCM, crosses over the surface of the SCM, and courses to the parotid gland and inferior part of the auricle.

Exposure of the Internal Carotid Artery Distal to the Bifurcation

- Key structures that lie superior to the carotid bifurcation are the posterior belly of the digastric muscle, the hypoglossal nerve, crossing veins from the SCM to the internal jugular vein, and muscular arterioles of the posterior branches of the external carotid artery (ECA) (**FIGURE 6**).
- The hypoglossal nerve is identified safely using a posterolateral to anteromedial dissection of the ICA. Moving cephalad, the hypoglossal nerve is dissected free from the medial surface of the digastric muscle. Crossing artery and veins of the SCM often tether this nerve closer to the bifurcation. Meticulous identification and controlled division of these tethering vessels will enable mobilization of the nerve. Tracing the course of the descending branch of the ansa cervicalis back to the hypoglossal itself provides positive confirmation of the location and course of the nerve (**FIGURE 7**).

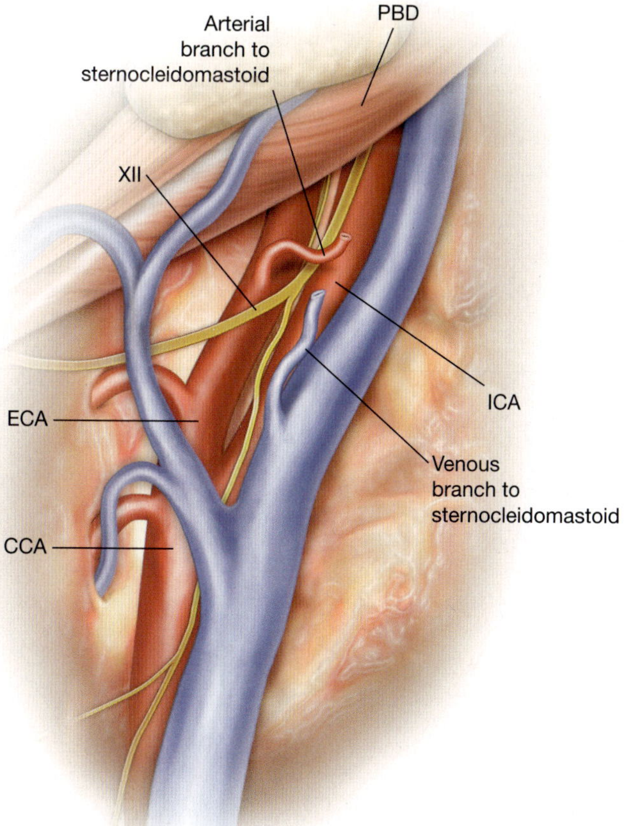

FIGURE 6 • Once the carotid sheath is entered, exposure of the distal internal carotid artery (ICA) from an anterior approach begins with identification and dissection of the hypoglossal nerve (XII), the posterior belly of the digastric muscle (PBD), and the crossing veins and arteries to the sternocleidomastoid muscle. CCA, common carotid artery; ECA, external carotid artery.

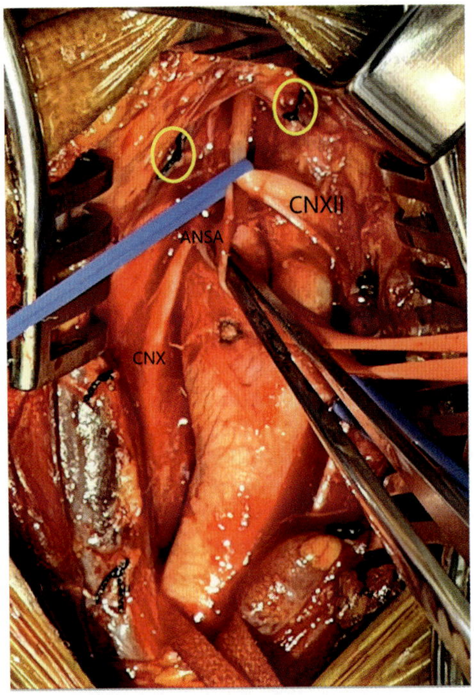

FIGURE 7 ● To further facilitate hypoglossal mobilization, the occipital artery coming off the external carotid artery has been ligated and divided. The ansa cervicalis (ANSA) can be ligated to further mobilize the hypoglossal nerve for distal carotid exposure.

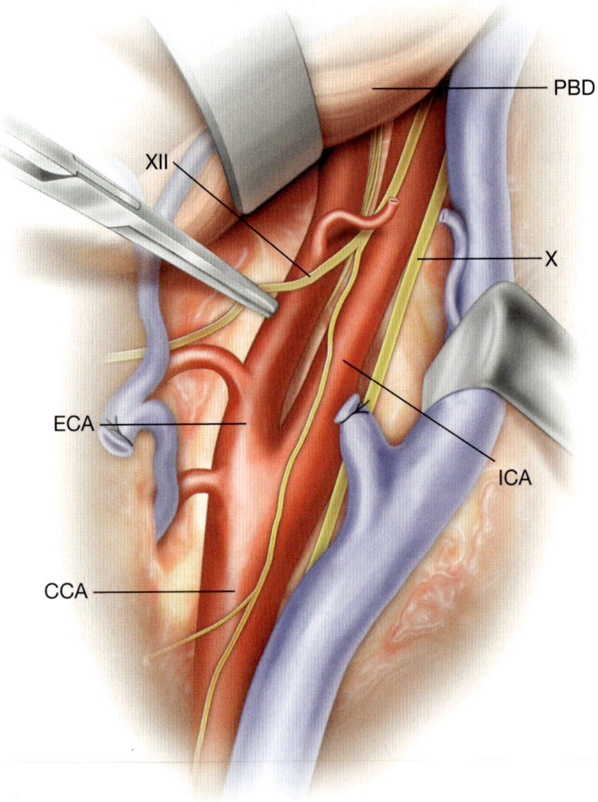

FIGURE 8 ● Mobilization of the hypoglossal nerve (XII) allows exposure of the distal internal carotid artery (ICA). CCA, common carotid artery; ECA, external carotid artery; PBD, posterior belly of the digastric muscle.

- The posterior digastric muscle belly may be retracted or divided as required for exposure, following release of the adherent hypoglossal nerve.
- Additional cephalad exposure at this juncture requires division of the occipital branch of the ECA. This further releases the hypoglossal nerve. This maneuver also requires division of the styloid musculature (styloglossus, stylopharyngeus).
- Continued cephalad dissection exposes the glossopharyngeal nerve, seen as a single or double trunk crossing the ICA anteriorly and coursing posterior to the external carotid. Care must be taken in separating the hypoglossal and glossopharyngeal nerves, as small motor fibers exiting the vagus nerve also course in this plane. Damage to these nerves or the glossopharyngeal can cause swallowing dysfunction. Classically, injury to the glossopharyngeal nerve in this region may impair the ability of the soft palate to rise sufficiently with swallowing to prevent nasopharyngeal liquid reflux.
- When these steps are safely completed, the ICA may be adequately exposed for reconstruction up to the level of C2 (**FIGURE 8**). Further exposure to the level of C1 following this course requires styloidectomy and/or preoperative mandibular subluxation.
- Distal dissection may also be facilitated by mobilization of the parotid gland and facial nerve. This is most safely accomplished with assistance from otolaryngologists or craniomaxillofacial surgeon. To provide this method of exposure, the skin incision is carried cephalad, anterior to the ear (**FIGURE 9**). This enables mobilization of the parotid gland superiorly and medially.

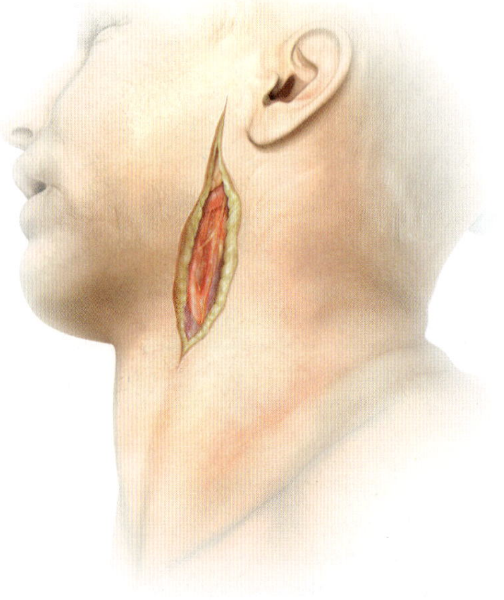

FIGURE 9 ● If further exposure of the internal carotid artery (ICA) is required and mandibular subluxation is not feasible, incision can be carried in front of the ear for mobilization of the parotid gland.

- The parotid fascia is entered and the branches of the facial nerve are dissected, identified, and protected before dividing the posterior belly of the digastric muscle.
- Care is again taken to identify the glossopharyngeal nerve and the motor fibers of the vagus nerve (**FIGURE 10**).
- Distal control of the ICA at high C1-C2 level may require specialized instrumentation. Small detachable occluding clamps (such as the Heifetz or Yasargil clips) may provide improved exposure compared to traditional "handled" vascular clamps in this region. When used, however, care must be taken to avoid clamp dislodgement in this crowded and moving field, which when it does happen, it usually does so at the maximally inconvenient time.
- As an alternative to distal clamp control, short occluding intraluminal catheters can be used, such as a #2 Fogarty embolectomy catheter with stopcock. Extreme care must be taken in positioning and deploying embolectomy balloons in this area, however, as inflation within the petrous portion or overinflation in any region may precipitate dissection, arterial rupture, or thrombosis. Only the lowest amount of inflation required to prevent back-bleeding should be used. The carotid artery is thin-walled at this level and easily traumatized by balloon inflation. Late complications also include pseudoaneurysm or arteriovenous fistula formation. The inflated catheter should be secured to prevent its migration. Stay sutures may be placed in the distal carotid to maintain access should control be lost due to reflux of the balloon from the distal artery or balloon puncture during suture closure of the anastomosis.

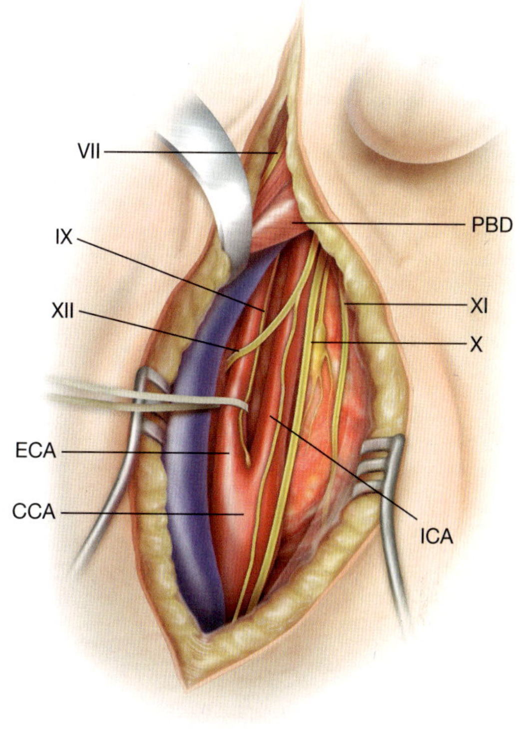

FIGURE 10 ● Once the parotid fascia is entered, the branches of the facial nerve (VII) are identified followed by the division of the posterior belly of the digastric muscle (PBD). CCA, common carotid artery; ECA, external carotid artery. Dissection is then carried anterior to the internal carotid artery (ICA) from the hypoglossal nerve (XII) distally to identify the glossopharyngeal nerve (IX). Motor fibers from the vagus nerve (X) are carefully identified and preserved.

RETROJUGULAR APPROACH TO THE DISTAL INTERNAL CAROTID ARTERY

Retrojugular Dissection

- A third approach to the distal ICA is provided by retrojugular access. The internal jugular (IJ) vein angles anteriorly as it ascends from the base of the neck to the base of the skull and overlies the distal ICA as the artery approaches the transverse process of C1.
- Using the posterior approach, dissecting behind the IJ vein, obviates the need for hypoglossal exposure and relocation, as that nerve passes anteriorly over the ICA. This approach is ideal when performing bypass rather than endarterectomy for an extensive ICA lesion.

Identification of the Spinal Accessory Nerve

- The retrojugular dissection uses the same incision as other approaches to the distal internal carotid, with the incision made longitudinally, anterior to the SCM muscle.
- Using this approach, it is essential to identify the spinal accessory nerve where it exits 2 to 3 cm below the edge of the mastoid process, anterior to the SCM. The SCM is fully mobilized to facilitate this exposure.
- Once the spinal accessory nerve is identified and isolated, the IJ vein is dissected along its posterior border. The vagus nerve is identified and reflected anteriorly. With the vein and vagus nerve mobilized anteriorly, the hypoglossal nerve remains anterior to the distal ICA (**FIGURE 11**).

Identification of the Superior Laryngeal Nerve

- In the retrojugular space, the ICA can be dissected along its posterior lateral wall superiorly whereupon the superior laryngeal nerve will be encountered exiting the vagus nerve and looping around the distal ICA. Often, the superior cervical ganglion can be identified just lateral to this looping point (**FIGURE 12**).
- For added exposure, the nerve is carefully lifted from the ICA adventitia.

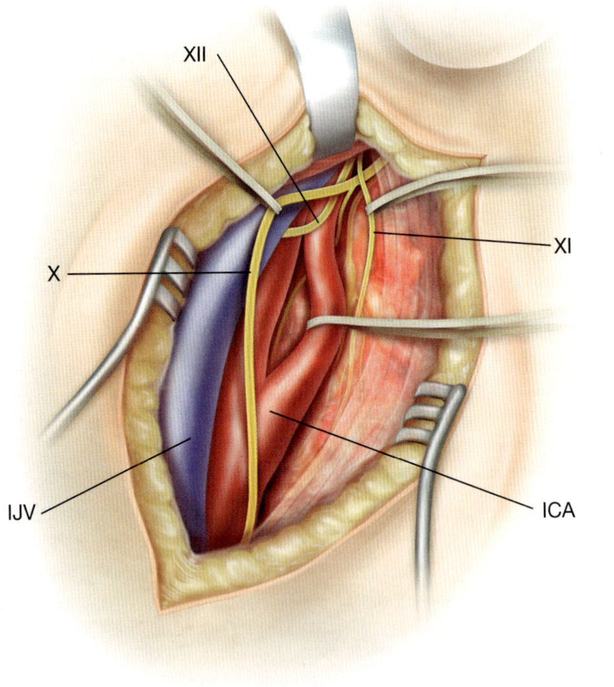

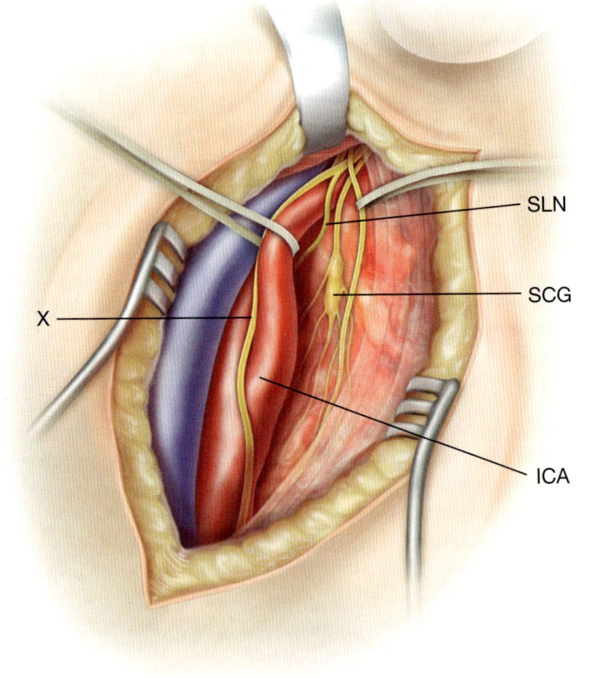

FIGURE 11 • Retrojugular exposure of the internal carotid artery (ICA): Dissection is carried behind the internal jugular vein (IJV) and the vagus nerve (X) mobilized anterior to the ICA. Care is taken in identifying the spinal accessory nerve (XI) at the superior aspect of the dissection. This approach avoids mobilization of the hypoglossal nerve (XII) as the plane of dissection remains posterior to the nerve.

FIGURE 12 • At the distal aspect of this retrojugular space, the internal carotid artery (ICA) will be looped by the superior laryngeal nerve (SLN) as it comes off the vagus nerve (X). Often, the superior cervical ganglion (SCG) serves as a landmark for where the SLN emanates.

PEARLS AND PITFALLS

Indications	▪ Make note of significant radiation or surgery to the neck, which may inform the choice of procedure (surgery vs CAS). ▪ Make certain the patient's cranial nerve status is documented, especially in the setting of prior neck operations.
Imaging	▪ High-resolution cross-sectional imaging (CTA/MRA) is essential for anticipating complex exposures and strategizing reconstructive techniques. ▪ The status of the circle of Willis should be defined in the course of preoperative planning.
Technique	▪ For lesions extending to the C1-C2 cervical spine, consider at a minimum nasotracheal intubation. ▪ In extreme situations, mandibular subluxation may provide critical additional degrees of freedom. ▪ Mandibular dislocation is not recommended and should not be performed to assist carotid surgery. ▪ *Knowledge of cranial nerve anatomy is the most important determinant of success as these are the structures most vulnerable to injury.* ▪ Any neural tissue crossing anterior to the carotid bifurcation and the ICA should *not* be divided. ▪ Mobilization of diseased arterial segments, including the carotid bifurcation, should be avoided and handling minimized prior to heparinization. ▪ Anterior distal ICA exposure is dependent on the extent to which the hypoglossal nerve can be safely mobilized. ▪ Posterior, retrojugular exposure requires early identification of the spinal accessory nerve and anterior reflection of the vagus nerves to visualize the superior laryngeal nerve encircling the distal internal carotid. ▪ Balloon occlusion may facilitate far distal carotid control, but overadvancement and overinflation are real risks that must be considered. ▪ Placement of stay sutures on the distal ICA will facilitate control maneuvers.

POSTOPERATIVE CARE AND COMPLICATION MANAGEMENT

- Cranial nerve injury during distal carotid exposure is the most frequently encountered complication. Most of these nerve injuries are transient; however, permanent deficits are more likely to occur with distal exposures.[1] The majority of these injuries are due to excessive retraction; therefore sharp dissection of the nerve and vessels, avoiding direct handling of any nerve tissue by grasping perineural tissue for retraction, and removal of excessive tension on nerves by detaching them from the surrounding tissues are recommended preventative strategies.
- If the endpoint of the CEA remains questionable despite the use of adjunct maneuvers, endovascular rescue should be considered.[9] Intraoperative CAS can be performed by extending the skin incision inferiorly to allow for placement of a vascular sheath in the supraclavicular common carotid artery.
- Following carotid revascularization, the immediate postoperative care is focused on close neurologic surveillance. Patients are recovered typically in an intensive care unit or monitored setting to facilitate ready identification of evolving neurologic deficits.
- Careful blood pressure monitoring and management is also essential. Following carotid revascularization, patients need to avoid the extremes of blood pressure, which may lead to development of hemodynamic stroke and cerebral reperfusion syndromes that can result in devastating intracerebral hemorrhage.
- Immediate postoperative (<24 hours) neurologic deficits should be assumed to be thromboembolic in nature, most commonly associated with a technical (surgical) error. Further imaging studies are unlikely to alter decision-making and should not delay immediate re-exploration. Neurologic deficits arising later in the postoperative period (>24 hours) may be due to intracranial hemorrhage; in these cases, computed tomography (CT) or magnetic resonance (MR) imaging may assist the decision-making process and should be considered when etiologic circumstances are less certain.
- Bleeding complications following carotid surgery are rare but potentially serious or fatal. These typically occur during the first several hours after surgery or even later, particularly in patients resuming anticoagulation therapy for existing conditions early in the postoperative period. Recognition and expeditious control of the airway is of utmost importance as a wound hematoma develops, as cord and airway edema rapidly worsen in response to reduced venous and lymphatic drainage. Reopening a carotid incision prior to anesthetic induction may facilitate emergency endotracheal intubation; however, this dramatic maneuver is best performed in a controlled environment with resuscitation equipment available should complications ensue. Ideally, preparations are made for wound decompression as endotracheal intubation is being attempted, with the wound being opened as a last step maneuver prior to emergency cricothyroidotomy. Cord edema in these circumstances may be profound, however, and visualization may not improve sufficiently after hematoma evacuation to enable orotracheal or nasotracheal intubation. Therefore, cricothyroidotomy may become necessary in extreme circumstances, and all carotid surgeons should be facile in this maneuver as a matter of course.

OUTCOMES

- Surgical outcomes of distal carotid exposure are dependent on the nature of disease vs lesion extent. Equivalent surgical mortality and neurologic outcomes are seen in patients undergoing CEA regardless of the extent of disease involvement.[1,10] Permanent cranial nerve injuries, however, are more realized with higher lesions. When distal carotid/skull base exposure appears to be necessary to safely manage an occlusive lesion, consideration should again be given to CAS as a lower risk alternative technique to open endarterectomy or interposition grafting.[10]
- Data describing the outcome of distal (base of skull) carotid reconstruction and bypass for aneurysmal disease or tumors are based on more limited, institution-specific case series. In these circumstances, outcomes are more difficult to benchmark. One recent series reported that one of five patients requiring a distal ICA bypass for aneurysm repair suffered a stroke; 60% suffered varying degrees of cranial nerve deficit.[11] The largest experience reported to date is that of Sessa et al,[12] who reported a 3% and 6% rate of perioperative stroke and restenosis at 1 year, respectively.

COMPLICATIONS

- Cranial nerve injury
- Stroke
- Horner syndrome
- Seroma
- Infection

REFERENCES

1. Vang S, Hans SS. Carotid endarterectomy in patients with high plaque. *Surgery*. 2019;166(4):601-606. doi:10.1016/j.surg.2019.06.017. Epub 2019 Aug 9. PMID: 31405580.
2. Attigah N, Hyhlik-Dürr A, Hakimi M, Allenberg JR, Böckler D. Der hohe Zugang zur Arteria carotis interna [High exposure of the distal internal carotid artery]. Article in German. *Chirurg*. 2010;81(2):155-159. doi: 10.1007/s00104-009-1784-y. PMID: 19711019.
3. North American symptomatic carotid endarterectomy trial. Methods, patient characteristics, and progress. *Stroke*. 1991;22:711-720.
4. Endarterectomy for asymptomatic carotid artery stenosis. Executive Committee for the asymptomatic carotid atherosclerosis study. *JAMA*. 1995;273:1421-1428.
5. Randomised trial of endarterectomy for recently symptomatic carotid stenosis: final results of the MRC European Carotid Surgery Trial (ECST). *Lancet*. 1998;351:1379-1387.
6. Weiss MR, Smith HP, Patterson AK, Weiss M. Patient positioning and nasal intubation for carotid endarterectomy. *Neurosurgery*. 1986;19(2):256-257.
7. Takigawa T, Yanaka K, Yasuda M, Asakawa H, Matsumaru Y, Nose T. Head and neck extension-fixation with a head frame for exposure of the distal internal carotid artery in carotid endarterectomy–technical note. *Neurol Med Chir (Tokyo)*. 2003;43:271-273. discussion 273, 2003.
8. Capoccia L, Montelione N, Menna D, et al. Mandibular subluxation as an adjunct in very distal carotid arterial reconstruction: incidence of peripheral and cerebral neurologic sequelae in a single-center experience. *Ann Vasc Surg*. 2014;28:358-365.

9. Tameo MN, Dougherty MJ, Calligaro KD. Carotid endarterectomy with adjunctive cephalad carotid stenting: complementary, not competitive, techniques. *J Vasc Surg*. 2008;48(2):351-354. doi:10.1016/j.jvs.2008.03.054. PMID: 18644483.
10. Kondo T, Ota N, Göhre F, et al. High cervical carotid endarterectomy-outcome analysis. *World Neurosurg*. 2020;136:e108-e118. doi: 10.1016/j.wneu.2019.12.002. Epub 2019 Dec 9. PMID: 31830599.
11. Eliason JL, Netterville JL, Guzman RJ, et al. Skull base resection with cervical-to-petrous carotid artery bypass to facilitate repair of distal internal carotid artery lesions. *Cardiovasc Surg*. 2002;10:31-37.
12. Sessa CN, Morasch MD, Berguer R, et al. Carotid resection and replacement with autogenous arterial graft during operation for neck malignancy. *Ann Vasc Surg*. 1998;12:229-235.

Chapter 6 Repair of Internal and External Carotid Injury

Melike N. Harfouche and Rosemary A. Kozar

DEFINITION

- Penetrating neck trauma is classified into zones, traditionally applied to anterior wounds of the neck.
- Zone I is defined as any injury from the sternal notch to the cricoid cartilage, zone II is any injury from the cricoid cartilage to the angle of the mandible, and zone III is any injury from the angle of the mandible to the base of the skull[1] (**FIGURE 1**).
- Blunt cerebrovascular injuries can occur to either the carotid artery or the vertebral arteries and develop from intimal trauma due to rapid acceleration/deceleration injuries or direct blunt force injury to the neck.
- In these cases, injury to the carotid artery usually occurs in the region in proximity to the petrous portion, where the artery is relatively fixed.
- Blunt carotid injury rarely requires operative intervention, and if so, it is usually treated with an endovascular approach. On the other hand, penetrating injuries to the carotid artery frequently mandate operative exploration.

DIFFERENTIAL DIAGNOSIS

- Penetrating trauma to the neck can involve vascular structures, but it can also involve the aerodigestive tract. It is important to consider laryngeal, tracheal, and esophageal injuries in the differential diagnosis.

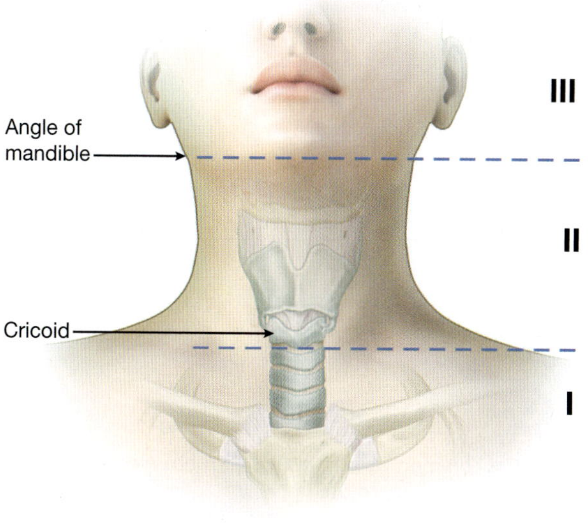

FIGURE 1 • Zones of the neck. The neck is divided into three zones: Zone III is above the angle of the mandible, Zone II is between the angle of the mandible and the cricoid cartilage, and Zone I is below the cricoid cartilage. (Reprinted with permission from Roon AJ, Christensen N. Evaluation and treatment of penetrating cervical injuries. *J Trauma*. 1979;19(6):391-397.)

- Injuries to the thoracic inlet (zone I) can involve other vascular structures, namely the subclavian arteries and veins and the innominate artery and veins.
- Injuries to the base of the skull can extend into intracranial structures.
- Missiles carry more kinetic energy than stab wounds and travel further distances. In these cases, it is important to have a wide differential diagnosis as to the body cavities and associated structures that may be injured, as they may not be limited to the structures within the neck.[2]

PATIENT HISTORY AND PHYSICAL FINDINGS

- Clinical findings of vascular injury to the neck are divided into hard signs and soft signs (**TABLE 1**).
- Hard signs of vascular injury mandate operative exploration; the surgical approach is dictated by the zone of injury (see below).
- Soft signs of vascular injury require investigation with imaging modalities, namely computed tomography angiography (CTA) or digital subtraction angiography (DSA).
- Crepitus in the neck is usually indicative of a tracheal injury, which may also present with severe hypoxia and rapid decompensation requiring orotracheal intubation or a surgical airway.
- Esophageal injuries rarely present with crepitus and are usually insidious. In some cases, hematemesis may occur.

IMAGING AND OTHER DIAGNOSTIC STUDIES

- In the absence of penetration of the platysma and no soft signs of vascular injury, no further imaging and a short period of observation is appropriate.
- A plain anteroposterior X-ray of the neck can be performed in the trauma bay to evaluate for subcutaneous emphysema. A lateral X-ray can provide additional information regarding missile trajectory.
- In the absence of hard signs of vascular injury mandating direct operative exploration, patients with soft signs of vascular injury should have further imaging.
- Traditionally, the gold standard test to evaluate for vascular injury in the neck was DSA; however, due to improvements in CT technology and speed of performance, CTA has largely replaced DSA as the imaging modality of choice to evaluate for vascular injury in the neck.[3] It has a sensitivity of 79%-100% and a specificity of 61%-100%.[4] **FIGURE 2** demonstrates a penetrating injury to the carotid artery at the thoracic inlet.
- Bronchoscopy can be performed to evaluate for injuries to the trachea or main bronchi. If this is being performed on an intubated patient, the endotracheal tube must be withdrawn

to the level of the vocal cords to adequately assess the entire trachea.

SURGICAL MANAGEMENT

- Patients with vascular injuries to the neck can deteriorate rapidly and require emergent intubation.
- It is important to anticipate potential airway loss and intubate patients prophylactically rather than wait for deterioration. Remain vigilant and communicate clearly with your anesthesiology and/or emergency room staff to ensure the patient is intubated safely and appropriately.
- Be prepared to perform emergent cricothyroidotomy if orotracheal intubation cannot be achieved.

Preoperative Planning

- Injuries to vascular structures within the thoracic inlet (Zone I) usually require sternotomy or thoracotomy to provide adequate exposure.
- Injuries to zone III are rarely amenable to direct surgical exploration and usually require endovascular techniques.
- Injuries to zone II can be exposed directly through a neck incision.

Table 1: Hard and Soft Signs of Vascular Injury to the Neck

Hard signs	Soft signs
Active bleeding	Neurologic deficit
Expanding or pulsatile hematoma	Nonpulsatile hematoma or venous oozing
Thrill/bruit	History of significant bleeding

- Communicate the planned procedure to the operating room staff, including surgical approach and any additional equipment that may be required.
- Consider requesting a bronchoscopy and/or endoscopy cart.
- Ask for blood products to be immediately available.

Positioning

- Patients should be placed supine with the neck rotated 45° away from the side of injury. Cervical spine injuries resulting from blunt trauma should be ruled out prior to neck rotation. If a cervical spine fracture is present, the neck should be immobilized in a midline position.
- A towel or padding underneath the shoulders may assist with improved exposure of the neck structures.
- Both arms should remain extended away from the body, to allow for access to the chest if needed, and the patient should be placed in a sitting position to bring the operative field closer.

Setup

- In general, the entire chest and neck should be prepped into the field to allow for sternotomy or thoracotomy if needed. If additional injuries have not been ruled out, a wide prep of chin to knees should be performed.
- If there is a documented zone II injury based on preoperative imaging, the entire neck from slightly above the angle of the mandible to the upper sternum should be prepped. If there is any concern for esophageal or tracheal injury, both sides should be prepped in the event an extension anteriorly needs to be performed or the contralateral side needs to be explored.
- The upper sternum, earlobe, and jaw should be draped into the field.

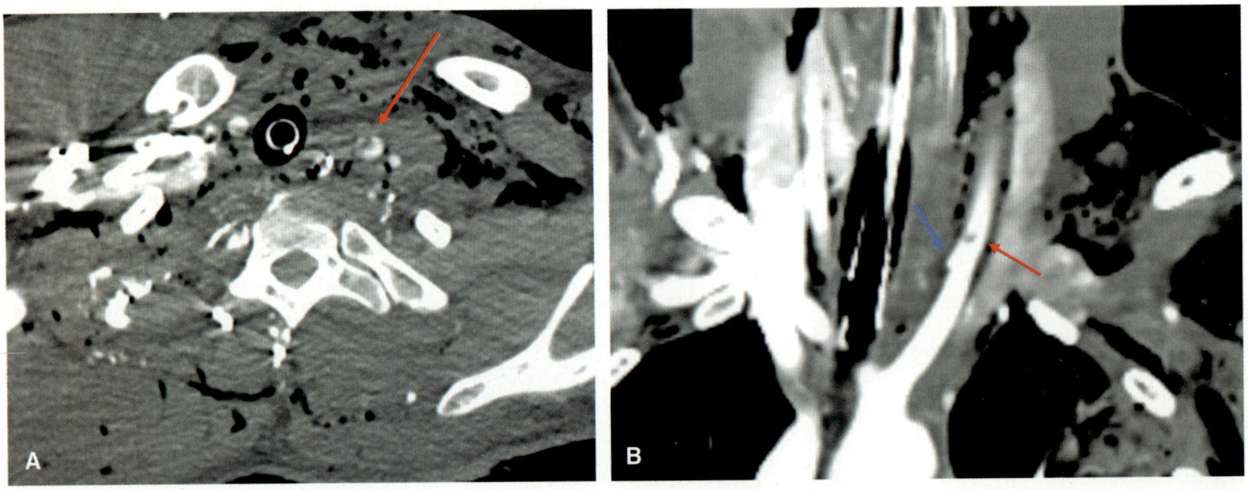

FIGURE 2 • Computed tomography scan of the neck demonstrating injury to the common carotid artery. Gunshot wound to the left neck, resulting in injury to the common carotid artery at the thoracic inlet, as well as an injury to the upper left lobe of the lung and an esophageal injury. **A,** The vascular injury is demonstrated by an intimal flap on the axial view (*red arrow*). **B,** The coronal view demonstrates an associated pseudoaneurysm (*blue arrow*) and an intimal flap (*red arrow*).

INCISION

- Mark out the angle of the mandible to the sternal notch (**FIGURE 3**).
- The incision should be made anterior to the sternocleidomastoid muscle (SCM), extending from the angle of the mandible to the sternal notch. The incision should be generous, to allow for adequate exposure for both proximal and distal control of the carotids.

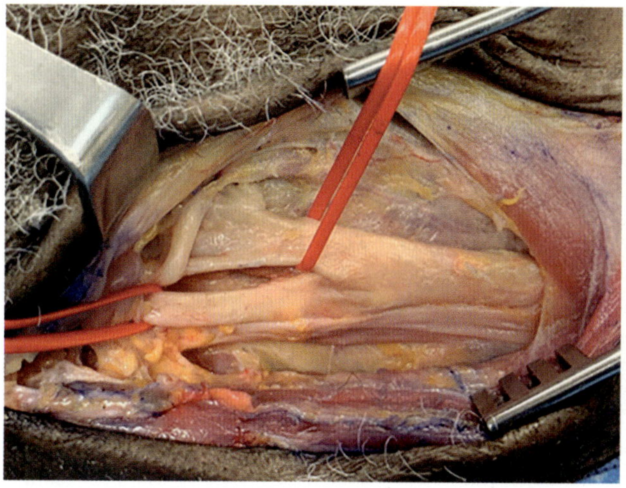

FIGURE 3 • Incision for neck exploration. The incision should typically extend from the angle of the mandible to the sternal notch.

EXPOSURE OF THE NECK

- The dissection should proceed through the platysma muscle, below which the SCM is visible.
- Continue the dissection anterior to the SCM, taking care to protect the parotid gland which is located at the superior most border of the incision. The first structure to be identified is the internal jugular vein, located lateral and superficial to the carotid sheath (**FIGURE 4**). A small venous branch crossing medially from the internal jugular vein is the facial vein, which can be ligated and transected. This vein usually lies immediately anterior to the bifurcation of the carotid artery. This will expose the carotid sheath, a thin structure overlying the carotid artery.

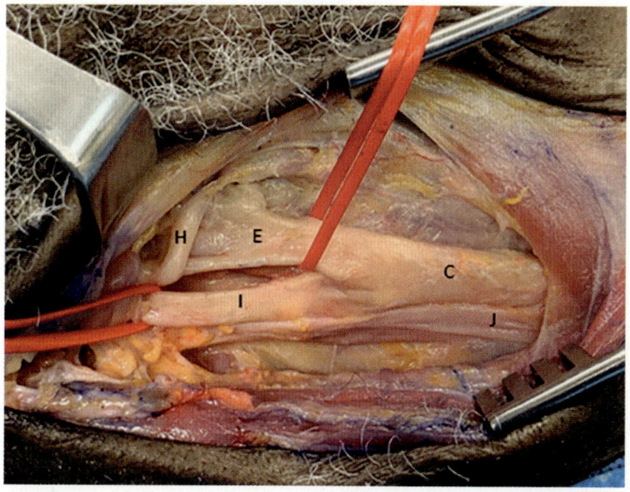

FIGURE 4 • Exposure of the carotid artery. Shown in this figure is the common carotid as it branches into the internal and external carotid. Also shown are the internal jugular vein and the hypoglossal nerve.C, common carotid artery; E, external carotid artery; H, hypoglossal nerve; I, internal carotid artery; J, internal jugular vein.

- Continue dissection through the carotid sheath, exposing the common carotid artery (CCA) (**FIGURE 4**). Dissect the CCA circumferentially and encircle it with a vessel loop, attaining proximal control. If there is significant bleeding preventing adequate visualization, direct pressure can be applied over the area of maximum bleeding while proximal control of the CCA is achieved.
- Identify and protect the vagus nerve (**FIGURE 5**), which is located in the carotid sheath and runs along the CCA. As dissection is continued cranially, the bifurcation of the internal carotid artery (ICA) and the external carotid artery (ECA) will be identified, the latter of which courses medially and gives off the superior thyroidal artery as its first branch (**FIGURE 4**). Circumferentially dissect and encircle each branch with a vessel loop. Take care to identify and preserve the hypoglossal nerve, which crosses transversely over the internal and external carotid arteries (**FIGURE 4**).

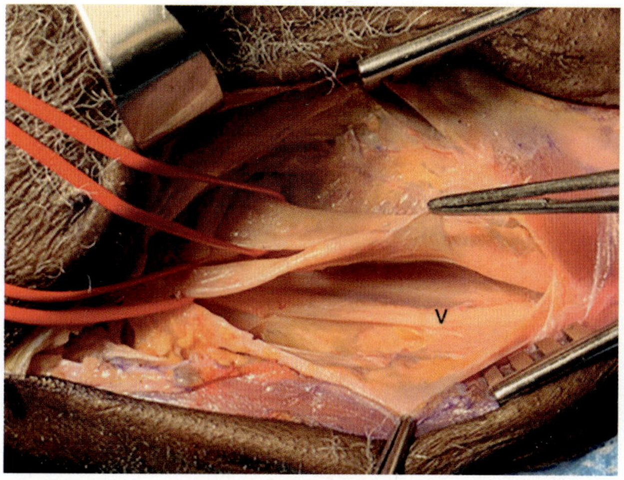

FIGURE 5 • Vagus nerve.

MANAGEMENT OF THE VASCULAR INJURY

- The use of systemic unfractionated heparin is generally recommended for complex repairs if not prohibited by associated injuries.
- Management of the vascular injury is dictated by the extent of the injury and the physiologic status of the patient. If the patient is hypothermic, coagulopathy, and acidotic (pH < 7.2), then damage control surgery should be performed. In this case, the fastest method that can achieve hemorrhage control should be performed.
- A small laceration of the CCA can be repaired with either a continuous or interrupted 5-0 Prolene suture. Larger injuries may need to be controlled with a temporary shunt if expedient hemorrhage control is required in an unstable patient as part of damage control surgery (**FIGURE 6**). In stable patients with brisk back bleeding, routine shunting is generally not needed. Although any tubular structure can serve as a shunt, commonly used shunts for the carotid artery are Argyle, Javid, and Pruitt-Inahara shunts. Once the physiologic derangements have been corrected, the patient should be taken back to the operating room for definitive repair (**FIGURE 7**).
- A similar approach can be used for repair of the ICA. In rare cases where gaining control of the ICA distal to the injury cannot be achieved due to its anatomic location, subluxation of the mandible can be performed to gain better exposure. However, this maneuver will only expose an additional 1-2 cm of vessel. If distal control cannot be achieved, temporary insertion and inflation of a Fogarty balloon into the injury tract can control bleeding.
- If primary, tension-free repair of either the ICA or CCA injury cannot be achieved, a saphenous vein or bovine pericardial patch can be applied to bridge the defect. If the artery must be replaced due to extensive tissue loss, a 6-mm polytetrafluoroethylene (Gore-Tex) graft or saphenous vein can be used as a conduit depending on vessel size. In these cases, an end-to-end interposition of the conduit should be performed.
- Simple injuries to the ECA can be repaired primarily, but in cases of complex injuries the artery can be ligated without consequence. Prior to ligation, ensure that the vessel is the ECA by identifying the presence of branches, which the ICA does not have.

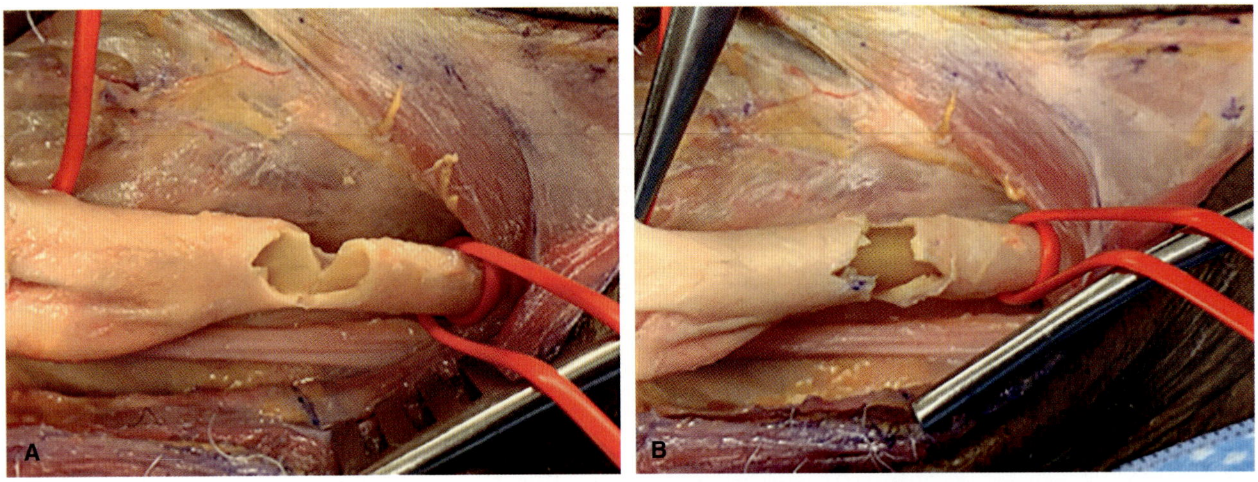

FIGURE 6 • Injury to common carotid artery. The left image **(A)** shows a large injury to the common carotid artery. The right image **(B)** shows temporary control with a shunt.

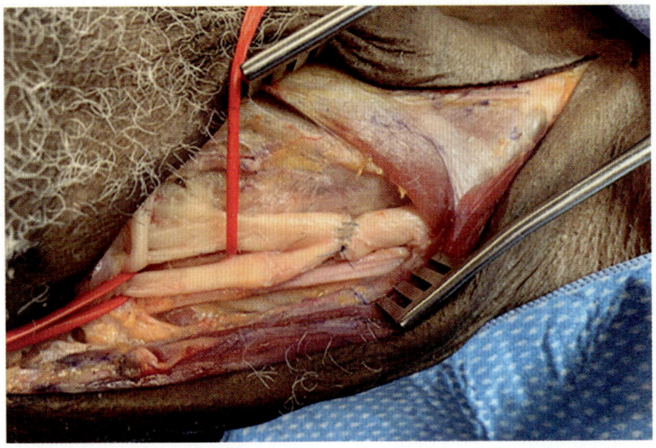

FIGURE 7 • Definitive repair of an injury to the common carotid artery.

PEARLS AND PITFALLS

- Patients with zone II injuries and hard signs of vascular injury (pulsatile bleeding, expanding hematoma) should proceed directly to the operating room.
- Principles of proximal and distal control pertain to the carotid arteries.
- Obtaining proximal and distal control prior to opening a hematoma is the preferred approach.
- When in doubt, the chest and bilateral neck areas should be included in the operative field. Prep out the contralateral neck if there is concern for aerodigestive tract injury that might require bilateral neck exploration.

POSTOPERATIVE CARE

- Patients should be closely monitored for the first 24 hours after surgery, preferably in an intensive care unit. Cross-clamping of the carotid artery places the patient at risk for cerebral ischemia.
- Once the patient is awake, a full neurologic assessment should be performed and documented.

COMPLICATIONS

- **Nerve injury:** Injuries to the vagus nerve may cause vocal cord dysfunction but will likely not impede breathing unless bilateral injury occurs. Patients with hoarseness postoperatively should be monitored closely for airway compromise and intubated early if there are any concerns.
- **Bleeding:** Patients should be monitored closely for evidence of ongoing bleeding, including hematoma development, shunt dislodgement, or missed injuries. As the patient is rewarmed and the acidosis corrected, vessels that were previously under vasospasm may relax and start bleeding. If this occurs, the patient should be taken back to the operating room expediently.
- **Stroke:** This is uncommon in most patients with penetrating injury to the carotid arteries but can occur in patients who have atherosclerotic carotid disease resulting in plaque dislodgement, or those who have little to no contralateral cerebral flow from the circle of Willis causing abrupt cessation of flow when the carotid artery is clamped. Stroke rate is higher in ICA injuries compared to CCA injuries.[5] In order to reduce the risk of stroke, minimize manipulation of the carotid artery and duration of clamp time.

REFERENCES

1. Roon AJ, Christensen N. Evaluation and treatment of penetrating cervical injuries. *J Trauma*. 1979;19(6):391-397.
2. Low GM, Inaba K, Chouliaras K, et al. The use of the anatomic "zones" of the neck in the assessment of penetrating neck injury. *Am Surg*. 2014;80(10):970-974.
3. Inaba K, Munera F, McKenney M, et al. Prospective evaluation of screening multislice helical computed tomographic angiography in the initial evaluation of penetrating neck injuries. *J Trauma Inj Infect Crit Care*. 2006;61(1):144-149.
4. Ibraheem K, Wong S, Smith A, et al. Computed tomography angiography in the "no-zone" approach era for penetrating neck trauma: a systematic review. *J Trauma Acute Care Surg*. 2020;89(6):1233-1238.
5. Ramadan F, Rutledge R, Oller D, Howell P, Baker C, Keagy B. Carotid artery trauma: a review of contemporary trauma center experiences. *J Vasc Surg*. 1995;21(1):46-55; discussion 55-56.

SECTION II: Management of the Thoracic Outlet

Chapter 7 Vertebral Transposition Techniques and Stenting

Mark D. Morasch

DEFINITION

- Treatment for occlusive lesions involving the origin of the vertebral artery (V1 segment) is undertaken to relieve posterior brain circulation ischemia, otherwise known as vertebrobasilar insufficiency. Revascularization options include open surgical and endovascular techniques. The most common operation is a proximal vertebral to common carotid transposition. Endoluminal treatment includes balloon angioplasty and (typically) stenting.

DIFFERENTIAL DIAGNOSIS

- Other medical conditions mimicking posterior circulation ischemia include postural hypotension, cardiac arrhythmias, anemia, brain tumors, and benign vertiginous states. A thorough investigation consists of ruling out (1) inner ear pathology, (2) cardiac arrhythmias, (3) internal carotid artery stenosis/occlusion, and (4) complications of excessive blood pressure control (**TABLE 1**).
- Evaluation of patients with posterior circulation ischemia requires defining the precise circumstances that elicit symptoms. Vertigo, instability, and occasional loss of consciousness often accompany positional changes and standing in older individuals due to reduced sympathetic venous tone. This is particularly common in patients with diabetes. The presence of orthostatic hypotension should be evaluated as a common alternative cause for vertebrobasilar symptoms. Any decreases in basilar artery perfusion pressure may precipitate hemodynamic symptomatology, with or without concomitant vertebral occlusive disease.
- The next most common cause of brainstem ischemia is reduced cardiac output. When suspected, evaluation includes 24-hour Holter monitoring and echocardiography. In patients with vertebrobasilar insufficiency, palpitations may be noted with the onset of symptoms. Transesophageal echocardiography may be necessary to rule out structural heart issues.
- Inner ear pathology, including rare cerebellopontine angle tumors, produces symptoms suggestive of vertebrobasilar insufficiency. Benign vertiginous states should also be considered. Physical examination can alert the physician to the possibility of subclavian steal syndrome in patients with differences in brachial blood pressure greater than 25 mm Hg or with diminished left upper extremity pulses. Reversed flow in the ipsilateral vertebral artery demonstrated on duplex scanning is pathognomonic for subclavian steal physiology and subclavian steal syndrome in patients with appropriate symptoms at rest or following exercise in the ipsilateral upper extremity.
- Patients may relate symptoms of vertebrobasilar insufficiency to positional changes, including turning or extending their head. These dynamic symptoms usually appear when turning the head to one side. In this circumstance, symptoms may be elicited by extrinsic compression of the dominant or sole vertebral artery (in the case of unilateral occlusion) by adjacent arthritic bone spurs.[1]

Table 1: Nonvascular and Cardiac Conditions That Mimic Vertebrobasilar Ischemia

Cardiac arrhythmia
Pacemaker malfunction
Cardioemboli
Antihypertensive medications
Labyrinthine dysfunction
Cerebellopontine angle tumors
Cerebellar degeneration
Myxedema
Electrolyte imbalance
Hypoglycemia

PATIENT HISTORY AND PHYSICAL FINDINGS

- In general, ischemic mechanisms in vertebrobasilar insufficiency can be categorized as hemodynamic or embolic. Symptoms of vertebrobasilar insufficiency include dizziness, vertigo, drop attacks, diplopia, perioral numbness, alternating paresthesia, tinnitus, dysphasia, dysarthria, and ataxia. When two or more of these symptoms are present, vertebrobasilar ischemia is more likely to be the inciting cause. Unlike other regions of the brain, strokes in the posterior circulation territory occur due to large artery occlusive diseases.
- Patients with "hemodynamic" ischemia experience transient vertebrobasilar symptoms due to inadequate vertebral artery inflow or collateral circulation. Symptoms are typically short lived, repetitive, somewhat predictable, and rarely result in stroke. Postural hypotension may precipitate serious traumatic injury, however, when patients lose their balance with standing.
- Embolic events may also precipitate vertebrobasilar ischemia as well as cerebellar and brainstem infarction. Microemboli from the heart, aortic arch, or any arteries leading directly to the basilar artery may arise from atherosclerotic lesions, intimal defects, repetitive trauma, fibromuscular dysplasia lesions, aneurysms, or dissections. Although much less

common than hemodynamic vertebrobasilar insufficiency, when present, microemboli are much more likely to cause fatal events or debilitating infarcts.[2-4]

- Timing of the onset of symptoms following positional changes may help differentiate vertebrobasilar insufficiency from labyrinthine disorders. In the latter circumstance, rapid head movement invokes immediate symptoms. In the case of vertebrobasilar insufficiency, however, a short delay usually precedes the onset of symptoms, including nystagmus.

IMAGING AND OTHER DIAGNOSTIC STUDIES

Duplex ultrasound, an otherwise excellent tool for the assessment of extracranial cerebrovascular disease, has limitations in the diagnosis of vertebral artery pathology. Direct visualization of the second portion is obscured by the transverse processes of C2-C6. As previously mentioned, however, duplex imaging reliably identifies subclavian steal physiology, as well as detects proximal velocity increases consistent with orificial vertebral or proximal subclavian stenosis.[5]

- Magnetic resonance imaging (MRI) provides safe, noninvasive, and detailed evaluation of the aortic arch and great vessels, the extracranial and intracranial arterial vasculature, as well as the presence of mass lesions, fluid collections, or parenchymal defects in the posterior fossa. Contrast-enhanced magnetic resonance angiography (MRA), with three-dimensional reconstruction and maximum image intensity techniques, provides excellent image quality in high resolution (**FIGURE 1**). As in other applications, however, in low-flow circumstances, excessive signal dropout may result in overestimation of lesion severity based on signal intensity alone.
- In contrast to computed tomographic (CT) imaging, transaxial MRI readily diagnoses both acute and chronic brain infarctions in the posterior fossa. Brainstem infarctions are typically small and as such may be overlooked with noncontrast CT imaging. Brain MRI is performed in symptomatic patients prior to vertebral artery intervention to identify infarctions when they are present and provide baseline images for future comparison.
- Evaluation of vertebral anatomy via catheter-based, contrast arteriography requires acquisition of images in multiple projections to fully evaluate the entire extent of both vertebral arteries. Evaluation begins with the aortic arch to determine the origin of the bilateral vertebral arteries. Anomalous origin of the left vertebral artery, arising directly from the aorta proximal to the left subclavian, is present in 6% of patients. Much less frequently, the right vertebral artery originates from the innominate or right common carotid artery. This anomaly often accompanies an aberrant right subclavian artery, which itself may precipitate symptoms of dysphagia lusoria.
- Usually, right and left posterior oblique projections are sufficient to comprehensively evaluate the V1 (first) vertebral artery segment from the origin to the transverse process of C6. In most patients, the left artery is usually dominant, but a number of normal variants may be encountered, including congenital atresia of either vertebral artery.
- The vertebral artery origin may not be visualized adequately with either duplex ultrasonography or MRA. Oblique projections are required during arteriography due to superimposition of the subclavian artery over the vertebral origin. Additional projections, including craniocaudal tube angulation, may also be required to optimize visualization. The presence of a poststenotic dilatation in the first centimeter of the vertebral artery is a clue that should prompt further projections to isolate the origin from the overlying subclavian artery.
- Dynamic arteriography, incorporating provocative positioning, may be required to assess the possibility of extrinsic vertebral artery compression. Finally, delayed imaging may demonstrate reconstitution of patent distal extracranial vertebral arteries through cervical collaterals when the origin initially appears occluded.

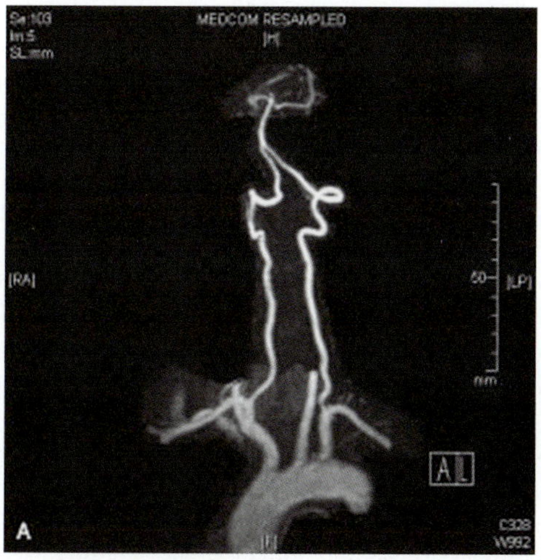

FIGURE 1 • Vertebral MRA (with the carotid image subtracted).

SURGICAL MANAGEMENT

- Some degree of vertebral artery orificial stenosis is present in 20% to 40% of patients with other manifestations of cerebrovascular disease.[2] A number of operative approaches will satisfactorily address V1 segment disease and orificial stenosis.[6,7] Vertebral transposition or repositioning of the origin of the vertebral artery onto the adjacent common carotid artery is the most common. Endoluminal dilatation, with or without stenting, is also appropriate in selected circumstances.

Vertebral to Common Carotid Transposition

- General endotracheal anesthesia is preferred. Positioning supine, with the back of the table slightly elevated toward a chair position with the head rotated away from the planned incision site facilitates additional deep mediastinal exposure when required.
- Proximal vertebral artery exposure is similar to that required for subclavian-to-carotid transposition. One fingerbreadth above the clavicle, a transverse incision is created directly over the two heads of the sternocleidomastoid muscle (SCM). Between the SCM heads, the omohyoid muscle is identified and divided. Lateral retraction of the internal jugular vein and vagus nerve exposes the carotid sheath medially. Maximal proximal carotid artery exposure, facilitated by positioning of the primary operator at head of the patient, is necessary to ensure an optimal result (**FIGURE 2**).
- The sympathetic ganglia are identified running behind and parallel to the carotid artery. On the left side, the thoracic duct is divided between ligatures to minimize lymphatic leaks. The proximal end should be doubly ligated, avoiding

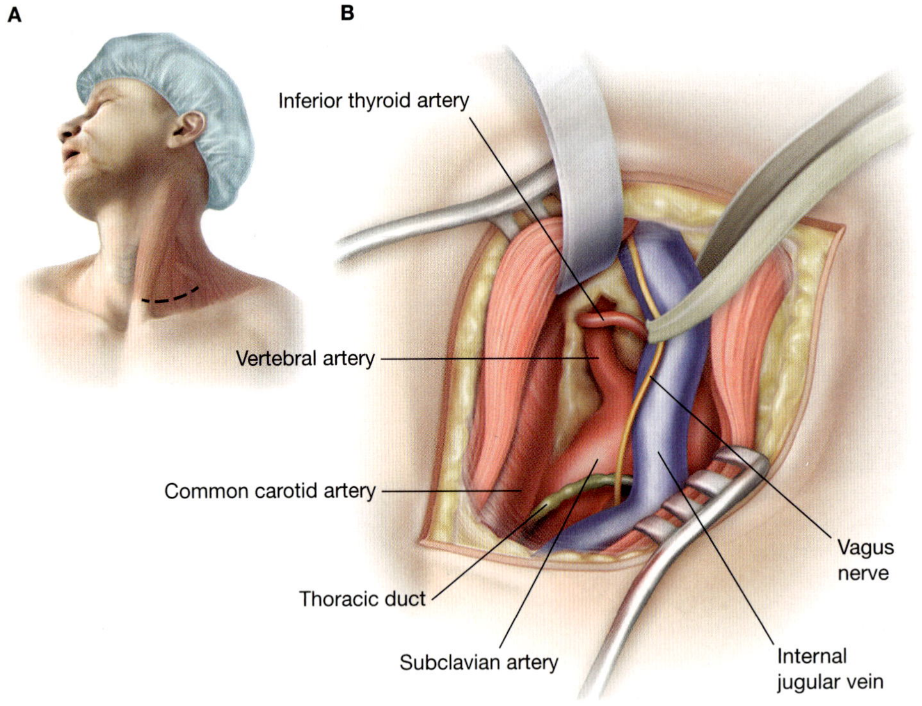

FIGURE 2 • **A,** Access to the proximal vertebral artery between the sternocleidomastoid muscle bellies. **B,** Transposition of the proximal vertebral artery to the posterior wall of the common carotid artery.

transfixion sutures. Accessory lymph ducts—often seen on the right side—should also be ligated and divided when identified. The entire dissection is confined medial to the prescalene fat pad covering the scalenus anticus muscle and phrenic nerve. These latter structures are left unexposed lateral to the field. The inferior thyroid artery, running transversely across the field, is also ligated and divided.

- The vertebral vein is next identified emerging from the angle formed by the longus colli and scalenus anticus and overlying the vertebral artery and, at the bottom of the field, the subclavian artery. Unlike its sister artery, the vertebral vein has branches. It is ligated in continuity and divided. Below the vertebral vein lies the vertebral artery. It is important to identify and avoid injury to the adjacent sympathetic chain. The vertebral artery is dissected superiorly to the tendon of the longus colli and inferiorly to its origin in the subclavian artery. The vertebral artery is freed from the sympathetic trunk resting on its anterior surface without damaging the trunk or the ganglionic rami. Preserving the sympathetic trunks and the stellate or intermediate ganglia resting on the artery usually requires freeing the vertebral artery from these structures, and after dividing its origin, the latter is transposed anterior to the sympathetics.
- Once the artery is fully exposed, an appropriate site for reimplantation in the common carotid artery is selected. The patient is systemically anticoagulated with intravenous heparin. The distal portion of the V1 segment of the vertebral artery is clamped below the edge of the longus colli with a microclip placed vertically to indicate the orientation of the artery and to avoid axial twisting during its transposition. The proximal vertebral artery is closed by transfixion with 5-0 polypropylene suture immediately above the stenosis at its origin. The artery is divided at this level, and its proximal stump is further secured with a hemoclip. The artery is then brought to the common carotid artery and its free end is spatulated for anastomosis.
- The carotid artery is then crossclamped. An elliptical 5- to 7-mm arteriotomy is created in the posterolateral wall of the common carotid artery with an aortic punch. The anastomosis is performed in open fashion with a continuous 6-0 or 7-0 polypropylene suture while avoiding any tension on the vertebral artery, which tears easily. Before completion of the anastomosis, any slack in the suture is tightened appropriately with a nerve hook, standard flushing maneuvers are performed, and the suture is tied to reestablish flow (**FIGURE 3**).

Vertebral Artery Angioplasty and Stent Placement

- In the past decade, endovascular treatment of vertebral artery disease has gained increasing acceptance. For endovascular intervention, patients are pretreated with dual antiplatelet therapy (aspirin and clopidogrel). The procedure is usually performed with local anesthesia and conscious sedation, enabling continuous neurologic monitoring of the patient. The patients are positioned supine and prepped to allow percutaneous entry into the chosen access vessel. Most cases are performed from a femoral approach (93%), although transbrachial (3%) and transradial (5%) access has also been used as noted in one recent review.[8] The stenotic lesions are crossed and then dilated with 0.014- or 0.018-in guidewires and small coronary-diameter balloons. If a stent is chosen, these are usually bare metal type, but drug elution has also been used. The same 0.014- or 0.018-in guidewires are used as platforms over which the stents are delivered and then deployed. Postdeployment angioplasty may be necessary in selected cases. Procedures can be performed with or without the assistance of embolic protection, although most vertebral arteries are too small to accommodate most distal protection devices.

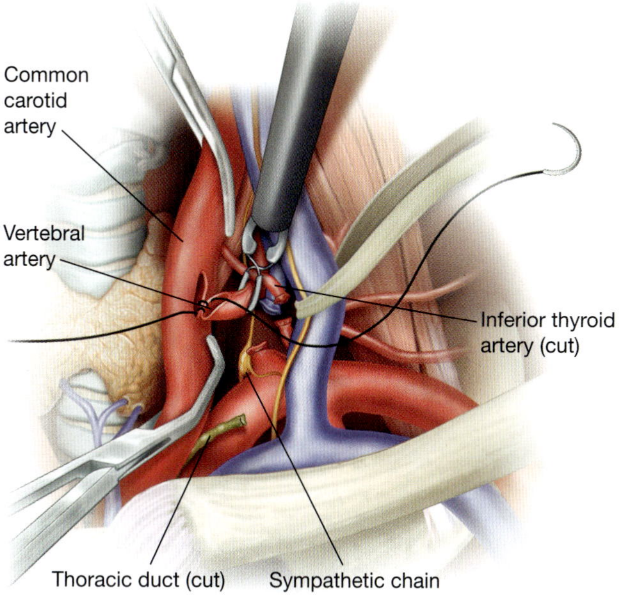

FIGURE 3 • Proximal vertebral-to-common carotid transposition.

PEARLS AND PITFALLS

Placement of incision	■ It is important to place the incision medially enough to dissect between the heads of the sternocleidomastoid. An approach lateral to this structure will make the transposition challenging, if not impossible, to complete.
Orientation	■ Enough of the V1 segment of the vertebral artery, up to near where it disappears into the transverse process of C6, needs to be mobilized. Also, plan ahead and see where on the carotid is best to reimplant the vertebral before creating the carotid arteriotomy.
Closure	■ A drain is usually helpful, especially on the left side where the thoracic duct crosses the exposure, just in case a tie comes off of a large lymphatic. The drain allows for early diagnosis of this complication.

POSTOPERATIVE CARE

- Following surgical transposition, absent significant lymphatic drainage from the wound, the patient may be safely discharged on the first or second postoperative day. Similarly, after endoluminal therapy, patients are kept overnight to ensure neurologic stability.

OUTCOMES

- After proximal vertebral-to-common carotid transposition, patency rates at 5 and 10 years equal or exceed 95% and 91%, respectively. When selected appropriately, more than 80% of patients will experience symptomatic relief following proximal surgical reconstruction.[9]
- Appropriate reconstruction and subsequent reperfusion of the brainstem in patients experiencing hemodynamic vertebrobasilar symptoms may also improve hypertension management.
- Overall, retrospective reviews suggest that endoluminal vertebral artery intervention is reasonably safe, although a selection bias exists. A 2005 Cochrane review identified 313 interventions for vertebral artery stenosis, with just over half using stent placement as part of the treatment. The technical success rate was 95%, and the 30-day stroke and death rate was 6.4%.[10]
- Despite high technical success rates, vertebral artery angioplasty alone, especially when used for the treatment of disease at the origin of the vessel, appears to have an unacceptably high rate of restenosis. Adjuvant stent placement adds to the clinical durability but adds potential morbidity such as malposition or potential fracture. In their series of 105 patients who underwent endovascular stenting for symptomatic vertebral artery disease, Jenkins et al[11] achieved 100% radiographic improvement (residual stenosis ≤30%). The authors reported immediate (30-day) periprocedural risk of death of 1% and periprocedural complication rate of 4.8%. Complications included transient ischemic attack, flow-limiting dissection, hematoma, and catheter-access-site problems. At 1 year of follow-up, six patients had died and five had experienced a vertebrobasilar stroke, and at approximately 2.5 years of follow-up, 70% of patients remained symptom-free, but 13% of patients had restenosis requiring retreatment.[11]
- A recent systematic review of the available literature noted a weighted mean technical success rate of 97%. The authors estimated mean periprocedural stroke and death rate from combined angioplasty and stenting to be around 1.1%.

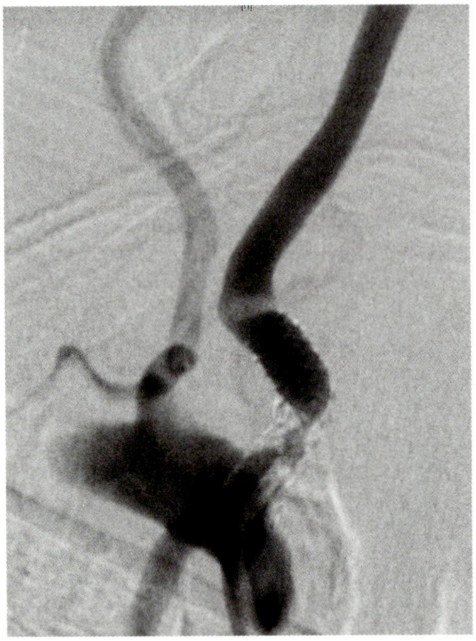

FIGURE 4 • Vertebral artery stent with fracture and in-stent restenosis. (Reprinted from Cronenwett JL, Johnston KW, eds. *Rutherford's Vascular Surgery*. 7th ed. Saunders; 2010. Copyright © 2010 Elsevier. With permission.)

Transient ischemic events occurred in 1.5% of patients. Recurrent symptoms occurred in 8% of patients within a reported range of follow-up of 6 to 54 months and greater than 50% restenosis developed in 23% of the subset of patients who underwent follow-up imaging.[8]

COMPLICATIONS

- Proximal vertebral to common carotid transposition has been reported to have a combined stroke and death rate of 0.9%.[9] Among patients undergoing this operation, in one report, there were no deaths or strokes in those who underwent only a vertebral reconstruction. Berguer and coauthors reported four instances of immediate postoperative thrombosis (1.4%). Three of the four patients had vein grafts interposed between the vertebral artery and the common carotid because of a short V1 segment. The grafts kinked and thrombosed. Other complications that are particular to proximal reconstruction include vagus and recurrent laryngeal nerve palsy (2%), Horner syndrome (8.4%-28%), lymphocele (4%), and chylothorax (0.5%).
- Periprocedural risks for angioplasty and stenting include access complications, distal embolization and stroke, arterial rupture, stent malposition, and vessel thrombosis or dissection. Later, restenosis and stent fracture are not uncommon (**FIGURE 4**).

REFERENCES

1. Bauer R. Mechanical compression of the vertebral arteries. In: Berguer R, Bauer R, eds. *Vertebrobasilar Arterial Occlusive Disease: Medical and Surgical Management*. Raven; 1984:45-71.
2. Caplan LR, Wityk RJ, Glass TA, et al. New England medical center posterior circulation registry. *Ann Neurol*. 2004;56:389-398.
3. Caplan L, Tettenborn B. Embolism in the posterior circulation. In: Berguer R, Caplan L, eds. *Vertebrobasilar Arterial Disease*. Quality Medical; 1992:52-65.
4. Pessin M. Posterior cerebral artery disease and occipital ischemia. In: Berguer R, Caplan L, eds. *Vertebrobasilar Arterial Disease*. Quality Medical; 1992:66-75.
5. Berguer R, Higgins R, Nelson R. Noninvasive diagnosis of reversal of vertebral-artery blood flow. *N Engl J Med*. 1980;302:1349-1351.
6. Edwards WH, Mulherin JL Jr. The surgical approach to significant stenosis of vertebral and subclavian arteries. *Surgery*. 1980;87:20-28.
7. Roon AJ, Ehrenfeld WK, Cooke PB, et al. Vertebral artery reconstruction. *Am J Surg*. 1979;138:29-36.
8. Antoniou GA, Murray D, Georgiadis GS, et al. Percutaneous transluminal angioplasty and stenting in patients with proximal vertebral artery stenosis. *J Vasc Surg*. 2012;55:1167-1177.
9. Berguer R, Flynn LM, Kline RA, et al. Surgical reconstruction of the extracranial vertebral artery: management and outcome. *J Vasc Surg*. 2000;31:9-18.
10. Coward LJ, Featherstone RL, Brown MM. Percutaneous transluminal angioplasty and stenting for vertebral artery stenosis. *Cochrane Database Syst Rev*. 2005;2005(2):CD000516.
11. Jenkins JS, Patel SN, White CJ, et al. Endovascular stenting for vertebral artery stenosis. *J Am Coll Cardiol*. 2010;55(6):538-542.

Chapter 8

Neurogenic Thoracic Outlet Syndrome Exposure and Decompression: Supraclavicular

Robert W. Thompson and Esmaeel Reza Dadashzadeh

DEFINITION

- Thoracic outlet syndrome (TOS) is a group of conditions caused by compression of one of the neurovascular structures that serve the upper extremity.[1-3] Neurogenic TOS (NTOS) is the most frequent of these, occurring in 85% to 90% of patients. It is caused by compression and irritation of the brachial plexus nerves within the supraclavicular scalene triangle and/or underneath the pectoralis minor muscle tendon in the subcoracoid space (**FIGURE 1**). NTOS tends to occur between the ages of 15 and 40 years and typically results in neck and upper extremity pain, paresthesia, and functional limitations. Although relatively uncommon, clinical recognition and appropriate treatment of NTOS are crucial to prevent disability in young active individuals.
- The causes of NTOS include anatomical variations (anomalous scalene musculature, aberrant fibrofascial bands, and/or cervical ribs) and previous neck or upper extremity injury, which has resulted in scalene/pectoralis muscle spasm, fibrosis, and other pathological changes. These muscular alterations, in turn, lead to compression and irritation of the adjacent brachial plexus nerves. The presence of a cervical rib is often cited as a predisposing factor in the development of NTOS; however, few patients with NTOS (approximately 10%) exhibit a definable cervical rib and the development of NTOS symptoms is rare, even in patients with a cervical rib, in the absence of additional injury.[4]
- NTOS often occurs in individuals engaged in occupational or recreational activities that involve repetitive overhead use of the arms and/or heavy lifting and may develop following various types of injury (eg, motor vehicle collisions or falls upon the outstretched arm). It may also arise as a consequence of low-grade repetitive strain injury (eg, prolonged keyboard use), poor posture, and dysfunctional shoulder girdle mechanics.
- Surgical treatment for NTOS may be effectively accomplished by several different approaches, including transaxillary first rib resection and anterior (supraclavicular) decompression. The supraclavicular approach has long been a mainstay in the surgical treatment of NTOS, providing excellent exposure for

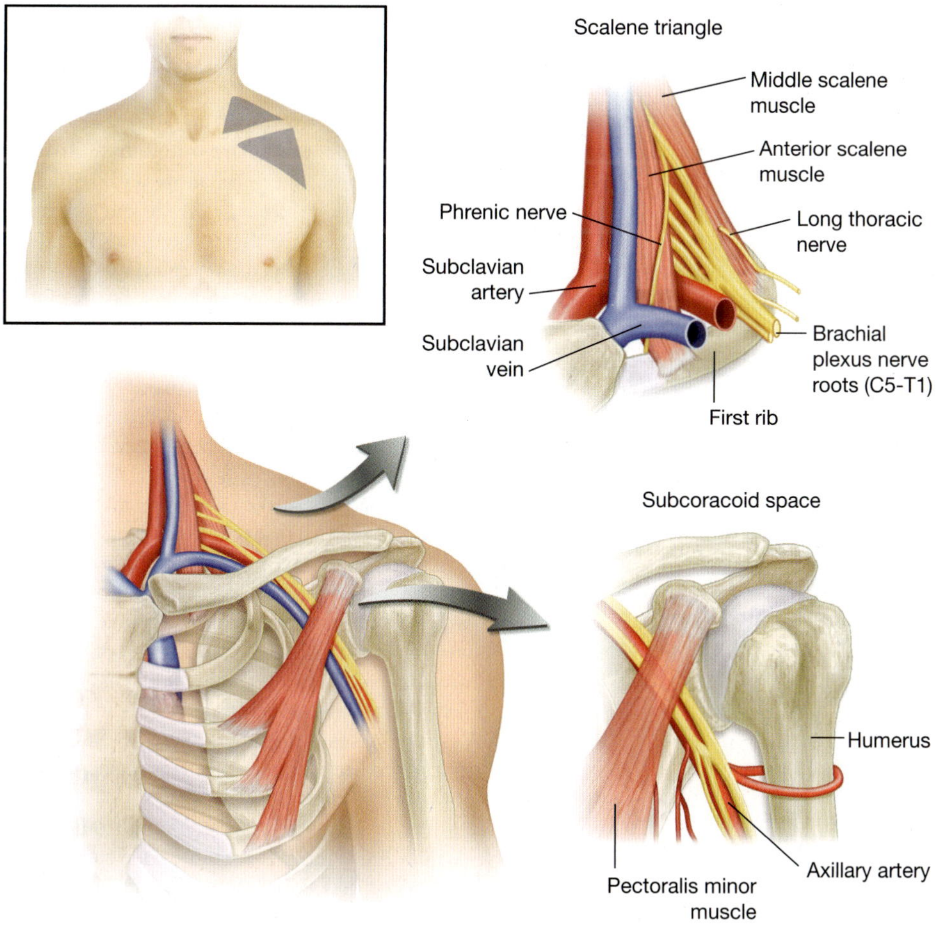

FIGURE 1 • Anatomy of the thoracic outlet, with emphasis on the supraclavicular scalene triangle and the infraclavicular subcoracoid space.

safe and definitive decompression of the relevant neurovascular structures and the flexibility to manage the entire spectrum of circumstances that may be encountered.[5-7]

DIFFERENTIAL DIAGNOSIS

- NTOS produces symptoms that can mimic or overlap those observed in other upper extremity neurological and musculoskeletal disorders, producing a particularly broad differential diagnosis (**TABLE 1**).[2,8-10] Clinical evaluation requires differentiation of NTOS from other cervical-brachial syndromes and optimal selection of patients for different forms of treatment.
- NTOS should be readily differentiated from venous TOS, which produces marked arm swelling, cyanotic discoloration, and distention of subcutaneous veins around the shoulder and chest wall, and often presents with axillary-subclavian vein "effort thrombosis" (Paget-Schroetter syndrome).[2] NTOS should also be distinguished from arterial TOS, which causes either fixed subclavian artery obstruction, resulting in cramping muscular fatigue with arm use similar to intermittent claudication, or poststenotic subclavian artery aneurysm formation, which can cause thromboembolism, hand ischemia, rest pain, and/or digital ulceration and necrosis.[2]
- Some patients with NTOS exhibit severe upper extremity pain and hypersensitivity, with digital swelling and discoloration, suggesting the presence of sympathetic nerve overactivity. In such cases, the possibility of reflex sympathetic dystrophy (complex regional pain syndrome) should be considered and evaluated using a temporary cervical sympathetic (stellate ganglion) anesthetic block.

PATIENT HISTORY AND PHYSICAL FINDINGS

- Symptoms attributable to brachial plexus nerve compression include pain, numbness, and tingling (paresthesia) in the neck, shoulder, arm, and hand. The distribution of symptoms in the hand often extends beyond that expected for either the median or ulnar nerves, involving all fingers. Patients with NTOS attributable to compression at the pectoralis minor tendon often describe upper anterior chest and axillary pain. The intensity of symptoms of NTOS can vary with the extent of upper extremity activity and is usually reliably exacerbated with arm elevation and abduction.[2,8-10]
- Many patients with NTOS have relatively mild symptoms, with a slow gradual progression interspersed by occasional exacerbations. Others exhibit a steady progression in the severity of symptoms leading to increasing and significant disability. Hand muscle weakness and atrophy (Gilliatt-Sumner hand) are rare and occur when there is particularly advanced and longstanding brachial plexus compression, associated with a cervical rib or other bony anomaly.
- Physical examination of patients with NTOS usually reveals well-localized tenderness to palpation over the supraclavicular scalene triangle and/or the infraclavicular subcoracoid space, associated with reproduction of upper extremity symptoms[2,8-10] (**FIGURE 2**).
- Most patients with NTOS exhibit rapid reproduction of upper extremity symptoms with provocative positional maneuvers, such as the upper limb tension test or the 3-minute elevated arm stress test (**FIGURE 2**). Positional dampening of the radial artery pulse at the wrist during arm abduction and external rotation (Adson test) is nonspecific and inaccurate and is not useful in establishing or excluding a diagnosis of NTOS.[2,11]
- Physical examination should include assessment for potential cervical spine degenerative disease and peripheral nerve compression (carpal tunnel and cubital canal syndromes), as well as any evidence of arterial or venous compromise to the upper extremity. Signs of upper extremity sympathetic overactivity should also be sought (mild digital swelling and discoloration, and skin hypersensitivity or allodynia).
- Documentation of patient-reported symptoms and quantification of the level of disability prior to treatment are facilitated by the use of various survey forms and other outcome measurement tools, such as the Disabilities of the Arm, Shoulder and Hand and quality-of-life instruments.[2,9,10,12] Repeated use of these instruments at various intervals before and following treatment has become increasingly important to assess the outcomes of different management strategies.[13]

Table 1: Differential Diagnosis of Neurogenic Thoracic Outlet Syndrome

Acromioclavicular arthropathy	Fibromyalgia and fibromyositis
Arterial atheroembolism	Nerve sheath neoplasm
Brachial plexus (stretch) injury	Pancoast tumor (lung apex)
Carpal tunnel syndrome (median nerve)	Parsonage-Turner syndrome
Cervical dystonia	Psychogenic syndrome
Cervical spine degenerative arthritis	Radial nerve compression (extensor forearm)
Complex regional pain syndrome	Raynaud syndrome
Cervical spine degenerative disc disease	Rotator cuff tendinitis
Cervical spine (muscular) strain	Scleroderma
Cubital canal syndrome (ulnar nerve)	Vasculitis

IMAGING AND OTHER DIAGNOSTIC STUDIES

- Although imaging and other diagnostic studies may provide helpful ancillary information, there are none with sufficient sensitivity or specificity to confirm or exclude the diagnosis of NTOS. Identification of NTOS thereby remains a clinical diagnosis dependent on experienced pattern recognition.[14]
- Plain anteroposterior chest radiographs may be useful to determine the presence or absence of a cervical rib. Other types of imaging studies of the brachial plexus are not specifically helpful in diagnosis or planning treatment (**FIGURE 3**).
- Conventional electrophysiological tests (electromyography and nerve conduction studies) are often performed to exclude peripheral nerve compression disorders or cervical radiculopathy. These tests are usually negative or nonspecific in NTOS and cannot be used to establish or exclude the diagnosis.[2]
- Vascular laboratory studies (Duplex ultrasound) are often performed to detect alterations in upper extremity blood flow that can be attributed to subclavian artery compression during arm elevation. However, positional subclavian artery compression may only be an incidental and unrelated vascular finding and does not establish a diagnosis of NTOS, nor does it represent arterial TOS. Vascular laboratory studies do not assess brachial plexus compression and are therefore of little specific value in the evaluation of patients with suspected NTOS.[11]
- Imaging-guided anterior scalene muscle and/or pectoralis minor muscle blocks with a local anesthetic can provide support for the clinical diagnosis of NTOS.[15-18] A positive block, characterized by a temporary relief or improvement in the presenting symptoms, is almost always attributable to NTOS. A positive

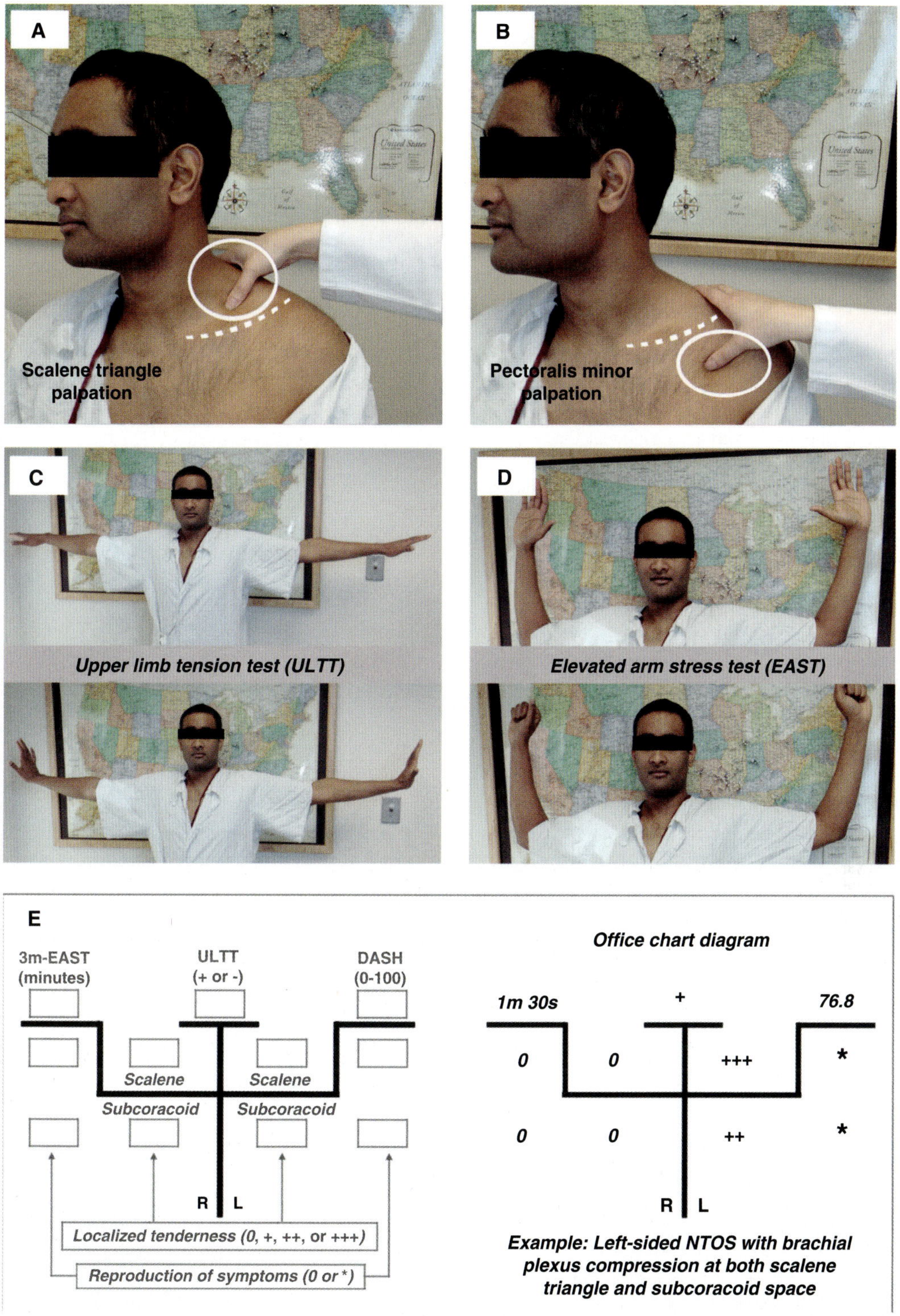

FIGURE 2 • Physical examination reveals localized tenderness to palpation over the supraclavicular scalene triangle **(A)** and/or the infraclavicular subcoracoid space **(B)**. The upper limb tension test (ULTT) **(C)** and the 3-minute elevated arm stress test (EAST) **(D)** utilize provocative positional maneuvers that rapidly elicit reproduction of upper extremity symptoms in patients with neurogenic thoracic outlet syndrome (NTOS). An office chart diagram is used to easily summarize physical examination findings for patients being evaluated for NTOS **(E)**.

muscle block can also help predict the reversibility of symptoms with treatment and is therefore useful in prognosis. In contrast, a negative anterior scalene/pectoralis minor muscle block is not sufficiently interpretable to exclude a diagnosis of NTOS or to preclude consideration of patients for surgical treatment.

- Initial treatment for NTOS is based on physical therapy to relieve scalene/pectoralis minor muscle spasm, improve postural disturbances, enhance functional limb mobility, strengthen associated shoulder girdle musculature, and diminish repetitive strain exposure in the workplace.

Incorrect approaches to physical therapy can result in worsening of symptoms and premature failure of conservative management. In most patients with mild NTOS or with symptoms of short duration, significant improvement is usually observed within the initial 4 to 6 weeks of physical therapy. Because NTOS is often a chronic condition subject to occasional "flare-ups" of acute symptoms (often related to overuse activities or new injury), such patients should continue regular physical therapy exercises during long-term follow-up. Patients that have not improved with an appropriate trial of physical therapy and other conservative measures are considered candidates for surgical treatment.[2,13]

SURGICAL MANAGEMENT

- Supraclavicular decompression (scalenectomy, first rib resection, and brachial plexus neurolysis) is a recommended treatment option when there is (1) a sound clinical diagnosis of NTOS, (2) substantial disability (symptoms interfering with daily activities and/or work), and (3) an insufficient response to targeted physical therapy.[5-7,13,19] Supraclavicular decompression is also ideal for patients with persistent or recurrent symptoms of NTOS following a previous operation, when there has been no response to appropriate conservative measures.

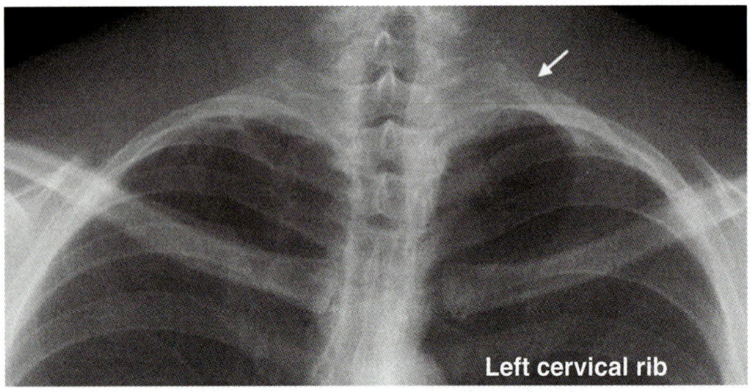

FIGURE 3 ● A left-sided cervical rib identified by plain chest radiography (*arrow*).

- For patients with symptoms of NTOS referable to the subcoracoid space, pectoralis minor tenotomy is an important addition to supraclavicular thoracic outlet decompression. Pectoralis minor tenotomy may also be performed as an isolated procedure when the subcoracoid space is the dominant location of nerve compression symptoms.[20,21]
- Surgical treatment should be staged for patients with bilateral NTOS. The initial supraclavicular decompression, with or without pectoralis minor tenotomy, is performed on the side with the most severe symptoms or for the dominant upper extremity. If contralateral symptoms persist or progress, supraclavicular decompression on the second side may be recommended at least 6 to 12 weeks later. Normal phrenic nerve function should be verified on the side of the previous procedure, by chest fluoroscopic examination, before proceeding with a contralateral operation.

Preoperative Planning

- The supraclavicular surgical site is marked in the preoperative holding area, being sure to include the subcoracoid space if concomitant pectoralis minor tenotomy is planned. Prophylactic antibiotics are administered within an hour of the planned procedure.
- An erector spinae plane local anesthetic block is placed in the preoperative holding area as a useful adjunct to help manage postoperative pain.[22]

Positioning

- After the induction of general endotracheal anesthesia, the patient is positioned supine with the head of the operating table elevated 30°. The neck is extended and turned to the opposite side, a small inflatable pillow is placed behind the shoulders, and the neck, chest, and affected upper extremity are prepped into the field. The arm is wrapped in stockinette to permit free range of movement during the operation and then held comfortably across the abdomen (**FIGURE 4**). Lower extremity sequential compression devices are used for thromboprophylaxis. Neuromuscular blocking agents are not used following the initial induction of anesthesia.

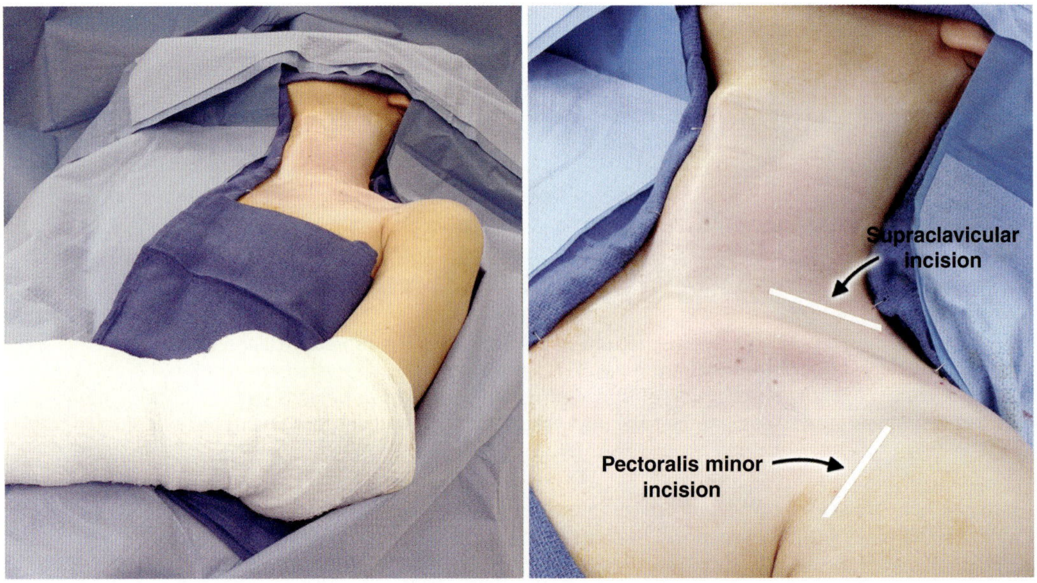

FIGURE 4 ● Patient position and planned incisions for left-sided supraclavicular thoracic outlet decompression with pectoralis minor tenotomy.

SUPRACLAVICULAR DECOMPRESSION

Incision and Mobilization of the Scalene Fat Pad

- A transverse neck incision is made parallel to and just above the clavicle, beginning at the lateral edge of the sternocleidomastoid muscle and extending to the anterior edge of the trapezius muscle. The incision is carried through the subcutaneous layer, the platysma muscle is divided, and subplatysmal flaps are developed to expose the scalene fat pad. The sternocleidomastoid muscle is retracted medially, but is not divided (**FIGURE 5**).
- One of the keys to simplifying the supraclavicular exposure is proper mobilization and lateral reflection of the scalene fat pad. This begins with the detachment of the fat pad along the lateral edge of the internal jugular vein and the superior edge of the clavicle, with ligation of small blood vessels and lymphatic tissues. The thoracic duct, usually observed near the junction of the internal jugular and subclavian veins on the left side (a prominent accessory thoracic duct may also exist on the right side), may be ligated and divided. The omohyoid muscle is routinely divided (**FIGURE 5**).
- The scalene fat pad is progressively elevated in a medial to lateral direction, by gentle fingertip dissection over the surface of the anterior scalene muscle. The phrenic nerve is observed passing in a lateral to medial direction as it descends along the muscle surface. Gentle manipulation of the phrenic nerve produces a "dartle" (diaphragmatic startle) response.

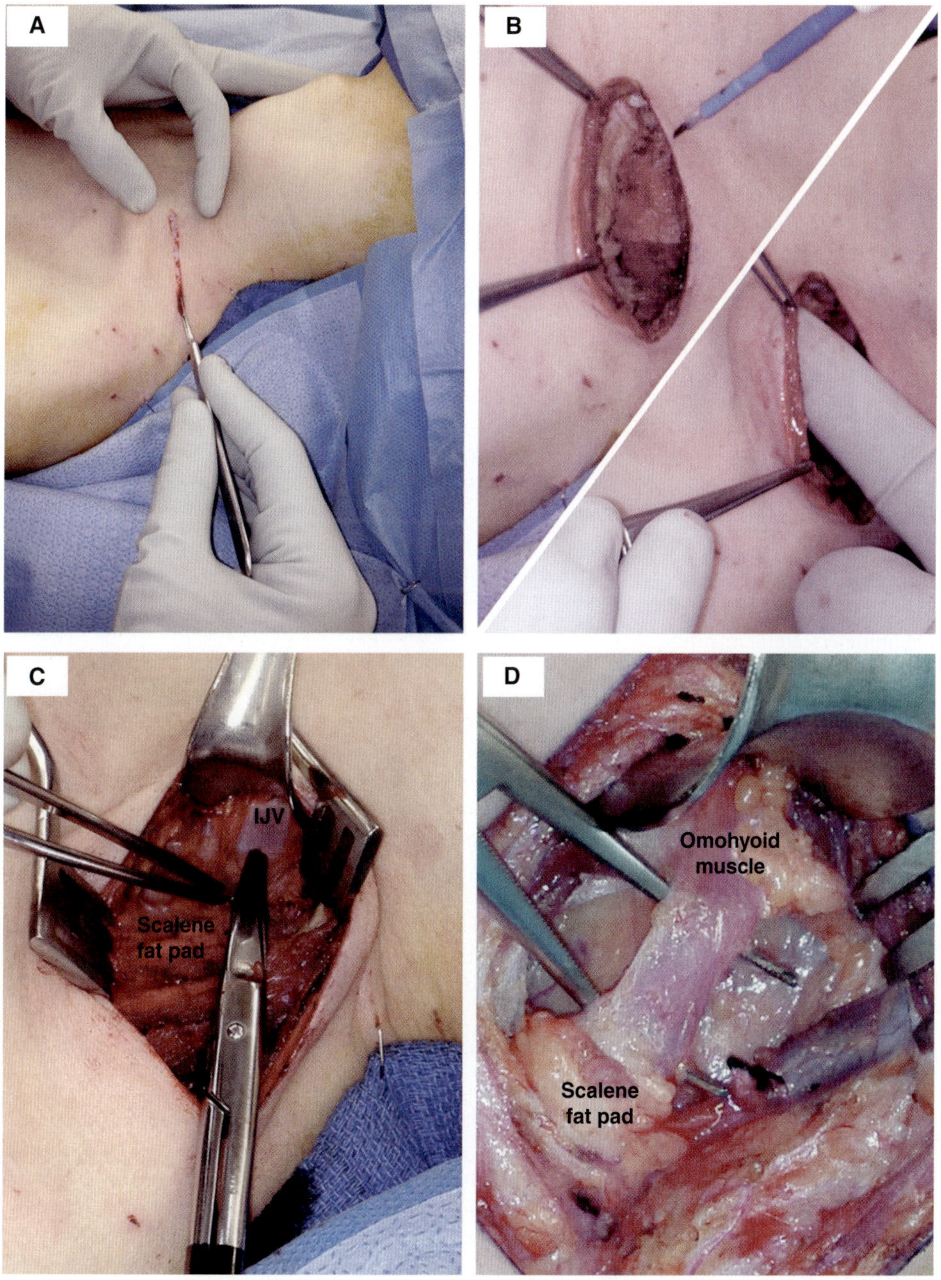

FIGURE 5 • The skin incision is made just above and parallel to the clavicle, extending from the lateral border of the sternocleidomastoid muscle to the anterior border of the trapezius muscle **(A)**. Subplatysmal flaps are created to expose the underlying scalene fat pad **(B)**. The scalene fat pad is mobilized, beginning with its medial attachments to the internal jugular vein (IJV) **(C)**, and the omohyoid muscle is divided **(D)**.

Table 2: Critical Views Obtained During Supraclavicular Thoracic Outlet Decompression

1. View of the operative field after lateral reflection of the scalene fat pad with visualization of the internal jugular vein, anterior scalene muscle, phrenic nerve, brachial plexus, subclavian artery, middle scalene muscle, and long thoracic nerve.
2. View of the lower part of the anterior scalene muscle where it attaches to the first rib with space sufficient to allow a finger to pass behind the anterior scalene muscle and in front of the brachial plexus and subclavian artery prior to division of the anterior scalene muscle insertion from the top of the first rib.
3. View of the upper part of the anterior scalene muscle at the level of the C6 transverse process in relation to the C5 and C6 nerve roots prior to division of the anterior scalene muscle origin.
4. View of the insertion of the middle scalene muscle on the first rib with each of the five nerve roots of the brachial plexus and the subclavian artery retracted medially and the long thoracic nerve retracted laterally prior to division of the middle scalene muscle insertion from the top of the lateral first rib.
5. View of the posterior neck of the first rib with the T1 nerve root passing from underneath the rib to join the C8 nerve root to form the inferior trunk of the brachial plexus prior to division of the posterior first rib.
6. View of the anterior portion of the first rib with placement of the rib shears medial to the scalene tubercle prior to division of the anterior first rib.

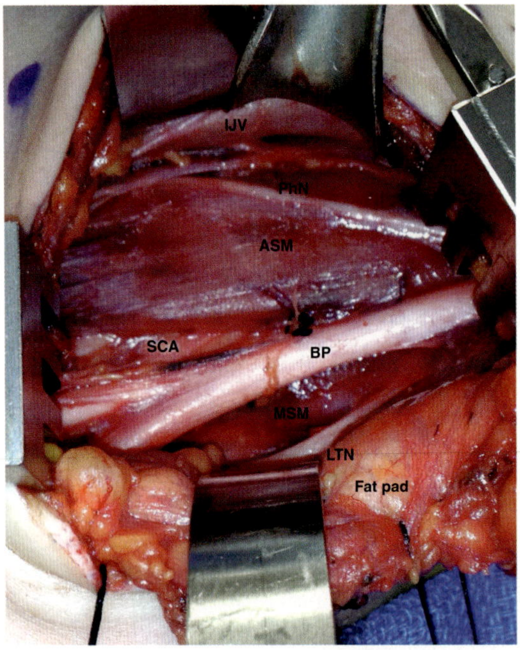

FIGURE 6 • Following lateral reflection of the scalene fat pad, direct visualization is obtained of the internal jugular vein (IJV), anterior scalene muscle (ASM), phrenic nerve (PhN), brachial plexus (BP), subclavian artery (SCA), middle scalene muscle (MSM), and long thoracic nerve (LTN).

- Upon further lateral rotation of the scalene fat pad, the brachial plexus nerve roots (posterior and lateral to the anterior scalene muscle) and the middle scalene muscle (behind the brachial plexus) are brought into view. The lateral aspect of the first rib is palpated and visualized, and the long thoracic nerve is identified as it emerges from the body of the middle scalene muscle to course past the lateral part of the first rib. The scalene fat pad is then held in position with several silk retraction sutures and the exposure is maintained with a Henley self-retaining retractor (using the third arm to hold the edge of the sternocleidomastoid muscle). The resulting exposure represents the first and most important of six "critical views" to be obtained during supraclavicular decompression (**TABLE 2**) (**FIGURE 6**).

Anterior Scalenectomy

- Attention is turned to the insertion of the anterior scalene muscle on the first rib. At the lower lateral edge of the anterior scalene muscle, the subclavian artery and brachial plexus are carefully mobilized until a fingertip can easily pass behind the muscle just above the first rib, thereby displacing the neurovascular structures posterolaterally. Blunt fingertip dissection is continued behind the muscle to its medial edge, taking care to avoid the phrenic nerve. Once the insertion of the anterior scalene muscle onto the first rib has been isolated under direct vision to protect the phrenic nerve, the subclavian artery, and the brachial plexus, it is sharply divided from the anterior surface of the bone with scissors (**FIGURE 7**).
- The end of the divided anterior scalene muscle is elevated and its attachments to the underlying extrapleural fascia are sharply divided (electrocautery is not used to avoid inadvertent nerve injury). Muscle fibers extending from the posterior surface of the muscle often pass around the subclavian artery to form a tethering "sling" and should also be resected to fully release the artery. Any scalene minimus muscle fibers found to be present (passing between the roots of the brachial plexus) are divided as the anterior scalene muscle is mobilized. As the anterior scalene muscle is lifted further, it is passed underneath and medial to the phrenic nerve, and its posterior attachments are divided with direct visualization and protection of the upper brachial plexus nerve roots. Dissection of the muscle is carried superiorly to its origin on the C6 transverse process, which is easily palpated in the upper aspect of the operative field (the apex of the "scalene triangle"). The anterior scalene muscle is then divided with scissors from its origin on the transverse process under direct vision and the entire muscle is removed, with a typical specimen weighing 5 to 10 g. Any minor bleeding from the edge of the divided muscle origin is controlled with small polypropylene sutures rather than electrocautery, given the proximity of the nerve roots (**FIGURE 7**).
- Anomalous fibrofascial bands may be observed after anterior scalene muscle resection, typically passing in front of the lower brachial plexus nerve roots. These structures are also resected as they are encountered to ensure thorough decompression and full nerve root mobility.

Mobilization of the Brachial Plexus and Middle Scalenectomy

- The brachial plexus nerve roots are next separated from the front edge of the middle scalene muscle. Blunt fingertip dissection along the lateral aspect of the nerves is used to extend the exposure deeper, to the inner curve of the first rib and the extrapleural space, and a small malleable retractor is placed between the brachial plexus nerves and the middle

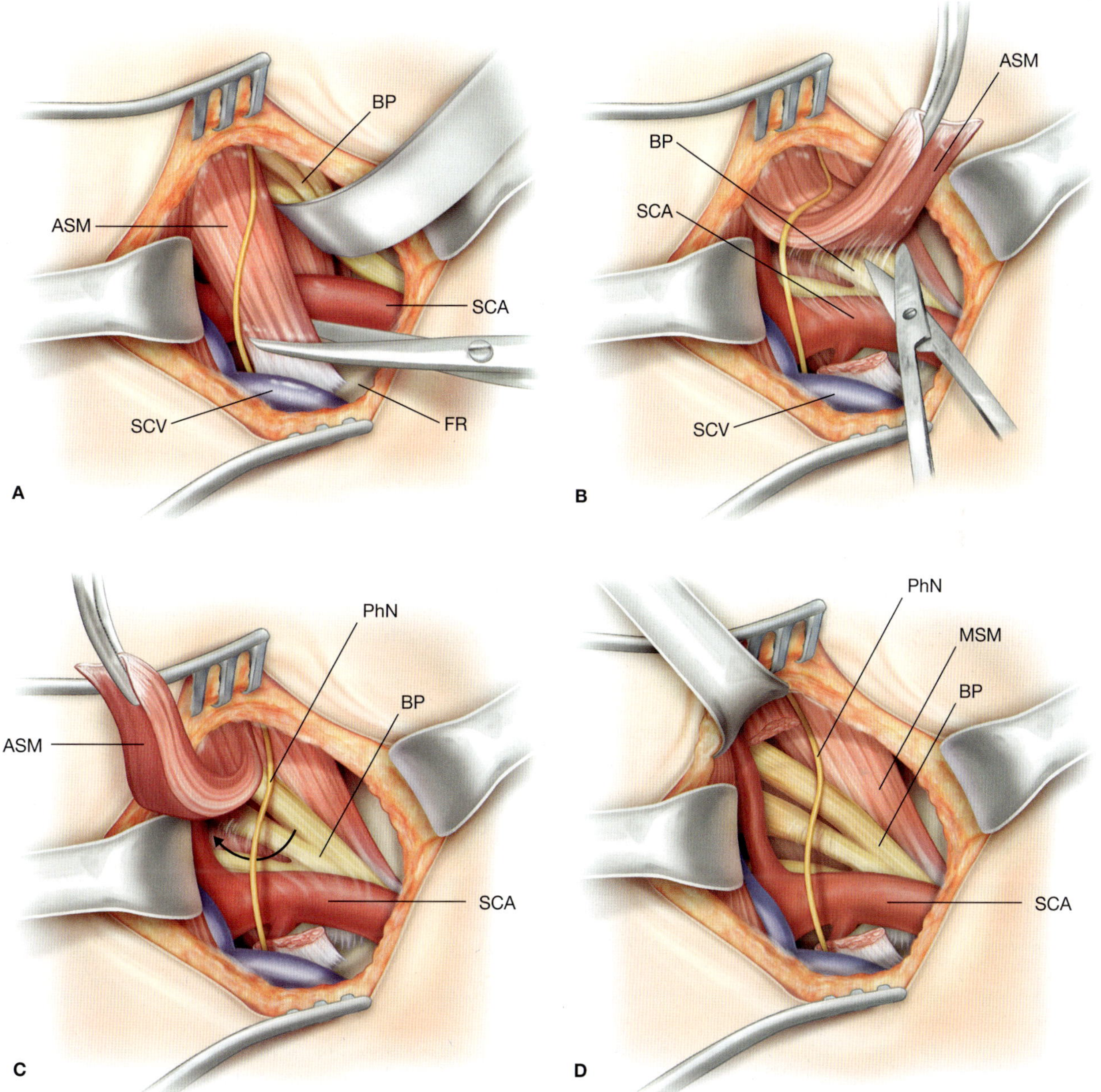

FIGURE 7 • The anterior scalene muscle (ASM) insertion is isolated by displacing the underlying subclavian artery (SCA) and brachial plexus (BP), using blunt fingertip dissection behind the muscle, and the muscle is sharply divided from the top of the first rib (FR) **(A)**. The end of the divided anterior scalene muscle is lifted and sharply dissected free of structures lying behind the muscle, including the subclavian artery **(B)**. As it is mobilized, the anterior scalene muscle is passed underneath and to the medial side of the phrenic nerve (PhN) **(C)**. The dissection is carried up to the level of the C6 transverse process, where the anterior scalene muscle can be safely divided from its origin and removed **(D)**. MSM, middle scalene muscle; SCV, subclavian vein.

scalene muscle. With gentle medial retraction of the brachial plexus, each nerve root from C5 to T1 is sequentially identified (**FIGURE 8**).

- The transverse cervical artery and vein should be ligated and divided where they pass through the brachial plexus and middle scalene muscle as they are at risk for avulsion during retraction.
- A second malleable retractor is placed lateral to the middle scalene muscle and first rib, to displace the long thoracic nerve posteriorly. The oblique attachment of the middle scalene muscle along the top of the posterolateral first rib is exposed. This muscle insertion is carefully divided from the surface of the bone with the electrocautery, using a periosteal elevator as the dissection proceeds posteriorly, extending to a point on the first rib that is parallel with the underlying T1 nerve root. The bulk of the middle scalene muscle anterior to the long thoracic nerve is then sharply excised, with a typical specimen weighing 3 to 8 grams (**FIGURE 9**). Minor bleeding

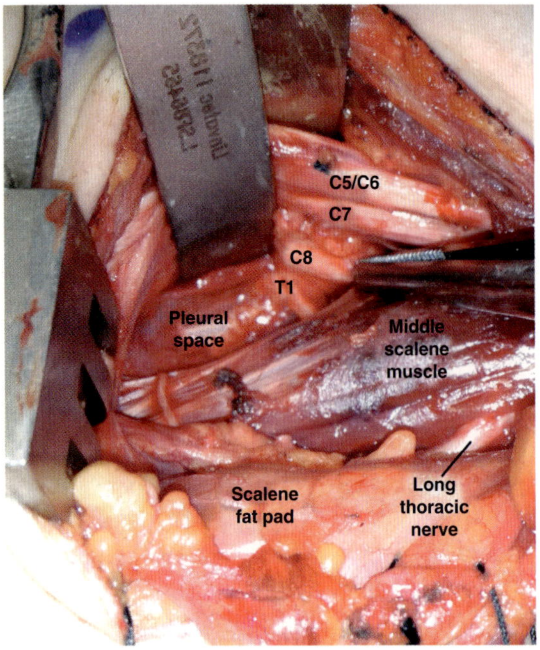

FIGURE 8 • The brachial plexus is separated from the anteromedial border of the middle scalene muscle down to the level of the first rib and extrapleural fascia and gently retracted medially to visualize all five nerve roots (C5 to T1).

from the cut edge of the middle scalene muscle should be controlled with figure-of-eight silk sutures rather than the electrocautery, to avoid thermal injury to the C8 nerve root or long thoracic nerve.

First Rib Resection

- Once the scalenectomy has been completed, the intercostal muscle attached to the lateral edge of the first rib is separated from the bone with the electrocautery. The first rib is fully exposed posteriorly, where the T1 nerve root emerges from underneath the bone to join the C8 nerve root in forming the lower trunk of the brachial plexus. A large right-angle clamp is passed underneath the posterior neck of the first rib and gently spread to detach additional intercostal tissues. A modified Stille-Giertz rib cutter is inserted around the neck of the first rib. After verifying protection of the C8 and T1 nerve roots, the bone is sharply divided. A Kerrison bone rongeur is used to smooth the posterior end of the bone, to a level medial to the underlying T1 nerve root, and the end of the bone is sealed with bone wax (**FIGURE 9**).
- The free end of the divided posterior first rib is elevated, and blunt fingertip dissection is used to separate the remaining extrapleural fascia and intercostal muscle attaching to the undersurface of the rib, progressing anteriorly to the level of the scalene tubercle (the previous site of attachment of the anterior scalene muscle). No effort is made to avoid opening the pleura during first rib resection, as the opened pleural space will allow better drainage of postoperative fluids away from the brachial plexus (which might otherwise promote perineural adhesions).
- The soft tissues underneath the clavicle, including the subclavian vein, are elevated with a small Richardson retractor. The posterior first rib is displaced inferiorly with fingertip pressure to open the anterior costoclavicular space, and the subclavian artery and brachial plexus are displaced laterally with a small malleable retractor. The Stille-Giertz rib cutter is placed around the anterior first rib, immediately medial to the scalene tubercle (**FIGURE 10**). The first rib is then divided under direct vision, and the intact specimen is extracted from the operative field (**FIGURE 11**). The remaining anterior end of the first rib is remodeled to a smooth surface with a bone rongeur, to a level well underneath the clavicle. Oxidized cellulose fabric (Surgicel, Ethicon, Inc.) is placed within the bed of the resected first rib as a topical hemostatic agent.
- Cervical ribs arise within the plane of the middle scalene muscle, posterior to the brachial plexus and subclavian artery, and anterior to the long thoracic nerve. Incomplete cervical ribs typically have a ligamentous extension to the first rib, whereas complete cervical ribs attach to the lateral first rib in the form of a true joint. The posterior portion of a cervical rib is thereby readily encountered during dissection of the middle scalene muscle and is divided in a manner similar to the posterior first rib. The anterior attachment of the cervical rib is then divided and the bone is removed, prior to first rib resection. When there is a true joint between a complete cervical rib and the first rib, the anterior portion of the cervical rib is left attached while the first rib resection is completed, and the two are removed together as a single specimen (**FIGURE 11**).

Brachial Plexus Neurolysis

- The last step of supraclavicular decompression is to fully mobilize each of the individual nerve roots contributing to the brachial plexus. Each nerve root from C5 to T1 is meticulously dissected free of any adherent perineural fibrous scar tissue that might impair mobility (external neurolysis). Inspection of the most proximal aspect of the C8 and T1 nerve roots will often reveal a small fibrofascial band overlying these nerves, which should be specifically sought out and resected. This step of the operation is not considered complete until each of the five nerve roots and three trunks of the brachial plexus has been completely cleared throughout its course in the operative field (**FIGURE 12**).

Drain Placement and Closure

- Upon the completion of supraclavicular decompression, the apex of the pleural membrane is opened to promote postoperative drainage of fluid into the chest cavity, away from the brachial plexus. A #19 closed suction drain is placed through a separate stab wound into the operative field, placed posterior to the brachial plexus with its tip extending into the posterior pleural space. To minimize postoperative perineural fibrosis, the brachial plexus is loosely wrapped with either a bioresorbable polylactide film (SurgiWrap; Mast Biosurgery) or a gluteraldehyde-free preparation of decellularized bovine pericardium membrane (Photofix; CryoLife, Inc.), held in place with several 5-0 polypropylene sutures. The scalene fat pad is restored to its anatomic position overlying the brachial plexus and held in place with several tacking sutures to the edge of the sternocleidomastoid muscle and to the periclavicular subcutaneous fascia. The platysma muscle layer is reapproximated with interrupted sutures and the skin is closed with an absorbable subcuticular stitch.

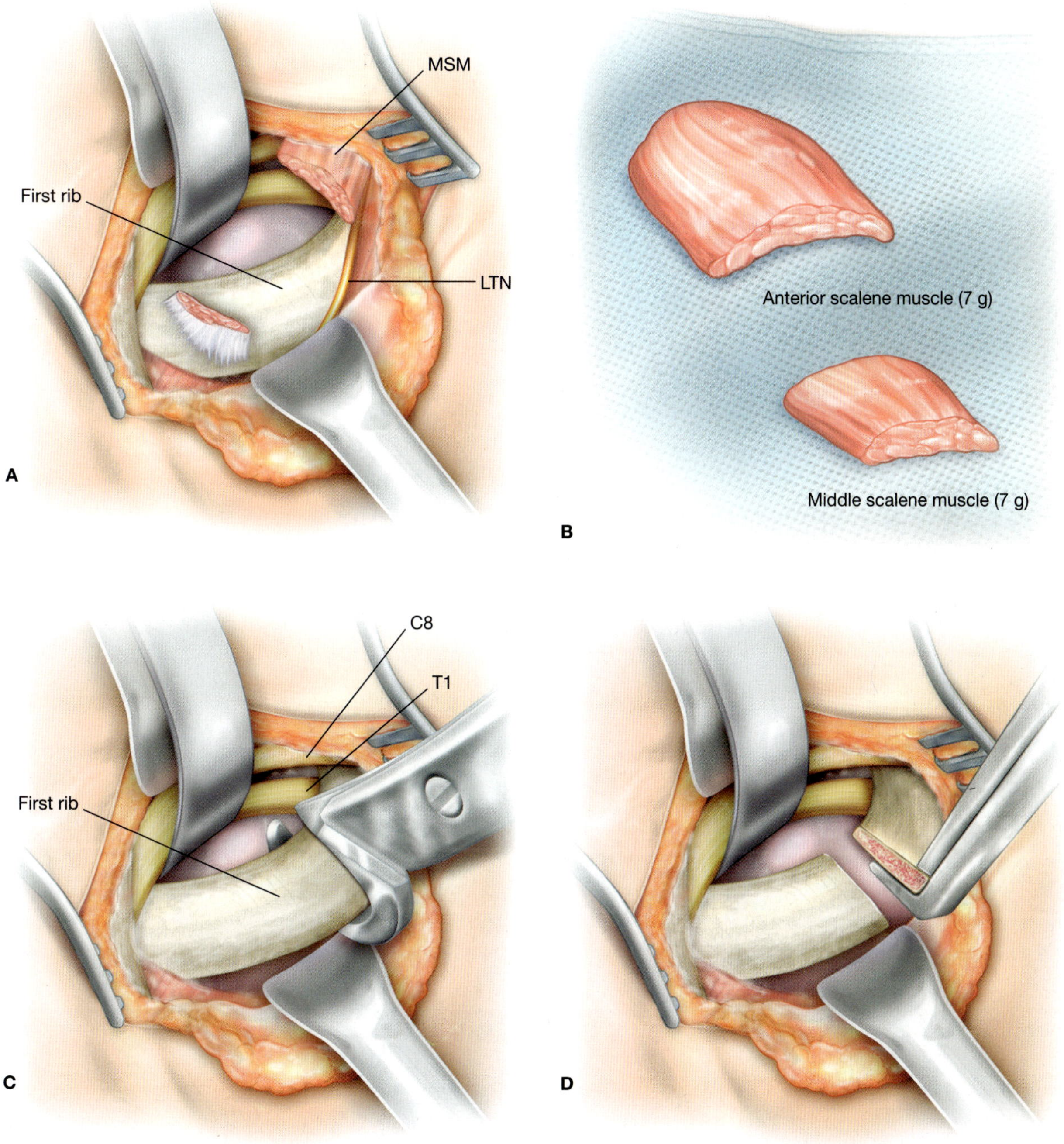

FIGURE 9 • After detaching the middle scalene muscle (MSM) from the top of the posterolateral first rib using the electrocautery, the muscle tissue lying anterior to the long thoracic nerve (LTN) is excised **(A)**. Typical operative specimens of the anterior and middle scalene muscles **(B)**. The posterior first rib is exposed with visualization of the C8 and T1 nerve roots, and the rib is divided with a modified Giertz-Stille rib cutter **(C)**. The posterior edge of the first rib is further remodeled with a Kerrison rongeur to obtain a smooth edge, immediately medial to the T1 nerve root **(D)**.

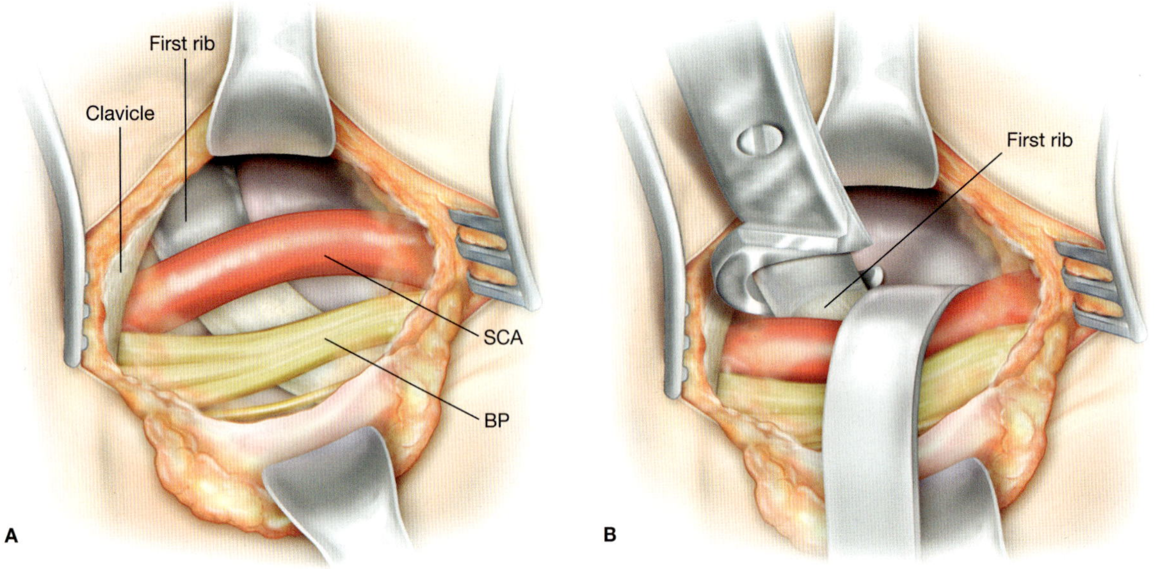

FIGURE 10 • With the posterior end of the first rib pushed downward to open the anterior costoclavicular space, the anterior portion of the first rib is exposed underneath the clavicle and the subclavian vein **(A)**. The subclavian artery (SCA) and brachial plexus (BP) are protected, and the anterior first rib is divided with a rib cutter immediately medial to the scalene tubercle **(B)**.

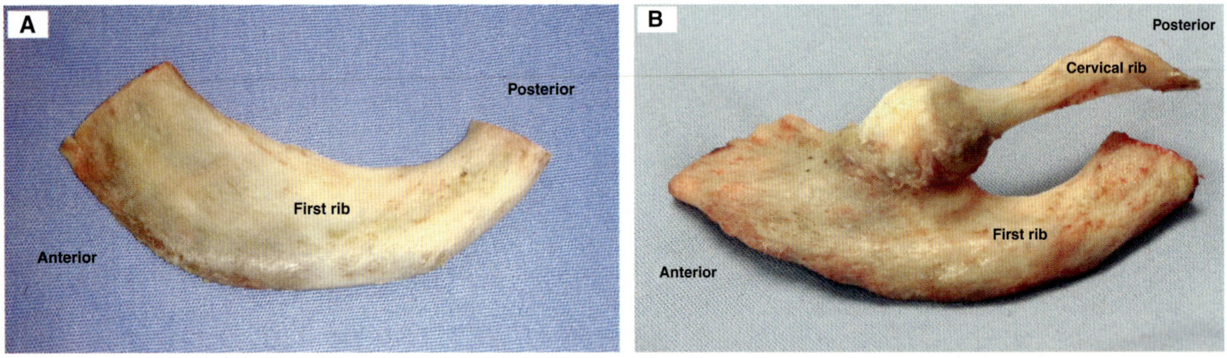

FIGURE 11 • Operative specimens following first rib resection **(A)** and following combined resection of a cervical rib and first rib **(B)**.

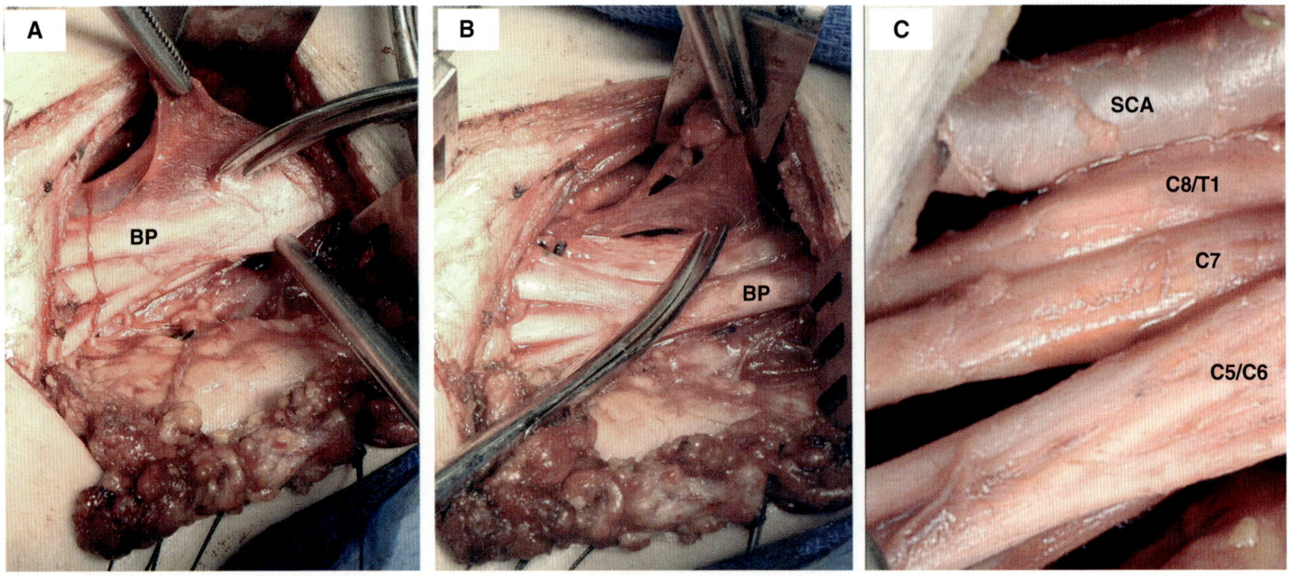

FIGURE 12 • Fibrous scar tissue is removed from each of the brachial plexus (BP) nerve roots and trunks by external neurolysis **(A-C)**. SCA, subclavian artery.

PECTORALIS MINOR TENOTOMY

Incision and Exposure

- A short vertical incision is made in the deltopectoral groove, beginning at the level of the coracoid process. The deltoid and pectoralis major muscles are gently separated and the plane of deeper dissection is carried medial to the cephalic vein. The lateral edge of the pectoralis major muscle is gently lifted with a small Deaver retractor, and the plane underneath the muscle is separated from the underlying fascia by blunt fingertip dissection. The fascia over the pectoralis minor muscle is exposed, where the muscle can be easily identified by palpation (**FIGURE 13**).

Division of the Pectoralis Minor Muscle Tendon

- The pectoralis minor muscle tendon is identified where it extends from the anterior chest wall to the coracoid process. The fascia along its medial border is opened and the muscle is encircled using blunt fingertip dissection. The fascia along the lateral border of the pectoralis minor muscle is opened to ensure its separation from the short head of the biceps muscle, which also inserts on the coracoid process. Taking care to protect the underlying neurovascular bundle, the pectoralis minor tendon is then elevated with umbilical tape or rubber tubing and its insertion on the coracoid process is exposed with a small Richardson retractor. A finger is placed behind the muscle to prevent thermal injury to the neurovascular structures and the insertion of the pectoralis minor tendon is divided with electrocautery. After the pectoralis minor muscle has been divided, the lower edge will retract inferiorly to release any compression of the neurovascular bundle (**FIGURE 14**).
- The remaining clavipectoral fascia is also incised to the level of the clavicle, along with any other anomalous fascial bands that might be present over the brachial plexus, such as Langer axillary arch, but no further dissection of the brachial plexus nerves or the axillary vessels is performed. The wound is irrigated and closed in layers without a drain.

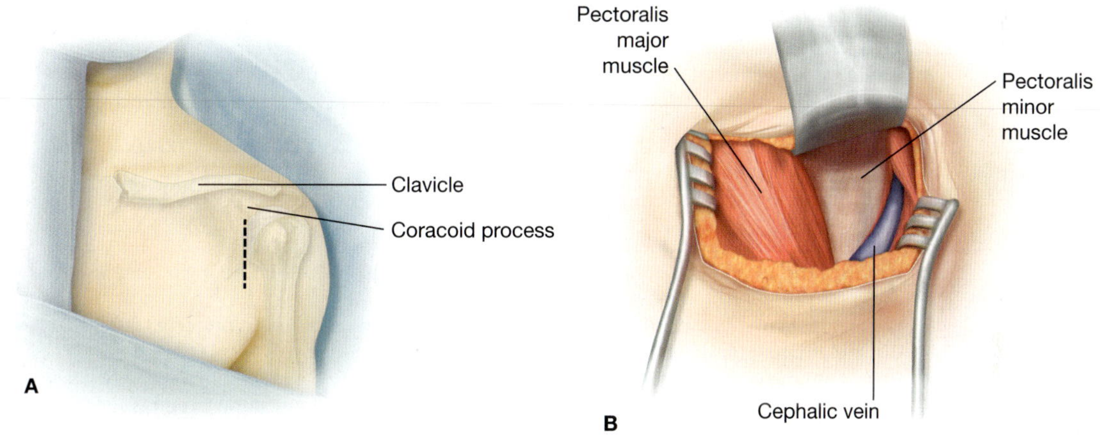

FIGURE 13 • Pectoralis minor tenotomy is performed through a short vertical incision in the deltopectoral groove, just below the coracoid process **(A)**. The plane of dissection is carried medial to the cephalic vein, and the pectoralis major muscle is lifted to expose the fascia over the pectoralis minor muscle **(B)**.

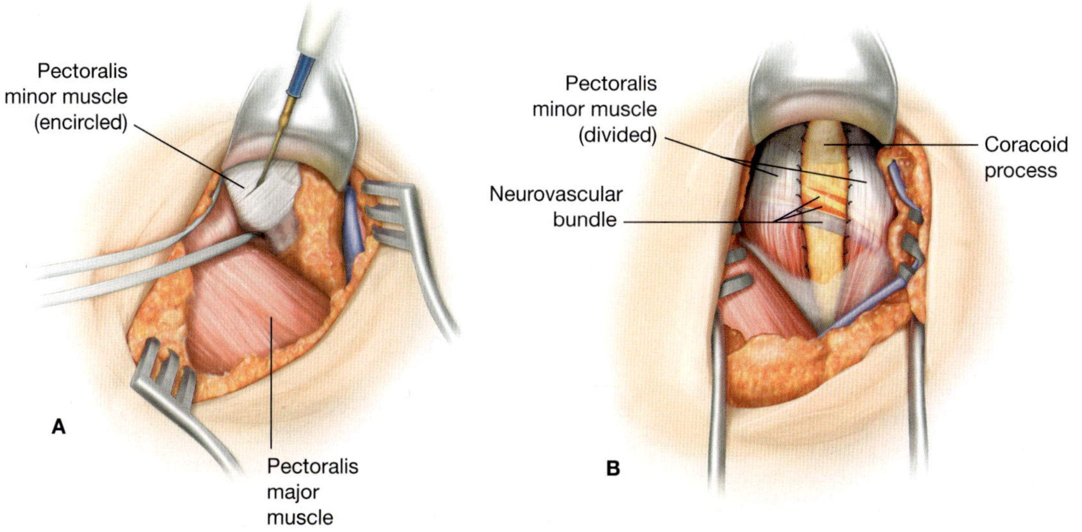

FIGURE 14 • The pectoralis minor muscle is encircled near its insertion on the coracoid process and then divided with the electrocautery **(A)**. The retracted edge of the divided pectoralis minor muscle is oversewn with a continuous suture **(B)**.

PEARLS AND PITFALLS

Indications	■ Operative treatment of NTOS should be based on a sound clinical diagnosis, a substantial level of disability, and failure of symptoms to improve with an adequate trial of conservative management. ■ Imaging studies, electrophysiological tests, and vascular laboratory examinations add little in the evaluation of NTOS, but may be useful in excluding other conditions. ■ A positive anterior scalene muscle block is a useful adjunct to support the clinical diagnosis of NTOS and indicates a strong likelihood of responsiveness to surgical treatment. ■ Assess the potential contribution of brachial plexus compression at the level of the subcoracoid space and include pectoralis minor tenotomy if present.
Mobilization of the scalene fat pad	■ Avoid division of the sternocleidomastoid muscle. ■ Proper mobilization and lateral reflection of the scalene fat pad is a key step in simplifying supraclavicular exposure for thoracic outlet decompression. This permits the critical view to be obtained in which all of the relevant structures can be visualized in the same operative field (internal jugular vein, phrenic nerve, anterior scalene muscle, brachial plexus, middle scalene muscle, first rib, and long thoracic nerve). ■ Ligate and divide the thoracic duct if necessary to prevent postoperative lymph leak. ■ Visualize and protect the phrenic nerve.
Anterior scalenectomy	■ Divide all fibers passing from the posterior aspect of the anterior scalene muscle to the subclavian artery and extrapleural fascia. ■ Divide any scalene minimus muscle encountered. ■ Pass the anterior scalene muscle underneath the phrenic nerve to facilitate dissection of the muscle up to its superior origin on the C6 transverse process.
Mobilization of the brachial plexus	■ Visualize all five nerve roots and three trunks of the brachial plexus. ■ Ligate and divide the transverse cervical vessels where they pass through the brachial plexus and middle scalene muscle.
Middle scalenectomy	■ Visualize and protect the long thoracic nerve. ■ Control minor bleeding from the cut edge of the muscle with silk sutures rather than the electrocautery.
First rib resection	■ Visualize the T1 and C8 nerve roots at the level of the posterior first rib, prior to division of the bone, to avoid nerve injury. ■ Remove a small segment of the divided posterior first rib to facilitate fingertip dissection underneath the remaining lateral and anterior portions of the bone. ■ Do not try to avoid opening the pleura. ■ Divide the anterior first rib at a level immediately medial to the scalene tubercle, underneath the clavicle and subclavian vein, while protecting the subclavian artery and brachial plexus. ■ Resect any cervical rib present along with the first rib.
Brachial plexus neurolysis	■ Thoroughly remove fibrous scar tissues from around each nerve root (C5 to T1) and trunk of the brachial plexus, to avoid one of the causes of persistent symptoms. ■ Resect any small fibrofascial bands overlying the proximal aspect of the C8 and T1 nerve roots.
Drain placement and closure	■ Wrap the brachial plexus to minimize perineural fibrosis. ■ Place a closed suction drain behind the brachial plexus with its tip extending into the pleural space.
Pectoralis minor tenotomy	■ Include pectoralis minor tenotomy as part of the supraclavicular decompression if there are concomitant symptoms of NTOS referable to the subcoracoid space. ■ Divide the pectoralis minor tendon close to its insertion on the coracoid process. ■ It is not necessary to place a separate drain in the subcoracoid space.

POSTOPERATIVE CARE

- An upright chest radiograph is performed in the recovery room and each morning for 3 days, and any small air or pleural fluid collections are observed with the expectation of spontaneous resolution. Postoperative analgesia is provided by patient-controlled intravenous opiates, until adequate pain control is achieved by oral medications alone. Oral narcotics, a muscle relaxant, and a nonsteroidal anti-inflammatory agent are routinely prescribed at hospital discharge and for at least several weeks following surgery. Postoperative hospital stay is typically 4 to 5 days. The closed suction drain is removed when its output is less than 50 to 100 mL/d, usually 3 to 4 days after surgery.
- Physical therapy is resumed the day after surgery to maintain range of motion and limit muscle spasm. The patient is allowed to use the extremity as tolerated, with no use of a sling or other restraint. Physical therapy is continued after hospital discharge, with advice to avoid excessive reaching

overhead or heavy lifting with the affected upper extremity, and other activities that might result in muscle strain, spasm and significant pain in the sternocleidomastoid, trapezius, and other neck muscles. Further rehabilitation is overseen by a physical therapist with expertise in the management of NTOS, usually in conjunction with a physical therapist located near the patient, emphasizing a gradual steady return to normal use of the upper extremity.

- The majority of patients are permitted cautious light-duty work activities by 4 to 6 weeks. Restrictions on upper extremity activity are progressively lifted between 6 and 12 weeks, when recovery from surgery is typically considered complete. Patients are seen in follow-up every 3 months in the first year to assess long-term results. Physical therapy and other aspects of care are continued as long as necessary to achieve an optimal level of function.

OUTCOMES

- In properly selected patients with disabling NTOS, approximately 85% to 90% can expect a substantial improvement in symptoms and increased functional use of the upper extremity within several months of supraclavicular decompression.[5-7,13,19] This estimate is higher in those who exhibited a positive anterior scalene/pectoralis minor muscle block prior to treatment. Factors that tend to diminish responsiveness to treatment include extremely longstanding (>5 years) and debilitating symptoms, widespread pain syndromes, multiple previous operations (cervical spine, shoulder, or peripheral nerves), depression, older age (>50 years), and preexisting use of opiate pain medications.[13,19]
- Patients with longstanding NTOS often display residual symptoms that may not be completely eliminated by thoracic outlet decompression. While these symptoms may be tolerable and are expected to gradually improve, the surgeon must provide continuing support and reassurance during the prolonged period of recovery and rehabilitation.
- Patients in the adolescent age group (<21 years) tend to have even better outcomes than adults, based on assessment of patient-reported survey instruments and postoperative use of opiate pain medications.[19] Patients that have been selected for isolated pectoralis minor tenotomy can exhibit early outcomes similar to those of patients that have undergone combined supraclavicular decompression and pectoralis minor tenotomy, but require ongoing follow-up for recurrent symptoms to determine if supraclavicular decompression may be warranted at a later time.[20,21]
- Recurrent symptoms of NTOS that warrant reoperation occur in 5% to 6% of patients, usually within the first 2 years of treatment. Reoperations for NTOS are generally performed using the supraclavicular approach, because this provides the most complete exposure of the anatomy with the greatest margin of safety.[23,24] Following lateral reflection of the scalene fat pad, the brachial plexus nerve roots are carefully exposed and mobilized. Great care must be taken during this dissection to avoid nerve and blood vessel injury, given the dense fibrous scar tissue that is usually present within the operative field. Any structures that were retained at the initial operation are then resected, including the scalene muscles, anomalous fibrofascial bands, and/or the first rib. A complete brachial plexus neurolysis is performed and the nerves are protected with a biological wrap and soft tissue coverage with the scalene fat pad.

COMPLICATIONS

- Persistent pain, numbness, and/or paresthesias
- Postoperative bleeding, localized hematoma, or hemothorax
- Wound infection (cellulitis or abscess)
- Pleural effusion (serosanguinous)
- Persistent lymph leak, chylothorax
- Brachial plexus nerve dysfunction (temporary or sustained)
- Phrenic nerve dysfunction (temporary or sustained)
- Long thoracic nerve dysfunction (temporary or sustained)
- Recurrent NTOS

REFERENCES

1. Thompson RW. Thoracic outlet syndrome: neurogenic. In: Sidawy AN, Perler BA, eds. *Rutherford's Vascular Surgery and Endovascular Therapy*. 9th ed. Elsevier; 2018:1619-1638.
2. Illig KA, Donahue D, Duncan A, et al. Reporting standards of the Society for Vascular Surgery for thoracic outlet syndrome. *J Vasc Surg*. 2016;64(3):e23-e35.
3. Illig KA, Thompson RW, Freischlag JA, et al, eds. *Thoracic Outlet Syndrome (TOS)*. 2nd ed. Springer Nature; 2021.
4. Sanders RJ, Hammond SL. Management of cervical ribs and anomalous first ribs causing neurogenic thoracic outlet syndrome. *J Vasc Surg*. 2002;36(1):51-56.
5. Reilly LM, Stoney RJ. Supraclavicular approach for thoracic outlet decompression. *J Vasc Surg*. 1988;8:329-334.
6. Sanders RJ, Hammond SL. Supraclavicular first rib resection and total scalenectomy: technique and results. *Hand Clin*. 2004;20:61-70.
7. Thompson RW, Ohman JW. Surgical techniques: operative decompression using the supraclavicular approach for neurogenic thoracic outlet syndrome. In: Illig KA, Thompson RW, Freischlag JA, et al, eds. *Thoracic Outlet Syndrome (TOS)*. 2nd ed. Springer Nature; 2021:265-285.
8. Sanders RJ, Hammond SL, Rao NM. Diagnosis of thoracic outlet syndrome. *J Vasc Surg*. 2007;46(3):601-604.
9. Jordan SE, Ahn SS, Gelabert HA. Differentiation of thoracic outlet syndrome from treatment-resistant cervical brachial pain syndromes: development and utilization of a questionnaire, clinical examination and ultrasound evaluation. *Pain Physician*. 2007;10(3):441-452.
10. Thompson RW. Diagnosis of neurogenic thoracic outlet syndrome: 2016 consensus guidelines and other strategies. In: Illig KA, Thompson RW, Freischlag JA, et al, eds. *Thoracic Outlet Syndrome (TOS)*. 2nd ed. Springer Nature; 2021:67-97.
11. Goeteyn J, Pesser N, van Sambeek MRHM, Thompson RW, van Neunen BFL, Teijink JAW. Duplex ultrasound studies are neither necessary or sufficient for the diagnosis of neurogenic thoracic outlet syndrome. *Ann Vasc Surg*. Published online November 11, 2021. doi:10.1016/j.asvg.2021.09.048
12. Balderman J, Holzem K, Field BJ, et al. Associations between clinical diagnostic criteria and pretreatment patient-reported outcomes measures in a prospective observational cohort of patients with neurogenic thoracic outlet syndrome. *J Vasc Surg*. 2017;66(2):533-544.
13. Balderman J, Abuirqeba AA, Pate C, et al. Physical therapy management, surgical treatment, and patient-reported outcomes measures in a prospective observational cohort of patients with neurogenic thoracic outlet syndrome. *J Vasc Surg*. 2019;70:832-841.
14. Raptis CA, Sridhar S, Thompson RW, Fowler K, Bhalla S. Imaging of the patient with thoracic outlet syndrome. *Radiographics*. 2016;36(4):984-1000.
15. Jordan SE, Machleder HI. Diagnosis of thoracic outlet syndrome using electrophysiologically guided anterior scalene blocks. *Ann Vasc Surg*. 1998;12(3):260-264.
16. Torriani M, Gupta R, Donahue DM. Sonographically guided anesthetic injection of anterior scalene muscle for investigation of neurogenic thoracic outlet syndrome. *Skeletal Radiol*. 2009;38(11):1083-1087.

17. Braun RM, Shah KN, Rechnic M, Doehr S, Woods N. Quantitative assessment of scalene muscle block for the diagnosis of suspected thoracic outlet syndrome. *J Hand Surg Am*. 2015;40(11): 2255-2261.
18. Weaver ML, Hicks CW, Fritz J, Black JHIII, Lum YW. Local anesthetic block of the anterior scalene muscle increases muscle height in patients with neurogenic thoracic outlet syndrome. *Ann Vasc Surg*. 2019;59:28-35.
19. Caputo FJ, Wittenberg AM, Vemuri C, et al. Supraclavicular decompression for neurogenic thoracic outlet syndrome in adolescent and adult populations. *J Vasc Surg*. 2013;57(1):149-157.
20. Sanders RJ, Rao NM. The forgotten pectoralis minor syndrome: 100 operations for pectoralis minor syndrome alone or accompanied by neurogenic thoracic outlet syndrome. *Ann Vasc Surg*. 2010;24:701-708.
21. Vemuri C, Wittenberg AM, Caputo FJ, et al. Early effectiveness of isolated pectoralis minor tenotomy in selected patients with neurogenic thoracic outlet syndrome. *J Vasc Surg*. 2013;57(5):1345-1352.
22. Guffey R, Abuirqeba AA, Wolfson M, et al. Erector spinae plane block versus perineural local anesthetic infusion for postoperative pain control after supraclavicular decompression for neurogenic thoracic outlet syndrome: a matched case-control comparison. *Ann Vasc Surg*. Published online August 26, 2021. doi:10.1016/j.avsg.2021.05.067
23. Ambrad-Chalela E, Thomas GI, Johansen KH. Recurrent neurogenic thoracic outlet syndrome. *Am J Surg*. 2004;187(4):505-510.
24. Jammeh ML, Ohman JW, Vemuri C, Abuirqeba AA, Thompson RW. Anatomically complete supraclavicular reoperation for recurrent neurogenic thoracic outlet syndrome: clinical characteristics, operative findings, and long-term outcomes. *Hand (NY)*. Published online January 27, 2021. doi:10.1177/1558944720988079

Chapter 9

Neurogenic Thoracic Outlet Syndrome Exposure and Decompression: Transaxillary

Gabriela Velazquez-Ramirez, Lauren N. West-Livingston, Misty D. Humphries, and Julie Ann Freischlag

DEFINITION

- In 1821, Sir Astley Cooper recognized the constellation of neurovascular symptoms involving the thoracic outlet. Ochsner called this the *scalenus anticus syndrome* in 1936 and described the presence of muscle abnormalities secondary to repetitive trauma. The first report of symptoms consistent with this condition was conveyed by Rogers in 1949. Rob and Standeven narrowed down the characterization in 1958. Peet assigned this condition its contemporaneous moniker *thoracic outlet syndrome* (*TOS*) in 1966.[1-4]
- TOS is a condition defined as a group of disorders that involve compression of one or more of the neurovascular structures contained within the thoracic outlet.[5]
- There are three important anatomic spaces that are part of the thoracic outlet: the scalene triangle, the costoclavicular space, and the pectoralis minor space.
  - Scalene triangle—this space is bordered by the anterior scalene muscle, the middle scalene muscle, and the first rib. Important anatomical structures that traverse this space include the brachial plexus and subclavian artery. Cervical ribs may impede on this space, causing compression leading to TOS.[6]
  - Costoclavicular space—this is the space between the clavicle and first rib. Important anatomical structures found in this space include the subclavian artery, the subclavian vein, and the brachial plexus. This is the most common site of compression of the subclavian vein.
  - Pectoralis minor space—this is the space between the anterior pectoralis minor and the posterior chest wall. This is a common site of compression causing neurovascular TOS.[7]
- From the surgeon's point of view the thoracic outlet can be visualized as an anatomic triangle: the two sides being the anterior and middle scalene muscles with the first rib serving as the base of the triangle. The scalene muscles, which originate from the lower cervical spine, may hypertrophy with repetitive neck motion or minor trauma. This hypertrophy is believed to contribute to compression of thoracic outlet structures.
- TOS is subdivided into three discrete etiologies[5,8]: neurogenic, venous, and arterial. In this chapter, we will focus on transaxillary exposure decompression for neurogenic TOS.
  - Neurogenic (over 90% of cases)
  - Venous (3%-5% of cases)
  - Arterial (1%-2% of cases)
- Appropriate classification of the type of TOS is important in guiding perioperative management, as well as surgical approach. This chapter focuses on transaxillary decompression and first rib resection for neurogenic TOS.

PATIENT HISTORY AND PHYSICAL FINDINGS

- A careful history and physical examination enables proper classification of TOS.
- **Neurogenic TOS**, which is more prevalent in women, include paresthesia, pain, and impaired strength in the affected shoulder, arm, or hand along with occipital headaches and neck discomfort.[9] There is commonly an antecedent history of hyperextension neck injury or repetitive neck trauma. Patients frequently manifest tenderness on palpation in the supraclavicular fossa over the anterior scalene muscle. A careful vascular physical examination should confirm the presence of normal circulation.[5,10]
  - Three physical examination maneuvers support the diagnosis of neurogenic TOS:
    - Rotation of the neck and tilting of the head to the opposite side elicit pain in the affected arm.
    - The upper limb tension test, in which the patient first abducts both arms to 90° with the elbows in a locked position, then dorsiflexes the wrists, and finally tilts the head to the side. Each subsequent step imparts greater traction on the brachial plexus, with the first two positions causing discomfort on the ipsilateral side and the head-tilt position causing pain on the contralateral side.
    - During the elevated arm stress test (EAST), the patient raises both arms directly above the head and repeatedly opens and closes the fists. Characteristic upper extremity symptoms arise within 60 seconds in patients with neurogenic TOS.
- **Venous TOS** is also called Paget-von Schroetter syndrome or effort vein thrombosis when the entrapped subclavian vein has progressed to thrombosing. Patients typically present with acute onset of dull aching pain of the upper extremity associated with arm edema and cyanosis. Paresthesias may be present but are due to hand swelling instead of thoracic outlet nerve involvement. A history of strenuous and repetitive work or athletics involving the affected extremity is common, and most patients are young. Some patients will present less acutely with nonthrombotic subclavian vein occlusion or stenosis manifested by intermittent swelling with activity. Regardless, the etiology of venous TOS is mechanical, and treatment is ultimately aimed at eliminating not only the venous obstruction but also the muscular bands and ligaments that have entrapped and damaged the vein.[5]
- **Arterial TOS** typically presents in one of the three ways: (1) asymptomatic, (2) arm claudication, and (3) critical ischemia of the hand. The majority of these patients have a cervical rib, which may or may not be fused to the first rib and is most commonly posterior to the subclavian artery.[6] The etiology is chronic repetitive injury to the subclavian artery as it exits the thoracic outlet. This injury may cause subclavian artery stenosis but more commonly leads to ectasia or a true aneurysm.[11]
  - In asymptomatic patients, a pulsatile mass or supraclavicular bruit can be detected on physical examination.

  - Arm claudication is caused by areas of stenosis which may be static due to long-standing repetitive injury or dynamic, occurring only with arm abduction or extension.
  - Critical ischemia is due to emboli of fibrin platelet aggregates that originate from an ulcerated mural thrombus in the aneurysmal segment.

DIFFERENTIAL DIAGNOSIS

- Carpal tunnel syndrome
- Ulnar nerve compression
- Rotator cuff tendinitis
- Pectoralis minor syndrome
- Cervical spine strain
- Cervical disc disease
- Cervical arthritis
- Brachial plexus injury
- Fibromyositis

PREOPERATIVE EVALUATION AND OTHER DIAGNOSTIC STUDIES

- Preoperative presentation of neurogenic TOS may be classic; however, it is always important to obtain a good history specifically looking for history of neck trauma or known cervical disease. In these cases, magnetic resonance imaging (MRI) is a valuable study.[12]
- A chest X-ray will show presence of cervical ribs as well as other bony abnormalities that could be contributing to the neurogenic presentation. This is imperative to determine if the cervical rib is complete or incomplete.
- Duplex ultrasound of the subclavian artery or vein may be needed in instances of combined types of TOS. This would specifically evaluate for subclavian artery aneurysm as well as patency of subclavian vein. Preoperative physical therapy should be attempted for at least 8 weeks in all patients with a diagnosis of neurogenic TOS. The aims of therapy are to improve posture and achieve greater range of motion. Patients with persistent symptoms of neurogenic TOS despite physical therapy merit surgical intervention. At least 60% of patients will improve with physical therapy and lifestyle alterations.
- A radiographically guided anterior scalene block with local anesthetic (lidocaine) injection may provide a few hours of symptomatic relief. Patients with suspected neurogenic TOS often present with a wide constellation of physical complaints, not all of which are directly attributable to the disorder. A scalene block not only helps confirm the diagnosis but also simulates the expected postoperative result, especially in older patients.[13] This provides the patient and the surgeon reassurance that surgical intervention will be of benefit and demonstrates which symptoms can be reliably expected to improve.
- Other options include Botox (Allergan, Irvine, CA) injection which takes approximately 2 weeks to effect symptom improvement and can be done several times. This may provide symptomatic relief for 2 to 3 months, allowing participation in physical therapy. Importantly, not all TOS patients respond to Botox. This practice is most helpful in patients who have had cervical spine fusions or shoulder operations as it allows them to strengthen the muscles of their neck and back, which may alleviate the TOS symptoms.
- Nerve conduction studies are typically normal in neurogenic TOS but may be useful in ruling out nerve compression such as carpal tunnel or cubital compression syndrome.

SURGICAL MANAGEMENT

Surgical Approach

- The transaxillary decompression is our preferred approach due to its low-risk profile and documented improvement in patients' quality of life.[4,5] This approach effectively decompresses the thoracic outlet and is generally reserved for patients with neurogenic or venous TOS.
- If vessel reconstruction is anticipated, a different approach should be considered as the transaxillary approach limits vessel exposure.

Surgical Anatomy

- The subclavian artery and the five nerve roots (C5–T1) to the brachial plexus are located within the thoracic outlet. The artery courses anterior to the brachial plexus nerve roots and exits the mediastinum in its course over the first rib behind the posterior border of the anterior scalene muscle. The cervical spine nerve roots join to form the initial trunks of the brachial plexus within the thoracic outlet and are located posterior to the subclavian artery. Subsequent merging and branching of these trunks into divisions, cords, and terminal nerves occurs outside the thoracic outlet.
- Other significant nerves within the thoracic outlet are the phrenic and long thoracic nerves.
  - The phrenic nerve receives fibers from C3–C5 and courses in a descending oblique direction from the lateral to the medial edge of the middle portion of the anterior scalene muscle. The phrenic nerve approaches the mediastinum posterior to the subclavian vein.
  - The long thoracic nerve, composed of nerve fibers from C5 to C7, passes through the center of the middle scalene muscle and heads toward the chest wall to innervate the serratus anterior muscle.
- The subclavian vein technically does not course through the thoracic outlet. It passes over the first rib anterior to the anterior scalene muscle. However, the middle segment of the vein remains susceptible to compression between the anteromedial first rib, clavicle, and the subclavius muscle (**FIGURE 1**). Hypertrophy of the subclavius muscle and tendon may occur in athletes and is often implicated in venous TOS.
- Several anatomic anomalies are relevant to the surgeon, as they predispose patients to the development of TOS.

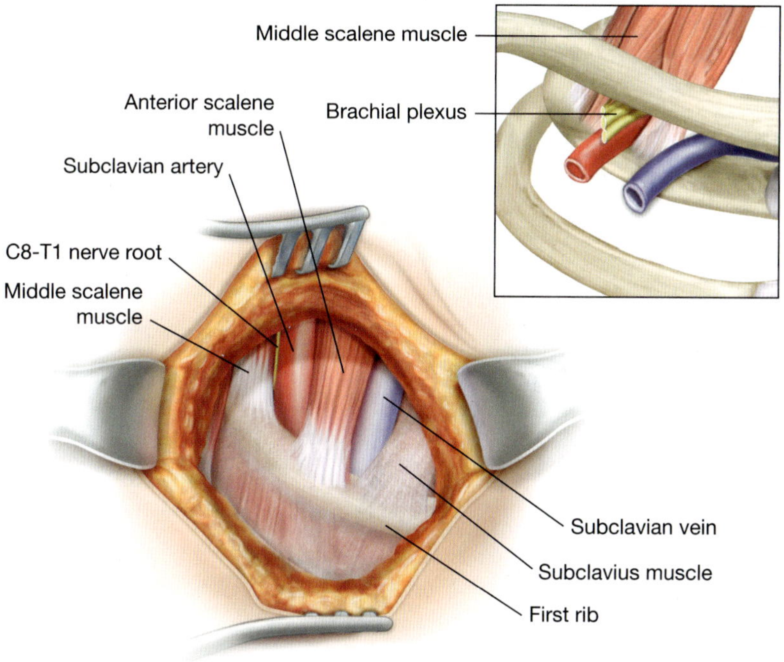

FIGURE 1 • Right-sided thoracic outlet anatomy from the surgeon's perspective as viewed through the operative field in a transaxillary approach. *Inset*, normal anatomic relationships of important thoracic outlet structures.

- The most common is a cervical rib, and a preoperative chest radiograph is adequate for its detection. When present, cervical ribs appear as extensions of the transverse process of C7. Cervical ribs may be complete or partial, with the anterior end attaching to the first rib or floating freely. Additionally, the anterior end may be fibrous and not calcified and thus not completely visualized on chest radiograph. By rigidly confining the thoracic outlet, cervical ribs render the neurovascular structures more prone to compression. Although present in the general population with an incidence of 0.5% to 1%, they are found in 5% to 10% of all TOS patients. A recent meta-analysis demonstrated that while the prevalence of a cervical rib in healthy patient populations was roughly 1%, the prevalence in individuals with TOS was 29.5%. Furthermore, 51.3% of symptomatic patients with a cervical rib had vascular TOS, while 48.7% had neurogenic TOS.[6]
- A prominent C7 transverse process or bifid first rib is also associated with TOS.

Anesthesia

- TOS surgeries are performed under general anesthesia, though since the case is relatively short, a Foley catheter is often not needed.
- Neuromuscular blocking agents should be limited at the time of induction due to proximity of the surgical procedure to the brachial plexus.
- Of note, a pectoralis block can be done after surgery is completed for postoperative pain control purposes.

Positioning

- General endotracheal anesthesia is induced and sequential compression devices are applied.
- The patient is then moved to the lateral decubitus position with affected arm up.
- A bean bag is used to hold the patient and axillary roll should be placed under the down arm. Patient is padded properly to protect bony prominences.
- The entire arm is prepped into the field, we use the Machleder retractor which is extremely helpful.
  - Care should be taken to pad the dependent axilla and support the head. The sterile field incorporates the arm, axilla, and shoulder.
- An adjustable Machleder arm support is affixed to the operating table with the vertical support bar attached to the operating table at the level of the patient's chin.
  - Generous padding around the patient's arm prior to placement in the arm holder protects the median and ulnar nerves from compression as they cross the elbow joint (**FIGURE 2**).

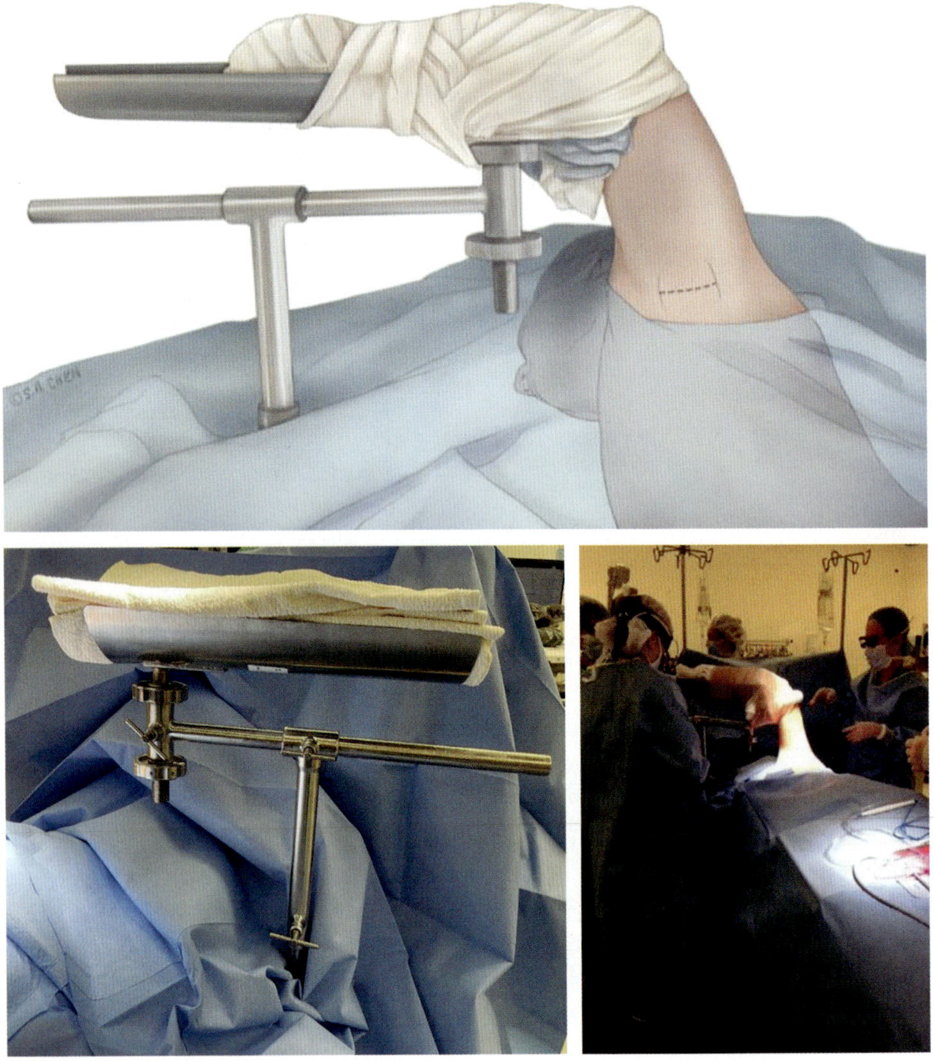

FIGURE 2 • An illustration and photograph depicting proper patient positioning for right transaxillary first rib resection and use of the Machleder arm support with generous padding to prevent compression nerve injury. A padded axillary roll is placed under the dependent axilla, and the patient is stabilized in the left lateral decubitus with the aid of a bean bag. The *dashed line* indicates the preferred location of the skin incision.

TECHNIQUES

INCISION AND EXPOSURE

- After securing the arm in the retractor, the surgeon identifies the anterior border of the latissimus dorsi muscle and the posterior surface of the pectoralis major muscle.
- A transverse skin line incision should be made in the inferior axillary hairline extending between these two muscle borders.
- Electrocautery is used to divide the subcutaneous tissue until thin areolar tissue superficial to the chest wall is encountered. A self-retaining Cerebellar or Weitlaner retractor is then inserted into the wound. Upon encountering the chest wall—and if in the correct anatomic plane—gentle blunt dissection with the surgeon's fingers or a pair of Kittner or peanut dissectors easily separates the soft tissues from the chest wall. Once the chest wall is encountered, the arm is lifted in the retractor system and the connective tissue over the thoracic outlet is bluntly dissected. Raising the Machleder arm support allows for optimal access to the first rib and the thoracic outlet. The arm is lifted with the retractor at 15-minute intervals, releasing the arm down intermittently prevents any nerve stretching injury. The intercostobrachial nerve is located in the second intercostal space. Although frequently difficult to avoid, care should be taken not to impart excess traction as injury results in numbness or dysesthesia of the medial aspect of the proximal arm.
- The aid of fiber optic–lighted Deaver retractors facilitates visualization during this portion of the dissection. Alternatively, the surgeon should wear a headlight (**FIGURE 3**).
- The first rib is identified near its insertion at the sternoclavicular joint and generally encountered higher than anticipated. A Kittner or peanut dissector is then used to gently sweep away the loose fibrous tissue overlying the first rib partially exposing the brachial plexus, subclavian artery and vein, and scalene muscles. There is occasionally a small branch of the subclavian artery that must be ligated and divided in order to fully expose the operative field.
- The next step is to fully expose the rib. Depending on the patient's anatomy, it generally is the easiest to first clear off the intercostal muscles laterally. A periosteal elevator works

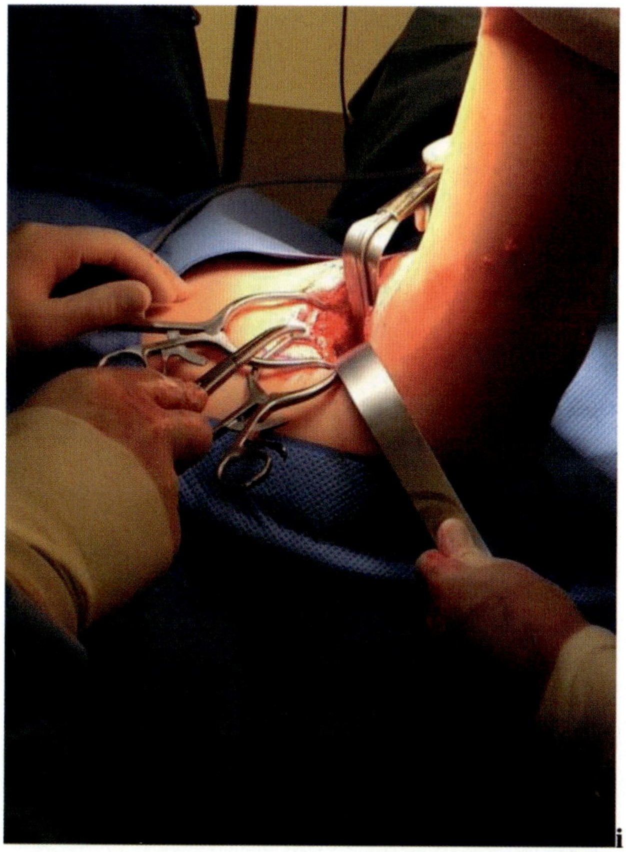

FIGURE 3 • A lighted retractor and Deaver retractor are used to give good visualization of the surgical field.

best, but any type of long elevator may be used (**FIGURE 4**). The dissection proceeds in the anterior and posterior directions until all the intercostal muscle attachments are divided from the rib. The elevator can then be used to elevate the first rib, thus separating the rib from the underlying parietal pleura. This mobilization should continue from behind the brachial plexus in the posterior direction to beyond the subclavian vein in the anterior direction.

- Attention is then directed to the superior border of the first rib, where the periosteal elevator is used to bluntly detach the scalene medius fibers from the rib. The long thoracic nerve courses along the lateral edge of the scalene medius muscle but is generally not visualized. Avoiding sharp dissection and closely adhering to the surface of the rib during blunt dissection prevents injury to the long thoracic nerve.
- The anterior scalene muscle should now be clearly identified as it arises from the medial superior aspect of the first rib (**FIGURE 5**). A right-angled clamp is passed behind the anterior scalene muscle Neurogenic Thoracic Outlet Syndrome Exposure and Decompression: Transaxillarynear its insertion on the scalene tubercle. Gently lifting the anterior scalene with the right-angled clamp protects the subclavian artery as it courses posterior to the muscle (**FIGURE 6**). It is important to free several centimeters of the muscle prior to dividing it with Metzenbaum scissors (**FIGURE 7**). This maneuver facilitates resection of a portion of the anterior scalene muscle, which has been shown to reduce recurrence rates when compared with division at its insertion point on the rib.
- Lastly, the subclavius muscle will appear as a crescent-shaped ligamentous attachment to the first rib adjacent to the subclavian vein. With care not to injure the subclavian vein, the subclavius muscle is sharply divided with scissors.

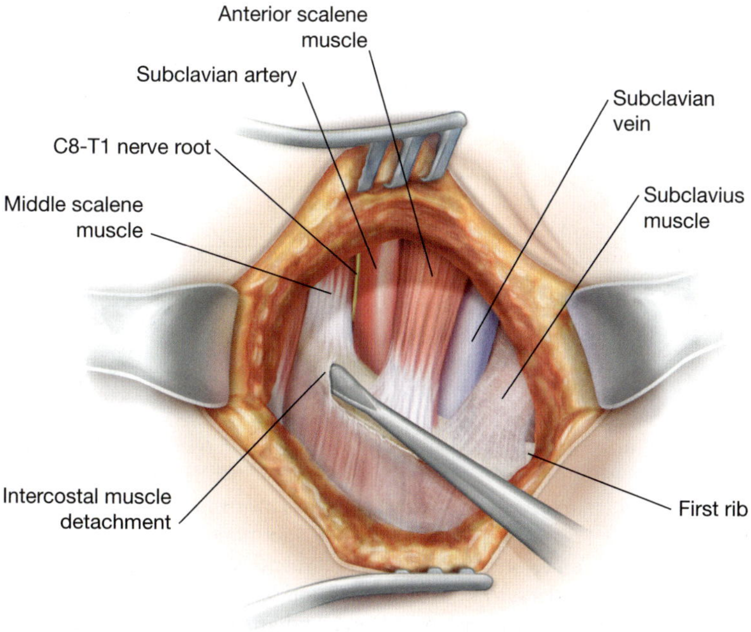

FIGURE 4 • A periosteal elevator is used to dissect along the superior surface of the first rib in order to divide intercostal muscle attachments.

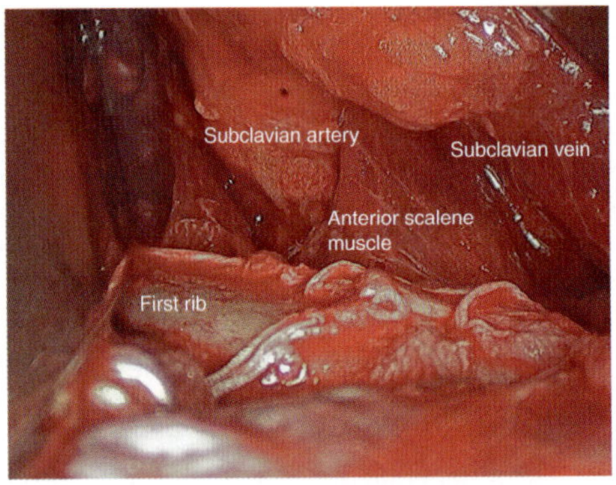

FIGURE 5 • An image of the gross anatomy from a close-up perspective of the right-sided thoracic outlet. The important relationships between the first rib, anterior scalene muscle, and subclavian vessels can be seen. (Reprinted from Arnaoutakis G, Freischlag JA, Reifsnyder T. Transaxillary rib resection for thoracic outlet syndrome. In: Cambria R, Chaikof E, eds. *Atlas of Vascular and Endovascular Surgery: Anatomy and Technique*. Elsevier; 2014:193-203. Copyright © 2014 Elsevier. With permission.)

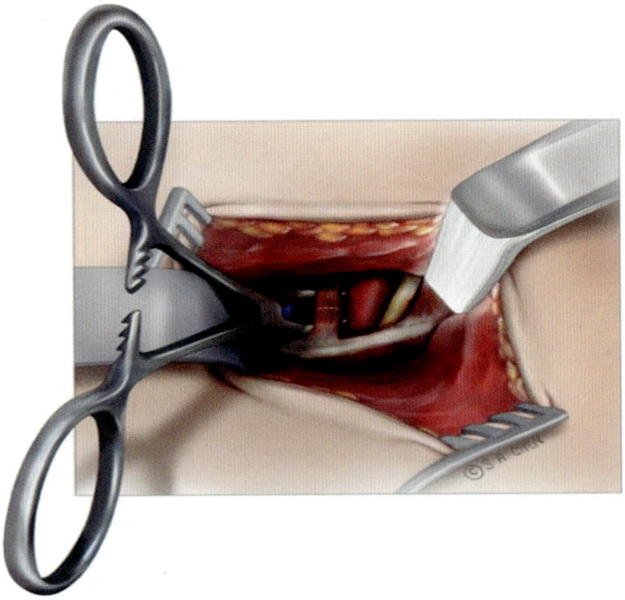

FIGURE 6 • A right-angled clamp is insinuated behind the anterior scalene muscle. Gentle elevation pulls the muscle away from the underlying subclavian artery, thereby protecting the artery prior to dividing the muscle with scissors. The subclavius muscle is a crescent-shaped ligamentous attachment to the first rib adjacent to the subclavian vein. The subclavius muscle is sharply divided with scissors with care not to injure the subclavian vein. (Images illustrated by S.A. Chen, made for Dr. Julie Freischlag, http://www.sarahachen.com/.)

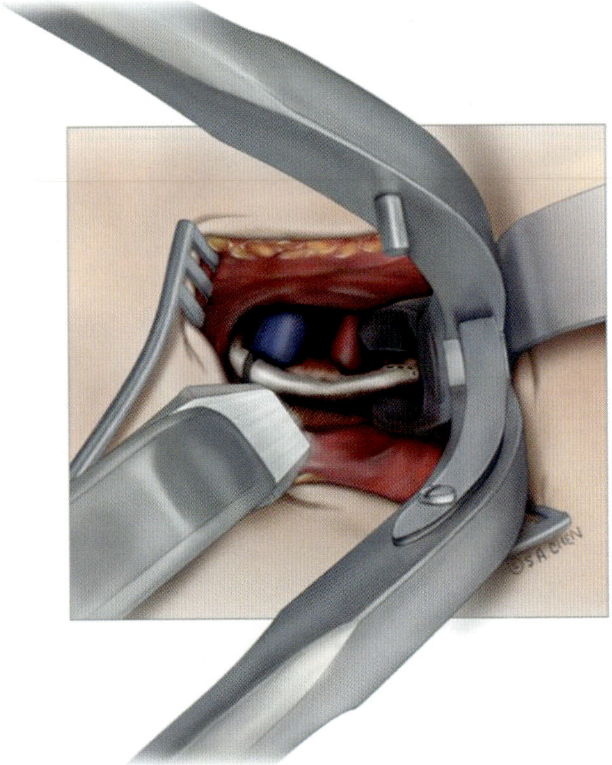

FIGURE 7 • The first rib is seen in the illustration of a left first rib resection. Metzenbaum scissors are used to sharply divide the anterior scalene muscle, with the right-angled clamp elevating the muscle to protect the subclavian artery as it courses behind the muscle. The divided ends of the tendinous anterior scalene fibers can be seen. (Images illustrated by S.A. Chen, made for Dr. Julie Freischlag, http://www.sarahachen.com/.)

RIB RESECTION

- Once the subclavius and anterior scalene muscles are divided and the rib completely mobilized, a periosteal elevator can be used again to free up the reminder intercostal muscle fibers along the lateral aspect of the first rib, and a bone cutter is then used to divide the rib. Generally, it is divided anteriorly and then posteriorly; however, the patient's body habitus may make the reverse order easier (**FIGURE 8**).
- In its anterior extent, the rib is divided adjacent to the subclavian vein, and in the posterior direction, it is divided just anterior to the brachial plexus; this ensures that the nerve roots are not inadvertently injured. The rib is then removed. It is important to always identify the tips of the bone cutter so that they are free of other structures to prevent injuries.
- A bone rongeur is used to remove residual rib and to smooth the cut ends until there is no residual nerve impingement. A Ross retractor or similar instrument may be used to protect the nerves during use of the rongeur (**FIGURE 9**).

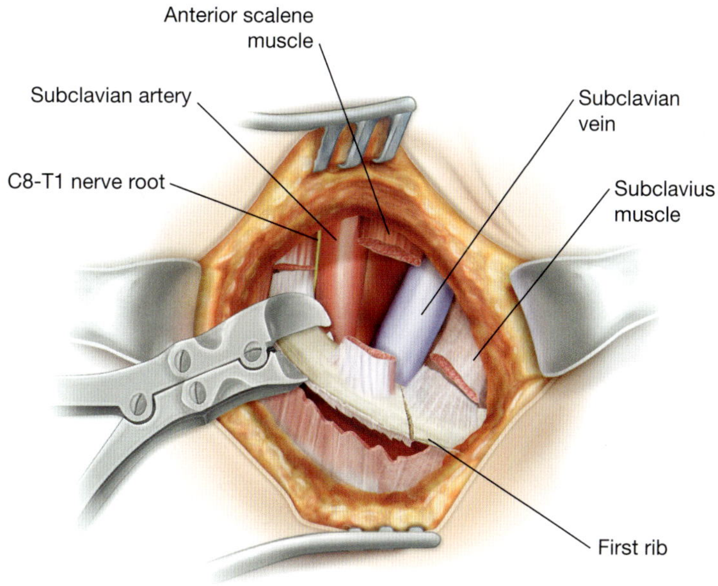

FIGURE 8 • A bone cutter is used to divide the first rib in its anterior and posterior direction. Once removed, the rongeur is used to achieve smooth rib edges.

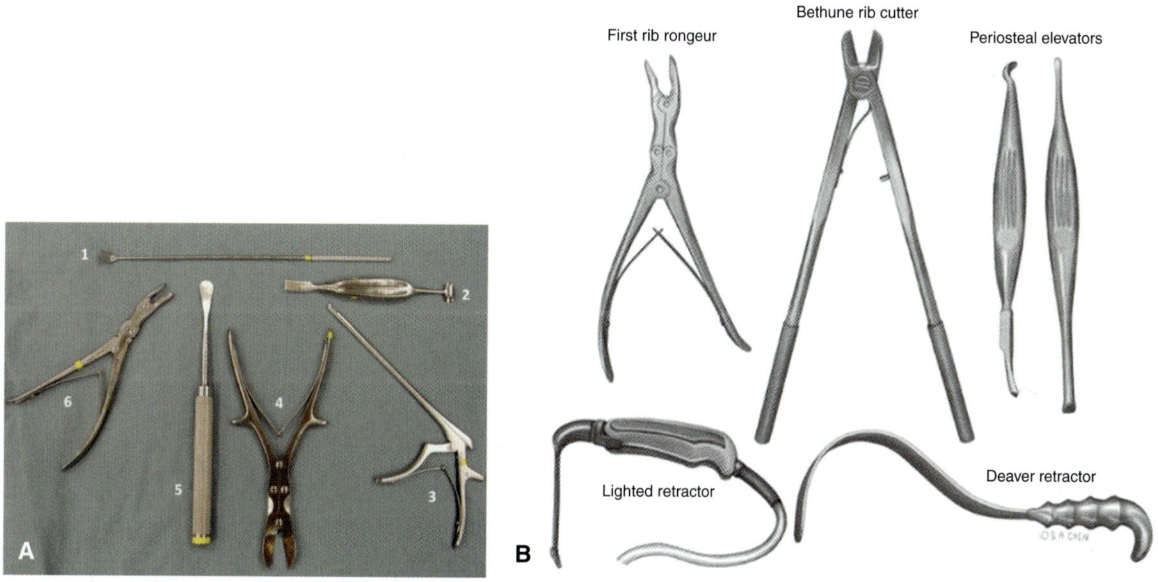

FIGURE 9 • **A,** From the top of the image in the clockwise direction, the instruments depicted are *(1)* Roos retractor, *(2)* Alexander periosteotome, *(3)* Kerrison punch upbiting instrument, *(4)* double-action bone cutter, *(5)* Cobb periosteal elevator, and *(6)* Rongeur. **B,** From the top of the image in the clockwise direction, the instruments depicted are (1) first rib rongeur, (2) Bethune rib cutter, (3) periosteal elevators, (4) Deaver retractor, (5) lighted retractor. **A,** (Reprinted from Arnaoutakis G, Freischlag JA, Reifsnyder T. Transaxillary rib resection for thoracic outlet syndrome. In: Cambria R, Chaikof E, eds. *Atlas of Vascular and Endovascular Surgery: Anatomy and Technique.* Elsevier; 2014:193-203. Copyright © 2014 Elsevier. With permission.)

- It is important to ensure that the rib be removed all the way to the spine, and that there are no residual fibers from the anterior scalene muscle crossing beneath the subclavian artery and inserting onto the thickened surface at the apex of the pleura, known as Sibson fascia. Any such fibers should be identified and divided (**FIGURE 10**).
- New approaches to TOS surgery have been described in the literature, such as rib-sparing scalenectomy.[14] Recent advances in technology include robotic first rib resections. Recent studies demonstrate symptom relief as well as less frequent complications with the robotic approach relative to the supraclavicular approach, though further investigation is necessary into this emerging approach.[15,16] We continue to advocate for complete decompression of the thoracic outlet with first rib resection and scalenectomy.

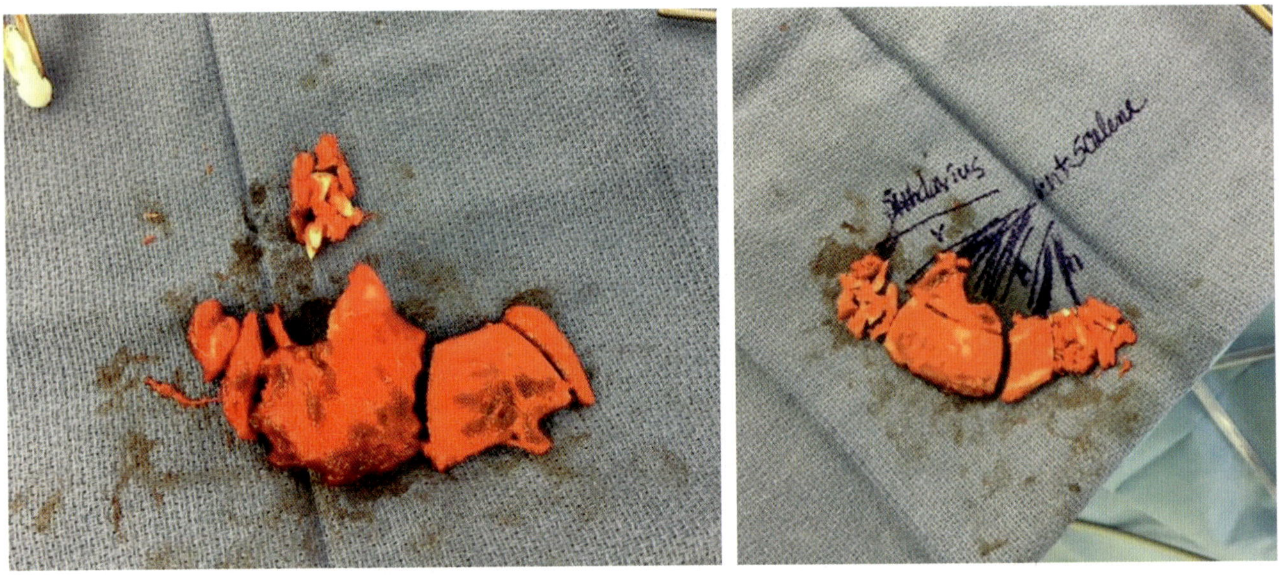

FIGURE 10 • Resected rib labeled with previous anatomical attachments and relationships.

CLOSURE

- The surgical field is next inspected for bleeding. Temporarily packing the wound reliably controls minor bleeding. The wound is then reinspected, and hemostasis is completed with judicious use of electrocautery.
- The wound is then filled with saline. Several positive pressure ventilations are administered with saline left in the wound to assess for an air leak indicative of a postoperative pneumothorax. If an air leak is present, a small caliber (12 French [Fr]) chest tube is warranted prior to closure.
- If the irrigation drains into the pleural space but there is no air leak, the pleura has been breached, but a chest tube may not be necessary. In this situation, a 12-Fr or 14-Fr red rubber catheter is placed into the bed of the first rib and attached to gentle suction. The Machleder arm holder is lowered to facilitate a tension-free closure. The subcutaneous fascia is then closed around the tube. While suction is applied to the red rubber catheter, the anesthesia team provides a sustained Valsalva and the fascial suture is tied as the suction tube is rapidly removed. This maneuver generally avoids a clinically significant postoperative pneumothorax.
- Closure is performed with absorbable 2-0 suture in the fascia and a 4-0 subcuticular skin closure.

PEARLS AND PITFALLS

Operative mantra	▪ Look twice and cut once. Always double-check placement of the bone cutters before dividing the first rib.
Incorrect diagnosis	▪ A successful operation hinges on an accurate preoperative diagnosis. A thorough history and physical and the anterior scalene block help to identify patients likely to benefit from first rib resection.
Brachial plexus injury	▪ Proper positioning and careful retraction help prevent excessive traction and injury to the brachial plexus.
Misidentification of the first rib	▪ During initial exposure, the second rib is often mistaken for the first rib. The cephalad surface of the first rib is flat unlike the second, which is more concave.
Incomplete first rib resection	▪ Incomplete first rib resection has been associated with recurrent TOS. After cutting and removing the rib, take your time to trim back the ends with the rongeur.
Hemostasis	▪ To keep a clean operative field, pack a 4 × 4 gauze into the wound, lower the arm retractor, and wait a couple of minutes. This often aids in hemostasis.

POSTOPERATIVE CARE

- A chest X-ray is obtained in the recovery room only in instances when a chest tube was placed or there was a pleural tear identified.
  - Small, clinically asymptomatic pneumothoraces may be observed with a follow-up chest X-ray the next morning.
- Postoperative pain control is one of the most important aspects of postoperative care.
- Patients are typically discharged from the hospital when adequate oral analgesia has been achieved.
- Activity is restricted by the amount of postoperative pain. Occasionally, a sling is required for patient comfort, but it is preferable to have the arm as mobile as tolerated.
- Physical therapy should be prescribed after 2 weeks in all patients undergoing transaxillary first rib resection, regardless of the cause, to restore range of motion and strength.

OUTCOMES

- Improvement after surgery for neurogenic TOS is somewhat subjective and based on the patient's perception of disability before and after decompression. Improvement in symptoms exceeds 90%.[17,18]
- Over time, the durability of these results may decrease, reinforcing the need for close follow-up of these patients beyond 2 years.[19,20]
- Factors that predict surgical failure include major depression, chronic symptoms, work-related injury, lack of response to anterior scalene muscle blocks, and a short segment of divided anterior scalene muscle.[21]
- The Quick Disabilities of the Arm, Shoulder, and Hand (QuickDASH) survey and the Cervical-Brachial Symptom Questionnaire (CBSQ) have increasingly been used to evaluate symptoms and functions preoperatively and postoperatively.[22,23]

CONTRAINDICATIONS AND COMPLICATIONS

Contraindications

- The primary contraindication to the transaxillary approach is vascular reconstruction. Scher class 2 and 3 subclavian artery aneurysm reconstructions are specifically contraindicated in the transaxillary approach, due to the inability to repair the subclavian vein with patch angioplasty.
- While dialysis access maintenance is not an absolute contraindication to the transaxillary approach, this surgical procedure should be approached with caution in this setting.

Vascular Injury

- A national query identified injury to the subclavian vessels as the most common complication following transaxillary rib resection for neurogenic TOS, occurring in 1% to 2% of cases.[24,25]
- Patients experiencing a vascular injury have greater lengths of stay as well as increased hospital charges.
- It is difficult to obtain proximal control of these vessels from the transaxillary approach, and therefore, the surgeon should exercise extreme caution when dissecting near these vessels.
- The prevalence of vascular injury is equal in the transaxillary and supraclavicular surgical approaches.[26]

Nerve Injury

- Major nerve injury has been traditionally regarded as the most common complication following surgery for TOS. However, large contemporary series disprove this belief, with rates of brachial plexus injury for patients undergoing transaxillary first rib resection approaching 0%.[20,24]
- Temporary or permanent numbness of the upper medial arm due to excessive traction or division of the intercostobrachial nerve occurs in up to 10%. Frequently, these symptoms will improve over time.
- Transient brachial plexus injury is more common in the transaxillary approach than in the supraclavicular approach, but not in a statistically significant fashion.[26]

Pneumothorax

- This complication occurs in 2% to 10% of patients.[20] Accordingly, an upright chest X-ray is routinely performed in the recovery room.
- Radiographically detected pneumothoraces only require a chest tube if symptomatic or enlarging.
- Adhering closely to the inferior surface of the first rib during blunt dissection will help protect against postoperative pneumothorax.
- The prevalence of pneumothorax is equal between the transaxillary and supraclavicular surgical approaches.[26]

Persistent Pain

- Persistent pain and symptoms are more common in the transaxiallary approach compared to the supraclavicular approach in a statistically significant fashion.[26]

Recurrence

- Symptoms of TOS recur in 10% to 20% of patients.[27-29]
- There may be functional impairment despite clinical improvement of symptoms.[30]
- Two intraoperative factors are known to reduce recurrence rates.
  - Resecting a significant portion (2-3 cm) of the anterior scalene muscle as opposed to simply dividing it at its insertion point
  - Ensuring that the posterior edge of the first rib is resected sufficiently so as to leave as short a rib stump as technically feasible
- Patients with spontaneous recurrence compared to those that are reinjured have worse outcomes when reoperation is performed.

REFERENCES

1. Roos DB. Transaxillary approach for first rib resection to relieve thoracic outlet syndrome. *Ann Surg*. 1966;163:354-358.
2. Kaplan J, Kanwal A. "*Thoracic Outlet Syndrome*." *StatPearls*. StatPearls Publishing; 2020. https://www.ncbi.nlm.nih.gov/books/NBK557450/.
3. Li N, Dierks G, Vervaeke HE, et al. Thoracic outlet syndrome: a narrative review. *J Clin Med*. 2021;10(5):962.
4. Chang MC, Kim DH. Essentials of thoracic outlet syndrome: a narrative review. *World J Clin Cases*. 2021;9(21):5804.
5. Jones MR, Prabhakar A, Viswanath O, et al. Thoracic outlet syndrome: a comprehensive review of pathophysiology, diagnosis, and treatment. *Pain Ther*. 2019;8(1):5-18.
6. Henry BM, Vikse J, Sanna B, et al. Cervical rib prevalence and its association with thoracic outlet syndrome: a meta-analysis

of 141 studies with surgical considerations. *World Neurosurg.* 2018;110:e965-e978.
7. Hussain MA, Aljabri B, Al-Omran M. *Vascular thoracic outlet syndrome.* In *Seminars in Thoracic and Cardiovascular Surgery.* Vol 28, No. 1. WB Saunders; 2016:151-157.
8. Illig KA, Rodriguez-Zoppi E, Bland T, Muftah M, Jospitre E. The incidence of thoracic outlet syndrome. *Ann Vasc Surg.* 2021;70:263-272.
9. Ferrante MA, Ferrante ND. The thoracic outlet syndromes: Part 1. Overview of the thoracic outlet syndromes and review of true neurogenic thoracic outlet syndrome. *Muscle Nerve.* 2017;55(6):782-793.
10. Povlsen S, Povlsen B. Diagnosing thoracic outlet syndrome: current approaches and future directions. *Diagnostics.* 2018;8(1):21.
11. Vemuri C, McLaughlin LN, Abuirqeba AA, Thompson RW. Clinical presentation and management of arterial thoracic outlet syndrome. *J Vasc Surg.* 2017;65(5):1429-1439.
12. Raptis CA, Sridhar S, Thompson RW, Fowler KJ, Bhalla S. Imaging of the patient with thoracic outlet syndrome. *Radiographics.* 2016;36(4):984-1000.
13. Lum YW, Brooke BS, Likes K, et al. Impact of anterior scalene lidocaine blocks on predicting surgical success in older patients with neurogenic thoracic outlet syndrome. *J Vasc Surg.* 2012;55:1370-1375.
14. Johansen K. Rib-sparing scalenectomy for neurogenic thoracic outlet syndrome: early results. *J Vasc Surg.* 2021;73(6):2059-2063.
15. Kocher GJ, Zehnder A, Lutz JA, Schmidli J, Schmid RA. First rib resection for thoracic outlet syndrome: the robotic approach. *World J Surg.* 2018;42(10):3250-3255.
16. Burt BM, Palivela N, Cekmecelioglu D, et al. Safety of robotic first rib resection for thoracic outlet syndrome. *J Thorac Cardiovasc Surg.* 2021;162(4):1297-1305.
17. Roos DB. The place for scalenectomy and first-rib resection in thoracic outlet syndrome. *Surgery.* 1982;92:1077-1085.
18. Peek J, Vos CG, Ünlü Ç, van de Pavoordt HD, van den Akker PJ, de Vries JP. Outcome of surgical treatment for thoracic outlet syndrome: systematic review and meta-analysis. *Ann Vasc Surg.* 2017;40:303-326.
19. Rochlin DH, Gilson MM, Likes KC, et al. Quality-of-life scores in neurogenic thoracic outlet syndrome patients undergoing first rib resection and scalenectomy. *J Vasc Surg.* 2013;57:436-443.
20. Altobelli GG, Kudo T, Haas BT, et al. Thoracic outlet syndrome: pattern of clinical success after operative decompression. *J Vasc Surg.* 2005;42:122-128.
21. Axelrod DA, Proctor MC, Geisser ME, et al. Outcomes after surgery for thoracic outlet syndrome. *J Vasc Surg.* 2001;33:1220-1225.
22. Beaton DE, Wright JG, Katz JN; Upper Extremity Collaborative Group. Development of the QuickDASH: comparison of three item-reduction approaches. *JBJS.* 2005;87(5):1038-1046.
23. Ruopsa N, Ristolainen L, Vastamäki M, Vastamäki H. Neurogenic thoracic outlet syndrome with supraclavicular release: long-term outcome without rib resection. *Diagnostics.* 2021;11(3):450.
24. Thompson RW. *Complications of surgery for thoracic outlet syndrome.* In *Vascular and Endovascular Complications.* CRC Press; 2021:233-245.
25. Chang DC, Rotellini-Coltvet LA, Mukherjee D, et al. Surgical intervention for thoracic outlet syndrome improves patient's quality of life. *J Vasc Surg.* 2009;49:630-635; discussion 635-637.
26. Hosseinian MA, Loron AG, Soleimanifard Y. Evaluation of complications after surgical treatment of thoracic outlet syndrome. *Korean J Thorac Cardiovasc Surg.* 2017;50(1):36.
27. Mingoli A, Feldhaus RJ, Farina C, et al. Long-term outcome after transaxillary approach for thoracic outlet syndrome. *Surgery.* 1995;118:840-844.
28. Mingoli A, Sapienza P, di Marzo L, et al. Role of first rib stump length in recurrent neurogenic thoracic outlet syndrome. *Am J Surg.* 2005;190:156.
29. Sanders RJ, Haug CE, Pearce WH. Recurrent thoracic outlet syndrome. *J Vasc Surg.* 1990;12:390-398; discussion 398-400.
30. Peek J, Vos CG, Ünlü Ç, Schreve MA, Van de Mortel RH, De Vries JP. Long-term functional outcome of surgical treatment for thoracic outlet syndrome. *Diagnostics.* 2018;8(1):7.

Chapter 10 Venous and Arterial Thoracic Outlet Syndrome

Kathryn Lambeth DiLosa and Misty D. Humphries

DEFINITION

- Venous thoracic outlet syndrome (vTOS), also known as effort thrombosis or Paget-Schroetter syndrome, involves repetitive subclavian vein compression resulting in endothelial injury and intermittent stasis. This damage ultimately contributes to acute thrombosis of the axillosubclavian veins. The external compression of the vein occurs between the clavicle/subclavius muscle from above, the first rib inferiorly, and the anterior scalene muscle insertion (**FIGURE 1**).
- Arterial thoracic outlet syndrome (aTOS) is the least common form of TOS, accounting for less than 1% of overall cases. Extrinsic subclavian artery compression results in poststenotic dilatation, aneurysmal degeneration, and subsequent distal embolization.[1] In aTOS, the arterial compression is caused by bony or muscular abnormalities including a cervical rib, anomalous first rib, anterior or middle scalene muscle bands, or hypertrophic callus from a healed clavicular injury or fracture.[2] The higher preponderance of cervical ribs in women translates to an increased incidence of aTOS among women.[3]

DIFFERENTIAL DIAGNOSIS

- Patients with vTOS present with upper extremity swelling and a differential diagnosis is elicited by a thorough history. Secondary axillosubclavian thrombosis due to iatrogenic catheterization or prior instrumentation of the upper extremity veins is far more common and should be considered first. In patients who do not perform repetitive overhead movements or play high-performance sports, malignancy or underlying hypercoagulable state should be ruled out.[4,5]
- In patients with hand or digit ischemia, a thorough workup for a cardiogenic source should be sought before assigning the etiology to aTOS. Cardiac etiology is far more common than embolization of thrombus from a subclavian aneurysm due to underlying aTOS. Paradoxical emboli, a patent foramen ovale, axillary artery branch aneurysms, congenital vascular abnormalities, or traumatic injuries/arterial dissection of the axillosubclavian arterial system should be ruled out.

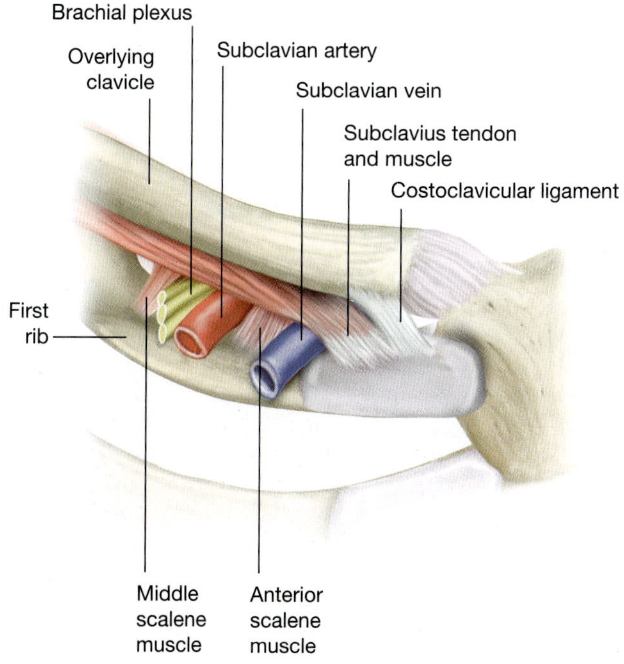

FIGURE 1 ● Normal structures in the thoracic outlet that can contribute to venous compression.

PATIENT HISTORY AND PHYSICAL FINDINGS

- Patients with vTOS are often young men, healthy, and athletically inclined who present with the abrupt onset of unilateral arm swelling in their dominant arm after repetitive, strenuous use for sport, work, or recreation.[6] Athletes who require their arms to hyperabduct and extend repeatedly, such as swimmers and baseball pitchers, are most commonly affected. The characteristic swelling present in the shoulder, arm, and hand and can be accompanied by aching, throbbing, or tightness that worsens with activity. The severity of venous thrombosis also correlates with symptomatology. Because most patients are otherwise young and healthy, orthopedic causes such as strain, muscle pull, or joint injury are often considered initially. Range of motion in the affected extremity can be impeded due to discomfort, further suggesting, albeit incorrectly, a musculoskeletal cause. Cyanosis of the affected extremity, chest wall venous collaterals, or progressively worsening symptoms indicate a vascular etiology and should prompt referral to a TOS comprehensive care center. On exam, the arm will appear edematous, tender to palpation, warm, and often has visible superficial collaterals that track onto the anterior chest wall (**FIGURE 2**).
- aTOS patients present with mild to severe hand ischemia arising from embolization. Frequently, there is long-standing embolization leading to small vessel thrombosis and this can manifest as digital ischemia or present with splinter hemorrhages. The diagnosis is often delayed as these patients have no typical atherosclerotic risk factors and are frequently young and athletic. A bruit or pulsatile mass may be palpable in the supraclavicular fossa and a bony prominence in that region may imply the presence of a cervical rib or muscular abnormality. Symptoms often are gradual and unnoticed by patients until the vessels thrombose or there is embolization to the brachial bifurcation and the patient presents with critical upper extremity ischemia.

IMAGING AND OTHER DIAGNOSTIC STUDIES

- Patients with suspected vTOS should undergo duplex ultrasound of the affected extremity. Depending on the chronicity of the lesion, well-developed collaterals can be mistaken for the subclavian vein. Color flow duplex, phasicity of flow with respiration, and augmentation with provocative maneuvers can all aid in confirming the diagnosis of deep venous thrombosis (DVT). An experienced vascular sonographer and interpreter can make the diagnosis with a high degree of accuracy based on the duplex alone. Cross-sectional imaging with magnetic resonance imaging (MRI) or computed tomography (CT) venography is rarely needed or indicated in the workup of vTOS. Catheter-based venography can confirm diagnosis and document the extent of vTOS while allowing for thrombolysis and reduction of clot burden; however, long-term studies have not supported that thrombolysis improves outcomes after first rib resection.[7]

- Patients presenting with digital ischemia suspicious for aTOS should undergo plain radiographic imaging to assess for a cervical rib (**FIGURE 3**). Digital photoplethysmography (PPG) of the bilateral upper extremities can be performed to visualize blood flow to each finger and can rule out Raynaud type etiologies but offers no anatomic evaluation of the artery for aneurysmal degeneration. When combined with provocative arm elevation, PPG will demonstrate dampening of waveforms, though this is nonspecific for the diagnosis of aTOS.[5] Similar results can be observed with duplex ultrasound when combined with provocative maneuvers. It is imperative to also understand that subclavian artery compression can be seen in up to a quarter of the population, and simple arterial compression is not diagnostic of aTOS.[6] CT angiography (CTA) of the neck or chest and upper extremity provides the most definitive visualization of the subclavian artery and thoracic outlet, confirming the presence of the cervical rib, delineating the amount of thrombus in the subclavian aneurysm, and documenting the proximal and distal vasculature for preoperative planning (**FIGURE 4A** and **B**). Arm elevation with CTA can obscure the course of the artery, thus should be done only in combination with neutral position imaging. While magnetic resonance angiography (MRA) can also be used to identify aTOS, the longer imaging acquisition times and bony artifact can fail to delineate the specific arterial anatomy for surgical planning.

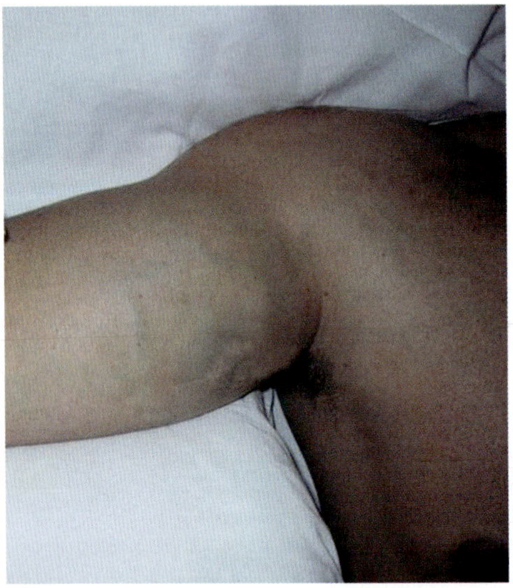

FIGURE 2 • Physical exam appearance of a patient with venous TOS and venous collaterals from long standing subclavian vein compression.

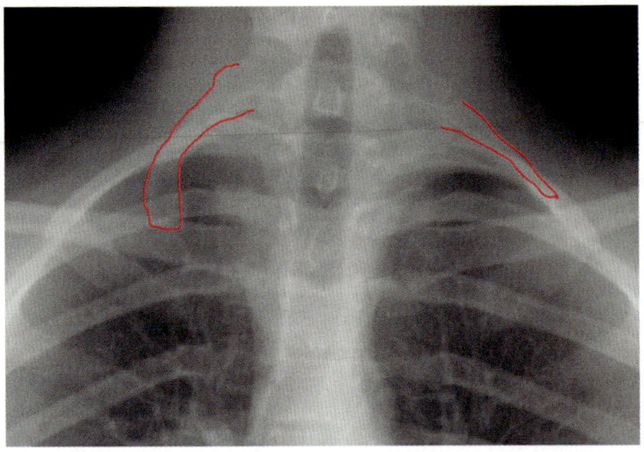

FIGURE 3 • Young patient with bilateral asymmetric cervical ribs (outlined in red).

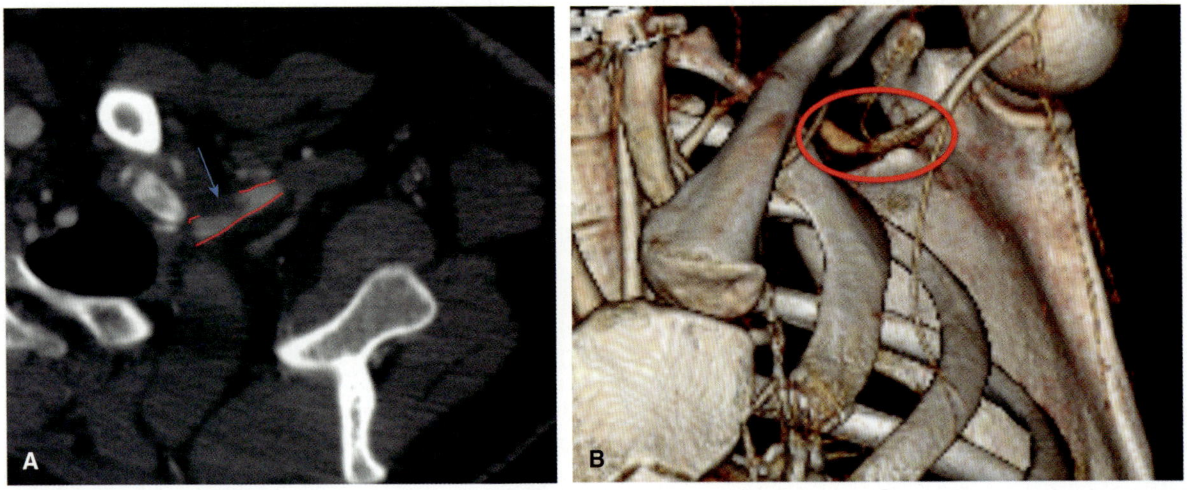

FIGURE 4 • **A,** Axial CT image of a left subclavian artery aneurysm (outlined in red) with evidence of thrombus (*blue arrow*). **B,** Three dimensional rendering of the left subclavian artery aneurysm (*red circle*) in relation to the left cervical rib and first rib.

COMPREHENSIVE CARE MODELS

- Chronic pain symptoms are common with neurogenic TOS, but outcomes for patients undergoing treatment for TOS have been shown to be better and more consistent when patients receive care from a coordinated care center.[8] Comprehensive TOS centers are more likely to use tools that adhere to the Society for Vascular Surgery Reporting Standards and collect long-term outcomes for patients with TOS, which are necessary for further advances in treatment methods.[9] These centers are also able to provide tailored pre and postoperative care for optimal recovery and prevention/ management of recurrent symptoms.

SURGICAL MANAGEMENT

Preoperative Planning

- Patients with mild to moderate vTOS symptoms can be managed with anticoagulation.[10] Young patients and high-performance athletes have better long-term outcomes with surgical decompression of the thoracic outlet.[11] When patients present with severe symptoms of swelling, pain, and numbness, thrombolysis should be performed. Successful thrombolysis can involve a combination of chemical and mechanical thrombectomy and is effective in decreasing clot burden and reducing long-term sequelae of upper extremity chronic DVT (**FIGURE 5A** and **B**).[12] Technical details of thrombolysis are well described and can be performed with minimal morbidity.
- Definitive therapy after thrombolysis involves thoracic outlet decompression, consisting of anterior scalenectomy, resection of the subclavius tendon, first rib resection, and venolysis. Venous reconstruction is an option, but with increased endovascular techniques; this is frequently not necessary.
- The timing of surgery after thrombolysis remains somewhat controversial and is limited by anecdotal reports and various surgeon biases. Successful outcomes can be achieved with definitive thoracic outlet decompression performed during the same hospitalization as the thrombolysis and up to 3 months after.[10] Management of anticoagulation during this time also impacts decisions about planning surgery, as intolerance to blood thinners or difficulty with maintaining adequate anticoagulation can affect the urgency of the required definitive decompression. The use of direct oral anticoagulants (DOACs) has limited most intolerance issues previously seen with anticoagulation.[13]
- aTOS in the presence of an ipsilateral cervical rib and a subclavian aneurysm is an indication for definitive surgical decompression and arterial reconstruction. Preoperative planning consists mainly of ensuring adequate and healthy vasculature proximal and distal to the aneurysmal segment, determining an appropriate bypass route, and choosing a conduit. Extra-anatomic bypass via a carotid-subclavian or carotid-axillary with interval ligation may be necessary, depending on the size and length of the subclavian aneurysm and extent of vascular thrombosis. Direct repair of the subclavian aneurysm with interposition grafting can be accomplished when there is a short segment aneurysm that limits itself to the visualized region in the supraclavicular fossa. Endovascular techniques such as stent grafting in the setting of aTOS are generally not recommended, given the young age of the typical patient, the compression that can occur from scarring even after surgical decompression, and the likely desire to resume prior activities in the postoperative period.

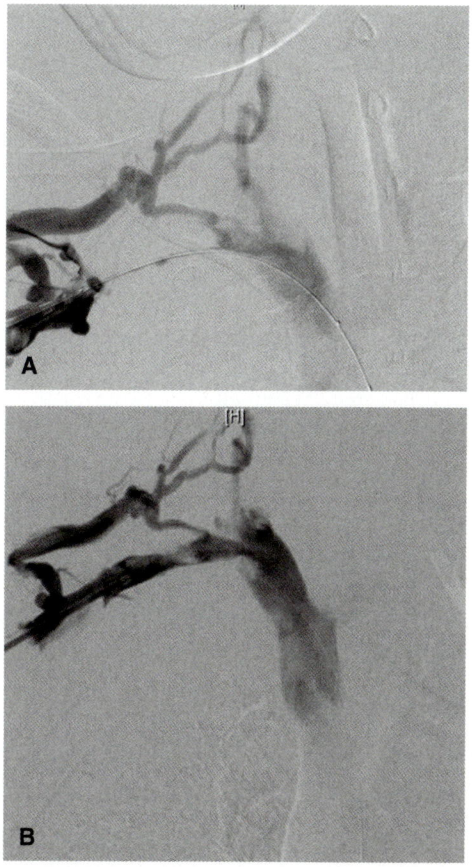

FIGURE 5 • **A,** Initial venogram demonstrating right axillosubclavian occlusion with large collateral development. Wire was passed through this region and pharmacomechanical thrombolysis initiated. **B,** Follow-up venogram 24 hours later with resolution of majority of thrombus load. Vein still shows signs of disease and scarring particularly in the region of compression.

Positioning

- vTOS decompression can be achieved through an infraclavicular, paraclavicular, or transaxillary approach. The approach determines patient positioning. For the infraclavicular and paraclavicular approach, the patient is positioned supine with a small roll between the shoulder blades. The head of the bed is elevated to 30° to decrease venous return and the face turned away from the operative side. For the transaxillary approach, the patient is positioned laterally on a bean bag with the affected arm up. An axillary roll is placed underneath the arm that is down. In all approaches, the affected arm is prepped into the field so that it can be moved around to evaluate for residual compression. This affords anterior visualization of the first rib and particularly the subclavius muscle. The entire ipsilateral neck, shoulder, arm (and axilla for transaxillary), and anterior chest wall are prepped into the field as well as a region on the lateral chest wall should there be a small postprocedural pneumothorax necessitating a chest tube. For the transaxillary approach, the arm is placed in a sterile Machleder retractor after it is wrapped with Kerlix for padding (**FIGURE 6**).

- The approach for the treatment of aTOS is dependent on the potential need for subclavian artery reconstruction. A supraclavicular or combined supra and infraclavicular approach is used when arterial bypass is required, and the patient is positioned as above. When the subclavian artery is not damaged, but a cervical rib is identified, a transaxillary approach can be considered. When arterial reconstruction with a venous conduit is planned, preparations should be made for saphenous or femoral vein harvesting.

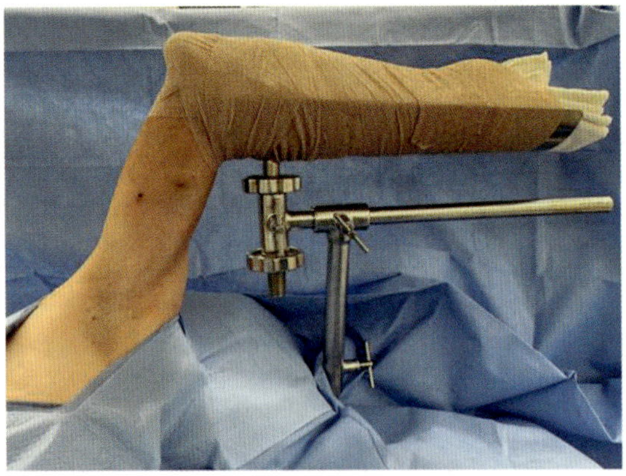

FIGURE 6 • Positioning of the arm in the Machleder retractor for transaxillary first rib resection.

VENOUS TOS

Infraclavicular Approach

- A 5-cm transverse incision is made one fingerbreadth below the clavicle, starting along the edge of the sternum extending laterally. The dissection is carried through the subcutaneous tissue and pectoralis fascia to expose the upper fibers of the pectoralis major muscle (**FIGURE 7**). Gentle spreading between muscle fibers in this region exposes the anteromedial quadrant of the axillary fat pad and allows easy palpation of the first rib. Handheld or self-retaining retractors can be placed to fully expose the most anterior portion of the first rib beneath a layer of axillary fat (**FIGURE 8**).
- Once the first rib is visualized, cautery is used to separate the inferior intercostal musculature from the rib. This dissection is carried superolateral along the C-curve of the rib (**FIGURE 9**). The lung pleura will be visualized immediately beneath the rib and care should be taken to not injure lung parenchyma. Along the inferior portion of the clavicle, the subclavius tendon is taken down with cautery to free up the anterior portion of the first rib from the overhanging clavicle. The costoclavicular ligament may also need to be taken down, as it can be a cause of venous compression.[14] Following along the superior aspect of the first rib, the anterior scalene fibers are also sharply taken down and further superior dissection takes place along the lateral edge of the first rib until palpation of the subclavian artery is noted. Often, moving the arm in a superior position facilitates more superior exposure of the first rib near the artery.

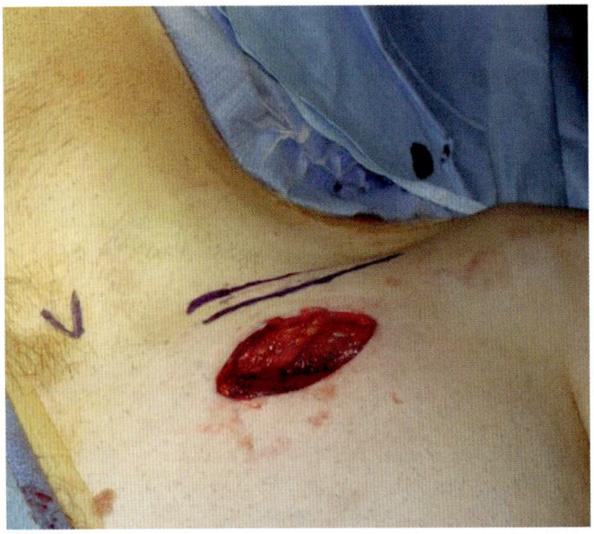

FIGURE 7 • Infraclavicular incision is made one fingerbreadth below clavicle.

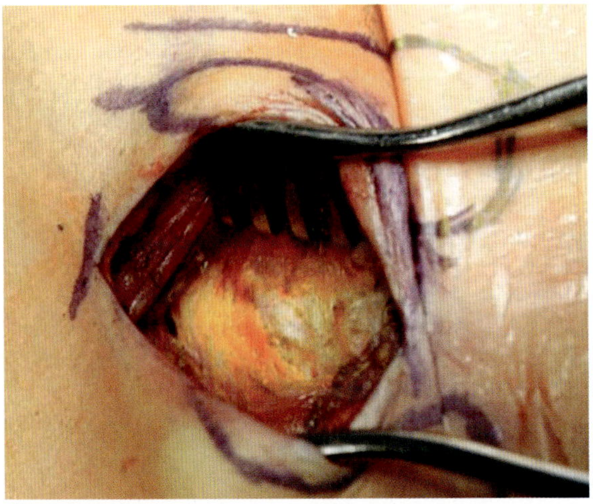

FIGURE 8 • Incision is carried down through pectoralis fascia, then the muscle fibers are split until axillary fat that covers the first rib is reached.

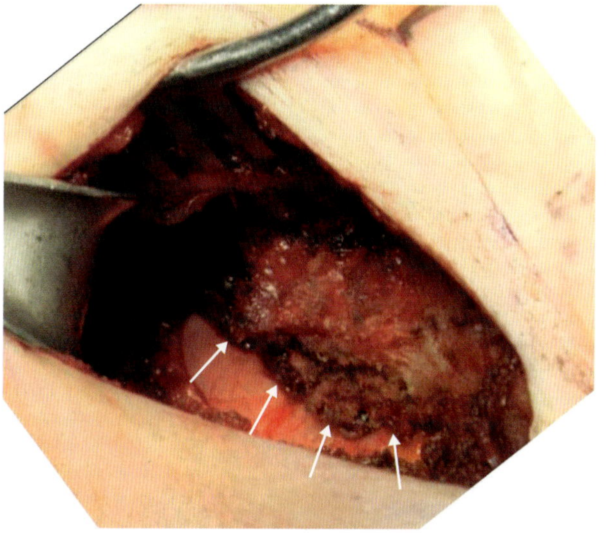

FIGURE 9 • Further dissection around the 1st rib involves sharp dissection of intercostal musculature along inferior aspect of first rib (*arrows*).

- When the rib is clear on its superior, lateral, and inferior edge, a rib cutter can be inserted superiorly, taking care to visualize the jaws, and then the superior cut is made in the rib. The inferior cut is done near the manubrial junction, commonly with a power saw. As the rib is pulled away from the body, sharp cautery can be used to facilitate hemostasis of individual muscle fibers (intercostals, anterior and middle scalene) holding the first rib in place.
- Care should be taken to ensure that no anterior rib remnants remain, as this increases the risk for recurrent venous symptoms. Posterior rib remnants can result in the development of neurogenic symptoms as a result of brachial plexus compression.[11] Following surgical decompression, as many as 20% of patients may experience persistent recurrent symptoms, most commonly the result of residual first rib remnant left behind during the index operation.[12]

Transaxillary Approach (**FIGURE 10**)

- The external landmarks are marked out on the skin, including the pectoralis major muscle and the latissimus dorsi muscle. A skin incision is created 2 fingerbreadths from the apex of the axilla just above the base of the hairline between the two muscles. The subcutaneous tissues are dissected down to the chest wall using a combination of blunt dissection and electrocautery. The arm is then elevated in the retractor (**FIGURE 10A** and **B**).
- Using a peanut on a long Pean clamp, the tissues are dissected following the subclavian vein down to the thoracic outlet. The subclavius muscle/tendon attachments that come down to the first rib, anterior scalene, and subclavian artery are dissected as well. With the vein protected, once the subclavius tendon is dissected it can be cut with scissors. Next, the anterior scalene muscle is incised by passing a right angle clamp posterior and cutting the muscle piece by piece until the entire muscle is cut (**FIGURE 10C**).
- A periosteal elevator is used to free the intercostal muscles along the lateral aspect of the first rib. A smaller elevator is then passed under the rib to dissect the pleura away from the rib, allowing the rib to be cut anteriorly. The middle scalene muscle fibers are then dissected off the rib with the elevator. Once the posterior rib is free of muscle, a Bethune rib cutter can be used to cut the posterior rib, with care taken to ensure the inferior trunk of the brachial plexus is protected (**FIGURE 10D**).
- The residual rib is removed with a first rib rongeur both anteriorly and posteriorly. Once the rib is removed completely, the pleura is tested for a tear by instilling saline in the wound and having a Valsalva maneuver performed by the anesthesia team. If a tear is present, a 19 French Blake drain can be placed under direct visualization.

Endovascular Venous Treatment/Venous Reconstruction

- With the rib removed from the infraclavicular approach, the vein is often palpable in a bed of tissue and muscle fibers immediately below the clavicle. Venolysis consists of freeing up these muscle fibers to expose the vein (**FIGURE 11**). More proximal exposure of the vein can be accomplished via a transmanubrial extension of the infraclavicular incision to the center of the sternum and vertically up to the sternal notch (**FIGURE 12**). This can be necessary to obtain adequate vascular control for patching of chronically diseased venous segments. When a strictured segment of vein is localized, saphenous vein or bovine pericardial patching provides an excellent strategy for the restoration of luminal diameter and can be performed with adequate proximal and distal control of the vein under direct visualization (**FIGURE 13**).
- If an intraoperative venogram is to be performed, the arm is placed on an arm board out to the side and ultrasound guidance is used to access the basilic vein following decompression. In the event the basilic vein is thrombosed, a brachial vein should be accessed. This provides direct access for treatment of the axillary and subclavian vein. Once a sheath is placed, venography is performed to identify the area of stenosis within the vein. The stenosis is crossed with a Glidewire using a Bern or KMP style catheter for support. A working wire is then positioned in the superior vena cava to allow for balloon angioplasty.

Closure

- Careful attention should be paid to the bone edge for hemostasis, as well as the region of the vein after venolysis and/or reconstruction.
- If the pleura or lung parenchyma has been injured, a round drain (19F Blake) can be placed in the pleural space under direct visualization.

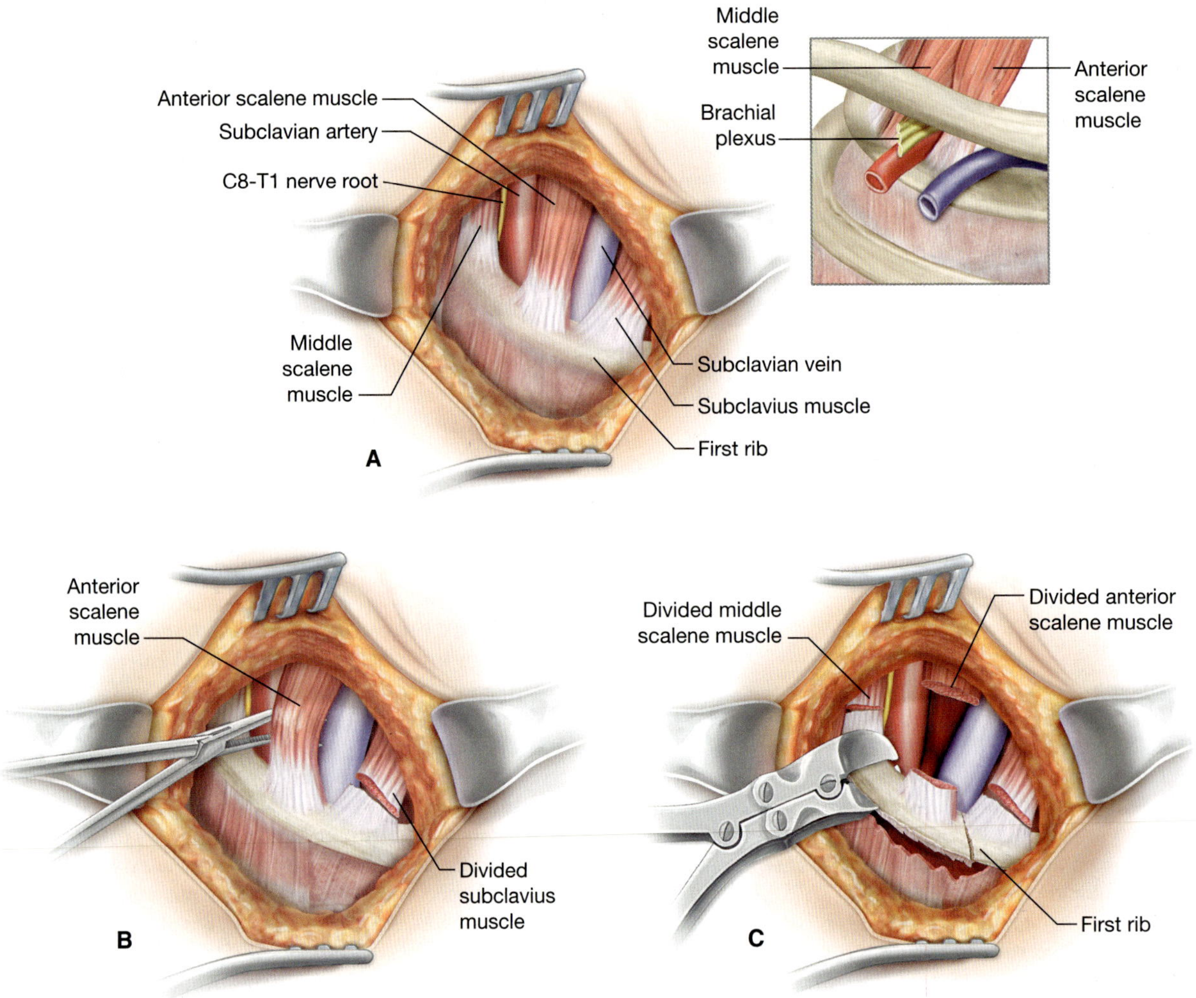

FIGURE 10 • **A,** Transaxillary view of the relationship of the subclavian artery and vein with the scalene muscles. **B,** The anterior scalene is transected using a right angle and Bovie cautery to free up the first rib. The subclavian artery and vein are identified and preserved. The brachial plexus nerve roots are seen laterally in this view directly behind the middle scalene muscle. **C,** A periosteal elevator is used to free the intercostal muscles along the lateral aspect of the first rib. A smaller elevator is then passed under the rib to dissect the pleura away from the rib, allowing the rib to be cut anteriorly. The middle scalene muscle fibers are then dissected off the rib with the elevator. Once the posterior rib is free of muscle, a Bethune rib cutter can be used to cut the posterior rib, with care taken to ensure the inferior trunk of the brachial plexus is protected.

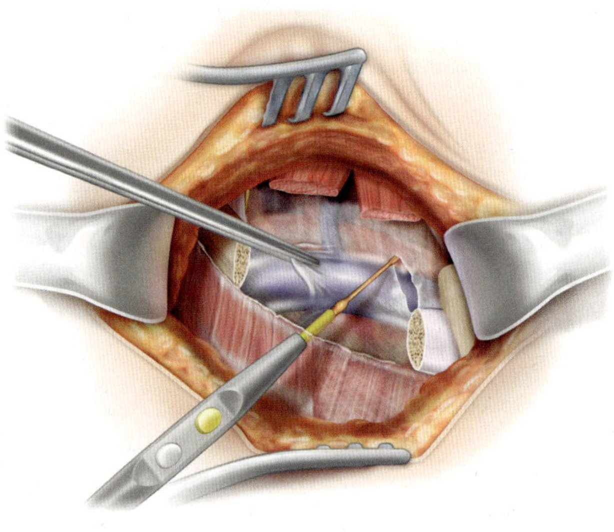

FIGURE 11 • After first rib is resected, careful dissection around vein with venolysis and takedown of fibers surrounding vein allows adequate visualization to check for stenotic regions.

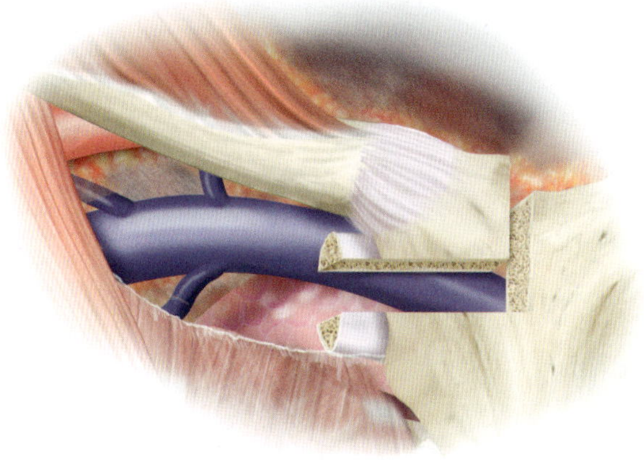

FIGURE 12 • If more proximal exposure is needed to clamp for control, extension of the incision into the manubrium and toward sternal notch allows wider visualization of the origin of subclavian vein and junction with jugular into the innominate.

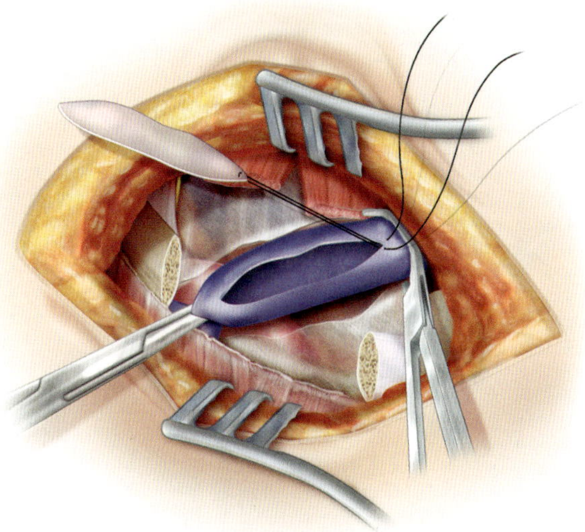

FIGURE 13 • Stenotic region of the subclavian vein repaired with patch venoplasty using greater saphenous vein.

ARTERIAL THORACIC OUTLET SYNDROME

Supraclavicular Approach

- A 7-cm incision is made one fingerbreadth above the clavicle, starting lateral to the palpable edge of the sternal head of the sternocleidomastoid muscle and carried through the platysma. This exposes the clavicular head of the sternocleidomastoid, which is transected with a cuff to sew back together later, exposing the anterior scalene fat pad (**FIGURE 14**). The fat pad is dissected along three borders, inferiorly, laterally, and medially, to allow it to swing northward to expose the anterior scalene muscle and the phrenic nerve (**FIGURE 15**). When operating on the left side, extra care is taken to visualize the thoracic duct when present, which is suture ligated to prevent a postoperative chyle leak if it becomes injured.
- With the phrenic nerve slung and protected, transection of the anterior scalene muscle off the superior edge of the first rib is accomplished with the use of electrocautery. Care is taken to stay on the bone during this portion so as not to injure the underlying subclavian artery. After the inferior

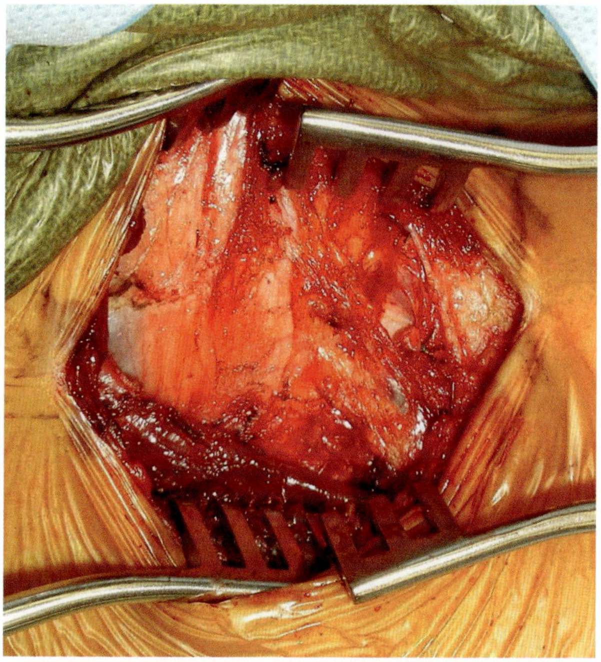

FIGURE 14 • Supraclavicular incision one fingerbreadth above the clavicle continues after transecting clavicular head of the sternocleidomastoid and exposure of the anterior scalene fat pad.

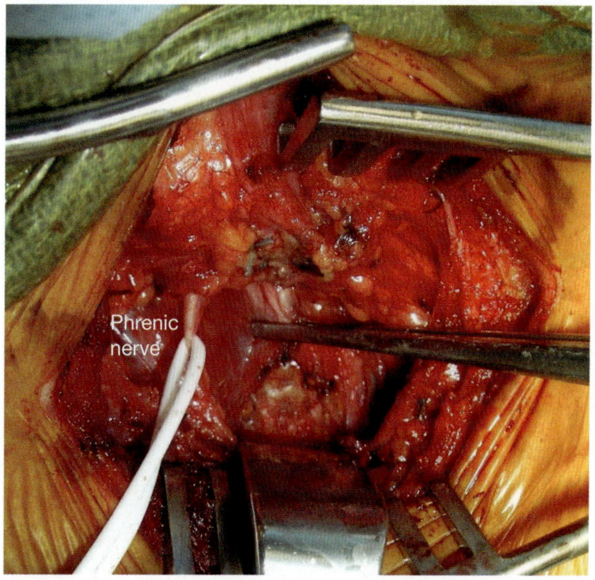

FIGURE 15 • With the scalene fat pad retracted superiorly, the anterior scalene muscle and phrenic nerve are clearly seen. The nerve is slung with a silastic loop.

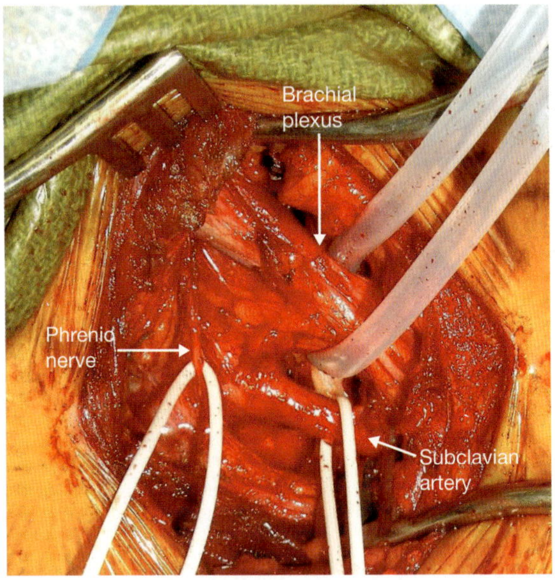

FIGURE 16 ● The first rib is cleared on both sides of the subclavian artery and the brachial plexus fibers, which are all slung to allow easy mobilization.

edge of the anterior scalene is removed, a portion of muscle can be transected to allow room for further visualization and subsequent dissection around the brachial plexus (**FIGURE 16**). The long thoracic nerve is identified laterally, and the brachial plexus structures are slung with a thick silastic loop.

- A cervical rib, when present, is often visualized at this time, with abnormal vasculature or musculature surrounding it, and can be fused to the first rib (**FIGURE 17**). Care is taken to dissect nerves and vessels away from the abnormal rib or its osseous portions that may not have been visualized on radiography.
- The first rib is visualized by maneuvering the subclavian artery and the nerve bundle back and forth while dissecting middle scalene fibers and intercostal musculature off the rib (**FIGURE 16**). This can be done sharply, with bipolar cautery, or by using a periosteal elevator. One should avoid the use of monopolar cautery in this area as it is likely to transmit to the brachial plexus or phrenic nerve.
- When the rib is clear from the region inferior to the subclavian artery and superior to the upper aspect of the brachial plexus, a power saw can be used to transect the rib. If there is a fused portion of the cervical rib, it should be removed as a single piece (**FIGURE 18**) to assure that all bony abnormalities have been freed up to allow for adequate decompression.
- The pleura is inspected to ensure there is no injury. If an injury is present, any air should be evacuated with a red rubber catheter underwater while the fat pad is replaced over the outlet. A small 7 flat Jackson Pratt drain can then be placed.

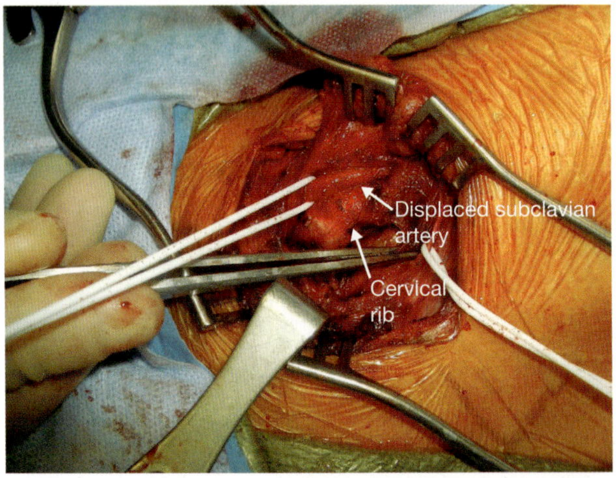

FIGURE 17 ● In this case, a fused cervical rib to the first rib is prominently tenting up the subclavian artery and brachial plexus fibers.

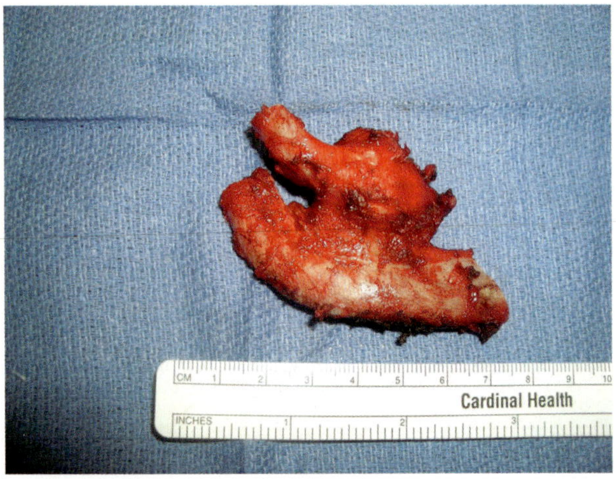

FIGURE 18 ● Removal of the congenitally fused cervical rib to the first rib as an en bloc piece, allowing the neurovascular bundle to return to its normal position without being kinked or displaced.

Arterial Reconstruction

- Subclavian aneurysm resection, when needed, consists of appropriate bypass principles and replacement with an autogenous or prosthetic interposition graft or extra-anatomic bypass of carotid to distal subclavian or carotid to axillary graft. Typical sizes and types required for prosthetic grafts include 6- or 8-mm ringed polytetrafluoroethylene (PTFE) or Dacron.

PEARLS AND PITFALLS

Indications	▪ vTOS definitive therapy consists of prompt diagnosis, venography with thrombolysis, and appropriate selection of patients to undergo thoracic outlet decompression. ▪ aTOS patients often present with ischemic hand symptoms that will have some delay in management due to a wide differential. Efforts should be directed toward decreasing long-term sequelae by limiting ischemic time. Abnormal bony or muscular anatomy along with the presence of subclavian aneurysmal disease requires definitive repair including thoracic outlet decompression and arterial reconstruction.
Preoperative workup	▪ Venography and pharmacomechanical thrombolysis provide the optimal reduction of clot burden to restore functional venous patency in patients with vTOS. Timing of rib resection and definitive thoracic outlet decompression are somewhat variable, and the approach should be individualized. ▪ aTOS patients should undergo plain radiography to search for a cervical rib and CTA to determine the portions of the diseased subclavian artery that might require reconstruction.
Patient setup	▪ Prepping the affected arm in the vTOS patients affords the ability to move the arm and, from the infraclavicular approach, gain access to the rib that is responsible for venous compression. ▪ For cervical rib resection and arterial revascularization, the supraclavicular approach gives numerous options for reconstructive purposes as well as the possibility of the carotid artery as an inflow source for bypass.
Infraclavicular approach	▪ Visualization of the subclavius tendon and its fibers, as well as the costoclavicular ligament, is paramount in decompressing the region that compresses the subclavian vein in vTOS. ▪ Liberal patching of the subclavian vein and extensive venolysis provide the best long-term patency results after vTOS decompression.
Supraclavicular approach	▪ Carefully mobilizing the anterior scalene fat pad allows good visualization of the anterior scalene muscle and phrenic nerve. ▪ When performing left-sided supraclavicular TOS decompression, one must be careful to identify and ligate the thoracic duct to prevent a postoperative chyle leak. ▪ Slinging the subclavian artery and brachial plexus fibers allows gentle traction back and forth to expeditiously dissect free the entire first rib.
Transaxillary Approach	▪ When using a transaxillary approach, the phrenic nerve course is typically separate from the anterior scalene muscle above the level of the operative field. However, if it isn't separate, it may be injured when transecting the muscle. ▪ If the inferior trunk of the brachial plexus is adherent to the first rib, this can result in injury to the nerve during resection.

POSTOPERATIVE CARE

- At the conclusion of the procedure, patients are extubated. If there was no evidence of pleural tear by Valsalva at the time of surgery, a chest x-ray is not needed. For patients with a chest drain due to pleural injury, a chest x-ray is obtained. If a chest drain was placed for a pleural injury, it can be connected to a Pleur-evac. At 12 hours, we typically convert this to water seal unless an air leak is identified. The drain is removed on postoperative day 1.
- Patients do not need a sling for their arms. They are given range-of-motion exercises immediately to encourage strengthening and lessen compressive scar tissue formation. Patients with a transaxillary or infraclavicular incision can safely be discharged on postoperative day 1. Most patients will require a taper of muscle relaxant and opioid narcotics for pain control. Patients with a supraclavicular or paraclavicular incision should have their drains removed once it is clear that there is no evidence of a thoracic duct leak and can typically be discharged on postoperative day 2.
- Anticoagulation for vTOS patients is usually resumed 2 to 3 days postoperatively at home. If patients are to return for postoperative venography and venoplasty, there is no need to hold anticoagulation for this procedure.[15]
- Anticoagulation is not always needed for aTOS patients, especially if arterial reconstruction is performed. If the patient initially presented with arterial ischemia, it may be reasonable to continue the patient on anticoagulation. If the patient did not present with ischemia, but a reconstruction was performed, appropriate antiplatelet therapy should be initiated postoperatively.

OUTCOMES

- Patients treated for vTOS with lysis and subsequent thoracic outlet decompression have a very low recurrence rate of thromboembolic disease. Morbidity and mortality are minimal, as these are often young and healthy patients, but typically include wound issues and bleeding given the need for anticoagulation. Satisfactory quality of life scores and return to full function are reported in the 80% to 90% range, and most patients can be counseled to expect a near full return to sports.[16]
- aTOS and the cervical rib patients often have the most dramatic recovery, as they are often the most symptomatic at presentation. Results are uniformly positive with the resolution of ischemic hand symptoms and lack of significant disease recurrence.

COMPLICATIONS

- The most common perioperative complications related to both forms of thoracic outlet decompression revolve around lung injury and wound issues. Pneumothoraces are often self-limited and treated effectively with chest tubes. Wound complications can include chyle leaks, seromas, and skin breakdown. Most of these are managed expectantly.
- Brachial plexus injuries may also occur. These injuries are most commonly a function of not recognizing important anatomic structures or not providing sufficient exposure to eliminate collateral damage during rib transection and removal. Finally, scar tissue or first rib remnants can contribute to the development of persistent vTOS symptoms or the onset of new neurogenic TOS symptoms in up to a fifth of patients.
- Timing of restarting anticoagulation in vTOS patients can lead to postoperative bleeding, which can manifest as delayed hemothorax. The cause of this bleeding is often related to recent thrombolysis and raw surfaces of muscle and cut bone, and this has led to the general recommendation of holding anticoagulation until 2 to 3 days following surgery.

CONCLUSION

Though accounting for approximately 1% and 5% of all TOS cases, respectively, arterial and venous TOS can be effectively managed with minimal long-term morbidity and mortality.[15] In conjunction with a thorough history and physical exam, noninvasive imaging typically provides sufficient evidence to confirm the diagnosis in symptomatic patients, successfully ruling out more common diagnoses on the differential. More severe forms of vTOS and symptomatic aTOS should be evaluated for surgical decompression with lysis or vessel reconstruction to prevent long-term morbidity. Multiple approaches can be used to facilitate decompression of the thoracic outlet and revascularization of the extremity, with the optimal approach for each patient ultimately determined by preoperative imaging. Vascular surgeons remain the optimal caretaker of this unique population, with the knowledge and skill set to manage these patients most effectively. Comprehensive care centers are best situated to provide all-encompassing care both before and after surgery, along with safe and complete decompression of the thoracic outlet when surgery is indicated.

REFERENCES

1. Illig KA, Rodriguez-Zoppi E, Bland T, Muftah M, Jospitre E. The incidence of thoracic outlet syndrome. *Ann Vasc Surg*. 2021;70:263-272. doi:10.1016/j.avsg.2020.07.029
2. Sanders RJ, Pearce WH. The treatment of thoracic outlet syndrome: a comparison of different operations. *J Vasc Surg*. 1989;10(6):626-634. doi:10.1016/0741-5214(89)90005-0
3. Davidoviovi:626-634. doi:10.1016/0741-5214(89)9IB. Arterial complications of thoracic outlet syndrome. *Am Surg*. 2009;75(3):235-239.
4. Cassada DC, Lipscomb AL, Stevens SL, Freeman MB, Grandas OH, Goldman MH. The importance of thrombophilia in the treatment of Paget-Schroetter syndrome. *Ann Vasc Surg*. 2006;20(5):596-601. doi:10.1007/s10016-006-9106-z
5. Likes K, Rochlin D, Nazarian SM, Streiff MB, Freischlag JA. Females with subclavian vein thrombosis may have an increased risk of hypercoagulability. *JAMA Surg*. 2013;148(1):44-49. doi:10.1001/jamasurgery.2013.406
6. Illig KA, Doyle AJ. A comprehensive review of Paget-Schroetter syndrome. *J Vasc Surg*. 2010;51(6):1538-1547. doi:10.1016/j.jvs.2009.12.022
7. Guzzo JL, Chang K, Demos J, Black JH, Freischlag JA. Preoperative thrombolysis and venoplasty affords no benefit in patency following first rib resection and scalenectomy for subacute and chronic subclavian vein thrombosis. *J Vasc Surg*. 2010;52(3):658-662; discussion 662-663. doi:10.1016/j.jvs.2010.04.050
8. Lee JT, Dua MM, Chandra V, Hernandez-Boussard TM, Illig KA. RR18. Surgery for thoracic outlet syndrome: a nationwide perspective. *J Vasc Surg*. 2011;53(6):100S-101S. doi:10.1016/j.jvs.2011.03.195
9. Illig KA, Donahue D, Duncan A, et al. Reporting standards of the Society for Vascular Surgery for thoracic outlet syndrome. *J Vasc Surg*. 2016;64(3):e23-e35. doi:10.1016/j.jvs.2016.04.039
10. Goss SG, Alcantara SD, Todd GJ, Lantis JC. Non-operative management of paget-Schroetter syndrome: a single-center experience. *J Invasive Cardiol*. 2015;27(9):423-428.
11. Lee JT, Karwowski JK, Harris EJ, Haukoos JS, Olcott C. Long-term thrombotic recurrence after nonoperative management of Paget-Schroetter syndrome. *J Vasc Surg*. 2006;43(6):1236-1243. doi:10.1016/j.jvs.2006.02.005
12. Molina JE, Hunter DW, Dietz CA. Paget-Schroetter syndrome treated with thrombolytics and immediate surgery. *J Vasc Surg*. 2007;45(2):328-334. doi:10.1016/j.jvs.2006.09.052
13. Vedovati MC, Tratar G, Mavri A, Pierpaoli L, Agnelli G, Becattini C. Upper extremities deep vein thrombosis and DOAC treatment: a prospective cohort study. *Eur Heart J*. 2020;41(suppl 2). doi:10.1093/ehjci/ehaa946.2407
14. Gu G, Liu J, Lv Y, et al. Costoclavicular ligament as a novel cause of venous thoracic outlet syndrome: from anatomic study to clinical application. *Surg Radiol Anat*. 2020;42(8):865-870. doi:10.1007/s00276-020-02479-7
15. Ann Freischlag JA. Decade OF excellent outcomes after surgical intervention: 538 patients with thoracic outlet syndrome. *Trans Am Clin Climatol Assoc*. 2018;129:88-94.
16. Chandra V, Little C, Lee JT. Thoracic outlet syndrome in high-performance athletes. *J Vasc Surg*. 2014;60(4):1012-1017; discussion 1017-1018. doi:10.1016/j.jvs.2014.04.013

SECTION III: Thoracic and Suprarenal Aortic Exposure and Treatment

Chapter 11

Exposure and Open Surgical Reconstruction in the Chest: The Thoracoabdominal Aorta

Enrico Rinaldi, Diletta Loschi, and Germano Melissano

DEFINITION

- A thoracoabdominal aortic aneurysm (TAAA) involves the aorta at the diaphragmatic crura and extends variable distances proximally and/or distally from this point (**FIGURE 1**).[1] TAAAs can be classified in terms of their causes, the two most common being medial degeneration and dissection.
- Open treatment of TAAAs consists of graft replacement with reattachment of the main aortic branches: The inclusion technique was introduced by S. E. Crawford in the 1970s and refined by subsequent surgeons in the following decades. TAAA repair, especially in extensive aortic disease, is associated with greater operative risk than repair of other aortic segments. The main sources of morbidity are spinal cord (SC) ischemia and renal as well as respiratory and cardiac complications.
- Experienced surgical centers now report lower mortality and morbidity rates for TAAA repair,[2] largely due to multimodal approaches to reduce surgical trauma and maximize organ protection.[3]

IMAGING AND OTHER DIAGNOSTIC STUDIES

- To plan the best possible treatment strategy for each patient, the preferred modality is computed tomographic arteriography. The acquisition of computed tomography (CT) data has benefited from spectacular progress, including multirow detectors, higher rotation and translation speeds with reduced scan times (single breath-hold), cardiac cycle synchronization, and better postprocessing capabilities.
- Digital Imaging and Communications in Medicine (DICOM) slices of adequate thickness (≤1 mm) should be postprocessed on a digital workstation using a multiplanar reformatting tool to visualize a scan in which angulation matches that of the aorta or the vessel under investigation (**FIGURE 2**).
- Beyond analysis of aortic diameter and the extent of pathologic involvement, reformatted images are particularly useful for evaluating the presence, extension, and characteristics of dissection and thrombus, particularly at proposed

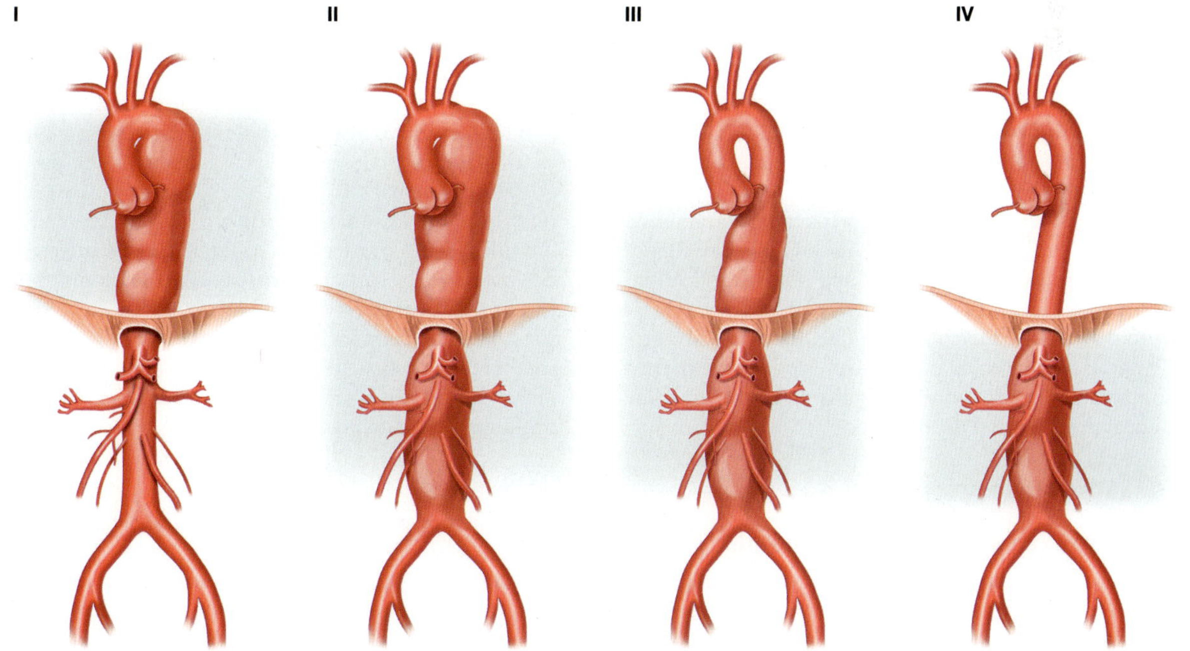

FIGURE 1 • An aneurysm is defined as thoracoabdominal when the highlighted region is involved. Crawford classification was developed to improve stratification of perioperative paraplegia risk. Subclassifications include the following: Extent I includes the thoracic and abdominal aorta, from the left subclavian artery to the level of the renal arteries; Extent II includes the entire descending aorta from the level of the left subclavian artery to the aortic bifurcation; Extent III includes aorta beginning at the T6 level extending to the bifurcation or lower; Extent IV includes the entire abdominal aorta starting at the level of the diaphragm (T12) to the aortic bifurcation or lower.

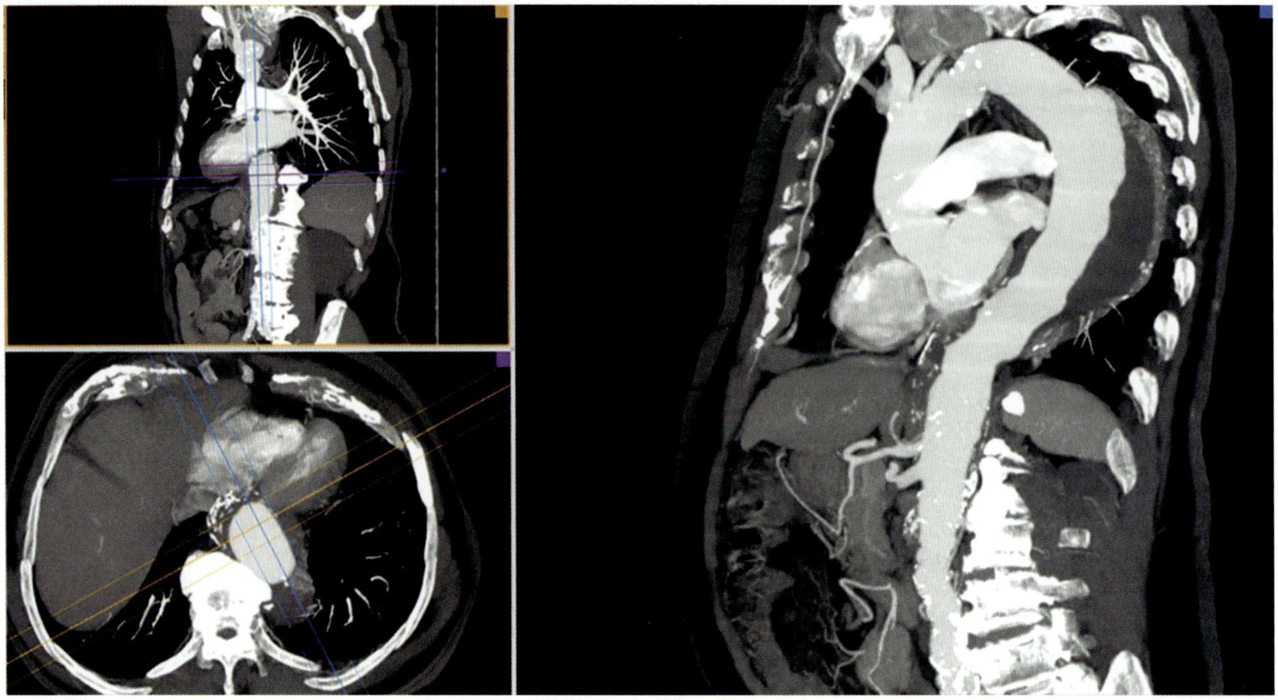

FIGURE 2 • Multiplanar reformatting tools allow the sagittal reconstruction to properly follow the major axis of the thoracic aorta. In this reformatted image, the entire thoracoabdominal aorta is included despite significant tortuosity.

sites of clamp placement and the infradiaphragmatic aorta when direct aneurysm cannulation is considered for distal aortic perfusion. The exact location and geometry of aortic branches is obtained to reveal possible anatomic variations or anomalies, which are particularly common at the level of the renal arteries and arch vessels. Vessel patency is also routinely evaluated; in particular, obstruction of the superior and inferior mesenteric artery and the hypogastric arteries and dominance of one vertebral artery are assessed.

- Three-dimensional rendering tools produce realistic imaging of the anatomic structures that expand anatomic understanding including, for instance, the most appropriate intercostal space to perform thoracotomy (**FIGURE 3**).
- Perioperative SC ischemia may precipitate paraparesis or paraplegia. Prior knowledge of the SC arterial supply informs both procedural planning and risk stratification. During the last 2 decades a progressively increasing experience with noninvasive imaging techniques has allowed a better identification of preoperative patient-specific risk criteria for SC perfusion impairments, giving the possibility to tailor the surgical procedure[4] (**FIGURE 4**).

SURGICAL MANAGEMENT

Preoperative Workup and Patient Optimization

- Preoperative transthoracic echocardiography is a satisfactory noninvasive screening method to evaluate both valvular and biventricular function. Stress testing identifies patients who require coronary catheterization and possible intervention.[5] Electrocardiographically (EKG) gated CT has emerged as a less invasive method of visualizing coronary anatomy. For severe, symptomatic coronary disease requiring percutaneous transluminal angioplasty prior to aneurysm repair, use of drug-eluting stents requiring prolonged double antiplatelet therapy should be avoided to reduce subsequent perioperative bleeding.
- The use of estimated glomerular filtration rate (eGFR), rather than serum creatinine levels alone, is recommended to assess renal function.[6] Based on the eGFR metric, chronic kidney disease (CKD) has been shown to be a strong predictor of death following open or endovascular thoracic aneurysm repair, even in patients without other clinical evidence of preoperative renal disease.[7]
- Pulmonary function evaluation with arterial blood gases and spirometry is used to evaluate the respiratory reserve of all patients undergoing open surgery of the descending aorta. In patients with a forced expiratory volume in 1 second (FEV_1) of less than 1 L and a partial pressure of carbon dioxide (PCO_2) greater than 45 mm Hg, operative risk may be improved by cessation of cigarette smoking, treatment of chronic bronchitis (if present), weight loss, and participation in a supervised exercise program for a period of up to 6 months prior to surgery. However, in patients with aneurysm-related symptoms, this type of respiratory rehabilitation may not be practical or possible.

POSITIONING

- After inserting a cerebrospinal fluid drainage (CSFD)[8] catheter into the subarachnoid space between L2 and L3 or L3 and L4 (**FIGURE 5**), the patient is turned to a right lateral decubitus position, with the shoulders at 60° and the hips flexed back to 30°.
- Preparation should allow for access to the entire left thorax, abdomen, and both inguinal regions. Patient position is maintained with a moldable beanbag attached to a suction line for vacuum creation. A circulating water mattress is placed between the beanbag and the patient in order to modify body temperature as necessary.

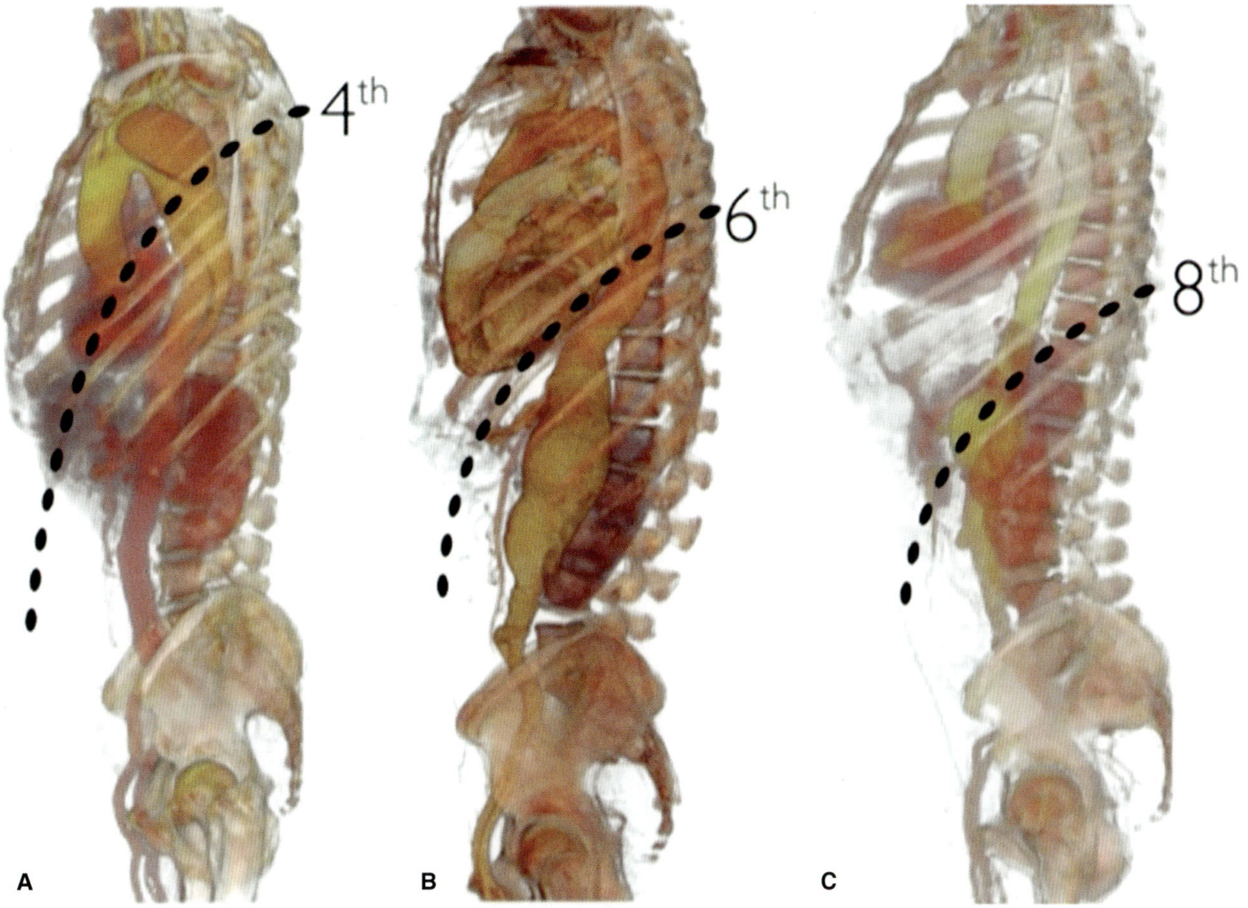

FIGURE 3 • Beyond aortic imaging, computed tomography provides extensive anatomic information to guide exposure and surgical decision making. In case of Extent I thoracoabdominal aortic aneurysm (TAAA) **(A)**, a surgical access through the 4th intercostal space may be performed while an incision in the 6th intercostal space could be done in case of Extent III TAAA **(B)**. For an Extent IV TAAA **(C)**, a lower access through the 8th intercostal space is generally performed.

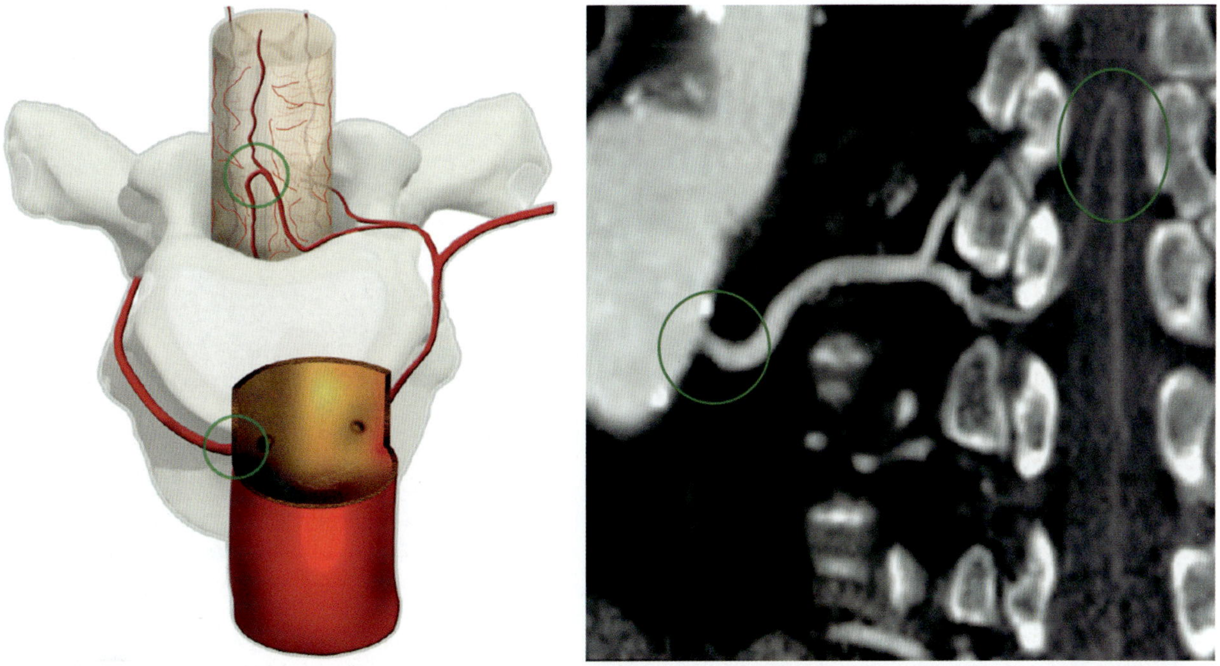

FIGURE 4 • With preoperative computed tomography, using postprocessing tools, the whole path of the arterial feeder to the spinal cord (arteria radicularis magna) can be visualized, from the aorta to the anterior spinal artery.

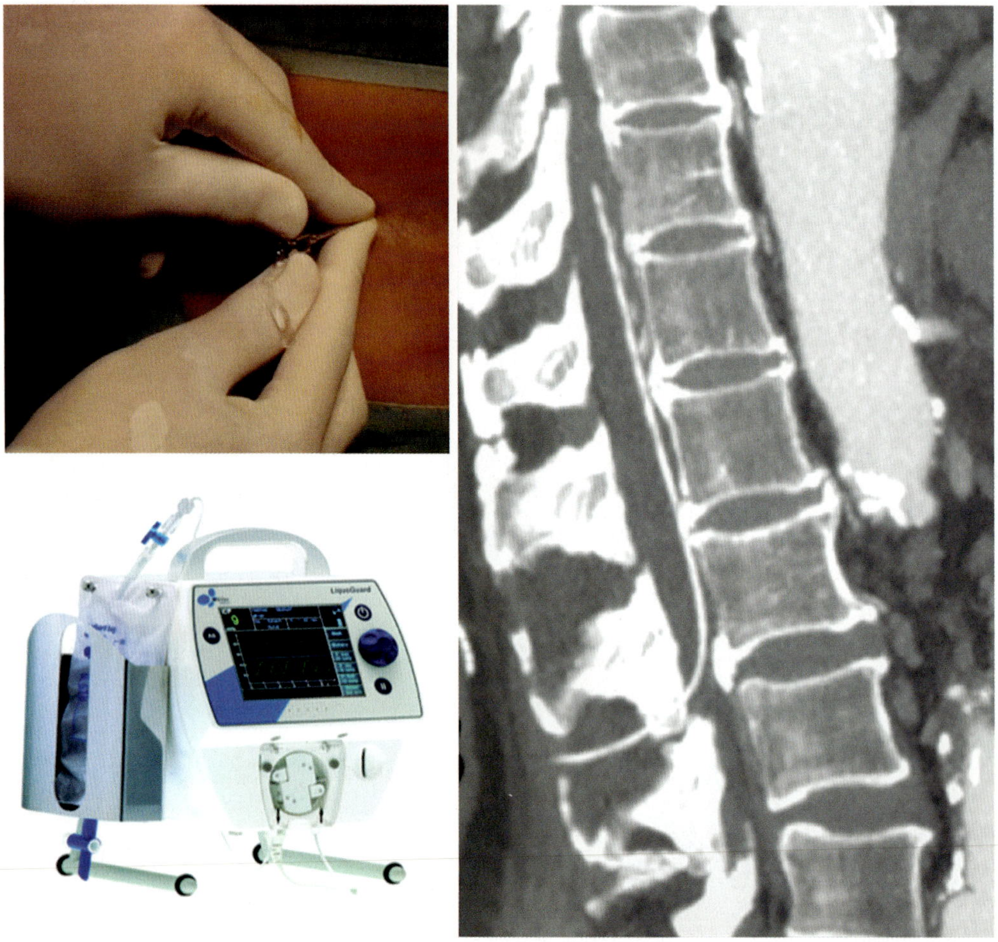

FIGURE 5 • Once the dura has been punctured with the introducer needle, a drainage catheter is inserted 8 to 10 cm along the intradural space. The catheter is then connected to a pressure transducer, and the fluid is drained to keep the pressure below 10 cm H_2O. Automated systems are available for this purpose.

THORACOPHRENOLAPAROTOMY

- The thoracic incision varies in length and level, depending on exposure requirements. Usually, the 5th, 6th, or 7th intercostal space is employed according to the aneurysm anatomy. The posterior section of the ribs is gently spread to reduce thoracic wall trauma and fractures; anterolaterally, the incision curves gently as it crosses the costal margin to minimize subsequent tissue necrosis (**FIGURE 6**). The pleural space is entered after single right lung ventilation is initiated. Monopulmonary ventilation is maintained throughout thoracic aorta replacement.
- Thoracotomy incisions are painful and can lead to postoperative complications, such as pulmonary atelectasis and infections. Successful postoperative pain management allows early patient mobilization and may contribute to shorter hospital length of stay. Common analgesic methods include opioid pain medications and epidural catheters. Side effects of opioid use, including respiratory, central nervous system, and bowel function depression, are not uncommon.[9] In order to reduce the postoperative pain in patients undergoing TAAA open repair, electromyography-guided cryoablation of intercostal nerves has been introduced in some high volume centers. Cryoanalgesia induces a Wallerian degeneration of the axons within the intercostal nerve,[10,11] and its benefits in terms of postoperative pain relief after thoracotomies performed for general thoracic procedures are reported in the literature.[12-15] CryoICE (AtriCure, Inc, Mason, OH) is a nitrous oxide cryoablation probe originally indicated for cryoablation of the heart for arrhythmias and was approved for

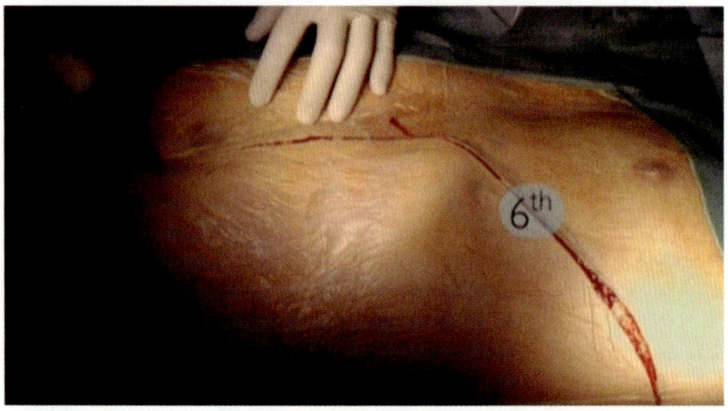

FIGURE 6 • Prepping and draping for thoracoabdominal aortic aneurysm. Posterolateral aspects of the left thorax, abdomen, and left groin are included in the sterile operatory field. Thoracophrenolaparotomy in the 6th intercostal space, please note the gentle curvature of the line indicating the skin incision to avoid flap necrosis.

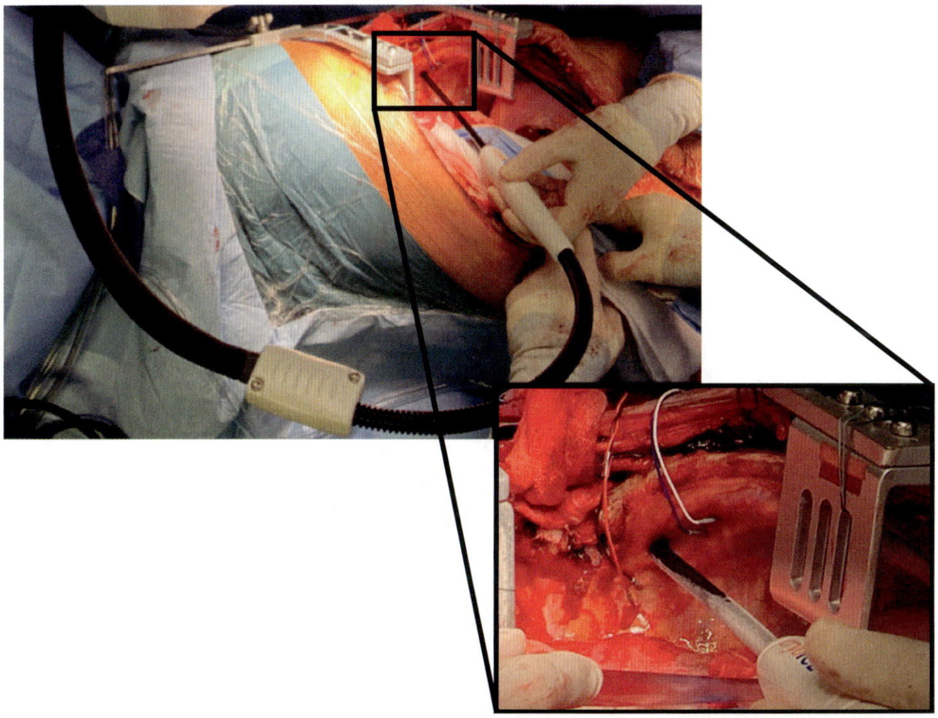

FIGURE 7 ● CryoICE is a nitrous oxide cryoablation probe used to induce a Wallerian degeneration of the axons within the intercostal nerve in order to reduce thoracic postoperative pain. Cryoablation may be performed under electromyography-guidance in order to assess the effective ablation.

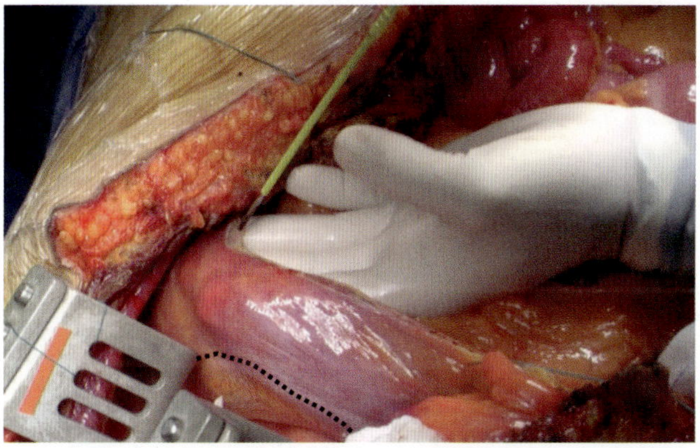

FIGURE 8 ● The diaphragm is circumferentially divided, for several centimeters near its peripheral attachment to the anterior chest wall sparing the phrenic center (dotted line).

intercostal nerve cryoanalgesia by the US Food and Drug Administration in 2015. Two recent studies reviewed the operative technique and the intraoperative and postoperative outcomes in patients undergoing TAA and TAAA repairs with and without cryoanalgesia to evaluate its efficacy and feasibility.[16,17] In both studies, opioid use was significantly reduced in the cryoanalgesia group; incidence of other major postoperative complications was similar in both groups. This procedure required additional 20 to 25 minutes, but it did not increase postoperative complications.[16,17] Prospective investigations and long-term follow-up are needed in order to understand the efficacy of this technique (**FIGURE 7**).

- Paralysis of the left hemidiaphragm contributes to postoperative respiratory failure; therefore, a limited circumferential rather than radial section of the diaphragm is routinely performed, sparing the phrenic center. Under favorable anatomic conditions, this approach reduces respiratory weaning time[18] (**FIGURE 8**).

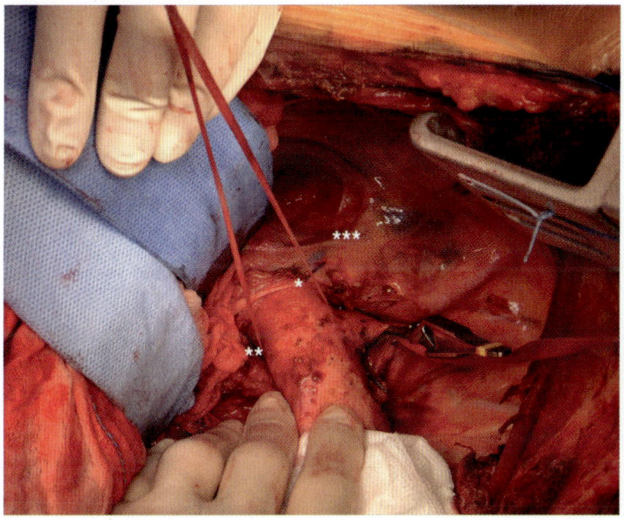

FIGURE 9 ● The vagus nerve (*) and the origin of the recurrent laryngeal nerve (**) are mobilized and identified to prevent injury during aortic clamping maneuvers or suture placement. The phrenic nerve is also identified (***). In this case, an aortic cross-clamping between left carotid and subclavian artery is required, so prior selective clamping of the left subclavian artery is performed before arch manipulation to prevent possible embolization.

- Special care must be taken when isolating the proximal aneurysm neck. The insertion of a large caliber esophageal probe makes it easier to distinguish the esophagus at this level. The vagus nerve and the origin of the recurrent laryngeal nerve must also be identified because they can also be damaged during isolation and clamping maneuvers (**FIGURE 9**). Identification and clipping of some "high" intercostal arteries can sometimes facilitate the preparation for the proximal anastomosis, thus reducing aortic bleeding (**FIGURE 10**).

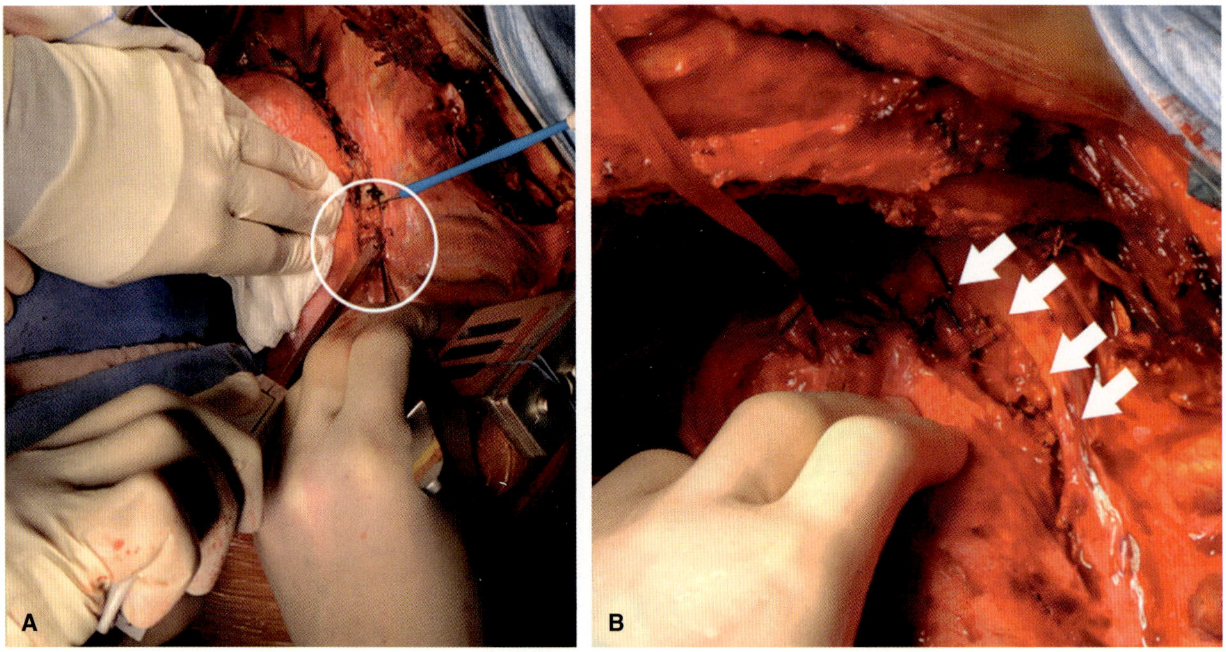

FIGURE 10 ● "High" noncritical intercostal arteries are identified during thoracic aortic exposure. These arteries are selectively clipped **(A)** in order to prevent back bleeding after the aortotomy. **B,** In this patient, four intercostal arteries were clipped at proximal thoracic aortic level.

- The upper abdominal aortic segment is exposed via a transperitoneal approach; after entering the peritoneum, medial visceral rotation is performed to retract the left colon, spleen, and left kidney anteriorly and to the right (**FIGURE 11**). Use of a transperitoneal approach allows direct assessment of the abdominal organs at the end of procedure. Extra care must be taken to avoid damage to the spleen, which is particularly prone to bleeding after capsular injuries regardless of size.

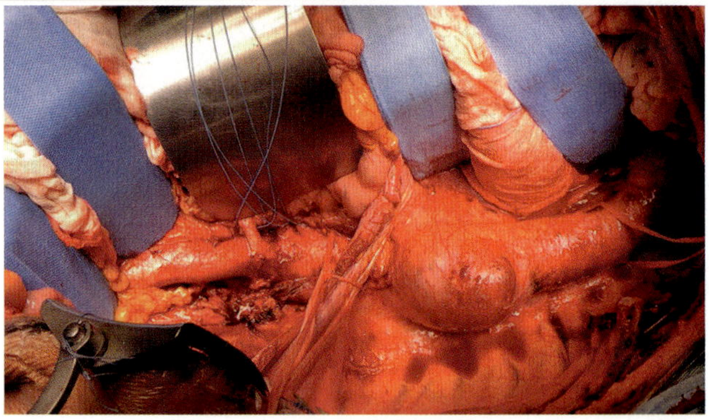

FIGURE 11 ● After thoracic aortic exposure, the abdominal aorta is also exposed throughout medial visceral rotation. With this approach, the origins of celiac trunk, superior mesenteric artery, and also left renal artery are identified and exposed.

DISTAL AORTIC PERFUSION

- Cross-clamping of the descending thoracic aorta produces immediate and significant increases in left ventricular afterload, myocardial oxygen consumption, and visceral and renal ischemia. Techniques incorporating distal aortic perfusion with left heart bypass (LHBP) have significantly improved outcomes in thoracic aortic surgery.[19] In preparation for LHBP and aortic cross-clamping, low-dose intravenous heparin is administered. If cessation of pump support is anticipated during the case, additional heparin should be administered at that time to provide full anticoagulation.
- The upper left pulmonary vein is usually cannulated for inflow of oxygenated blood, which is routed through a centrifugal pump (Bio-Medicus) into the left femoral artery. A "Y" connector included in the circuit provides two occlusion/perfusion catheters (9-Fr) for selective visceral perfusion when needed (**FIGURE 12**).

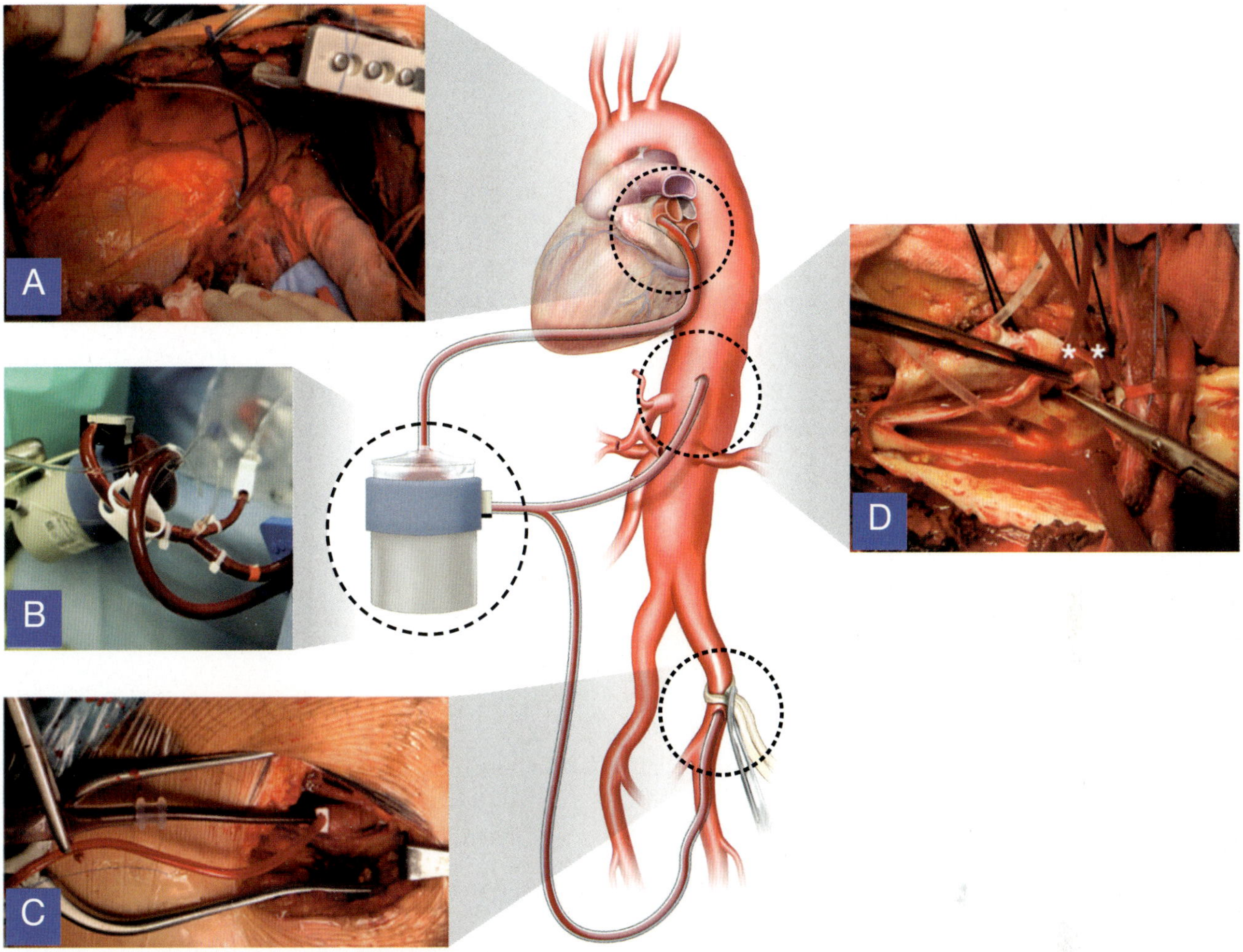

FIGURE 12 • Schematic view of Left Heart Bypass (LHBP). A 20-Fr cannula is inserted in left superior pulmonary vein for the arterial blood drainage **(A)**. Through a centrifugal pump (Bio-Medicus) **(B)**, the oxygenated blood is routed into the left femoral artery for synchronous proximal and distal perfusion using a nonocclusive femoral cannula (14-18-Fr) **(C)**. **D,** A "Y" connector provides two occlusion/perfusion catheters (9-Fr) for selective visceral perfusion with blood (*).

AORTIC REPAIR

- Once the neck of the TAAA is isolated and controlled between clamps, the descending thoracic aorta is transected and separated from the esophagus (**FIGURE 13**). The graft is sutured proximally to the descending thoracic aorta using 2-0 polypropylene suture in a running fashion. The anastomosis is reinforced with Teflon felt (individual pledgets or single strip) (**FIGURE 14**). An additional aortic clamp is applied onto the abdominal aorta above the celiac axis before the proximal aortic clamp is removed (sequential cross-clamping).
- Intercostal artery reimplantation into the aortic graft plays a critical role in SC protection. Patent intercostal arteries from T7 to L2 are temporarily occluded to prevent back-bleeding/maximize cord perfusion pressure[20] and then selectively reattached to the graft by means of aortic patch or graft interposition (**FIGURE 15**). When ready, the distal clamp is moved below the renal arteries and the aneurysm is opened across the diaphragm. The centrifugal pump maintains visceral perfusion (400 mL per minute) following insertion of the 9-Fr irrigation-perfusion catheters (LeMaitre Vascular) into the celiac trunk and the superior mesenteric artery. Cold perfusion of Custodiol[21] (histidine-tryptophane-ketoglutarate) is directed into the renal arteries (**FIGURE 16**). For visceral artery reimplantation, a fenestration is created in the graft and the visceral vessels are reattached as a single patch. Usually, the left renal artery is reconnected with an 8-mm polyester interposition graft. If creation of the visceral patch requires retaining a large segment of native aorta, we prefer to place a multibranched graft instead. This prosthesis, although somewhat more time-consuming, significantly reduces the risk of recurrent aortic patch aneurysm (**FIGURES 17** and **18**). Finally, the distal end-to-end anastomosis with the distal aorta is performed, the graft flushed, and clamps removed.

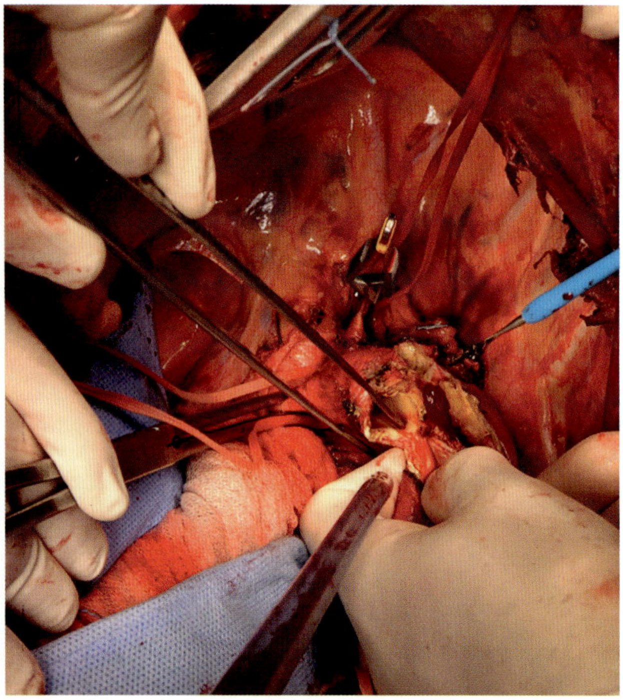

FIGURE 13 • The proximal descending thoracic aorta is controlled and completely transected to avoid accidental injury to the adjacent esophagus.

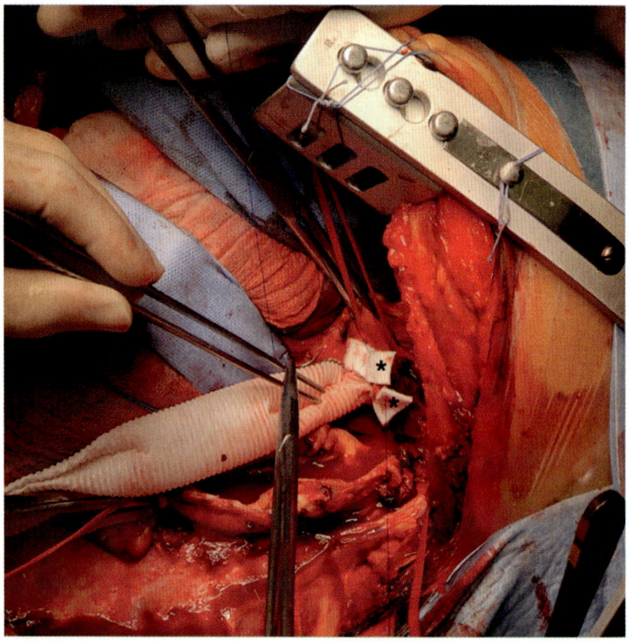

FIGURE 14 • The proximal anastomosis is routinely reinforced with a Teflon strip (*).

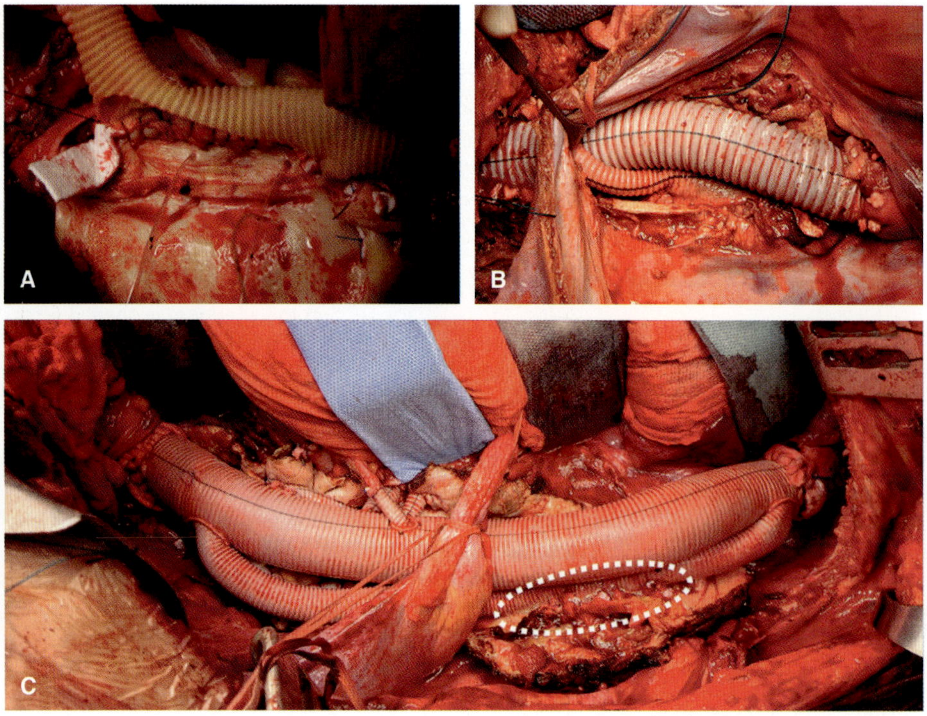

FIGURE 15 • Critical intercostal arteries reattachment. Here visualized are three different techniques: **(A)** an aortic island including the origin of several intercostal arteries is reattached to a fenestration created on the aortic graft; **(B)** intercostal arteries are reattached selectively to the graft via 6/8-mm interposition grafts. **C,** Another possible way to reattach critical intercostal arteries is represented by the "loop graft." A 14/16-mm is anastomosed proximally and distally to the aortic graft. A fenestration is created in this loop graft to reattach the origin of multiple intercostal arteries (*dotted circle*).

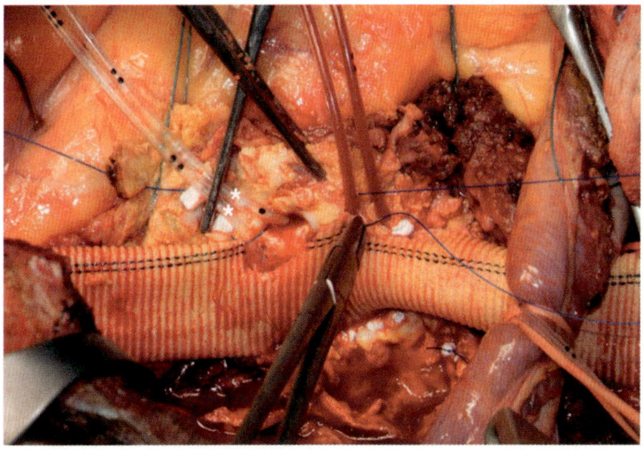

FIGURE 16 • Visceral arteries perfusion with blood, renal perfusion with cold Custodiol solution (*) during branch artery reattachment.

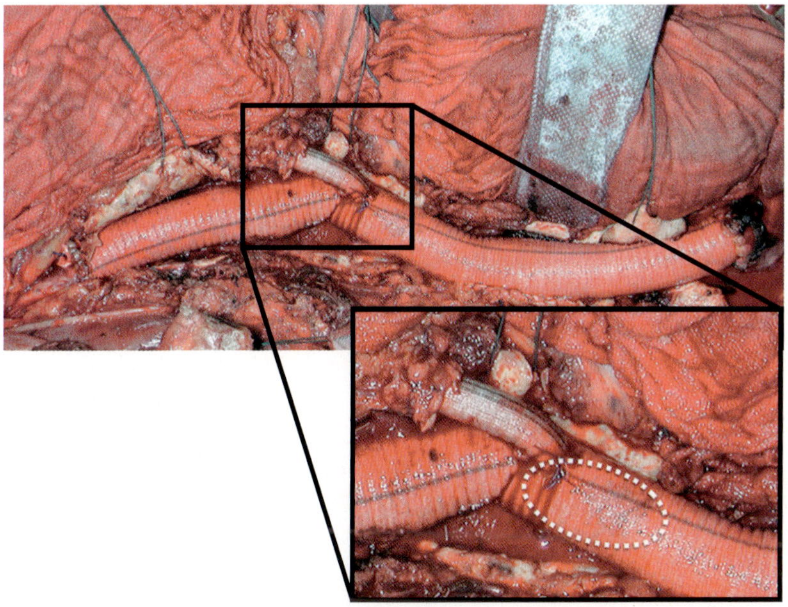

FIGURE 17 • If creation of the visceral patch requires retaining a large segment of native aorta, a separate reattachment of the left renal artery may be performed. Celiac trunk ostia, superior mesenterica ostia, and right renal artery ostia are reattached using a standard Carrel patch (dotted circle) while a selective 6/8-mm bypass is used to reattach the left renal artery. This configuration significantly reduces the risk of recurrent aortic patch aneurysm.

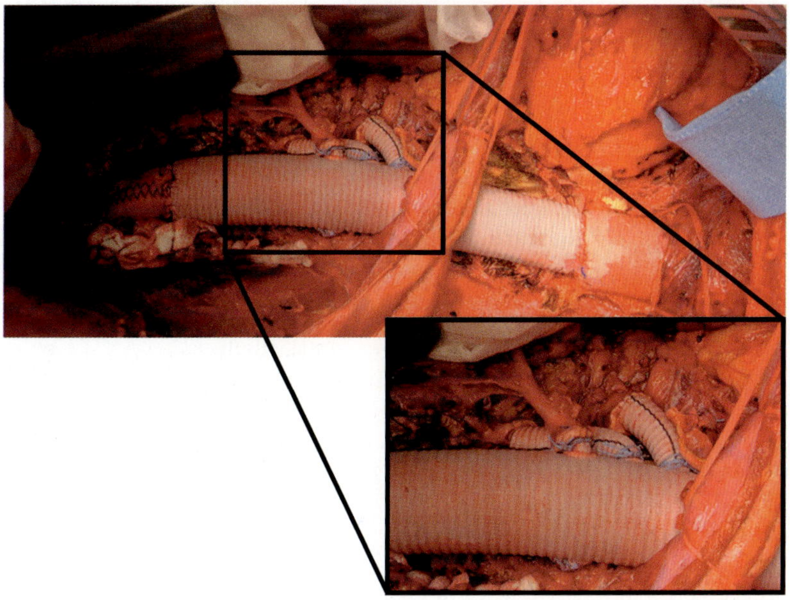

FIGURE 18 • Visceral vessels and renal arteries could be reattached also separately by means of multibranched grafts. These prosthesis are used to reduce as much as possible the aortic native tissue and prevent recurrent aortic aneurysm formation, especially in patients with connective tissue disorders. In the white box, the selective reattachment of celiac trunk, superior mesenteric artery, and left renal artery are highlighted while the right renal artery bypass is located posteriorly and covered by the aortic graft. At the end of the aortic repair, radiopaque markers may be placed at the origin of the bypasses for an easier identification in case of possible late endovascular procedure.

RENAL PROTECTION

- Acute kidney injury (AKI) is a common complication in TAAA repair.[22-24] The incidence of postoperative AKI after TAAA repair varies depending on the patient's preoperative status and comorbidities, the surgical technique, and the disease extension. The duration of renal ischemia in determining the risk of postoperative AKI in aortic surgery is also important. Scores for postoperative AKI have been developed in order to objectively stratify the risk.[25-28] Postoperative AKI not only impairs renal function, but also confers a higher risk of morbidity and mortality in both the short- and long term, including an increased incidence of CKD at follow-up.[29-31] During TAAA open repair, temporary interruption of blood flow to the kidney is required, and the reduction of oxygenation after clamping in the proximal tubular cells induces an intracellular reduction of ATP and an increase in lactate. Prevention of renal hypoperfusion by maintaining both adequate cardiac output and mean arterial pressure (MAP) has been reported as effective in decreasing the incidence of postoperative AKI. Preventive pharmacological strategies have been also reported in the literature by the European Society of Intensive Care.[32] End-organ ischemia can be also prevented or reduced by means of perfusion strategies, such as active distal perfusion by partial cardiopulmonary bypass or LHBP during aortic cross-clamping. Selective renal perfusion during suture time may prevent ischemia/reperfusion injury.[33] Historically warm blood perfusion is the closest approach to physiologic perfusion that prevents cell membrane injury and intracellular edema; however, it requires a more complex setting in extracorporeal blood circuits and provides nonpulsatile blood flow. Until recently, clinical practice mainly involved crystalloid perfusion. Retrospective analysis of postoperative renal function in patients treated with renal cooling with crystalloid reported AKI in 7.6% of patients, temporary dialysis in 2%, and permanent dialysis in 0.66%.[34] Some studies reported renal damage with lactated Ringer solution.[35,36] Custodiol (Dr. Franz-Kohler Chemie GmbH, Bensheim, Germany) is another solution for organ protection, similar to intracellular fluid. Recently a single-center, randomized, double-blind, phase IV prospective study compared the efficacy of renal perfusion with Custodiol vs enriched Ringer solution during TAAA open repair.[37] A significantly lower AKI rate was found in patients who received Custodiol compared with patients who received Ringer solution for renal perfusion during open TAAA repair.

CLOSURE

- The entire aortic repair is inspected (**FIGURE 19**). All exposed aortic branch pulses are palpated after derotation and replacement of the abdominal viscera. Any bleeding or kinking of the aortic branches is addressed at this juncture. The atrial and femoral cannulae are removed; the purse-string sutures are tied and reinforced. Anticoagulation is reversed with protamine. The crus of the diaphragm is reapproximated to restore the aortic hiatus and the left hemidiaphragm loosely sutured with a running polypropylene suture. The left lung is temporarily inflated to check for air leakage.
- A closed suction abdominal drain is placed next to the aortic graft in the left retroperitoneal space, and two chest tubes are placed in the posteroapical and basal pleural space. Absorbable pericostal sutures are placed to approximate the ribs, and two steel wires are used to stabilize the costal margin. The lung is inflated, and the correct expansion of all the segments is carefully checked; the pericostal and diaphragmatic sutures are tightened and ligated. The steel wires are twisted and buried in the cartilaginous costal margin. The abdominal fascia is closed with a running suture. The abdominal and thoracic drains are connected to suction. The serratus and latissimus dorsi muscles are approximated with separate absorbable sutures. Subdermal layer is sutured, and the skin is closed with staples.

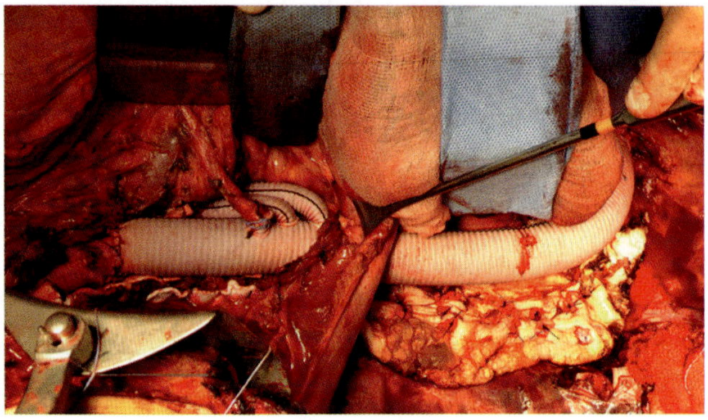

FIGURE 19 • Final repair of a type II thoracoabdominal aortic aneurysm with selective reimplantation of visceral and renal vessels using a multibranched graft.

PEARLS AND PITFALLS

Indications	■ Aortic diameter and aneurysm morphology ■ Signs and symptoms of acute aortic syndrome
Preoperative planning	■ Level of intercostal incision ■ Graft selection ■ Identification of accessory renal arteries and other visceral anomalies (eg, horseshoe kidney) ■ Potential need for multibranch graft vs Carrel patch

Surgical access	▪ Avoid skin flap necrosis ▪ Rib section ▪ Intercostal nerves cryoablation ▪ Limited phrenotomy (circumferential diaphragmatic incision) ▪ Transperitoneal approach ▪ Careful and limited lung manipulation ▪ Nonocclusive femoral cannulation
Technical adjuncts for organ protection	▪ SC drainage ▪ LHBP ▪ Sequential aortic clamping ▪ Critical intercostal artery reattachment ▪ Visceral perfusion from LHBP cannulas ▪ Renal perfusion with cold Custodiol

POSTOPERATIVE CARE

- The main focus of immediate postoperative management is the early detection of neurologic or cardiovascular complication as prompt intervention may prevent substantial long-term morbidity. As soon as baseline blood pressure and body temperature are restored, sedation is lightened regardless of ventilatory status. When SC or cerebral neurologic injury is suspected, CT imaging is performed immediately to address the possibility of intracranial or intradural SC hematoma. In case of paraparesis or paraplegia, MAP is chemically maintained above 80 mm Hg, CSFD is drained in order to lower the cerebrospinal fluid pressure below 10 mm Hg, and methylprednisolone (1 g bolus followed by 4 g per 24 hours continuous infusion) and 18% mannitol (5 mg/kg, four times a day) are administrated.
- If malperfusion develops in the lower limbs, renal or visceral circulation, efforts should be made to restore normal circulation immediately. For a precise visualization of visceral organ perfusion, emergency arteriography (catheter-based or CT) is required.
- Blood pressure fluctuations, including recalcitrant hypertension, is common in the early postoperative period, especially in the chronically hypertensive patient; prompt attention should be paid to regulating the MAP in a physiologic range. Immediate intervention may be required to reduce the risk of anastomotic bleeding, especially in the setting of dissection.
- In uncomplicated cases, drainage tubes are removed at 36 to 48 hours postoperatively, whereas the intrathecal CSFD catheter is removed usually after 72 hours. A prolonged requirement for ventilatory support is not unusual, especially after emergency operations, in patients with significant blood loss and after longer periods of circulatory arrest (if necessary for concurrent arch or ascending aortic reconstruction). In case of severe CKD, transient temporary renal replacement therapy may also be necessary in the early postoperative period.

COMPLICATIONS

- Bleeding
- Multiorgan failure
- Dialysis
- Paraplegia
- Stroke
- Death
- Aneurysm recurrence

REFERENCES

1. Johnston KW, Rutherford RB, Tilson MD, et al. Suggested standards for reporting on arterial aneurysms. Subcommittee on reporting standards for arterial aneurysms, Ad Hoc committee on reporting standards, society for vascular surgery and North American chapter, international society for cardiovascular surgery. *J Vasc Surg.* 1991;13:452-458.
2. Coselli JS, Bozinovski J, LeMaire SA. Open surgical repair of 2286 thoracoabdominal aortic aneurysms. *Ann Thorac Surg.* 2007;83:S862-S864.
3. MacArthur RG, Carter SA, Coselli JS, et al. Organ protection during thoracoabdominal aortic surgery: rationale for a multimodality approach. *Semin Cardiothorac Vasc Anesth.* 2005;9:143-149.
4. Melissano G, Civilini E, Bertoglio L, et al. Angio-CT imaging of the spinal cord vascularisation: a pictorial essay. *Eur J Vasc Endovasc Surg.* 2010;39:436-440.
5. Kieffer E, Chiche L, Baron JF, et al. Coronary and carotid artery disease in patients with degenerative aneurysm of the descending thoracic or thoracoabdominal aorta: prevalence and impact on operative mortality. *Ann Vasc Surg.* 2002;16:679-684.
6. Stevens LA, Coresh J, Greene T, et al. Assessing kidney function—measured and estimated glomerular filtration rate. *N Engl J Med.* 2006;354:2473-2483.
7. Mills JLSr, Duong ST, Leon LR Jr, et al. Comparison of the effects of open and endovascular aortic aneurysm repair on long-term renal function using chronic kidney disease staging based on glomerular filtration rate. *J Vasc Surg.* 2008;47:1141-1149.
8. Cina CS, Abouzahr L, Arena GO, et al. Cerebrospinal fluid drainage to prevent paraplegia during thoracic and thoracoabdominal aortic aneurysm surgery: a systematic review and meta-analysis. *J Vasc Surg.* 2004;40:36-44.
9. Senturk M. Acute and chronic pain after thoracotomies. *Curr Opin Anaesthesiol.* 2005;18:1-4.
10. Nelson KM, Vincent RG, Bourke RS, et al. Intraoperative intercostal nerve freezing to prevent postthoracotomy pain. *Ann Thorac Surg.* 1974;18:280-285.
11. Evans PJ, Lloyd JW, Green CJ. Cryoanalgesia: the response to alterations in freeze cycle and temperature. *Br J Anaesth.* 1981;53:1121-1127.
12. Law L, Rayi A, Derian A. *Cryoanalgesia.* In: *StatPearls* [Internet]. StatPearls Publishing; 2021.
13. Momenzadeh S, Elyasi H, Valaie N, et al. Effect of cryoanalgesia on post-thoracotomy pain. *Acta Med Iran.* 2011;49(4):241-245.
14. Maiwand O, Makey AR. Cryoanalgesia for relief of pain after thoracotomy. *Br Med J.* 1981;282:1749-1750.
15. Khanbhai M, Yap KH, Mohamed S, et al. Is cryoanalgesia effective for post-thoracotomy pain? *Interact Cardiovasc Thorac Surg.* 2014;18(2):202-209.
16. Clemence J Jr, Malik A, Farhat L, et al. Cryoablation of intercostal nerves decreased Narcotic usage after thoracic or thoracoabdominal aortic aneurysm repair. *Semin Thorac Cardiovasc Surg.* 2020;32(3):404-412.

17. Tanaka A, Al-Rstum Z, Leonard SD, et al. Intraoperative intercostal nerve cryoanalgesia improves pain control after descending and thoracoabdominal aortic aneurysm repairs. *Ann Thorac Surg*. 2020;109(1):249-254.
18. Engle J, Safi HJ, Miller CCIII, et al. The impact of diaphragm management on prolonged ventilator support after thoracoabdominal aortic repair. *J Vasc Surg*. 1999;29(1):150-156.
19. Schepens MA. Left heart bypass for thoracoabdominal aortic aneurysm repair: technical aspects. *Multimed Man Cardiothorac Surg*. 2016;2016:mmv039.
20. Etz CD, Homann TM, Plestis KA, et al. Spinal cord perfusion after extensive segmental artery sacrifice: can paraplegia be prevented? *Eur J Cardio Thorac Surg*. 2007;31(4):643-648.
21. Schmitto JD, Fatehpur S, Tezval H, et al. Hypothermic renal protection using cold histidine-tryptophan-ketoglutarate solution perfusion in suprarenal aortic surgery. *Ann Vasc Surg*. 2008;22(4):520-524.
22. Rocha RV, Lindsay TF, Friedrich JO, et al. Systematic review of contemporary outcomes of endovascular and open thoracoabdominal aortic aneurysm repair. *J Vasc Surg*. 2020;71(4):1396-1412.e12.
23. Coselli JS, Lemaire SA, Preventza O, et al. Outcomes of 3309 thoracoabdominal aortic aneurysm repairs. *J Thorac Cardiovasc Surg*. 2016;151(5):1323-1337.
24. Waked K, Schepens M. State-of the-art review on the renal and visceral protection during open thoracoabdominal aortic aneurysm repair. *J Vis Surg*. 2018;4:31.
25. Yuan SM. Acute kidney injury after cardiac surgery: risk factors and Novel biomarkers. *Braz J Cardiovasc Surg*. 2019;34(3):352-360.
26. Mehta RH, Grab JD, O'Brien SM, et al. Bedside tool for predicting the risk of postoperative dialysis in patients undergoing cardiac surgery. *Circulation*. 2006;114(21):2208-2216.
27. Ma MX, Chang Q, Yu CT, et al. Risk factors for acute renal failure after thoracoabdominal aortic aneurysm surgery. *Zhongguo Yi Xue Ke Xue Yuan Xue Bao*. 2020;42(2):147-153.
28. Pannu N, Graham M, Klarenbach S, et al. A new model to predict acute kidney injury requiring renal replacement therapy after cardiac surgery. *CMAJ (Can Med Assoc J)*. 2016;188(15):1076-1083.
29. Chertow GM, Burdick E, Honour M, et al. Acute kidney injury, mortality, length of stay, and costs in hospitalized patients. *J Am Soc Nephrol*. 2005;16(11):3365-3370.
30. Zeng X, McMahon GM, Brunelli SM, et al. Incidence, outcomes, and comparisons across definitions of AKI in hospitalized individuals. *Clin J Am Soc Nephrol*. 2014;9(1):12-20.
31. Doyle JF, Forni LG. Acute kidney injury: short-term and long-term effects. *Crit Care*. 2016;20(1):1-7.
32. Joannidis M, Druml W, Forni LG, et al. Prevention of acute kidney injury and protection of renal function in the intensive care unit: update 2017—expert opinion of the Working Group on Prevention, AKI section, European Society of Intensive Care Medicine. *Intensive Care Med*. 2017;43(6):730-749.
33. Wynn MM, Acher C, Marks E, et al. Postoperative renal failure in thoracoabdominal aortic aneurysm repair with simple cross-clamp technique and 4°C renal perfusion. *J Vasc Surg*. 2015;61(3):611-622.
34. Aftab M, Coselli JS. Renal and visceral protection in thoracoabdominal aortic surgery. *J Thorac Cardiovasc Surg*. 2014;148(6):2963-2966.
35. Lemaire SA, Jones MM, Conklin LD, et al. Randomized comparison of cold blood and cold crystalloid renal perfusion for renal protection during thoracoabdominal aortic aneurysm repair. *J Vasc Surg*. 2009;49(1):11-19.
36. Köksoy C, LeMaire SA, Curling PE, et al. Renal perfusion during thoracoabdominal aortic operations: cold crystalloid is superior to normothermic blood. *Ann Thorac Surg*. 2002;73(3):730-738.
37. Kahlberg A, Tshomba Y, Baccellieri D, et al. CURITIBA Investigators. Renal perfusion with histidine-tryptophan-ketoglutarate compared with Ringer's solution in patients undergoing thoracoabdominal aortic open repair. *J Thorac Cardiovasc Surg*. 2021:S0022-5223(21)00408-6.

Chapter 12

Thoracic Aortic Stent Graft Repair for Aneurysm, Dissection, and Traumatic Transection

Elizabeth Leigh George and Jason T. Lee

DEFINITION

- In 1994, Dake and colleagues[1] at Stanford University were the first to report the use of custom-designed thoracic aortic stent-grafts for the treatment of descending thoracic aortic aneurysms in patients deemed high risk for conventional open surgery. Each of these devices was delivered through peripheral arterial access, usually the femoral arteries, and, when successful, would exclude the aneurysm from systemic pressurization and possible rupture. This groundbreaking minimally invasive technique thereby avoided many of the physiologic insults associated with open surgery, including the need for thoracotomy, aortic cross-clamping, reperfusion injury, and acute hemodynamic changes.
- Results from the first multicenter US Food and Drug Administration–sponsored trial for thoracic aortic stent-grafts demonstrated significantly less perioperative mortality, respiratory failure, renal insufficiency, and spinal cord ischemia in patients after thoracic endovascular aortic repair (TEVAR) compared with a matched cohort of patients undergoing open descending thoracic aortic aneurysm repair.[2]
- After now nearly 3 decades of surgeon experience and endovascular technologic advancement, TEVAR has evolved to serve as a primary treatment strategy for an increasingly diverse group of acute and chronic aortic pathologies including thoracic aortic aneurysms, dissections, and traumatic transections.

DIFFERENTIAL DIAGNOSIS

- Depending on the type and extent of pathology, TEVAR may include the use of fenestrated or branched stent grafts, advanced snorkel/chimney/periscope or parallel graft techniques, or the need for hybrid debranching procedures. The decision to treat thoracic aortic pathology with stent grafts is based on individual patient comorbidity burden, detailed analysis of thoracic aortic anatomy, and physician experience.
- Acute thoracic aortic pathologies often present with chest pain and therefore must be considered in the workup for acute coronary syndrome. The ubiquitous use of computed tomography angiography (CTA) scanning for pain, shortness of breath, trauma, and to "rule out" many pathologies has led to an increase in the recognition of thoracic aortic pathology potentially benefitting from TEVAR technology.

PATIENT HISTORY AND PHYSICAL FINDINGS

- Thoracic aortic aneurysms (TAAs) are defined as localized (saccular) or diffuse (fusiform) dilation of 50% or more relative to the diameter of the adjacent normal-sized aorta. Common risk factors for aneurysmal degeneration include smoking, hypertension, chronic obstructive pulmonary disease, atherosclerosis, and connective tissue disorders. Indications for repair of descending TAAs are similar to those for conventional open repair: maximum aortic diameter greater than 6 cm, rapid aneurysmal growth (>5 mm of growth over 6 months), or symptoms such as persistent chest or back pain, rupture, or dissection. Most TAAs are diagnosed following routine imaging ordered for other reasons, and patients are typically asymptomatic when being considered for treatment.
- Aortic dissection occurs when an intimal tear in the aorta causes blood to flow between the layers of the wall of the aorta and most often presents as tearing chest pain that radiates to the back. Potential etiologic factors leading to aortic dissection include poorly controlled acute or chronic hypertension, connective tissue disorders, trauma, or vasculitis. Medical management of uncomplicated type B thoracic aortic dissection serves as the current standard of care, although there are high-risk anatomic and clinical factors that tend to favor more aggressive interventional therapy. These practice guidelines stem from the results of the INvestigation of STEnt grafts in patients with type B Aortic Dissection (INSTEAD) trial, the first prospective, multicenter randomized trial comparing optimal medical therapy (eg, blood pressure control) with TEVAR for uncomplicated type B dissection, and the follow-up INSTEAD-XL trial.[3,4] The first trial demonstrated no significant improvement in 2-year survival or adverse event rates with TEVAR despite favorable aortic remodeling, but the 5-year follow-up data with landmark analysis in INSTEAD XL trial suggest improved long-term survival in patients undergoing TEVAR. In contrast, for patients with complicated type B dissections involving rupture, malperfusion (eg, visceral or limb ischemia), or refractory back pain despite optimal medical management, TEVAR is indicated. The goal of TEVAR in this setting is to cover, or exclude, the primary entry tear and re-expand the true lumen while promoting thrombosis of the false lumen.
- Traumatic aortic transection results from a high-velocity or deceleration injury to the aorta. The tethering of the aorta by the ligamentum arteriosum makes this site most susceptible to shearing forces during sudden deceleration. A high index of suspicion is necessary to help make the diagnosis. Trauma workups most often involve whole-body CT scanning, which allows rapid triage for possible treatment. CTA commonly demonstrates an irregular outpouching beyond the takeoff of the left subclavian artery at the aortic isthmus, which corresponds to the presence of an aortic pseudoaneurysm caused by the traumatic event. Extent of blunt traumatic aortic injury and the corresponding physiologic insult may range from clinically occult intimal injury to life-threatening complete transection and rupture (**FIGURE 1**).[5]

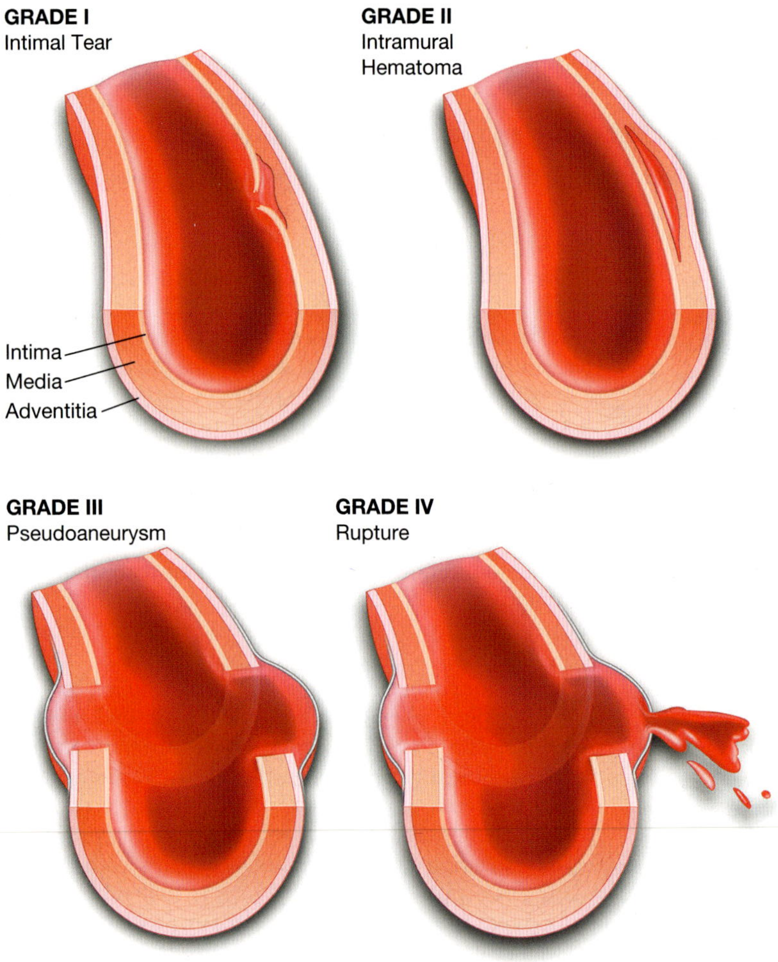

FIGURE 1 • Society for Vascular Surgery classification of blunt traumatic aortic injury. (Adapted from Lee WA, Matsumura JS, Mitchell RS, et al. Endovascular repair of traumatic thoracic aortic injury: clinical practice guidelines of the Society for Vascular Surgery. *J Vasc Surg*. 2011;53(1):187-192. Copyright © 2011 Society for Vascular Surgery. With permission.)

Early diagnosis and endovascular treatment is generally recommended for those presenting with a traumatic aortic transection, particularly when there is a contour abnormality visualized on cross-sectional imaging.

IMAGING AND OTHER DIAGNOSTIC STUDIES

- Transesophageal echocardiography (TEE) may serve as a useful imaging tool, particularly in the setting of acute thoracic aortic pathology. TEE can confirm the presence of aortic dissection, distinguish between types A and B dissections, identify involvement of supra-aortic vessels, and assess for contained rupture.
- High-resolution CTA with three-dimensional reconstructive software allows for the most complete anatomic analysis, including details regarding aneurysm morphology, diameter, dissection flap characterization, thrombus burden, calcification, angulation, and branch vessel orientation.
- Familiarity and routine usage of three-dimensional software on dedicated workstations and the ability to customize measurements provide an accurate road map to guide endovascular strategy, device selection, intraoperative maneuvers to best visualize pathology, and stent graft sizing.

SURGICAL MANAGEMENT

Preoperative Planning

- Patients scheduled for elective TEVAR undergo routine preoperative cardiac evaluation. Based on cardiovascular risk profile, symptomatology, and presence of electrocardiogram abnormalities, selected patients may need to undergo further evaluation in the form of an exercise stress test, dobutamine stress echocardiography, or Persantine thallium stress testing. Coronary angiography is pursued in cases involving extensive or symptomatic coronary artery disease.
- Aortic transections or symptomatic dissections and aneurysms should have early and aggressive blood pressure control using intravenous beta-blocker or calcium channel blocker medications. After obtaining a reliable clinical examination, refractory chest, back, or abdominal pain should be treated with narcotic analgesics.
- Renal protective strategies should be employed preoperatively to minimize the risk of contrast-induced nephropathy. Intravenous hydration is initiated preoperatively and, in the setting of baseline renal insufficiency, may warrant early hospital preadmission.
- Suspected blunt aortic injury should prompt a referral to a level I trauma center to facilitate early evaluation by an

endovascular specialist and other pertinent members of a multidisciplinary trauma team.

- Anesthetic choice is based on institution comfort, and can consist of general, regional, or local during TEVAR cases. Prophylactic lumbar cerebrospinal fluid (CSF) drainage is considered in every case based on the relative risk of spinal cord ischemia, hemodynamic status, and acuity of clinical presentation. Arterial monitoring is often performed via a right radial artery approach. Peripheral intravenous lines are typically adequate; however, more intensive central venous monitoring may be required in cases involving unstable traumatic transections, patients with significant baseline cardiovascular comorbidities, or any case involving hemodynamic instability.
- Preoperative imaging should be heavily scrutinized for the adequacy of iliofemoral access anatomy. An iliac conduit may be required in cases involving small-caliber, tortuous, or heavily calcified access vessels and can be done via a flank incision for an open bypass graft or via endovascular techniques with covered stenting of the iliac vessels.
- Numerous variables have been identified as risk factors for the development of spinal cord ischemia after TEVAR. Given that hypoperfusion represents the primary etiology of spinal cord injury following TEVAR, commonly cited risk factors involve those relating to the extent of impairment or exclusion of the collateral perfusion to the spinal cord. The European Collaborators on Stent/Graft Techniques for Aortic Aneurysm Repair (EUROSTAR) investigators reported results from the largest multicenter registry to date (N = 606).[6] In the EUROSTAR registry, the incidence of spinal cord ischemia was 2.5% and independent risk factors included left subclavian artery coverage without revascularization (odds ratio [OR], 3.9; P = .037), concomitant open abdominal aortic surgery (OR, 5.5; P = .037), and the use of three or more stent grafts (OR, 3.5; P = .043). Staging of TEVAR coverage for thoracoabdominal endovascular procedures should also be considered to allow for spinal conditioning.
- Based on the principle that spinal cord perfusion pressure is approximated by the difference between the mean arterial pressure (MAP) and CSF pressure, placement of a prophylactic lumbar drain has the potential to increase spinal cord perfusion pressure by decreasing CSF pressure and may be beneficial in select patients at high risk for spinal cord ischemia. Percutaneous drainage of CSF is performed by inserting a silastic catheter 10 to 15 cm into the subarachnoid space through a 14-gauge Tuohy needle at the L3-L4 vertebral interspace. The open end of the catheter is attached to a sterile closed-circuit reservoir, and the lumbar CSF pressure is measured with a pressure transducer zero-referenced to the midline of the brain. Lumbar CSF can be drained continuously or intermittently in the operating room to achieve target CSF pressures of 10 to 12 mm Hg. Postoperatively, intermittent or continuous CSF drainage can be continued in the intensive care unit for CSF pressures exceeding 10 mm Hg or at the first sign of lower extremity weakness. In the absence of neurologic deficits, the lumbar CSF drainage catheter can be clamped 24 hours post procedure followed by continued monitoring of CSF pressure together with serial neurologic assessments. The CSF drain can then be removed at 48 hours after operation. Although prophylactic or therapeutic lumbar CSF drainage has an established record of safety, complications have been reported to occur in approximately 1% of patients, which may include neuraxial hematoma, subdural hematoma, catheter fracture, meningitis, intracranial hypotension, chronic CSF leak, and spinal headache.

Selection and Sizing of Thoracic Stent Graft

Landing Zones

- Proximal and distal landing zones must be of sufficient length (usually at least 2 cm) to enable safe and accurate deployment bracketing the area of thoracic aortic pathology, which often includes the subclavian artery proximally or the celiac artery distally.
- Intentional coverage of the left subclavian artery is sometimes required due to a very proximal extent of aortic pathology, especially transections. Left subclavian artery revascularization may be required in select cases. The celiac artery rarely requires intentional coverage.
- Significant tortuosity, circumferential mural thrombus, and extensive calcification can compromise the proximal or distal landing zone, thereby predisposing to inadequate fixation and subsequent development of endoleak or migration. Site of proximal and distal landing zones should be selected to minimize the impact of these anatomic features, even if it requires extending the length of aortic coverage.
- A variety of anatomic measurements are taken from preoperative CTA imaging to assist in the sizing and selection of the thoracic stent-graft (**FIGURE 2**). Interventionalists should be proficient in accurate sizing and measuring of key thoracic aortic locations that influence device selection and ultimately determine patient outcomes.

Sizing of Stent Grafts

- The degree of stent graft oversizing can vary based on the indication for intervention. Stent-grafts are generally oversized by 10% to 20% based on the aortic diameter at the proximal and distal fixation sites for aneurysmal disease. Insufficient oversizing for the treatment of TAAs may predispose to inadequate exclusion and the potential for endoleak or migration. Aggressive oversizing, on the other hand, increases the risk for stent graft collapse, graft thrombosis, access arterial injury, and potential for peri- or postprocedural iatrogenic retrograde type A dissection.
- Chronic type B dissections are frequently characterized by a thick, nonmobile dissection flap, or septum, that separates true and false lumens into concave or convex discs of flow lumen. Such dissection flaps have limited compliance; therefore, minimal or no oversizing may be required to achieve a suitable proximal or distal seal.
- Aortic transections frequently occur in young trauma patients with normal or minimally diseased aortas. As such, minimal oversizing is needed to achieve an adequate seal and only recently did device manufacturers create devices meant for smaller-diameter aortas. Note also that underresuscitated patients on admission will have smaller aortic diameters on their CTA.
- Currently available stent-grafts range in diameter from 18 to 46 mm. Given the traditional 10% to 20% rule of device oversizing, these devices are designed to safely treat aortas with landing zones ranging from 16 to 43 mm in diameter.

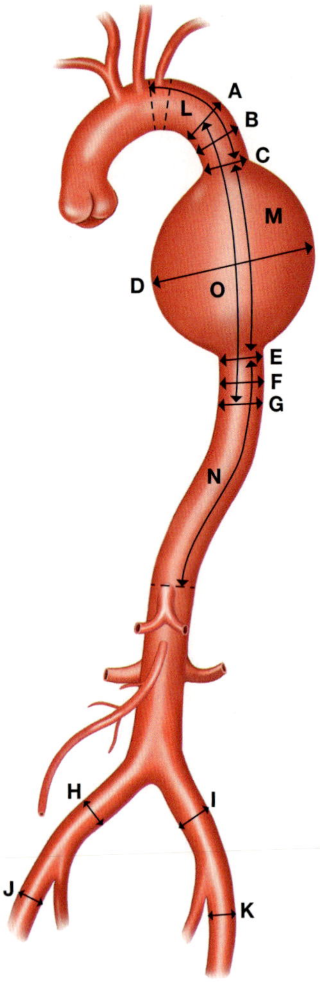

A

Measurements to be taken during the pretreatment assessment of isolated lesions are described below:

A, B, C. Proximal aortic neck diameter (minimum of 1 cm apart)
D. Maximum lesion diameter
E, F, G. Distal aortic neck diameter (minimum of 1 cm apart)
H. Right common iliac artery diameter
I. Left common iliac artery diameter
J. Right external iliac/femoral artery diameter
K. Left external iliac/femoral artery diameter
L. Distance between the left subclavian/left common carotid artery and the proximal end of the lesion (minimum of 2 cm)
M. Length of the lesion measured along the greater curvature of the flow lumen
N. Distance between the distal end of the lesion and the celiac axis (minimum of 2 cm)
O. Total treatment length

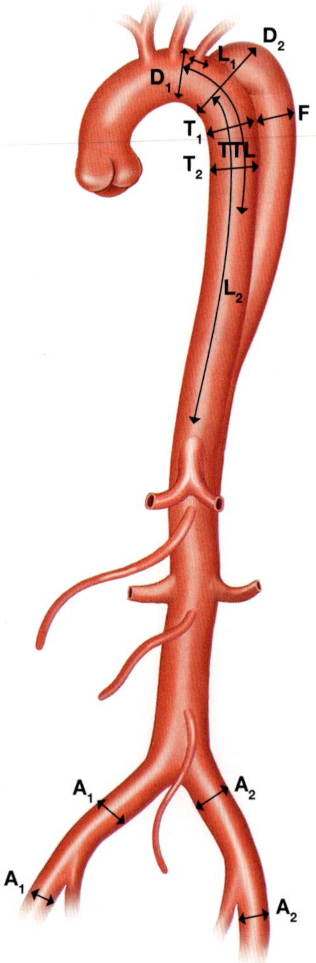

B

Measurements to be taken during the pretreatment assessment of dissections are described below:

D1. Diameter at proximal extent of proximal landing zone (must be in nondissected aorta)
D2. Maximum transverse aortic diameter (combined true and false lumen)
T1. Maximum true lumen diameter in DTA
T2. Minimum true lumen diameter in DTA
F. Maximum false lumen diameter in DTA
A1. Right access vessel diameter (common iliac, external iliac, femoral)
A2. Left access vessel diamter (common iliac, external iliac, femoral)
L1. Proximal landing zone length from proximal end of primary entry tear to left subclavian or left common carotid
L2. Distal neck length from distal end of primary entry tear to celiac
TTL. Total treatment length from left subclavian or left common carotid

FIGURE 2 • Anatomic measurements to assist in thoracic stent graft device sizing and selection for the treatment of aneurysms **(A)** and dissections **(B)**. DTA, descending thoracic aorta.

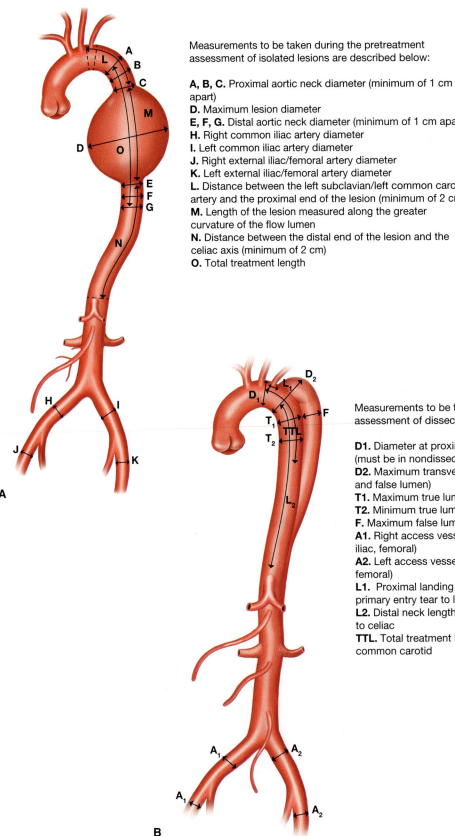

Access Vessel Anatomy

- Current thoracic aortic stent-grafts require large-caliber delivery systems, ranging from 16 to 26 Fr in outer diameter. Depending on the manufacturer, some systems come with their own delivery systems. Small, tortuous, and heavily calcified iliofemoral arteries may prohibit sheath advancement and predispose to access site–related complications, including groin hematoma, dissection, or rupture.
- Careful evaluation of access vessel anatomy on preoperative imaging should be performed to assess the caliber, tortuosity, thrombus burden, and extent of calcification of the iliofemoral arteries. Such anatomic information will serve as the basis for deciding laterality of femoral access as well as to determine the need for an iliac conduit.
- Serial dilation may be attempted for patients with small iliofemoral vessels. Iliac atherosclerotic lesions may be pretreated with balloon angioplasty and/or stent-grafting (often with an iliac limb or peripheral stent-graft) to facilitate sheath advancement and introduction of the thoracic stent graft components.
- Iliac conduits serve as a safe and reliable technique to circumvent issues related to suboptimal access vessel anatomy. From either flank incision, a retroperitoneal exposure provides visualization of the common iliac artery or distal abdominal aorta. A 10- or 12-mm Dacron graft is commonly used as the conduit of choice. The conduit can be modified by creating a patch at the distal end to further facilitate the delivery of a large-caliber sheath and enable additional degrees of torqueability (**FIGURE 3**). This modification involves creating a patch by cutting the Dacron graft along its long access, thereby enlarging the transition zone from the graft to artery.

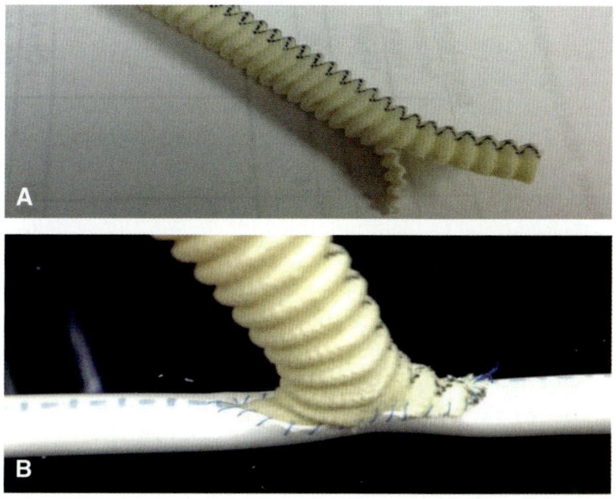

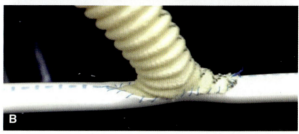

FIGURE 3 • **A,** A 10-mm Dacron conduit bisected longitudinally to create a sewing patch. **B,** Dacron iliac conduit sewn to native iliac artery allows easy mobility of the conduit at multiple angles of entry for large-caliber device or sheath. (Reprinted from Lee JT, Lee GK, Chandra V, et al. Comparison of fenestrated endografts and the snorkel/chimney technique. *J Vasc Surg*. 2014;60(4):849-857. Copyright © 2014 Society for Vascular Surgery. With permission.)

EARLY PROCEDURAL CONSIDERATIONS

Positioning

- The C-arm is typically configured in the "head" position. The left arm may be abducted to 75° to 90° and circumferentially prepped into the field if an embolization or snorkel/chimney procedure involving the left subclavian artery is anticipated. Axillary access can also be used and allows for the arms to be tucked. Some interventionalists prefer the right arm approach based on the design of their hybrid suite. The chest, abdomen, and bilateral groins should be prepped. As frequently only one groin access is required for the performance of a routine TEVAR, laterality of the operator position may vary based on surgeon preference or anticipated access site location.

Establishing Vascular Access

- The ipsilateral femoral artery is accessed either percutaneously or from an open exposure. Secondary access may be obtained from the contralateral femoral artery or brachial artery as needed for a 5-Fr sheath and flush catheter. Surgical exposure is obtained from a small oblique incision at the level of the inguinal ligament. The common femoral artery is exposed, with proximal control obtained at the level of the external iliac artery and distal control at the level of the femoral bifurcation or proximal superficial femoral and profunda femoral arteries. Heavy calcification may require preemptive endarterectomy and patch angioplasty to facilitate safe sheath placement.
- The femoral artery is punctured using a standard micropuncture set, and if arterial access is obtained percutaneously, a sheathogram is performed to confirm adequate puncture site location (mid–common femoral artery). A standard-length Bentson wire is inserted into the aorta through micropuncture sheath and exchange for a 7-Fr sheath is then performed using Seldinger technique. Wire exchange is then done for a 260-cm stiff Lunderquist wire. The Lunderquist wire should have a flexible, curved proximal end that should be advanced under fluoroscopy across the aortic arch to abut the aortic value. The location of the distal end of the Lunderquist wire should be marked on the operating table, and this wire position should be maintained throughout the procedure.
- Over the stiff Lunderquist wire platform, the 7-Fr sheath is removed and serial dilators are advanced to gradually enlarge the subcutaneous tract and arteriotomy site to accommodate either the stent-graft device itself or a larger 16- to 26-Fr introducer sheath required for device delivery.
- After placement of the larger sheath, systemic heparin is administered at a dose of 100 U/kg (goal activated clotting time of >250 seconds). Concomitant traumatic injuries, particularly intracranial hemorrhage, may alter the dose or decision to administer heparin.

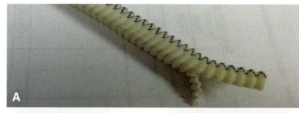

INITIAL AORTOGRAM

- A 5-Fr 100-cm Omniflush or pigtail catheter is inserted into the aorta and advanced to the level of the aortic arch. This catheter may be advanced via a contralateral 5-Fr sheath or it may be inserted into an additional ipsilateral 5-Fr sheath placed distal to the arteriotomy for the main body delivery sheath.
- If satisfied with stent graft sizing based on available preoperative imaging, the thoracic aortic stent graft may be advanced over the Lunderquist wire and be positioned in the proximal to midportion of the thoracic aorta prior to initial aortogram.
- Optimal angiographic imaging of the aortic arch is obtained by placing the fluoroscopic C-arm in a left anterior oblique orientation, often 35° to 65°, and can be optimized by referencing the preoperative CTA. The location of the supra-aortic vessels, particularly the left subclavian artery, should be noted and marked on viewing monitors (**FIGURE 4A**). Many new advances with image overlay techniques have further allowed accurate stent-graft deployment and savings on branch catheterization time and radiation.
- Intravascular ultrasound (IVUS) is an important adjunct in cases involving dissection to assist in the identification of true and false lumens, as well as to gain additional information on aortic diameter, branch vessel location, and morphology of proximal and distal landing zones. IVUS also aids in limiting intravenous contrast exposure in those patients with baseline impaired renal function.
- If necessary to guide distal extent of stent graft placement, the celiac artery is best imaged from a full lateral projection. Additional structures to note are large, patent intercostal arteries at the level of the aortic hiatus. Efforts should be made to avoid covering these if at all possible during the course of the repair.

Device Deployment

- Precise proximal positioning of the stent graft is facilitated by either marking the location of the left subclavian artery on the viewing screen and/or using the road-mapping feature

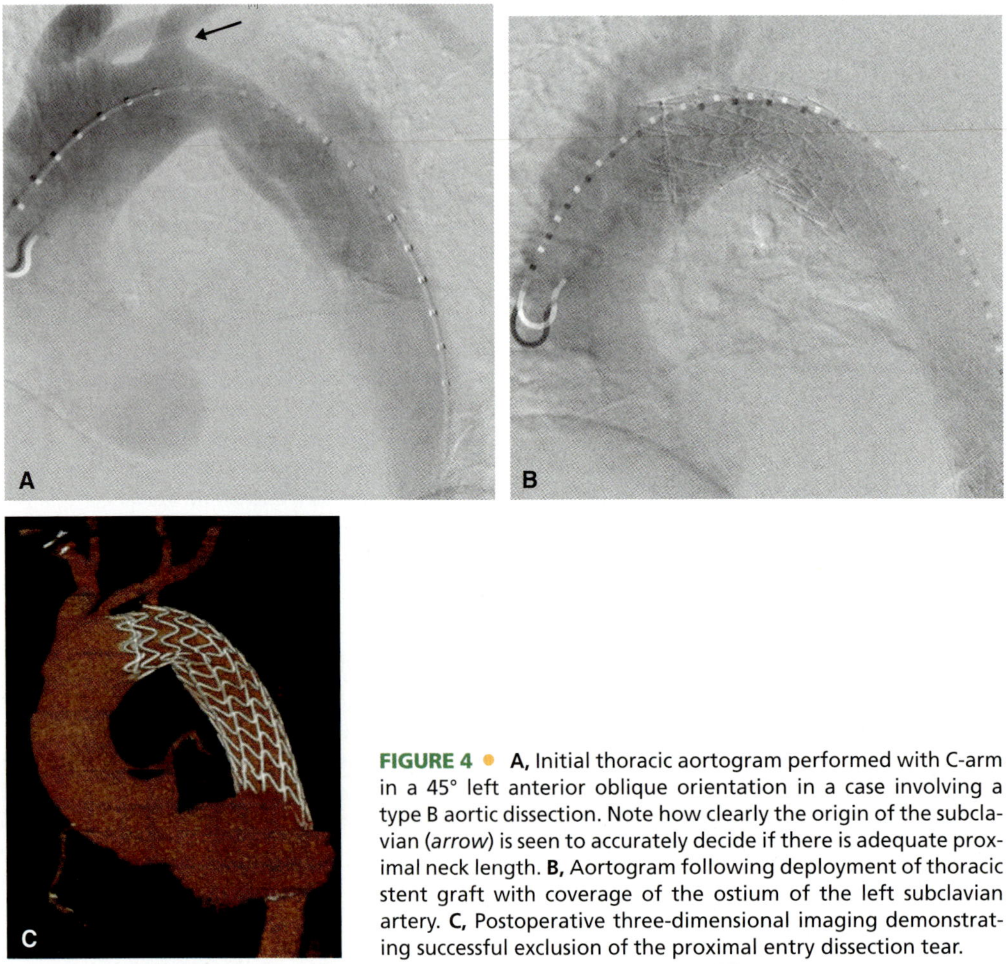

FIGURE 4 • **A,** Initial thoracic aortogram performed with C-arm in a 45° left anterior oblique orientation in a case involving a type B aortic dissection. Note how clearly the origin of the subclavian (*arrow*) is seen to accurately decide if there is adequate proximal neck length. **B,** Aortogram following deployment of thoracic stent graft with coverage of the ostium of the left subclavian artery. **C,** Postoperative three-dimensional imaging demonstrating successful exclusion of the proximal entry dissection tear.

and/or using image overlay. The distal radiopaque line of the endotracheal tube seen on fluoroscopy at about 45° left anterior oblique can sometimes correlate to the position of the left common carotid artery, thereby serving as a convenient landmark in unstable cases requiring left subclavian artery coverage when bleeding must be expeditiously controlled.

- Immediately prior to stent graft deployment, systemic arterial blood pressure is reduced below 100 mm Hg to reduce risk of caudal migration.
- The stent-grafts are generally deployed in a proximal-to-distal sequence. However, a distal-to-proximal sequence may be preferred in cases involving precise deployment near the celiac artery or in aortas with significant diameter taper and a larger proximal landing zone compared with the distal landing zone (where devices of different diameter may need to be stacked up on each other).
- Deployed endografts will naturally extend toward the outer curvature of the aorta, and precision deployment is facilitated by gently providing forward traction on the wire toward the outer curve during deployment. This maneuver also facilitates straightening out of the transverse arch, which can be helpful in minimizing the "bird-beaking" effect at the proximal graft margin, where the device may not fully oppose to the "inner" aortic wall. Bird beaking, when present, can predispose to proximal type I endoleaks, endograft collapse, and potential aortic occlusion. Newer next-generation conformable devices and device modifications have significantly reduced this risk.
- Additional graft components are added, when necessary, by exchanging the first device over the Lunderquist wire. A minimum overlap of 5 cm between pieces is recommended to ensure adequate apposition and minimize risk of junctional (type III) endoleak.

Balloon Molding

- Balloon molding is often required in cases involving TAAs. Under fluoroscopic guidance, a noncompliant molding balloon (Coda [Cook Medical, Bloomington, IN, USA] or Tri-Lobe [W. L. Gore, Flagstaff, AZ, USA]) is advanced up to the proximal edge of the stent-graft and balloon molding is performed in a proximal-to-distal sequence. Balloon molding should be performed at the proximal and distal fixation sites, as well as at areas of stent-graft overlap in those cases requiring multiple stent-grafts.
- Aggressive ballooning can cause component fracture and aortic injury, and care must be taken during inflation with constant visualization and knowledge of the tension applied to the balloon.
- Balloon molding is not typically required in cases involving aortic dissection or transection, particularly in cases where no obvious endoleak is visualized. Balloon molding may increase risk for iatrogenic retrograde type A conversion if performed in a region of friable or fragile aorta and is generally not recommended during dissection cases.

COMPLETION AORTOGRAM

- After stent-graft deployment, the pigtail catheter is withdrawn along the outside of the deployed device(s) over a wire to below the level of the stent-graft. The catheter is then readvanced over a wire within the stent-graft lumen and positioned at the level of the aortic arch.
- Additional aortograms may be performed at this time as necessary in order to ensure adequate stent-graft position and patency of the supra-aortic and celiac arteries and to assess for the presence of endoleaks.

REMOVAL OF SHEATH AND ARTERIOTOMY CLOSURE

- In cases involving percutaneous access, the two previously placed Perclose ProGlide devices are used to close the arteriotomy site(s) (see Chapter 25 for details). If open surgical exposure was obtained, proximal and distal vascular control is obtained in the respective groin. All wires and sheaths are removed. The arteriotomy is closed transversely using a polypropylene suture in either a running continuous or interrupted fashion. Antegrade and retrograde flushing maneuvers should be performed prior to completion of the arteriotomy closure.

LEFT SUBCLAVIAN ARTERY REVASCULARIZATION

- Endovascular procedures that require coverage of the left subclavian artery have the potential to increase the risk of spinal cord injury by compromising blood flow to the ipsilateral vertebral artery, an important collateral pathway for arterial flow to the anterior spinal artery. Subclavian artery revascularization therefore serves as an additional strategy to decrease the risk of spinal cord ischemia in select patients deemed high risk.
- Techniques to revascularize the left subclavian artery include transposition of the subclavian onto the left carotid artery or left carotid–subclavian bypass grafting with subsequent embolization of the left subclavian artery proximal to the bypass graft (**FIGURE 5**). These revascularization procedures may be performed as part of a staged repair or at the time of TEVAR. Laser in situ fenestrations and purpose-specific single side branch grafts are currently being studied as an alternative to extra-anatomic open revascularization.
- The existing clinical evidence to support the efficacy of routine left subclavian artery revascularization remains controversial; there are advocates for routine revascularization, selective revascularization, or no revascularization. A meta-analysis of published studies showed a trend toward increased risk of spinal cord ischemia when the left subclavian artery was covered, suggesting a potential benefit for left subclavian artery revascularization, but the finding was not statistically significant.[5-7]

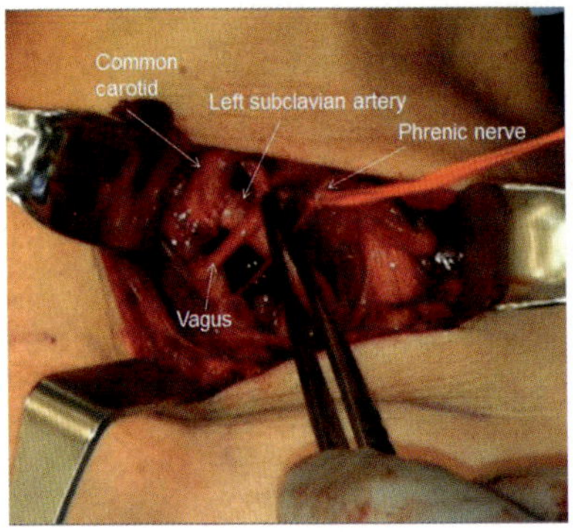

FIGURE 5 ● Left subclavian artery transposition is performed by ligating the left subclavian artery proximal to the vertebral artery and moving it cephalad in order to perform an end-to-side anastomosis between the left subclavian and left common carotid arteries. Alternatively, a Dacron graft can be used as a left carotid–subclavian bypass.

SPECIAL CONSIDERATIONS BASED ON AORTIC PATHOLOGY

Aortic Dissection

- The primary goal of TEVAR for the treatment of dissection is coverage of the proximal entry tear (**FIGURE 6A** and **B**). Stent-graft sizing is based on the diameter of the adjacent nondissected thoracic aorta. Minimal or no oversizing of the stent graft is recommended.
- In acute type B dissections, the septum is relatively mobile and compliant. Therefore, the diameter of the small true lumen in the dissected portion often returns to normal diameter following successful exclusion of the proximal entry tear.
- Chronic dissections have thicker, less compliant septa, which may limit expansion of the true lumen despite adequate entry tear coverage. Often, these patients have chronic false lumen aneurysmal dilation, and entry tear and fenestration covering serve simply to decrease false lumen pressurization and promote thrombosis.
- IVUS serves as a useful adjunct in dissection cases, both in terms of initial identification of true and false lumen, as well as assisting in precise positioning of the device.
- The placement of a distal noncovered stent in the manner of the STABLE trial in theory can lead to positive remodeling, and current outcomes are still in mid-term.[8]

Aortic Transection

- Traumatic aortic injuries are typically located along the inner curve of the proximal descending thoracic aorta (**FIGURE 7**). Given the proximal location, left subclavian artery coverage is sometimes needed.[5]
- In the absence of concomitant hemorrhage or brain injury, routine heparin is recommended.
- Trauma patients are frequently hypovolemic and, as a result, may have an underdistended aorta on preoperative cross-sectional imaging. Initial cross-sectional imaging can underestimate true aortic morphology at the region of the subclavian by as much as 10% to 20%. In such settings, IVUS may assist in more accurate stent graft sizing performed in vivo.[9]

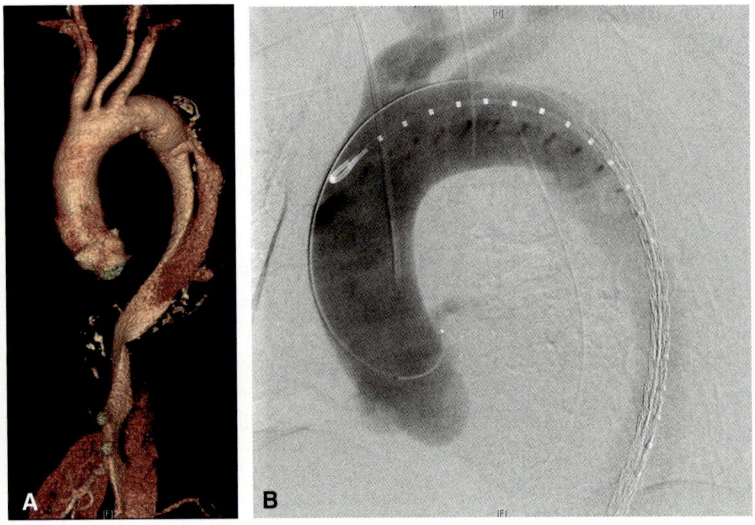

FIGURE 6 ● **A,** CTA reconstruction demonstrating complex thoracoabdominal aortic dissection with proximal entry tear located in the proximal descending thoracic aorta. **B,** Initial aortogram documenting position of the supra-aortic arteries. Note the stent graft has been advanced into approximate position but is not yet deployed.

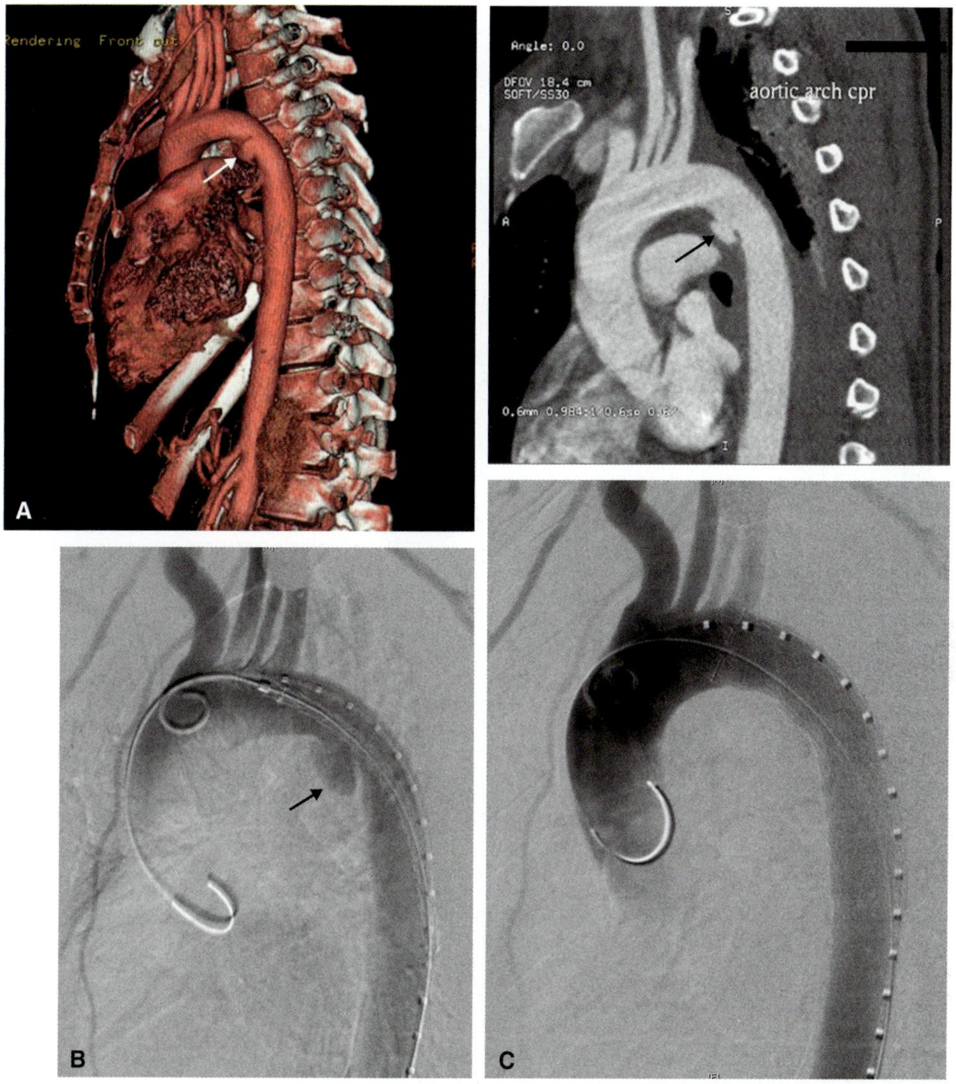

FIGURE 7 • **A,** Three-dimensional reconstructed images showing the presence of traumatic aortic transection at the level of the ligamentum arteriosum (*arrow*). **B,** Aortogram showing focal outpouching (*arrow*) along the inner curve of the proximal descending thoracic aorta, correlating to the traumatic transection observed on preoperative imaging. Note that the stent graft has been advanced into the proximal descending thoracic aorta but is not yet deployed. **C,** Aortogram following thoracic stent graft deployment with successful exclusion of the transection site.

PEARLS AND PITFALLS

Indications	▪ TEVAR follows general recommendations for elective repair of descending thoracic and thoracoabdominal aortic aneurysms and should be offered to good anatomic risk patients with aneurysms >6 cm. ▪ Patient selection should take into account the need for regular interval clinical and radiologic follow-up in order to monitor for stent-graft–related complications and endoleaks.
Preoperative workup	▪ High-quality imaging and ability to configure three-dimensional reconstructive software are essential for successful preoperative planning and device selection. ▪ Pre- and perioperative hydration is a central part in the protection from contrast-induced nephropathy. ▪ Patients should be stratified according to baseline risk of spinal cord ischemia. A prophylactic lumbar drain should be considered in those at high risk.
Patient setup	▪ A hybrid endovascular suite provides optimal opportunity for accurate imaging and capability to perform necessary open surgical exposure or repair of access-related complications. ▪ Anticipated adjunct procedures, including left subclavian artery embolization or revascularization, may require prepping the left neck and/or arm into the surgical field.

Thoracic aneurysms	▪ Oversizing of stent-grafts by 10%-20% and balloon molding are generally recommended in order to maximize proximal and distal fixation. ▪ Proximal and distal landing zones should be relatively free of stenosis, calcification, and thrombus to maximize durability of this minimally invasive technology.
Type B dissection	▪ Accurate identification of true and false lumen is essential prior to deployment of the stent-graft. IVUS is a useful adjunct in this setting to confirm true or false lumen position. ▪ Aggressive oversizing of stent-grafts is not recommended in patients with aortic dissection. Balloon molding is generally reserved only for those with type I or III endoleak on completion angiography and not against the region where there is a mobile septum.
Traumatic transection	▪ Routine heparin is recommended unless contraindicated by concomitant intracranial or solid organ injury. ▪ Similar to dissections, aggressive oversizing and balloon molding is not routinely performed during the treatment of transections.

POSTOPERATIVE CARE

- Patients are typically extubated if they had a general anesthetic immediately following the procedure unless prohibited by concomitant physiologic insults (eg, hemodynamic instability, trauma patient).
- Intensive care unit monitoring is required for patients who require a lumbar drain for 24 to 48 hours. Immediate and frequent neurologic assessments are critical in the early perioperative period to assess for spinal cord ischemia. Raising MAP goals are an additional way to minimize risk of cord ischemia.
- Durability of TEVAR is reliant on routine imaging to evaluate for stent-graft–specific complications postoperatively. Follow-up chest CTA and plain x-rays are typically obtained at 1, 6, and 12 months and at intervals thereafter. Consideration should be made between balancing risks for cumulative lifetime iodinated contrast and radiation exposure vs the necessity for serial graft monitoring. In stable patients, chest x-rays may suffice to confirm device position, with CT scanning reserved for those with migration suggested by CT or evidence of progressive aortic enlargement or onset of recurrent symptoms such as chest pain.

OUTCOMES

- The largest published series, which has reported 1-year follow-up, included 443 patients treated with TEVAR for a variety of indications, both emergent and elective, as follows: TAA (n = 249), thoracic aortic dissection (n = 131), traumatic aortic injury (n = 50), and false anastomotic aneurysm (n = 13).[10] Technical success was achieved in nearly 90% of patients, with an all-cause mortality among patients treated for aortic aneurysm and aortic dissection of 20% and 10%, respectively. In the most recent analysis of Medicare data, TEVAR for aneurysm has the best long-term survival after traumatic injury, with outcomes slightly worse in TAA and dissection, which has the highest reintervention rate.[11]
- No randomized trials comparing TEVAR with open surgery have been published to date. However, multiple nonrandomized comparisons suggest equivalent or better outcomes with TEVAR. In a single-center, retrospective study of over 700 patients who underwent either TEVAR or open surgery, mortality was not significantly different at 30-day (5.7% vs 8.3%, respectively) or 1-year (15.6% vs 15.9%, respectively) follow-up.[12] Two smaller studies demonstrated a reduction in 30-day perioperative mortality with TEVAR compared with open surgery (1.9% vs 5.7%).[13,14]

COMPLICATIONS

- Stroke continues to be a common complication following TEVAR and is associated with significant in-hospital mortality. Recent clinical series have reported an incidence of stroke after TEVAR to range from 2% to 8%.[15,16] The underlying mechanisms contributing to acute ischemic stroke after TEVAR and the temporal relationship of stroke to the procedure are not completely understood. However, the constellation of preoperative risk factors, neurologic examinations, and patterns of brain infarction observed in these patients has led most investigators to conclude that cerebral embolization and ischemic events are the primary mechanisms for perioperative stroke in TEVAR.[6,16,17] Embolic events are related to instrumentation of the aortic arch in patients with severe atheromatous disease, whereas ischemia is a result of the planned or inadvertent endovascular coverage of supra-aortic vessels. Flushing of devices is even thought to potentially contribute to embolic debris that can lead to cerebrovascular compromise.
- Spinal cord ischemia and subsequent acute or delayed paraplegia represents the most devastating complication of TEVAR. The pathogenesis of spinal cord injury after TEVAR is likely multifactorial but still poorly understood. The deployment of thoracic stent-grafts results in rapid complete exclusion of varying lengths of segmental collateral vessels without the ability to surgically reimplant or revascularize the intercostal arteries. Stent deployment and catheter manipulation can predispose patients to dislodgement of thrombotic or atheromatous debris from the aortic wall into segmental vessels, with subsequent distal embolization and occlusion of arteries supplying the spinal cord. Moreover, endovascular coverage of the left subclavian artery may compromise spinal cord perfusion in patients with a dominant left vertebral artery, solitary vertebral artery, carotid artery disease, or an incomplete circle of Willis. Access site injuries to the iliofemoral vessels may further increase the risk of spinal cord ischemia by compromising collateral flow to the anterior spinal artery through the hypogastric and pelvic vascular plexus. Lastly, pharmacologic measures aimed

at decreasing arterial blood pressure to enhance accuracy of device deployment in cases involving difficult aortic anatomy may lead to hypotension similar to that observed in open surgery.

- Due to the large sheath sizes required for the delivery of thoracic stent-grafts, small-diameter, tortuous, or heavily calcified access vessels can predispose to iliofemoral arterial injury. Postoperative CTA often documents arterial dissections and injury that can be followed with noninvasive duplex and managed expectantly until patients have claudication-like symptoms.
- Endoleaks are a relatively common finding after TEVAR, affecting nearly 15% of patients in the early or late postoperative periods. Type I or III endoleaks typically require additional stent placement or balloon molding in order to improve proximal, distal, or junctional fixation. Most type II endoleaks observed on completion angiogram or early follow-up cross-sectional imaging will resolve spontaneously. Persistent type II endoleaks, especially those with aneurysm sac expansion or failure to adequately seal a proximal entry tear or transection, warrant additional intervention. Retrograde flow from intercostal or left subclavian arteries can be treated using coil embolization or vascular plug placement.

REFERENCES

1. Dake MD, Miller DC, Semba CP, et al. Transluminal placement of endovascular stent-grafts for the treatment of descending thoracic aortic aneurysms. *N Engl J Med*. 1994;331:1729-1734.
2. Bavaria JE, Appoo JJ, Makaroun MS, et al. Endovascular stent grafting versus open surgical repair of descending thoracic aortic aneurysms in low-risk patients: a multicenter comparative trial. *J Thorac Cardiovasc Surg*. 2007;133:369-377.
3. Nienaber CA, Rousseau H, Eggebrecht H, et al. Randomized comparison of strategies for type B aortic dissection: the INvestigation of STEnt Grafts in Aortic Dissection (INSTEAD) trial. *Circulation*. 2009;120:2519-2528.
4. Nienaber CA, Kische S, Rousseau H, et al. Long-term results of the randomized investigation of stent grafts in aortic dissection trial. *Circ Cardiovasc Interv*. 2013;6:407-416.
5. Lee WA, Matsumura JS, Mitchell RS, et al. Endovascular repair of traumatic aortic injury: clinical practice guidelines of the Society for Vascular Surgery. *J Vasc Surg*. 2011;53:187-192.
6. Buth J, Harris PL, Hobo R, et al. Neurologic complications associated with endovascular repair of thoracic aortic pathology: incidence and risk factors. A study from the European Collaborators on Stent/Graft Techniques for Aortic Aneurysm Repair (EUROSTAR) registry. *J Vasc Surg*. 2007;46:1103-1110.
7. Rizvi AZ, Murad MH, Fairman RM, et al. The effect of left subclavian artery coverage on morbidity and mortality in patients undergoing endovascular thoracic aortic interventions: a systematic review and meta-analysis. *J Vasc Surg*. 2009;50:1159-1169.
8. Lombardi JV, Gleason TG, Panneton JM, et al. STABLE II clinical trial on endovascular treatment of acute, complicated type B aortic dissection with a composite device design. *J Vasc Surg*. 2020;71:1077-1087.
9. Pearce BJ, Jordan W. Using IVUS during EVAR and TEVAR: improving patient outcomes. *Semin Vasc Surg*. 2009;22:172-180.
10. Leurs LJ, Bell R, Degrieck Y, et al. Endovascular treatment of thoracic aortic diseases: combined experience from the EUROSTAR and United Kingdom Thoracic Endograft registries. *J Vasc Surg*. 2004;40:670-679.
11. Ho VT, Itoga NK, Tran K, et al. Mid-term survival after thoracic endovascular aortic repair by indication in the medicare population. *J Am Coll Surg*. 2021 01;232(1):46-53.e2.
12. Greenberg RK, Lu Q, Roselli EE, et al. Contemporary analysis of descending thoracic and thoracoabdominal aneurysm repair: a comparison of endovascular and open techniques. *Circulation*. 2008;118:808-817.
13. Matsumura JS, Cambria RP, Dake MD, et al. International controlled clinical trial of thoracic endovascular aneurysm repair with the Zenith TX2 endovascular graft: 1-year results. *J Vasc Surg*. 2008;47(2):247-257.
14. Bavaria JE, Appoo JJ, Makaroun MS, et al. Endovascular stent grafting versus open surgical repair of descending thoracic aortic aneurysms in low-risk patients: a multicenter comparative trial. *J Thorac Cardiovasc Surg*. 2007;133:369-377.
15. Feezor RJ, Martin TD, Hess PJ, et al. Risk factors for perioperative stroke during thoracic endovascular aortic repairs (TEVAR). *J Endovasc Ther*. 2007;14:568-573.
16. Gutsche JT, Cheung AT, McGarvey ML, et al. Risk factors for perioperative stroke after thoracic endovascular aortic repair. *Ann Thorac Surg*. 2007;84:1195-1200.
17. Fattori R, Nienaber CA, Rousseau H, et al. Results of endovascular repair of the thoracic aorta with the talent thoracic stent graft: the talent thoracic retrospective registry. *J Thorac Cardiovasc Surg*. 2006;132:332-339.

Chapter 13 Arterial Injury

Lisbi del Valle Rivas Ramirez, Natalie M. Wall, and Paula Ferrada

DEFINITION

- Thoracic vascular injury can result from both blunt and penetrating trauma, most common being the latter. Blunt thoracic vascular trauma is rare, contributing less than 5% of traumatic vascular injuries. While penetrating trauma can involve a multitude of arterial structures within the chest, blunt thoracic vascular trauma most commonly affects the aorta and innominate arteries.[1]
- Blunt thoracic aortic injury (BTAI) accounts for 1.5% of all thoracic trauma and is associated with high prehospital mortality. For those patients who survive to hospital arrival, mortality nears upward of 50%.[2-4] Mechanism of BTAI involves substantial high-impact force, most commonly an abrupt deceleration resulting in vascular injury at the level of the aortic isthmus.[2,5] Blunt injury sustained by such force typically leads to compromise and subsequent tearing of the vessel's intima and media, resulting in formation of a dissection plane along the artery. As the intimal injury progresses to involve the vessel's adventitia, pseudoaneurysm or free rupture can occur.[2] It is this reported mechanism of injury that must make the clinician mindful of elevated mean arterial pressures and aggressive fluid resuscitation, both of which may expedite this process and ultimately worsen outcomes.
- Much like blunt aortic injury, penetrating injury to the thoracic great vessels is associated with high prehospital mortality, nearing 50%. The literature places operative mortality between 5% and 40%, dependent on factors such as initial patient acuity and concomitant injuries.[6]

PATIENT HISTORY AND PHYSICAL FINDINGS

- Workup for blunt thoracic arterial injuries should begin with an examination performed in accordance with advanced trauma life support guidelines, with initial focus on performing a thorough primary survey, ensuring adequate airway, breathing, and circulation. Indicators of major chest trauma in the setting of high-velocity impact such as steering column markings on the chest, massive hemothorax, diaphragmatic injury, pulse discrepancies between upper and/or lower extremities, tracheobronchial or esophageal injuries, and fractures of the first or second rib, manubrium, and scapula should heighten suspicion of blunt aortic injury.[2,4] Chief complaints associated with major chest trauma are nonspecific and may not necessarily be present upon patient arrival. Likewise, up to 50% of hemodynamically stable patients may have no initial physical examination evidence of blunt thoracic vascular injury.[4]
- In the case of penetrating thoracic arterial injury, physical examination findings may include overt external hemorrhage through an obvious penetrating tract or internal hemorrhage leading to hemothorax, hematoma, or cardiac tamponade. Much like in the case of blunt trauma, these patients may also present with pseudoaneurysms or intimal flaps indicative of arterial compromise. While distal pulses may be absent, the presence of such does not exclude severe arterial injury and impending catastrophe.[7]

DIFFERENTIAL DIAGNOSIS

- Chest radiograph may demonstrate widened mediastinum, absence of aortic knob, apical cap, loss of aortopulmonary window, left hemothorax, tracheal deviation, or fractures of the bony structures noted above.[2,4] While chest radiograph may provide further evidence of suspicion, the gold standard of diagnosis remains computed tomography angiography (CTA) for the clinically stable patient.[2-4] Transesophageal echocardiogram may be performed to aid in diagnostic confirmation.[2] CTA is a useful adjunct in further identifying injury pattern and structural involvement. Patients with hemodynamic instability are taken directly to the operating room for surgical exploration.[6]
- The surgical approach is largely dependent on which anatomical structure(s) is/are involved in the injury. Given this, structural assessment with radiographic evaluation is preferable to aid in operative planning if the patient's hemodynamics allow for such.

SURGICAL MANAGEMENT

Approach

- Management of thoracic vascular injury can vary from nonoperative management to open or endovascular approach. The preferred method depends on clinical presentation, type of injury, hemodynamic stability, among other factors. Nonoperative management can be done in hemodynamically stable patients with small intimal injuries. Endovascular repair is a suitable option if the patient is stable and angiography is readily available, whereas in unstable patients, open repair is the best option.

SUBCLAVIAN INJURY

- Exposure of the subclavian artery is challenging for many reasons: its location in a very small space, proximity to other important neurovascular structures, and presence in a confined bony thorax. Exposure can also take a significant amount of time when the patient is hemorrhaging, and it can require very morbid incisions. The open approach to the subclavian artery injury depends on the side of the injury and location. Supraclavicular or infraclavicular incisions are often necessary. For proximal control of the right subclavian artery injury, median sternotomy is the best approach. The left subclavian artery can be approached from a high (2nd-3rd intercostal space) left anterior thoracotomy. Claviculectomy is rarely necessary and carries significant morbidity[8] (**FIGURE 1**).
- A combination of clavicular incision with a median sternotomy is often necessary for more proximal injuries to the subclavian vessels.

Supraclavicular Incision

- On the left side the subclavian artery courses posterior and deep; therefore, this incision works better for the right subclavian.
- Incision is made parallel to the medial half of the clavicle, 1 cm above.
- The platysma and the sternocleidomastoid attachment to the clavicle are divided to expose the internal jugular vein.
- The anterior scalene muscle is exposed identifying and preserving the phrenic nerve, which runs anterior to the muscle.
- The anterior scalene muscle is divided 1 cm above the clavicle to expose the subclavian artery.

Infraclavicular Incision

- Incision starts at the inferior border of the center of the clavicle and runs lateral in the clavipectoral groove.
- The pectoralis major muscle is exposed after the incision goes through the skin and subcutaneous tissue. The muscle is then either split along its fibers' direction or divided 2 cm from its humeral insertion. If the exposure seems to be adequate we avoid dividing the muscle.
- The pectoralis minor is divided exposing the subclavian/axillary artery. The brachial plexus is in close relationship with the artery, and the vein runs inferior to the artery (**FIGURE 2**).

"Trapdoor" Incision

- For injuries of the left subclavian artery a "trapdoor" incision is described.
- It is a combination of a supraclavicular incision, a midline sternotomy across the manubrium and upper portion of the sternum, and an anterior left thoracotomy on the 3rd or 4th intercostal space (**FIGURE 3**).

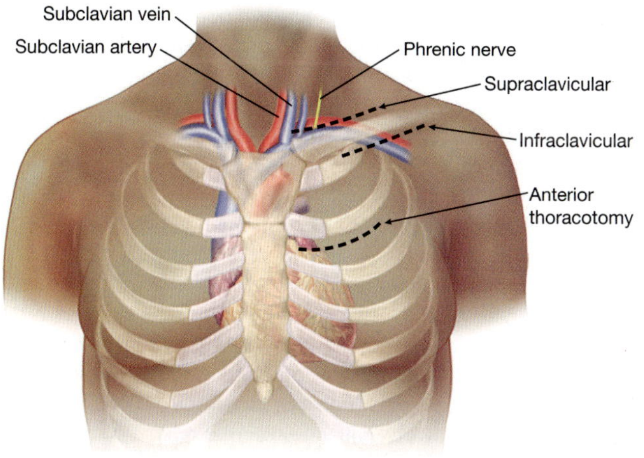

FIGURE 1 • Subclavian vessels exposure.

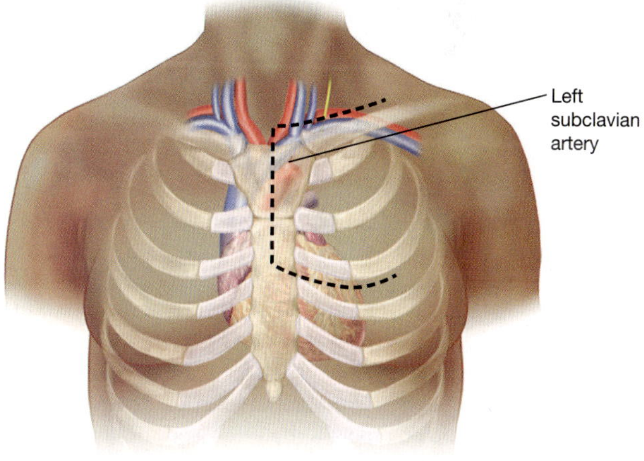

FIGURE 2 • Infraclavicular exposure.

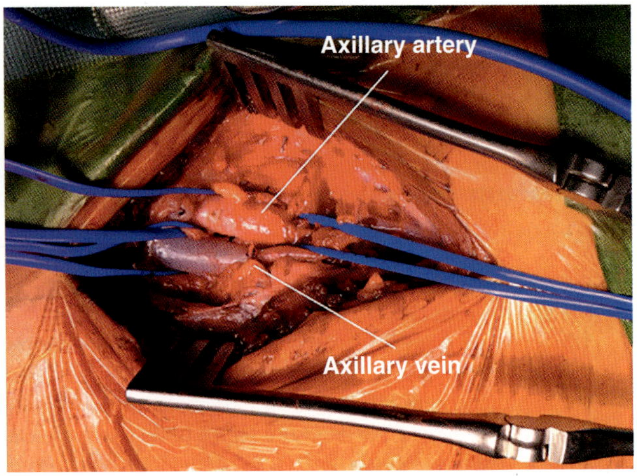

FIGURE 3 • "Trapdoor" incision.

BLUNT AORTA INJURY

- Classification of blunt aortic injury is noted in **TABLE 1**.
- While the traditional approach to operative management of blunt thoracic arterial injury involved open repair, endovascular management has replaced this as the gold standard of care.[9] Data demonstrate lower mortality associated with endovascular vs open repair of BTAI.[2,3] Open repair with systemic anticoagulation is associated with mortality rates ranging from 24% to 42%. While the risk of paraplegia, a feared complication of open repair, decreased with routine use of cardiopulmonary bypass (3% vs 7%), studies noted a subsequent increase in hemorrhagic complications given systemic anticoagulation required for circuit initiation. The benefits of endovascular repair compared with open repair for blunt aortic injury include the absence of a thoracotomy incision and its associated recovery, no single-lung ventilation requirement, less systemic anticoagulation, no cross-clamping, and markedly less estimated blood loss.[3,10]
- Initial medical management consists of blood pressure and heart rate control, allowing for "permissive hypotension" as to not expedite aortic injury and potential catastrophe.[2] Esmolol is the first-line drug of choice for blood pressure management given its quick time of onset and short half-life allowing for easy titration.
- When operative repair is indicated, understanding of the patient's anatomy is essential for an endovascular approach. A small aortic arch can pose a challenge, specifically in young patients when this is the most common. Volume depletion can also lead to undersizing the graft, which can be helped by using intravascular ultrasound. Arterial access is obtained in the common femoral arteries percutaneously or by cutdown or iliac conduit. Aortogram is performed to confirm the anatomy and define the landing zones for the device. The endograft is advanced into approximate position over a stiff wire, and the position is confirmed with repeat angiography. The device is deployed at that time with subsequent completion aortogram performed to confirm that the injury has been excluded. The left subclavian artery may need to be covered by the graft for an adequate landing zone, depending on the location of the lesion. When this is the case, it will need to be determined preprocedure if the patient possesses a dominant left vertebral artery circulation.[11]

Table 1: Blunt Aortic Injury Grading Scale

Grade		Management
GRADE 1	Intimal tear	Can be managed nonoperatively, tends to resolve on own
GRADE 2	Intramural hematoma	Medical vs operative, if imaging demonstrates advancement of injury > delayed repair
GRADE 3	Pseudoaneurysm	Endovascular repair (endografting); delayed repair > immediate if stable
GRADE 4	Free rupture	Immediate repair, most do not survive to hospital

OUTCOMES

- There is growing evidence about the use of endovascular techniques in the management of vascular injuries, particularly interesting in the management of subclavian injuries.[12] A recent multicenter review showed that management of subclavian arterial injuries still requires a wide variety of open exposures, especially for the control of active hemorrhage. Endovascular repair was used in a small percentage of cases, who were hemodynamically stable, with the most common injury type being intimal tear and pseudoaneurysm.[13]
- Outcomes between open and endovascular management of subclavian injuries has been compared. Endovascular repair, when feasible, was associated with improved mortality and lower complication rates. Long-term outcomes were not reported.[14]

REFERENCES

1. Mattox KL, Feliciano DV, Burch J, Beall AC, Jordan GL, Debakey ME. Five thousand seven hundred sixty cardiovascular injuries in 4459 patients: epidemiologic evolution 1958 to 1987. *Ann Surg.* 1989;209(6):698-707. doi:10.1097/00000658-198906000-00007
2. Mouawad NJ, Paulisin J, Hofmeister S, Thomas MB. Blunt thoracic aortic injury - concepts and management. *J Cardiothorac Surg.* 2020;15(1):1-8. doi:10.1186/s13019-020-01101-6
3. De Mestral C, Dueck A, Sharma SS, et al. Evolution of the incidence, management, and mortality of blunt thoracic aortic injury: a population-based analysis. *J Am Coll Surg.* 2013;216(6):1110-1115. doi:10.1016/j.jamcollsurg.2013.01.005
4. Mattox KL. Thoracic vascular trauma. *J Vasc Surg.* 1988;7(5):725-729. doi:10.1016/0741-5214(88)90031-6
5. Sevitt S. The mechanisms of traumatic rupture of the thoracic aorta. *Br J Surg.* 1977;64(3):166-173. doi:10.1002/bjs.1800640305
6. O'Connor JV, Scalea TM. Penetrating thoracic great vessel injury: impact of admission hemodynamics and preoperative imaging. *J Trauma Inj Infect Crit Care.* 2010;68(4):834-837. doi:10.1097/TA.0b013e3181b250df
7. Wall J, Granchi T, Liscum K, Mattox KL. Penetrating thoracic vascular injuries. *Surg Clin North Am.* 1996;76(4):749-761. doi:10.1016/s0039-6109(05)70478-3
8. McKinley AG, Abdool Carrim AT, Robbs JV. Management of proximal axillary and subclavian artery injuries. *Br J Surg.* 2000;87(1):79-85. doi:10.1046/j.1365-2168.2000.01303.x
9. Scalea TM, Feliciano DV, DuBose JJ, Ottochian M, O'Connor JV, Morrison JJ. Blunt thoracic aortic injury: endovascular repair is now the standard. *J Am Coll Surg.* 2019;228(4):605-610. doi:10.1016/j.jamcollsurg.2018.12.022
10. Takagi H, Kawai N, Umemoto T. A meta-analysis of comparative studies of endovascular versus open repair for blunt thoracic aortic injury. *J Thorac Cardiovasc Surg.* 2008;135(6):1392-1395. doi:10.1016/j.jtcvs.2008.01.033
11. Farber MA, Mendes RR. Endovascular repair of blunt thoracic aortic injury: techniques and tips. *J Vasc Surg.* 2009;50(3):683-686. doi:10.1016/j.jvs.2009.01.009
12. White R, Krajcer Z, Johnson M, Williams D, Bacharach M, O'Malley E. Results of a multicenter trial for the treatment of traumatic vascular injury with a covered stent. *J Trauma Inj Infect Crit Care.* 2006;60(6):1189-1195. doi:10.1097/01.ta.0000220372.85575.e2
13. Walker PA, May AC, Mo J, et al. Multicenter review of robotic versus laparoscopic ventral hernia repair: is there a role for robotics? *Surg Endosc.* 2018;32(4):1901-1905. doi:10.1007/s00464-017-5882-5
14. Branco BC, Boutrous ML, DuBose JJ, et al. Outcome comparison between open and endovascular management of axillosubclavian arterial injuries. Presented at the 2015 Vascular Annual Meeting of the Society for Vascular Surgery, Chicago, Ill, June 17-20, 2015. *J Vasc Surg.* 2016;63(3):702-709. doi:10.1016/j.jvs.2015.08.117

Chapter **14**

Retroperitoneal Abdominal Aortic Exposure for Visceral Aortic Endarterectomy

Matthew W. Mell

DEFINITION

- Occasionally, patients may present with visceral aortic occlusive disease that is not conducive to endovascular repair or amenable to open repair through a transabdominal approach. Open thoracoabdominal surgical revascularization of the mesenteric or renal arteries remains a useful alternative for revascularization of symptomatic visceral artery occlusive disease.
- "Coral reef aorta" is one such example (**FIGURE 1**), whereby the atherosclerotic disease is calcified and encompasses the visceral aorta, extending into the celiac axis, superior mesenteric artery, and renal arteries. For this and related conditions, a thoracoretroperitoneal approach will provide adequate exposure to perform a transaortic endarterectomy to successfully restore flow to the visceral vessels and distal aorta. It has been shown that endarterectomy provides equivalent or superior durability to other open surgical approaches.[1]

Patient History and Physical Findings

- Patients to be considered for this procedure generally present with signs and symptoms of mesenteric ischemia, including postprandial abdominal pain, food fear, weight loss, and nausea, vomiting, or diarrhea. Persistent postprandial pain may lead to food fear in 30% to 50% of patients who ameliorate symptoms by avoiding meals.[2] Weight loss, thought to be due to both decreased caloric intake and reduced nutrient absorption, is present in nearly all patients and can be substantial. Diarrhea may be present in up to 30% of patients, and occurs because of intestinal malabsorption and subsequent increased osmotic load (REF).
- Renovascular hypertension accounts for only 1% of patients with hypertension. Suggestive clinical presentations may include refractory hypertension, hypertension with retinal artery hemorrhage, acute decompensation of otherwise stable hypertension, or flash pulmonary edema. Severe stenosis of the visceral aorta may manifest as bilateral claudication. Asymptomatic visceral artery stenosis is common; as such, the presence of symptoms is a requisite to recommending repair.
- It is imperative to perform and document a baseline vascular exam for postoperative comparison.

DIFFERENTIAL DIAGNOSIS

- The differential diagnosis of chronic mesenteric ischemia is broad, and includes peptic ulcer disease, acute cholecystitis and biliary colic, acute mesenteric ischemia, biliary obstruction, cholangitis, cholecystitis, gastritis, chronic pancreatitis, diverticulitis, irritable bowel syndrome, inflammatory bowel disease and others. It is not uncommon for there to be a delay in the diagnosis of chronic mesenteric ischemia in part due to its non-specific symptoms and its relative low incidence compared with other conditions.

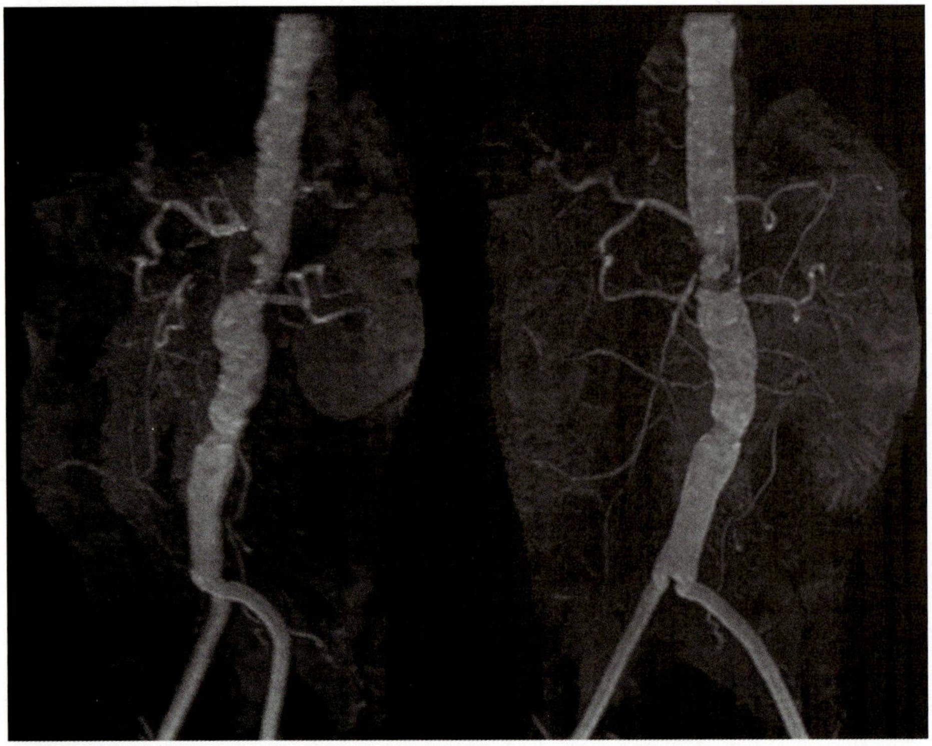

FIGURE 1 • AP and oblique view of a coral reef aorta, with severe stenosis of the celiac origin and left renal artery origin, segmental occlusion of the superior mesenteric artery, and occluded right renal artery.

- Similarly, the differential diagnosis for hypertension is broad, and other more common causes of hypertension should be considered before attributing it to renal artery stenosis.

IMAGING AND OTHER DIAGNOSTIC STUDIES

- Duplex ultrasound and physiologic testing can identify significant stenosis of the visceral vessels as well as compromise of the lower extremity perfusion.
- Elevated plasma renin levels are consistent with symptomatic renal artery stenosis.
- High-definition computed tomographic angiography (CTA) has typically been performed as part of the workup of symptoms and to rule out other causes of abdominal pain, weight loss, nausea/vomiting, or diarrhea. CTA will confirm the anatomic disease and is essential in operative planning. Relevant information in addition to ruling out other causes includes the extent and degreed of atherosclerotic disease, the presence of occluded arteries, and the quality of the thoracic and abdominal aorta in regard to safe cross-clamping.
- Angiography is generally not required but can be helpful if the CTA cannot confirm the absence of completely occluded visceral arteries. For symptomatic patients with occluded visceral arteries, endarterectomy would not be the procedure of choice. For this anatomic pattern, an antegrade or retrograde bypass may be a more suitable option.

SURGICAL MANAGEMENT

Preoperative Planning

- When considering a thoracoabdominal approach, certain factors should be considered. Previous retroperitoneal surgery or left thoracic surgery or severe illness may preclude safe access.
- Cardiac and pulmonary function should be assessed prior to surgery. Severe pre-existing pulmonary disease may lead to pneumonia, ventilator dependence, or other pulmonary complications associated with thoracotomy. Cardiac function will need to be adequate to tolerate aortic cross-clamping at the supraceliac location.
- Many patients with severe visceral occlusive disease have had significant weight loss with an abnormally low body mass index (BMI), which provides for a technically more straightforward dissection; however, an increased BMI should not in itself be considered a contraindication to a thoracoretroperitoneal approach, as with positioning an abdominal pannus generally falls away from the incision and does not impede exposure.

Positioning

- Patients undergoing aortic endarterectomy should have adequate central intravenous access, a bladder catheter, and an arterial line (preferably place in the right arm). The need for transesophageal echocardiography and double-lumen endotracheal tube should discussed in collaboration with the anesthesia team. If it is not used a nasogastric or orogastric tube should be placed. A double lumen endotracheal tube may improve access to the thoracic aorta for cross-clamping. If exposure of only the distal thoracic aorta is required, a single lumen endotracheal tube with gentle retraction of the left lower lobe may provide sufficient exposure for cross-clamping.
- After monitoring lines have been placed and induction of general anesthesia, the patient should be positioned in a modified left lateral decubitus position, with the left arm supported over the right arm and the hips positioned as flat as possible (**FIGURE 2**). A beanbag or rolled towels placed on each side of the patient will stabilize the position. The hips should be placed over the break of the table which will improve exposure when the break is utilized. The goal of positioning is to have wide access to the entire left chest, scapula, abdomen, retroperitoneum, and both groins. Cell-saver suction should be used. Baseline vascular pulse exam should be confirmed.

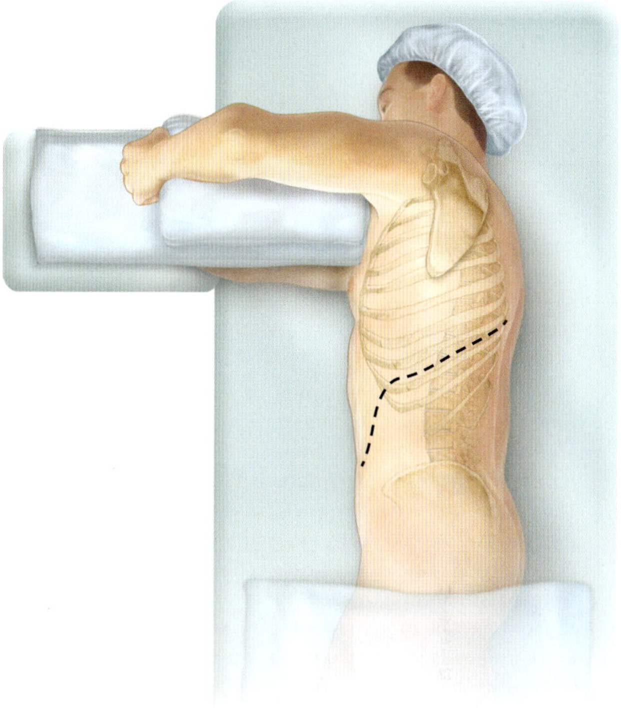

FIGURE 2 • Patient position for thoracoabdominal exposure with incision in the 8th intercostal space (dotted line). Positioning is supported with a beanbag and right axillary roll.

OPERATIVE DETAILS

- The surgeon stands on the patient's left side. After positioning, the ribs can generally been counted from below to identify the 8th intercostal space. An oblique incision is made incorporating this space, from the lateral border of the rectus sheath at or just cephalad of the umbilicus to the mid- or posterior axillary line. The incision is carried down through Scarpa fascia with electrocautery.
- For the abdominal portion of exposure, the external oblique, internal oblique, and transversus abdominal muscles are divided with electrocautery, stopping at the preperitoneal layer. This layer can frequently be identified by a layer of yellow fat just deep to the abdominal muscles. With this approach, the peritoneum should not be entered and can be repaired with absorbable sutures if it is entered inadvertently.
- The retroperitoneal approach is developed with blunt dissection, first by working centrally and inferiorly to identify the psoas muscle. Laterally, the dissection is continued behind Gerota fascia, lifting the left kidney up (**FIGURE 3**). The peritoneum may be more adherent in the left upper quadrant, and care needs to be taken as it is taken off the diaphragm to avoid entry into the peritoneum or injury to the spleen. As exposure of the retroperitoneal space is developed the aorta will be exposed, as well as the left renal artery.
- For the thoracic exposure, the dissection is carried down to the latissimus dorsi. This muscle can be divided, or preserved by dissecting along its anterior border, developing a plane deep to the muscle, and retracting it posteriorly. Preserving the latissimus dorsi will add time to the dissection and save time from the closure, and may improve pain and pulmonary toilet postoperatively. The serratus anterior muscle is divided along its fibers, and the chest wall is exposed. At this time, the correct intercostal space can be confirmed. If more proximal thoracic aortic exposure is required, a more proximal intercostal space can be used.
- The chest is then entered by incising the intercostal space, which is opened posteriorly to the spinae erector muscles and anteriorly through the costal margin where the exposure is joined with retroperitoneal dissection.
- The inferior pulmonary ligament is identified and divided along its length to facilitate retraction of the left lower lobe. The thoracic aorta can then be dissected for proximal control. Circumferential control may not be necessary, and if obtained the esophagus and intercostal arteries must be avoided. The esophagus will be behind the aorta with this approach and can be avoided by palpating the TEE probe or NG tube during the dissection. The thoracic exposure is facilitated by cutting the eighth and or ninth ribs posteriorly and placing a Burford or Finochietto retractor.
- For complete exposure of the visceral aorta, the diaphragm should be divided circumferentially from the costal margin to the aortic hiatus (**FIGURE 4**). An effective approach is to start the division at the costal margin once the peritoneum has been dissected off the diaphragm and the costal margin divided. It is important to leave a rim of 2 to 4 cm attached to the chest wall and enough of the free edge dissected free to facilitate closure at the end of the case. Dividing the median arcuate ligament from the left chest will facilitate complete division of the diaphragm.

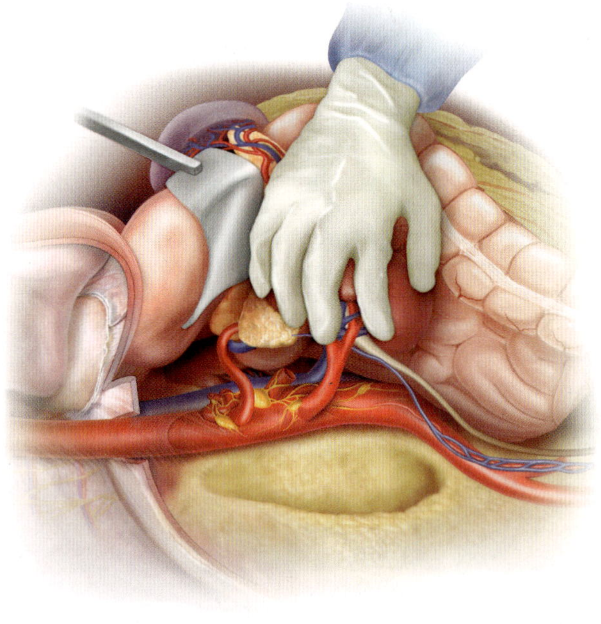

FIGURE 3 • Exposure of the visceral aorta with left kidney rotated anteriorly. This approach allows for additional exposure of the proximal superior mesenteric artery.

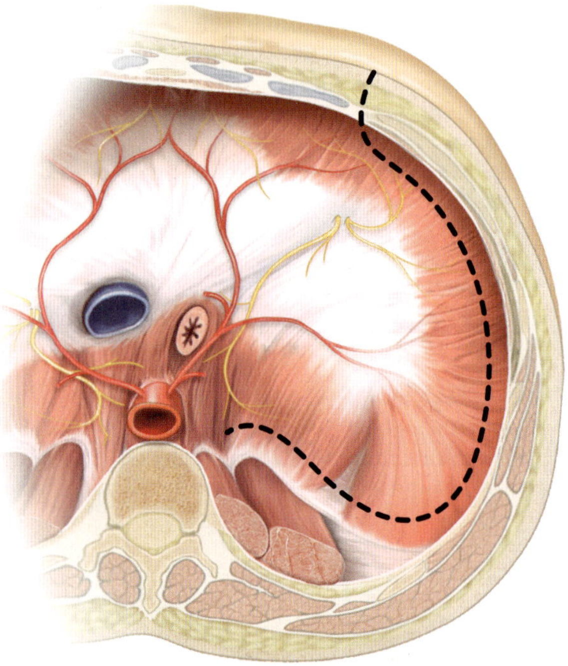

FIGURE 4 • The diaphragm is incised circumferentially (dotted line) to protect the phrenic nerve and thereby preserve diaphragmatic function. A 1 to 2 cm cuff of diaphragm is left attached to the chest was to aid in closure.

- With complete exposure of the visceral aorta the left renal artery, superior mesenteric artery (SMA), and celiac axis (CA) are addressed. If not already identified, the left renal artery is dissected and circumferentially controlled with a silastic loop. Depending on the extent of the atherosclerotic disease of the SMA and CA, a decision can be made to dissect these vessels and control them with silastic loops. If this is not performed, control can be obtained with occlusion balloons once the aorta is opened.
- At this point, the patient is given heparin (100 U/kg) to obtain an activating clotting time (ACT) of 250 to 300 seconds to be maintained throughout the cross-clamp, and 25 to 50 g of mannitol. After allowing for adequate circulation time, proximal and distal aortic clamps are placed.
- A longitudinal trap door incision is made in the aorta. This can be placed either anterior or posterior to the left renal artery orifice. Renal arteries should be cooled with 300-400 mL 4 °C saline for protection of renal function if not precluded by the plaque burden. The nondiseased left renal artery, SMA and CA are controlled with silastic loops or vascular clamps. A nondiseased right renal artery is controlled with an occlusion balloon. Control of diseased vessels requiring endarterectomy should not be initially obtained unless it can be done distal to the disease.
- The endarterectomy begins in the diseased aorta; it is performed circumferentially first at the proximal extent and then the distal extent. The plaque is transected sharply to obtain a satisfactory transition. The proximal transition generally does not require tacking sutures; distally the transition can be tacked with 5-0 prolene sutures if needed.
- The dissection plane is carried into the affected visceral vessels (**FIGURE 5**). At times, endarterectomy of these vessels may be simplified by first removing the aortic plaque, leaving postage stamp-sized aortic plaque at the orifices of the visceral vessels. This technique allows for endarterectomy of the branch vessels without the burden of the large aortic plaque and better control of the endarterectomy with feathering of the endpoints. As the atherosclerotic disease generally does not extend deep into the visceral vessels, the endpoint is generally easily obtained. If the feathering is inadequate, the plaque can be excised sharply and the transition tacked with 7-0 prolene sutures.
- When the endarterectomy is complete, there may be significant back-bleeding from the visceral arteries or lumbar arteries. Lumbar vessels, if they were occluded prior to the endarterectomy, can safely be suture-ligated for hemostasis without concern of spinal cord ischemia. Those that were patent should be preserved if possible. Significant back-bleeding from the left renal artery can be controlled with a vascular clamp or silastic loop. Back-bleeding from the right renal artery can be controlled with an occlusion balloon. Back-bleeding from the SMA and CA can be controlled with either technique. Control of these vessels also will protect from embolization when forward flow is re-established.
- The aortic incision is then closed directly with 3-0 or 4-0 running prolene, supported with pledgets if needed. Patch repair is generally not required. The shafts of the balloon occlusion catheters can be incorporated temporarily in the closure. Prior to completing closure, the visceral vessels and distal aorta are individually back flushed, and the proximal aorta is flushed. Flow is established serially to the visceral arteries and then distal aorta.
- Communication with the anesthesia team is key when preparing to re-establish antegrade flow, as blood pressure support will likely be required with volume and pressors. Flow should be established gradually to avoid uncontrolled hypotension.
- With closure complete the repair is inspected for hemostasis, and adequate flow in all vessels is confirmed with palpation and Doppler ultrasound. If concerns are present for the visceral vessels, intraoperative duplex can be performed to identify any anatomic obstruction to flow. Abnormalities if noted can be addressed with a variety of techniques, including embolectomy for thrombosis/embolization, excision with or without tacking for endothelial flaps, placement of visceral stents under direct vision, or bypass. If there is concern for

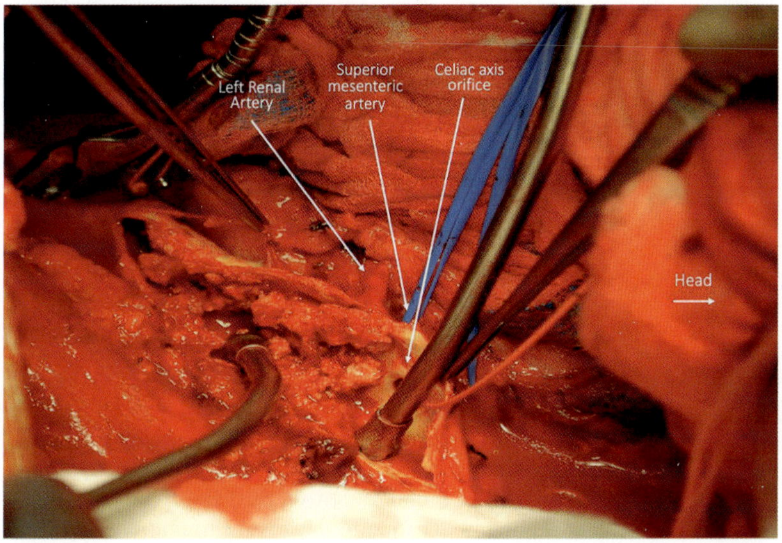

FIGURE 5 • Intraoperative exposure and endarterectomy of a coral reef aortic plaque.

intestinal ischemia, the peritoneum can be opened and inspected directly.

- Once reconstruction is deemed adequate, heparin is reversed with an appropriate dose of protamine. Retractors are released and the operating table break is flattened. Two drains are placed through separate incisions in the thoracic cavity, one inferiorly and the other at the apex. The diaphragm is closed with PDS suture from the aortic hiatus to the costal margin. Usually, this can be done is a running fashion, at times facilitated with interrupted sutures reapproximating the costal margin. Absorbable interrupted sutures are placed to reapproximate the chest wall. The left lobe is inflated and the chest closed. This step may facilitate completing the diaphragmatic closure.
- The serratus anterior is reapproximated as is the latissimus dorsi if it was divided. The abdominal wall muscles are closed in layers. Scarpa fascia is reapproximated and the skin is closed.

PEARLS AND PITFALLS

Location of other visceral arteries	■ Identifying the left renal artery early can be helpful in orienting to the location of the other visceral arteries, and to identify and expose the infrarenal aorta for exposure and distal cross-clamping.
Exposure	■ If possible the retroperitoneal and thoracic exposure can be performed simultaneously by two teams. This strategy will allow for a more efficient dissection and provide for better exposure of the visceral aortic segment. ■ Self-retaining retractor systems will aid with exposure. Each (Buckwalter, Omni, Martin arm, etc.) has its benefits and limitations, and the decision of which to choose should be at the discretion, comfort, and human resources of the surgical team.
Positioning	■ With the patient in a lateral decubitus position, knowledge for the directionality of the visceral arteries will facilitate their safe exposure. The left renal artery origin will be directed toward the operating surgeon and toward the ceiling with the kidney retracted anteriorly, and will be found just caudal to where the median arcuate ligament was divided (ie, more cephalad than might be expected). The SMA and CA will be found on the anterior aortic surface, traveling up and away from the operating surgeon.
Equipment and tools	■ Compliant occlusion balloons with a stopcock are a convenient tool for direct endoluminal control of the visceral arteries. They can be left in place until the aortotomy closure is complete by placing throws on each size of the balloon shaft. Balloons can be slid out afterward, and any suture line bleeding from gaps caused by the balloon occlusion catheters can be repaired with interrupted prolene sutures.

POSTOPERATIVE CARE

- In addition to routine postoperative care, there are specific areas of focus when recovering these patients. This includes early and aggressive fluid resuscitation, as third-spacing may be significant in the first 48 hours. Generous urine output may not accurately reflect fluid status, as with the mannitol and the supraceliac clamping, urine output may reflect the osmotic load as well as mild nonoliguric acute kidney injury. It is common for the serum creatinine to rise over the first 2 days before trending to normal. When third-space fluid is mobilized, fluid requirements will decrease, and diuresis may be necessary.
- Routine vascular checks should be performed to confirm no decline from baseline. Patients with significant aortic lumen compromise can be expected to have an improved vascular exam postoperatively.
- Mesenteric revascularization after severe compromise can lead to hyperactive peristalsis, sometimes while the incision is still open. Under these circumstances, serial examination for bowel sounds in the first 24 hours can provide clues to the continued patency of the revascularization. Serial lactate levels can also be checked. Although immediate postoperative lactate levels are elevated, they should return to normal as the patient is warmed and resuscitated. Coagulation parameters may also be elevated initially in response to blood loss and transient hepatic ischemia. These parameters should be monitored and corrected for active bleeding; normal values are usually present by the first postoperative day.
- Chest tubes should be kept in place until any air leaks resolve and drainage decreases to less than 50 mL per shift, nasogastric tube removed with return of function, and bladder catheter until diuresis is complete and close monitoring of urine output is no longer necessary.

COMPLICATIONS

- In addition to the complications associated with a thoracoabdominal incision, complications specific to this procedure include embolization or thrombosis of the visceral arteries or embolization to the lower extremities.

- Thrombosis of a renal artery, unless it is quickly identified, generally leads to irreversible renal infarct.
- Thrombosis of the SMA or celiac artery may be asymptomatic; however, signs and symptoms of intestinal ischemia warrant urgent evaluation with CTA and intervention, either operative or endovascular depending on the anatomic defect, the interval between the index operation and the complication, and the likelihood of compromised bowel.
- Acute kidney injury is a potential but uncommon complication.[3-5] Contributing factors include hypoperfusion, hypovolemia, or renal artery thrombosis. Workup includes duplex ultrasound to identify reversible causes of acute kidney injury.
- While possible, spinal cord ischemia is unlikely with this procedure. As such, a spinal drain is typically not required unless there are other concerns such as subclavian artery occlusion or severe aortoiliac disease for compromised preoperative spinal cord circulation. Postoperative neurologic checks should be performed, focusing on both proximal and distal motor function of the lower extremities.

REFERENCES

1. Mell MW, Acher CW, Hoch JR, Tefera G, Turnipseed WD. Outcomes after endarterectomy for chronic mesenteric ischemia. *J Vasc Surg*. 2008;48(5):1132-1138.
2. ter Steege RW, Sloterdijk HS, Geelkerken RH, Huisman AB, van der Palen J, Kolkman JJ. Splanchnic artery stenosis and abdominal complaints: clinical history is of limited value in detection of gastrointestinal ischemia. *World J Surg*. 2012;36(4):793-799. doi:10.1007/s00268-012-1485-4. PMID: 22354487; PMCID: PMC3299959.
3. Kasirajan K, O'Hara PJ, Gray BH, et al. Chronic mesenteric ischemia: open surgery versus percutaneous angioplasty and stenting. *J Vasc Surg*. 2001;33(1):63-71.
4. Rapp JH, Reilly LM, Qvarfordt PG, Goldstone J, Ehrenfeld WK, Stoney RJ. Durability of endarterectomy and antegrade grafts in the treatment of chronic visceral ischemia. *J Vasc Surg*. 1986;3(5):799-806.
5. Weibull H, Bergqvist D, Bergentz SE, Jonsson K, Hulthen L, Manhem P. Percutaneous transluminal renal angioplasty versus surgical reconstruction of atherosclerotic renal artery stenosis: a prospective randomized study. *J Vasc Surg*. 1993;18(5):841-850; discussion 850-842.

Chapter 15

Hybrid Revascularization Strategies for Visceral/Renal Arteries

Benjamin W. Starnes

DEFINITION

- The term "hybrid" in vascular surgery traditionally refers to the use of *both* traditional open surgical and endovascular techniques for remedy of the vascular condition (**FIGURE 1**).
- Two hybrid approaches are described in this chapter:
  - Complete visceral debranching and endovascular tube graft repair
  - Partial visceral debranching and physician-modified fenestrated endovascular repair

DIFFERENTIAL DIAGNOSIS

- Paravisceral aortic aneurysms may develop due to the following conditions:
  - Degenerative aneurysm
  - Aortic dissection
  - Mycotic aneurysm
  - Paraanastomotic juxtarenal aneurysm
  - Connective tissue disorders (Marfan syndrome)
  - Behçet syndrome

PATIENT HISTORY AND PHYSICAL FINDINGS

- The majority of patients are asymptomatic and the diagnosis is made with imaging done for other reasons. Some patients will complain of mild to moderate abdominal and low back pain. Severe and unrelenting pain should raise the index of suspicion for a mycotic process which, if confirmed, would make hybrid approaches prohibitive.

IMAGING AND OTHER DIAGNOSTIC STUDIES

- Contrast-enhanced, axial thin-slice computed tomography arteriography (CTA) is the current standard for imaging paravisceral aneurysms. Detailed information can be gathered regarding the precise origin of the celiac, superior mesenteric artery (SMA), and renal arteries (**FIGURE 2**).
- Other important findings on CTA should be as follows:
  - Size and quality of access vessels for delivery of endovascular devices (>7 mm)
  - Location of left renal vein
  - Aberrant anatomy (eg, replaced right hepatic artery)
  - Quality of gastroduodenal artery for possible celiac artery ligation or sacrifice
  - Renal cortical thickness

SURGICAL MANAGEMENT

- Indications for repair include aortic aneurysms of more than 5.5 cm, symptoms, or evidence of rapid expansion (>0.5 cm per 6 months).

Preoperative Planning

- As formal open repair would often include a bicavitary incision (chest and abdomen, as in a formal thoracoabdominal repair), the standard preoperative assessment should focus on the patient's fitness to undergo major vascular surgery. This includes assessment of the heart, lung, and kidney function and reserve.

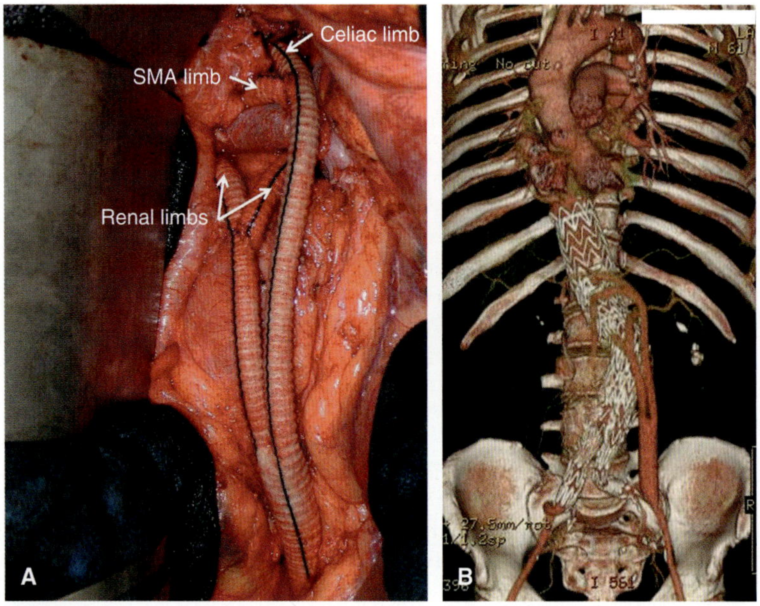

FIGURE 1 • "Hybrid repair" refers to the use of both traditional open surgical and endovascular techniques to manage the same problem. SMA, superior mesenteric artery. **A,** Intraoperative photo. **B,** Postoperative computed tomography arteriography after completed repair.

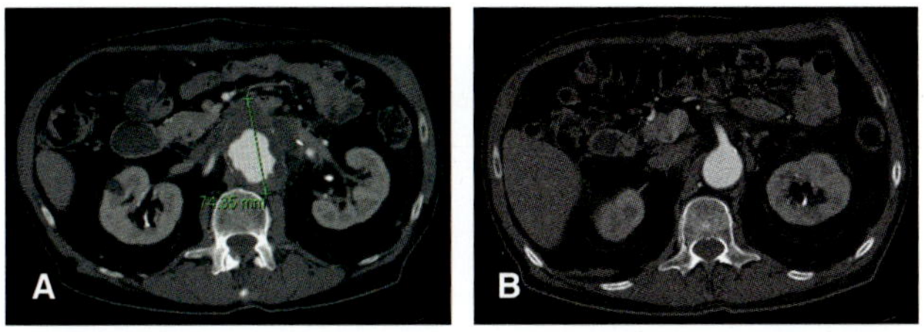

FIGURE 2 Computed tomography arteriography axial images depicting **(A)** a 7.4-cm paraanastomotic juxtarenal aortic aneurysm and **(B)** a healthy aortic segment in the region of the superior mesenteric artery.

Positioning

- Proper and precise positioning should be as follows (**FIGURE 3**):
  - Patient supine on standard operating room (OR) table or imaging table
  - Hair properly clipped over entire abdomen and both groins
  - Both arms tucked (option to have right arm at 90° if planning brachial access)
  - Foley under one leg and padded

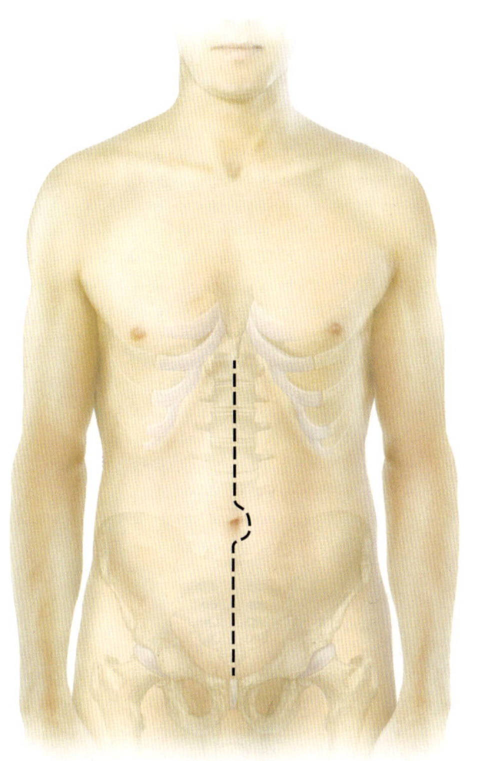

FIGURE 3 • Depiction of positioning and intended incision in the midline.

COMPLETE VISCERAL DEBRANCHING AND ENDOVASCULAR TUBE GRAFT REPAIR—STAGE 1

First Step—Exposure

- Standard midline laparotomy and positioning of retractor system.
- Upon entry into the abdomen, the falciform ligament is divided between clamps and ligated. The triangular ligaments above the liver are divided to facilitate adequate exposure/retraction while minimizing risk of hepatic capsular injury, anticipating systemic anticoagulation later in the procedure.
- A nasogastric tube is positioned in the stomach to provide temporary decompression. The common hepatic artery is identified following division of the gastrohepatic ligament and traced back to origin of celiac artery. Once identified, the target artery is encircled with a silastic vessel loop. Space is created along the left side of the aorta with blunt/finger dissection, beginning at the level of the celiac artery, to create the retrograde bypass tunnel posterior to the pancreas (**FIGURE 4**).
- The colon and omentum are lifted in a cephalad direction, the small bowel swept to the patient's right and packed in moist towels. Self-retaining retractors (Omni or Bookwalter) should be positioned at this juncture to maintain exposure, with care taken to appropriately pad the retractor blades as necessary.
- The third and fourth portions of the duodenum are mobilized to the right following division of the ligament of Treitz, exposing the anterior surface of the aorta. The inferior mesenteric vein is ligated and divided as well and the dissection continued along the proximal aorta until the left renal vein is clearly identified (**FIGURE 5**).
- Widely mobilize the left renal vein sharply and encircle with a moist umbilical tape. The self-retaining renal vein retractor blade is used to retract the left renal vein cephalad as necessary to facilitate further exposure.
- The origin of the renal arteries is identified by careful posterolateral dissection around the aorta, just cephalad of the overlying renal vein. Exposure on the right is complicated somewhat by the overlying inferior vena cava/left renal vein confluence. At least 2 cm of renal artery should be exposed bilaterally. Encircle the renal arteries with silastic vessel loops. On the left, fingers dissect bluntly along the aorta in a cephalad fashion to complete the retropancreatic tunnel for the celiac limb of the bypass graft.
- The SMA is identified next by palpation within the base of the small bowel mesentery, directly anterior to the pancreas. Doppler ultrasonography may assist identification when the pulse is faint. Once identified, a 3-cm segment of SMA is isolated as proximal as possible to the root of the mesentery. Beginning with the middle colic artery, multiple mesenteric arteries quickly branch from the SMA as it emerges from the pancreas, underscoring the need for proximal identification and isolation. The SMA is controlled with vessel loops.
- The next step is to prepare the donor artery for hybrid bypass. The specific artery—most commonly the common or external iliac arteries—should be selected from the preoperative imaging study. The retroperitoneum is opened directly over

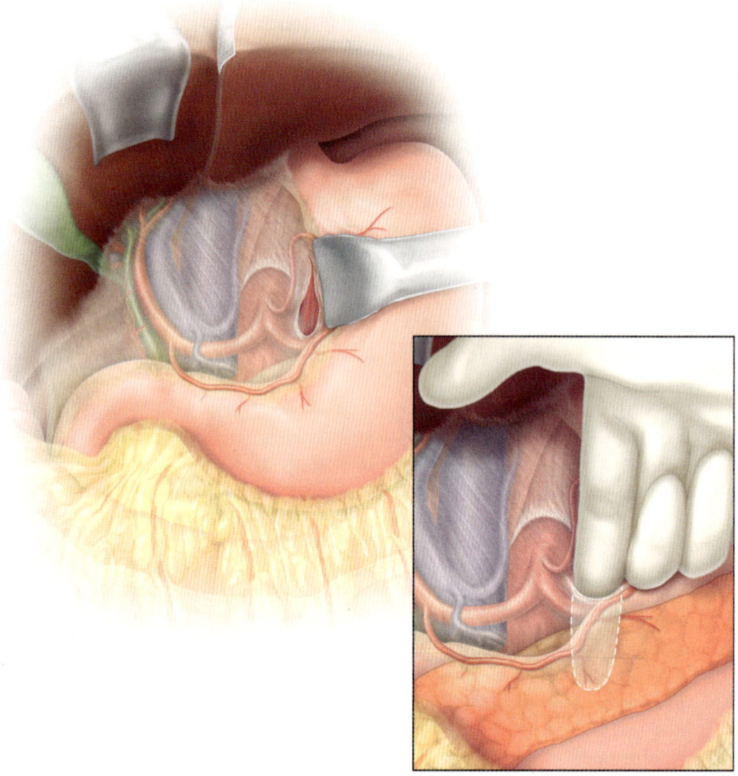

FIGURE 4 • Drawing of exposure of the celiac artery through the lesser sac. Note the blunt finger dissection along the left side of the aorta and behind the pancreas.

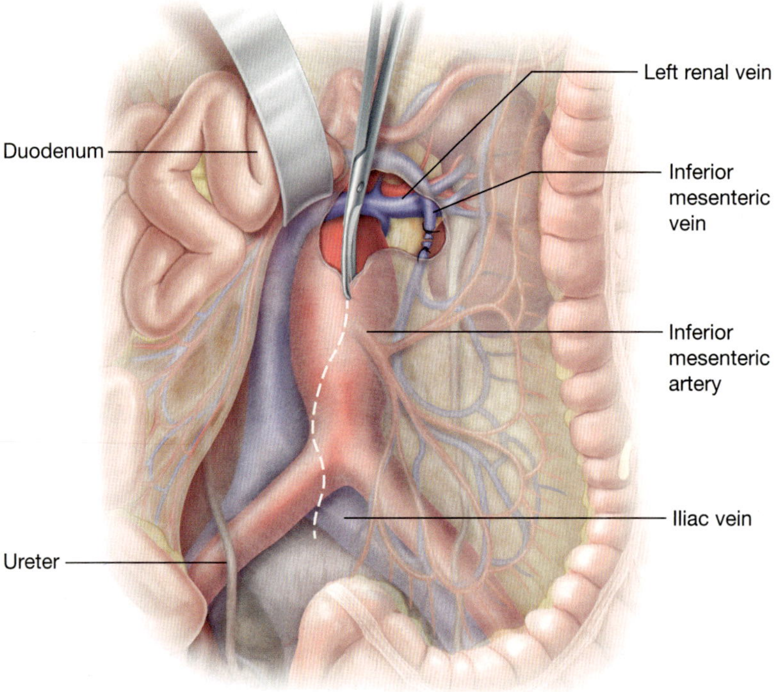

FIGURE 5 • Drawing of exposure of the left renal vein and anterior surface of the aortic aneurysm. Dashed line depicts intended incision line to avoid nervi erigentes.

the selected donor artery, which is exposed while protecting the adjacent ureter. Alternatively, donor artery exposure may be achieved via medial-visceral rotation, developing the entire retroperitoneal plane on the left. The latter approach provides the added benefit of exclusion of the graft from the viscera and abdominal contents once the viscera are returned to their original position. This maneuver adds significantly more time to the case, however, and contributes to increased blood loss. Graft coverage can also be obtained without developing the entire retroperitoneal plane, either via direct tunneling along the preferred course of the graft or creation of an omental tongue affixed directly to the graft.

Second Step—Anticoagulation

- Systemic anticoagulation is achieved with a bolus injection of unfractionated heparin, 50 U/kg. Monitoring activated clotting time is a useful method of maintaining adequate anticoagulation during the procedure.

Third Step—Multivisceral Bypass

- Trifurcated grafts exist for the purpose of facilitating multivessel hybrid revascularization, but the use of these is limited by the tendency of the middle limb to occlude when "squeezed" between the outside limbs during graft routing and abdominal closure. In most circumstances, a standard 12 × 7 bifurcated, collagen-impregnated knitted polyester graft provides excellent conduits for bilateral renal revascularization, with a separate 8-mm limb connected to the celiac and SMA. Examples of bypass graft configurations are shown in **FIGURES 6** and **7**.
- The proximal (iliac/inflow) anastomosis is completed first with running 4-0 or 5-0 polypropylene suture.
- The next anastomosis to be completed should be one anticipated to be the technically most difficult, given exposure and graft routing issues. Most commonly, this is the right renal artery. This is divided following placement of a large clip at the origin. The appropriate graft limb is pulled to length and anastomosed end-to-end with 5-0 polypropylene suture. The limb and artery are flushed just prior to completion of the graft, after which the clamps are released to reperfuse the kidney. Following this sequence, warm renal ischemia time is generally less than 12 minutes. The stump of the right renal artery is then suture ligated; avoid clip dislodgement. Note: Excessive traction on the confluence of the left renal vein and vena cava may cause caval injury and massive hemorrhage during preparation and completion of the right renal artery anastomosis. Retractor positioning needs to account for potential venous injury during exposure and significantly relaxed following completion of the anastomosis.
- The left renal anastomosis is completed in nearly identical fashion, minus many of the exposure limitations present on the right.
- The SMA graft is carefully sized to length so that it follows a "C"-shaped configuration without kinking. Inflow can be obtained either from the many bodies of the graft or either of the completed renal limbs. The SMA graft anastomosis is completed end-to-side with interrupted or running 5-0 polypropylene suture. The end-to-side arteriotomy length is 1.5 to 2 times the width of the bypass graft (12-16 mm). Alternatively, end-to-end anastomotic configuration may reduce the likelihood of graft kinking depending on final configuration. Following completion of the anastomosis, the proximal SMA is ligated with a large clip or circumference suture. Again, ischemia time should be under 10 to 12 minutes.
- Typically, following SMA and renal graft completion, repositioning of the retraction system is necessary to reobtain and optimize celiac artery exposure. Prior to reexposing the celiac, a vascular clamp is repassed through the retropancreatic tunnel left of the aorta. This position is then maintained until the transverse colon and mesocolon are reduced to their usual location. This reexposes the "looped" celiac and common hepatic arteries previously isolated in the lesser sac. The

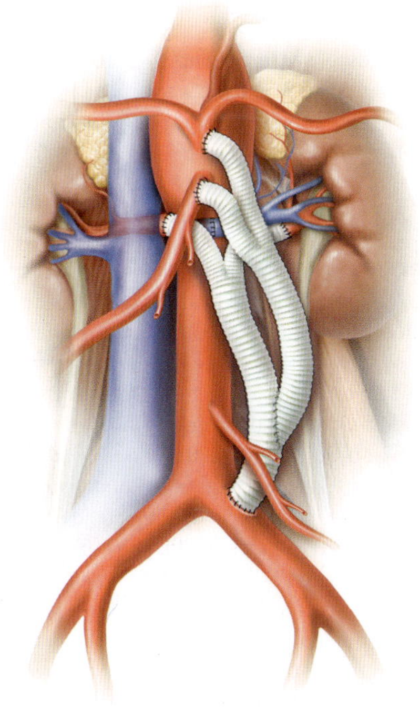

FIGURE 6 • Drawing of a four-vessel debranching based on the left common iliac artery. Note that the left renal vein was divided in this case, and subsequently repaired, for better exposure of the renal arteries.

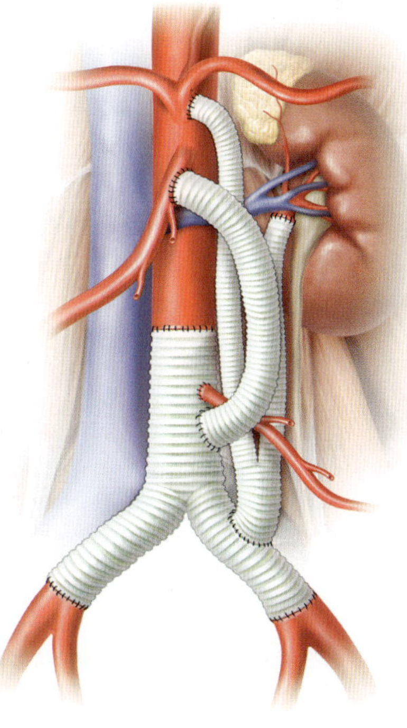

FIGURE 7 • Aortobiiliac and subsequent debranching for a patient with a solitary left kidney and infrarenal aneurysm.

clamp tip exiting the retrohepatic tunnel is identified, and a moist umbilical tape is pulled through the tunnel. Following this, the celiac limb is tied to the umbilical tape, which is then pulled cephalad behind the pancreas and into position for either end-to-end or end-to-side anastomosis. Care again needs to be taken to optimize limb routing and length to minimize risk for kinking.

- After coverage of remaining exposed graft limbs with omentum or parietal peritoneum as appropriate, standard abdominal closure is performed.

COMPLETE VISCERAL DEBRANCHING AND ENDOVASCULAR TUBE GRAFT REPAIR—STAGE 2

First Step—Percutaneous Access

- Following the "debranching" procedure described in stage 1, endovascular aneurysm repair (EVAR) may be performed either at the same setting or within several weeks of the initial procedure. The risk of potential aneurysm rupture associated with a staged approach needs to be balanced with the additional operative risk inherent in the longer anesthetic time required to complete both stages in one sitting. For the EVAR procedure itself, standard percutaneous access to an appropriately sized access vessel is obtained using Seldinger technique and a wire advanced into the aorta under fluoroscopic guidance. In our practice, this is most commonly obtained percutaneously, using ultrasound guidance and preplacement of polypropylene suture prior to dilation of the access sites (also known as the "preclose" Perclose technique) (Abbott Vascular Inc., Redwood City, CA).[1] An 11-Fr standard sheath is placed into the common femoral artery and flushed with heparinized saline. Wire advancement from the femoral artery to the aortic arch must be visualized radiographically throughout its course, as the wire may preferentially enter the debranching graft and cause end-organ injury or hemorrhage without real-time position monitoring and guidance.

Second Step—Stiff Wire Exchange

- After wire advancement to the transverse aortic arch, standard wire exchange technique is used to position a 0.035-in stiff (eg, Lunderquist, Cook Medical, Bloomington, IN) wire through the abdominal and thoracic aorta. Optimal final wire positioning is at/just distal to the left subclavian artery orifice.

Third Step—Intravascular Ultrasound

- An 8.2-Fr Visions catheter (Volcano Therapeutics, Irvine, CA) is used to confirm appropriate proximal and distal landing zones for endovascular graft placement. The optimal graft size and configuration is determined by analysis of CTA images reformatted and visualized on a dedicated 3D image workstation (AquariusNet, TeraRecon, Inc., San Mateo, CA). Graft diameter should be oversized by 10% to 15% for this application.
- During advancement of the device, the origin of the debranching graft can also be visualized either through fluoroscopic confirmation of a metallic clip placed during the debranching procedure or under intravascular ultrasound (IVUS) real-time guidance. Using IVUS, the position of the IVUS catheter is marked on the fluoroscopic monitor when the catheter itself recognizes the orifice of the debranched graft. Alternatively, a contrast power injection can be performed through an appropriately positioned arteriographic catheter with 30 mL of contrast injected at 15 mL per second to confirm the proximal and distal landing zones.

Fourth Step—Endograft Deployment

- The endovascular graft is deployed following device-specific instructions for use (IFU), covering the native origins of the visceral vessels and excluding the aortic aneurysm. The femoral arteriotomy is then closed.

PARTIAL VISCERAL DEBRANCHING AND PHYSICIAN-MODIFIED ENDOVASCULAR REPAIR—STAGE 1

First Step—Exposure

- Standard midline laparotomy and positioning of retractor system.
- Upon entry into the abdomen, the falciform ligament is divided between clamps and ligated. The triangular ligaments above the liver are divided to facilitate adequate exposure/retraction while minimizing the risk of hepatic capsular injury, anticipating systemic anticoagulation later in the procedure.
- A nasogastric tube is positioned in the stomach to provide temporary decompression. The common hepatic artery is identified following division of the gastrohepatic ligament and traced back to origin of celiac artery. Once identified, the target artery is encircled with a silastic vessel loop. Space is created along the left side of the aorta with blunt/finger dissection, beginning at the level of the celiac artery, to create the retrograde bypass tunnel posterior to the pancreas.
- The colon and omentum are lifted in a cephalad direction, the small bowel swept to the patient's right and packed in moist towels. Self-retaining retractors (Omni or Bookwalter) should be positioned at this juncture to maintain exposure, with care taken to appropriately pad the retractor blades as necessary.
- The third and fourth portions of the duodenum are mobilized to the right following division of the ligament of Treitz, exposing the anterior surface of the aorta. The inferior mesenteric vein is ligated and divided as well and the dissection continued along the proximal aorta until the left renal vein is clearly identified.
- Widely mobilize the left renal vein sharply and encircle with a moist umbilical tape. The self-retaining renal vein retractor blade is used to retract the left renal vein cephalad as necessary to facilitate further exposure.
- The origin of the renal arteries is identified by careful posterolateral dissection around the aorta, just cephalad of the overlying renal vein. Exposure on the right is complicated somewhat

by the overlying inferior vena cava/left renal vein confluence. At least 2 cm of renal artery should be exposed bilaterally. Encircle the renal arteries with silastic vessel loops. On the left, finger dissect bluntly along the aorta in a cephalad fashion to complete the retropancreatic tunnel for the celiac limb of the bypass graft.

- The SMA is identified next by palpation within the base of the small bowel mesentery, directly anterior to the pancreas. Doppler ultrasonography may assist identification when the pulse is faint. Once identified, a 3-cm segment of SMA is isolated as proximal as possible to the root of the mesentery. Beginning with the middle colic artery, multiple mesenteric arteries quickly branch from the SMA as it emerges from the pancreas, underscoring the need for proximal identification and isolation. The SMA is controlled with vessel loops.
- The next step is to prepare the donor artery for hybrid bypass. The specific artery—most commonly the common or external iliac arteries—should be selected from the preoperative imaging study. The retroperitoneum is opened directly over the selected donor artery, which is exposed while protecting the adjacent ureter. Alternatively, donor artery exposure may be achieved via medial-visceral rotation, developing the entire retroperitoneal plane on the left. The latter approach provides the added benefit of exclusion of the graft from the viscera and abdominal contents once the viscera are returned to their original position. This maneuver adds significantly more time to the case, however, and contributes to increased blood loss. Graft coverage can also be obtained without developing the entire retroperitoneal plane, either via direct tunneling along the preferred course of the graft or creation of an omental tongue affixed directly to the graft.

Second Step—Anticoagulation

- Systemic anticoagulation is achieved with a bolus injection of unfractionated heparin, 50 units/kg. Monitoring activated clotting time is a useful method of maintaining adequate anticoagulation during the procedure.

Third Step—Multivisceral Bypass

- Trifurcated grafts exist for the purpose of facilitating multivessel hybrid revascularization, but the use of these is limited by the tendency of the middle limb to occlude when squeezed between the outside limbs during graft routing and abdominal closure. In most circumstances, a standard 12 × 7 bifurcated, collagen-impregnated knitted polyester graft provides excellent conduits for bilateral renal revascularization, with a separate 8-mm limb connected to the celiac and SMA. Examples of bypass graft configurations are shown in **FIGURES 6** and **7**.
- The proximal (iliac/inflow) anastomosis is completed first with running 4-0 or 5-0 polypropylene suture.
- The next anastomosis to be completed should be one anticipated to be the technically most difficult, given exposure and graft routing issues. Most commonly, this is the right renal artery. This is divided following the placement of a large clip at the origin. The appropriate graft limb is pulled to length and anastomosed end-to-end with 5-0 polypropylene suture. The limb and artery are flushed just prior to completion of the graft, after which the clamps are released to reperfuse the kidney. Following this sequence, warm renal ischemia time is generally less than 12 minutes. The stump of the right renal artery is then suture ligated; avoid clip dislodgement. Note: Excessive traction on the confluence of the left renal vein and vena cava may cause caval injury and massive hemorrhage during preparation and completion of the right renal artery anastomosis. Retractor positioning needs to account for potential venous injury during exposure and significantly relaxed following completion of the anastomosis.
- The renal anastomosis is completed in nearly identical fashion, minus many of the exposure limitations present on the right.

PARTIAL VISCERAL DEBRANCHING AND PHYSICIAN-MODIFIED ENDOVASCULAR REPAIR—STAGE 2[2]

First Step—Creation of a Fenestrated Graft for the Celiac and Superior Mesenteric Artery

- The appropriate endovascular device is chosen according to standard IFU sizing guidelines, typically incorporating 10% to 15% oversizing. The sterile graft is unsheathed on a dedicated sterile table in the OR and marked with the relative locations (length from proximal end and clockface measurements) of the celiac and SMA fenestrations as previously determined via TeraRecon workstation analysis. Minor adjustments are allowed to minimize strut overlap of planned fenestration locations. Fenestrations in the polyester endograft fabric are created with a disposable ophthalmic cautery to minimize fraying. The fenestrations are outlined and reinforced with 15-mm gold Amplatz Gooseneck snares (ev3 Endovascular, Inc., Plymouth, MN). These are hand sewn into place using 4-0 Prolene suture in a double row circumferentially (**FIGURE 8**). Diameter-reducing ties were then used to constrain the device along its posterior border (opposite the SMA and or celiac fenestration at 6-o'clock) by rerouting the existing proximal trigger wire through and through the graft material at the midportion of each of the top two Z stents. The constraining ties are then tied down into place over the trigger wire. The entire graft is then wetted with heparinized saline and then reloaded into the existing sheath.

Second Step—Percutaneous Access

- Standard percutaneous access to an appropriately sized access vessel is obtained using Seldinger technique. The initial guidewire is advanced into the aorta under fluoroscopic guidance. In our practice, this is most commonly obtained percutaneously, using ultrasound guidance and preplacement of polypropylene suture prior to dilation of the access sites (also known as the "preclose" Perclose technique) (Abbott Vascular Inc., Redwood City, CA).[1] An 11-Fr standard sheath is placed into the

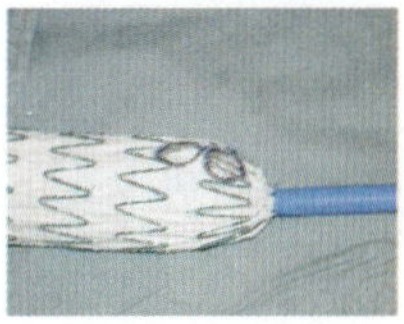

FIGURE 8 Photograph of a thoracic endograft with two fenestrations created for the celiac (struts present) and superior mesenteric artery (strut free), prior to resheathing and deployment.

common femoral artery and flushed with heparinized saline. Wire advancement from the femoral artery to the aortic arch must be visualized radiographically throughout its course, as the wire may preferentially enter the debranching graft and cause end-organ renal injury, rupture of Gerota fascia, and retroperitoneal hemorrhage without real-time position monitoring and guidance.

Third Step—Stiff Wire Exchange

- A standard 4-Fr or 5-Fr catheter is used to perform a wire exchange to a stiff 0.035-in Lunderquist wire (Cook Medical, Bloomington, IN). The wire is positioned so that its tip is just distal to the left subclavian artery.

Fourth Step—Marking of the Target Vessels and Graft Deployment

- A contrast power injection can be performed with 10 mL of contrast injected at 25 mL per second to mark the precise origins of the celiac and SMA (**FIGURE 9**). The modified graft is positioned over the target vessels, oriented, and deployed.

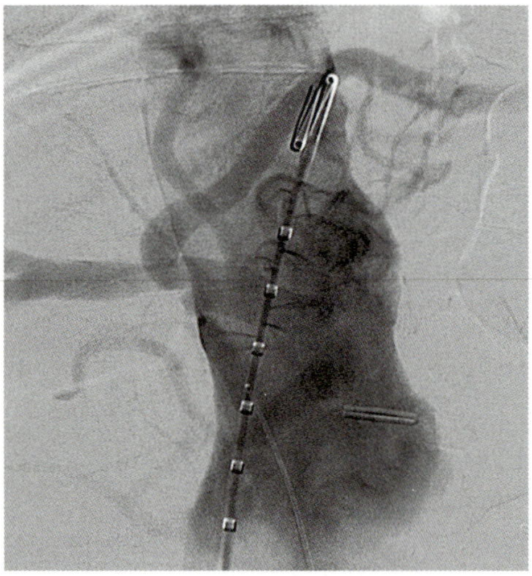

FIGURE 9 Note the double densities depicting the origins of the celiac and superior mesenteric artery on this flush aortogram.

Fifth Step—Cannulation of the Target Vessels

- An 18-Fr sheath is advanced from the contralateral groin and into the distal graft over a stiff wire. Two 7-Fr Raabe sheaths (Cook Medical, Bloomington, IN) are advanced together through the 18-Fr sheath. Working through these sheaths, the SMA and celiac vessels are selected through the fenestrations using standard catheter and guidewire techniques, with the sheaths ultimately advanced into the target vessels over stiff wires.
- After sheath advancement and confirmation of target vessel acquisition, the main body is distended flush with the surrounding aorta with a molding balloon (eg, Coda, Cook Medical, Bloomington, IN). This inflation represents the final opportunity to distend the endograft in the region of the visceral stents. Lateral positioning of the image intensifier guides stent placement into the SMA and celiac arteries (typically 8- to 9-mm stents; **FIGURE 10**). **FIGURE 11** shows follow-up computed tomography imaging of a patient 1 year after successful treatment with this technique.

Sixth Step—Access Site Closure

- The access sites are closed with the previously placed sutures.

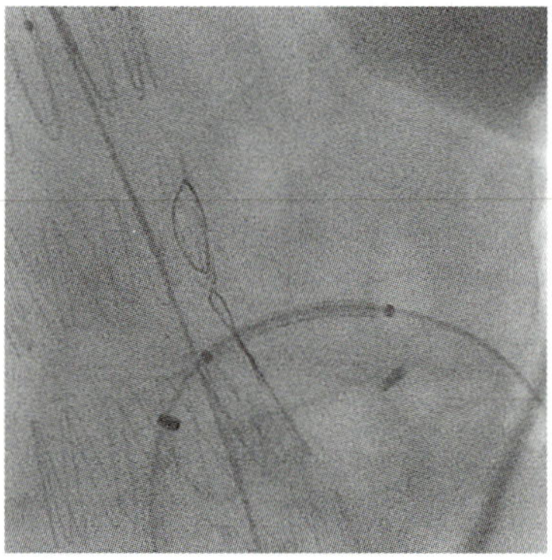

FIGURE 10 Lateral image depicting placement of a covered balloon-expandable stent into the superior mesenteric artery prior to deployment.

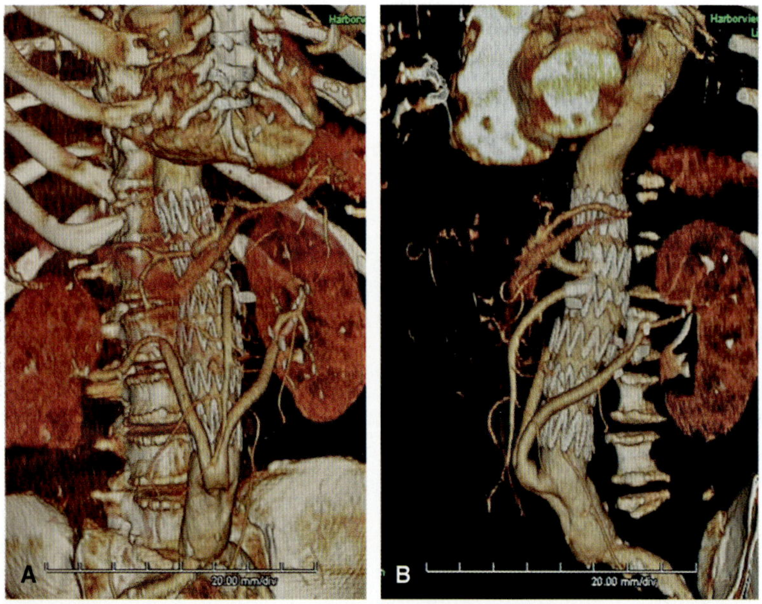

FIGURE 11 **A** and **B,** Follow-up computed tomography images of a patient successfully treated with partial visceral debranching and physician-modified endovascular fenestrated repair.

PEARLS AND PITFALLS

Choice of operating room (OR) table	■ Use standard OR tables for open surgical procedures and imaging tables for image-guided or hybrid procedures. Advanced planning is essential to optimize outcome. Never sacrifice exposure!
Exposure of common iliac artery	■ Identify and protect the ureter.
Placement of wires after debranching procedure	■ Pass guidewires under continuous fluoroscopic guidance following debranching. An advancing aortic wire may preferentially enter and traverse the debranching graft, causing end-organ injury, disorientation, and possible endograft maldeployment if not recognized.
Timing of stent graft balloon molding during fenestrated EVAR	■ Always seat the endograft with balloon inflation prior to placement of visceral bridging stents. Instrumentation or distention of the fenestrated endograft following branch vessel stenting may compromise stent positioning, integrity, and patency.

POSTOPERATIVE CARE

- Open aortic debranching procedures are not benign; almost all patients will require intensive care postprocedure. Spinal drainage is used selectively for aortic coverage extending more than 10 cm cephalad to the celiac artery. Postoperative anuria or persistent acidosis/rising lactate require immediate investigation to prove branch vessel patency.

OUTCOMES

- Contemporary hybrid debranching procedures for complex abdominal aortic aneurysmal disease are associated with a 13% operative mortality rate, 2% permanent paraplegia rate, and 1% stroke rate.[3]
- Hybrid approaches offer the advantage of versatility, avoidance of extensive operative exposures, and potentially offer a broader range of therapies to a patient population that would not otherwise be considered for aortic surgical repair.

COMPLICATIONS

- Access-related complications
- Hemorrhage requiring transfusion
- Paraplegia
- Stroke
- Renal failure
- Death

REFERENCES

1. Starnes BW, Andersen CA, Ronsivalle JA, et al. Totally percutaneous aortic aneurysm repair: experience and prudence. *J Vasc Surg*. 2006;43(2):270-276.
2. Starnes BW, Quiroga E. Hybrid-fenestrated aortic aneurysm repair: a novel technique for treating patients with para-anastomotic juxtarenal aneurysms. *Ann Vasc Surg*. 2010;24(8):1150-1153.
3. Starnes BW, Tran NT, McDonald JM. Hybrid approaches to repair of complex aortic aneurysmal disease. *Surg Clin North Am*. 2007;87(5):1087-1098, ix.

Chapter **16**

Parallel Stenting for Visceral and Renal Protection During Complex Endovascular Aneurysm Repair

Matthew John Rossi and Javairiah Fatima

INTRODUCTION

- Endovascular aortic repair has been well established as a safe, and minimally invasive treatment for patients with anatomically suitable infrarenal aortic aneurysms.[1] Open repair and in select cases hybrid repair has traditionally been reserved for those with more complex anatomy including juxtarenal, pararenal, and thoracoabdominal aortic aneurysms. Over the past couple of decades, significant technological advances have occurred in the realm of endovascular aortic surgery to offer endovascular repair even in patients with such complex anatomy.
- Use of fenestrated and branched technology (F-/B-EVAR) has been a breakthrough to address complex aortic aneurysms while maintaining perfusion to the visceral and renal vessels. However, most of these devices require a lead time for customization to the individual patient anatomy or are currently still in trial phase with limited access, or to those with physician-sponsored investigational device exemptions, leaving a need for alternate techniques. One of these alternate approaches is the parallel graft technique (snorkels and chimneys) utilizing immediately available devices that can be readily used even in urgent or emergent settings. This technique encompasses placement of stents in the renal and visceral arteries that are extended parallel to the main aortic endograft to allow perfusion into the branches from above or below the excluded aneurysm.[2] Additionally, parallel stenting can be helpful as a bail out technique in inadvertent coverage of a renal artery during EVAR.[3]

DEFINITIONS

- Antegrade parallel stenting, or chimneys, extend cranially above the endograft (**FIGURE 1**) while retrograde parallel stenting, also known as periscopes, extend caudally below the endograft (**FIGURE 2**). Complex thoracoabdominal aneurysms may require thoracic coverage in conjunction with chimneys or snorkels; this type of repair is referred to as a snorkel sandwich (**FIGURE 3**).[4]

PATIENT HISTORY AND PHYSICAL FINDINGS

- Most aortic aneurysms are detected incidentally on imaging performed for other indications. Once diagnosed, repair is done prophylactically to prevent rupture, which can be fatal in over 90% of patients. In patients presenting in an elective setting, physiologic and anatomic considerations are the primary determinants of optimal repair for each patient. A thorough discussion should be held with the patient of the prophylactic nature of repair, risks, and benefits of continued surveillance vs open, hybrid, or various techniques of endovascular repair. It is important that patients understand what the undertaking entails perioperatively and in the long term, including need for continued imaging surveillance and potential future reinterventions. A discussion of the off-label use of the endografts as well as the anticipated radiation exposure should be had, and informed consent documented.

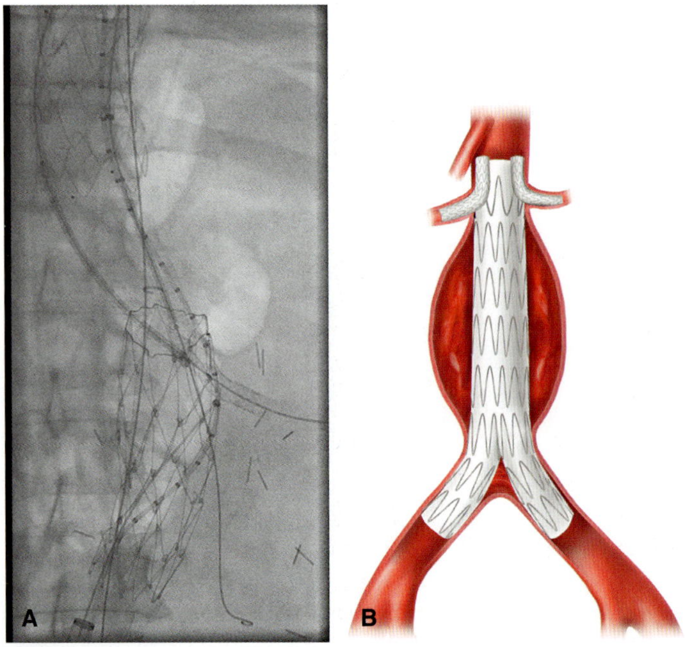

FIGURE 1 • Antegrade Parallel Stenting (Chimney) Repair with one renal stent, and superior mesenteric stent cannulation in preparation for stent placement. **A,** Placement of two renal chimneys for repair of a juxtarenal aortic aneurysm **(B)**.

- All patients should undergo history and physical exam, and evaluation of their comorbidities. A full cardiopulmonary evaluation should be undertaken to establish the patient's risk profile. Evaluation of potential renal or liver insufficiency is also necessary.

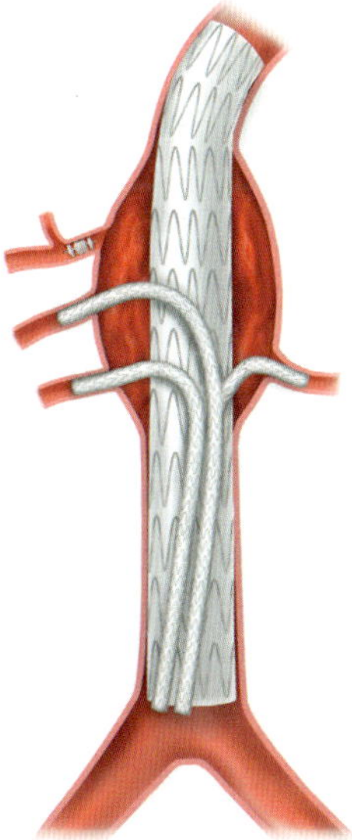

FIGURE 2 • Retrograde Parallel Stenting (Periscope) Repair with a superior mesenteric and two renal stents and Amplatzer plug in the celiac axis.

IMAGING AND OTHER DIAGNOSTIC STUDIES

- Computed tomography angiography (CTA) of chest, abdomen, and pelvis with 1 to 2 mm slices is essential with virtual aortic reconstruction to allow for precise determination of lengths, diameters, angulation, and quality of the aortic landing zones and target vessels. It can help predict and plan for pitfalls and anatomic challenges preoperatively. The CTA is imported into three-dimensional reconstruction software for creation of centerline of flow to allow for precise anatomic evaluation and accurate operative planning and endograft selection.
- Given the use of axillary access for antegrade cannulation of target vessels, CTA should include upper extremity access vessels to look for kinks, dissection, aneurysm, or diseased artery that would preclude their use.

SURGICAL MANAGEMENT

Preoperative Planning

- Detailed review of preoperative imaging with 3D reconstruction and precise measurements must be completed ahead of time. A well-planned case is crucial for successful execution. A healthy, parallel aortic segment should be identified to provide an appropriate proximal seal zone. Thereafter, all necessary measurements of visceral and renal vessel diameters, lengths to branch points, and distances from planned proximal seal zone should be taken. An operative plan should be drawn out with any potential pitfalls discussed. Excessive tortuosity, calcifications, or thrombus burden

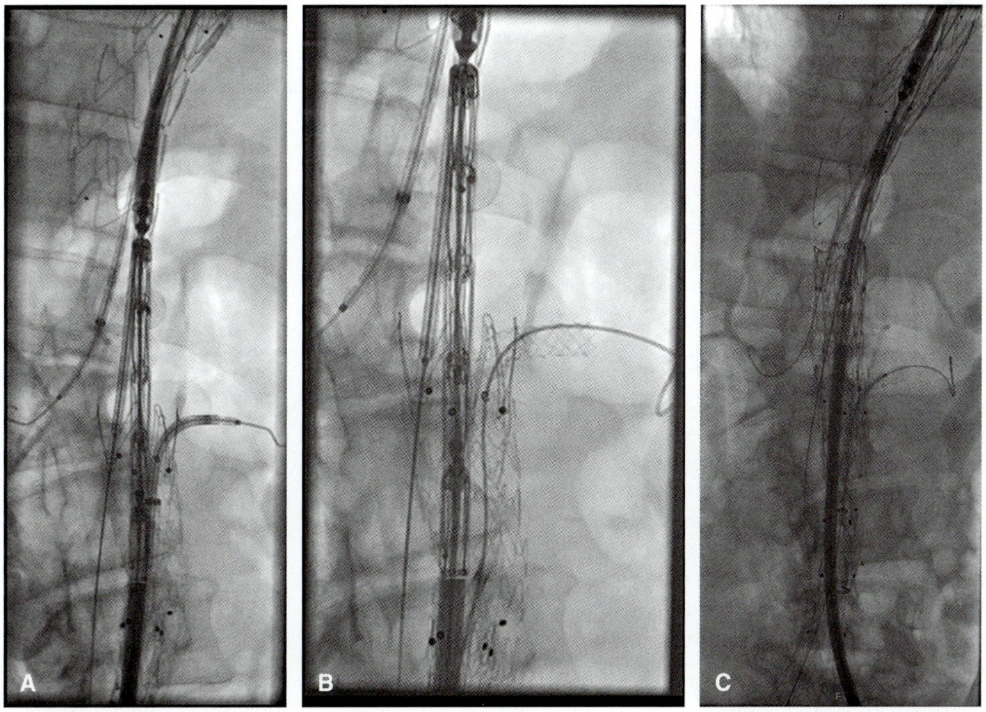

FIGURE 3 • **A,** Pre-deployment placement of celiac antegrade and left renal retrograde stents **(B)** Post-deployment of left renal retrograde stent **(C)**. Complex thoracoabdominal aneurysms may require thoracic coverage in conjunction with chimneys and snorkels; this type of repair is referred to as a snorkel sandwich.

confer a formidable risk of stroke or distal embolization, rendering endovascular intervention prohibitive.

- The natural history of the aorta is to progressively degenerate, thus the plan should allow for room for proximal extension if needed in the future. Longer seal length will decrease the likelihood that the patient will require future intervention for a type Ia endoleaks. Given this likelihood, most parallel stenting procedures include the visceral vessels.
- Typically 25% to 30% oversizing to a healthy aortic segment is considered when selecting the aortic endograft to account for fabric infolding around the chimney/snorkel stent grafts. There are several carefully determined formulae that have been suggested to optimize seal and minimize gutter leaks.[5] It is also important for the renal arteries to be 4 to 8 mm in diameter to establish anatomic feasibility. An upward going renal artery is not amenable to chimney and is fraught with complications such as kinks and thrombosis with loss of renal artery. Such vessels would be best served by retrograde parallel stenting or prior debranching.

Operative Room Setup

- A hybrid room fixed imaging setup with CT fusion technology is ideal for complex aortic cases. This technology allows the preoperative imaging to overlay the images obtained intraoperatively, and can be used to delineate the anatomy and target vessels. Use of these tools minimizes the need for cine runs and significantly reduces contrast volume and radiation. Cone-beam CT should be considered at the end of procedures prior to removal of access sheaths to identify and address any kinks or suboptimal modular or stent architecture, thus preventing future reintervention.[6]
- Anesthesia/OR team: At our institution, a dedicated team of cardiovascular anesthesiologists are involved in all complex aortic cases. General anesthesia is preferred by our group given the length of the procedure, the ability to better control respiration during distal subtraction angiography, and often due to the need for access via axillary cutdown. Finally, the need for a spinal drain should be considered, especially if a long length of thoracic coverage is anticipated or any segment of aorta has been previously covered or replaced.[7,8]
- Intraoperative neurophysiologic monitoring of spinal cord somatosensory and motor-evoked potentials should be performed for elective cases and when available for nonelective cases when covering large segments of thoracic aorta, for early detection and intervention of spinal cord ischemia.
- A dedicated aortic scrub technician/nurse with knowledge and familiarity with the devices, procedure, and the surgeon's workflow allows the operation to proceed smoothly.

Positioning

- The patient is positioned supine with both arms tucked with the C-arm coming from the patient's left and the ability to position it at the patient's head as well. If two or more visceral/renal vessels will require access, then a right or left axillary cutdown is performed, depending on which offers the most trackability of sheaths to the descending thoracic aorta. There are conflicting data on whether right sided access to the arch confers a higher risk of stroke. In general, the optimal side for sheath trackability is chosen.[9,10]
- The patient is prepped from neck to knees, with a large piece of Ioban used to cover the prepped area, followed by draping in a sterile fashion. The primary operator is positioned on the patient's right with the second surgeon or first assistant at the head to facilitate axillary exposure and sheath/wire manipulations. Alternatively, when a left axillary approach is used, a sterile table may be directed laterally from the patients left arm to aid in maintaining sterility of the wires, catheters, and sheaths.

TECHNIQUES

ANTEGRADE PARALLEL STENTING IN EVAR

Axillary Artery Access

- A 5-cm transverse incision is created 2 fingerbreaths below the mid clavicle. After dividing the subcutaneous tissue and pectoral fascia, the fibers of the pectoralis major are bluntly separated. Underneath, the clavipectoral fascia is divided. Approximately 5 to 6 cm of the axillary artery should be isolated, taking care to obtain control without damaging a branch.
- Starting proximally at 2-o'clock on the artery, micropuncture access is obtained and a purse-string suture using 4-0 polypropylene is placed. Approximately 15 mm distally and positioned in tandem to the first purse-string suture at 12-o'clock on the artery, the second access site is secured with a purse-string suture followed by the third at 10-o'clock (**FIGURE 4**). Alternatively, a 10-mm Dacron conduit can be sutured directly onto the axillary artery and access obtained through the conduit.
- A Cobra 2 catheter (Angiodynamics, Netherlands) is used to direct a Glidewire into the descending thoracic aorta, which can then be switched out under catheter protection to a stiffer wire such as an Amplatz (Cook, Bloomington, IN) to upsize to 6- or 7-French sheaths of appropriate length to

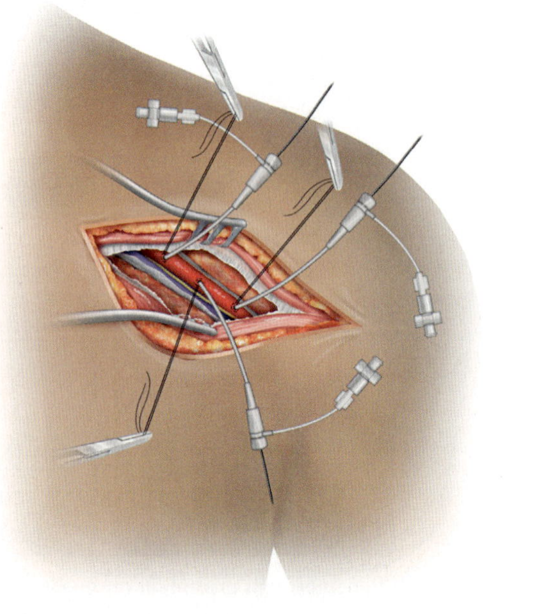

FIGURE 4 • Axillary cutdown with three strategically placed tandem access sites with Prolene purse-string sutures.

extend to the visceral/renal vessels. The patient is then systemically heparinized for a goal activated clotting time (ACT) of greater than 250 seconds. This is accomplished by ACT measurements every 30 minutes with appropriate redosing of IV unfractionated heparin.

Endograft Deployment

- Bilateral femoral artery access is obtained percutaneously under ultrasound guidance using a micropuncture kit. Perclose Proglide devices are placed for eventual closure. The access is then upsized to the appropriate sheath size for the main body of the selected device.
- While any endograft can be used for the main body, AFX (Endologix Irvine, CA) deserves a mention as the presence of the fabric outside of the stents in AFX, allows bellowing into the gutters than are inevitably formed with the use of the parallel stenting technique.
- Should you choose another endograft, the next step in the procedure is cannulation of the renal/visceral vessels.

Renal/Visceral Cannulation and Stent Positioning

- The appropriate length (typically 90 cm) 6- or 7-French sheath is advanced to the visceral segment. It is at this point that if the advanced software and C-arm is available, that a cone-beam CT scan is taken intraoperatively. Bony landmarks are then matched to the preoperative CTA imaging to allow for fusion of contrasted preoperative CT to overlay the bony landmarks to delineate the aortic, renal, and visceral anatomy, facilitating cannulation with less contrast and radiation. When CT fusion is not available, a digital subtraction angiography (DSA) is performed at the level of the visceral aorta, with the c-arm positioned at an angle perpendicular to the ostium of the desired vessel.
- Next, the target vessels are selectively catheterized using a selection catheter and a hydrophilic Glidewire (Terumo, Sunrise, FL). The Glidewire is exchanged for a Rosen wire (Cook, Bloomington, IN) with a floppy tip for renals and an Amplatz wire (Cook, Bloomington, IN) for mesenteric vessels (**FIGURE 5**). The sheaths are then advanced into the branch vessels and the catheters removed after angiographic confirmation of successful cannulation and vessel patency.
- If the parallel graft involves the celiac axis, it is not uncommon to establish the adequacy of gastroduodenal artery collaterals and then cover the celiac artery, precluding the need for a fourth parallel stent; one may consider placing an Amplatzer plug (Abbott) to prevent type II endoleaks in this setting. When this is performed, it is done prior to placement of parallel stents.
- A wide array of balloon expandable covered stents and self-expanding stent grafts are available to choose from for visceral and renal vessels. An ideal stent graft should offer a low-profile delivery system, incorporating flexibility

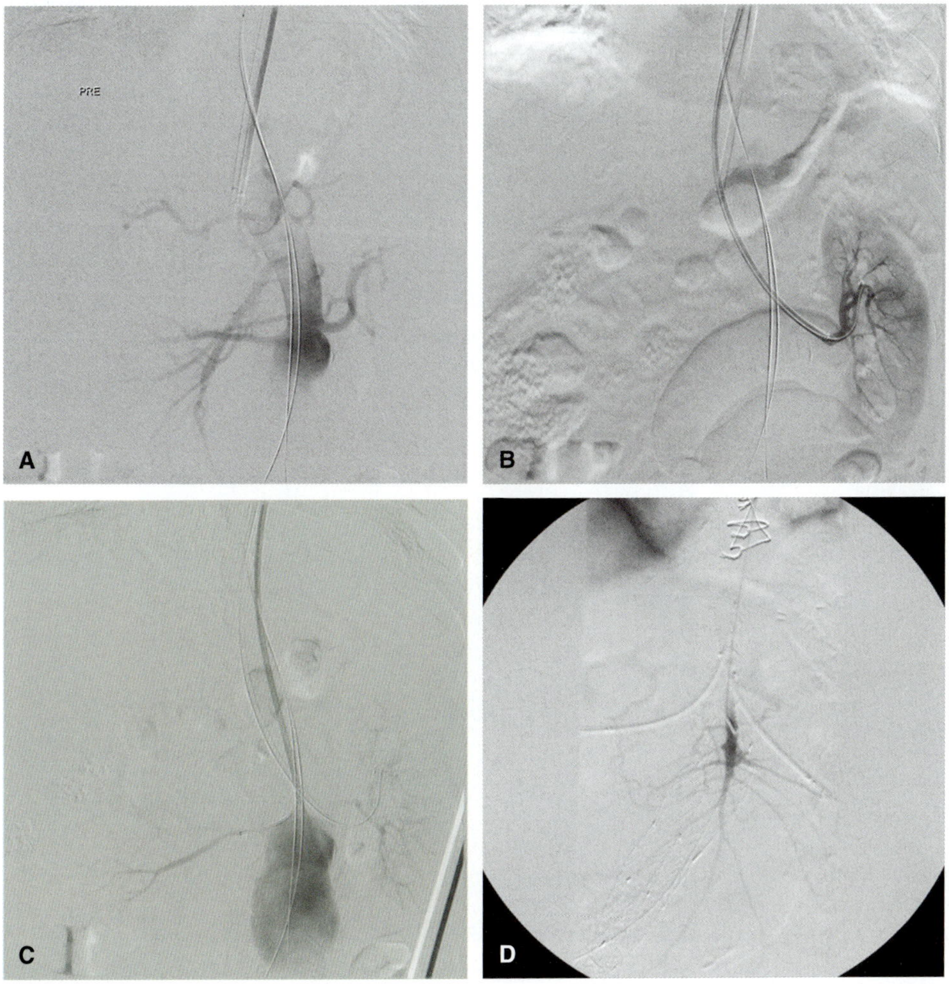

FIGURE 5 • Angiography demonstrating pararenal aortogram. **A,** Selective catheterization of left renal artery with placement of a Rosen wire **(B)**, Selective catheterization of right renal artery with placement of a Rosen wire **(C)**, Selective catheterization of superior mesenteric artery **(D)**.

to conform to a wide range of target vessels and angulations. It is important to have a stent that can accommodate a wide range of diameters and lengths with minimal foreshortening, allowing predictable and precise stent deployment. Additionally, high radial strength with resistance to kinking is critical to achieve long-term patency, and resist migration, minimizing risk of endoleak.

- Viabahn (Gore, Flagstaff, AZ) offers high flexibility and kink-resistance; however, when high radial strength is needed as in tight orificial lesions, balloon expandable covered stents such as VBX (Gore, Flagstaff, AZ) or iCAST (Atrium Medical, USA) are advantageous given their increased radial strength as well as their ability to customize to a larger diameter with postdilatation. Additionally, the bidirectional deployment mechanism of Viabahn makes it suboptimal in short landing zones such as with early target vessel branching, where a balloon expandable stent graft may have a more predictable deployment. Ultimately, it is largely surgeon preference and experience that dictate the choice of stent graft.
- For renal/visceral stents, a minimum of 1.5 cm of length from the ostium should be covered to allow for appropriate fixation. Angiography is used to identify target vessel branches, which should be preserved whenever possible.

Endograft Positioning and Parallel Stent Deployment

- Once all the target vessel stent grafts are positioned within their respective sheaths, the main body aortic device is advanced and deployed at the desired level of seal. The sheaths of the branches are carefully walked back over the positioned stent grafts and the branch vessels stents are simultaneously deployed with caution to ensure the chimneys extend at least 1 cm proximal to the main body to maintain patency. With the balloons within parallel grafts still inflated, a CODA balloon is inflated in the aortic graft to achieve molding of the endograft fabric around the stent grafts (**FIGURE 6**). The CODA balloon is deflated prior to deflation of the chimney stent grafts to avoid inadvertent crushing of the renal/visceral stents.
- Once the entirety of the aortic endograft is deployed completion angiogram is done to ensure adequacy of repair and to look for any endoleaks, kinking, or crushing of the parallel stents. The initial run is done with the wires in place in case a type 1a endoleak is present or there is visceral/renal malperfusion. Evaluation for brisk filling of the distal renal, superior mesenteric, and celiac axis branch vessels should be performed without any stiff wires to insure adequate run off and evaluate for stent graft patency as they remodel and conform to the native anatomy. A high-resolution x-ray shot should be performed to evaluate satisfactory stent architecture and overlap (**FIGURE 7**). A cone-beam CT with or without contrast is a useful tool for 3D evaluation of the repair.
- Removal of the axillary and femoral sheaths with cinching of previously placed sutures allows for straight forward closure of the access sites. After removal of all sheaths, inspection for distal pulses is performed and documented.

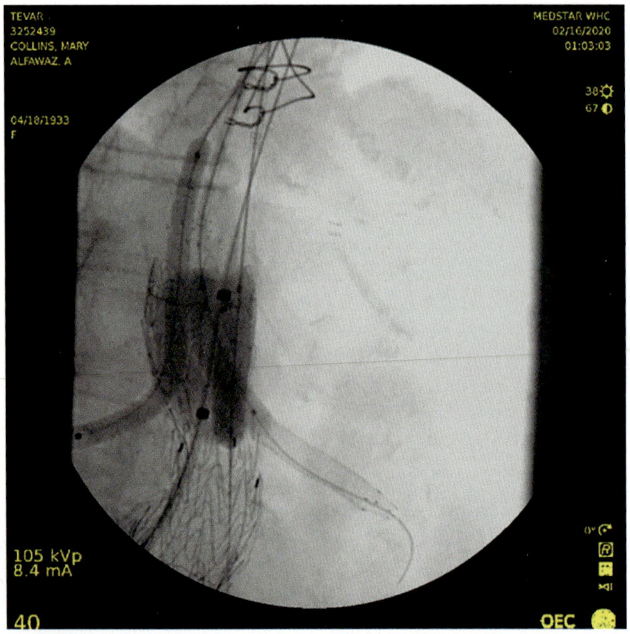

FIGURE 6 • Inflation of CODA and parallel stents to allow for molding of stents.

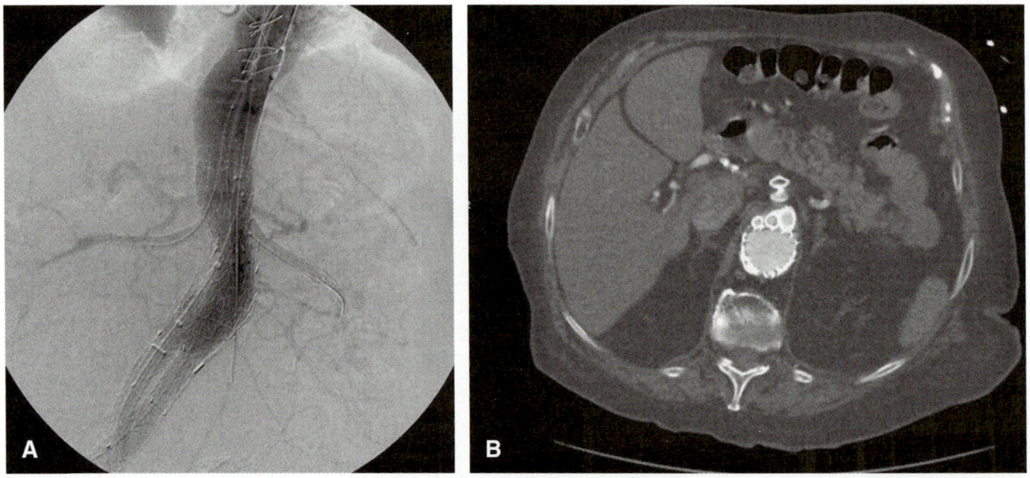

FIGURE 7 • High resolution of completion angiogram demonstrating patency of all stent grafts and target vessels. **A,** Postoperative CT scan demonstrating celiac plug with 3 vessel snorkel repair **(B)**.

RETROGRADE PARALLEL STENTING IN EVAR

Femoral Access

- A periscope is a parallel stent positioned in a retrograde fashion alongside the aortic endograft. Femoral access is obtained under ultrasound guidance on the anterior surface of the common femoral artery. If there is concern for inadequate access or a significant underlying burden of disease, placement of an iliac conduit using 10-mm Dacron graft should be considered. After access is obtained, systemic anticoagulation is achieved with intravenous unfractionated heparin dosed to an ACT of at least 250 seconds.
- Access for cannulation is dependent on the size of the stents to be placed. Perclose sutures should be placed preemptively. A large bore sheath can be used to allow up to two or three smaller 6-Fr sheaths for cannulation of the branch vessels. If 7-Fr sheaths are required, placement of an external conduit with separate access of conduit for each sheath is preferred. Once adequate access is obtained, the branch vessels are cannulated as previously described. A hydrophilic Glidewire is exchanged for a stiffer wire and the sheath is advanced. Once branch sheaths are in place, stent grafts are advanced to their appropriate location as outlined above with same principles for positioning, and an adequate length of stent graft extended into the target vessel (minimum of 15 mm of apposition with the target vessel).
- The main endograft is advanced into the aorta, positioned at the appropriate level, and deployed with the sheaths still in place. The sheaths are slowly withdrawn, and the periscope stents are deployed. If the stents fall short of the end of the aortic graft, they should be extended with additional covered stents. With balloons inflated in all the parallel stents, a CODA balloon is inflated to mold the main endograft around the stents. Extension of the main body proximally to exclude the thoracic aneurysm or pathology is then completed. Finally, completion angiography is performed with similar principles as described above.

PEARLS AND PITFALLS

Chronic aortic dissection	■ A small true lumen diameter was initially considered a relative contraindication to parallel grafting, mostly due to concerns with possible stent-graft collapse, disruption of the septum, and difficulty to cannulate the vessels. This dogma has largely been debunked with increasing experience showing high technical success even in the presence of a compressed true lumen[11] (**FIGURE 8**).

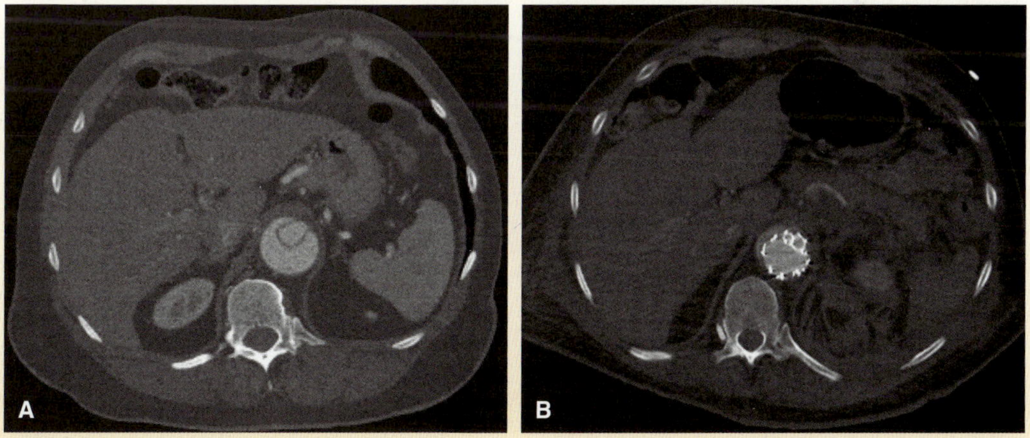

FIGURE 8 • Chimney in aneurysms secondary to chronic aortic dissection; Initial preoperative CT scan demonstrating a compressed true lumen. **A,** Postoperative CT scan demonstrating a fully expanded true lumen with chimneys **(B)**.

Severely calcified or tortuous access vessels	▪ The limitations for standard TEVAR/EVAR are also applied to these endografts. Approximately 10%-20% of patients may require conduits. Most aortic devices require delivery systems with outer diameter of 20-25 Fr, requiring 7-9 mm of healthy external iliac artery diameter. In the setting of severe tortuosity, calcification, narrowing, or prior stents, a planned iliac conduit offers a suitable alternative to avoid inadvertent disruption of the iliac arteries. In addition to iliac artery access, brachial and axillary artery access should be assessed for dissection, narrowing or aneurysmal degeneration that can impact suitability as access vessels.
Short or early branching of the target branch artery	In cases of early branching or a solitary kidney with a short angulated renal artery, one may consider single vessel surgical debranching prior to endovascular repair of the aortic aneurysm.

POSTOPERATIVE CARE

- Almost all of our parallel stenting cases are admitted to the ICU postoperatively. This allows for hourly neurovascular and hemodynamic assessments for at least 24 hours. Our spinal cord protection protocol includes withholding of certain perioperative hypertensive medications (long-term beta blockers are continued), perioperative cerebrospinal fluid (CSF) drainage, perioperative mean arterial pressure maintenance ≥90 mm Hg, maintenance of hemoglobin to ≥10 g/dL intra- and postoperatively, as well as a steroid bolus in patients with any changes in intraoperative somatosensory and motor evoked potentials.
- Frequent laboratory checks are performed including troponin, lactate, CBC, and BMP. Close monitoring of urine output is continued with any sign of oliguria brought to the attention of the surgeon. When a patient has been neurologically intact for 24 hours, the spinal drain is clamped. After 6 to 24 hours of a stable neurologic exam depending on length of thoracic coverage, the drain is removed. The patient is discharged on aspirin and clopidogrel and a follow up CTA is performed within 1 month, followed by CTA or combination of noncontrast CT with duplex evaluation at 6 months, 1 year, and annually thereafter.

COMPLICATIONS

- Gutter leaks: Type I endoleaks that occur along the space between the main endograft and parallel stents are termed gutter leaks. These are best avoided by having an adequate length of overlap, at least 2 to 3 cm between the aortic wall, main endograft, and chimney grafts. Most gutter leaks resolve spontaneously within a year of implantation without evidence of sac expansion.[12]
- Kinked or crushed parallel stents: Kinked or crushed parallel stents can occur if the molding sequence is not followed. It is best to keep all wires in the branch vessels until after the completion angiogram to address this issue. This circumstance can occur if there is a long length of self-expanding stent as well. Typically, placement of a bare metal stent within the self-expanding stent can remediate this situation.

OUTCOMES

- The most comprehensive registry evaluating parallel stenting is the PERICLES registry.[13] Type IA endoleaks were noted in approximately 10% of patients intraoperatively. However, after intervention most are resolved prior to leaving the operating room. Ischemic stroke or TIA occurred in approximately 2% to 3% of patients in the PERICLES study. No patients suffered spinal cord ischemia. Two percent of patients suffered access complications requiring intervention. Two percent of patients suffered a postoperative myocardial infarction and 12% of patients suffered an AKI including 1.8% that required temporary or permanent dialysis. Of the 517 patients with parallel stenting, 2.5% required reintervention for an occluded chimney.[2,14]

CONCLUSION

- Parallel stenting has yielded acceptable short and midterm outcomes in carefully selected patients with complex aortic aneurysms that are not within the realm of repair using commercially available devices, or in urgent/emergent situations where access to a clinical trial device or a custom-made device is not an option.

REFERENCES

1. The UK EVAR Trial Investigators. Endovascular versus open repair of abdominal aortic aneurysm. *N Engl J Med*. 2010;362:1863-1871.
2. Donas K, Lee JT, LAchat M, Torsello G, Veith F. Collected world experience about the performance of the snorkel/chimney endovascular technique in the treatment of complex aortic pathologies: the PERICLES registry. *Ann Surg*. 2015;262(3):546-553.
3. Tanious A, Wooster M, Jung A, Nelson PR, Back M, Shames ML. Endovascular management of proximal fixation loss using parallel stent grafting techniques to preserve visceral flow. *Ann Vasc Surg*. 2017;42:169-175.
4. Kansagra K, Kang J, Taon M, et al. Advanced endografting techniques: snorkels, chimneys, periscopes, fenestrations, and branched endografts. *Cardiovasc Diagn Ther*. 2018;8(suppl 1):S175-S183.
5. Kölbel T, Carpenter SW, Taraz A, Taraz M, Larena-Avellaneda A, Debus ES. How to calculate the main aortic graft-diameter for a chimney-graft. *J Cardiovasc Surg*. 2016;57(1):66-71.
6. Doelare S, Smorenburg S, van Schaik T, et al. Image fusion during standard and complex endovascular aortic repair, to fuse or not to fuse? A meta-analysis and additional data from a single-center retrospective cohort. *J Endovasc Ther*. 2021;28(1):78-92. doi:10.1177/1526602820960444.
7. Scali S, Kim M, Kubilis P, et al. Implementation of a bundled protocol significantly reduces risk of spinal cord ischemia after branches or fenestrated endovascular aortic repair. *J Vasc Surg*. 2018;67(2):409-423.e4.
8. Sulzinski M; Rossi MJ; Alfawaz A, et al. Optimization of factors for the prevention of spinal cord ischemia in thoracic endovascular aortic repair. *Vascular*. 2022;30(2):199-205.
9. Meertens M, Lemmes C, Oderich G, Schurink G, Mees B. Cerebrovascular complications after upper extremity access for complex aortic interventions: a systematic review and meta-analysis. *Cardiovasc Intervent Radiol*. 2020;43:186-195.

10. Plotkin A, Ding L, Han S, et al. Association of upper extremity and neck access with stroke in endovascular aortic repair. *J Vasc Surg*. 2020;71(5):1602-1609.
11. Kitagawa A, Greenberg RK, Eagleton MJ, Mastracci TM, Roselli EE. Fenestrated and branched endovascular aortic repair for chronic type B aortic dissection with thoracoabdominal aneurysms. *J Vasc Surg*. 2013;58(3):625-634. doi:10.1016/j.jvs.2013.01.049
12. Ullery B, Tran K, Itoga N, Dalman RL, Lee JT. Natural history of gutter-related type Ia endoleaks after snorkel/chimney EVAR. *J Vasc Surg*. 2017;64(4):981-990.
13. Taneva GT, Lee JT, Tran K, et al. Long-term chimney/snorkel endovascular aortic aneurysm repair experience for complex abdominal aortic pathologies within the PERICLES registry. *J Vasc Surg*. 2021;73(6):1942-1949. doi:10.1016/j.jvs.2020.10.086
14. Li Y, Hu Z, Bai C, Liu J, Zhang T, Ge Y et al. Fenestrated and chimney technique for juxtarenal aortic aneurysm: a systematic review and pooled data analysis. *Sci Rep*. 2016;6:2.

Chapter 17 Branched and Fenestrated Endovascular Stent Graft Techniques

Peter J. Rossi

- Endovascular repair of abdominal aortic aneurysms depends on specific anatomic constraints regarding infrarenal neck length and angulation in order to accommodate commercially available infrarenal devices. Fenestrated and branched endografts were introduced to enable minimally invasive repair of complex juxtarenal and suprarenal aortic aneurysms.[1] These devices incorporate reinforced fenestrations or directional branches, permitting incorporation of visceral and renal artery origins into the proximal endograft seal zone without compromising end-organ perfusion or aneurysm exclusion.[2] Devices can be manufactured to patient-specific specifications, or commercially available devices can by modified by the surgeon prior to being reconstrained and implanted. This chapter summarizes the technical features of endovascular aneurysm repair using fenestrated and branched stent grafts for pararenal and thoracoabdominal aortic aneurysms (TAAAs).

DEFINITION

- The term *fenestrated repair* refers to deployment of an endograft featuring custom orifices created and reinforced at precise locations around the aortic endograft to enable branch artery access, cannulation, and placement of a bridging stent graft during aneurysm exclusion. Fenestration sites are selected from analysis of patient-specific cross-sectional image data to enable exclusion of aneurysms with short or angled infrarenal necks. Graft design may be aided by three-dimensional reconstruction, and in some cases three-dimensional printing, of the aneurysm.[3] In general, the target arteries (renal or mesenteric) must arise from normal aorta to enable fenestrated repair. As a rule, fenestrations must be able to deploy flush with the aortic wall to ensure adequate aneurysm exclusion. "Alignment" stents (covered or uncovered, depending on individual patient circumstance) are deployed as needed to prevent target artery malperfusion as a consequence of misalignment between the fenestration and target artery orifice.
- *Branched repair* refers to endovascular aneurysm exclusion employing covered stents to directly connect the main lumen of the endograft to the target visceral artery. These devices enable repair of aneurysms involving or extending proximal to the origins of the renal or visceral vessels (eg, type IV TAAAs). Some distance must be present between the main body of the endograft at full deployment and the aortic wall at the target visceral artery orifice. Branched stent grafts are currently available in two distinct configurations:
  - *Fenestrated branches* arise from reinforced fenestrations bridged by balloon-expandable covered stents.
  - *Directional or cuffed branch* devices feature appended fabric cuffs, precisely located to enable straight, helical, down- or upgoing guidewire egress, target vessel cannulation, and deployment of bridging covered stents. Self-expanding flexible nitinol stents are usually employed for this purpose.
- Physician-modified endograft refers to back table modification of a commercially available endograft (thoracic or abdominal) which is subsequently reconstrained before being introduced into the patient. This technique is not approved for general use by the US Food and Drug Administration (FDA) and generally should be used within the confines of an ongoing clinical trial.

DIFFERENTIAL DIAGNOSIS

- Most aneurysms are degenerative (previously characterized as "atherosclerotic").
- Other etiologies include infection (eg, mycotic aneurysms), inflammation (eg, inflammatory aneurysm or aortitis), development of penetrating ulcers or asymmetric saccular enlargement, connective tissue disorders (eg, Marfan syndrome), and related aortic pathologies (dissection or intramural hematoma).

PATIENT HISTORY AND PHYSICAL FINDINGS

- Aortic aneurysms are asymptomatic prior to rupture and are diagnosed incidentally or during screening. The Society for Vascular Surgery (SVS) recommends elective aneurysm repair at a size greater than 5.5 cm for males and greater than 5 cm for females or enlargement greater than 5 mm in 6 months.[4]
- In up to 10% of patients, aneurysms may be accompanied by periaortic inflammation and resultant retroperitoneal fibrosis involving adjacent structures, including the duodenum and ureters.[5] These patients may present with abdominal or back pain, fatigue, malaise, or low-grade fever even at relatively small diameters. The SVS recommends repair of aneurysms where symptoms are attributable to the aneurysm regardless of size.[4]
- A comprehensive history should be obtained to fully appreciate the potential natural history of each patient's disease, including a full assessment of cardiovascular risk factors, current smoking habits, and a family history of aneurysm disease or connective tissue disorders.
- Evaluation of perioperative clinical risk emphasizes cardiac, pulmonary, and renal functional status and reserve, including baseline laboratory testing, noninvasive cardiac stress testing, pulmonary function assessment, and carotid duplex ultrasonography when indicated.

DIAGNOSTIC IMAGING

- Preprocedural aortic imaging studies provide fundamental and necessary guidance for endovascular repair strategies of all types. Aneurysm morphology is best analyzed through acquisition of high-resolution computed tomography angiography (CTA) datasets.[3] CTA with submillimeter slice acquisition is recommended for optimal acquisition, allowing three-dimensional reformatting techniques, maximum intensity projections, and volume rendering.

- Stent grafts are currently custom-made to conform to patient anatomy, based on estimates of longitudinal distance, axial clock position, arc lengths, and angles derived from centerline of flow measurements.
- Anatomic limitations to be considered include difficult iliac access, excessive aortic tortuosity or angulation,[6] visceral artery occlusive disease, and anatomic variants including multiple accessory renal arteries or early renal branch bifurcation.

STENT GRAFT DESIGN

- Device planning starts with selection of the proximal landing zone based on "healthy" aorta. The proximal landing zone should include at least a 2-cm length of "normal," noncalcified, parallel aortic wall and at least 25 to 30 mm of proximal seal for endovascular TAAA treatment.[7] The outer-to-outer aortic diameter should be more than 18 mm and less than 32 mm for pararenal aneurysms and more than 18 mm and less than 38 mm for TAAAs.[8] Landing zone diameter should be no larger than the diameter of the next most proximal aortic segment.
- Fenestrated stent grafts are currently manufactured with three fenestration options: small and large circles and more proximal scallops (**FIGURE 1A**). *Small fenestrations* are 6 × 6 mm or 6 × 8 mm, created without crossing struts and reinforced by circumferential nitinol rings. *Large fenestrations*' diameters are 8, 10, or 12 mm and may incorporate stent struts crossing the edge or middle of the circular defect, limiting space available for alignment stents. *Scallops* are contoured indentations along the upper edge of the main body endograft fabric, 10 mm wide and ranging in height from 6 to 12 mm, depending on individual patient anatomy.[9]
- Device designs vary with aneurysm extent. For pararenal aneurysms, 70% of patients are adequately treated with two small fenestrations for the renal arteries and a scallop for the superior mesenteric artery (SMA),[9] though increasing the number of fenestrations to 3 or 4 to increase the proximal seal has been shown to improve the proximal seal from an average of 26 mm up to an average of 48 mm.[7] Suprarenal and type IV TAAAs typically require four fenestrations (no scallops). Extensive TAAAs (types I to III) need directional branches, particularly if the aortic diameter is relatively large or aneurysmal at the level of the visceral arteries. The combination of directional branches for celiac and SMA management with fenestrations for the renal arteries is increasingly popular.

SURGICAL MANAGEMENT

Ancillary Tools

- These procedures require advanced endovascular skills and a comprehensive inventory of applicable catheters, balloons, and stents (**TABLE 1**). Dedicated training in fenestrated and branched techniques is highly recommended for physicians already experienced in endovascular disease management and ancillary procedures including renal and visceral artery disease management.

Perioperative Measures

- Patients with difficult aneurysm anatomy, chronic kidney disease, or advanced age are preadmitted for bowel preparation and intravenous hydration with bicarbonate infusion. Oral acetylcysteine is no longer routinely recommended to minimize risk of periprocedural renal dysfunction following administration of iodinated contrast and should be used on a case-by-case basis.[10]

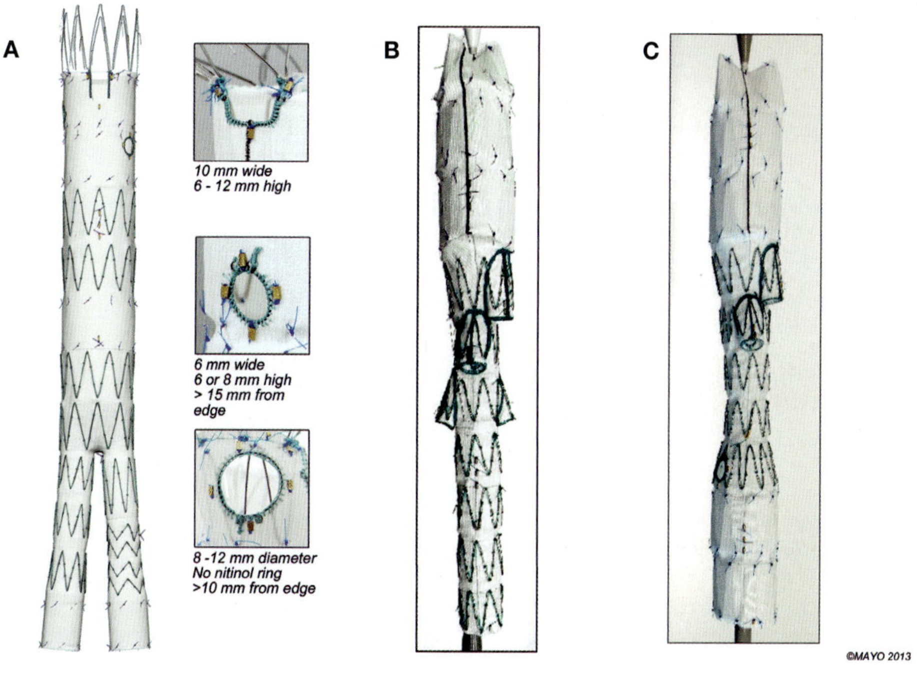

FIGURE 1 • **A,** There are three types of fenestrations that can be manufactured: small, large, and scallop fenestrations. The fenestrated stent graft consists of a proximal fenestrated tubular component, a distal bifurcated universal component, and a contralateral iliac limb extension. **B,** The Cook Zenith stent graft lineage. **C,** Newer design with two straight downgoing branches and two fenestrations.

- Hybrid, fixed imaging platforms are essential for optimal results of these complex procedures. Most are performed using general endotracheal anesthesia; local or regional anesthesia may be sufficient in select cases.
- Intraoperative blood salvage systems ("cell saver") are recommended for difficult cases and all TAAAs. The creation of large, impermeable pockets within dependent portions of the surgical drapes will facilitate pooling and collection via the cell saver.
- The use of iodinated contrast is minimized by avoidance of power injector digital subtraction angiography runs during device implantation and side stent placement. Whenever possible, hand injections of dilute contrast are used to locate the side branches. Completion aortography is obtained only after all stents are positioned and post-dilated, again using diluted contrast (50%).
- To minimize contrast, use of onlay computed tomography (CT) images is recommended. In experienced hands, branch vessel precatheterization adds little to the overall procedure time.
- Spinal drainage should be strongly considered in high-risk patients including Crawford extent I-III aneurysms, previous open or endovascular infrarenal aortic repair, "shaggy" aorta, hypogastric artery occlusion, and left subclavian artery occlusion.[11]

Positioning

- Patients are positioned supine with the imaging unit oriented from the head of the table. Both arms are tucked for repair of pararenal aneurysms requiring up to three fenestrations.
- Brachial artery access is used in patients treated by directional branches or those who need four fenestrations.

Table 1: List of Ancillary Tools Recommended for Physicians Performing Fenestrated Stent Graft Procedures

Category	Manufacturer	Application
Sheaths		
20-Fr to 24-Fr Check-Flo sheath (30 cm)	Cook Medical, Bloomington, IN	Femoral access for multivessel catheterization
6-Fr or 7-Fr Ansel sheath (55 cm, flexible dilator)	Cook Medical, Bloomington, IN	Femoral access for branch artery stenting
6-Fr or 7-Fr TourGuide steerable sheath	Medtronic, Minneapolis, MN	Femoral access for branch artery stenting
7-Fr or 8-Fr Raabe sheath (90 cm long)	Cook Medical, Bloomington, IN	Brachial access for branch artery stenting
12-Fr Ansel sheath (55 cm, flexible dilator)	Cook Medical, Bloomington, IN	Brachial access for tortuous aortic arch to facilitate branch artery stenting
5-Fr Shuttle sheath (90 cm)	Cook Medical, Bloomington, IN	Branch artery access during difficult arch
Catheters		
Kumpe or Berenstein catheter 5-Fr (65 cm)	Multiple	Selective vessel catheterization
Kumpe or Berenstein catheter 5-Fr (100 cm)	Multiple	Selective vessel catheterization
C1 catheter 5-Fr (100 cm)	Multiple	Selective vessel catheterization
MPA catheter 5-Fr (125 cm)	Multiple	Selective vessel catheterization
MPB catheter 5-Fr (100 cm)	Multiple	Selective vessel catheterization
Van Schie 3 catheter 5-Fr (65 cm)	Cook Medical, Bloomington, IN	Selective vessel catheterization
Vertebral catheter 4-Fr (125 cm)	Multiple	Selective vessel catheterization
VS1 catheter 5-Fr (80 cm)	Multiple	Selective vessel catheterization
Simmons I catheter 5-Fr (100 cm)	Multiple	Selective vessel catheterization
Diagnostic flush catheter 5-Fr (100 cm)	Multiple	Diagnostic angiography
Diagnostic pigtail catheter 5-Fr (100 cm)	Multiple	Diagnostic angiography, selective vessel catheterization
Quick-cross catheter 0.014 in to 0.035 in (150 cm)	Phillips Medical	Selective vessel catheterization
Renegade catheter (150 cm)	Boston Scientific, Minneapolis, MN	Selective vessel catheterization
Guide catheters		
LIMA guide 7 Fr (55 cm)	Cordis Corporation, Bridgewater, NJ	Precatheterization
Internal mammary (IM) guide 7 Fr (100 cm)	Multiple	Selective vessel catheterization
MPA guide 7 Fr (100 cm)	Multiple	Selective vessel catheterization
Balloons		
10 mm × 2 cm angioplasty balloon	Multiple	Proximal stent flare
12 mm × 2 cm angioplasty balloon	Multiple	Proximal stent flare
5 mm × 2 cm angioplasty balloon	Multiple	Advance sheath over balloon
Wires		
Bentson wire 0.035 in (150 cm)	Multiple	Initial access
Soft glidewire 0.035 in (260 cm)	Multiple	Target vessel catheterization
Stiff glidewire 0.035 in (260 cm)	Multiple	Target vessel catheterization
Rosen wire 0.035 in (260 cm)	Multiple	Branch artery stenting
1-cm tip Amplatz wire 0.035 in (260 cm)	Multiple	Branch artery stenting
Lunderquist wire 0.035 in (260 cm)	Multiple	Aortic stent graft
Glidegold wire 0.018 in (180 cm)	Multiple	Target vessel catherization
Stents		
iCAST stent grafts 5-10 mm	Atrium, Hudson, NH	Branch artery stenting
Gore VBX balloon-expandable stent grafts, 6-8 mm	Gore Medical, Phoenix, AZ	Branch artery stenting
LifeStream balloon-expandable stent grafts, 5-10 mm	Becton-Dickinson, Franklin Lakes, NJ	Branch artery stenting
Balloon-expandable stents 0.035 in	Multiple	Branch artery stenting or reinforcement
Self-expandable stents 0.035 in	Multiple	Distal branch artery stenting
Self-expandable stents 0.014 in	Multiple	Distal branch artery stenting

LIMA, left internal mammary artery; MPA, main pulmonary artery; VS1, Van Schie 1.

The left arm is abducted and prepped in the surgical field up to the axilla. A working sterile side table is oriented in the same axis of the abducted arm for optimal support of necessary wires and catheters.

- Electrocardiogram (EKG) leads, urinary catheter, and other monitoring cables and lines should be taped or secured so that they are not in the path of the X-ray beam of the fluoroscopic unit and do not impede movement of the C-arm gantry.

Arterial Access

- Access is established in the femoral arteries. Patients with small, calcified, or stenotic iliac arteries may require creation of an iliac conduit for safe device delivery.
- Total percutaneous femoral access is the preferred approach in patients with noncalcified arteries or mild posterior plaque. Appropriately applied standard "preclosure" with suture-mediated closure devices allows hemostasis in 99% of femoral arteries with a 30-day complication rate of 3.1% per artery.[11] When femoral arteries are small, calcified, or bifurcate close to the inguinal ligament, standard surgical exposure and access is obtained. Proximal and distal control is obtained using vessel loops.
- The left brachial artery is surgically exposed via small longitudinal incision in the upper arm, just proximal to the origin of the deep brachial artery. Likewise, percutaneous axillary access with standard preclosure may be utilized when anatomically feasible.
- Intravenous heparin (80-100 U/kg) is administered immediately after femoral and brachial access is established. An activated clotting time longer than 250 seconds is maintained throughout the procedure with frequent rechecks every 30 minutes. Prior to deployment of the stent graft, diuresis is induced with intravenous mannitol and/or furosemide.

ENDOVASCULAR REPAIR USING FENESTRATED STENT GRAFTS

- Fenestrated–branched repair is currently performed using the Cook Zenith stent graft lineage. Newer designs by Medtronic (Valiant), Terumo (Anaconda), and Cook Medical (p-Branch) remain under clinical investigation. A four-branched device (Gore TAMBE) is under investigation as well.
- The Cook Zenith fenestrated stent graft consists of a proximal fenestrated tubular component, a distal bifurcated universal component, and a contralateral iliac limb extension (**FIGURE 1A**). The fenestrated tubular component is custom-made to fit the patient's anatomy. Four to 8 weeks are required for manufacturing and delivery in the United States.
- Bilateral percutaneous femoral access is established under ultrasound guidance; each femoral puncture is preclosed using two Perclose devices. Bilateral 8-Fr sheaths are introduced to the external iliac arteries over Benson guidewires (Cook Medical, Bloomington, IN). The guidewires are exchanged to 0.035-in soft glidewires and Kumpe catheters, which are advanced to the ascending aorta and exchanged for stiff 0.035-in Lunderquist guidewires (Cook Medical, Bloomington, IN).
- Choice of access site is dependent on tortuosity and vessel diameter. Provided there are no issues with both iliac arteries, the branches are performed via the right femoral approach, whereas the fenestrated and bifurcated devices are introduced via the left femoral approach. A 20-Fr (two fenestrations) or 22-Fr (three fenestrations) Check-Flo sheath (Cook Medical, Bloomington, IN) is introduced via the right femoral approach (**FIGURE 2A**). The valve of the Check-Flo sheath has four leaflets, which are accessed by two short 7-Fr sheaths at 2- and 7-o'clock positions.
- Precatheterization of the renal arteries is performed using 0.035-in soft glidewires and 5-Fr Kumpe or C1 catheters (Cook Medical, Bloomington, IN), which are supported by 7-Fr left internal mammary artery (LIMA) guide catheters (**FIGURE 2B**). Alternatively, onlay fusion CTA is recommended to minimize contrast use. Generally, for two-vessel fenestrated endograft, precatheterization is not necessary with the use of onlay fusion techniques.
- The fenestrated stent graft is oriented extracorporeally, introduced via the left femoral approach, and deployed with optimal apposition between the fenestrations and the target catheters.
- Proper device orientation, using the anterior and posterior markers, is essential. It is useful to deploy the first two or three stents and then rotate the imaging unit laterally, confirming alignment. The device should be deployed slightly higher than what is anticipated, with lowest of the four radiopaque markers in the fenestration at the upper edge of the renal artery. The diameter-reducing wire on the fenestrated component allows for some rotational and cranial–caudal movement to optimize alignment following initial deployment.
- After deployment of the fenestrated component, if precatheterization has been used, each catheter is removed from its target artery and used to sequentially regain target vessel access through the respective fenestration (**FIGURE 2C**). In most cases, when alignment is carefully confirmed prior to attempted cannulation, the target vessel is accessed without difficulty. When access is challenging, catheterization of the fenestration may be facilitated by the use of a steerable sheath (ie, 6-Fr Tour Guide [Medtronic, Minneapolis, MN]).
- After the target vessel is catheterized, soft glidewire is removed and hand injection is used to confirm location. The glidewire is exchanged for a 0.035-in Rosen guidewire (Cook Medical, Bloomington, IN). The Rosen guidewire has a floppy J tip, reducing the risk of branch renal artery perforations. When additional support is required, the Amplatz guidewire (Cook Medical, Bloomington, IN) with 1-cm soft tip can be used.
- After the Rosen or stiff guidewire of choice is positioned, a 7-Fr Ansel sheath with flexible dilator is advanced. If there is difficulty to advance the sheath, an undersized balloon may be used as a dilator to facilitate advancement.
- Once the sheath is in position, an alignment stent is positioned under protection of the sheath with the tip of the stent just beyond the tip of the sheath (**FIGURE 2D**).

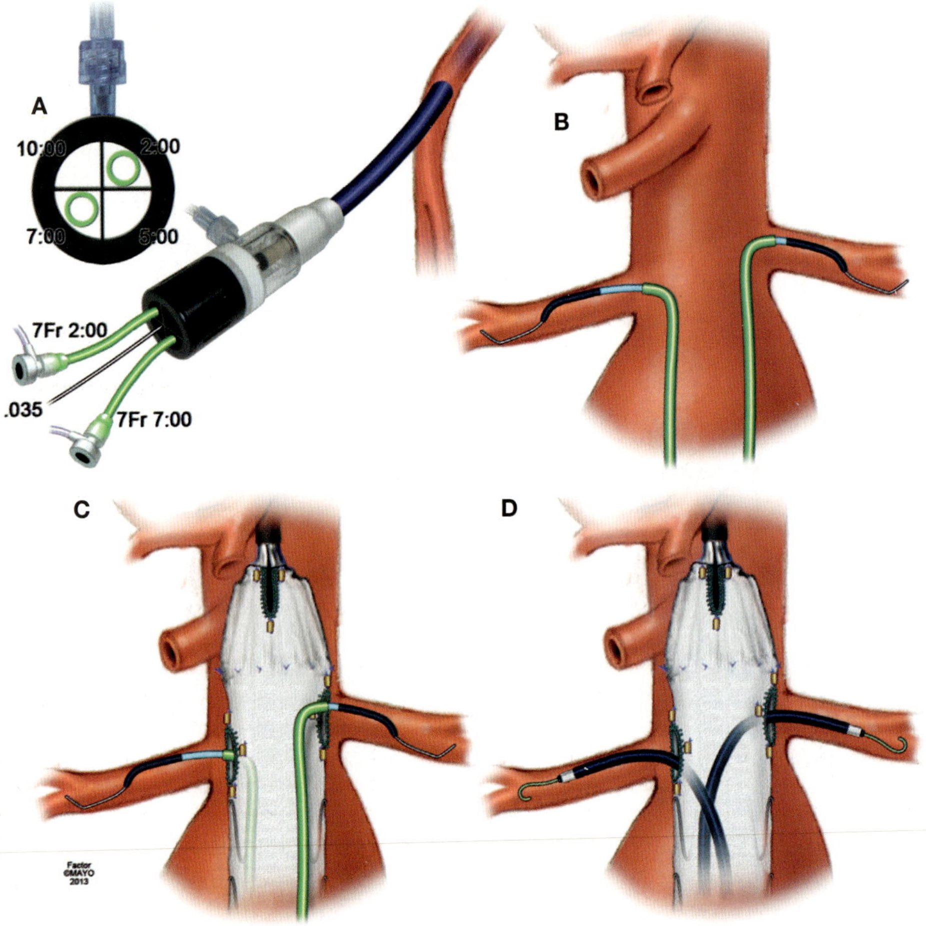

FIGURE 2 • **A,** A 20-Fr (two fenestrations) or 22-Fr (three fenestrations) Check-Flo sheath is introduced via the right femoral approach. **B,** Precatheterization of the renal arteries. **C,** Sequentially regain access into the fenestrated component, fenestration, and target vessel. **D,** An alignment stent is advanced under protection of the sheath. (A, Used with permission of Mayo Foundation for Medical Education and Research, all rights reserved.)

- For repairs requiring two or three vessel fenestrations, the target vessels are accessed sequentially using femoral approach. For those requiring four fenestrations, the celiac axis is accessed via brachial approach using a preloaded catheter, which is placed through the celiac fenestration and exits the stent graft via an access scallop at the top of the device.
- The diameter-reducing tie on the fenestrated segment is removed after all the target arteries are accessed and secured by 7-Fr hydrophilic sheaths.
- The top cap of the device is advanced forward to deploy the uncovered fixation stent (**FIGURE 3A**). The top cap is retrieved prior to deployment of the alignment stents.
- After the top cap and dilator are removed, the proximal landing zone is gently dilated using a compliable balloon such as the Coda balloon (Cook Medical, Bloomington IN, **FIGURE 3B**). It is critical that the balloon dilatation is performed prior to placement of alignment stents, or alternatively, each stent has to be protected by separate balloons.
- The alignment stents are sequentially deployed following removal of the diameter-reducing tie, retrieval of the top cap, and balloon dilatation of the neck. **The sequence of stent deployment is renal arteries followed by SMA and celiac axis**. Prior to each stent deployment, the position of the stent is confirmed by hand injection. The stent is deployed 3 to 5 mm into the aorta (**FIGURE 3C**) and flared using a 10 mm × 2 cm balloon (**FIGURE 3D**). A completion angiography of each branch is performed using hand injection after direct injection of 100 to 200 μg of nitroglycerin to minimize spasm.
- Following placement of the alignment stents, a distal bifurcated stent graft is oriented, advanced, and deployed with preservation of the ipsilateral internal iliac artery. The dilator of the bifurcated device may encroach the contralateral renal stent or the SMA stent. In these cases, it is useful to leave a 10-mm balloon ready to be inflated in the renal stent to prevent damage (**FIGURE 4A**, *inset*). The minimum overlap between the bifurcated and the fenestrated component is two full-length stents (17 mm each), but ideally, more than three full stents is recommended to minimize risk of component separation (**FIGURE 4B**).[12,13] After deployment of the bifurcated device, the dilator is removed with care to avoid damage or dislodgement of the renal stents.
- The contralateral gate is catheterized using a soft glidewire and 5-Fr catheter (**FIGURE 4B**). Access is confirmed by 360° catheter rotation. The glidewire is exchanged for a 0.035-in Lunderquist guidewire. Limited iliac angiography using contralateral oblique views with hand injection. The contralateral limb extension is deployed with preservation of the internal iliac artery (**FIGURE 4C**).
- A completion cone beam CT angiography of the aorta and iliac arteries is obtained using power injection to demonstrate patency of the visceral arteries, main body, iliac limbs, and iliac arteries.

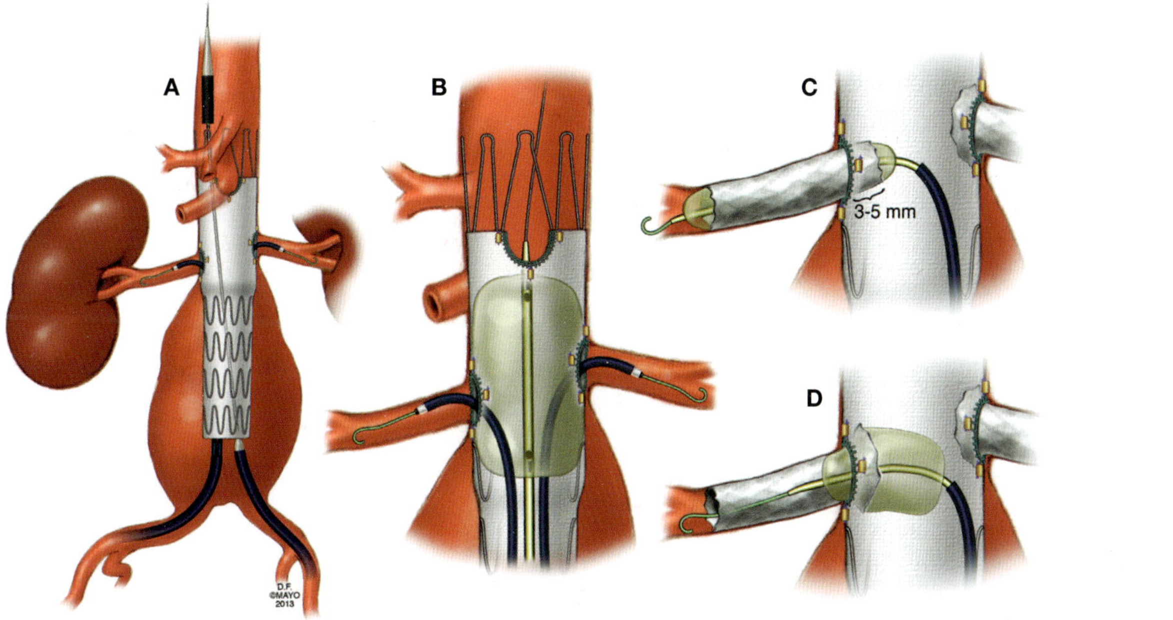

FIGURE 3 • **A,** The top cap of the device is advancing forward allowing deployment of the uncovered fixation stent. **B,** The proximal landing zone is gently dilated using a compliable balloon. Stent deployed 3 to 5 mm into the aorta **(C)** and flared using a 10 mm × 2 cm balloon **(D)**.

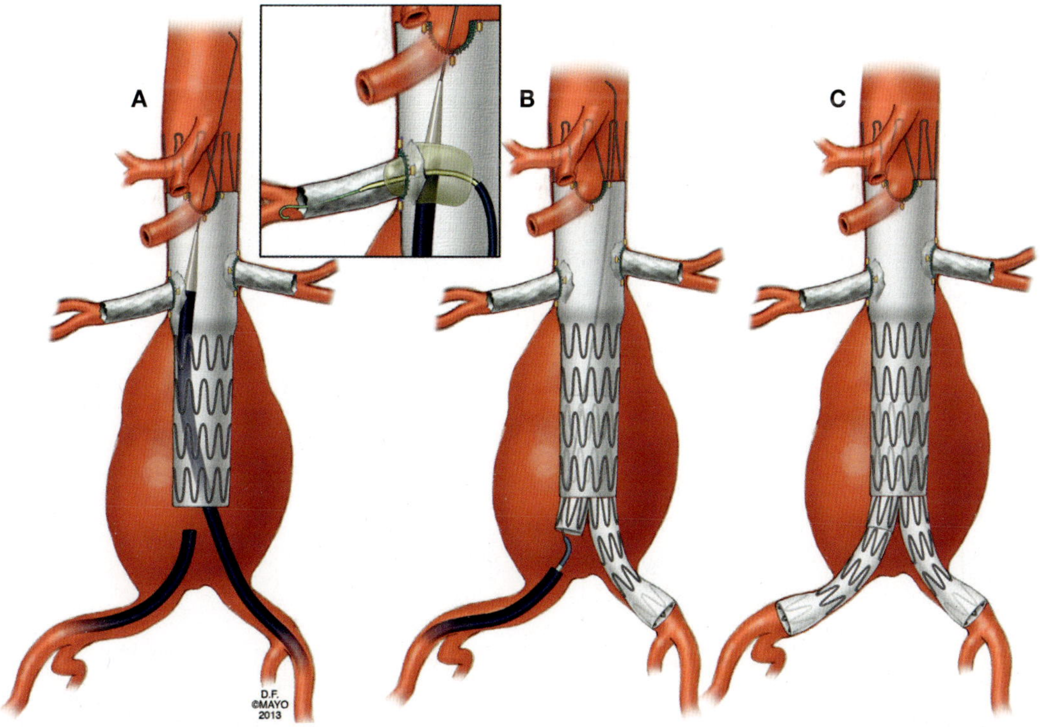

FIGURE 4 • To avoid the dilator of the bifurcated device encroaching the contralateral renal stent or the superior mesenteric artery stent, leave a 10-mm balloon ready to be inflated in the renal stent (**A,** *inset*). **B,** The minimum overlap between the bifurcated and the fenestrated component is more than two full-length stents. **C,** The contralateral limb extension is deployed with preservation of the internal iliac artery.

ENDOVASCULAR REPAIR USING MULTIPLE DIRECTIONAL BRANCHES (MULTIBRANCH T-BRANCH STENT GRAFT)

- Directional branches created with presewn cuffs are currently available from Cook Zenith stent graft lineage on an investigational use basis (**FIGURE 1B**). A four-vessel multibranch stent graft design (T-branch) remains under investigation for treatment of TAAAs.
- The extent of repair varies depending on the proximal extension of aneurysm within the thoracic aorta. The procedure is performed using bilateral femoral and left brachial approach. In general, the repair starts with deployment of a proximal thoracic TX2 stent graft (Cook Medical, Bloomington, IN) followed by deployment of the T-branch stent graft (Cook Medical, Brisbane, Australia) and distal bifurcated component and contralateral limb extension. The self-expandable stents are placed into the four branches following deployment of all aortic components. The critical steps are reviewed as follows:
- Bilateral femoral and left brachial arterial access is obtained (**FIGURE 5A**). A proximal thoracic stent graft is deployed if needed depending on aneurysm extent.

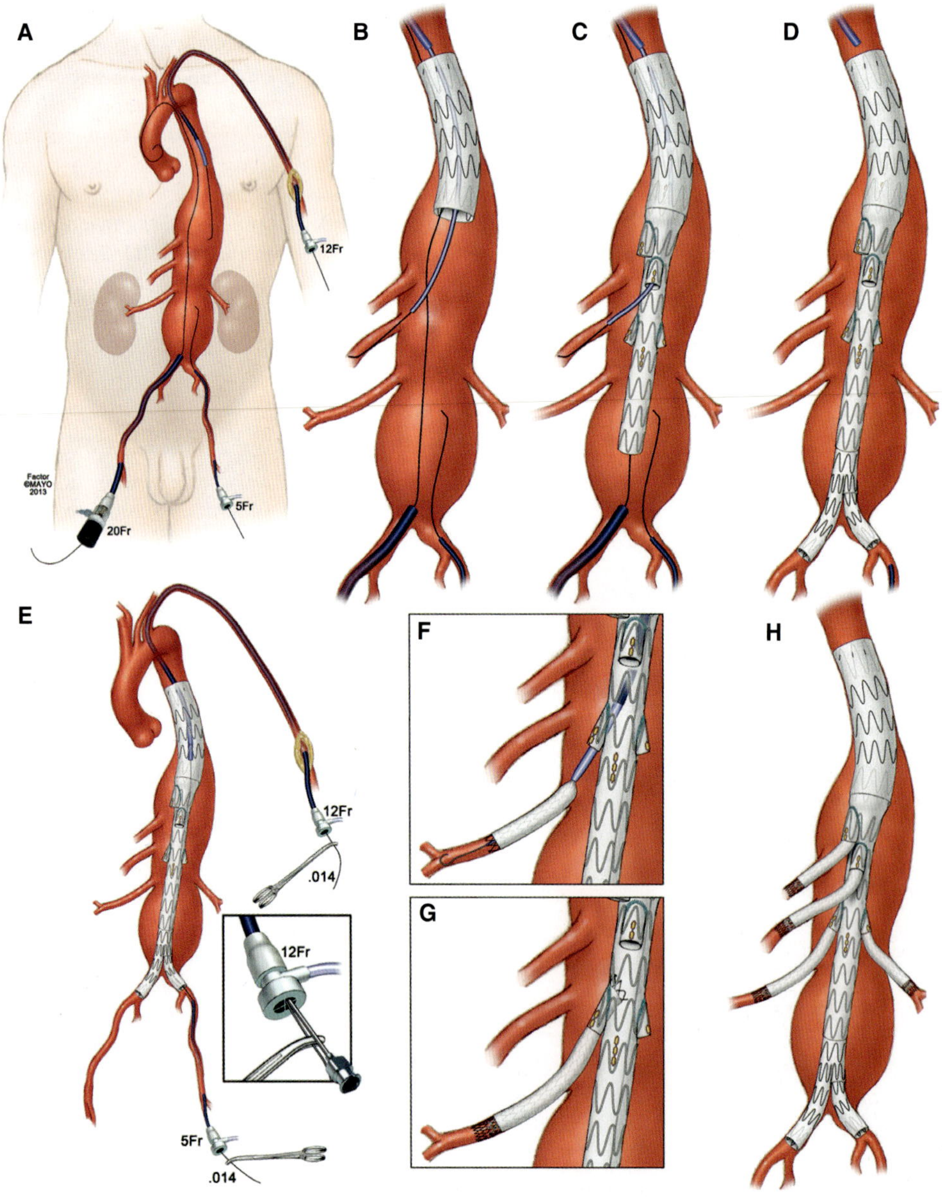

FIGURE 5 ● **A,** Endovascular repair using multiple directional branches is performed using bilateral femoral and left brachial approach. Deployment of proximal thoracic TX2 stent graft **(B)**, followed by deployment of the T-branch stent graft **(C)**, and distal bifurcated component and contralateral limb extension **(D)**. The femoral arteries may be closed, restoring flow into the lower extremities; maintain access into one of the femoral arteries using a 5-Fr sheath (**E**, *inset*). **F** and **G**. 9-Fr 80-cm flexor sheath is advanced into the target vessel, followed by placement of a self-expandable stent graft. **H,** Complete procedure. (A, B, F, and G Used with permission of Mayo Foundation for Medical Education and Research, all rights reserved.)

- Precatheterization of the renal arteries is not required, but it is critical that the distal edge of the directional branch is deployed above its intended target vessel. To guide deployment of the T-branch component, the SMA is precatheterized via the brachial approach (**FIGURE 5B**).
- The T-branch stent graft is oriented extracorporeally, introduced via the femoral approach, and deployed with the directional branches located proximal to its intended target vessel (**FIGURE 5C**).
- Deployment of the distal universal bifurcated stent graft and contralateral iliac extension are identical to what was described in the fenestrated technique (**FIGURE 5D**).
- The femoral arteries are closed at this point, restoring flow into the lower extremities. It is useful to maintain access into one of the femoral arteries with a 5-Fr sheath (**FIGURE 5E**, *inset*). This maneuver allows passage of a 0.014-in guidewire from the left brachial artery to femoral artery. The guidewire is clamped in both ends, which locks the 12-Fr sheath in place and provides support for deployment of the side branches.
- The 12-Fr Ansel I sheath (Cook Medical, Bloomington, IN) is advanced via the left brachial approach and positioned inside the T-branch component in the descending thoracic aorta (**FIGURE 5E**). At this point, a 0.014-in guidewire is advanced through and through from the left brachial to femoral artery, preventing movement of the 12-Fr sheath in the aortic arch.
- Each side branch is individually catheterized in a sequential fashion, starting with the renal arteries (**FIGURE 5F**) followed by the SMA and celiac axis. A 5-Fr main pulmonary artery (MPA) or Kumpe catheter (Cook Medical, Bloomington, IN) is used to access the directional branch and target vessel. Once the vessel is catheterized, the soft glidewire is exchanged for a stiff guidewire (Rosen or short-tip Amplatzer, Cook Medical, Bloomington, IN), which is positioned in the target vessel.
- A 9-Fr 80-cm flexor sheath (Cook Medical, Bloomington, IN) is advanced coaxially within the 12-Fr sheath into the target vessel.
- Each target vessel is stented with a self-expandable stent graft (**FIGURE 5F**). The stent graft should be oversized by 1 to 2 mm and should provide at least 2 cm of distal landing zone in the target vessel, extending 3 to 5 mm into the aortic lumen of the T-branch device.
- To prevent kinks in the transition of the stent graft to the target artery, each self-expandable stent graft is reinforced by a second self-expandable uncovered stent, which is deployed 1 cm beyond the distal edge of the stent graft (**FIGURE 5G**). Selective completion angiography is obtained for each sequential branch.
- A completion angiography of the arch and thoracoabdominal aorta is obtained after all matting stent grafts are deployed (**FIGURE 5H**).

ENDOVASCULAR REPAIR USING TWO DIRECTIONAL BRANCHES AND TWO FENESTRATIONS (TWO BRANCH–TWO FENESTRATED STENT GRAFT)

- A design with directional branches for the celiac and SMA and fenestrations for the renal arteries has been widely used at the Cleveland Clinic.[14] A design with two straight downgoing branches and two fenestrations has been used (**FIGURE 1C**). The advantage of the latter is the ability to provide short, transversely oriented branches for the renal arteries.
- The same principles already described for fenestrated stent grafts are applied with respect to device design, planning, and arterial access.
- Bilateral femoral access and left brachial artery access are needed (**FIGURE 6A**). The right femoral access is used for precatheterization of the renal arteries. The left brachial access is used for the celiac axis and SMA (**FIGURE 6B**).
- A proximal thoracic TX2 stent graft (Cook Medical, Bloomington, IN) is deployed first, depending on proximal extension of the aneurysm (**FIGURE 6A**).
- After the renal arteries and SMA are precatheterized, the fenestrated–branched stent graft is oriented extracorporeally, introduced via the femoral approach and deployed with perfect apposition between the renal fenestrations and the target renal arteries (**FIGURE 6B**).
- The celiac and SMA branch are accessed using preloaded catheters and glidewires, which are snared via the left brachial approach (**FIGURE 6B**).
- Each catheter is sequentially removed from the renal arteries and used to regain access into the fenestrated component, renal fenestration, and target renal artery (**FIGURE 6C**). Hydrophilic sheaths and alignment renal stents are advanced as previously described.
- The preloaded catheters in the SMA and celiac branch allow advancement of a 0.035-in soft glidewire, which is snared via the left brachial approach (**FIGURE 6B**). A sheath and catheter are advanced into the celiac branch. Following access into the celiac axis, a 0.035-in Amplatz guidewire is placed.
- The SMA is accessed using similar steps, and after access is established with Amplatz guidewire, a 9-Fr sheath is advanced to allow positioning of a self-expandable stent graft.
- Once all four vessels are catheterized and sheaths are positioned into the renal arteries and SMA, the diameter-reducing tie is removed, allowing complete expansion of the fenestrated–branched component (**FIGURE 6D**).
- Sequential target artery stenting is performed using balloon-expandable covered stents for the renal fenestrated branches (**FIGURE 6E**, *inset*) and self-expandable stent grafts for the SMA and celiac axis (**FIGURE 6E**, *inset*). Selective branch angiography is performed after each branch stent is placed.
- Deployment of distal bifurcated component and contralateral iliac limb extension is identical to what has been described for fenestrated stent grafts (**FIGURE 6F**).

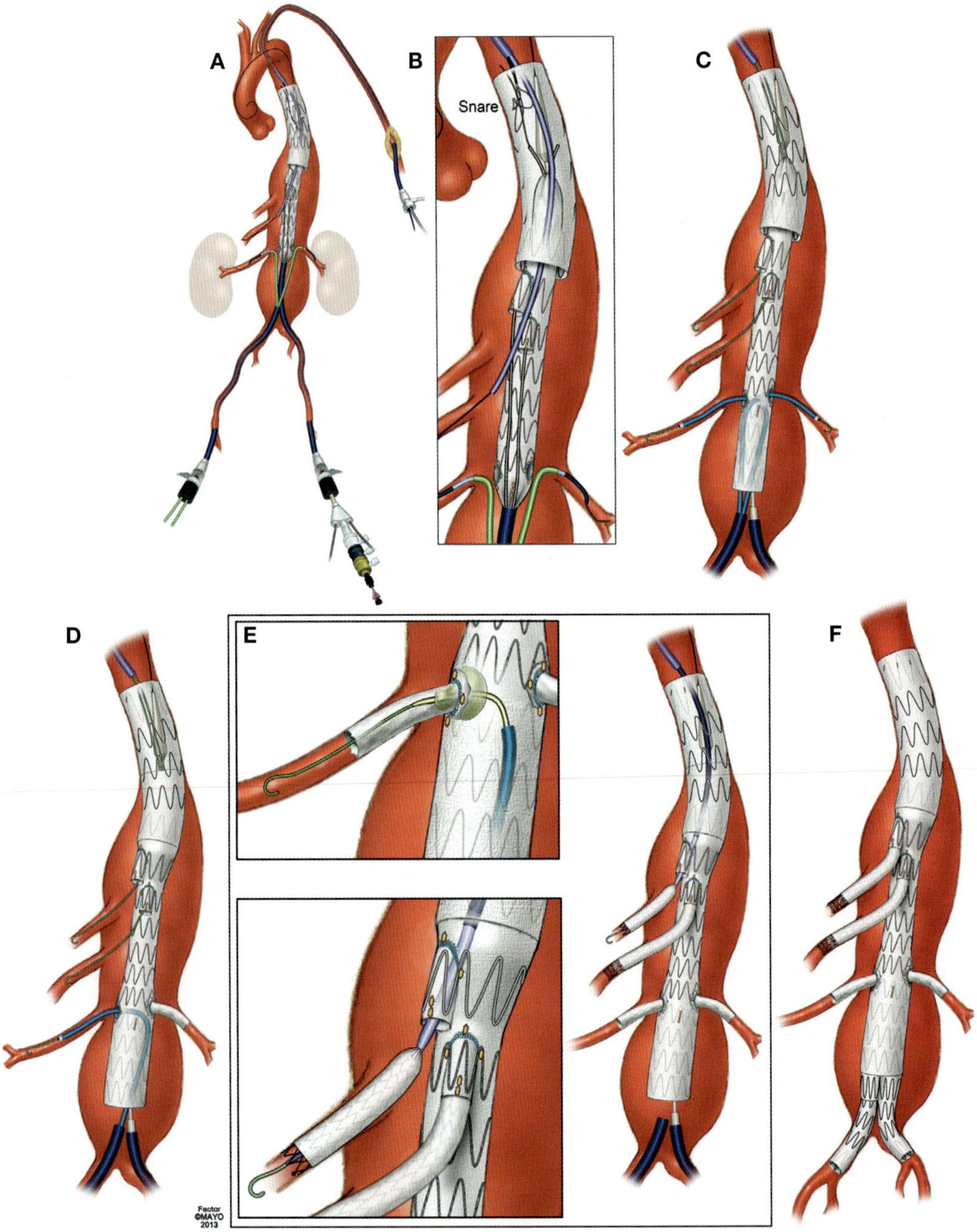

FIGURE 6 • **A,** Bilateral femoral access and left brachial artery access is needed. **B,** After the renal arteries and superior mesenteric artery (SMA) are precatheterized, the fenestrated–branched stent graft is oriented extracorporeally, introduced via the femoral approach. The celiac and SMA branch are accessed using preloaded catheters and glidewires, which are snared via the left brachial approach. **C,** Regain access into the fenestrated component, renal fenestration, and target renal artery. **D,** Complete expansion of the fenestrated–branched component. Sequential target artery stenting is performed using balloon-expandable covered stents for the renal fenestrated branches and self-expandable stent grafts for the SMA and celiac axis (**E,** *inset*). **F,** Deployment of distal bifurcated component and contralateral iliac limb extension.

PEARLS AND PITFALLS

Preoperative evaluation	▪ Complete history and physical examination with emphasis on cardiovascular risk factors, family history of aneurysm disease, and connective tissue disorders. ▪ Preoperative medical evaluation focused on cardiac, pulmonary, and renal performance. ▪ Aortic imaging with CTA allows detailed analysis of aneurysm morphology for stent graft design and procedure planning.
Arterial access	▪ Iliac conduits are recommended in patients with small, diseased, or excessively tortuous iliac arteries. ▪ Pelvic perfusion with maintenance of internal iliac artery flow decreases risk of spinal cord injury.
Stent graft implantation	▪ Precise stent graft design and implantation are critical aspects of the procedure. ▪ Minimize use of iodinated contrast by avoiding contrast aortography during device implantation. ▪ Precatheterization and/or onlay CT allows precise device implantation with minimal need of angiography. ▪ Fenestrations are typically accessed via the femoral approach and stented using balloon-expandable covered stents. ▪ Directional branches are accessed via the brachial approach and stented using self-expandable stent grafts.
Misaligned fenestrations	▪ Excessive tortuosity in the iliac or visceral segment may cause misalignment of fenestrations and difficult target vessel catheterization. ▪ Rotation of the device, which is constrained by a diameter-reducing tie, and use of balloon displacement or curved catheters allow successful catheterization in most cases.
Branch perforation or dissection	▪ Small, diseased, and tortuous visceral arteries are prone to perforation or dissection, particularly if an Amplatz guidewire is needed to provide more support. ▪ Careful attention to detail and minimizing guidewire manipulation with close attention to the tip of the guidewire help prevent this complication.
Stent kinks	▪ Branch tortuosity may lead to kinks within the side stents. ▪ This should be immediately recognized and treated by placement of a second self-expandable stent to prevent branch occlusion.

POSTOPERATIVE CARE

- Length of stay averages 2 to 3 days for endovascular repair of pararenal aneurysms and 4 to 5 days for TAAAs.
- Cerebrospinal fluid drainage, if used, is discontinued on postoperative day 2, after a 6-hour clamp trial and documentation of normal coagulation profile.
- Oral diet is resumed the day after the operation for uncomplicated cases requiring two to three fenestrations, but it is typically withheld for 1 or 2 days for difficult cases or those requiring four fenestrations or branches.
- Cone beam CTA is obtained at the completion of stent graft deployment in the operating room, which may reveal a technical issue requiring intervention in up to 31% of patients.[15] Follow-up includes clinical examination and imaging (CTA and ultrasound) in 6 to 8 weeks, every 6 months during the first year, and yearly 1 year, and early thereafter.
- Patients are started on aspirin indefinitely. Clopidogrel is not recommended unless there is a specific concern with one of the side branches because of small size (<4 mm), occlusive disease, or dissection. Clopidogrel should be avoided early after extensive TAAA repair because of risk of delayed spinal cord injury and paraplegia, which may necessitate replacement of the spinal drain.

OUTCOMES

- Branched and fenestrated aortic repairs have become more common and devices continue to evolve. The European Society for Vascular and Endovascular Surgery has recommended B/FEVAR over open repair of pararenal and TAAAs in patients with appropriate anatomy.[16] Short-term and mid-term outcomes have been good for these devices, with perioperative death rates of 0.9%, 5-year freedom from aortic-related mortality of 98%, and 64% freedom from reintervention at 5 years.[17] Freedom from reintervention is lower in patients undergoing F/BEVAR to treat type Ia endoleak after failed infrarenal EVAR.[18]
- Technical success is high for endovascular repair using fenestrated stent grafts, with branch artery preservation successful in up to 99.2% of vessels for extent IV TAAA and pararenal AAA, and 98.5% in extent I-III TAAA.[17]
- Up to 20% of patients undergoing F/BEVAR may require a secondary intervention for endoleak (type I or type III), highlighting the need for life-long postoperative surveillance.[17]
- Likelihood of reintervention for branch artery instability (type Ic endoleak or loss of patency) becomes more likely with increasing extent of repair.[19] Mastracci and associates have reported a freedom from branch-related complications of 84% at 5 years.[20]

COMPLICATIONS

Intraprocedural Complications

- ***Fenestration misalignment***: Neck angulation, tortuosity, and errors of design or implantation can lead to misalignment between the fenestration and the target vessel. Several maneuvers can be used to overcome misalignment between the fenestration and the vessel. Initially, the catheter and guidewire are rotated to "probe" the aortic wall in search for the vessel. To maintain access into the fenestration, a 7-Fr Ansel sheath is advanced into the fenestration and secured by a 0.018-in guidewire, whereas a 5-Fr "buddy" catheter (eg, Van Schie [VS] 3) is used to locate the renal artery. In patients with downgoing or stenosed renal arteries, it may be difficult to advance the catheter over a soft glidewire. The catheter and glidewire may bounce up into the top cap, providing support for the catheter to be advanced deep into the renal artery.

- Diameter-reducing ties are located posteriorly, which may result in the fenestrations being pulled slightly more posterior than its intended location. A useful maneuver is to gently rotate each fenestration, usually anteriorly. Other maneuvers are rarely needed but included use of reverse-curved catheters (eg, Omni-Select or SOS) for downgoing vessels or vessels that are originating from the lower part of the fenestration, microcatheters, and balloon displacement of the main stent graft. The latter is rarely needed but may provide more room for catheter manipulations.
- ***Branch perforation or dissection***: Branch vessel perforation and/or dissection can be prevented by meticulous technique, visualization of the tip of the wire, and avoiding wire manipulations. The guidewire should not be positioned in small terminal branches, which are prone to perforate or dissect. It should be visualized and stabilized during exchanges manipulations, avoiding forward or retrograde movement. If perforation occurs, it should be immediately recognized and treated using a microcatheter and coil embolization. Dissections within the main renal artery can be treated by placement of a self-expandable stent.
- ***Endoleaks***: Type II and type IV endoleaks may occur and should be left untreated. Type I and type III endoleaks occur in up to 8% of patients with proper selection of a healthy landing zone and adequate planning.[21] In the event of a type Ia endoleak, the proximal neck may be redilated, but all the alignment stents need to be protected by separate balloons. Type III endoleaks may result from inadequate flare, lack of apposition, use of bare metal stent, or inadequate length into the aorta.
- ***Stent kinks or narrowing***: Kinks are preventable and can be anticipated from careful review of vessel anatomy by CTA. These remain a cause of reintervention or branch vessel loss if not recognized. Short stents (<2 cm) tend to avoid bends and the mid- or distal portion of the renal artery, which has greater respiratory motion. The right renal may have a posterior orientation from its course behind the inferior vena cava. If a kink is anticipated by CTA or is evident by completion angiography, a self-expandable stent should be placed. Kinks or narrowing may also result from inadequate flare, strut compression, and ostial disease. In these cases, angioplasty or stenting with a reinforcing balloon-expandable stent may be recommended.

Postoperative Complications

- Spinal cord injury
- Stroke
- Cardiac events (myocardial infarction, arrhythmias, congestive heart failure)
- Pulmonary complications (pneumonia, prolonged ventilation, tracheostomy)
- Gastrointestinal complications (ileus, pancreatitis, cholecystitis)
- Systemic inflammatory response (fever, leukocytosis, thrombocytopenia)
- Renal function deterioration
- Access-related problems (bleeding, thrombosis, pseudoaneurysm)

ACKNOWLEDGEMENT

We gratefully acknowledge the contributions of Gustavo S. Oderich and Karina S. Kanamori as portions of their chapter were retained in this revision.

REFERENCES

1. Park JH, Chung JW, Choo IW, et al. Fenestrated stent-grafts for preserving visceral arterial branches in the treatment of abdominal aortic aneurysms: preliminary experience. *J Vasc Interv Radiol*. 1996;7(6):819-823.
2. Nordon IM, Hinchliffe RJ, Holt PJ, et al. Modern treatment of juxtarenal abdominal aortic aneurysms with fenestrated endografting and open repair—a systematic review. *Eur J Vasc Endovasc Surg*. 2009;38(1):35-41.
3. Coles-Black J, Barber T, Bolton D, Chuen J. A systematic review of three-dimensional printed template-assisted physician-modified stent grafts for fenestrated endovascular aneurysm repair. *J Vasc Surg*. 2021;74:296-306.
4. Chaikof EL, Dalman RL, Eskandari MK, et al. The Society for Vascular Surgery practice guidelines on the care of patients with an abdominal aortic aneurysm. *J Vasc Surg*. 2018;67:2-77.
5. Ketha SS, Warrington KJ, McPhail IR. Inflammatory abdominal aortic aneurysm: a case report and review of the literature. *Vasc Endovasc Surg*. 2014;48:65-69.
6. Squizzato F, Oderich GS, Balachandran P, Tenorio ER, Mendes BC, De Martino RR. Effect of aortic angulation on the outcomes of fenestrated-branched endovascular aortic repair. *J Vasc Surg*. 2021;74:372-382.
7. Katsargyris A, Marques de Marino P, Verhoeven EL. Graft design and selection of fenestrations vs. branches for renal and mesenteric incorporation in endovascular treatment of pararenal and thoracoabdominal aortic aneurysms. *J Cardiovasc Surg*. 2019;60:35-40.
8. Mendes BC, Oderich GS, Correa MP, et al. Endovascular repair of complex aortic pathology. *Curr Surg Rep*. 2013;1(2):67-77.
9. Greenberg RK, Sternbergh III WC, Makaroun M, et al. Intermediate results of a United States multicenter trial of fenestrated endograft repair for juxtarenal abdominal aortic aneurysms. *J Vasc Surg*. 2009;50(4):730-737.
10. Aucoin VJ, Eagleton MJ, Farber MA, et al. Spinal cord protection practices used during endovascular repair of complex aortic aneurysms by the US Aortic Research Consortium. *J Vasc Surg*. 2021;73:323-330.
11. Bradley NA, Orawiec P, Bhat R, Pal S, Suttie SA, Flett MM, Guthrie GJK. Mid-term follow-up of percutaneous access for standard and complex EVAR using the ProGlide device. *Surgeon*. doi:10.1016/i.surge.2021.03.005
12. Dowdall JF, Greenberg RK, West K, et al. Separation of components in fenestrated and branched endovascular grafting—branch protection or a potentially new mode of failure? *Eur J Vasc Endovasc Surg*. 2008;36(1):2-9.
13. Wang SK, Lemmon GW, Gupta AK, et al. Aggressive surveillance is needed to detect endoleaks and junctional separation between device components after zenith fenestrated aortic reconstruction. *Ann Vasc Surg*. 2019;57:129-136.
14. Barrett T, Khwaja A, Carmona C, et al. Acute kidney injury: prevention, detection, and management. Summary of updated NICE guidance for adults receiving iodine-based contrast media. *Clin Radiol*. 2021;76:193-199.
15. Mezzetto L, Mastrorilli D, Abatucci G, et al. Impact of cone beam computed tomography in advanced endovascular aortic aneurysm repair using latest generation 3D c-arm. *Ann Vasc Surg*. 2021;78:132-140. doi:10.1016/j.avsg.2021.04.035

16. Wanhainen A, Verzini F, Van Herzeele I, et al. Editor's choice – European Society for Vascular Surgery (ESVS) 2019 clinical practice guidelines on the management of abdominal aorto-iliac artery aneurysms. *Eur J Vasc Endovasc Surg*. 2019;57:8-93.
17. Oderich GS, Tenorio ER, Mendes BC, et al. Midterm outcomes of a prospective, nonrandomized study to evaluate endovascular repair of complex aortic aneurysms using fenestrated-branched endografts. *Ann Surg*. 2021;274:491-499.
18. Hostralich A, Mesnard T, Soler R, et al. Prospective multicentre cohort study of fenestrated and branched endografts after failed endovascular infrarenal aortic aneurysm repair with type Ia endoleak. *Eur J Vasc Endovasc Surg*. 2021;62:540-548.
19. Diamond KR, Simons JP, Crawford AS, et al. Effect of thoracoabdominal aortic aneurysm extent on outcomes in patients undergoing fenestrated/branched endovascular aneurysm repair. *J Vasc Surg*. 2021;74:833-842.
20. Mastracci TM, Greenberg RK, Eagleton MJ, et al. Durability of branches in branched and fenestrated endografts. *J Vasc Surg*. 2013;57(4):926-933; discussion 933.
21. Edman NI, Schanzer A, Crawford A, et al. Sex-related outcomes after fenestrated-branched endovascular repair for thoracoabdominal aortic aneurysms in the US Fenestrated and Branched Aortic Research Consortium. *J Vasc Surg*. 2021;74:861-870.

SECTION IV: Visceral and Renal Artery Disease Management

Chapter 18

Stenting, Endografting, and Embolization Techniques: Celiac, Mesenteric, Splenic, Hepatic, and Renal Artery Disease Management

Mohamed A. Zayed and Ronald L. Dalman

DEFINITION

- The content discussed in the following text presupposes familiarity with basic wire and catheter-based endovascular techniques. For a summary of such techniques, the reader may refer to excellent existing references.[1]
- Various occlusive and/or aneurysmal disease processes in renal and visceral arteries may necessitate endovascular interventions (**TABLE 1**).
- Progressive renal artery stenosis (RAS) or occlusion may predispose to renovascular hypertension (RVH; most common form of secondary hypertension) and ischemic nephropathy.[2] Aortic atherosclerosis at the ostia or proximal renal artery accounts for two-thirds of cases.[3] Fibromuscular dysplasia (FMD) also causes progressive serial stenoses throughout the renal arteries and may also predispose to RVH. FMD occurs most commonly in younger female patients.[4]
- Acute mesenteric ischemia (AMI) and chronic mesenteric ischemia (CMI) are life threatening but fortunately rate conditions (1 in 1000 and 1 in 100,000 hospital admissions, respectively).[5,6] The infrequent nature of symptomatic mesenteric ischemia may be due to the rich collateral supply derived from the celiac, superior, and inferior mesenteric arteries. CMI most commonly develops following progressive atherosclerotic occlusion of two or more mesenteric arteries, with the superior mesenteric artery (SMA) being the most critical of the three. Arterial embolization, leading to acute occlusion of the celiac artery or SMA, more commonly is associated with AMI.[6] In rare circumstances, in critically ill patients, impaired intestinal perfusion due to arterial vasospasm may occur in the absence of thromboembolic occlusion.
- Extra- and intraparenchymal renal artery branch aneurysms occur with a reported autopsy incidence between 0.01% and 0.7% and may arise from various disease etiologies.[7] Overall, the risk of acute clinical evolution (rupture or thrombosis) is low but may be increased during pregnancy, with high resultant maternal and fetal mortality. The risk of progression/rupture, as is the case in most visceral artery aneurysms, is presumed to decline significantly following menopause.
- Aneurysms of the celiac artery, SMA, and their branches are also infrequent and associated with varying etiologic entities. Splenic artery aneurysms are the most common (60%), followed by aneurysms in the hepatic (20%), superior mesenteric, and celiac arteries, in that order.[8,9] Syndromes such as polyarteritis nodosa or Kawasaki disease may be associated with aneurysms in various segments of the mesenteric arterial circulation. Guidelines for intervention vary,[10] depending on aneurysm location, rate of enlargement, symptom status, and demographic considerations: age, gender, and menstruation status.

Table 1: Renal/Visceral Arterial Disease

Causes of renal/visceral artery stenosis or occlusion	• Atherosclerosis • Fibromuscular dysplasia • Dissection • Coarctation syndromes • Extrinsic compression • Vasculitis • Hypercoagulable state
Causes of renal/visceral artery aneurysm	• Extension of aortic aneurysmal disease • Atherosclerotic degeneration • Blunt or penetrating trauma • Fibromuscular dysplasia • Connective tissue disorder • Iatrogenic injury

PATIENT HISTORY AND PHYSICAL FINDINGS

- RVH, with or without concurrent evidence of ischemic nephropathy, is seen in less than 50% of individuals manifesting severe RAS.[2,3] Hypertension in children, new onset hypertension in individuals younger than 30 or older than 55 years old, or accelerated hypertension should prompt suspicion for the presence of RAS. Older patients with RVH/RAS typically manifest other stigmata of systemic vascular disease, including coronary and cerebrovascular disease, in addition to peripheral vascular disease. In patients with severe bilateral RAS, renal failure may be exacerbated with recent initiation of an angiotensin-converting enzyme (ACE) inhibitor.[11] Acute exacerbations of poorly controlled RVH may manifest with "hypertensive crisis," flash pulmonary edema, or neurologic symptoms ranging from headache to seizure and stroke. Physical examination may reveal severe elevation of both systolic and diastolic blood pressures, abdominal bruits, and other manifestations of peripheral arterial occlusive disease.

- Patients with CMI are typically elderly and have a prior history of symptomatic vascular disease. Like RAS/RVH patients, CMI rarely is present without other signs and symptoms of advanced vascular disease, including aortic and mesenteric branch arterial calcification on plain x-ray films of the abdomen. Symptoms produced by CMI are frequently nonspecific and intermittent, leading to delayed diagnosis and disease progression. Classical symptoms usually include postprandial dull/crampy midepigastric abdominal pain, progressive weight loss, and "food fear" with decreased caloric intake.[12] Findings on physical examination are usually noncontributory, similar to those related to advanced peripheral arterial disease (eg, absent pedal pulses); patients frequently are malnourished and cachectic. Abdominal auscultation frequently reveals hyperactive bowel sounds, and a bruit may sometimes be auscultated.
- AMI presents more dramatically, with sudden onset of abdominal pain, often in patients suffering acute embolic occlusion of the SMA. Although pain may seem out of proportion to objective physical examination findings initially, progressive tenderness to palpation and ultimately peritoneal signs develop in parallel with diminishing bowel viability. Clinical status also rapidly deteriorates, with progressive metabolic acidosis, shock, and multisystem organ failure.[6]
- Patients with renal artery aneurysms (RAAs) may provide a history of trauma, arterial dissection, syndromic vascular conditions, connective tissue disorders, or RAS. The majority of RAAs are asymptomatic at the time of diagnosis, identified as incidental findings on cross-sectional imaging studies ordered for unrelated indications. Specific associated historical and physical findings are rare but may include acute onset hypertension, abdominal distension, flank pain, hematuria, syncope, and shock. Occasionally, an abdominal pulsatile mass is present on physical examination.[7] Although not always fatal, RAA rupture, particularly those in segmental branches, frequently predisposes to renal infarction and resultant decrease in glomerular filtration capacity.
- Patients with aneurysms of the celiac and SMAs and derived branches may manifest with a history of arterial dissection, trauma, pancreatitis, or other local inflammatory processes or infections. One-third of patients may also have aneurysmal disease in other segments of their arterial anatomy.[8] As is the case with RAAs, patients rarely present with symptoms other than rupture, which itself is also rare. Free rupture may result in hemoperitoneum, hematobilia, or life-threatening gastrointestinal hemorrhage. The risk of rupture is highest with hepatic (20%-44% of mesenteric arterial aneurysm ruptures) and splenic artery aneurysms, the latter notoriously at risk during the third trimester of pregnancy.[13,14] Presence of a splenic artery aneurysm recognized during pregnancy should prompt consideration of immediate repair, regardless of the status of the pregnancy.[15]

IMAGING AND OTHER DIAGNOSTIC STUDIES

- Renal artery disease assessment usually begins with duplex ultrasonography, which has a reported sensitivity of 86% to 93%, specificity of 98%, and overall accuracy of 96%.[16] Duplex criteria used to diagnose more than 60% RAS include an arterial peak systolic velocity of more than 180 to 200 cm per second, a ratio of renal artery to aortic peak systolic velocity of more than 3.5, or acceleration time between onset and peak of systole of more than 100 m per second. Kidney length and resistive indexes derived from parenchymal insonation may also provide important insight into the presence, nature, and severity of end-organ disease.
- Similarly, duplex ultrasound provides a useful, noninvasive method of assessing for the presence of chronic mesenteric occlusive disease.[17] In the celiac artery, peak systolic velocities of more than 200 cm per second provides a sensitivity and accuracy for detecting a greater than 70% stenosis of 87% and 82%, respectively. In the SMA, peak systolic velocities of more than 275 cm per second provides a sensitivity and accuracy for detecting a greater than 70% stenosis of 92% and 96%, respectively.
- Computed tomography angiography (CTA) is the current gold standard for confirming the presence, severity, and extent of occlusive mesenteric vascular disease. CTA-derived images also provide insights into the potential underlying mechanism of occlusion, including FMD, associated dissection, evidence of inflammation/infection, or thromboembolic occlusion. Moreover, three-dimensional reconstructions generated from CTA datasets also provide valuable guidance for preprocedural planning. In emergent circumstances, such as those associated with suspected AMI, CTA usually represents the "go-to" diagnostic test.
- For patients with contrast allergies or other contraindications to computed tomography (CT) scanning, magnetic resonance angiography (MRA) may provide a suitable alternative, particularly for initial diagnosis and screening purposes. Overall resolution of MRA is not equal to that of CTA, and in some circumstances may not provide sufficient detail for the precise surgical or interventional planning.

SURGICAL MANAGEMENT

Patient Selection

- Appropriate patient selection for endovascular intervention is paramount and dependent on therapeutic indication, anatomy, patient comorbidities, and acuity of the disease process. In the following text, we discuss considerations for patients with renal/mesenteric arterial occlusive disease, followed by considerations for patients with renal/mesenteric arterial aneurysmal disease.
- For RAS, the indication for endovascular intervention is contingent on severity of stenosis, the presence and severity of presumed resulting hypertension, and extent of residual glomerular filtration capacity. For RAS, there is no accepted indication currently for "prophylactic" intervention. Endovascular intervention is considered only in patients with severe hypertension, who have failed medical management with at least three concurrent antihypertensive medications or have demonstrated progressive loss of renal

function due to ischemic nephropathy in the setting of more than 60% RAS. The future role for endovascular intervention in treating RVH has been called into question by level I data demonstrating only modest reductions in blood pressure following renal artery stenting.[18]

- Patients with critical stenosis or occlusion of at least two mesenteric arteries, in the setting of signs and symptoms consistent with CMI, are also potential candidates for endovascular management. Patients with atypical symptoms who may meet anatomic criteria for mesenteric occlusive disease often experience disappointing results following endovascular intervention.
- Given the compromises inherent in management of AMI, often in the setting of uncertain bowel viability, hybrid open and endovascular approaches may represent the safest and most expeditious option. Particularly in regard to "acute-on-chronic" occlusion of the proximal SMA, with a patent distal segment preserved by collateral flow, surgical exposure at celiotomy enables distal SMA cannulation and sheath placement. Standard angiographic techniques are then employed to cross the occlusive proximal lesion in a retrograde fashion, with subsequent angioplasty and stenting performed to restore pulsatile antegrade flow.[19] We have employed this technique reliably under a variety of challenging clinical conditions with consistently good results.
- In patients with disease in multiple mesenteric arterial segments and symptoms concerning for mesenteric ischemia, SMA revascularization, either via endovascular or open surgical approaches, represents the most reliable and effective method for resolving critical mid- and distal gut ischemia. Decompressive laparotomy should always be considered as an essential adjunct in these circumstances, regardless of revascularization method used, to facilitate selective resection of nonviable bowel if needed and limit the noxious effects of abdominal compartment syndrome in these already compromised patients.
- In comparison, the safety and use of primary inferior mesenteric artery (IMA) endovascular intervention remains controversial in patients with disease in multiple mesenteric arteries. Recent series report relatively frequent procedure-related complications and poor outcomes following attempted IMA intervention.[20] These results may in part be due to the progressive nature of occlusive vascular disease in the most distal aortic segment at the level of the IMA and resulting difficulty in resolving significant ostial stenoses with even high-pressure angioplasty techniques.
- The criteria for elective repair of asymptomatic RAAs are controversial. Recommendations vary for intervention based on aneurysm diameter, also taking into account the size of the parent artery, extent of mural calcification, and rate of enlargement, if available. Consensus exists regarding treatment for all aneurysms larger than 3 cm in diameter.[21,22] Similarly, patients with intact but symptomatic true aneurysms, recent-onset false (pseudo-) aneurysms, and aneurysms resulting from associated FMD are also typically repaired promptly, given their presumed higher risk of rupture. RAAs in women of childbearing age with plans for future pregnancies are usually repaired, when recognized, at almost any size. Less agreement is present for RAAs larger than 2 cm but smaller than 3 cm in diameter, with treatment recommendations often customized based on individual circumstances.
- There are no set size criteria for visceral artery aneurysm repair. Although larger aneurysms are thought to have an increased potential risk of rupture, small visceral artery aneurysms are also known to rupture and manifest with life-threatening hemorrhage. Therefore, most visceral aneurysms larger than 2 cm should be repaired when identified. This recommendation does not necessarily apply to poststenotic arterial dilations (not true aneurysms) and distal SMA aneurysms. The latter are generally best managed by embolization and/or resection of the dependent loops of adjacent small intestine. In most circumstances, ruptured visceral artery aneurysms are best managed by open or hybrid approaches, allowing for assessment of bowel or end-organ ischemia in conjunction with restoration of arterial flow.

Preoperative Planning

- Prior to attempted repair or exclusion, aneurysm location and access issues should be precisely determined via cross-sectional imaging studies. Luminal plaque, thrombus burden, associated aneurysms, and pre-existing dissections should also be noted. Finally, target vessel diameter should be determined at several intervals before, within, and after the lesion of interest to optimize coil, stent, and graft selection.
- The preferred method of critical renal artery ostial lesion management is by balloon-expandable stent placement. In rare circumstance, angioplasty predilation may be required to advance the appropriate stent through the renal ostia and across the stenotic lesion. Renal artery stents range from 10 to 30 mm in length and 4 to 7 mm in diameter. Transfemoral approaches to the renal artery are generally preferred due to the shorter distance to target, smaller imaging fields, and abundant availability of purpose-specific instrumentation. However, cephalad angulation of the renal artery origins relative to the aorta, the presence of extensive infrarenal aortoiliofemoral arterial occlusive disease, or significant iliac artery tortuosity may favor consideration of the left brachial artery and descending thoracic aorta as the preferred route of access.
- For the treatment of mid- to distal RAS in the setting of FMD, angioplasty alone is generally the preferred treatment modality. Either transfemoral or transbrachial approaches may be considered, depending on the considerations noted earlier. Care must be taken to minimize procedural trauma with precise determination of target artery diameter and selection of appropriately sized instruments (sheaths, balloons, and stents). Poor planning or ill-considered procedural technique may precipitate arterial dissection, thrombosis, and renal infarction.
- Depending on the degree of lesional calcification, the extent of associated juxtaostial aortic occlusive disease, lesion length, and associated target vessel tortuosity, balloon- or self-expanding stent grafts may be chosen for luminal reconstitution and may provide improved long-term patency in the proximal SMA.[23] Cannulation of either the celiac or SMA may be achieved from both femoral and brachial approaches. However, in emergent or extenuating circumstances, left brachial access often proves more expeditious and effective. This is particularly true in the setting of high-grade ostial

stenosis or occlusion, where brachial access and antegrade aortic sheath placement may provide improved guidewire, sheath, and crossing catheter pushability and trackability.

- Successful wire cannulation of ostial SMA and celiac lesions may require "telescoping" techniques with different sheath and wire combinations (see in the following text). This is also true of attempts to deploy devices in the mid- and distal splenic artery, where a triaxial catheter and sheath combination extending into the target lesion is frequently most effective. Given the short and often tortuous nature of the celiac artery, stable sheath placement is challenging, often representing the most difficult aspect of the procedure.
- Similar principles are used when treating aneurysms of renal and visceral arteries, including precise catheter positioning and stable sheath support. Aneurysm size, location, neck anatomy, and extent of tortuosity of feeding target vessels impact the strategy of repair. For example, for large retropancreatic splenic artery aneurysms, coil embolization of the aneurysm sac (preferably with large-end-first or nesting coils) prior to covered stent placement across the ostium of the aneurysm is necessary to ensure long-term procedural success. For precise embolization of shallow or wide-necked aneurysms, adjuncts such as distal balloon occlusion with deployment of detachable coils may be necessary. For more accessible aneurysms with a wide-based aneurysm neck, bare metal stenting may be performed across the ostium of the aneurysm first, followed by placement of coils through the open interstices of the stent to keep the coils localized to the area of interest. Branch artery aneurysms usually occur at bifurcation points and are accompanied by small, well-defined necks and are ideally suited for embolization with microcoils (0.018–in catheter compatible) delivered through a triaxial delivery system.
- The preferred size/shape of embolization devices or covered stents may be either accurately estimated from a preprocedural CT arteriogram or determined at the time of angiographic imaging and sheath placement. Based on these measurements, coil and plug diameters may be oversized by 20% of the target vessel diameter. The length of coils selected is derived from the anticipated arterial lumen surface area that requires embolization. Similarly, the length of vascular plugs selected depends on the target artery to be embolized and the estimated luminal flow. For example, higher flow arteries, such as those proximal to arteriovenous fistulae, usually need more extensive coverage to ensure definitive occlusion. Both self-expanding and balloon-expandable stent grafts are available. The former are also typically oversized by 20%, and the latter are usually sized 1 mm greater than the target artery diameter. Attention should be given to the sheath selection to ensure adequate diameter and length. The device-specific instructions for use (IFU) should be consulted in all circumstances prior to use of occlusion devices, or more generally, any endovascular device with the potential risk for significant vascular injury.
- Depending on their specific location, some visceral artery aneurysms may be embolized without specific end-organ ischemic injury. However, embolization of distal aneurysms, such as those located within the splenic hilum, may result in splenic infarction, further bleeding, or abscess formation. Therefore, splenectomy remains a viable alternative method of splenic artery aneurysm management for many patients. Appropriate vaccinations should be administered with sufficient lead time to allow for an appropriate immunization response prior to elective splenic artery embolization procedures or planned splenectomy.

Operating Room Setup

- Procedures may be performed in an angiography suite, or in an operating room, equipped with a floating-point carbon fiber, radiolucent operating table; fluoroscopy platform; and monitor-viewing bank. However, for precise visceral artery interventions requiring steep oblique/lateral imaging and higher fluoroscopic kilovolt (kV), portable systems in the operating room setting may not provide sufficient image clarity and resolution. Under these circumstances, use of a fixed-imaging system, either in an angiography suite or hybrid operating room, will maximize the likelihood of success.
- For the majority of elective renal and visceral artery interventions, conscious sedation with a combination of short-acting analgesic and sedative agents will provide adequate patient comfort, immobility, and optimal imaging parameters. Standard patient safety measures for conscious sedation, including supplemental oxygen, standard monitoring, and availability of resuscitation equipment should be employed in compliance with local hospital policy. However, general anesthesia is clearly indicated to facilitate treatment of AMI, urgent/emergent management of aneurysm rupture, and/or hemorrhage potentially requiring bowel resection or open conversion.
- For the most part, all renal and visceral artery endovascular interventions can be performed with the patient in the supine position. The left arm may be positioned out at 90° to allow for transbrachial interventions. If a transfemoral intervention is planned, the patient's arms may be extended over the head to aid with image clarity; however, most patients can only tolerate this for certain time periods prior to fatigue. Placing the patient in a 30° rotation to the right, on bolsters placed behind the left flank, at the time of the procedure, will facilitate "true lateral" position to localize and cannulate the origin of the SMA without requiring the image intensifier and radiation source to be in full horizontal position and limiting operator access to the patient as a result.
- In addition to a full array of complementary wires, catheters, and sheaths, premounted balloon-expandable stents and stent grafts should be available, including in low-profile platforms (0.014 in or 0.018 in). Appropriate sizes of coils and plugs should also be identified and readily available.

RENAL ARTERY ANGIOPLASTY AND STENTING

First Step

- For arterial access, a retrograde transfemoral approach is usually selected; however, antegrade transbrachial access may improve accessibility and sheath stability in the presence of significant abdominal/pelvic girth, significantly down-sloping renal arteries, or tortuosity/obstruction of the distal aorta or iliac arteries.
- Arterial access is usually obtained percutaneously using standard Seldinger technique. Bedside ultrasound may facilitate precise placement. Once an interventional sheath access is placed, intravenous unfractionated heparin is administered to maintain an activated clotting time (ACT) of more than 250 seconds.

Second Step

- Wire access to the pararenal aorta may be achieved with 0.035-in guidewire. A 4- or 5-French (Fr) flush catheter is advanced over the guidewire to approximately the level of the first lumbar vertebral body.
- If renal function permits, a complete aortoiliac arteriogram in anterior–posterior image intensifier orientation should be performed to assess both the renal arteries and renal accessory arteries. A power injector should be used for the road map aortogram, using a high injection rate (eg, 15-20 mL per second) and low volume (eg, 10-15 mL). Breath-holding instructions should be given to the patient or the assisting anesthesiologist to allow for aortogram acquisition during end expiration. Glucagon (0.25-2 mg intravenous; approximately 10 minutes preprocedure) can also be administered to diminish intestinal motility and enhance arterial visualization.
- A magnified angiogram can be repeated in areas of interest and intended treatment. For better visualization of the renal artery, the image intensifier should be oriented with a few degrees in cranial and lateral obliquity ipsilateral to the renal artery of interest.
- Intraoperative angiographic measurements are obtained to confirm device selection. A marked flush catheter or radiopaque ruler may facilitate accurate angiographic measurements.

Third Step

- A stiff 0.035-in guidewire (ie, Amplatz, Rosen) is placed in the pararenal aorta to facilitate advancement of a 45-cm 8-Fr renal dilation guide catheter (RDC), or 6-Fr RDC sheath (ie, Terumo Pinnacle destination or Cook Ansel Flexor). The sheath dilator tip should not be advanced into the target vessel to avoid compromise of the residual vessel lumen.
- Wire cannulation of the renal artery is the essential first step. Depending on the angle of entry at the orifice, a number of different catheter tip shapes may facilitate successful renal cannulation (Sos 1 or 2, Cobra, Vanchi, etc.). Once cannulated, the sheath tip is advanced immediately adjacent to, but not across, the renal artery orifice (**FIGURE 1**). A 0.014-in or 0.018-in stiff guidewire with a floppy or hydrophilic tip is then employed to probe across areas of severe stenosis, through a reverse curve or angled catheter, depending on the optimal angle for access. Alternatively, a 0.035-in guidewire, with improved handling and radiopacity, may provide suitable trackability for less critical stenoses.
- Once access is achieved, the wire should be advanced to a secondary branch to optimize positional stability. Care should be taken to maintain wire tip visualization in the field of view, particularly when using hydrophilic guidewires, as they can easily perforate parenchymal arterioles when advanced too

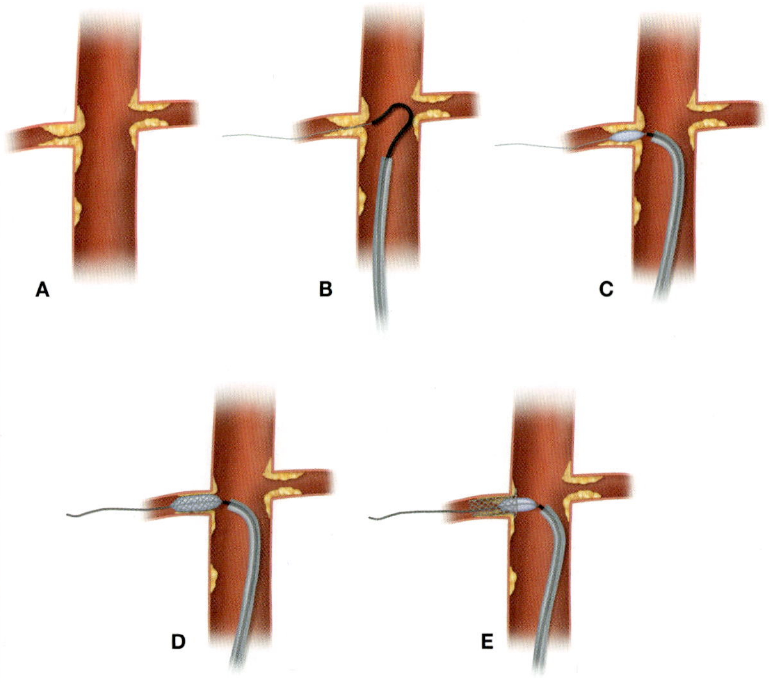

FIGURE 1 • **A,** Pararenal aorta demonstrating high-grade stenosis at the right renal artery orifice. **B,** Cannulation of the right renal artery with a 0.014-in or 0.018-in Glidewire guided by a curved-tip catheter. Wire and catheter cannulation system are stabilized by a 6-Fr sheath. The cannulating wire is advanced into the distal right renal artery to provide additional stability to the system. **C,** The right renal artery orifice stenosis is predilated with a low-profile, small-diameter balloon. **D,** Using sheath support for stability, an appropriately sized balloon-expandable stent is deployed across the stenosis and is protruding 1 mm into the aortic lumen. **E,** While maintaining cannulation system, protruding edge of the stent is flared into the aortic lumen with an appropriate compliant angioplasty balloon.

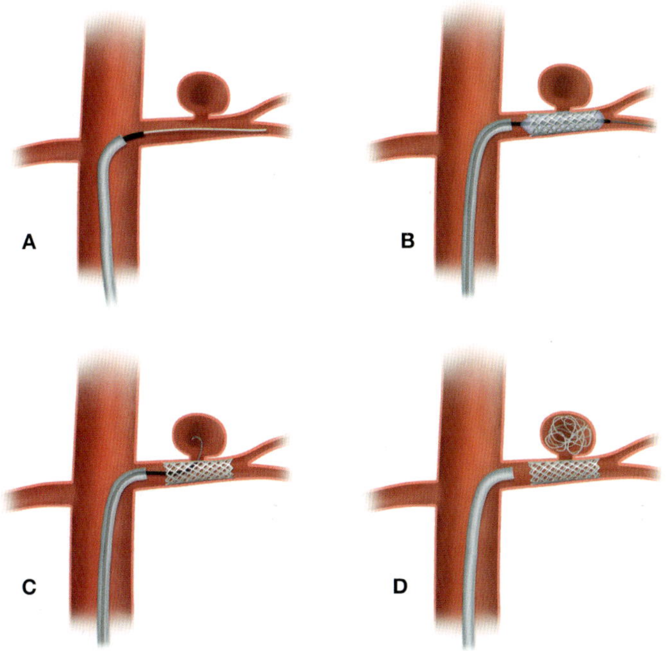

FIGURE 2 • **A,** Left renal artery has an associated saccular aneurysm. Cannulation of the left renal artery is facilitated with an angled guidewire and curved-tip catheter. The cannulation system is stabilized by an appropriately sized sheath. **B,** A bare metal stent is deployed across the origin of the left RAA. **C,** A telescoping technique is used to cannulate the aneurysm sac through an interstice of the bare metal stent. Sheath tip is advanced to the renal artery orifice and catheter is advanced up to the inner luminal wall of the bare metal stent to stabilize and facilitate cannulation of the aneurysm sac. **D,** Appropriately sized coils are deployed into the aneurysm sac through the stent interstices.

far into the segmental renal circulation. Parenchymal perforation may precipitate intra- or extracapsular hematoma formation, renal hemorrhage, and circulatory collapse unless immediately recognized and corrected.

Fourth Step

- Prior to renal artery stenting, predilation may be necessary to provide sufficient luminal space for delivery of the crimped stent/delivery catheter (**FIGURE 1**). A 2- to 4-mm low-profile, semicompliant, or coronary balloon compatible with a 0.014-in or 0.018-in system can be used for this purpose. Care needs to be taken to maintain wire position during subsequent stent exchange; loss of wire position here can preclude stent delivery or precipitate luminal thrombosis if aortic and/or orificial atheroma is displaced by predilation.
- Using a low-profile 0.014-in or 0.018-in system (rapid exchange or over the wire [OTW]), a balloon-expandable stent (eg, Cordis Palmaz Blue, Boston Scientific Express SD, Cook Formula) is delivered across the lesion (**FIGURE 1**). The low-profile nature of these devices enables facile placement, as well as contrast delivery across the lesion to confirm appropriate position. Rapid exchange or monorail systems allow for shorter wire length, aiding procedural efficiency vis-à-vis catheter/wire/device exchanges. In contrast, OTW devices provide improved pushability and trackability across constricting lesions.
- For mid- or distal RAS, the shortest balloon-expandable stent length providing complete coverage should be selected. For mid- or distal RAAs, appropriate length self-expanding or balloon-expandable stent grafts should be selected to provide adequate pre- and postaneurysm renal artery sealing zones (**FIGURE 2**).
- Following stent placement under fluoroscopic guidance, the balloon should be deflated fully prior to its withdrawal to avoid movement or dislodging of the stent. Areas with substantial tortuosity may precipitate arterial kinking at the transition point between stented and nonstented segments. Excessive oversizing, or overinflation of stents mounted on semicompliant balloons, may promote renal artery injury, dissection, or thrombosis. Temptation to optimize the post-procedural angiographic image, potentially at the expense of vessel integrity or anticipated long-term patency, should also be avoided.
- For ostial renal artery lesions, the balloon-expandable stent should be positioned so that the aortic end is deployed approximately 1 mm into the aortic flow stream. The aortic edge of the stent can be "flared" outward with a repeat angioplasty using the distal edge of the same balloon (**FIGURE 1**).

Fifth Step

- After successful deployment, the sheath should only be withdrawn after the completion imaging encompassing the entire ipsilateral kidney is performed to confirm uniform perfusion and absence of parenchymal and/or capsular injury.
- Following withdrawal of the sheath from the renal orifice, while maintaining wire access, completion paraorificial aortography is performed to confirm stent positioning and target lumen diameter. Residual stenosis, kinking, or dissection should be confirmed to be absent prior to withdrawal of the wire.

VISCERAL ARTERY ANGIOPLASTY AND STENTING

First Step

- As previously noted, access considerations need to account for individual patient anatomy, operator experience and skill, available devices, potential complications, goals of treatment, and anticipated time of the procedure. Most internationalists prefer the transfemoral approach for visceral vascular access. However, proximal left brachial artery exposure and puncture often facilitates access to significantly down-sloping or tortuous mesenteric arteries.
- A 4- or 5-Fr sheath is placed in the arterial access site to facilitate advancement of a 4- or 5-Fr marked flush catheter to the paravisceral aorta.
- Intravenous unfractionated heparin is administered after sheath placement to achieve an ACT of more than 250 seconds.

Second Step

- After a standard aortogram, a magnified paravisceral aortogram can be performed with the image intensifier placed in a steep oblique or true lateral position to optimize localization and cannulation of the celiac artery and SMA origins.
- Care should also be taken here to visualize the major branches of the celiac artery and/or SMA. Attempts should be made to visualize the first significant branch of the SMA, usually the middle colic artery, to avoid inadvertent coverage and/or compromise of colonic arterial perfusion as a consequence of planned procedures.
- Visceral lesions of interest can be further characterized at this time by optimizing image intensifier obliquity. Accurate measurements are facilitated by marked flush catheter or radiopaque ruler placement.

Third Step

- After withdrawal of the flush catheter, a stiff guidewire and a long (90 cm), braided 6-Fr sheath (ie, Terumo Pinnacle destination, Cook Ansel Flexor) is advanced to the paravisceral aorta. Various angled sheath tips (ie, straight, angled hockey tip, curved) can be used depending on the degree of visceral artery angulation, aortic diameter, and access approach (femoral or brachial).
- Along with selected sheath, various guide catheter types (ie, angled, vertebral, cobra, RDC, or reverse curved SIM or Sos catheters) can be used to facilitate visceral artery cannulation.

Fourth Step

- An exchange-length, stiff 0.014-in or 0.018-in guidewire, with a floppy tip, is advanced through the preselected catheter and sheath combination. However, wire cannulation of a diseased visceral arteries orifice may be challenging. From the brachial approach, successful cannulation may be facilitated with sheath placement distal to the artery of interest, followed by gradual withdrawal of the sheath with the selected angled catheter inside the sheath protruding slightly outward. When the catheter "clicks" into place, an exploratory hydrophilic guidewire is then gently advanced to obtain luminal access. Once the lumen is cannulated, the guidewire is then advanced to a secondary visceral branch to facilitate catheter and sheath advancement, as indicated (**FIGURE 3**). Another cannulation strategy is to withdraw wire and catheter combinations from a stable sheath position across the anticipated vessel orifice area at various "clock" positions.
- For a "no-touch" technique, a shaped catheter or sheath tip is positioned luminally in direct proximity to the orifice of interest. A 0.014-in or 0.018-in hydrophilic guidewire is then

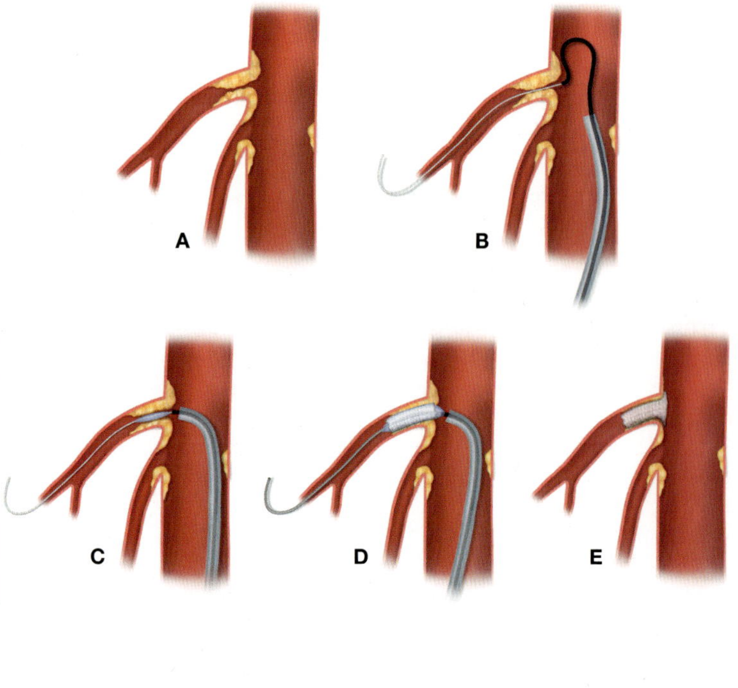

FIGURE 3 • **A,** High-grade stenosis of the proximal celiac artery origin. **B,** A curved-tip guide catheter is used to facilitate celiac artery cannulated with a 0.014-in or 0.018-in guidewire. The cannulation system is stabilized with distal advancement of the guidewire into a celiac artery branch, as well as maintaining a sheath in the aortic lumen. **C,** A low-profile, compliant predilation balloon may be advanced over the guidewire to dilate the stenosis and provide a tract for future stenting. **D,** An appropriately sized balloon-expandable covered stent graft is deployed across the stenosis while slightly protruding into the aortic lumen. **E,** Full stent apposition following deployment and proximal flaring of the stent graft at the prior stenosis site.

used to localize and facilitate cannulation. To improve trackability and pushability of the system, a stabilizing "buddy" stiff guidewire may also be advanced, when necessary, to "pin" the cannulation sheath to the opposite wall.

- When single-wire cannulation proves inadequate to support catheter and sheath advancement into the target vessel, placement of a second, or even third 0.014-in or 0.018-in wire, across the area of stenosis may facilitate successful catheter/sheath advancement.

Fifth Step

- An appropriately sized self-expanding or balloon-expandable stent graft is preferred for the treatment of visceral artery stenoses. Predilation of the tract may be necessary with a small, low-profile balloon to facilitate advancement of the balloon-expandable stent (**FIGURE 3**).
- The aortic end of a balloon-expandable stent used for the treatment of ostial or proximal visceral artery lesions should be positioned 1 mm into aortic flow lumen, and the stent edge should be flared out with the edge of an angioplasty balloon.
- Accuracy of deployment of self-expanding stent grafts can be improved with partial deployment of the stent while maintaining the cannulation sheath in the orifice of the visceral artery. Once the distal portion of the stent graft is accurately deployed, the remainder of the proximal stent graft can be unsheathed to allow for full deployment. An appropriately sized compliant balloon may then be subsequently used to fully mold the self-expanding stent graft to profile and/or slightly flare the aortic edge.
- For friable lesions, or lesions that may include fresh thrombus, consideration should be given to advancing and deploying balloons and stents over a filter wire (0.014-in eV3 SpiderFX embolic protection system). Although placement of a distal filter may not preclude all embolic sequelae, it may reduce the severity or significance of associated potential complications. This option may be particularly valuable in SMA interventions.

HYBRID REPAIR OF PROXIMAL MESENTERIC ARTERY STENOSIS/OCCLUSION

First Step

- In the setting of acute or acute-on-chronic mesenteric ischemia, where exploratory laparotomy is otherwise indicated to assess bowel viability, a hybrid retrograde catheterization approach is generally preferred. At laparotomy, surgical exposure of the superior mesenteric or celiac artery is obtained. To expose the celiac artery, the left triangular ligament is incised, the left hepatic lobe is retracted to the right, and the gastroesophageal junction is retracted to the left. Further caudal dissection along the surface of the aorta may be used to expose the SMA origin.
- For purposes of both embolectomy and hybrid retrograde catheterization, exposure of the proximal section/midsection of the SMA is preferentially obtained at the superior root of the small bowel mesentery (**FIGURE 4**). This location generally provides access four or more centimeters distal to the SMA orifice, which allows stable sheath positioning to facilitate retrograde cannulation and stenting. Distal to the lower margin of the pancreas, the length of the SMA is limited by early branching of the ileocolic artery and intestinal cascade, so relatively proximal positioning should be achieved to minimize excessive dilation/trauma to the vessel by the sheath.[19]

Second Step

- When embolic occlusion is present, embolectomy is performed gently through an anterior arteriotomy. The tapering nature of the SMA in this area requires gentle catheter withdrawal with gradual balloon deflation in order to avoid iatrogenic arterial damage, dissection, or thrombosis.
- Retrograde cannulation of an exposed distal segment of the target vessel provides optimal access for definitive endovascular intervention. In emergent conditions with compromised intestine, this approach is preferential to open revascularization strategies, which may require prosthetic graft placement following prolonged, extensive dissection of the mesentery and aortic root.
- Retrograde mesenteric cannulation is facilitated by placement of a longitudinal arteriotomy in the exposed distal segment of the target vessel. To reduce the risk of injury to the exposed artery during cannulation, the arteriotomy site is closed with a prosthetic or autogenous patch. The patch itself is then cannulated to facilitate sheath placement, angiogram, stent placement as well as expedited puncture site closure at the end of the procedure (**FIGURE 4**).
- Relatively long sheaths (20 cm or more) should be used during retrograde cannulation to ensure that the operator's hands are clear from the fluoroscopy field and minimize operator radiation exposure during catheterization maneuvers.[19]

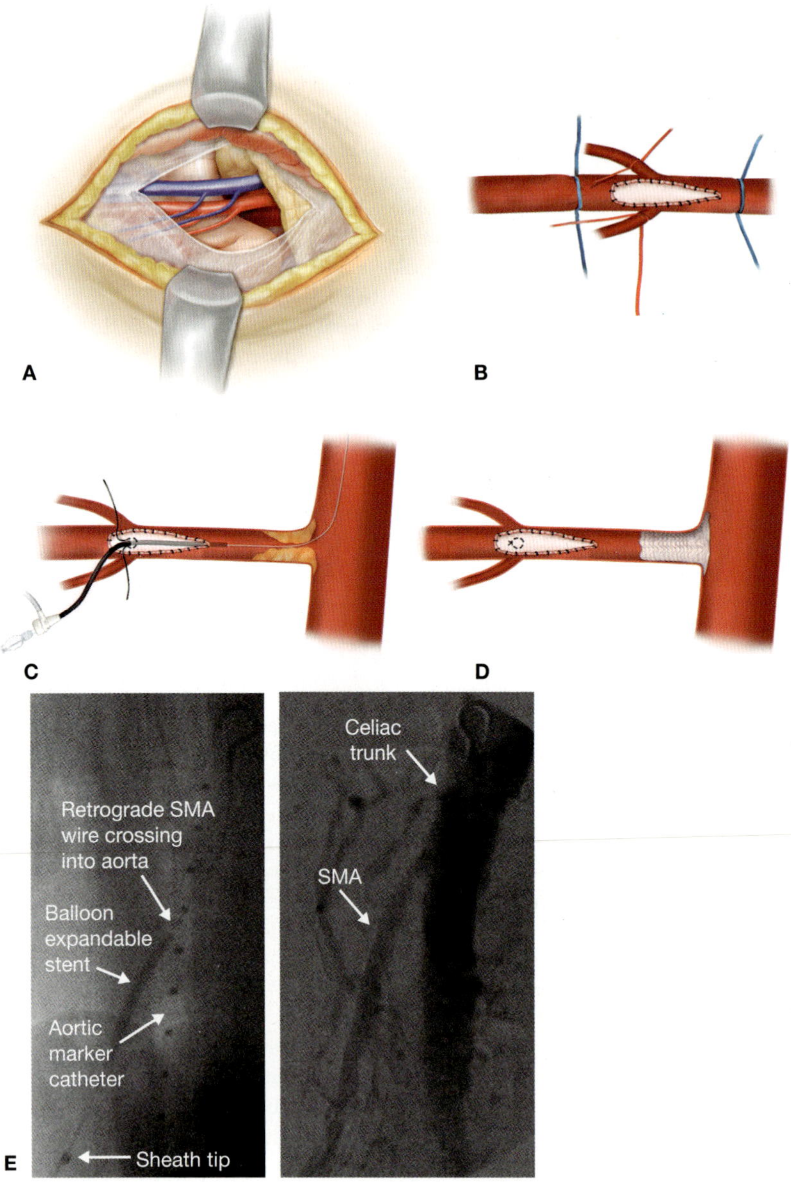

FIGURE 4 • **A,** Open exposure of the proximal SMA at the caudal portion of the mesenteric root. **B,** The proximal SMA, ~3 to 4 cm from its aortic origin, is circumferentially exposed while preserving its side branches. A longitudinal arteriotomy is created and thrombectomy is performed with patch angioplasty. **C,** Sheath is placed through a puncture in the angioplasty patch and arteriogram is performed to evaluate stenosis in the proximal SMA origin. **D,** A stent is deployed using fluoroscopic guidance at the SMA origin across the identified hemodynamic stenosis. The patch puncture site is repaired to maintain hemostasis. Ei. Retrograde access to SMA, with inflation of balloon expandable stent extending into aorta proximally, spanning length of proximal occlusive lesion. Eii. Completion mesenteric arteriogram from aortic injection, showing complete restoration of mesenteric arterial lumen and normal distal arterial perfusion. Retrograde mesenteric wire has been removed, and arteriotomy closed at the patch site in distal SMA.

RENAL OR VISCERAL ARTERY EMBOLIZATION

First Step

- Arterial access can be secured via either a left brachial artery or transfemoral approach, depending on the intended target vessel and its angulation relative to the aorta.
- For standard coil embolization, a 5- or 6-Fr sheath access will be adequate. However, if an occlusion device will be used, a larger sheath size may be required depending on device specifications.
- Systemic anticoagulation with intravenous unfractionated heparin is also commonly used during these procedures.

Second Step

- Angiographic characterization may require angiograms in multiple different obliquities to fully appreciate size, extent, and angulation of the lesion of interest, particularly those affecting secondary visceral branches. In the angiographic parlance, regarding the extent, severity, and profile of a luminal obstruction, "one view is no view."
- One should note the extent of vascular collateralization associated with the vascular segment that will be embolized.

Third Step

- A telescoping cannulation technique is usually used to enhance the positioning and stability of the embolization system. To perform this, a sheath is advanced as close to the target lesion as possible. A catheter is then extended from beyond the tip of the sheath and used to protrude into target lesion (**FIGURE 5**).
- Embolization of remote target lesions may require higher orders of telescoping. Placing a sheath into another larger sheath, or a 0.018-in microcatheter (ie, Codman Prowler, Cook CXI, BSCI Renegade) into a standard 0.035-in

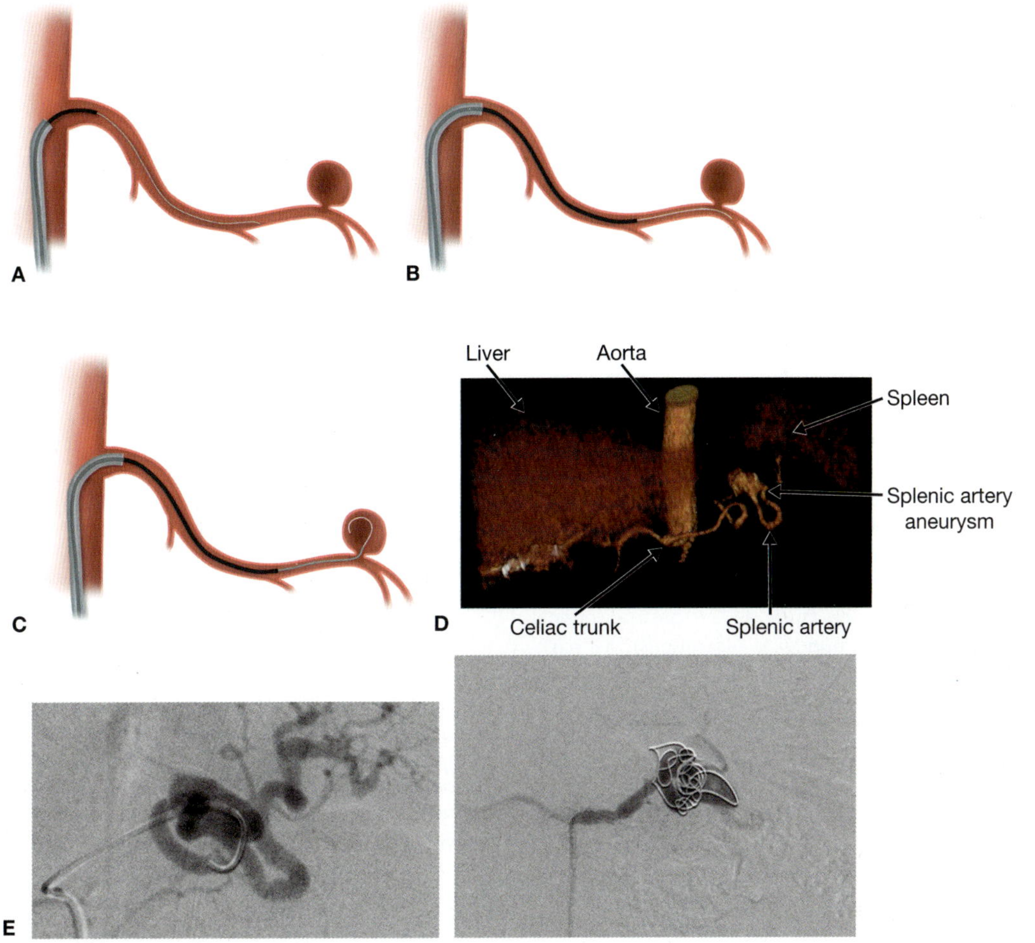

FIGURE 5 • **A,** Cannulation is attempted of a saccular visceral artery aneurysm. A sheath and angled catheter facilitate cannulation of the visceral artery origin with a guidewire. **B,** A 0.035-In catheter and guidewire negotiate proximal arterial tortuosity. **C,** A microcatheter is telescoped through the 0.035-in catheter to facilitate wire cannulation of the aneurysm. **D,** Three-dimensional abdominal CTA of a female with a mid-splenic artery saccular aneurysm. **E,** Selective splenic artery aneurysm pre- and postselective coiling.

guide catheter, can help access more challenging lesions (**FIGURE 5**). Alternating wire and microcatheter advancements may facilitate cannulation of smaller and more tortuous arteries (such as the superior and inferior gastroduodenal arteries [**FIGURE 6**]) and distal/hilar splenic artery.

- If possible, the cannulation catheter/microcatheter should be advanced into the lesion slightly further than the intended embolization site, because the system can draw back during deployment of coils or plugs.

Fourth Step

- Once the cannulation catheter is positioned in the target lesion, 0.018-in or 0.035-in coils are delivered sequentially into the target area through their respective catheters. For detached coils, the metal tube housing the coil is attached to the back end of the cannulation catheter, and the stiff end of a guidewire is used to push the coil out of its housing unit and into the catheter shaft. The floppy tip of the guidewire is then replaced into the catheter to push the coil along the entire shaft of the catheter and into the lesion (**FIGURE 5**). The stiff end of the guidewire should not be used to push the coil into the lesion because it can change the cannulating catheter tip shape and lead to instability in the cannulation system and maldeployment.
- Alternatively, small aneurysm may be occluded with detachable or nondetachable microcoils or ethylene vinyl alcohol copolymer. IFU are variable and should be referred to for recommended deployment techniques.
- When coil deployment can be accurately localized, and precise coil positioning is critical to the success of the procedure, large-to-small tapered coils should be used. When arterial blood flow is needed/required to carry part of the coil into the preferred deployment location, small-to-large tapered coils are preferred in this situation. Newer "nesting" coils will reform immediately into larger, obstructing profiles. Older tubular coils need to be advanced as they are being deployed to avoid simply lining the target artery without sufficient luminal obstruction. Attention to understanding what coils are in inventory, and how respective coil choices are optimally deployed, is essential for procedural success.

- For larger aneurysms or planned occlusion of an entire vessel lumen, a vascular plug (ie, AGA Medical Amplatzer I or II vascular plug) may be preferable and a more effective means for target embolization. However, plug placement usually requires stable sheath target artery cannulation. Amplatzer I and II vascular plugs are produced in diameters ranging between 4 and 22 mm and lengths ranging between 6 and 18 mm. Recommended device IFU should be consulted to ensure proper device selection and deployment. When sheath access cannot be withdrawn to enable plug deployment, catheter-delivered coils should be deployed instead.
- Once a coil or plug is delivered into a lesion, its position may be modified slightly by catheter tip advancement. This maneuver, when performed properly, maximizes the obstructive surface area and resulting coil thrombogenicity.
- When multiple coils or plugs are used, deployment should also be strategized and deliberate. For example, the first coil should be placed in the deepest part of the lesion (base of an aneurysm), whereas the last coil should be placed in the entry point of the lesion (neck of an aneurysm).
- For acutely bleeding vessels (such as the gastroduodenal arteries in the setting of duodenal ulcerations), a "back-door"–"front-door" approach ensures hemostasis. This involves occluding the culprit vessel pre and post the area of bleeding (**FIGURE 6**). Coiling only one side of the bleeding artery may prevent further access attempts while not providing sufficient vessel occlusion and hemostasis. Small bleeding pelvic arteries may similarly be embolized using a Gelfoam slurry slush preparation.[24] Recommended IFU should be consulted to ensure proper preparation and administration of these slurries.

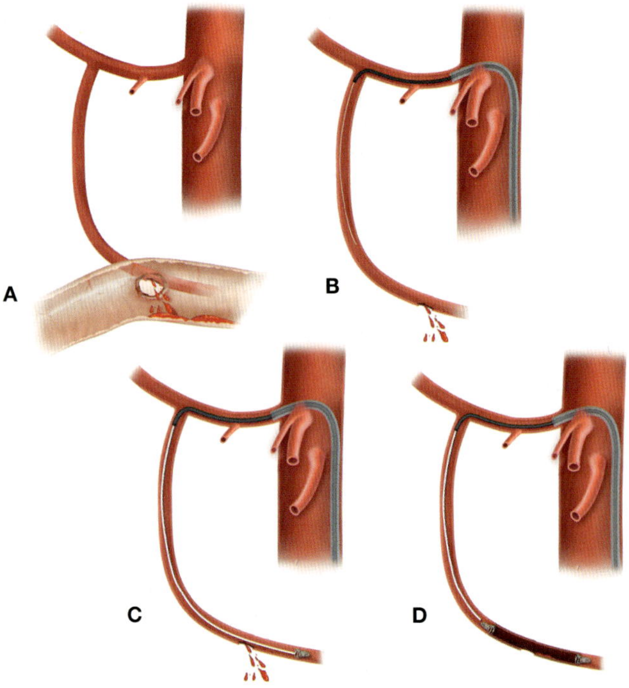

FIGURE 6 • **A,** Bleeding gastroduodenal artery with an associated duodenal ulceration. **B,** Sheath cannulation of the common hepatic artery branch of the celiac artery, followed by catheter cannulation of the gastroduodenal artery. **C,** Back-door deployment of an embolization coil distal to the angiographically identified bleeding point in the gastroduodenal artery. **D,** Subsequent "front-door" embolization of the feeding segment of the gastroduodenal artery.

Fifth Step

- It is customary to perform postembolization arteriography to confirm final coil/plug positioning. Residual flow will still be evident in the recently embolized vessel segment, because the patient generally remains heparinized during this period of the procedure. If uncertainty persists as to the adequacy of embolization, arteriography may be repeated following reversal of anticoagulation, taking into account increased risks of thrombosis/embolization around the delivery sheaths and catheters proximal to the targeted lesion.

PEARLS AND PITFALLS

Indications	▪ Preoperative imaging (duplex and CTA) should be reviewed in detail to ensure patient suitability and help plan out appropriate intervention. ▪ Combining information gathered from duplex and CTA is beneficial, especially in situations when the stenosis is overestimated due to heavy luminal calcification.
Vessel cannulation	▪ One should note the angulation of the target vessel relative to the aorta. Because this angle may vary with respiration, angiograms should be obtained while the patient is apneic (if intubated) or at end expiration. ▪ Generally, renal arteries and up-sloping visceral vessels may be easier to cannulate from a transfemoral artery approach. Down-sloping renal and visceral vessels may be easier to cannulate from a proximal left brachial artery puncture. ▪ Using an angulated, flexible, low-profile sheath system also aids in the cannulation process.
Angioplasty balloon selection	▪ Care should be taken in selecting appropriate size and types of balloons. ▪ Generally, only low-profile compliant balloons should be used for angioplasty interventions in the renal and visceral arteries. In rare circumstances, a noncompliant balloon may be used to help mold a stent graft to full profile. ▪ Diameter of angioplasty balloon should be estimated relative to adjacent normal vessel lumen. Oversizing is generally not necessary, and a smaller diameter balloon may be preferred when performing angioplasty across highly calcified lesions.

(Continued)

Stent selection	■ Care should also be taken in selecting appropriately sized stents for desired interventions. ■ Stent diameter should be estimated relative to normal vessel lumen diameter adjacent to target lesion to be treated and is generally oversized by approximately 1 mm. ■ Stent length should be estimated relative to the length of the target lesion while providing enough coverage into the adjacent normal vessel lumen (area of needed coverage is variable depending on type of lesion and intervention). ■ Oversized stents are prone to kinking and may risk damaging the target vessel. Undersized stents may lead to maldeployment, migration, and ineffective seal with adjacent vessel lumen. ■ Sometimes, the angioplasty balloon of a balloon-expandable stent gets stuck in the stent during its removal. In this situation, pulling the balloon risks misplacing or dislodging the stent from its desired location. Instead, the operator should ensure complete deflation of the balloon and attempt slowly advancing the balloon while rotating its catheter.
Coil/plug selection	■ Size of coils and plugs should be selected relative to lesion dimensions. Undersized coils and plugs risk migration to unintended vascular beds. ■ Stability of the embolization delivery system should be selected relative to the size of the embolization device. Larger embolization devices may cause instability in low-profile delivery systems.
Renal/visceral artery dissection	■ Sheath and large catheter cannulation of renal and visceral arteries should be avoided to prevent damage or dissection. ■ If a dissection occurs, angiographic evaluation is required to determine whether it is flow limiting. All flow-limiting dissections should be stented with an appropriately sized balloon-expandable stent.
Renal/visceral arterial spasm	■ Arterial spasms may be induced with vessel cannulation, angioplasty, or stenting. Younger patients are typically more prone for this. Arterial vasodilators, such as nitroglycerin or papaverine, may be infused into the vessel lumen by way of cannulation sheath or catheter to help relieve this. ■ The operator should be aware that papaverine may precipitate out of solution if mixed with heparin.
Renal capsular perforation or hematoma	■ This may be caused by inadvertent advancement of cannulating wire into the renal parenchyma. To avoid this complication, always keep the end of the wire in sight during sheath and device advancements over the wire. Also, avoiding the use of straight or angled-tip stiff Glidewires in this circumstance can decrease the risk of this complication. ■ Symptoms of renal capsular hematoma or perforation include abdominal pain and nausea, accompanied by a vasovagal response, which frequently requires aggressive resuscitation and stabilization maneuvers by the interventional team. ■ If this complication is encountered, maintain wire access (do not remove the offending wire) to facilitate a catheter exchange to provide access to coil placement and occlusion of the perforation site. Loss of wire access can further complicate this situation; however, as long as sheath access remains in the renal artery, the relevant segmental branches can be reaccessed for coil delivery.
Removal of malpositioned/misplaced devices	■ All attempts should be made to safely reposition malpositioned/misplaced stents, endografts, coils, or plugs. This may involve secondary cannulations, larger sheath placement, and balloon angioplasty with gentle directional force. ■ If endovascular retrieval or repositioning is unsuccessful, angiographic flow across malpositioned/misplaced devices should be evaluated. If arterial flow is clearly obstructed to unintended vital structures or may become a significant nidus for thrombosis or hemodynamic stenosis, open surgical removal may be indicated or attempted repositioning of devices in areas of less critical hemodynamic significance (eg, iliac arterial system).

POSTOPERATIVE CARE

- At the conclusion of the procedure, hemostasis is achieved with manual compression or, in cases requiring larger than 6-Fr sheath size, closure devices. Heparin reversal with protamine administration is also helpful unless anticoagulation is to be continued following the procedure.
- As is the case with all patients undergoing peripheral arterial intervention in our practice, patients are observed for a 6- to 24-hour period following device placement. During this period, access site hemostasis and ipsilateral pedal perfusion status is monitored periodically, along with hydration status/urine output and signs of unintended end-organ malperfusion.
- Patients treated with renal/visceral artery angioplasty or stenting receive exaggerated antiplatelet therapy in the immediate perioperative period. In our practice, we load patients with 300 mg of Plavix following the procedure, therapy continuing at 75 mg daily for 6 additional weeks.
- Postoperative surveillance of patients with renal/visceral artery interventions is necessary. Duplex evaluation of renal/visceral artery stents 1 to 3 months following intervention is usually recommended, followed by repeat duplex evaluation every 6 months for at least 1 to 2 years. Afterward, stents with no evidence of in-stent restenosis or de novo disease progression may be imaged at yearly intervals. Evidence of restenosis, either by end-organ dysfunction or surveillance

imaging studies, should prompt reevaluation and reintervention as necessary to maintain luminal patency and long-term success.

OUTCOMES

- Endovascular treatment of RAS has a reported technical success rate of 88% to 100%. Treatment effects on hypertension alone are quantitatively modest and inconsistent between studies.[25,26] Improvement in renal function is reported in approximately 25% of patients.
- Treatment of mesenteric occlusive disease has a reported technical success rate of 96%. Postoperative symptom improvement/resolution is reported in approximately 88% of treated patients. Primary patency is estimated at 65% to 92%, with primary assisted patency at 92% to 100%, and secondary patency at 99%.[27,28]
- Embolization and stent graft techniques for repair of renal and visceral artery aneurysms are limited to variably sized retrospective series but with acceptable technical success rates in appropriately selected patients.

COMPLICATIONS

- For renal artery interventions, complications most commonly arise from access site complications, contrast-induced nephropathy, or atheroembolization. Renal artery restenosis is reported between 5% and 66%, depending on duration of follow-up and criteria used for continued surveillance. The perioperative 30-day mortality is estimated at 0% to 5% and survival at 3 years is estimated at 74%.[29] Other less frequent complications include iatrogenic renal parenchymal perforation, capsular hematoma, arterial dissection, thrombosis, or distal plaque embolization into branch or accessory arteries.
- For mesenteric artery interventions, restenosis or occlusion of treated visceral vessels is documented in 10% to 27% of patients,[30] emphasizing the need for continued postprocedural surveillance. Less common complications include mesenteric artery perforation, dissection, or distal parenchymal embolization due to wire/catheter manipulation of areas with fresh thrombus or friable plaque. While treating branch artery aneurysms of the spleen, occasionally, portions of the splenic parenchyma may be lost due to coiling and branch occlusion, with attendant symptoms consistent with segmental splenic infarction.

REFERENCES

1. Schneider PA. *Endovascular Skills, Guidewire and Catheter Skills for Endovascular Surgery*. 3rd ed. Informa Healthcare; 2009.
2. Garovic VD, Textor SC. Renovascular hypertension and ischemic nephropathy. *Circulation*. 2005;112:1362-1374.
3. Hansen KJ, Edwards MS, Craven TE, et al. Prevalence of renovascular disease in the elderly: a population-based study. *J Vasc Surg*. 2002;36:443-451.
4. Beregi JP, Louvegny S, Gautier C, et al. Fibromuscular dysplasia of the renal arteries: comparison of helical CT angiography and arteriography. *AJR Am J Roentgenol*. 1999;172:27-34.
5. McMillan WD, McCarthy WJ, Bresticker MR, et al. Mesenteric artery bypass: objective patency determination. *J Vasc Surg*. 1995;21:729-740.
6. Stoney RJ, Cunningham CG. Acute mesenteric ischemia. *Surgery*. 1993;114:489-490.
7. Tham G, Ekelund L, Herrlin K, et al. Renal artery aneurysms. Natural history and prognosis. *Ann Surg*. 1983;197:348-352.
8. Messina LM, Shanley CJ. Visceral artery aneurysms. *Surg Clin North Am*. 1997;77:425-442.
9. Tessier DJ, Abbas MA, Fowl RJ, et al. Management of rare mesenteric arterial branch aneurysms. *Ann Vasc Surg*. 2002;16:586-590.
10. Chaer RA, Abularrage CJ, Coleman DM, et al. The Society for Vascular Surgery clinical practice guidelines on the management of visceral aneurysms. *J Vasc Surg*. 2020;72:3s-39s.
11. Hobbs SD, Thomas ME, Bradbury AW. Manipulation of the renin angiotensin system in peripheral arterial disease. *Eur J Vasc Endovasc Surg*. 2004;28:573-582.
12. Chang JB, Stein TA. Mesenteric ischemia: acute and chronic. *Ann Vasc Surg*. 2003;17:323-328.
13. Carr SC, Mahvi DM, Hoch JR, et al. Visceral artery aneurysm rupture. *J Vasc Surg*. 2001;33:806-811.
14. Dave SP, Reis ED, Hossain A, et al. Splenic artery aneurysm in the 1990s. *Ann Vasc Surg*. 2000;14:223-229.
15. Selo-Ojeme DO, Welch CC. Review: spontaneous rupture of splenic artery aneurysm in pregnancy. *Eur J Obstet Gynecol Reprod Biol*. 2003;109:124-127.
16. House MK, Dowling RJ, King P, et al. Using Doppler sonography to reveal renal artery stenosis: an evaluation of optimal imaging parameters. *AJR Am J Roentgenol*. 1999;173:761-765.
17. Moneta GL, Lee RW, Yeager RA, et al. Mesenteric duplex scanning: a blinded prospective study. *J Vasc Surg*. 1993;17:79-84.
18. Wheatley K, Ives N, Gray R, et al. Revascularization versus medical therapy for renal-artery stenosis. *N Engl J Med*. 2009;361:1953-1962.
19. Wyers MC, Powell RJ, Nolan BW, et al. Retrograde mesenteric stenting during laparotomy for acute occlusive mesenteric ischemia. *J Vasc Surg*. 2007;45:269-275.
20. Oderich GS. Current concepts in the management of chronic mesenteric ischemia. *Curr Treat Options Cardiovasc Med*. 2010;12:117-130.
21. Pfeiffer T, Reiher L, Grabitz K, et al. Reconstruction for renal artery aneurysm: operative techniques and long-term results. *J Vasc Surg*. 2003;37:293-300.
22. Panayiotopoulos YP, Assadourian R, Taylor PR. Aneurysms of the visceral and renal arteries. *Ann R Coll Surg Engl*. 1996;78:412-419.
23. Tallarita T, Oderich GS, Macedo TA, et al. Reinterventions for stent restenosis in patients treated for atherosclerotic mesenteric artery disease. *J Vasc Surg*. 2011;54:1422-1429.
24. Bauer JR, Ray CE. Transcatheter arterial embolization in the trauma patient: a review. *Semin Intervent Radiol*. 2004;21:11-22.
25. Corriere MA, Pearce JD, Edwards MS, et al. Endovascular management of atherosclerotic renovascular disease: early results following primary intervention. *J Vasc Surg*. 2008;48:580-587.
26. Tuttle KR, Chouinard RF, Webber JT, et al. Treatment of atherosclerotic ostial renal artery stenosis with the intravascular stent. *Am J Kidney Dis*. 1998;32:611-622.
27. Sharafuddin MJ, Olson CH, Sun S, et al. Endovascular treatment of celiac and mesenteric arteries stenoses: applications and results. *J Vasc Surg*. 2003;38:692-698.
28. Sivamurthy N, Rhodes JM, Lee D, et al. Endovascular versus open mesenteric revascularization: immediate benefits do not equate with short-term functional outcomes. *J Am Coll Surg*. 2006;202:859-867.
29. Yutan E, Glickerman DJ, Caps MT, et al. Percutaneous transluminal revascularization for renal artery stenosis: Veterans Affairs Puget Sound Health Care System experience. *J Vasc Surg*. 2001;34:685-693.
30. Brown DJ, Schermerhorn ML, Powell RJ, et al. Mesenteric stenting for chronic mesenteric ischemia. *J Vasc Surg*. 2005;42:268-274.

Chapter 19

Visceral Reconstruction to Facilitate Cancer Management: Celiac, Mesenteric, Splenic, Hepatic, and Renal Artery Disease Management

Arash Fereydooni and E. John Harris Jr.

DEFINITION

- This chapter assumes basic knowledge of surgical oncology principles and the management of patients with intra-abdominal tumor pathology. For further review of these topics, please refer to relevant background sources.[1]
- Advanced primary and recurrent abdominal malignant tumors may frequently involve adjacent arterial and venous structures. Surgical management may require curative en bloc tumor resection, with the goal of achieving negative macroscopic and microscopic margins. Adjunct vascular reconstruction may be necessary to achieve complete tumor removal.
- A wide variety of malignancies may develop in the peritoneal space and retroperitoneum. A representative range of pathologies involving intra-abdominal arterial and venous structures is summarized in **TABLE 1**.
- Primary vascular tumors are exceedingly rare, frequently mimic other oncologic disease processes, and may evolve slowly—leading to delay in diagnosis and treatment. Although most commonly arising from large vessels such as the aorta and vena cava, primary vascular tumors may also originate from distal branches of the iliac, mesenteric, and renal arteries. Classification systems (Wright/Salm classification) have broadly categorized primary vascular tumors as intimal (majority, 70%) and mural.[2]

Table 1: Range of Intra-abdominal Oncological Pathologies That Can Potentially Involve Arterial and Venous Structures

Arterial	
Aorta	Angiosarcoma,[a] paraganglioma, pheochromocytoma, leiomyosarcoma, rhabdomyosarcoma
Superior mesenteric artery	Adenocarcinoma, neuroendocrine carcinoma, adenosquamous carcinoma, cystadenocarcinoma
Iliac artery	Adenocarcinoma, leiomyoma, endometrial stromal carcinoma, fibrosarcoma, fibroma
Venous	
Inferior vena cava	Angiosarcoma,[a] adrenocortical carcinoma, teratoma, Wilms tumor, pheochromocytoma, neuroendocrine carcinoma, intestinal carcinoma, hepatocellular carcinoma
Renal vein	Renal cell carcinoma, adrenocortical carcinoma, pheochromocytoma
Portal vein	Adenoma, adenocarcinoma, cholangiocarcinoma, neuroendocrine carcinoma, hepatocellular carcinoma
Iliac vein	Intestinal carcinoma, leiomyoma, endometrial stromal carcinoma, fibrosarcoma, fibroma, transitional cell carcinoma, liposarcoma. leiomyosarcoma

[a]*Primary vascular tumor.*

PATIENT HISTORY AND PHYSICAL FINDINGS

- Patients with complex intra-abdominal oncologic pathology are best managed by a multidisciplinary care team at a tertiary care center. If tumor extension to adjacent vascular structures is suspected, surgical planning should include evaluation of potential revascularization options by a vascular surgeon.
- The initial assessment should include a thorough evaluation of the patient's presenting symptoms. This may include focal or regional abdominal pain resulting in tumor parenchyma pressing against adjacent structures. Patients may also present with gastrointestinal symptoms such as early satiety, nausea, and vomiting. Erosive gastrointestinal lesions may manifest with hematochezia, melena, or hematemesis. Constitutional flu-like symptoms, fevers, malaise, fatigue, night sweats, and muscle aches may also rarely present in patients with certain patients with rapidly expanding tumors.
- Depending on the primary site and tissue of origin, tumor-associated physical findings may not be obvious until relatively late in the disease process. Abdominal distension can result from increasing tumor volume or from serous ascites due to portal venous compression. Tumor mass effect or infiltration of the inferior vena cava (IVC) or iliac venous system may lead to unilateral or bilateral lower extremity edema, dilated abdominal wall veins, evidence of deep venous thrombosis (DVT), biliary symptoms, and renal insufficiency. Accordingly, physical examination should not only include a thorough abdominal exam with palpation of all nodal basins but also a complete vascular exam with evaluation of limb pulses, Doppler signals, and assessment of extent/grade of limb edema.
- Patients with primary vascular tumors, particularly ones with intimal expansion and growth, can present with evidence of venous or arterial embolization. Manifestations of recurrent venous pulmonary emboli include shortness of breath, respiratory distress, and hemodynamic changes including tachycardia and right heart failure. Depending on the volume of arterial emboli, symptoms can range from lower extremity pain to digital discoloration.

IMAGING AND OTHER DIAGNOSTIC STUDIES

- Tumor staging and classification systems are beyond the scope of this chapter. Please refer to other excellent references for tumor-specific staging modalities and requirements.[1,3]

- Patients deemed candidates for surgical resection by a multidisciplinary team should receive a high-resolution, thin-slice (at least 1 mm), multidetector computed tomography (MDCT) scan with intravenous contrast injection to allow for imaging during arterial, and venous phases. Image acquisition should allow for multiplanar sagittal, coronal, and three-dimensional reconstructions. This type of detailed imaging provides valuable information regarding tumor margins, suspected histologic subtype, and grade and can also help determine the morphology, patency, and extent of involvement of adjacent vascular structures.
- In situations where mesenteric venous thrombosis is visualized on MDCT, specific postprocessing protocols may be further implemented to improve clarity regarding the extent of thrombus burden and associated and/or resultant venous congestion.
- Adjunct imaging studies may also include magnetic resonance imaging (MRI), ultrasonography, and rarely angiography/venography. Particularly, in patients with concern for osseous or neurogenic tumor involvement, MRI may be particularly useful in defining tissue planes and tumor parenchyma boundaries. MRI also has a nearly 100% sensitivity for detecting intracaval tumor thrombus.
- Autogenous vascular conduit may be necessary for adequate revascularization, particularly following bowel resection and reconstruction. When anticipated, preoperative venous duplex scanning of the lower extremities will help document the presence and usage of superficial femoral vein as potential graft conduit. The presence of deep venous obstruction, either acute or chronic, may preclude venous harvest from that particular extremity. Similarly, the bilateral lower extremity greater saphenous veins should be evaluated for patency, diameter, and adequate length.
- Occasionally, preoperative or intraoperative transesophageal echocardiography may be needed to confirm the proximal extent of intracaval tumor thrombus visualized using other cross-sectional imaging modalities and determine whether the tumor thrombus is encroaching into the right atrium.[4]

SURGICAL MANAGEMENT

Patient Selection

- Whenever possible, the goal of surgical extirpation of abdominal solid organ tumors should be oncologic cure. This assumption presupposes tumor localization to a distinct anatomic region that will allow for resection with negative macroscopic and microscopic margins. Thus, the goals of the procedure should be clearly defined by sufficient preoperative high-quality anatomic cross-sectional imaging, multidisciplinary consultation, and discussions with the patient regarding the operative risks, benefits, expectant outcomes, and overall prognosis.[1,5]
- Abdominal solid organ tumors are traditionally considered unresectable when they involve the arterial or venous vasculature, are diffusely metastatic throughout the peritoneum or at remote sites, or involve the root of the mesentery or spinal cord to a significant extent. Patients with extensive tumor burden precluding resection may still be offered incomplete removal or debulking operations to potentially prolong survival and improve symptom palliation.[5]
- Equally as important as the anatomic considerations, preoperative patient functional status is a significant determinant of surgical eligibility. Performance assessments, such as outlined by the Karnofsky or Eastern Cooperative Oncology Group (ECOG) score, help predict patient-specific postoperative quality of life.[1,6] At our institution, patients who are bedridden at the time of initial assessment, severely disabled, or unable to independently perform activities of self-care are often not offered curative resection.
- Candidacy for intra-abdominal vascular reconstruction is also contingent on the extent of potential or preexisting vascular compromise. As such, we have typically attempted arterial reconstruction when tumors involve critical arterial structures such as the aorta, celiac artery and its branches, proximal superior mesenteric artery (SMA), common/external iliac artery, and the internal iliac artery in the setting of an embolized, occluded, or resected contralateral internal iliac artery. Similarly, venous reconstruction is also anticipated when tumor margins appear to include the vena cava, portal, superior mesenteric, common, and external iliac veins.

Preoperative Planning

- Items to consider in preoperative multidisciplinary review include the extent of planned gross surgical resection margins, the need for preoperative arterial or venous embolization, the need for other prophylactic procedures such as placement of ureteral stents or nephrostomy tubes, and the likelihood for intestinal resection and/or reconstruction.
- Ureteral stent placement should be considered in all patients who demonstrate evidence of ureteral obstruction, renal hydronephrosis, or urinary obstructive signs or symptoms from either tumor mass effect or invasion of urologic structures. Moreover, ureteral stents should also be considered in patients with pelvic tumors where there is potential concern of ureteral injury during resection of the tumor or during vascular reconstruction.
- A thorough review of detailed preoperative imaging will greatly facilitate proper conduit selection and preparation and, ultimately, a successful outcome. Particular attention should be directed to the length of vascular segment involved by adjacent tumor, the branch points and bifurcations present along this length, and which segments, if any, are circumferentially encased by tumor parenchyma.
- Attention should be paid as to whether planned resection will include vessels which are already occluded with adequate collateral circulation already in place or whether adjacent or contralateral vascular structures are capable of supplying adequate inflow and outflow. Vascular segments to be reconstructed should be patent and preserved to the greatest extent possible during the planned tumor resection.
- Endovascular embolization is the preferred method of preoperative vascular occlusion prior to open surgical resection. This strategy is commonly used for preoperative splenic artery/vein embolization prior to planned surgical splenectomy, internal iliac artery embolization prior to planned pelvic tumor resection, and renal artery/vein embolization prior to planned nephrectomy with or without the need for further exposure of the retrohepatic IVC. Moreover, retroperitoneal liposarcoma encompassing the abdominal aorta

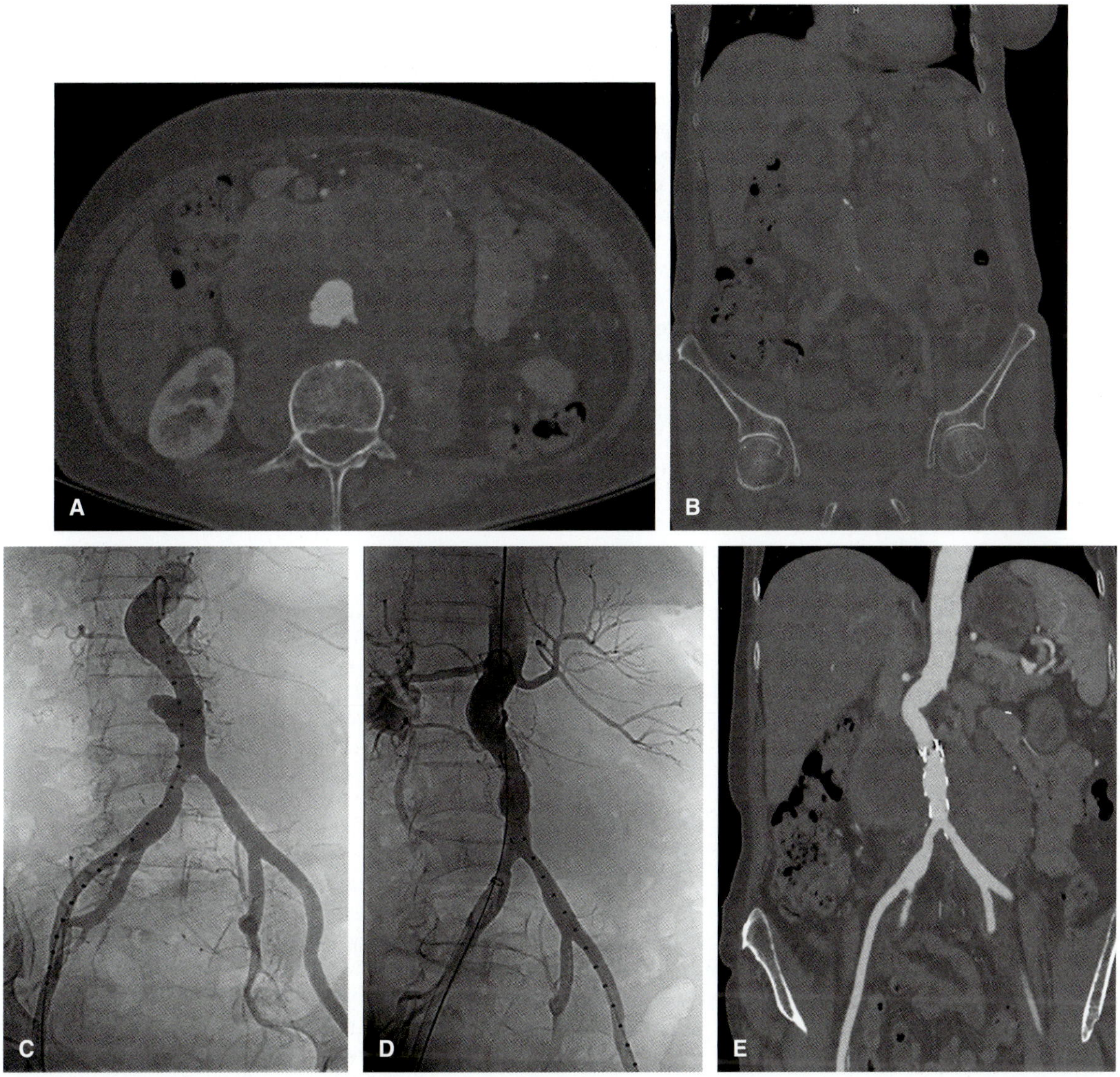

FIGURE 1 • **A** and **B,** Circumferential encasement of the infrarenal abdominal aorta by a bulky, heterogeneously enhancing retroperitoneal liposarcoma. Much of the infrarenal segment of the abdominal aorta extending into the bifurcation is encased by a large heterogenous retroperitoneal mass. Associated with this tumor is a saccular infrarenal abdominal aortic aneurysm within the tumor, **(C)** well-demonstrated on the diagnostic angiogram. **D,** Endovascular repair of the infrarenal abdominal aortic intratumoral pseudoaneurysm with an aortic cuff extender covering the aneurysmal segment of the aorta prior to neoadjuvant chemotherapy and surgical resection. **E,** Computed tomographic angiography demonstrating complete exclusion of the pseudoaneurysm with an aortic cuff endograft, with no evidence of endoleak.

may have associated saccular aneurysms within the tumor. Given the risk of degradation of the tumor and subsequent rupture of the aneurysm with neoadjuvant chemotherapy or surgical resection, the degenerated segment of the artery may be preemptively excluded (**FIGURE 1**). For this purpose, the preferred size of coils/plugs or endograft are estimated based on the diameter and length measurements of the target vessel on preoperative cross-sectional imaging and is typically oversized by up to 20% of the target vessel diameter. For additional details regarding visceral embolization techniques, refer to Chapter 18 (Stenting, Endografting, and Embolization Techniques). For additional details regarding endovascular abdominal aortic aneurysm repair, refer to Chapter 23 (Advanced Aortic Aneurysm Management: Endovascular Aneurysm Repair—Standard and Emergency Management). For additional details regarding internal iliac artery embolization techniques, refer to Chapter 24 (Advanced Aneurysm Management Techniques: Management of Internal Iliac Artery Aneurysm Disease).

- Aortoiliac arterial involvement often requires resection followed by reconstruction with patch angioplasty, interposition, or extra-anatomic bypass. Type of reconstruction and conduit type (autogenous venous allograft, cryopreserved homograft, or synthetic conduit) is contingent on the type of tumor, extent of vascular segment involvement, and degree to which intestinal reconstruction is also anticipated. In the latter case, when contamination by succus entericus is likely, autogenous femoral vein conduits for iliac artery reconstructions and IVC or spliced femoral vein conduits for aortic reconstructions are preferred. Alternatively, when not available, rifampin-soaked, gel-sealed knitted Dacron conduit may serve as a potential substitute with acceptable results.[7]

- Reconstruction of the celiac trunk, common hepatic artery, SMA, portal vein, and superior mesenteric vein (SMV) are similarly contingent on the extent of involvement of these structures with tumor pathology. Unless the artery in question is circumferentially involved, it is our preference to resect only the portion of vessel wall directly involved with tumor while preserving the remaining vessel architecture with patch repair. Autogenous venous conduit (using superficial femoral vein or greater saphenous vein or femoral vein) is preferred for vessel segments requiring interposition grafting.
- The mainstay of treatment of primary and secondary tumors of the IVC is surgical resection and reconstruction. The extent of reconstruction is contingent on the type of tumor, extent of caval involvement, and the anatomic segments involved. Adequate retrohepatic caval exposure is challenging and may require total vascular isolation of the liver to minimize blood loss during this maneuver. In circumstances where the IVC is chronically occluded with tolerable lower extremity edema and adequate renal function, ligation and resection without reconstruction should be considered. On the other hand, patients with recent occlusion of the IVC, few venous collaterals, notable lower extremity symptoms, or renal insufficiency should be considered for either interposition grafting or patch venoplasty.

Operating Room Setup

- Preoperative endovascular embolization procedures should be performed in an angiography suite or hybrid operating room. A full complement of compatible guidewires, catheters, sheaths, coils, and plugs should be available.
- Open tumor resection is best performed in an operating room setting with adequate space to facilitate the maneuvering of multiple surgical subspecialty teams and their necessary operative trays/equipment.
- Most intra-abdominal tumor resection and reconstruction procedures may be performed with the patient in the supine position. In the surgical field, the patient's lower extremities should be prepared for vein harvest if potentially necessary.
- In patients who require retrohepatic IVC exposure and reconstruction, the left lateral decubitus position should be employed to facilitate right thoracoabdominal exposure through the 8th or 9th rib interspace.
- Placement of ureteral stents will require initial positioning of the patient in lithotomy position and then subsequent repositioning of the patient to facilitate further planned surgical intervention.

TECHNIQUES

AORTIC RECONSTRUCTION

- For a discussion of the technical exposure of the paravisceral, pararenal, and infrarenal aorta, please refer to Chapter 22 (Advanced Aneurysm Management Techniques: Open Surgical Anatomy and Repair).

First Step

- The surgical exposure of an intra-abdominal tumor either directly adjacent or involving the aorta should aim to not only provide adequate exposure of tumor resection but also facilitate adequate proximal and distal arterial control. A traditional midline abdominal incision, extending from the xiphoid process to the pubis, can facilitate this in the majority of patients.
- In patients with wide costal margins or an anticipated need for wide parahepatic or parasplenic exposure, a bilateral subcostal incision may also be useful.
- For large abdominal tumors, renal tumors, or tumors with cephalad intra-abdominal extension to the level of the diaphragm, a lateral decubitus thoracoabdominal approach to facilitate both adequate tumor exposure and vascular proximal control and reconstruction is advised.

Second Step

- Proximal aortic control can often be obtained directly above the anticipated cephalad margin of the tumor. In this circumstance, via either retroperitoneal or transperitoneal approaches, the medial and lateral aortic margins are cleared for 2 to 3 cm proximal to the tumor margin. The exposed segment is inspected for lumbar vessel branches, which may be externally ligated as necessary to aid in exposure and control. A large, slightly curved vascular aortic clamp (eg, DeBakey aortic occlusion clamp) is best suited to obtain proximal aortic control.
- Supraceliac or suprarenal aortic exposure may be necessary for optimal control (**FIGURE 2**).
- For control of the supraceliac aorta, the peritoneal cavity is entered below the level of the xiphoid process. With cephalad retraction of the left lobe of the liver, the left triangular ligament of the liver is divided and the lesser sac is entered via a longitudinal incision in the gastrohepatic ligament. Care should be taken here to avoid injury to the esophagus (identified by aid of orogastric/nasogastric tube placement) or a replaced left hepatic artery. For additional exposure, the median arcuate ligament and the right crus may be divided (**FIGURE 2**).
- Suprarenal aortic control is obtained following circumferential dissection and mobilization of the left renal vein off the ventral surface of the aorta. Left renal vein inferior lumbar branches should be ligated to facilitate mobilization. In rare circumstances, the left renal vein may need to be ligated during this maneuver. When this is anticipated, existing collateral veins such as the left gonadal, adrenal, or lumbar should be intentionally preserved prior to division of the left renal vein.
- Infrarenal aortic exposure can be achieved either via transperitoneal or retroperitoneal approaches. If the tumor has pelvic extensions or if exposure/control of the right iliac system is anticipated, a transperitoneal approach may be preferable.

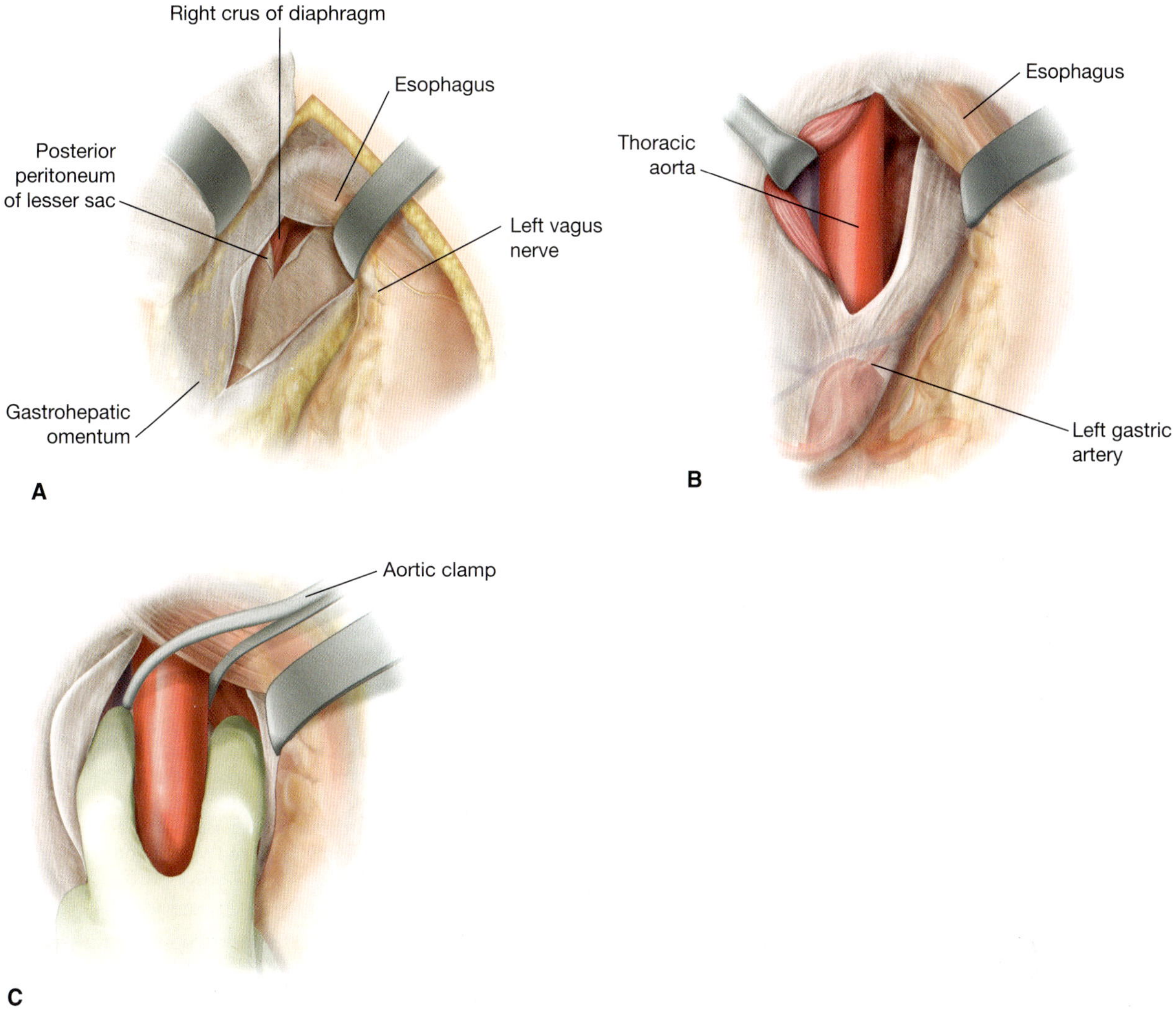

FIGURE 2 • Transabdominal exposure of the supraceliac aorta for proximal aortic control. **A,** The left lobe of the liver is retracted superiorly and to the patient's right. The distal esophagus is identified and gently retracted to the patient's left. A longitudinal incision is made in between these structures through the gastrohepatic ligament to enter the lesser sac. **B,** The posterior peritoneum and the right crus of the diaphragm can then be incised to expose the supraceliac aorta. **C,** Blunt digital dissection can aid with circumferential exposure of this aortic segment to allow for proximal control with vascular clamping.

Third Step

- Depending on the extent of aortic tumor involvement, durable repair may be achieved using either patch angioplasty or interposition grafting.
- Patch repair is commonly performed with a woven Dacron, bovine pericardium, or autogenous femoral vein. The patch is fashioned in a manner to facilitate a wide repair without narrowing the residual the aortic lumen. The anastomosis is usually performed with 4-0 Prolene sutures, in a running fashion, with one suture starting from each end of the patch repair. Depending on the age of the patient, presence and extent of retroperitoneal soilage by intestinal contents, and amount of retroperitoneal inflammation present, polyester pledgets may be required to minimize suture-related aortic injury and needle hole bleeding (**FIGURE 3**).
- Alternatively, when more extensive aortic segments are involved or the tumor cannot be safely mobilized circumferentially around the aorta, interposition grafting may be more appropriate. After resection, the residual aorta should be inspected for any intimal defects, tumor infiltration, or intraluminal thrombus. Once clean endpoints are determined, the interposition graft of choice can be brought to the field. Conduit choices include autogenous vena cava or spliced femoral veins, cryopreserved homogenous arterial conduit, or knitted or woven polyester and expanded polytetrafluoroethylene (ePTFE). Once selected, the proximal end is fashioned in a way to minimize diameter differences between the aorta and graft. The anastomosis is usually performed with a running 3-0 or 4-0 polypropylene suture. Once completed, the proximal clamp is temporarily released to allow the conduit to be routed in such a way to avoid redundancy, kinking, or twisting. After reclamping the graft (to avoid repeated aortic clamping), the distal anastomosis is completed in a similar fashion after sufficient proximal and distal flushing maneuvers (**FIGURE 4**).

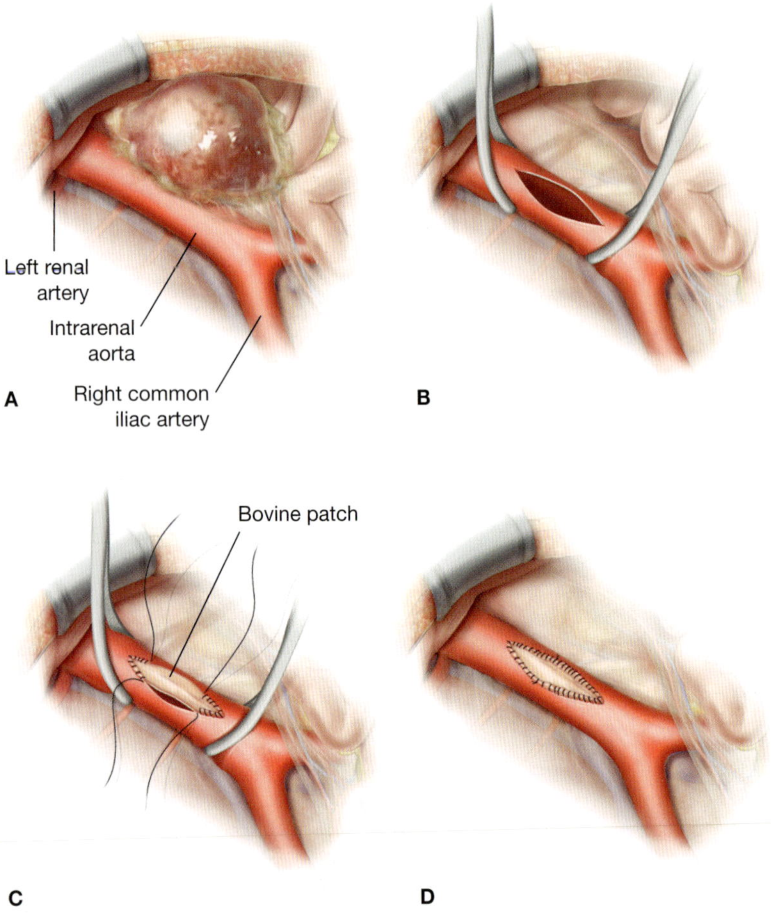

FIGURE 3 • Patch angioplasty repair of infrarenal aorta. **A,** Transabdominal exposure of the infrarenal abdominal aorta and adjacent tumor mass. **B,** Following proximal and distal aortic control, mass is removed along with associated aortic wall. **C** and **D,** Aortotomy repaired with a bovine pericardial patch.

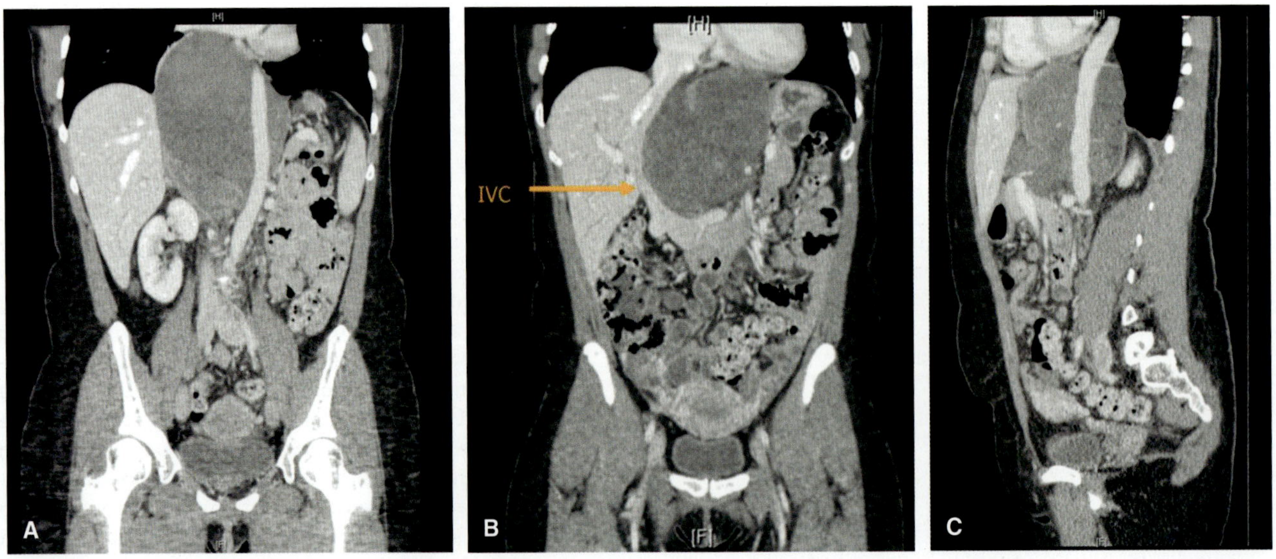

FIGURE 4 • Branched aortovisceral repair following resection of a large retroperitoneal thoracoabdominal myxoid sarcoma mass. **A,** Coronal abdominal computed tomography (CT) demonstrates large thoracoabdominal and mediastinal mass directly adjacent to major organ structures and the paravisceral aorta. **B,** CT demonstrates retroperitoneal portion of tumor mass displacing inferior vena cava toward the patient's right. **C,** Sagittal CT demonstrates circumferential involvement of the paravisceral aorta with the tumor mass. **D,** Left thoracoabdominal exposure reveals a large retroperitoneal mass extending proximally directly underneath the diaphragm. The supradiaphragmatic aorta **(E)**, proximal left renal artery **(F)**, and proximal superior mesenteric artery (SMA) **(G)** were all exposed to facilitate tumor resection and aortic branched repair. **H,** Aortic branch graft was constructed on the operative back table by attaching a 14-mm bifurcated Dacron graft to the side of a 16-mm Dacron tube graft. Following en bloc resection of the mass along with associated aortic segment **(I and J)**, the resected aortic segment was then repaired with the constructed graft. Branches were used for end-to-end anastomosis to the left renal artery and SMA.

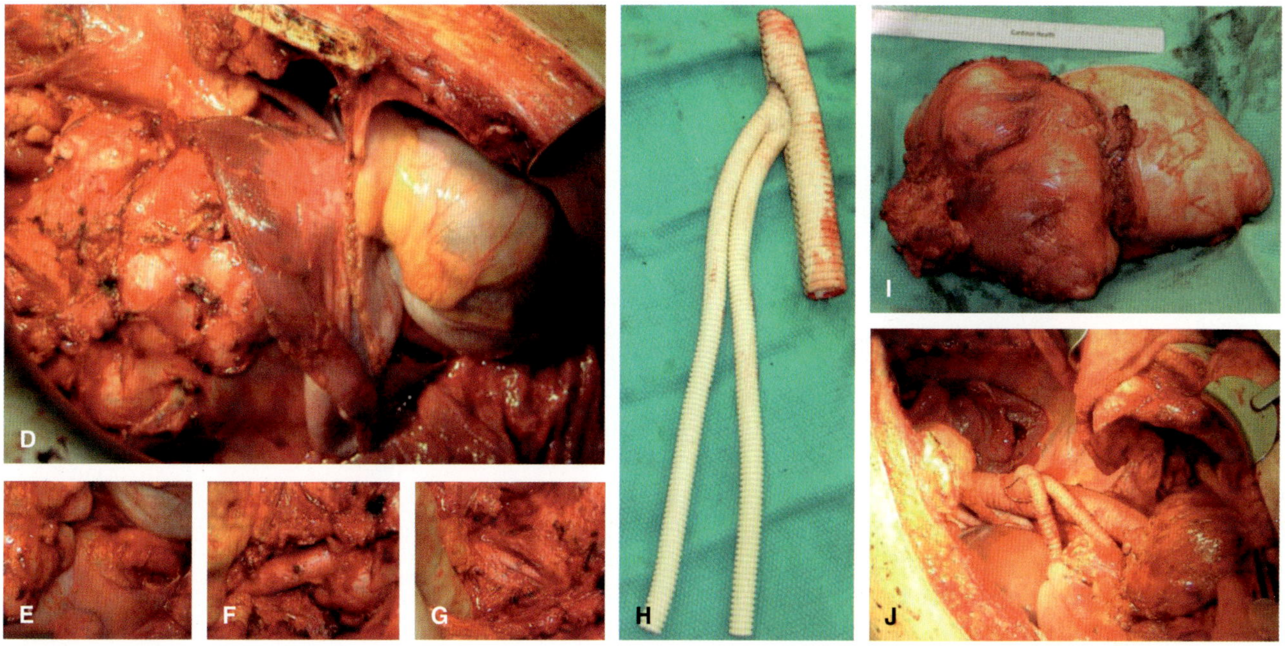

FIGURE 4 • Continued

- Autogenous tissue repairs of the aorta are preferred in circumstances where intestinal continuity has been interrupted. However, if autogenous tissue is not available or not adequate for use, gel-impregnated woven polyester graft material immersed in rifampin solution is the prosthetic conduit of choice. To achieve adequate coverage, the graft is immersed in 50 mL of normal saline containing 600 mg of rifampin for at least 30 minutes.
- If the paravisceral or pararenal aorta reconstruction is required, visceral and renal vessels can be reimplanted to the interposition aortic graft. Alternatively, a premanufactured or surgeon-modified branched aortic graft can be used to facilitate end-to-end anastomoses to the visceral or renal vessels following aortic interposition graft repair, with side limbs typically 6 to 8 mm in diameter (**FIGURE 4**).

SUPERIOR MESENTERIC ARTERY RECONSTRUCTION

First Step

- Exposure of the SMA, in situations where it is involved with the tumor, may be performed jointly with the surgical oncology team. Particularly in situations where the SMA is extensively involved, sufficient vascular control should be obtained prior to significant debulking or resection maneuvers.
- To expose the SMA at the base of the mesentery, the transverse colon and omentum are elevated while packing the small bowel to the right. The peritoneum is then incised at the base of the transverse mesocolon, taking care to identify and preserve the middle colic and jejunal arterial branches. Judicious cephalad retraction of the inferior border of the pancreas may also improve exposure (**FIGURE 5**).
- Alternatively, proximal SMA exposure may be gained laterally, following division of the ligament of Treitz and mobilization of the fourth portion of the duodenum. Visualization of the underlying SMA can be further enhanced with gentle retraction of the inferior border of the pancreas to the level of the left renal vein (**FIGURE 5**).
- The splanchnic nerves must be sharply excised to effectively elevate the SMA off the anterior aortic wall.

Second Step

- Reconstruction approach is dictated by the extent of tumor ingrowth. SMA involvement may be tangential or require segmental resection to achieve appropriate tumor margins.
- Partial SMA involvement may only require resection and reconstruction of one of the SMA walls. With arterial control established, the tumor tissue and involved SMA can be sharply resected en bloc. Following inspection to ensure a disease-free patent lumen, the arteriotomy is repaired with a patch angioplasty technique. Autogenous vein is the preferred patch material when available, especially following interruption of intestinal continuity. When alimentary tract continuity is not disrupted, bovine pericardial tissue, polytetrafluoroethylene (PTFE), or polyester patch may be used for repair. 6-0 Polypropylene monofilament suture is a good choice for arteriotomy closure and repair.

Third Step

- More extensive tumor involvement with the SMA may require segmental resection and interposition grafting. Variables to consider include the length of the defect, whether the SMA

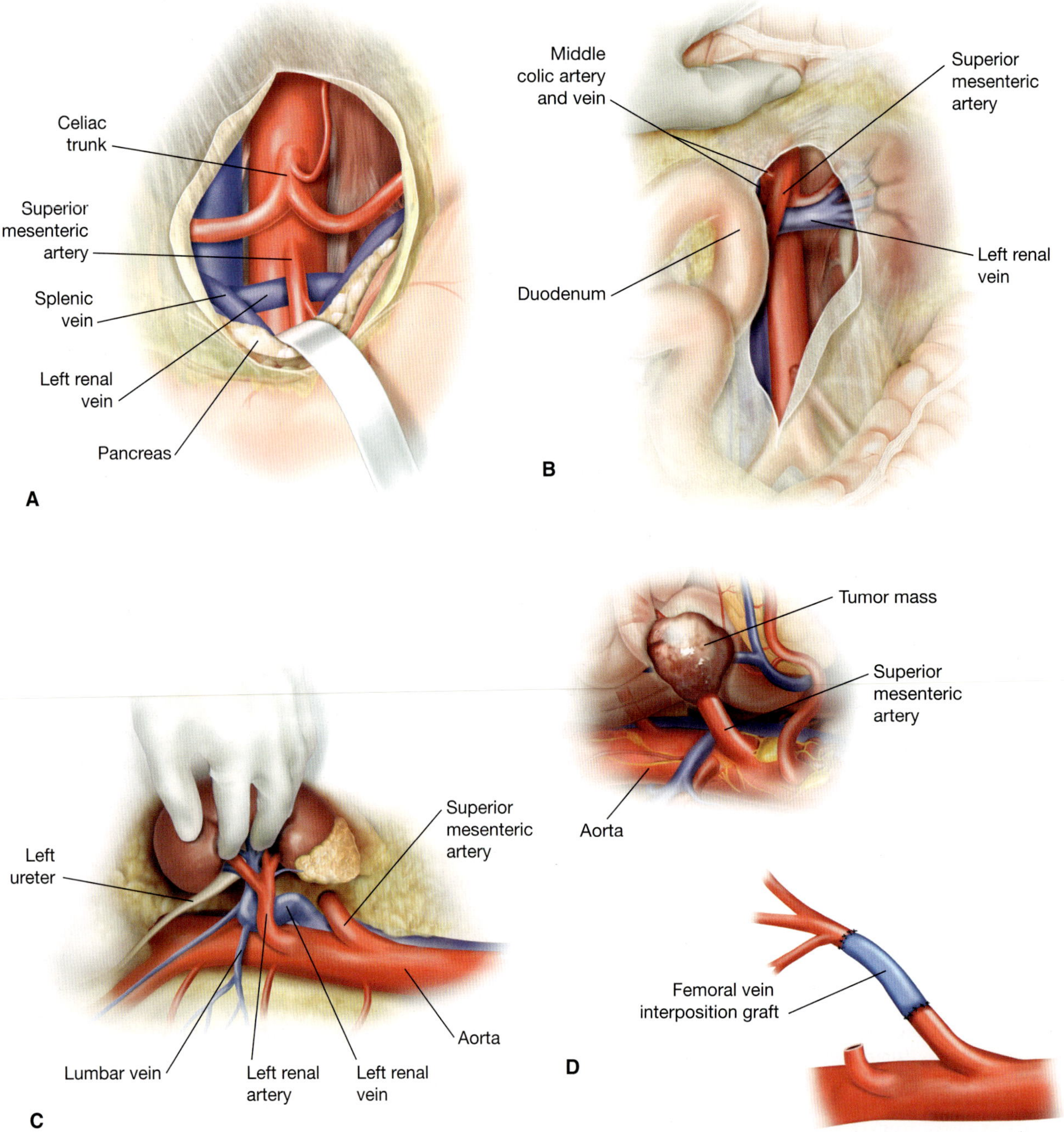

FIGURE 5 • Transabdominal exposure and reconstruction of the superior mesenteric artery (SMA). **A,** The origin of the SMA may be exposed with mobilization and gentle retraction of the superior border of the pancreas along with extended cephalad exposure of the aorta to the level of the celiac trunk. **B,** Alternatively, the SMA can be exposed from a lateral approach with division of the ligament of Treitz and right lateral mobilization of the fourth portion of the duodenum. **C,** Exposure can be enhanced with gentle cephalad retraction of the inferior border of the pancreas and ventral mobilization of the left kidney. Care should be taken to not avulse left renal vein lumbar, gonadal, or adrenal branches during mobilization of the left kidney. **D,** Tumor mass resection with associated segment of SMA. The arterial segment is repaired with an autogenous interposition greater saphenous vein graft.

origin is also involved, and conduit material available for repair.

- For short segment replacement, reversed greater saphenous vein is the preferred conduit for SMA grafting. Appropriately sized saphenous vein is usually harvested from the thigh, distended, and prepared for interposition. The tumor tissue is resected en bloc with the involved segment of SMA. Following confirmation of adequate margins, sequential end-to-end proximal anastomosis is performed. The graft is then brought to length while avoiding any twisting or kinking of the graft. The distal end-to-end anastomosis is then similarly performed. Spatulation of both the arterial endpoints and saphenous conduit may or may not be helpful, depending on size discrepancy.
- For long segment resections or resections involving the origin of the SMA, a long retrograde "question mark" graft, so named for its appearance on contrast arteriography following the procedure, is used to route arterial blood from the right iliac artery around the base of the mesentery to the distal SMA. Alternatively, an antegrade bypass from the supraceliac aorta may be tunneled posterior to the pancreas and brought out coaxially along the course of the distal SMA. Finally, when the SMA origin is involved but sufficient distal SMA is present to allow mobilization, the SMA may be reimplanted on the distal aorta if a disease-free segment can be identified by palpation or from assessment of preoperative imaging studies. For bypass options under these circumstances, cryopreserved arterial homograft or 6-mm polyester or externally supported PTFE are typically preferred conduits. Care is once again taken to avoid conduit twisting or kinking during placement or tunneling.
- Although a potential option, direct bypass from the region of the origin of the SMA to the distal mesenteric artery is problematic in that fashioning the bypass requires elevation of the mesentery, with the distal anastomosis positioned on the posterior aspect of the distal mesenteric artery. Although the graft may function well with the mesentery elevated, reduction of the intestines into the abdomen invariably causes graft conduit, autogenous or prosthetic, to kink and potentially thrombose. In this circumstance, it is almost impossible to fashion an interposition graft of appropriate length, so approaches such as retrograde grafting or reimplantation should be considered as preferred alternatives.

SUPERIOR MESENTERIC VEIN OR PORTAL VEIN RECONSTRUCTION

First Step

- Exposure of the portal vein is facilitated via entry of the peritoneal cavity and interruption of the umbilical vein and falciform ligament. The porta hepatis can be better visualized with cephalad retraction of the right lobe of the liver, downward retraction of the colonic hepatic flexure, and medial mobilization of the first and second portions of the duodenum. The portal vein is then easily identified in the right posterior border of the hepatoduodenal ligament. This exposure can be extended from the hilum of the liver to the head of the pancreas inferiorly. Inferiorly, care should be taken to identify and preserve the coronary vein and splenic vein (**FIGURE 6**).
- In most instances, the neck of the pancreas is divided as part of the tumor exposure and resection, which improves caudal exposure of the portal vein, splenic vein, and SMV.
- Exposure of the SMV can be achieved via exposure distal to the splenic vein confluence or via similar techniques used to expose the SMA. At the base of the transverse mesocolon, the SMV can be found lying to the right of the SMA near the midline. Multiple dense lymphatics overlying the vein often require careful dissection and meticulous control. Care should also be taken to identify and preserve the middle colic vein proximally and ventral venous tributaries distally (**FIGURE 6**).

Second Step

- The extent of tumor involvement with the SMV and portal vein is variable. Reconstruction is often required to preserve mesenteric outflow.
- Following establishment of vascular control, en bloc resection of the tumor and associated venous structures can be performed. Partial involvement is best managed via patch venoplasty. Preservation of an intact back wall of the splenic SMV confluence is often beneficial in maintaining the structural integrity of the bifurcation. SMV and portal vein patch venoplasty repairs can be performed using autogenous saphenous vein or bovine pericardium. A 6-0 polypropylene suture repair is used to close the vein, running or interrupted (**FIGURE 6**).
- Tumor involvement requiring complete resection of the portal vein or SMV will require interposition graft reconstruction. Interposition grafting with autogenous superficial femoral vein or cryopreserved venous homograft is preferred when intestinal resection and reconstruction is anticipated. Alternatively, 6- or 8-mm ringed PTFE when venous conduit is unavailable or inadequate. The distal end-to-end anastomosis is completed first, followed by the proximal end, with either interrupted or triangulated running sutures to prevent purse-stringing and anastomotic narrowing (**FIGURE 6**).

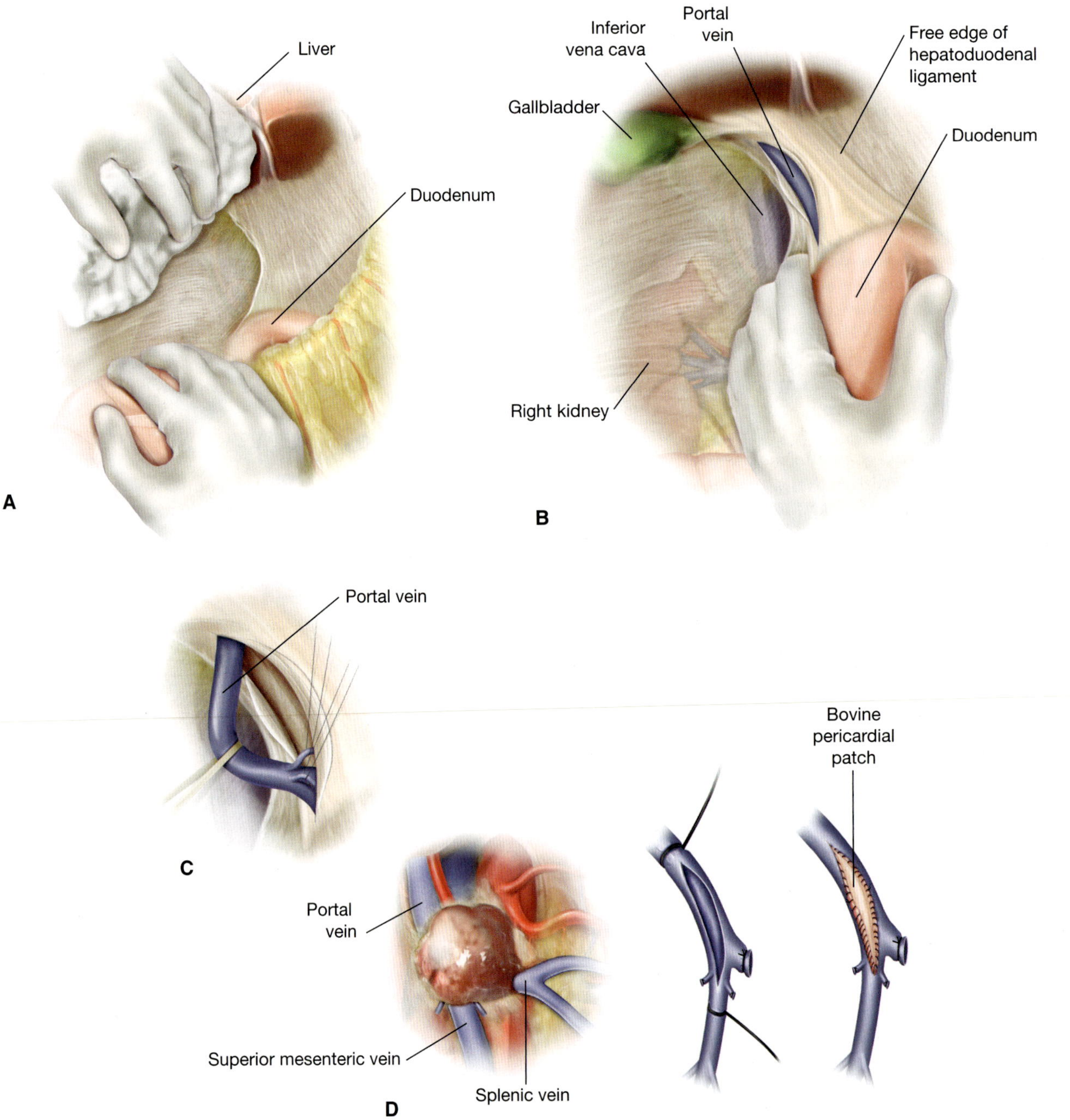

FIGURE 6 • Transabdominal exposure and reconstruction of the portal vein and superior mesenteric vein (SMV) confluence. **A,** With cephalad retraction of the right lobe of the liver, the posterior peritoneal attachments of the first and second portions of the duodenum may be visualized. **B,** The portal vein and proximal SMV may be exposed through a longitudinal incision along the lateral free aspect of the hepatoduodenal ligament. **C,** Venous tributaries draining into the portal vein and SMV confluence may be ligated to facilitate exposure and reconstruction of this venous segment. **D,** Tumor mass resection with associated ventral segment of the portal vein and SMV confluence and repair with a patch venoplasty using a bovine pericardial patch.

INFERIOR VENA CAVA RECONSTRUCTION

First Step

- Infrahepatic IVC exposure can be facilitated either through right retroperitoneal or transperitoneal exposure. Exposure is typically dictated by the extent of other planned intra-abdominal procedures and anticipated tumor resection margins.
- For right retroperitoneal exposure, the flank is elevated to 15° to 20° with the patient positioned in the supine position. A transverse incision can then be made extending from the rectus abdominis to the tip of the 11th or 12th rib. The external oblique, internal oblique, transversus abdominis muscles, and transversalis fascia are divided to create the retroperitoneal plane via blunt dissection. With judiciously placed self-retaining retractors, a 6-cm segment of the right lateral aspect of the pararenal and infrarenal vena cava may be easily exposed (**FIGURE 7**).

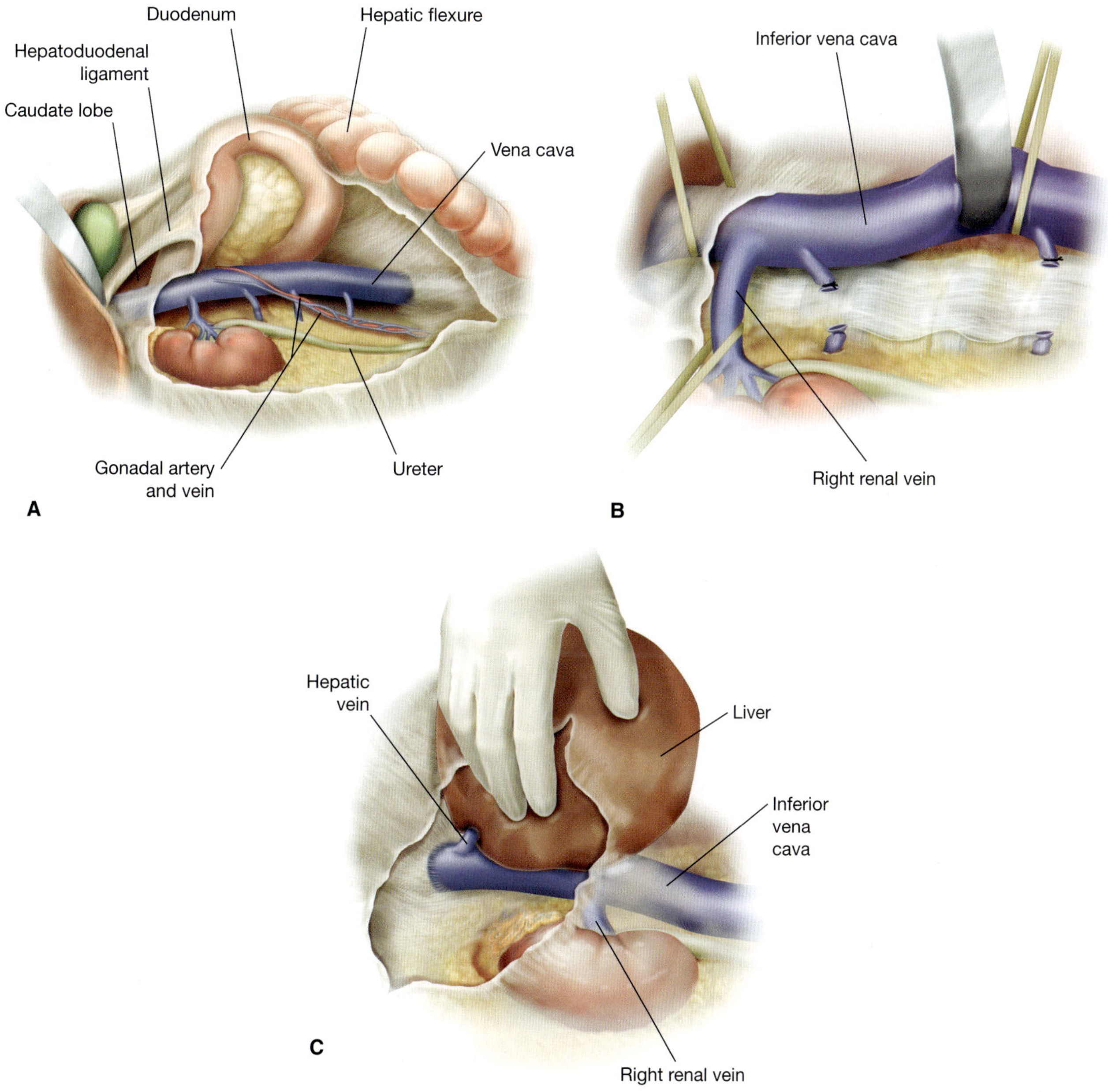

FIGURE 7 • Transabdominal exposure of the inferior vena cava (IVC) to facilitate operative reconstruction. **A,** An extended right retroperitoneal exposure of the IVC can be achieved with mobilization of the small bowel to the patient's left, division of the lateral peritoneal attachments of the right colon to allow its medial reflection, and division of the retroperitoneal attachments of the second and third portions of the duodenum. **B,** Posterolateral lumbar veins can be ligated to allow for full anterior mobilization of the IVC and facilitate circumferential control. **C,** The retrohepatic vena cava is visualized with medial mobilization of the right hepatic lobe. Small hepatic vein branches enter the IVC at this level and will require careful dissection and division to facilitate this segment of the IVC.

- For a transperitoneal exposure, either a midline laparotomy or bilateral subcostal incision will facilitate adequate exposure. Once the peritoneal space is entered, the small bowel is retracted to the left and the lateral peritoneal attachments of the right colon are divided. This facilitates medial mobilization of the right colon and mesentery and provides access to the retroperitoneal attachments of the second and third portions of the duodenum. Once these attachments are divided, the underlying vena cava can then be adequately exposed from the suprarenal level to the common iliac veins. Ligation and division of the ventral pararenal lymphatics, right lateral lumbar veins, and anterior crossing left gonadal vein will aid in caval mobilization during proximal and distal circumferential dissection. Vascular tapes may be placed around the proximal and distal exposed segments of the vena cava to facilitate vascular control. Care should be taken to not avulse medial lumbar veins with overaggressive mobilization of the vena cava during these maneuvers (**FIGURE 7**).
- For extended retrohepatic IVC exposure, a right thoracoabdominal incision may be performed with the patient positioned in a left lateral decubitus position. Once the peritoneal cavity is entered, the right triangular ligament and lateral and posterior peritoneal attachments to the right hepatic lobe can be divided. Medial retraction of the right hepatic lobe can then be performed to facilitate visualization of the lateral surface of the retrohepatic IVC (**FIGURE 7**). Hepatic compression here, especially following placement of self-retaining retractors, can increase hepatic congestion and ischemia and should be minimized to the greatest extent possible. In situations where caval visualization is not adequate despite optimal hepatic retraction, proximal extension or even division of the sternum may be necessary to facilitate safe exposure. Once adequate exposure is achieved, circumferential control can be achieved following ligation and division of small hepatic venous branches that course between the caudate lobe of the liver and the IVC in this region.
- The suprahepatic IVC can be exposed following ligation and division of the round ligament and wide division of the falciform and coronary ligaments. Caudal retraction of the bare dome of the liver facilitates visualization of the suprahepatic vena cava and at least two of the three main hepatic veins. Careful dissection of the areolar tissue surrounding these veins allows for circumferential exposure of each of these veins as well as this segment of the vena cava.

Second Step

- Once the vena cava is controlled both proximally and distally, the tumor mass can be dissected off other pertinent structures to facilitate en bloc resection. Systemic anticoagulation is accomplished with unfractionated heparin sulfate (100 U/kg intravenous infusion) and reversed with protamine sulfate, 1 mg/100 units of heparin, when vascular reconstruction or retraction is complete.
- Prior to removal of the tumor mass, the patient is placed in Trendelenburg position and vascular clamps positioned proximal and distal to the anticipated margins of resection. If the involved segment of the IVC is limited to only a few centimeters or one side wall, a long Satinsky side-biting vascular clamp may be used for partial caval occlusion (**FIGURE 7**).
- Acute occlusion of the suprarenal or retrohepatic IVC may induce profound hypotension due to significant preload reduction. In these circumstances, preemptive aggressive fluid resuscitation, gradual clamping of the vena cava, or partial occlusion may be better tolerated. Alternatively, venovenous bypass or atriocaval shunt placement may be necessary. Please refer to prior references for further details regarding preparation and placement of atriocaval shunts.[8,9]
- Specific isolation of the retrohepatic vena cava requires control of both the hepatic inflow and outflow. Inflow control is achieved with cross-clamping of the infrahepatic vena cava as well as with a Pringle maneuver (clamping of the hepatic artery and portal vein). Outflow control is achieved with suprahepatic or infradiaphragmatic clamping of the IVC.

Third Step

- The strategy for reconstruction is dictated by the extent of the IVC defect and the concomitant need for other vascular reconstructions. Typically, the vena cava is repaired, when necessary, following arterial reconstructions to decrease end-organ ischemia. The duration of caval occlusion should be limited to less than 30 minutes to minimize venous congestion and resultant ischemia.
- For small caval defects, primary repair may suffice when the lumen diameter is reduced by less than 50%. Otherwise, autogenous internal jugular vein or bovine pericardial patch repair may be incorporated into the repair. Lower extremity vein harvest is not preferred for caval reconstruction due to increased risk for distal thrombotic complications.
- For replacement of the IVC, when necessary, interposition graft using externally supported ePTFE is the preferred conduit. Following resection of the involved segment, the transected ends of the vena cava are inspected for any residual disease within the lumen. Controlled sequential flushing of the transected ends also ensures patency. The graft diameter is chosen to be deliberately smaller than the caval segment being replaced to promote higher velocities within the graft segment following reconstruction. The proximal anastomosis is completed first using either a running 4-0 or 5-0 Prolene suture. The distal anastomosis is then similarly performed with the patient in Trendelenburg position. Prior to completion of the distal anastomosis, proximal and distal clamps are sequentially removed, a Valsalva maneuver is induced by the anesthesiologist, and the graft is filled with heparinized saline while flushing is performed to minimize retained air and the risk for air embolization.
- External support rings are maintained to the greatest extent possible to avoid compression of the graft, including at midgraft segments where end-to-side anastomoses are necessary for renal vein or common iliac vein reimplantation. For repair of the confluence of the common iliac veins, we have successfully modified this procedure by incorporating a short segment of nonsupported bifurcated ePTFE graft into the repair. Externally supported ePTFE grafts are then sutured to the nonringed segment with ePTFE suture. The suture lines are then covered with BioGlue or sterile Dermabond to prevent suture line bleeding and the graft is then placed in situ (**FIGURE 8**).

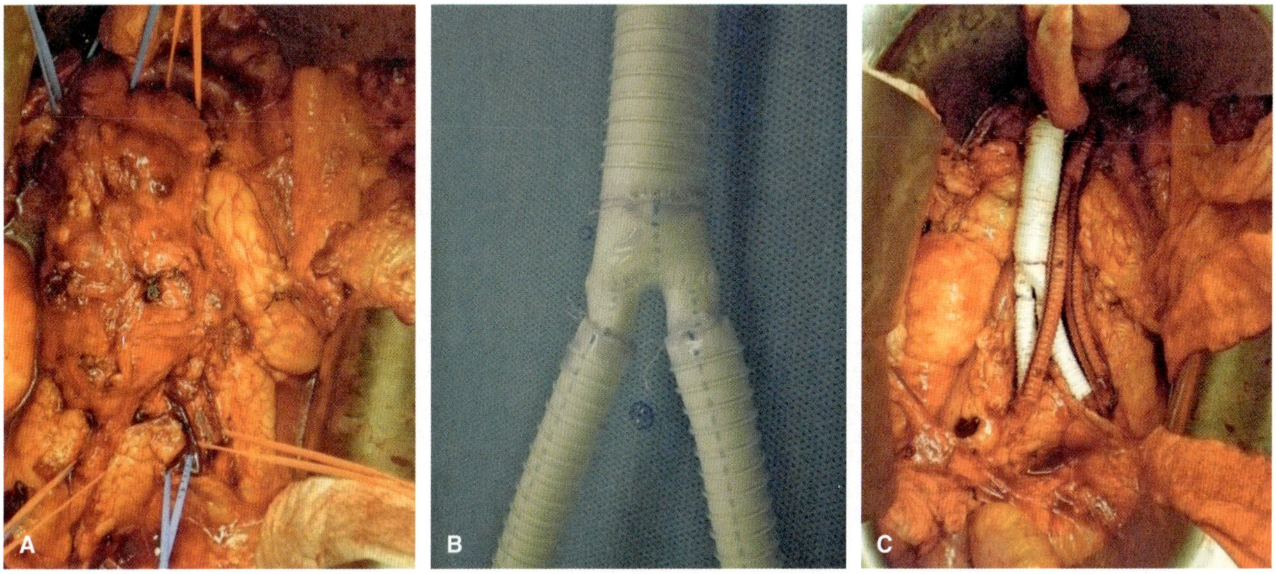

FIGURE 8 • Inferior vena cava (IVC) and aortic reconstruction in the setting of intra-abdominal resection of a large retroperitoneal high-grade leiomyosarcoma. **A,** Operative exploration demonstrated a large retroperitoneal mass with circumferential involvement with the infrarenal aorta and IVC. Proximal infrarenal aorta and distal bilateral common iliac arteries were circumferentially exposed and controlled. The proximal infrarenal IVC and distal left common iliac vein were also controlled. **B,** Back-table construction of a custom polytetrafluoroethylene (PTFE) bifurcated graft for reconstruction of the IVC. This was performed by suturing a 16-mm ringed PTFE graft to two 10-mm ringed PTFE grafts using a 6-0 Gore-Tex suture. The anastomosis was reinforced with Dermabond. **C,** Following tumor mass resection along with associated IVC, infrarenal aorta, and proximal bilateral common iliac arteries, the vena cava is reconstructed using the custom-constructed bifurcated PTFE graft. The resected aortoiliac segment was reconstructed using traditional techniques using a bifurcated Dacron graft.

PEARLS AND PITFALLS

Preoperative workup	■ It is imperative that a comprehensive plan for resection and vascular reconstruction be developed and agreed upon by all participating surgical specialties well in advance of the procedure. ■ Adequate preoperative evaluation will facilitate discussion of planned vascular reconstructions as well as the risks and anticipated outcomes of the procedure.
Intraoperative anticoagulation	■ The presence of adequate systemic anticoagulation prior to vascular occlusion is essential to the optimal outcome of the procedure. Anticoagulation may be delayed to minimize tumor bed bleeding during resection but should be established well in advance of planned vascular reconstruction. ■ An activated clotting time of greater than 250 seconds is recommended during vascular repairs to avoid thrombotic complications. Reversal of anticoagulation following completion of arterial repairs is also standard practice.
Arterial repairs	■ If the aorta is known to be involved with tumor, it is imperative that proximal control be established well proximal to the anticipated margin of resection. ■ To optimize outcome, the presence and extent of underlying vascular arterial disease should be fully appreciated. For example, complete aortoiliac or aortofemoral reconstruction may be necessary when significant atherosclerotic disease is present in the distal aorta (as an alternative to segmental patching or replacement). Similarly, endarterectomy of residual SMA or celiac artery diseased lumens may be necessary to optimize patency of patch or interposition graft repairs. ■ Attempts should be made to preserve as many SMA and celiac artery branches as possible during vascular reconstruction to maintain adequate bowel perfusion. This is particularly important if concomitant bowel resection is anticipated.

Venous repairs	■ In the setting of complete compression or occlusion of the IVC, the indications for reconstruction following resection may be less compelling. Reconstruction of chronically occluded iliac veins is generally not indicated under any circumstances during oncologic resections—particularly when patients are free preoperatively of significant lower extremity edema. ■ Air embolus is a significant potential complication of extensive venous reconstruction. The risk of air embolization may be minimized when repairs are performed with the patient in Trendelenburg position and with timely Valsalva induction by the anesthesiologist during retrograde flushing maneuvers prior to completion. If a large air embolus is suspected, blood can be aspirated directly from the vena cava or right atrium while the patient is maintained in Trendelenburg and left lateral decubitus position.
Renal vascular repairs	■ Right renal vein reconstruction and/or reimplantation to the vena cava is necessary because there is no adequate collateral venous outflow from the right kidney. During right renal vein reimplantation, the right renal artery should also be controlled and clamped to avoid venous congestion injury to the kidney. ■ Left renal vein can be sacrificed and ligated if the left adrenal and gonadal veins are intact. However, if left kidney venous outflow collaterals were ligated during exposure and reconstruction, the left renal vein should be preserved or reconstructed whenever possible.
Postoperative bleeding	■ In the immediate postoperative period, sudden or acute anemia, abdominal pain, abdominal distension, or hemodynamic instability should be approached with heightened awareness for possible intra-abdominal bleeding. ■ Particularly in patients with recent pancreatic reconstructions, bowel-associated leaks may compromise arterial/venous repairs and can lead to acute catastrophic bleeding requiring urgent intervention.
Methods to avoid lower extremity edema	■ Patients are prone to increased lower extremity edema following lower extremity venous harvest or intra-abdominal vena cava reconstructions. For these patients, lower extremity elevation in the immediate postoperative period is recommended. ■ Early compression therapy of the lower extremity can also significantly minimize the extent of lower extremity edema in the perioperative period. Arterial insufficiency should be ruled out prior to initiation of compression therapy to avoid compromise of already limited arterial inflow.

POSTOPERATIVE CARE

- Patients are typically managed in a monitored setting where periodic vascular examination is available and vasoactive agents are administered as necessary to maintain homeostatic arterial perfusion pressure.
- Intravenous fluid resuscitation is maintained in the short-term perioperative period until the patient resolves an anticipated course of intestinal ileus.
- All patients should be initiated and maintained on an antiplatelet agent, typically 325 mg aspirin daily.
- In patients who preoperatively received therapeutic anticoagulation, this should slowly be restarted 1 to 2 days following the patient's operation to minimize perioperative bleeding complications.
- Patients with large PTFE interposition caval grafts are typically anticoagulated for at least 6 months postoperatively and potentially lifelong depending on risk factors, history of prior DVT, and extent of reconstruction required to restore caval continuity.
- Early mobilization and DVT mechanical and/or chemical prophylaxis should be initiated as soon as safely possible in the postoperative period.

OUTCOMES

- Abdominal tumor resection with vascular reconstruction is feasible for many malignancies previously deemed unresectable.
- In a series of 47 patients who underwent IVC reconstruction with en bloc tumor resection, there was an 80% 5-year patency rate of the vascular reconstruction and a 45% 5-year survival.[10]
- In a series of 17 patients with SMA and portal vein reconstructions with pancreatic mass resection, there was an 88% primary patency rate. Two patients returned to the operating room for vascular-related complications. Eighty-two percent of patients were reported alive over follow-up period (4-48 months).[11]
- In a series of 120 patients undergoing vein resection, 41.7% had primary repair or patch venoplasty, 29.2% had primary anastomosis, and 29.2% had interposition graft. Around 28% of patients developed portal vein thrombosis, 26.5% of which happened in the preoperative period. Late thrombosis was often detected concurrently with local recurrence.[12]
- In a series of 35 patients who underwent pancreatectomy with arterial reconstruction, including 18 hepatic, 8 celiac, 3 splenic, 3 middle colic, 2 superior mesenteric, and 1 left renal artery, had an overall patency of 97% at a mean follow-up of 510 ± 184 days with 1 hepatic artery thrombosis.
- In a series of 14 patients receiving retroperitoneal sarcoma resection and major arterial and venous reconstruction, primary arterial patency was 58% and primary-assisted patency was 83%. Venous patency was 78%. Local recurrence occurred in 21% of patients and 5-year disease-free survival was 52%.[13]
- In a series of 141 patients who underwent resection of retroperitoneal soft tissue sarcomas with either major arterial or venous structure involvement, arterial continuity was retained in all patients and venous continuity was retained in 80%. Perioperative morbidity was 36% and mortality was 4%. Midterm arterial patency was 88.9% and venous patency was 93.8%. The overall 5-year patient survival was 66.7%.[14]

COMPLICATIONS

- Intraoperative bleeding
- Perioperative infection
- Thrombosis or occlusion of repair or graft site
- Venous air embolism
- Wound complications due to poor nutrition or possible radiation to operative field
- DVT from hypercoagulable state

REFERENCES

1. Feig BW, Ching CD. *The M.D. Anderson Surgical Oncology Handbook*. University of Texas MD Anderson Cancer Center; 2012.
2. Wright EP, Glick AD, Virmani R, Page DL. Aortic intimal sarcoma with embolic metastases. *Am J Surg Pathol*. 1985;9(12):890-897.
3. Amin MB, Greene FL, Edge SB, et al. The Eighth Edition AJCC Cancer Staging Manual: continuing to build a bridge from a population-based to a more "personalized" approach to cancer staging. *CA Cancer J Clin*. 2017;67(2):93-99.
4. Sigman DB, Hasnain JU, Del Pizzo JJ, Sklar GN. Real-time transesophageal echocardiography for intraoperative surveillance of patients with renal cell carcinoma and vena caval extension undergoing radical nephrectomy. *J Urol*. 1999;161(1):36-38.
5. Swallow CJ, Strauss DC, Bonvalot S, et al. Management of primary retroperitoneal sarcoma (RPS) in the adult: an updated consensus approach from the transatlantic australasian RPS working group. *Ann Surg Oncol*. 2021;28(12):7873-7888.
6. Ghosh J, Bhowmick A, Baguneid M. Oncovascular surgery. *Eur J Surg Oncol*. 2011;37(12):1017-1024.
7. Bandyk DF, Novotney ML, Johnson BL, Back MR, Roth SR. Use of rifampin-soaked gelatin-sealed polyester grafts for in situ treatment of primary aortic and vascular prosthetic infections. *J Surg Res*. 2001;95(1):44-49.
8. Baumgartner F, Scudamore C, Nair C, Karusseit O, Hemming A. Venovenous bypass for major hepatic and caval trauma. *J Trauma*. 1995;39(4):671-673.
9. Klein SR, Baumgartner FJ, Bongard FS. Contemporary management strategy for major inferior vena caval injuries. *J Trauma*. 1994;37(1):35-41; discussion 41-42.
10. Quinones-Baldrich W, Alktaifi A, Eilber F, Eilber F. Inferior vena cava resection and reconstruction for retroperitoneal tumor excision. *J Vasc Surg*. 2012;55(5):1386-1393.
11. Song TK, Harris EJ Jr, Raghavan S, Norton JA. Major blood vessel reconstruction during sarcoma surgery. *Arch Surg*. 2009;144(9):817-822.
12. Snyder RA, Prakash LR, Nogueras-Gonzalez GM, et al. Vein resection during pancreaticoduodenectomy for pancreatic adenocarcinoma: patency rates and outcomes associated with thrombosis. *J Surg Oncol*. 2018;117(8):1648-1654.
13. Tedesco MM, Norton JA, Cisco RM, Song TK, Harris EJ Jr. Pancreatic mass resection and revascularization. *J Vasc Surg*. 2010;52(2):530.
14. Schwarzbach MH, Hormann Y, Hinz U, et al. Clinical results of surgery for retroperitoneal sarcoma with major blood vessel involvement. *J Vasc Surg*. 2006;44(1):46-55.

Chapter 20 Open Renal Revascularization: Hepatorenal, Splenorenal, and Aortorenal Bypass

Fred Arthur Weaver and Gregory A. Magee

DEFINITION

- While the aorta is the most commonly used source of inflow for renal artery revascularization, the hepatic and splenic arteries can be used as an alternative inflow source when the aorta is severely diseased, occluded, or there is a hostile periaortic retroperitoneum. Patients with congestive heart failure may benefit from hepatic- or splenic-based revascularization as it minimizes the increase in cardiac afterload induced by aortic crossclamping, and these approaches have been shown to be durable alternatives to aorta-renal bypass. Alternative terms for hepatic- or splenic-based renal revascularization include hepatorenal, splenorenal bypass, splanchnorenal bypass, or extra-anatomic renal revascularization.

DIFFERENTIAL DIAGNOSIS

- Renal revascularization is most commonly performed to alleviate "resistant" renovascular hypertension. Resistant hypertension is defined as a systolic blood pressure greater than 140 mm Hg in patients on at least three antihypertensives, representing 5% to 10% of all hypertensives. A subset of these patients has secondary hypertension due to renal artery pathology or endocrine tumors. Alternative causes of resistant hypertension include:
  - Renal artery
    - Atherosclerosis
    - Aneurysm arteriovenous fistula
    - Fibromuscular dysplasia
    - Takayasu arteritis
    - Other vasculitidies involving the renal artery (eg, Behçet syndrome, polyarteritis nodosa)
    - Trauma
    - Aortic and/or renal artery dissection
  - Endocrine tumors associated with hypertension
    - Pheochromocytoma
    - Primary aldosteronism (Conn disease)
    - Cushing syndrome
    - Primary adrenal hyperplasia
    - Hyperthyroidism
    - Acromegaly

PATIENT HISTORY AND PHYSICAL FINDINGS

- Patient age: In younger patients, renovascular hypertension generally arises from nonatherosclerotic pathologies, such as Takayasu arteritis or fibromuscular dysplasia. In patients older than 50 years of age, atherosclerosis is the most common etiology.
- Associated risk factors are those typical for all occlusive arterial disease: tobacco use, diabetes, hyperlipidemia, and hypertension.
- Length of the hypertensive diathesis: Was the hypertension easily controlled for a period of time, with a recent increase in the difficulty of control? Is the hypertensive diathesis severe and recent in onset? If either is true, the patient is more likely to have secondary hypertension.
- Recognition of the systemic burden of the vascular disease present provides an important perspective on indications and treatment options. Many vascular maladies involve multiple vascular beds. Is there evidence of disease involving the carotid arteries, lower extremity arterial tree, and/or thoracic and abdominal aorta?
- A history of postprandial pain, significant unintentional weight loss, and food avoidance is suggestive of mesenteric occlusive disease.
- Prior pancreatitis may complicate attempts at splenic-based renal revascularization.
- Prior Hodgkin disease or other neoplasms requiring mantle or midline abdominal radiation.
- For general operative risk considerations, recognition and documentation of the presence of coronary artery disease, previous coronary stents, or surgical coronary revascularization as well as valvular disease and congestive heart failure are fundamental to surgical planning.
- Documentation of renal function as evidenced by increased serum creatinine, pedal edema, and recent requirement for renal replacement therapy.
- Recognition of prior aortic procedures, or intra-abdominal nonvascular procedures such as a retroperitoneal lymphadenectomy for testicular cancer, which would complicate retroperitoneal dissection and aortic exposure.
- Family history of syndromic aortic connective tissue disorders such as Marfan, Ehlers-Danlos, or Loeys-Dietz.
- The specific antihypertensive regimen in place prior to surgery needs to be verified and documented.
- To obtain the most accurate baseline measurement, the highest blood pressure obtained from either arm should be recorded and retained.
- A complete vascular examination must be performed, with particular attention paid to pulse deficits and bruits. In particular, diminished femoral pulses or an abdominal bruit may indicate significant aortic or branch vessel occlusive disease, potentially complicating revascularization plans. The presence of concomitant carotid bruits may suggest carotid occlusive disease that should be assessed prior to renal revascularization. The presence of an aortic aneurysm should be assessed by abdominal palpation.

IMAGING AND OTHER DIAGNOSTIC STUDIES

- Laboratory assessment of renal function should include, at a minimum, serum creatinine, blood urea nitrogen (BUN), and electrolytes. Baseline glomerular filtration rate can be estimated from creatinine level, age, sex, and race using the Modification of Diet in Renal Disease (MDRD) or the Chronic Kidney Disease Epidemiology Collaboration (CKD-EPI) equations.

- The co-occurrence of endocrine syndromes, such as pheochromocytoma or functional adrenal tumors that potentially contribute to resistant hypertension must be evaluated with appropriate serologic and/or urine studies prior to operative intervention.
- Renal artery duplex ultrasonography is performed to document existing renal artery disease, renal mass, and intraparenchymal renal blood flow indices. Hemodynamically significant renal artery stenosis (>60%) is determined by duplex-derived assessment of peak systolic velocity measurements across lesions. Baseline characteristics (ie, kidney size, velocity, spectral waveforms, and resistive indices) serve as reference points for future surveillance imaging following revascularization.
- Selective visceral and renal arteriograms are obtained to define normal and variant vascular anatomy, including lateral imaging of both the celiac and superior mesenteric arteries (**FIGURES 1** and **2**).
- Computed tomography (CT) angiography of the abdomen and pelvis, with arterial and venous phases, may provide additional useful information regarding the extent of existing aortic disease and other associated abdominal pathology (**FIGURES 3** and **4**). Catheter-based arteriography alone may not identify significant arterial wall disease or the presence of aneurysmal lesions. However, the expense, contrast load, and radiation associated with complementary arteriographic imaging modalities may not be justified or appropriate in every patient, so anatomic information obtained from these examinations should be integrated into the operative plan on an iterative basis. Preoperative, imaging-based planning is combined with direct intraoperative assessment to create the most effective and durable revascularization possible for each patient.
- Documentation of celiac, hepatic, splenic, and superior mesenteric artery patency is a mandatory prerequisite for hepatic- or splenic-based revascularization procedures. Significant stenosis of the celiac origin or hepatic or splenic artery occlusive disease will prevent successful renal revascularization from these arteries. Associated superior mesenteric artery disease also needs to be considered, particularly when the gastroduodenal artery provides significant collateral flow from the celiac artery to the mesenteric bed. Renal artery anatomy, including branch vessel involvement and the presence of multiple renal arteries must also be documented.
- Bilateral lower extremity vein mapping is also necessary to identify potential graft conduit. Standard vein mapping techniques, including imaging in a warm room with the patient

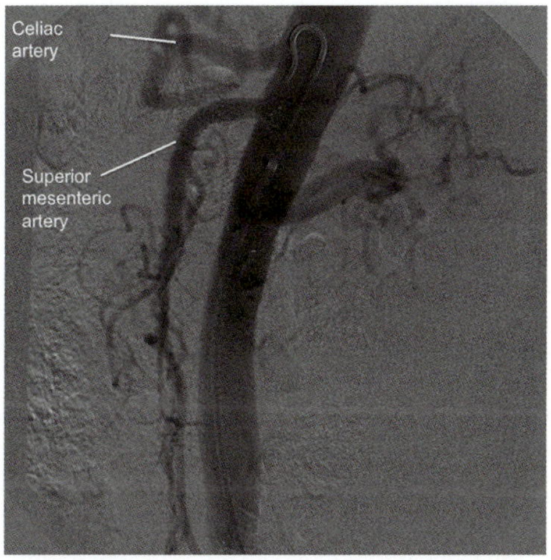

FIGURE 1 • Abdominal angiogram with lateral view shows a normal celiac artery.

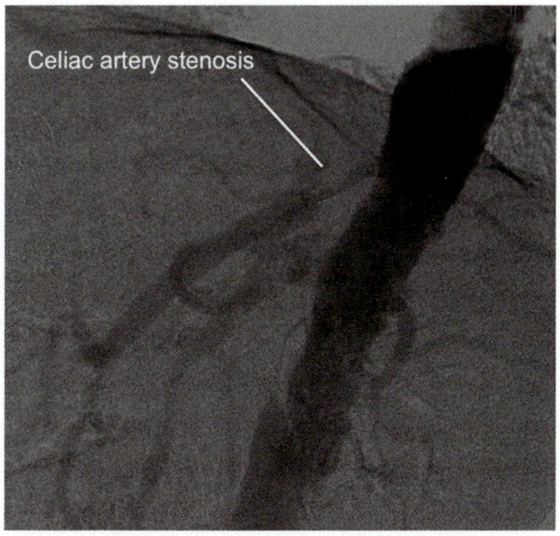

FIGURE 2 • Abdominal angiogram with lateral view shows a stenotic celiac artery.

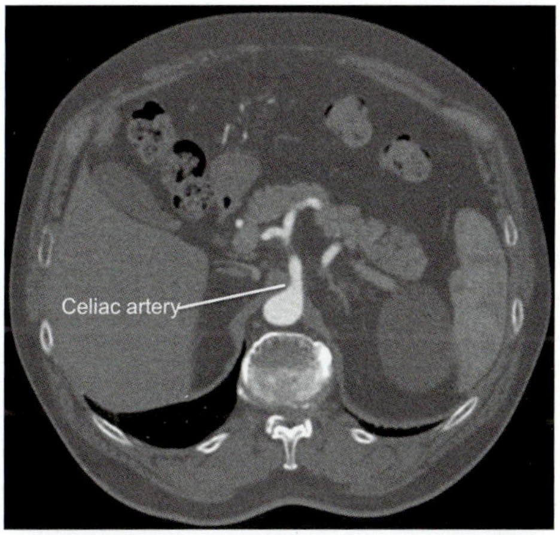

FIGURE 3 • Axial CT scan image shows a normal celiac artery origin.

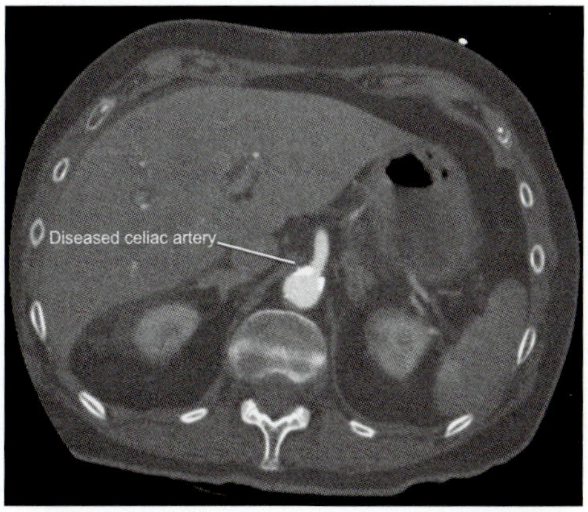

FIGURE 4 • Axial CT scan image shows a diseased celiac artery origin.

in reverse Trendelenburg position, should be employed to ensure accuracy and reproducibility.

- For selected patients, a more extensive preoperative evaluation for coronary artery or valvular disease should be considered. This may include both a transthoracic echocardiogram and cardiac stress evaluation. Selective pulmonary evaluation may be required in patients with chronic obstructive pulmonary disease (COPD)-associated respiratory compromise. Additional vascular assessments should be performed as indicated, including carotid duplex ultrasonography to access the significance of carotid bruits identified on physical examination.

SURGICAL MANAGEMENT

Preoperative Planning

- Aorta-renal bypass is the most direct and generally most expeditious approach.[1,2] However, extra-anatomic renal artery revascularization may be preferable in selected circumstances as previously noted.
- Review of preoperative imaging is performed to determine variant vascular anatomy, if present. Anatomical extent of the existing renal artery disease is assessed.
- The aorto-renal and hepatic-right renal bypasses require a conduit, preferably autogenous vein.
- The splenic-left renal bypass may be performed with or without graft conduit. The native splenic artery has sufficient length, usually to extend directly to the left renal artery, when fully mobilized. When necessary due to variant anatomy, or prior scarring around the pancreas, a venous conduit can also be employed.
- Planning for availability of duplex ultrasonography in the operating room will facilitate intraoperative confirmation of adequate target revascularization and renal perfusion.

Positioning

- Patient is placed in supine position with both arms tucked.
- A small bump is placed under the respective flank.
- The operative field is prepped from the nipples to the knees.

HEPATORENAL BYPASS

Placement of Incision

- Optimal access is gained through a right subcostal incision extending from the midline to the tip of the 12th rib. In large or obese patients, the medial extent of the incision can be extended across the midline as a chevron (**FIGURE 5**).
- When necessary, an upper midline incision may also provide sufficient exposure.

Hepatic Artery Exposure

- The hepatoduodenal ligament is exposed by retracting the right lobe of the liver cephalad.

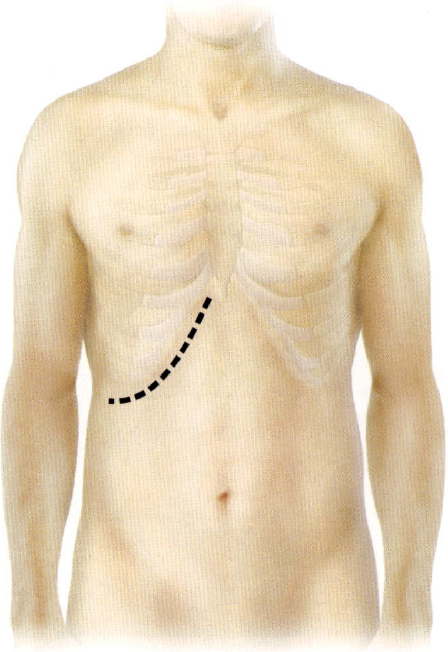

FIGURE 5 • Right subcostal incision extended to the tip of 12th rib.

- The right colon and duodenum are reflected anteriorly and to the left (Kocher maneuver). The small intestine is packed toward the pelvis with moist laparotomy pads.
- The hepatoduodenal ligament is incised longitudinally. The hepatic artery is located in the porta hepatis medial to the common bile duct (**FIGURE 6**).
- The gastroduodenal artery is identified as the first large branch coursing caudad and encircled with a silastic vessel loop. The gastroduodenal artery should be preserved in the presence of superior mesenteric artery occlusive disease as it provides important collateral circulation to the small intestines.
- The hepatic artery is controlled proximally and distally with silastic vessel loops (**FIGURE 7**).

Right Renal Artery Exposure

- The right colon and duodenum are reflected as detailed earlier to expose the inferior vena cava and right renal vein.
- The right renal artery is located posterior and superior to the main renal vein. Depending on its position, the renal vein is retracted either cephalad or caudad. To ensure the main renal artery is exposed, the dissection should be carried to its aortic origin. This requires medial retraction of the inferior vena cava and division of lumbar veins when necessary.
- The right renal artery is controlled using a silastic vessel loop.
- The main renal artery is exposed circumferentially and then distally to the three segmental renal artery branches. Each branch is identified and controlled with a silastic vessel loop. This is a critical operative maneuver that excludes the presence of branch disease and ensures a successful renal artery revascularization (**FIGURE 7**).

Distal Anastomosis

- The distal anastomosis is always performed first to take advantage of the additional degrees of freedom provided by the mobile graft.

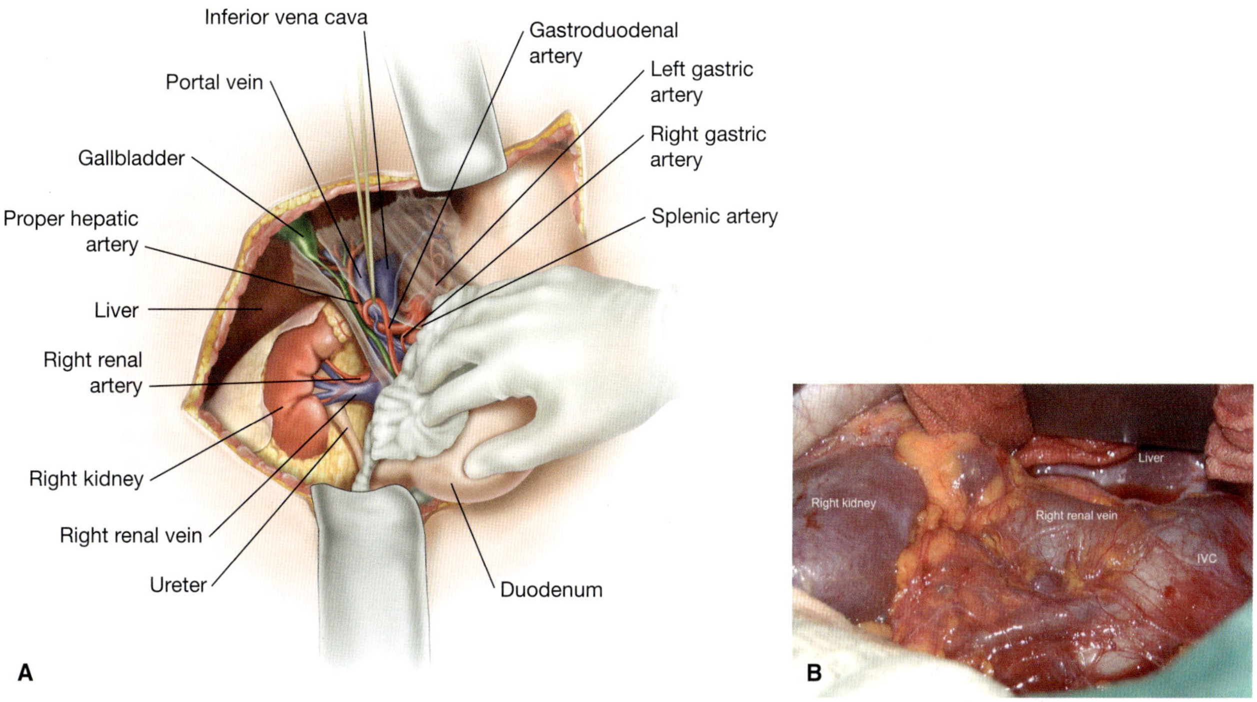

FIGURE 6 • **A** and **B,** Kocher maneuver with porta hepatis dissected. IVC, inferior vena cava.

- An appropriate length of great saphenous vein is harvested from the thigh. The patient is then heparinized with 100 U/kg intravenously. The vein itself is reversed before placement.
- The proximal renal artery is mobilized following its division from the aorta, at its origin. The proximal stump is oversewn with 5-0 polypropylene suture.
- The redundant renal artery is trimmed distally from its origin until the disease-free segment is reached. The mobile renal artery is then transposed anterior to the inferior vena cava.
- The vein graft and renal artery are spatulated and an end-to-end anastomosis is created with 6-0 polypropylene suture, tied at opposite ends of the anastomosis to prevent purse-stringing. Alternatively, depending on renal artery diameter, eight interrupted sutures may be distributed circumferentially around the lumen. The smaller the renal artery diameter, the more advantageous the interrupted technique. Loupe magnification is necessary to ensure optimal results regardless of which suture technique is chosen (**FIGURE 7**).
- Once the distal anastomosis is completed, the vein graft is oriented longitudinally to prevent twisting or kinking prior to completion of the proximal anastomosis.

Proximal Anastomosis

Hepatic artery

- Small vascular clamps or removal clips are used to control the proximal and distal hepatic artery.
- A longitudinal arteriotomy is made on the hepatic artery and extended using Potts scissors.
- The vein is spatulated and an end-to-side anastomosis is performed using polypropylene (**FIGURE 8A**).

Gastroduodenal artery

- The gastroduodenal artery may be used as an alternative inflow vessel if sufficiently large size (4-6 mm in diameter). This anastomosis may be performed either end-to-end or end-to-side, but prior to division of the gastroduodenal artery, consideration should be given toward its contribution to the mesenteric circulation (**FIGURE 8B**).

Intraoperative Duplex Ultrasonography

- We recommend insonation of the graft and both anastomoses using an appropriately sized 7-MHz scan head to ensure technical proficiency following completion of the reconstruction. In recent years, our practice has come to rely on duplex ultrasonography for intraoperative assessment of all small and medium size autogenous reconstructions, especially in light of the reduced frequency of such procedures in the era of endovascular and hybrid reconstructions. Renal artery reconstruction is unforgiving. Less than a technically perfect anastomosis can result in bypass graft stenosis or occlusion leading to either recurrent hypertension and/or a decrease in renal function.
- Spectral waveforms, velocities, and B-mode are all employed to detect technical errors requiring immediate repair.

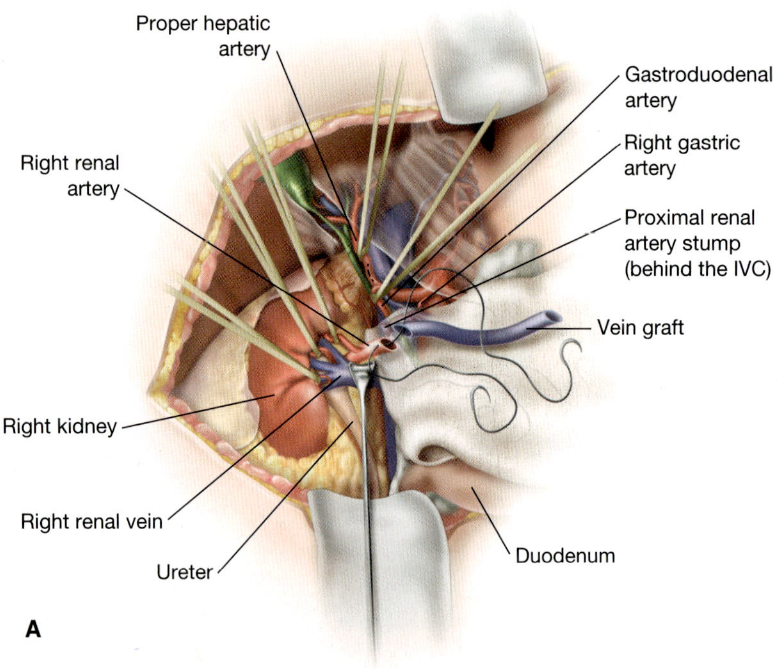

A

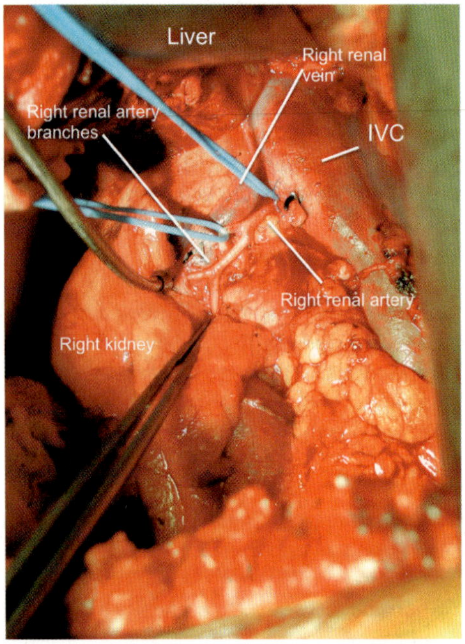

B

FIGURE 7 • **A and B,** Right renal artery and distal branches encircled with silastic loops. Distal anastomosis is performed first. IVC, inferior vena cava.

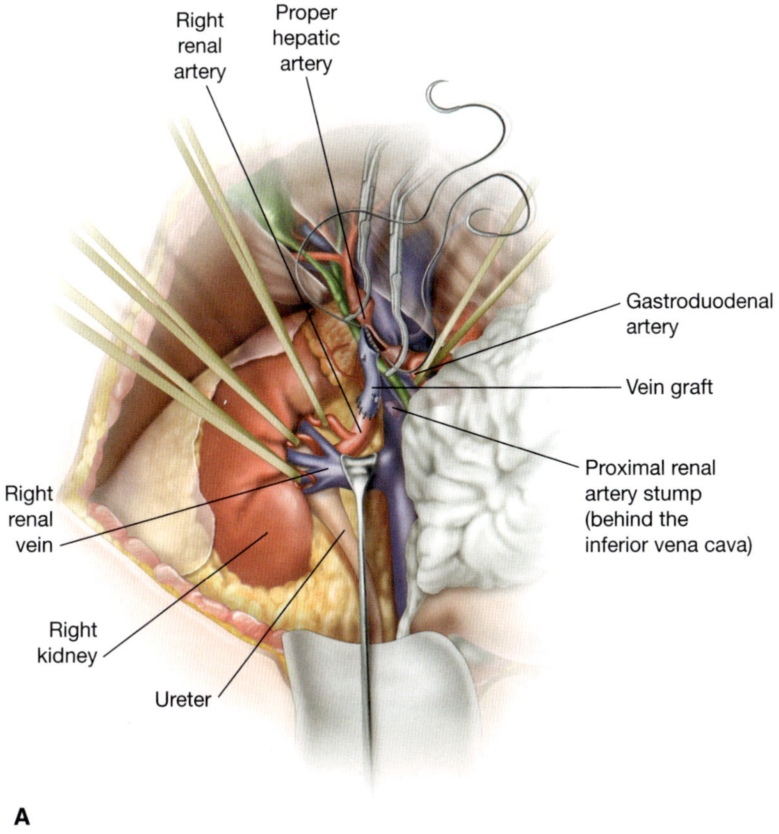

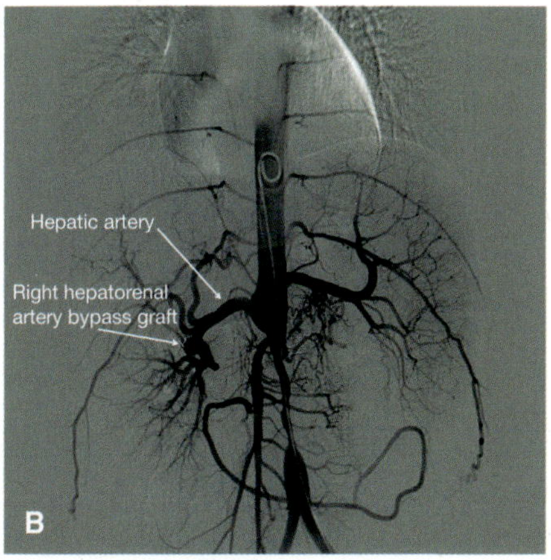

FIGURE 8 • **A,** Proximal Anastomosis. **B,** Anterior-posterior angiographic image demonstrates a hepatorenal artery bypass.

SPLENORENAL BYPASS

Placement of Incision

- Exposure is obtained through a left subcostal incision extending from the midline to the tip of the 12th rib. In large or obese patients, the medial extent of the incision can be extended across the midline as a chevron (**FIGURE 9**).
- As was the case on the right side, the upper midline incision may also provide sufficient access depending on body habitus, prior operations, and operator experience.

Splenic Artery Exposure

- The greater omentum is elevated exposing the transverse mesocolon. The ligament of Treitz is taken down and the inferior mesenteric vein is ligated and divided. The plane between the pancreas and kidney is entered and the pancreas is elevated. The splenic vein is embedded in the body of the pancreas—avoid injury during mobilization of the distal pancreas. The splenic artery should be palpable along the cephalad border of the pancreas. It is mobilized medially and laterally until sufficient length is obtained to fashion either transposition or support an autogenous vein conduit bypass (**FIGURE 10**).

Left Renal Artery Exposure

- After mobilizing the distal pancreas, the left renal vein is located just posterior and caudad.

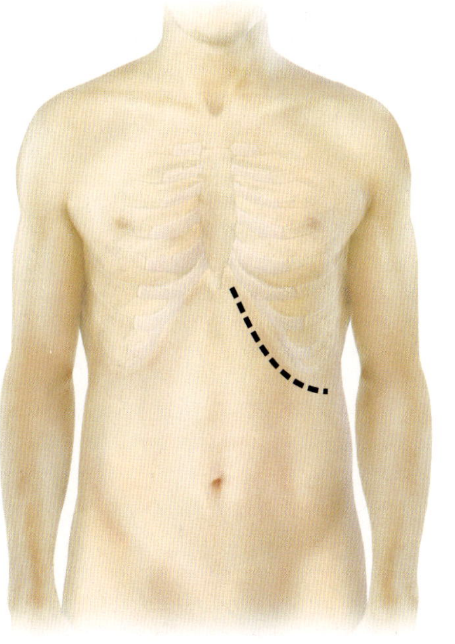

FIGURE 9 • Left subcostal incision extended to the tip of 12th rib.

- The left renal vein is circumferentially mobilized. This requires division of its nonrenal tributaries: the gonadal, adrenal, and renolumbar veins. Dividing these veins greatly enhances renal vein mobility, facilitating renal artery exposure.
- As previously described on the right, the left renal artery is dissected to its aortic origin and controlled with a silastic vessel loop. The distal artery and its three segmental branches are identified and encircled with silastic vessel loops. The importance of mobilization of the segmental branches is again emphasized (**FIGURE 11**).

Splenorenal Anastomosis

- The patient is heparinized with 100 U/kg of unfractionated heparin intravenously. The left renal artery is clamped

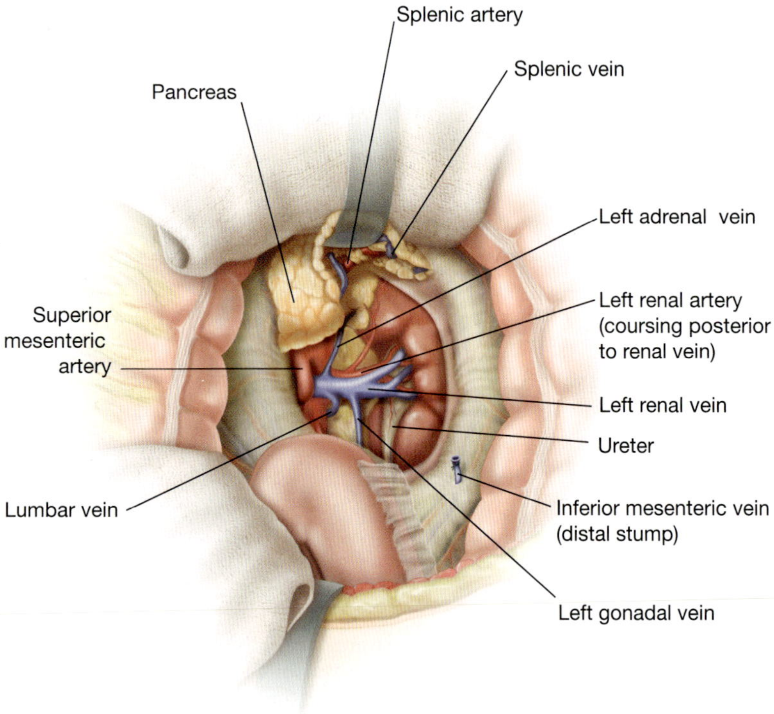

FIGURE 10 • Left renal artery and vein exposure. Division of the inferior mesenteric vein allows cephalad retraction of the retropancreatic plane, which allows visualization of the splenic artery.

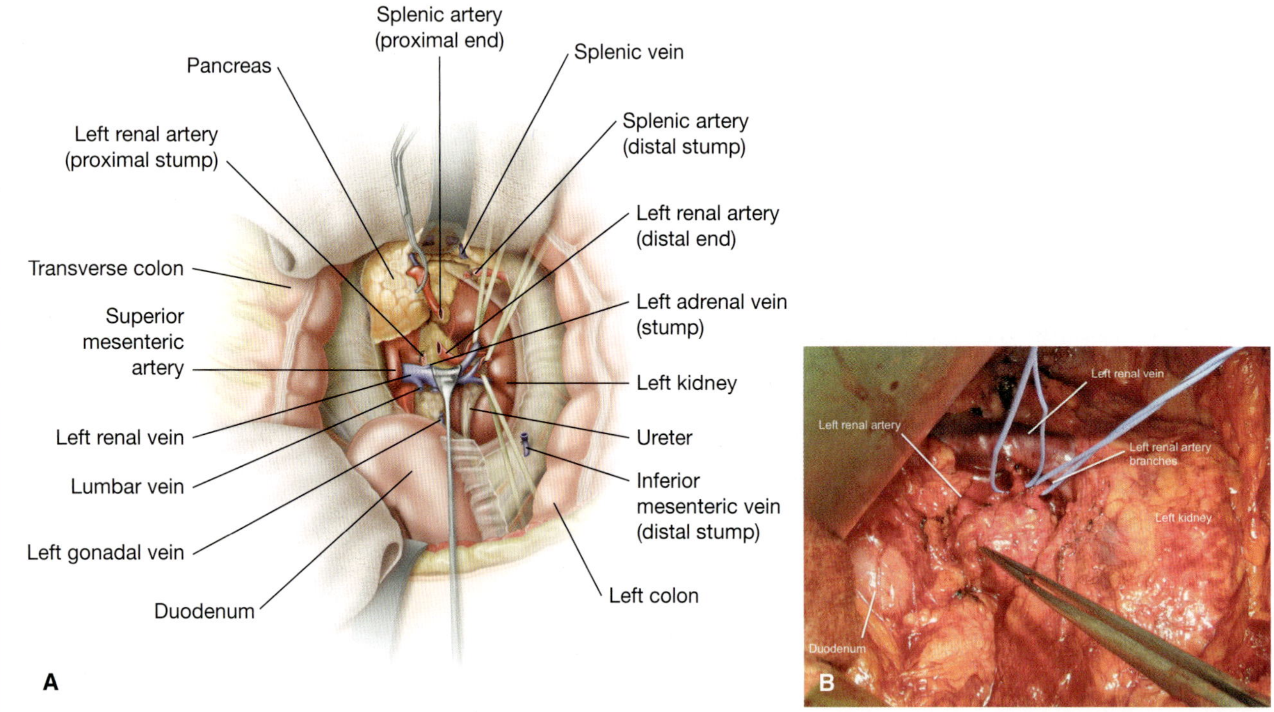

FIGURE 11 • **A and B,** The splenic artery and left renal artery are divided. The gonadal, adrenal, and lumbar veins are ligated and divided, allowing complete mobilization of the left renal vein.

at the origin and divided. The proximal renal stump is oversewn with 5-0 polypropylene suture. The distal main renal artery is spatulated distal to the existing renal artery disease. The mobilized splenic artery is divided with sufficient length to extend behind the pancreas to the left renal artery without undue tension. The distal splenic artery is oversewn.

- The mobilized splenic artery is spatulated and transposed end to end to the left renal artery, again with either running or interrupted polypropylene suture depending on the respective arterial diameters (**FIGURE 12**).
- Alternatively, when splenic artery length is insufficient, reversed saphenous vein may be employed as a bridge graft. Again, to optimize the degrees of freedom, the distal anastomosis is performed first, followed by an end-to-end or end-to-side anastomosis to the splenic artery. The vein graft is positioned posterior and inferior to the body of the pancreas.

Intraoperative Duplex Ultrasonography

- As described earlier.

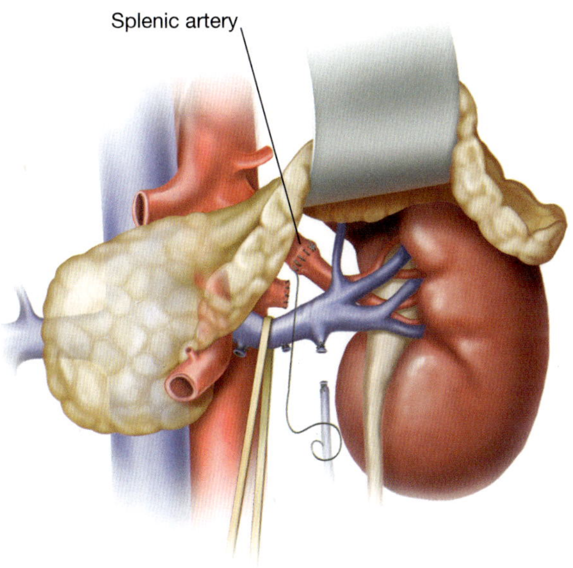

FIGURE 12 • Completed anastomosis between the splenic artery and left renal artery.

AORTORENAL BYPASS

Placement of Incision

- A subcostal incision is performed on the appropriate side as described earlier.
- A midline incision may be used if bilateral aortorenal bypasses are planned.

Infrarenal Aortic Exposure

- The infrarenal aorta is exposed circumferentially from the renal artery origins to above the aortic bifurcation.
- Beware of lumbar arteries when placing the aortic clamps.

Renal Artery Exposure

- As described earlier.

Distal Anastomosis

- As described earlier.

Aortorenal Anastomosis

- The aorta is cross clamped below the contralateral renal artery and above the aortic bifurcation with sufficient length to easily perform the anastomosis.
- A small arteriotomy is performed on the lateral aspect of the aorta and an aortic punch is used to create a round arteriotomy appropriately sized to the vein graft.
- The vein graft is spatulated and an end-to-side anastomosis is performed using polypropylene suture.

Intraoperative Duplex Ultrasonography

- As described earlier.

FINAL INSPECTION

With completion of the revascularization procedure, all anastomoses and oversewn renal artery origins are inspected for hemostasis. Heparin anticoagulation is reversed with protamine, in a quantity sufficient to normalize the activated clotting time (ACT). Palpation of the superior mesenteric artery (SMA) at the base of the mesentery is performed to confirm a pulse. Operative traction and/or pre-existing disease may compromise SMA flow or precipitate an occult dissection. If the SMA pulse is absent, or the intestinal viability is uncertain, mesenteric artery revascularization may be necessary.

PEARLS AND PITFALLS

Preoperative imaging	■ Surgical planning may require CT and catheter-based arteriography as complementary references. ■ Celiac artery stenosis is an absolute contraindication for hepatic- and splenic-based renal revascularization.
Preoperative vein mapping	■ Autogenous vein is the preferred conduit for renal revascularization. ■ Lower extremity vein mapping allows assessment for suitable conduit.
Exposure of the renal artery	■ Circumferential exposure of the entire main renal artery and the three segmental branches is imperative for placement of the renal anastomosis distal to existing disease.
Graft orientation	■ Longitudinal orientation needs to be confirmed repeatedly during graft placement. Excessive reliance on graft marking or "striping" as the sole method of orientation may lead to inadvertent kinking or twisting.
Intraoperative duplex	■ Completion duplex scanning is easy, quick, and invaluable in identifying technical errors, which may compromise graft patency and renal viability. ■ Unlike lower extremity bypass procedures, perioperative graft occlusion cannot typically be identified expeditiously to prevent end-organ compromise.

POSTOPERATIVE CARE

- Postoperative care typically involves central venous and arterial pressure monitoring in the intensive care unit (ICU) for the first 24 to 48 hours.
- Serial monitoring of serum creatinine, urine output, and acid-base status is essential in the early postoperative period. Unexplained changes in acid-base status or elevation of serum creatinine could indicate occlusion of the revascularization or mesenteric ischemia.
- Blood pressure is maintained in a physiologic range with vasoactive medications as necessary. Oral antihypertensives are resumed on postoperative day one and adjusted depending on the response to renal revascularization.
- Diet is resumed as bowel function returns; nasogastric suction is usually not required.
- Blood pressure and antihypertensive medication requirements may decrease after renal revascularization and should be adjusted prior to discharge.
- Diet is resumed as bowel function returns; nasogastric suction is usually not required.
- Follow-up surveillance duplex ultrasonography is performed at 6 and 12 months, then annually thereafter. Detected abnormalities suggesting stenosis of the renal reconstruction may be addressed with remedial endovascular intervention or surgical revision when indicated.

OUTCOMES

- Large case series documenting the outcomes following isolated hepatorenal and splenorenal artery bypass are sparse. Published results are derived from two relatively large series, generally demonstrating acceptable perioperative morbidity and mortality with improved renal function and blood pressure and durable patency.
- Moncure et al. reported 77 patients who underwent 79 procedures (29 hepatorenal and 50 splenorenal bypasses) for the treatment of renovascular hypertension and renal preservation. The perioperative mortality was 6%. Deterioration in renal function occurred on three occasions but only in patients with bilateral simultaneous repair. Cure or improvement in hypertension was observed in 52 of 63 patients. Renal function was preserved or improved in 67 of 77 patients.[3]
- Another series by Geroulakos et al. document similar outcomes with extra-anatomic renal artery revascularization for atherosclerotic renal artery disease. Forty-five hepatorenal and/or splenorenal bypasses were performed in 38 patients for the treatment of renovascular hypertension, renal preservation, or both. There was one postoperative death from myocardial infarction and two cases of early graft thrombosis. There was a significant decrease in postoperative mean serum creatinine as well as the average number of antihypertensives. Over a median follow-up of 33 months, there were 10 deaths, all from cardiac issues.[4]

COMPLICATIONS

- Bypass graft thrombosis
- Intestinal ischemia due to pre-existing disease or traction injury to the SMA during operative exposure
- Bleeding from the renal, hepatic, splenic, aortic anastomoses, ligated renal artery stump, and portal or splenic vein if injured
- Acute renal failure requiring temporary or permanent renal replacement therapy
- Pancreatitis, splenic infarction, and common bile duct injury
- Incisional hernia

REFERENCES

1. Benjamin ME, Dean RH. Techniques in renal artery reconstruction: part II. *Ann Vasc Surg*. 1996;10(4):409-414.
2. Weaver FA, Kumar SR, Yellin AE, et al. Renal revascularization in Takayasu arteritis–induced renal artery stenosis. *J Vasc Surg*. 2004;39:749-757.
3. Moncure AC, Brewster DC, Darling RC, et al. Use of the splenic and hepatic arteries for renal revascularization. *J Vasc Surg*. 1986;3:196-203.
4. Geroulakos G, Wright JG, Tober JC, Anderson L, Smead WL. Use of the splenic and hepatic artery for renal revascularization in patients with atherosclerotic renal artery disease. *Ann Vasc Surg*. 1997;11:85-89.

Chapter 21

Open Visceral Revascularizations for Ischemia: Superior Mesenteric Artery Embolectomy, SMA/Celiac Bypass/Endarterectomy

Robyn A. Macsata†, Benjamin Pomy, and Kellie R. Brown

DEFINITION

Acute/Subacute

- Acute mesenteric ischemia (AMI) is an uncommon, life-threatening, vascular and general surgical emergency effecting approximately 1 in 1000 patients annually. This disease is accompanied by significant morbidity and mortality following both endovascular and open surgical intervention.[1] The most common cause of AMI is secondary to an embolic event from a cardiac source, such as atrial fibrillation (**FIGURE 1**). Other causes include nonocclusive mesenteric ischemia (NOMI) and mesenteric venous thrombosis (MVT). NOMI is a result of a generalized low-flow state creating vasoconstriction to the mesenteric vessels in order to shunt blood to the more vital organs (heart and brain); treatment is of the underlying conditions and in some extreme circumstances catheter-directed vasodilatory agents. MVT is a result of a surrounding inflammatory event; treatment is directed at the involved organ, which may require removal (such as a cholecystectomy) and therapeutic anticoagulation. Both treatment of NOMI and MVT are outside the scope of this chapter.

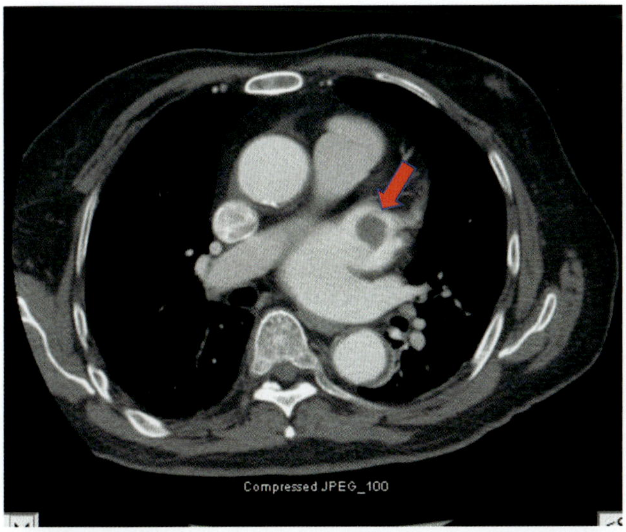

FIGURE 1 • Left atrial appendage thrombus (*red arrow*) in a patient who presented with SMA occlusion. (Courtesy of Dr. Benjamin Pomy, George Washington University.)

- Subacute mesenteric ischemia is secondary to in situ thrombus of preexisting mesenteric artery occlusive disease (MAOD) in the proximal superior mesenteric artery (SMA). This occurs secondary to either plaque rupture or a generalized low-flow state with resulting in situ thrombus formation.

Chronic

- Chronic mesenteric ischemia (CMI) presents with chronic postprandial pain and weight loss and can be difficult to diagnose due to its nonspecific presentation. CMI is caused by the inability to maintain adequate postprandial blood flow to the visceral organs due to atherosclerotic severe stenosis or occlusion of multiple visceral vessels, resulting in oxygen and metabolite supply and demand mismatch. This is a result of MAOD; however, the presence of MAOD alone does not always correlate with CMI symptoms.[2]

DIFFERENTIAL DIAGNOSIS

Acute/Subacute

The differential diagnosis for AMI is broad and includes many abdominal pathologies, which may present with peritonitis, such as:

- Appendicitis
- Cholecystitis
- Pancreatitis
- Diverticulitis
- Bowel obstruction
- Perforated ulcer disease

Chronic

The differential diagnosis for CMI is even more broad than that of AMI due to the often-vague nature of presentation. The differential for CMI includes:

- Gallstones
- Peptic ulcer disease
- Various food intolerances (celiac disease, etc.)
- Chronic pancreatitis
- Occult malignancy
- Inflammatory bowel disease
- Irritable bowel syndrome
- Functional abdominal pain

†Deceased

PATIENT HISTORY AND PHYSICAL FINDINGS

Acute/Subacute

- Patients commonly present to the emergency department with acute onset of severe abdominal pain. In some patients this pain may be accompanied by bloody diarrhea, and it is not uncommon for patients to report a large bowel movement immediately following symptom onset. Patients often will have a diagnosis of cardiac dysrhythmias, most commonly atrial fibrillation, and may have reported a missed dose of their anticoagulation.
- "Pain out of proportion" to physical examination is a hallmark of AMI; however, this may be absent in 20% to 25% of cases. Patients may rapidly decline and exhibit profound metabolic acidosis, sepsis, and multisystem organ failure. Patients with preexisting MAOD may have a history of CMI symptoms with postprandial abdominal pain and weight loss that then develops into acute peritonitis. This presentation is very often difficult to diagnose given the nonspecific nature of the symptoms. Presentation is otherwise similar to AMI, but slightly more insidious with a history of vague abdominal symptoms.[1]

Chronic

- Chronic mesenteric ischemia is typically diagnosed in elderly, frail patients, with a classic triad of symptoms: vague abdominal pain, weight loss, and "food fear." These patients often have nonspecific symptoms for a prolonged period of time. They realize their pain is related to eating, which leads to anorexia, significant weight loss, and chronic malnutrition. Patients with CMI usually undergo an extensive workup for other abdominal pathologies including occult malignancies, ulcer disease, and functional abdominal pain prior to being diagnosed with CMI.[2]

IMAGING AND OTHER DIAGNOSTICS

Acute/Subacute

- Diagnosis of both acute and subacute mesenteric ischemia is best performed with computed tomography angiography (CTA) (**FIGURE 2**). CTA is both sensitive and specific for acute arterial embolism, thrombosis, and MAOD and can evaluate the bowel for ischemia and necrosis.[3] CTA can then be used for either endovascular or open surgical operative planning, including need for possible bowel resection. Arteriogram is generally reserved for when endovascular treatment is planned.

Chronic

- Given the noninvasive nature and low cost, screening is done with duplex ultrasound (DUS) in the noninvasive vascular laboratory. Patients should be fasting before this procedure for better visualization of the vessels, to decrease bowel gas, and to assure a resting state. Patients without any mesenteric stenosis will have high resistance waveforms preprandial that become low resistance postprandial, and velocities will all be below 200 cm/s^2 in the celiac and below 275 cm/s^2 in the SMA. Patients with a greater than 70% celiac and/or SMA stenosis will have high resistance waveforms both pre- and postprandial, and velocities will be above 200 cm/s^2 in the celiac and 275 cm/s^2 in the SMA. CTA can be used to confirm the diagnosis, but most often patients progress straight to arteriogram, which is the gold standard for diagnosis and most commonly therapeutic as well.[4]

SURGICAL MANAGEMENT

Endovascular Options

- While out of scope of this chapter, it should be noted that endovascular strategies for mesenteric revascularization have become increasingly popular and, specifically for

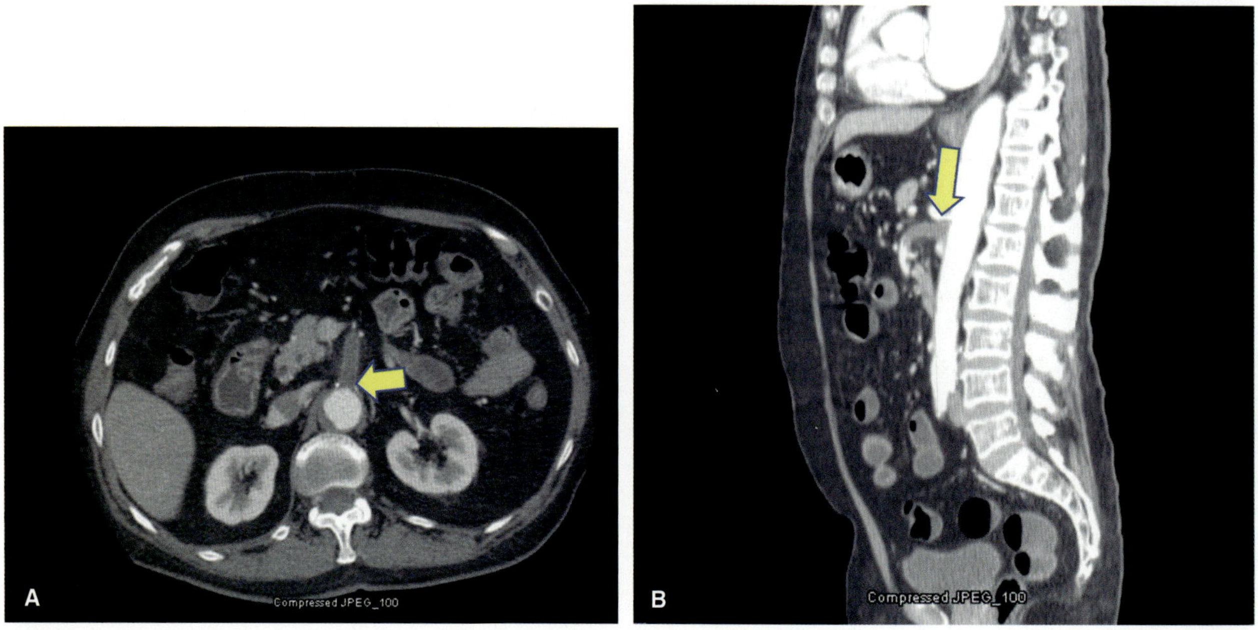

FIGURE 2 • Acute SMA occlusion (*yellow arrows*) at the vessel origin. **A,** Axial view. **B,** Coronal view. (Courtesy of Dr. Benjamin Pomy, George Washington University.)

CMI, have become first-line therapy. This is due to the minimally invasive nature of these interventions resulting in improved perioperative morbidity with a relative trade-off for decreased long-term patency and freedom from symptom recurrence.[4] Obviously, endovascular options for AMI are limited to cases when bowel ischemia has not progressed to the point of requiring bowel resection. Endovascular strategies for mesenteric revascularization include catheter-directed mechanical thrombectomies and thrombolysis to treat acute thrombus followed by angioplasty and/or stenting to treat any underlying chronic occlusive disease. Mesenteric angioplasty and stenting can also be employed alone in the setting of symptomatic CMI (see Chapter 15).

Acute/Subacute

Preoperative Planning

- Given the acute nature of their presentation and likelihood of underlying bowel ischemia, these patients are often septic and require ongoing aggressive resuscitation. This requires a full laboratory evaluation and type and cross for blood products. Once mesenteric thrombosis is identified by CTA, patients should be fully anticoagulated with full-dose intravenous (IV) heparin (70 U/kg) on the way to the operating room.

Positioning

- The patient should be placed on the operating table in supine position with at least one arm extended for anesthesia access for intravenous fluids and intra-arterial blood pressure monitoring. A nasogastric tube is placed for gastric decompression. A Foley catheter is placed for accurate urine monitoring. The patient is prepped and draped from the level of the nipples to the knees; this wide prep will allow harvesting of the greater saphenous vein (GSV) if needed for revascularization.

Chronic Mesenteric Ischemia

Preoperative Planning

- Given the prolonged nature of their presentation, these patients are often severely malnourished. Preoperative workup includes a full laboratory panel including liver enzymes and a full nutritional assessment. Improving preoperative nutrition via an oral route is often difficult given the underlying disease; preoperative total parenteral nutrition may be considered but has not been proven to show any benefit. Priority should be placed on revascularization, and the operation should not be delayed for nutritional optimization.
- In addition to nutritional concerns, patients with CMI should have undergone screening DUS (as described above) as well as either CTA or catheter-based angiography. These images are used to determine the optimal revascularization strategy (discussed in the sections that follow). If vein is to be used for bypass, patients should undergo vein mapping to ensure adequate length and caliber of GSV.

Positioning

- The patient is placed on the table in supine position with at least one arm extended to give the anesthesiologist access for intravenous fluids and intra-arterial pressure monitoring during the procedure. A nasogastric tube is placed for gastric decompression. A Foley catheter is placed to accurately measure urine output. A semi-lateral position with the patient's left side elevated with a shoulder roll to aid in accessing the retroperitoneum is an alternative option.

EMBOLECTOMY (WITH OR WITHOUT ENDARTERECTOMY AND PATCH ANGIOPLASTY):

- ***FIRST STEP—laparotomy, control contamination:*** A midline laparotomy is performed extending from the xiphoid process to the public tubercle; this gives wide access to the abdomen to perform bowel evaluation and dissection of the aorta and mesenteric vessels as needed. The bowel is thoroughly evaluated upon opening the abdomen, any frankly necrotic or perforated bowel is resected, and any questionably ischemic bowel management is delayed until after revascularization.
- ***SECOND STEP—identify and expose the SMA (FIGURE 3):*** The SMA is reached by packing the small bowel to the patient's right side and the transverse colon along with its mesentery cephalad, similar to exposure of an infrarenal abdominal aortic aneurysm. Given the nature of the event, the SMA pulse usually cannot be felt at the base of the mesentery. Nevertheless, a longitudinal incision is made at the base of the mesentery followed by sharp dissection to identify the SMA. Of note, there are many crossing veins as well as lymphatics throughout the mesentery that should be identified, tied, and transected on the way to the SMA. Once identified, the SMA can be traced back to its origin at the aorta as well as forward to its first branches beyond the thrombus. The main trunk of the SMA as well as its branches are dissected free from the surrounding mesentery and controlled with vessel loops to maintain proximal and distal control (**FIGURE 4A** and **B**).
- ***THIRD STEP—heparinize and perform thrombectomy (optional endarterectomy):*** The patient is rebolused with heparin as needed depending on the preoperative emergency dosing. The SMA is inspected to determine the level of disease present. If it feels as if only acute thrombus is present, a transverse arteriotomy is made just proximal to any branch point (**FIGURE 3**). Proximal and distal embolectomy is performed using a range of #2 to 4 Fogarty balloons; when proximal embolectomy is completed pulsatile arterial flow from the aorta should be reestablished. Distal thrombectomy may

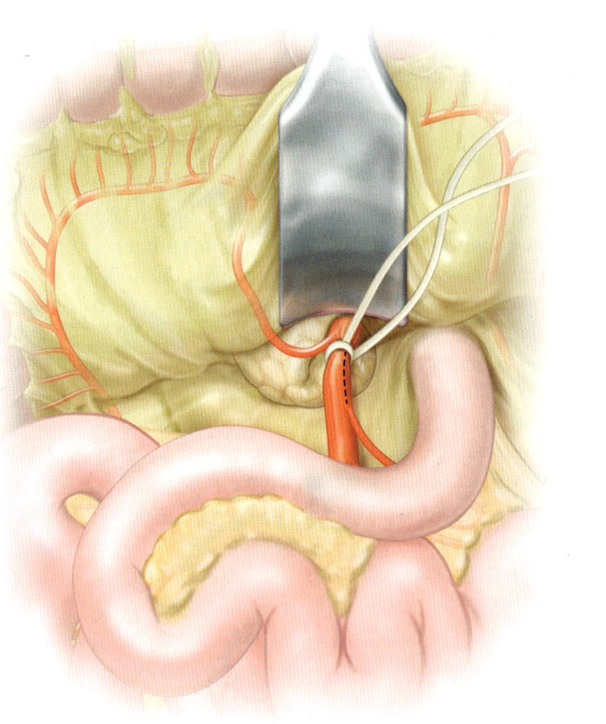

FIGURE 3 • Exposure of the SMA: The colon is retracted cephalad, and small bowel to the right. The base of the mesentery is incised, and the SMA is identified at the base of the mesentery.

require embolectomy of multiple branches. When complete there should be back bleeding from all involved vessels. The arteriotomy is then closed using two 6-0 Prolene sutures running toward each other and tied together.

- If underlying plaque is identified upon palpation of the SMA, a longitudinal arteriotomy is performed as opposed to a transverse arteriotomy. Following thrombectomy, as described above, an endarterectomy is performed to remove bulky atherosclerotic plaque from the SMA. To perform the endarterectomy, the longitudinal arteriotomy should extend from the proximal aspect to the distal aspect of the atherosclerotic disease, a plaque elevator is then used to elevate the calcified thrombus off the vessel media. Following plaque removal, the artery is thoroughly irrigated with heparinized saline to prevent further embolization of atherosclerotic debris, and the arteriotomy is closed using a patch angioplasty, usually with a bovine pericardial patch, or if contamination is significant, a GSV vein patch.
- ***FOURTH STEP—manage ischemic bowel, determine closure strategy:*** Once the revascularization is complete, bowel viability is once again assessed. Any frankly necrotic or perforated bowel that was not identified or removed prior to revascularization is resected. At this time, the surgeon should use their best judgment of the strategy for abdominal closure, need for a second-look operation, bowel anastomosis, etc. In general, a second look operation is advocated, and bowel reanastomosis is deferred until this second look, when a full appraisal of viability can be undertaken.

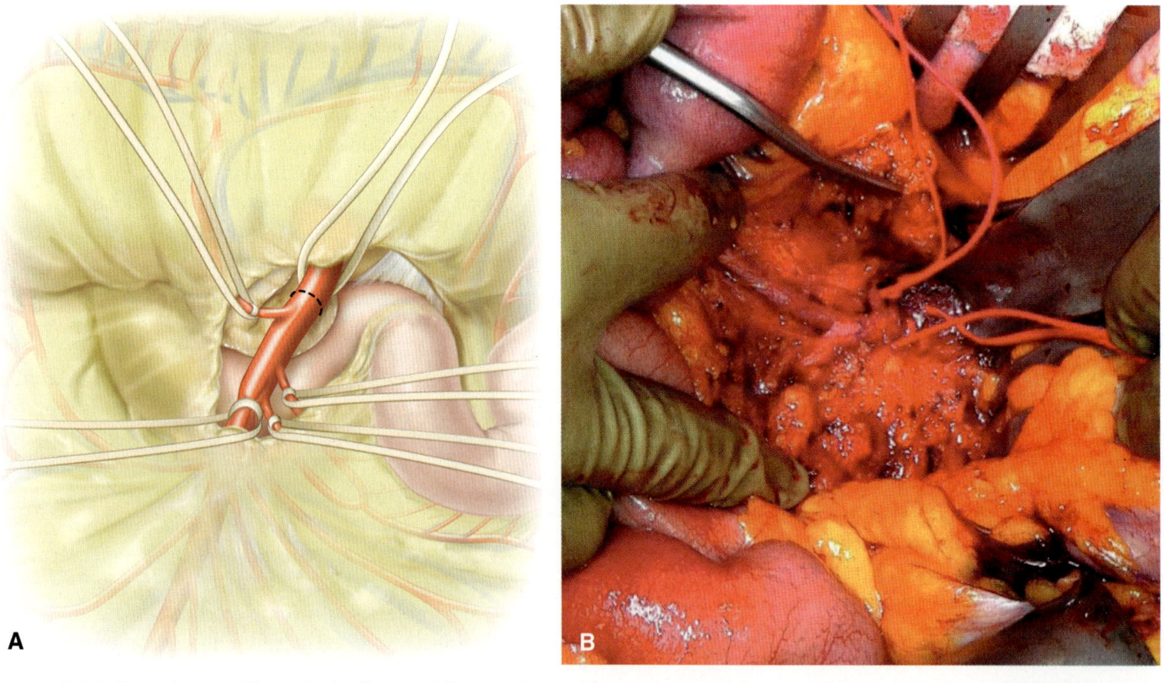

FIGURE 4 • SMA dissection. **A,** The SMA is dissected free and vessel loops are used to control branches. Transverse incision is made to facilitate embolectomy. **B,** Intraoperative picture of SMA exposed and controlled. (Courtesy of Dr. Kellie R. Brown, The Medical College of Wisconsin.)

CHRONIC MESENTERIC ISCHEMIA

Surgical Decision Making

- Similar to bypasses in the lower extremity, mesenteric revascularization does require careful operative planning with knowledge of the patient's anatomy. As with all vascular bypasses, one needs:
  - Inflow
  - Outflow
  - Conduit

The section that follows provides a brief discussion of the surgical decision-making process for each of these considerations.

Inflow: Antegrade vs Retrograde Bypass

- An arterial bypass to the mesenteric vessels may be performed either antegrade, with the supraceliac aorta as the source of inflow, or retrograde, with either the infrarenal aorta or right common iliac artery as the source of inflow. Benefits of an antegrade approach are a less diseased (atherosclerosis/calcium) inflow vessel and a shorter straighter bypass to the outflow vessels. However, dissection of the supraceliac aorta may be difficult and cross clamping of the aorta is often required, which comes with hemodynamic consequences. Occasionally, a partially occluding clamp (such as a Satinsky clamp) may be used; however, this is not always possible. Benefits of a retrograde approach include an easier dissection and avoiding cross clamping of the aorta (if the right common iliac artery is used as inflow). However, often these more distal vessels have atherosclerotic disease and may be calcified; furthermore, the bypass requires retrograde flow and can be fraught with kinking on its way to the outflow vessels. Ultimately, no differences in outcomes have been reported between an antegrade or retrograde approach to inflow; therefore, this is left up to the surgeon's best judgment and usually based on the unique anatomy and pathophysiology of the patient.[4]

Outflow: One-Vessel vs Two-Vessel Revascularization

- The main two sources of outflow for a mesenteric bypass are the celiac (often extended to the common hepatic artery) and SMA. When patients present with clinically symptomatic CMI, the SMA nearly invariably has a high-grade stenosis while the celiac artery may or may not also be involved. There are little data available to support the number of vessels to revascularize, and, while the theoretical advantage to multivessel revascularization is better long-term patency, outcomes in the literature appear equivocal. Therefore, revascularization strategy is often based on surgeon preference along with patient anatomy and comorbidities. In younger patients with a longer life expectancy, two-vessel bypasses should be considered if the anatomy presents itself, while in patients with a lower life expectancy and more comorbidities, one-vessel bypass is a valid option.[4]

Conduit: Prosthetic vs Autogenous

- The main conduit choices for mesenteric reconstruction are autogenous (commonly GSV), polytetrafluorethylene (PTFE), and Dacron. In the acute setting, with bowel ischemia and necrosis, autogenous conduits are preferred even for vein patches. This is to reduce the risk of graft infection from bacterial translocation or frank contamination. When performing a retrograde bypass in a clean field, a ringed graft is preferred to reduce the chance of kinking. Ultimately, there is no solid evidence to support optimal conduit choice for long-term patency, and the conduit choice is largely left up to surgeon experience and patient factors.[5]

SMA/CELIAC BYPASS (WITH OR WITHOUT SMA ENDARTERECTOMY)

- ***FIRST STEP—laparotomy:*** A midline laparotomy is performed extending from the xiphoid process superiorly to the public tubercle inferiorly; this allows for wide access to the abdomen including the supraceliac and infrarenal aorta, as well as all mesenteric vessels.
- ***SECOND STEP—isolate and control the inflow vessel***
  - ***Antegrade bypass: supraceliac aorta and celiac artery (FIGURE 5)***: The supraceliac aorta is exposed by retracting the small bowel and colon inferiorly, dividing the left triangular ligament, followed by mobilization and retraction of the left lobe of the liver. The lesser sac is entered by dividing the gastrohepatic ligament, the stomach is retracted inferiorly, and the esophagus is retraced to the patient's left. Here, the diaphragmatic crura are overlying the aorta and must be divided to reach the supraceliac aorta. Enough distance must be cleared in order to place clamps and perform an anastomosis. This dissection can then be taken down inferiorly to the celiac artery and its branches that require exposure as well.
  - ***Retrograde bypass: isolate and control the infrarenal aorta/common iliac artery:*** The infrarenal aorta and the right common iliac are exposed by retracting the small bowel to the patient's right side and the colon superiorly followed by opening of the retroperitoneum. The retroperitoneum dissection is extended up the base of the colon mesentery to the SMA, as described earlier. The celiac artery may also be exposed in this direction by continuing this dissection further superior. The aorta/iliac artery is controlled with side biting clamps while the mesenteric vessels are controlled with vessel loops.
- ***THIRD STEP—Isolate outflow vessel:*** If the celiac artery is to be revascularized, it is exposed in the same manner as the supraceliac aorta, with slightly further distal dissection to identify and free the celiac artery (**FIGURE 6**). If the celiac artery has a long segment occlusion, the hepatic artery can be used for outflow. The hepatic artery is exposed through the lesser sac by retracting the stomach inferiorly and incising the gastrohepatic peritoneum. The celiac artery is identified and the common hepatic can be found extending to the left (**FIGURE 6**). In nearly every instance of mesenteric bypass the SMA is revascularized, with or without the celiac artery (or hepatic artery). The SMA is exposed in a similar manner as with acute mesenteric ischemia, described above.

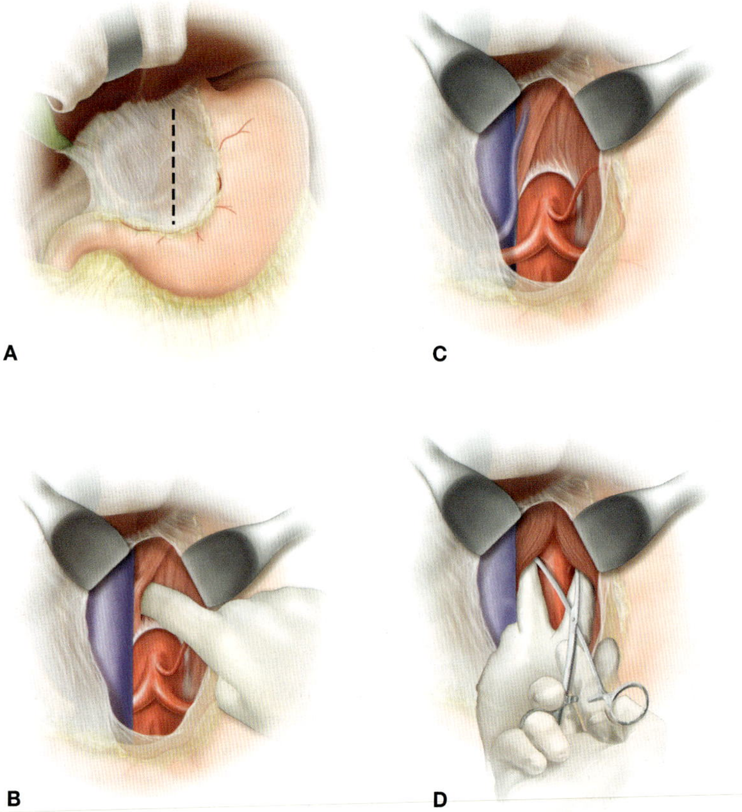

FIGURE 5 • Exposing the supraceliac aorta. **A,** Dotted line shows the location for division of the gastrohepatic ligament. **B,** Once the ligament is divided, the crus is encountered. **C,** Bluntly divide the fibers of the crus. **D,** Using fingers for retraction, control of the aorta can be gained with a clamp, although circumferential control is optimal.

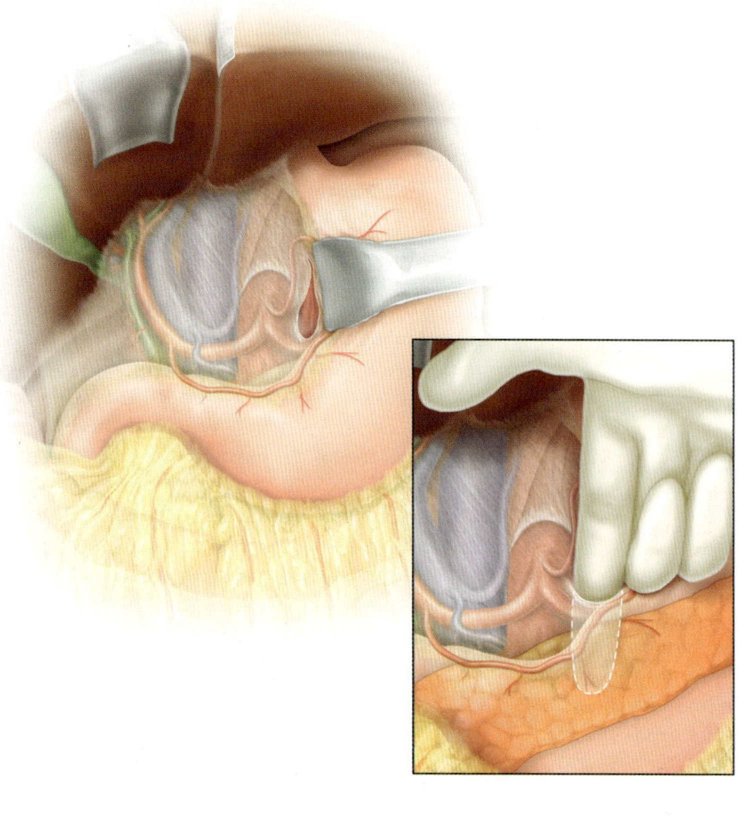

FIGURE 6 • Exposure of the hepatic artery is through the gastrohepatic peritoneum. The liver is retracted superiorly, and the stomach inferiorly. The peritoneum is incised to expose the celiac axis and the hepatic artery.

- ***FOURTH STEP—heparinize and perform revascularization:***
  - The patient is given an IV heparin bolus (70 mg/kg) for anticoagulation. If a one-vessel bypass is planned (most commonly to the SMA), a 6- or 8-mm Dacron tube graft is chosen, and if a two-vessel bypass is planned a 12 × 6 mm or 14 × 7 mm bifurcated Dacron graft is chosen (**FIGURE 7**). The proximal (inflow) anastomosis is sewn first to the aorta or iliac artery in an end-to-side fashion using running 5.0 Prolene sutures. Supraceliac inflow bypasses (antegrade) are tunneled under the pancreas to the SMA. The retropancreatic tunnel is created by careful blunt finger dissection posterior to the pancreas and anterior to the left renal vein. When tunneling care must be taken to assure there is no disruption of the underlying venous network. If a retropancreatic tunnel appears to be too dangerous then an anterior approach is also acceptable.
  - Infrarenal/common iliac bypasses (retrograde) are tunneled to the patient's left using a "lazy C" configuration passing a tunnel through the ligament of Treitz to the lateral aspect of the SMA and celiac arteries. This bypass can also be tunneled deep to the left renal pedicle in what is known as a "French bypass." At this time, the SMA is inspected to determine the need for endarterectomy prior to performing the anastomosis. If endarterectomy is required, this is performed as described above. If possible, the arteriotomy used for the endarterectomy can be used for the bypass anastomosis. The mesenteric (outflow) artery anastomosis is sewn in an end-to-side fashion using running 6.0 Prolene sutures. When performing a single-vessel bypass, priority should be placed on revascularizing the SMA unless the patient's anatomy dictates otherwise. In a two-vessel reconstruction, one limb of the graft is anastomosed to the SMA and the other to the celiac or hepatic artery. Prior to completing the anastomosis, the graft should be flushed and de-aired to prevent any distal embolization. It is of upmost importance to assure that there is no kinking of the conduit. This is especially critical in a retrograde bypass given the longer distance traveled and the "lazy C" configuration.

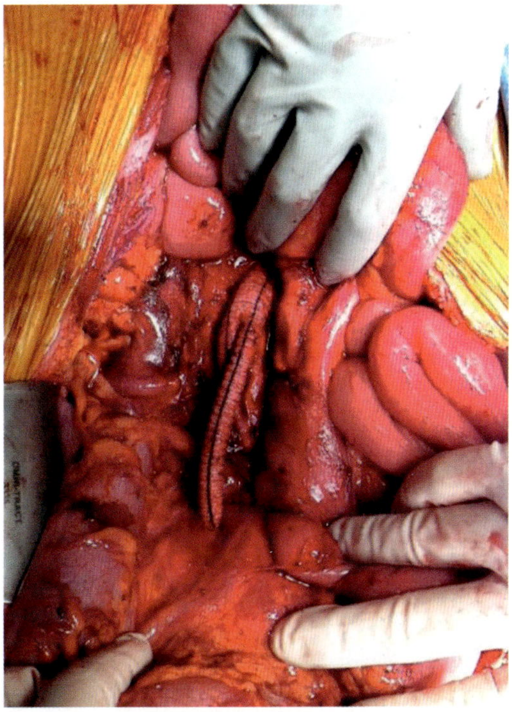

FIGURE 7 • Orientation of bifurcated antegrade graft to celiac and SMA. (Courtesy of Dr. Benjamin Pomy, George Washington University.)

- ***FIFTH STEP—inspect bowel and close the abdomen:*** After completing the revascularization, the bowel should be inspected to note any areas of ischemia. In some cases, there is graft exposed in the retroperitoneum, and the tongue of the omentum may be used to cover the graft to avoid any contact with the bowel. The abdomen is then closed in usual fashion.

PEARLS AND PITFALLS

Inflow dissection	▪ In order to gain access to the supraceliac aorta and successfully sew an anastomosis, appropriate exposure and retraction is imperative. This stresses the need for a full midline laparotomy extending to the xiphoid process superiorly. Given its mobile articulating arms and retractors, the Omni retractor system works best in this tight deep space.
▪ Outflow dissection	▪ When crossing the mesentery on the way to both the celiac and SMA, there are multiple crossing veins. Care should be taken to dissect carefully in this area to identify and ligate all crossing veins and prevent bleeding, which further disrupts visualization and will make dissection even harder. ▪ The left gastric artery is typically the smallest of the celiac axis and may be divided in order to enhance retraction and space to perform the anastomosis and tunneling.

▪ Embolectomy technique	▪ Fogarty catheter sizes range from 2 to 7 Fr (4-14 mm inflated balloon diameter); given the size of mesenteric vessels are about 1 cm, 3-4 French Fogarty catheters usually work best. An embolectomy catheter should pass clean with residual back bleeding at least twice before it is felt to be successful. ▪ When performing the proximal (aortic) embolectomy, it is imperative that the surgeon (or assistant) maintains proximal control on the SMA. As the thrombus is cleared there will be a torrential return of pulsatile flow from the aorta.
Endarterectomy technique	▪ A full arterial incision beyond the plaque in both directions assures a complete endarterectomy. The distal flap is going against the direction of blood flow and should be tacked in order to prevent recurrent thrombosis of the vessel.
Bypass technique	▪ When tunneling, consideration should always be made to the patient in different position, most importantly sitting up, when planning how to tunnel the bypass. ▪ These patients are often very thin, and consideration of how to cover the prosthetic bypass with minimal mesenteric fat should also be made when planning how to tunnel the bypass. If needed, a tongue of omentum can be pulled beneath the small bowel mesentery to cover the bypass graft.

POSTOPERATIVE CARE

Acute/Subacute

- Given their emergent/urgent preoperative presentation, extensive nature of the surgery, and possibility of ongoing bowel ischemia and reperfusion, the aggressive resuscitation begun in the emergency department and continued in the operating room must be maintained in a surgical intensive care unit postoperatively. Often these patients will require open abdomens to facilitate planned return to the operating room to reevaluate bowel viability. The details of this intensive and general surgical care are beyond the scope of this chapter but are imperative to avoid the significant mortality and morbidity rates associated with these presentations and procedures. Therapeutic systemic anticoagulation with intravenous heparin should be maintained to avoid recurrent thrombosis of mesenteric vessels; this allows for easier surgical management of anticoagulation if repeated surgeries are necessary. Lastly, given the likely cardiac incitement of the event, a full cardiac workup looking for source of embolism should also be completed during this critical time.

Chronic

- Even in the elective setting, this is a large surgery on patients with multiple comorbidities; furthermore, bowel reperfusion may still occur creating electrolyte abnormalities. Therefore, these patients should be monitored in surgical intensive care unit postoperatively. Chronic poor nutrition will reverse over an extended time after the patient is able to tolerate greater oral intake; poor nutrition at the time of the procedure may lead to poor wound healing, gastritis, and bowel anastomosis failure, which should all be anticipated. Given the chronic nature of the atherosclerotic disease, systemic anticoagulation is not necessary; however, antiplatelets for treatment of generalized atherosclerosis, particularly coronary artery disease, should be started once oral intake is tolerated.

OUTCOMES

Acute/Subacute

- Acute mesenteric ischemia carries a very high risk of perioperative mortality. Most series estimate perioperative mortality as high as 70%. There are little long-term data available for mortality in these patients; however, 1-year survival has been reported to be around 70% in recent years. The complication rates following revascularization for AMI have been reported as high as 60%. The most common complications following these operations are cardiac and pulmonary complications.[6]

Chronic

- As discussed above, open revascularization for chronic mesenteric ischemia is increasingly reserved as a second-line option due to relatively higher perioperative morbidity and mortality compared with endovascular therapy. Perioperative mortality after revascularization for CMI is estimated at approximately 6%. In some high-volume centers, the mortality has been shown to be around 1% to 3% for good-risk patients, but it can be as high as 20% in low-volume settings. Perioperative morbidity is similarly high and is estimated to be about 30% overall. The most common complications after these operations are pulmonary are cardiac complications, including prolonged mechanical ventilation, myocardial infarction, and cardiac arrest. Long-term symptom relief is excellent after open revascularization, approximately 76% at 5 years. Patency for SMA bypass is also excellent, with primary patency rates estimated at 85% to 90% at 3 years.[2]

COMPLICATIONS

Acute/Subacute

Graft/Surgical-Related Complications

- SMA dissection/stenosis and resulting reocclusion
- Anastomosis failure with hemorrhage
- Other surgical bleeding requiring transfusion
- Limb ischemia secondary to showering emboli
- Enterotomy/missed intestinal ischemia with peritonitis

Hemodynamic Complications

- Myocardial infarction/cardiac arrest
- Prolonged mechanical ventilation
- Acute renal insufficiency/acute renal failure
- Refractory shock with multiorgan system failure
- Death

Chronic

Graft/Surgical-Related Complications

- Graft kinking with occlusion
- SMA/celiac dissection with occlusion
- Graft infection
- Anastomosis failure with hemorrhage
- Enterotomy
- Limb ischemia secondary to showering atherosclerotic emboli
- Surgical wound infection/breakdown (poor nutritional status)

Hemodynamic Complications

- Myocardial infarction/cardiac arrest
- Prolonged mechanical ventilation
- Acute kidney injury/acute renal failure
- Refeeding syndrome
- Death

ACKNOWLEDGMENT

The authors would like to acknowledge the guidance and input of Dr. Robyn Macsata who sadly passed away prior to publication of this text.

REFERENCES

1. Wyers MC, Martin MC. *Acute mesenteric arterial disease-clinicalKey. Rutherford's Textbook of Vascular Surgery and Endovascular Therapy*. 9th ed. Elsevier Inc; 2019. doi:10.1016/B978-0-323-42791-3.00133-X
2. Oderich GS, Ribeiro M. *Chronic mesenteric arterial disease: clinical evaluation, open surgical and endovascular treatment. Rutherford's Textbook of Vascular Surgery and Endovascular Therapy*. 9th ed. Elsevier Inc; 2019. doi:10.1016/B978-0-323-42791-3.00132-8
3. Ginsburg M, Obara P, Lambert DL, et al. ACR Appropriateness Criteria® imaging of mesenteric ischemia. *J Am Coll Radiol*. 2018;15(11):S332-S340. doi:10.1016/j.jacr.2018.09.018
4. Huber TS, Björck M, Chandra A, et al. Chronic mesenteric ischemia: clinical practice guidelines from the society for vascular surgery. *J Vasc Surg*. 2021;73(1):87S-115S. doi:10.1016/j.jvs.2020.10.029
5. Foley MI, Moneta GL, Abou-Zamzam AM, et al. Revascularization of the superior mesenteric artery alone for treatment of intestinal ischemia. *J Vasc Surg*. 2000;32(1):37-47. doi:10.1067/mva.2000.107314
6. Ryer EJ, Kalra M, Oderich GS, et al. Revascularization for acute mesenteric ischemia. *J Vasc Surg*. 2012;55(6):1682-1689. doi:10.1016/j.jvs.2011.12.017

Chapter 22

Advanced Aneurysm Management Techniques: Open Surgical Anatomy and Repair

Harold Davis Waller and Mark F. Conrad

DEFINITION

- An aneurysm is defined as a permanent, focal dilation of an artery to a size that is greater than 50% of the normal or expected transverse diameter of the vessel. Although dimensions differ slightly for men and women, practically speaking the normal diameter for the abdominal aorta is 2 cm; therefore, the abdominal aorta is considered aneurysmal when it reaches 3 cm in the transverse dimension.
- A *fusiform* aneurysm is the symmetric enlargement of the entire vessel and is the most common type of abdominal aortic aneurysm (AAA). A *saccular* aneurysm is a focal outpouching of the vessel wall to one side and is much less common.
- Aneurysms may occur in virtually any vessel in the body but are most commonly seen in the infrarenal AAA. The *neck* is the length of normal aorta between the ostium of the inferior-most renal artery and the beginning of the aneurysmal aorta. The term *juxtarenal* is used to describe AAAs that do not involve the renal arteries but, due to their proximity to the inferior-most renal artery (<1 cm neck), require clamping above the renal arteries to complete the proximal aortic anastomosis. For a *suprarenal* aneurysm, at least one of the renal arteries arises from aneurysmal aorta, which implies the need for both a proximal clamp and renal artery reconstruction at the time of the repair (**FIGURE 1**). This chapter will focus on the indications and techniques for open repair of infrarenal and juxtarenal AAAs.
- The dreaded complication of AAA is rupture. Size and expansion rate are the two most important predictors of rupture, such that they guide the indication for repair in asymptomatic patients.[1]
- Other factors that increase rupture risk include female gender, a family history of aneurysms, smoking status (higher risk for current smokers vs never and former smokers), hypertension, and chronic obstructive pulmonary disease (COPD).[2-5]

PATIENT HISTORY AND PHYSICAL FINDINGS

- A thorough history and physical exam is imperative in the evaluation of a patient being considered for aneurysm repair.
- History of present illness: Determine how the aneurysm was found. Often, AAAs are an incidental discovery on an imaging test performed for another purpose. It is critical to ask about abdominal or back pain as these symptoms may be caused by a "symptomatic" aneurysm that would require more urgent repair.
- Past medical history: Patients with concomitant cardiac, lung, and/or renal disease tend to have more complications perioperatively and should be medically optimized prior to proceeding with elective repair. Although there is no broad recommendation for preoperative cardiac revascularization in asymptomatic patients, those with known cardiac disease or risk factors should be evaluated by a cardiologist as there is some recent evidence that certain subgroups of these high-risk patients may benefit from preoperative revascularization.[6,7]
- Family history: Approximately 15% to 20% of patients with AAA will have a first-degree relative with aneurysmal disease. Patients with AAA should be counseled to alert their siblings and children to this condition, so they may be screened appropriately.[3,8]
- Social history: Smoking has been linked to an increased risk of aneurysm formation and rate of expansion. Patients should be counseled on smoking cessation.
- Review of systems: In addition to the generalized systems review appropriate for all patients undergoing major surgery, particular attention should be directed to other vascular comorbidities. In particular, query about previous cerebrovascular accident (CVA) or transient ischemic attack (TIA) symptoms, amaurosis fugax, mesenteric ischemia, and lower extremity ischemic symptoms (claudication, rest pain, ulcers). Work up positive symptoms as appropriate.

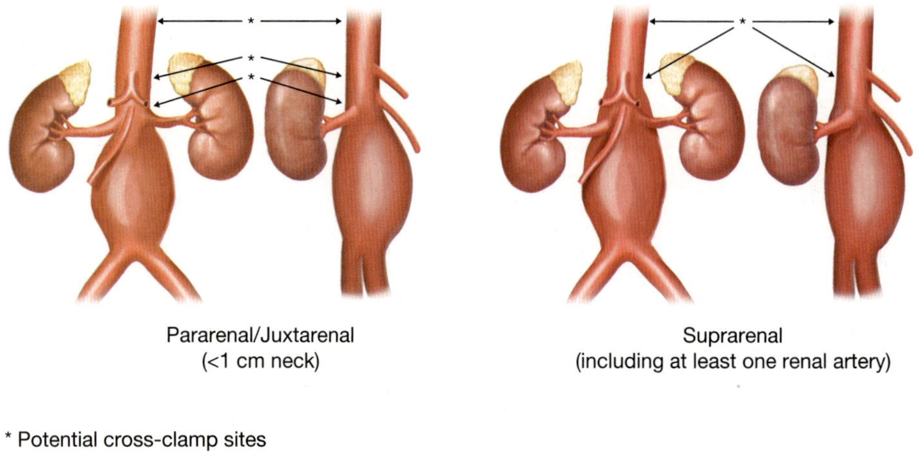

FIGURE 1 • Anatomic differences between a juxtarenal AAA, where the neck of normal aortic diameter is less than 1 cm, and a suprarenal AAA, where the takeoff of at least one renal artery arises from the aneurysm.

- On physical exam, perform a thorough abdominal exam noting the location of surgical scars, and be aware that the positive predictive value for localizing a small- to moderate-sized AAA on exam is poor. A small proportion (1%-10%) of patients with AAA will have a concomitant aneurysm elsewhere, so be cognizant that those patients with known AAA and a prominent femoral or popliteal pulse may need further imaging to exclude an aneurysm in these locations.[9]
- Conversely, patients who initially present with peripheral aneurysms such as femoral (85%) or popliteal aneurysms (60%) have a much higher rate of concomitant AAA and aortic screening should be performed in these patients.[9,10]

IMAGING AND OTHER DIAGNOSTIC STUDIES

- Of all imaging techniques used for AAA screening and surveillance, B-mode ultrasonography is the least expensive and safest with regard to radiation exposure. Currently, the U.S. Preventative Services Task Force (USPSTF) recommends a one-time abdominal ultrasound as a AAA screening test for all males between the ages of 65 and 75 years who have ever smoked and selective abdominal ultrasound screening based on risk factors for all males in this age range who have never smoked. Women aged 65 to 75 years who have never smoked and have no family history of AAA should not undergo any routine ultrasound screening for AAA. It is generally accepted that a negative screening ultrasound exonerates the patient from further screening or surveillance imaging, as the likelihood of new aneurysm development of clinical significance after the age of screening is extremely low. If a screening ultrasound detects a small aneurysm, yearly ultrasounds are indicated until the sac approaches a size where repair may be indicated, at which time further imaging with computed tomography (CT) is recommended.[9,11,12]
- Computed tomography angiography (CTA) provides a more accurate assessment of aneurysm size, extent, branch vessel proximity, and involvement (which is used to determine if the aneurysm is amenable to endovascular or open repair, and if open repair is to be done, where the proximal clamp should be applied) and is the test that should be used for planning open AAA repair. A thorough exam should include thin (1.5 cm or smaller) cuts of the chest, abdomen, and pelvis with contrast administered in the arterial phase (**FIGURE 2**).

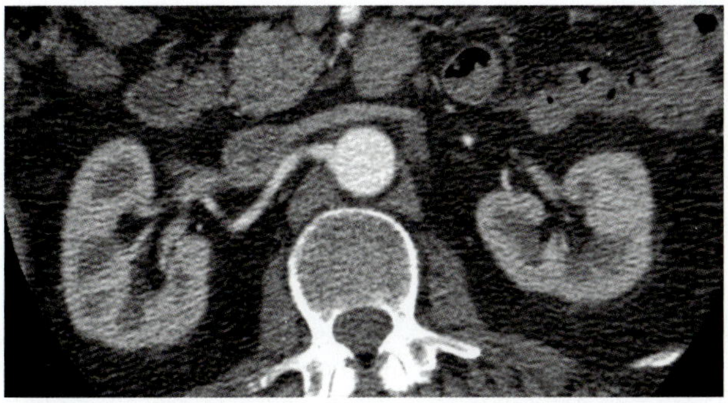

FIGURE 2 • Axial cut of a CTA showing the takeoff or the right renal artery and the more commonly seen renal vein lying anterior to the aorta.

- It is important to note the location of the aneurysm and its relationship to the renal arteries. Renal anatomy should be noted as well, including any accessory renal arteries, renal vein course, and the presence of a pelvic or horseshoe kidney. The renal vein usually travels anterior to the aorta, but a retroaortic renal vein should be noted as it will influence the operative approach to the aorta. Other venous anatomy, such as a duplicated or left-sided inferior vena cava (IVC), should be noted as well.

SURGICAL MANAGEMENT

- The decision to operate on an asymptomatic patient is based on three primary factors: the risk of aneurysm rupture, the risk associated with aneurysm repair, and the patient's life expectancy. The operative risk and overall life expectancy should be assessed. Assuming that a patient is fit to proceed with repair, size is currently our best predictor of rupture. The UK Small Aneurysm Trial and ADAM VA Trial recommend treatment for all patients with an infrarenal AAA larger than 5.5 cm in size, with consideration for repair in women with AAA of 5.0 cm given their higher risk of rupture and likely smaller baseline aortic size. These studies also support repair for those patients who have an increase in diameter of greater than 0.5 cm over a 6-month period (**TABLE 1**).[13,14]
- Although there are no large trials looking specifically at iliac aneurysms, repair is generally recommended when they reach 4 cm or greater in size. Iliac aneurysms are more often seen in patients with a concomitant aortic aneurysm and only a quarter of patients with iliac aneurysms will have isolated disease.
- All open repairs should be performed under general anesthesia. It is preferable for the anesthesia team to evaluate the patient prior to the day of surgery so that appropriate time for developing an anesthetic plan, lines, and other means of hemodynamic monitoring are allowed. The use of an epidural for pain control in the postoperative period is useful as it limits narcotic use and improves pulmonary toilet during the early postoperative period. In addition, arrangements should be made for autotransfusion given the unavoidable amount of intraoperative blood loss, which is often measured in liters.
- Preoperative understanding of the patient's individual anatomy is of the utmost importance. The surgeon must know the proximity of the aneurysmal aorta to the renal and visceral vessels and whether these branch vessels arise from the aneurysm, as this will determine where the proximal cross clamp will be applied. If at all possible, clamps should only be applied to nonaneurysmal aorta with minimal thrombus

Table 1: Indications for Repair of Abdominal Aortic Aneurysm

- Leak or frank rupture
- Size (5.5 cm in men, 5 cm in women for aortic aneurysm, and 4 cm for iliac aneurysms)
- Increase in size of >0.5 cm over a 6-mo period
- Symptomatic (pain, compression on adjacent structures)
- Dissection within aneurysm

or calcification to minimize risk of clamp injury or distal embolization of debris, and all aneurysmal aorta should be resected even if this means involvement of the visceral or iliac segment. One exception to this rule is the case where the aneurysm arises directly below the renal artery but does not involve the artery. In this instance, a cuff of aneurysmal tissue can be plicated into the anastomosis to avoid the need for an aortorenal bypass, which can lead to increased operative times, length of stay, and a decline in renal function.[15] If the aorta contains a significant amount of debris or there is little space between branch vessels, a more proximal clamp site in the supraceliac aorta should be considered. It is important to discuss the proposed clamp site with anesthesia preoperatively, as this will affect their management of the patient. The choice of clamp site should be made during the preoperative planning stage, as the intraoperative need to move the clamp higher is associated with adverse outcomes.[16]

- Planning for the distal anastomosis requires review not only of the aortic bifurcation but of the iliac arteries as well. If there is aneurysmal or occlusive disease within the iliac arteries, concurrent repair with a bifurcated graft may be appropriate; otherwise, the majority of AAAs are repaired with a tube graft to the iliac bifurcation. The type of distal anastomosis may predicate the method of distal control, which can be obtained with a single clamp across the bifurcation or both iliac origins, or occlusion balloons (Foley catheters or Pruitt occlusion balloons) for heavily diseased vessels.
- Key preoperative planning concerns are summarized in **TABLE 2**.

Table 2: Operative Planning

- Is a retroperitoneal or transperitoneal approach better?
- Where is the best location for proximal control? What are the alternatives should intraoperative findings preclude using this site?
- Will clamping cause renal or visceral ischemia?
- Will the renal or visceral arteries need to be reconstructed as part of the repair? If so, what size grafts should be used for the bypass?
- Where is the renal vein? Does it pass anteriorly or posterior to the aorta? Will the kidney be taken up or left down?
- How will distal control be obtained? Will reconstruction involve the iliac arteries or can the distal anastomosis be to the bifurcation?
- What size/type graft should be used?

TECHNIQUES

- There are two approaches for the open repair of the infrarenal or juxtarenal aortic aneurysm: transperitoneal or retroperitoneal approach (**FIGURE 3**). The approach used for an infrarenal AAA is based on several factors: body habitus (obese patients are often best approached via retroperitoneal incision), prior abdominal surgery (concern for intraperitoneal adhesions), and clamp sites; above the renal arteries may favor a retroperitoneal approach, whereas planned intervention on the right renal or iliac artery would be easily performed from a transperitoneal approach.

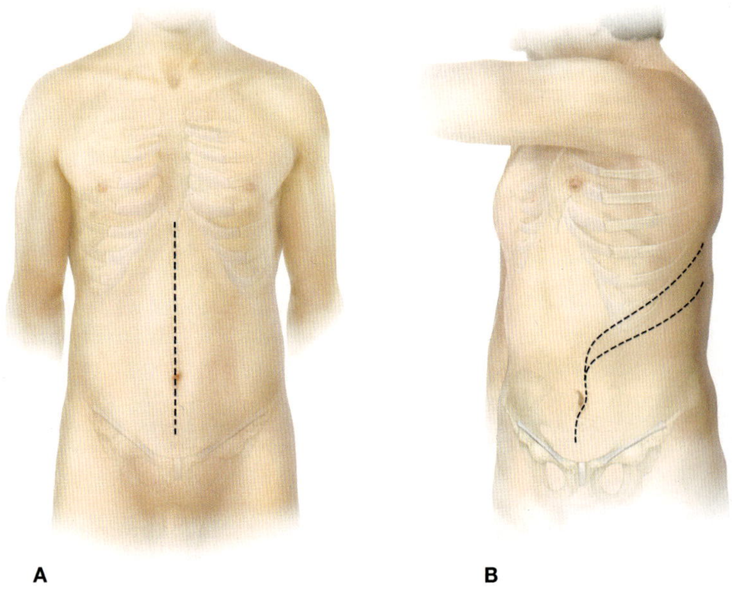

FIGURE 3 • Incision for the two approaches to aneurysm repair. **A,** Transperitoneal and **B,** retroperitoneal. The retroperitoneal approach can be modified for higher exposure on the visceral aorta.

TRANSPERITONEAL APPROACH

- Positioning: The patient is positioned supine on a standard operating room (OR) table with both arms extended. The operative field should include the nipple line superiorly to midthighs inferiorly to allow exposure for a high incision as well as groin access should the femoral vessels be needed. The hair is clipped and a towel is placed over the perineum. Any previous incisions within the operative field are marked. A Steri-Drape or Ioban is used to secure the drapes in position. Once fully prepped, check pulse volume recording (PVRs) and/or distal pulses to establish a baseline for distal perfusion.
- Incision: A generous midline incision from the xiphoid to the pubis is made and dissection is carried through the underlying tissue until the peritoneal cavity is entered (**FIGURE 3**). It may be necessary to extend the incision cephalad lateral alongside the xiphoid if higher exposure is needed, or in emergent situations such as a rupture where immediate supraceliac control is needed. A self-retaining retractor system should then be positioned. Our preference is the Omni retractor as the open configuration of the system does not limit the width of exposure.
- Dissection: The greater omentum and transverse colon are retracted cephalad and packed away in a moistened towel or lap pad on top of the patient's chest. The small bowel is retracted to the right and packed within a separate moistened towel. The small bowel is gently placed behind a self-retaining retractor, taking care not to compromise the superior mesenteric artery (SMA). This exposes the ligament of Treitz (LOT), which can be divided along the jejunum to the level of the aorta (**FIGURE 4**). Reposition the retractor to displace as much small bowel as possible out of the field, and take down the LOT with electrocautery, taking care not to injure the bowel. The inferior mesenteric vein is usually ligated during this dissection. This allows access to the infrarenal aorta where the overlying retroperitoneal tissue can be dissected-free. Depending on the proximal extent of aorta needed for an adequate cuff of the proximal anastomosis, an anterior renal vein may need to be mobilized cephalad and surrounded with a red rubber catheter or Penrose drain for easy manipulation during creation of the proximal anastomosis. In order to gain the best mobility, the gonadal, adrenal, and renal lumbar branches are ligated if necessary (**FIGURE 5**).
- Exposure of the supraceliac aorta (**FIGURE 6**): This maneuver is only needed in cases where high abdominal aortic exposure is needed, such as in a rupture. The left lobe of the liver must be retracted laterally by taking down the triangular ligament. Next, identify and dissect-free the gastroesophageal junction after dividing the gastrohepatic ligament, which is most expeditiously done by palpating for

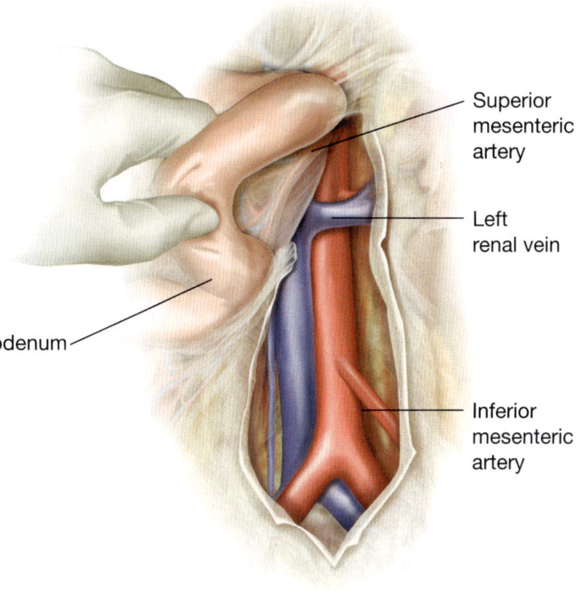

FIGURE 4 • Division of the ligament of Treitz (LOT). After reflecting the colon cephalad and the small bowel to the patient's right, the LOT can be divided to expose the infrarenal aorta.

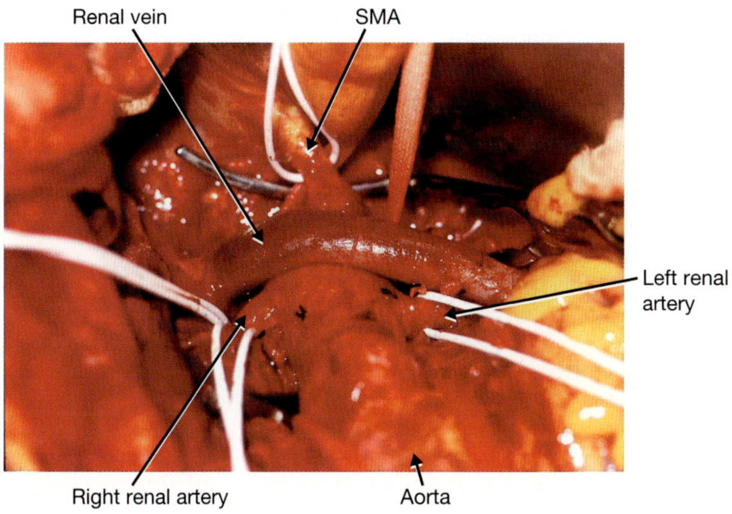

FIGURE 5 • (illustration and photo): Mobilization of the left renal vein. Cephalad or caudal mobilization of the left renal vein to expose the origin of the renal arteries. Ligation of several venous side branches may be needed for safe mobilization.

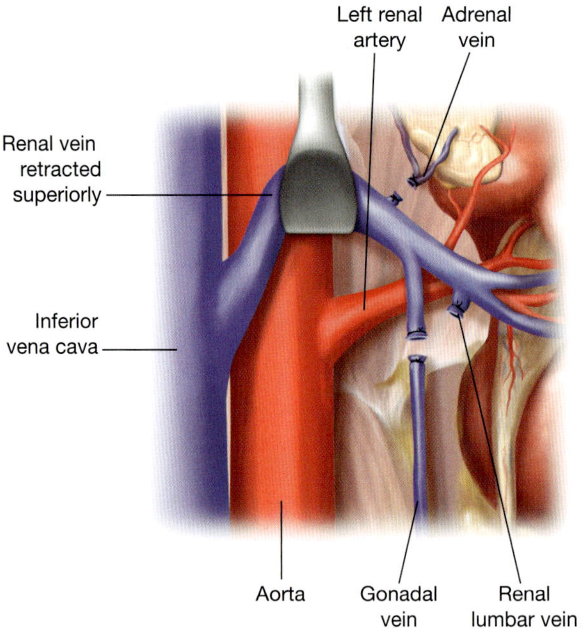

FIGURE 5 • (*continued*)

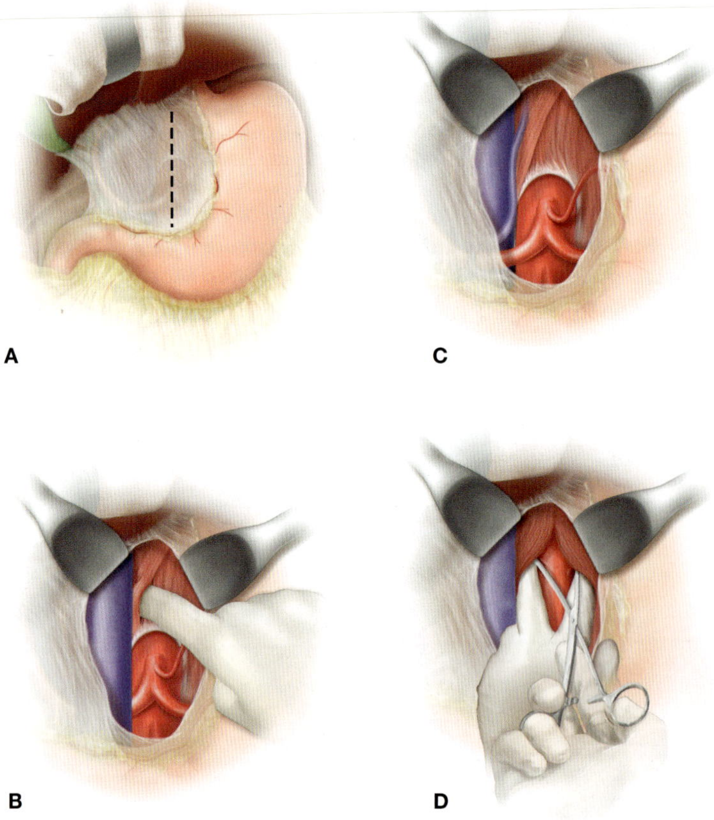

FIGURE 6 • Gaining control of the supraceliac aorta. **A,** *Dotted line* shows the location for division of the gastrohepatic ligament. **B,** Once the ligament is divided, the crus is encountered. **C,** Bluntly divide the fibers of the crus. **D,** Using fingers for retraction, control of the aorta can be gained with a clamp, although circumferential control is optimal.

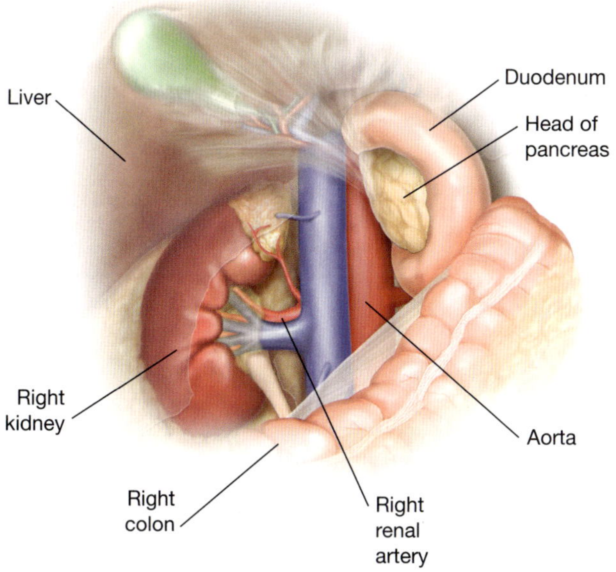

FIGURE 7 • Exposure of the aorta and right renal artery via right medial visceral rotation.

the nasogastric tube and applying caudal traction. Division of the gastrohepatic ligament must be performed with the cautious consideration that a replaced left hepatic artery could be coursing beneath this structure. The esophagus can then be retracted to the patient's left, which exposes the aorta. To obtain control, an aortic compressor can be used in extreme circumstances; however, dissection of the aorta circumferentially and surrounding the aorta with a shoestring (if the patient's condition allows) is preferable. This exposure, although useful when urgent supraceliac control is needed, will not allow access to the visceral segment of the aorta. In order to gain visceral exposure, a right or left medial visceral rotation should be incorporated into the dissection. The use of a right medial visceral rotation will allow access to the right renal artery, as well as placing the SMA on 90° tension, and is useful for exposing a clamp site in those patients with a juxtarenal aneurysm with very little room between the renals and SMA (**FIGURE 7**). The use of a left medial visceral rotation also allows for exposure to the entire visceral segment of the aorta as well as the left renal artery. In this approach, care must be taken to avoid injury to the spleen and tail of the pancreas. In patients where a supra-SMA or supraceliac clamp is planned, the retroperitoneal approach is preferable.

RETROPERITONEAL APPROACH

- Positioning: Once asleep, the patient is placed in the lateral position with the left side up at an approximately 60° angle (**FIGURE 8**). The right arm is extended on an armboard, being sure to leave room for an Omni or other self-retaining retractor post. The upper left arm should be placed on another armboard and padded to prevent neural injury. The bed is flexed at the patient's flank to open up the area between the ribs and the left anterior superior iliac spine. Position the legs so that the lower leg is straight and the upper leg is flexed at the knee. Pillows are used as padding

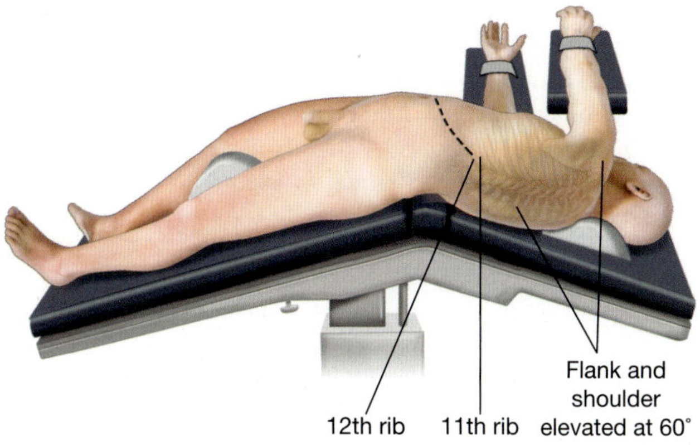

FIGURE 8 • Positioning for retroperitoneal incision.

between legs. A beanbag can be inflated to keep the patient in place, and we secure thick cloth tape over the shoulder to keep the patient on their side with the shoulders at 90° and the hips rotated posteriorly. If a bean bag is not available, blanket rolls can be used anteriorly and posteriorly to further secure the patient. All bony prominences and pressure points should be well padded to avoid injury. Ultimately, positioning should allow access to prep an operative field from the spine posteriorly to the umbilicus anteriorly and from the nipple line to the groins. Use clippers to remove hair within the prep area. Prep from the axilla and nipple line to the upper thigh. Mark all previous incisions and use a Steri-Drape or Ioban over the entire prepped area to secure the drapes. Once fully prepped, check pulse volume recording (PVR) and/or distal pulses/signals to establish a baseline for distal perfusion.

- Incision: Unless clamping is planned at or above the level of the SMA, a standard retroperitoneal incision over the 11th rib (10th interspace) will provide adequate exposure (**FIGURE 3**). Some practitioners confirm this location by ultrasound. Carry the incision from the posterior axillary line to the anterior border of the rectus. Avoid entry into the pleural cavity if possible by being cognizant that the further posterior the incision is commenced, the higher likelihood this will occur.
- Dissection: Carry the dissection through the underlying tissue, dividing the transversalis fascia, and enter the retroperitoneal space down to but not violating Gerota's fascia. This space can be more easily identified by resecting a distal segment of the 11th rib, as the transversalis fascia and transversus abdominal musculature insert along the inferior border of this rib. It is possible to stay entirely within a retroperitoneal plane during this dissection; however, if the peritoneum is violated the abdominal contents can be packed away with retractors, or the peritoneum can be immediately repaired with a running 3-0 chromic suture and the dissection continued in the retroperitoneum. The aorta is approached via an anterorenal (colloquially referred to as "leaving the kidney down") or retrorenal plane ("taking the kidney up") (**FIGURE 9**). Generally, the aorta is approached via a retrorenal approach unless there is a retroaortic renal vein or a need to access the SMA beyond its origin. As the retroperitoneal dissection continues, the left ureter should be identified, swept toward the midline, and placed behind a retractor to avoid injury during the aortic dissection. The left renal artery is identified and dissected back to its aortic origin.
- The renal lumbar vein should be identified and ligated to avoid injury and excessive bleeding. Once the origin of the renal artery is identified, a right angle clamp can be placed along the surface of the aorta and the overlying retroperitoneal tissue divided with electrocautery. It is imperative to get on the aorta and stay on the aorta to avoid excessive bleeding from the retroperitoneal tissue. The aorta is exposed to the bifurcation and can be dissected circumferentially here if a clamp site is planned; however, note the left iliac vein can course posterior to the bifurcation and should be avoided. It is often easier to expose an area of the left common iliac artery for clamping and control the right common iliac artery with an occlusion balloon from within. It is unwise to gain distal circumferential control of the iliac arteries in this situation as the iliac veins are often adherent to the posterior aspect of the artery and are easily injured. Also, limiting dissection of the left common iliac artery will minimize the risk of retrograde ejaculation in men, which occurs when the surround nerve plexus is disrupted. Pay particular attention to identifying and not injuring the ureters, which eventually cross anterior to the iliac vessels. Identify and isolate the inferior mesenteric artery (IMA) with a vessel loop. If necessary, by commencing the incision along a higher rib space, the dissection can be carried caudal to expose the entire visceral segment (**FIGURE 10**).

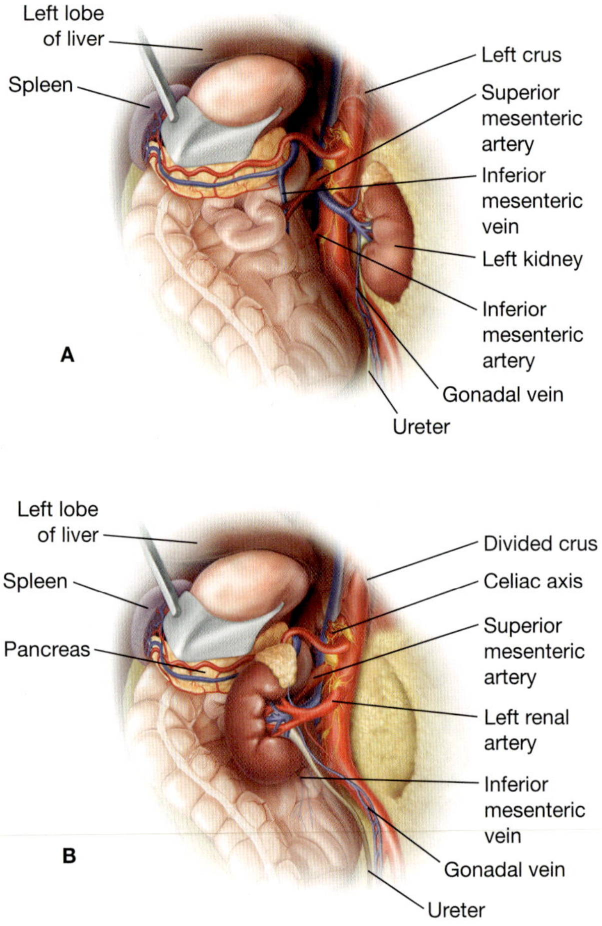

FIGURE 9 • The aorta can be approached in an anterorenal plane **(A)** or a retrorenal plane **(B)**.

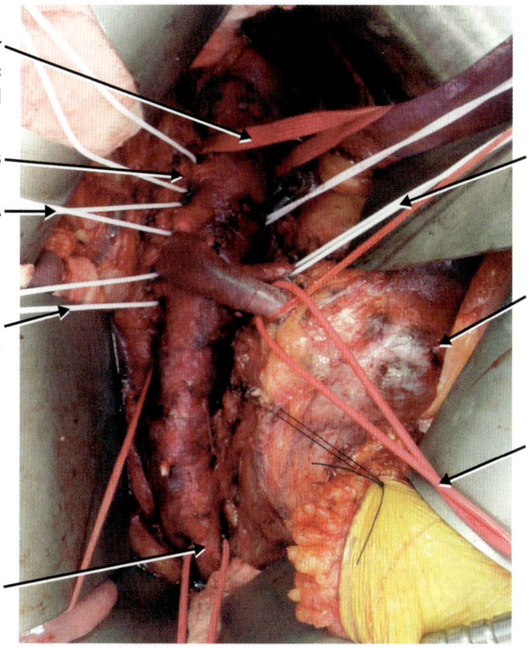

FIGURE 10 • Exposure of the entire abdominal aorta from a retroperitoneal approach. Here, the kidney is "left down" in an anterorenal plane. All vessels are surrounded with vessels loops.

AORTIC CLAMPING AND REPAIR

- When dissecting on the aorta, care must be taken to minimize aggressive manipulation and subsequent atheroembolization, particularly if preoperative imaging shows extensive mural debris. Regardless of approach, it is important during circumferential dissection of the aorta to avoid injury to the posterior lumbar arteries, which are usually paired. The posterior aortic dissection is performed with a blunt sweeping motion of your finger. If the tissue does not pull away from the aorta easily, it is likely due to the presence of a branch vessel. In this instance, the aorta is gently retracted and the dissection is continued sharply under direct vision. If the lumbar vessels are encountered and require ligation, carefully circumferentially dissect out the artery, tie the proximal side of the vessel, and use another tie or apply a double clip to the distal end prior to dividing.
- Choice of graft: There are several choices for conduit during open AAA repair. Generally, a polytetrafluoroethylene (PTFE) or Dacron tube graft is sewn from the proximal aorta to the bifurcation. The aorta can be measured for the appropriate graft with aortic sizers, but often, an estimation of size can be made from the preoperative CTA. Regardless, the majority of patients can be repaired with an 18- to 22-mm graft. In patients with extensive bifurcation or iliac disease, a bifurcated graft may be used. If this is the case, the proximal single lumen portion of the graft should be as short as possible to prevent kinking. In contemporary practice, we make this portion 3 to 4 cm to provide a seal zone if future endografting is necessary. Tunneling the limb to the femoral level should be done only in special circumstances, and if so, care must be taken to position the graft posterior to the ureter (**FIGURE 11**).

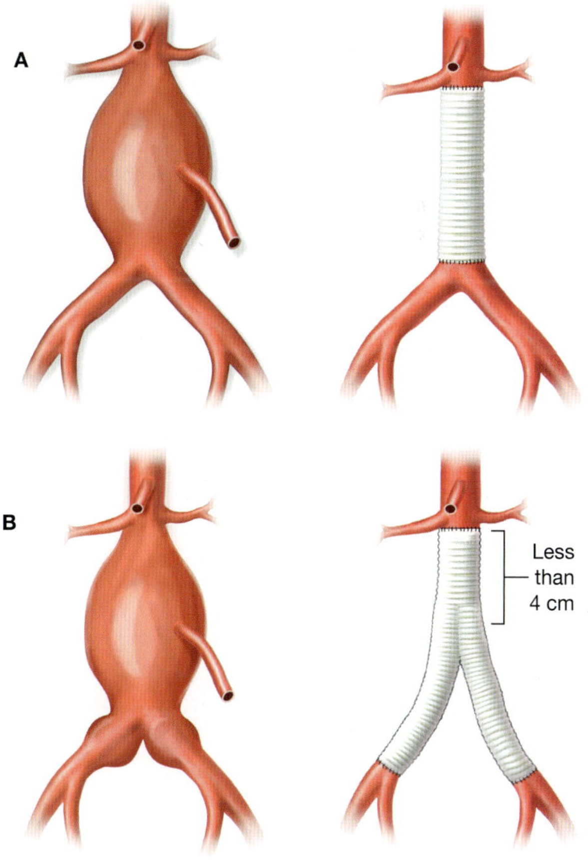

FIGURE 11 • **A,** Tube graft from infrarenal aorta to bifurcation and **(B)** bifurcated graft from infrarenal aorta to iliac or femoral vessels.

- Choosing the site of the proximal anastomosis: This will depend on the quality of the proximal neck of the aneurysm and the vicinity of the visceral vessels. In the most straightforward scenario, an adequate cuff of normal aorta is present below the renal arteries to allow for infrarenal clamping and an end-to-end anastomosis. In the event of a short infrarenal cuff, a suprarenal clamp can be used to provide space to sew. If the aneurysmal tissue extends to the visceral branches, or if there is significant atherosclerotic disease of the branches, a beveled anastomosis may be required, possibly including an endarterectomy of the origin of a branch vessel or a bypass to the left renal artery (**FIGURE 12**). When there is aneurysmal tissue to the level of the renal arteries, whether one employs a suprarenal clamp and plication of the aneurysm cuff with the graft sewn below the renal arteries or a beveled anastomosis with left renal artery bypass, there is no difference in the 3-year incidence of aneurysmal degeneration of the proximal anastomosis, change in long-term renal function, or mortality (**FIGURE 13**).[15] Overall, these considerations should be apparent based on careful review of preoperative imaging and planned well before clamping of the aorta. From the retroperitoneal approach, every effort should be made to incorporate the right renal artery into the anastomosis.
- In preparation for clamping, the patient should be systemically heparinized at a dose of 70 U/kg and heparin is allowed to circulate for 3 to 5 minutes. It is important to communicate with anesthesia prior to clamping and unclamping so they may anticipate and address subsequent hemodynamic shifts. Generally, the systemic pressure should be reduced in preparation for the proximal clamping. If the visceral segment is involved, bulldog clamps should be applied to the visceral vessels prior to aortic clamping to avoid embolization. The proximal clamp is then carefully applied and secured with a shoestring around the clamp. The aortic sac is then opened with electrocautery and heavy scissors proximally and distally. Mural debris should be carefully removed to identify all patent lumbar arteries. Distal control can then be obtained by internal balloon occlusion of each iliac with Foley catheters if external control was not previously obtained. All backbleeding lumbar vessels should be suture ligated with 2-0 silk in a figure-of-eight fashion. In heavily calcified aortas, focal endarterectomies may be necessary for effective ligation of each vessel.
- Sewing of the proximal anastomoses: There are several techniques to complete the anastomosis, and the choice is based on a combination of surgeon preference and tissue quality. Regardless of technique, however, the posterior row of sutures should be sewn first. Ensure that there is adequate exposure of the proximal aorta; this may require the use of a self-retaining retractor within the opened sac or stay sutures on the edges of the sac. Place the graft on the patient's chest upside down, so the posterior aspect of the graft lies anteriorly. If the posterior row is to be done in an interrupted fashion, the first mattress suture is placed in the middle of the graft from outside to inside, placing a snap on the needled ends of the sutures. Place four more mattress sutures, two on each side, working your way to the 3- and 9-o'clock positions on the graft. Care must be taken to ensure there are no gaps between sutures; all travel must be within a mattress stitch and not between stitches. Once all sutures are placed in the graft, begin placing the aortic sutures from inside to outside on the aorta. The proximal aorta is usually not completely transected and the posterior wall can be used to create a Creech bite that uses the aortic wall as a pledget. Once all sutures are placed, each individual stitch is pledgeted and tied down snugly. The anterior

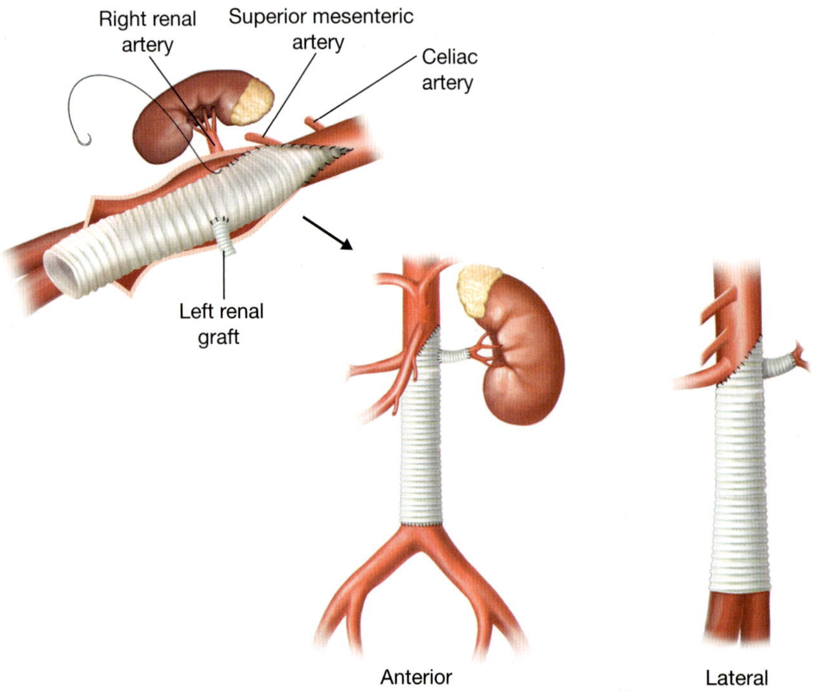

FIGURE 12 • Beveled anastomosis with bypass to the left renal artery. The suture line runs just inferior to the right renal artery.

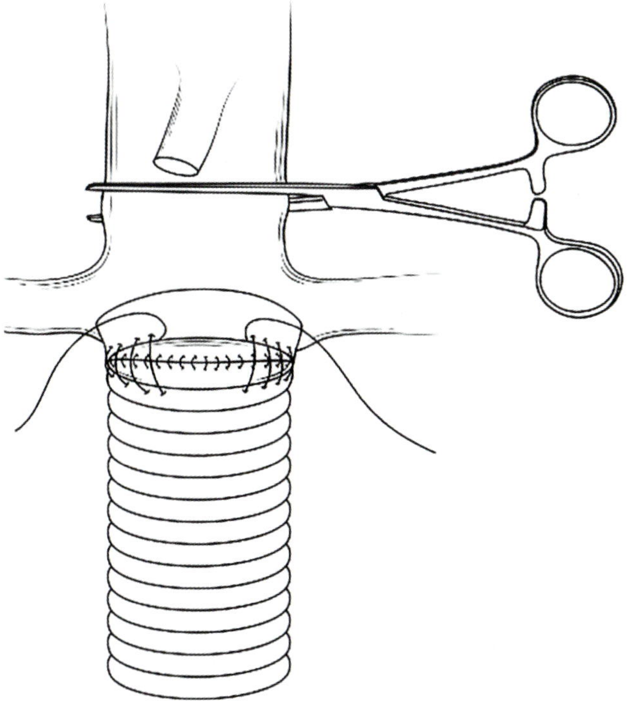

FIGURE 13 • Plicated aneurysm cuff (PLI) technique, in which aneurysm cuff is plicated on itself and cuff is sewn to the graft up to the level of the renal arteries.

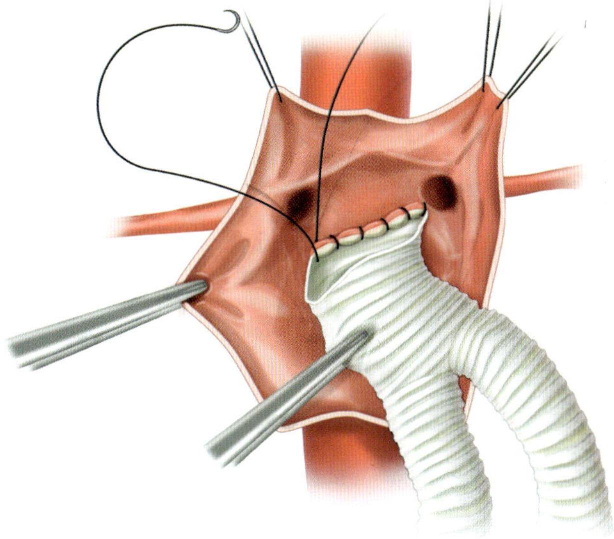

FIGURE 14 • Construction of the posterior row of the proximal anastomosis. Note that the anterior and lateral aspects of the aorta are divided but the posterior wall is left intact in this figure, using "Creech" suturing technique.

row is then completed, starting from each side and working your way to the center, such that the anterior-most stitch is the final stitch placed. These are also pledgeted and tied into place. Once the proximal anastomosis is completed, an atraumatic clamp should be applied to the body of the graft, and the proximal aortic clamp is slowly released to test for integrity of the repair. Any leaks in the suture line should be addressed at this time, particularly along the posterior row, as this will be inaccessible once the distal anastomosis is in place. It is unwise to attempt to place stitches on a fully perfused aorta, and the proximal clamp should be reapplied if pledgeted repair stitches are necessary. A running anastomosis can also be performed with a 3-0 Prolene and an atraumatic needle. The back row is again begun in the middle of the graft with deep Creech bites on the aorta. The graft can be parachuted in to make the suture line taut. The back row should be inspected to ensure that it is snug and additional sutures are used at the 3- and 9-o'clock positions to secure the back row and run to the top of the aorta (**FIGURES 14** and **15**).

- IMA implantation: Although the IMA can generally be ligated without clinical consequence, there are certain situations where it may be beneficial to reimplant the vessel to avoid bowel ischemic complications. Reimplantation generally is associated with excellent long-term patency and a low risk of large bowel ischemia. Patients with altered pelvic blood flow, such as those with prior gastrointestinal surgery or occluded hypogastric arteries, should especially be considered for IMA reimplantation. Furthermore, visual inspection of the sigmoid colon prior to closure should be done, and IMA reimplantation is performed if there appears to be any questionable viability of the bowel. Additionally, prior to IMA ligation, an assessment of back-bleeding (and thus the collateral circulation to the IMA territory) should be performed and reimplantation is considered in cases where the back-bleeding is poor.[17]

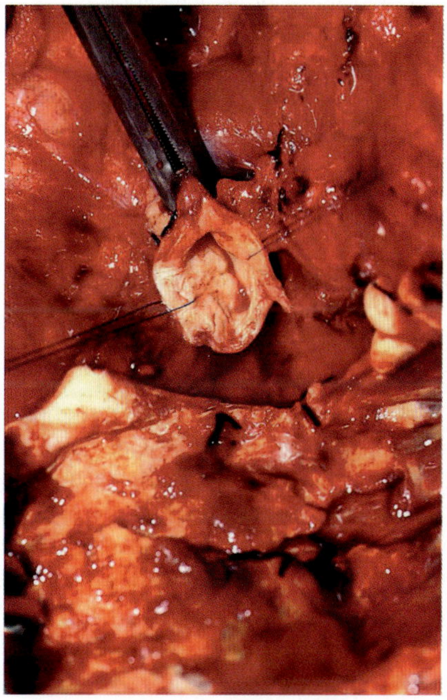

FIGURE 15 • Aortic cuff. The aorta can be totally transected and stay sutures applied in preparation for the anastomosis.

- Creating the distal anastomosis: After the proximal anastomosis is completed and hemostasis is ensured, the graft should be pulled taut to the location of the distal anastomosis (or anastomoses if a bifurcated graft is to be used).

The graft should be measured to ensure no redundancy or kinking occurs but should not be so tight as to put undue strain on the proximal anastomosis. The distal anastomosis can be performed in a running or interrupted fashion, as described previously. While sewing, the assistant should use a forceps to pull the graft distally to relieve tension on the anastomosis, which decreases the incidence of loose sutures.

- Flushing and unclamping: Just prior to the completion of the distal anastomosis, the graft needs to be flushed proximally and distally to remove any clot, air, and/or debris. After flushing, irrigate the graft with heparinized saline and complete the anastomosis. Once both anastomoses are completed, communicate with the anesthesiologist that the clamps are ready to be removed as they need to prepare to react to a possibly substantial drop in systemic blood pressure when the lower extremities are reperfused. It is more appropriate to tolerate a slightly longer clamp time and allow the anesthesiologist to regulate the blood pressure accordingly than to unclamp a hypotensive patient. As the surgeon slowly unclamps, the assistant can exert manual pressure at the level of the femoral arteries to encourage any debris to flush into the pelvis, which may tolerate embolization better due to the extensive collateral network. Pressure is then released from the femoral vessels and systemic pressure is monitored. If there is substantial hypotension, partial or complete reclamping may need to be performed to allow the anesthesia team time to optimize hemodynamics. Once unclamped, inspect the anastomosis and sac for bleeding. There may be new lumbar bleeding as a result of pelvic reperfusion that was not apparent during the graft placement. Diffuse oozing can be treated with hemostatic agents. Check pulses and Doppler signals in the iliac arteries and any clamped branch vessels, as well as distal pulses and/or PVRs. If lower extremity PVRs are significantly worse than the preoperative assessment, this should heighten concern for embolization and may warrant groin exploration and distal thrombectomy.
- Sac closure: This is especially important for the transperitoneal approach, as an uncommon but equally disastrous late complication from open aortic surgery is an aortoenteric fistula, which occurs when graft and/or anastomosis erodes into the bowel. To help prevent this complication, the walls of the now decompressed aortic sac should be closed over the graft and sewn in a running fashion with a long 3-0 silk or chromic suture. If there is insufficient sac to cover the graft, an omental flap can be mobilized and placed over the graft prior to returning the viscera to its anatomic location. The sac of the aorta can be a significant source of bleeding, so the cut edge of the sac should be cauterized to ensure hemostasis and persistent bleeding should be suture ligated prior to sac closure.
- Drainage and closure: If the pleural cavity was violated, drainage can be achieved by a red rubber suction catheter, placed during diaphragmatic repair, or chest tube placement. Additional placement of a closed suction Jackson-Pratt (JP) or Blake drain in the peritoneal or retroperitoneal (RP) cavity can be done on a selective basis; we generally place a drain if there was excessive mobilization near the tail of the pancreas raising concern for a potential pancreatic leak, or in coagulopathic patients. The spleen should be carefully inspected for injury, and we have a low threshold for splenectomy if there is any injury. The abdominal wall should then be closed in layers.

PEARLS AND PITFALLS

- Ideally, proximal clamp time should be less than 30 min. It is therefore imperative to have all tools and grafts ready and all team members briefed on the operative plan prior to clamping. If the clamp is suprarenal, complications begin with more than 40 min of ischemia. However, for an infrarenal clamp, the operator will have several hours if necessary to complete the anastomosis.
- Injury to the common iliac vein or distal IVC during dissection is a potentially lethal complication. This is a complication that is much better to avoid than to treat. If necessary, it is important to completely mobilize the vein and perform a primary repair under direct vision. Blind suturing in a bleeding field will only lead to disaster. If exposure cannot be obtained, it is acceptable to transect the overlying artery (aorta or iliac) to allow access to the vein.
- The ureters can be injured during both the transperitoneal or retroperitoneal approach. The ureters should always be identified prior to repositioning retractors or beginning a new dissection plane.

POSTOPERATIVE CARE

- Patients should be monitored in an intensive care unit (ICU) postoperatively with systolic blood pressure goals of 100 to 140 mm Hg for a straightforward infrarenal or juxtarenal repair. Blood pressure goals should be higher for thoracoabdominal repairs to promote spinal cord perfusion.
- Suitable patients should be extubated as early as possible, even in the OR if appropriate as early extubation decreases complications.[18]
- A nasogastric tube (NGT) is kept in place given the bowel manipulation and likelihood of ileus. We keep the NGT in for the first full postoperative day and although it is not imperative to maintain it until full return of bowel function, we will keep it in place an additional day if outputs are unusually high. We generally start standing rectal suppositories on the first postoperative day.
- If a chest tube is placed, we leave this to suction until removal, which is done when output is less than 150 mL per 24 hours and the chest x-ray (CXR) shows no large effusion.

- Postoperative mobilization should be done as soon as possible. These patients will require physical therapy and many will ultimately require inpatient rehab.

OUTCOMES

- Mortality for an elective, open infrarenal AAA repair is less than 5%, and although the risk increases for those with a juxtarenal or suprarenal repair, our recent experience shows that 30-day mortality in patients with juxtarenal repair is 2.5%. Mortality increases in the instance of an urgent or rupture to as high as 70%.[1,5]
- Patient-specific predictors of postoperative complications and mortality include older age, higher modified frailty index (mFI) score, COPD, chronic renal disease (creatinine >1.8), or history of myocardial infarction (MI)/congestive heart failure (CHF).[1,19]
- Operative-specific predictors of postoperative complications include long OR or clamp times, hypothermia, high blood turnover, and a high perioperative fluid requirement.
- Open aneurysm repair cases are becoming more complex as EVAR and its fenestrated counterparts are increasingly employed for elective cases. When employed in urgent situations and for explantation, perioperative mortality and complications increase. However, elective repair of complex aneurysms (juxtarenal and suprarenal) showed no long-term survival difference when compared to elective open infrarenal AAA repair.[20,21]

COMPLICATIONS

- Bleeding
- Infection
- Splenic injury (consider adding splenectomy to operative consent)
- Renal failure
- MI
- CVA
- Spinal cord ischemia (increased risk with suprarenal and thoracoabdominal repairs)
- Anastomotic breakdown
- Aortoenteric fistula
- Pancreatitis

REFERENCES

1. Brewster DC, Cronenwett JL, Hallett JW Jr, et al. Guidelines for the treatment of abdominal aortic aneurysms. Report of a subcommittee of the Joint Council of the American association for vascular surgery and Society for vascular surgery. *J Vasc Surg*. 2003;37:1106-1117.
2. Cronenwett JL, Sargent SK, Wall MH, et al. Variables that affect the expansion rate and outcome of small abdominal aortic aneurysms. *J Vasc Surg*. 1990;11(2):260-269.
3. Darling RC III, Brewster DC, Darling RC, et al. Are familial abdominal aortic aneurysms different? *J Vasc Surg*. 1989;10(1):39-43.
4. Strachan DP. Predictors of death from aortic aneurysm among middle-aged men: the Whitehall study. *Br J Surg*. 1991;78(4):401-404.
5. Tsai S, Conrad MF, Patel VI, et al. Durability of open repair of juxtarenal abdominal aortic aneurysms. *J Vasc Surg*. 2012;56(1):2-7.
6. McFalls EO, Ward HB, Moritz TE, et al. Clinical factors associated with long-term mortality following vascular surgery: outcomes from the Coronary Artery Revascularization Prophylaxis (CARP) Trial. *J Vasc Surg*. 2007;46(4):694-700.
7. Garcia S, Rider JE, Moritz TE, et al. Preoperative coronary artery revascularization and long-term outcomes following abdominal aortic vascular surgery in patients with abnormal myocardial perfusion scans: a subgroup analysis of the coronary artery revascularization prophylaxis trial. *Catheter Cardiovasc Interv*. 2011;77(1):134-141.
8. Van de Luijtgaarden KM, Bastos Gonçalves F, Hoeks SE, Majoor-Krakauer D, et al. Familial abdominal aortic aneurysm is associated with more complications after endovascular aneurysm repair. *J Vasc Surg*. 2014;59(2):275-282.
9. Chaikof EL, Brewster DC, Dalman RL, et al. SVS practice guidelines for the care of patients with an abdominal aortic aneurysm: executive summary. *J Vasc Surg*. 2009;50(4):880-896.
10. Dawson I, Sie RB, van Bockel JH. Atherosclerotic popliteal aneurysm. *Br J Surg*. 1997;84(3):293.
11. Johnston KW, Rutherford RB, Tilson MD, et al. Suggested standards for reporting on arterial aneurysms. Subcommittee on Reporting standards for arterial aneurysms, Ad Hoc Committee on Reporting standards, Society for vascular surgery and North American chapter, International Society for Cardiovascular surgery. *J Vasc Surg*. 1991;13(3):452-458.
12. US Preventive Services Task Force; Owens DK, Davidson KW, Krist AH, et al. Screening for abdominal aortic aneurysm: US preventive Services Task Force recommendation Statement. *JAMA*. 2019;322(22):2211-2218.
13. Lederle FA, Johnson GR, Wilson SE, et al. The aneurysm detection and management study screening program: validation cohort and final results. Aneurysm Detection and Management Veterans Affairs Cooperative Study Investigators. *Arch Intern Med*. 2000;160:1425-1430.
14. Lederle FA, Wilson SE, Johnson GR, et al. Immediate repair compared with surveillance of small abdominal aortic aneurysms. *N Engl J Med*. 2002;346(19):1437-1444.
15. Wang LJ, Tsougranis GH, Tanious A, et al. The removal of all proximal aneurysmal aortic tissue does not affect anastomotic degeneration after open juxtarenal aortic aneurysm repair. *J Vasc Surg*. 2020;71(2):390-399.
16. Green RM, Ricotta JJ, Ouriel K, DeWeese JA. Results of supraceliac aortic clamping in the difficult elective resection of infrarenal abdominal aortic aneurysm. *J Vasc Surg*. 1989;9(1):124-134.
17. Jayaraj A, DeMartino RR, Bower TC, et al. Outcomes following inferior mesenteric artery reimplantation during elective aortic aneurysm surgery. *Ann Vasc Surg*. 2020;66:65-69.
18. Zettervall SL, Soden PA, Shean KE, et al. Early extubation reduces respiratory complications and hospital length of stay following repair of abdominal aortic aneurysms. *J Vasc Surg*. 2017;65(1):58-64.
19. Barbey SM, Scali ST, Kubilis P, et al. Interaction between frailty and sex on mortality after elective abdominal aortic aneurysm repair. *J Vasc Surg*. 2019;70(6):1831-1843.
20. Fairman AS, Chin AL, Jackson BM, et al. The evolution of open abdominal aortic aneurysm repair at a tertiary care center. *J Vasc Surg*. 2020;72(4):1367-1374.
21. Deery SE, Lancaster RT, Baril DT, et al. Contemporary outcomes of open complex abdominal aortic aneurysm repair. *J Vasc Surg*. 2016;63(5):1195-1200.

Chapter 23 Advanced Aortic Aneurysm Management: Endovascular Aneurysm Repair—Standard and Emergency Management

Oonagh H. Scallan and Audra A. Duncan

DEFINITION

- Abdominal aortic aneurysm (AAA) is defined as abnormal dilatation of the abdominal aorta greater than 50% of the normal proximal segment, typically greater than 3 cm.
- The most common etiology of AAAs is degenerative, often also referred to as atherosclerotic. Other etiologies include inflammatory, dissection, trauma, developmental or congenital, and infectious.

DIFFERENTIAL DIAGNOSIS

- Most AAAs are asymptomatic and are identified incidentally during an exam for an unrelated pathology. The classic triad of symptoms in a patient with a ruptured aneurysm includes acute-onset abdominal or back pain, hypotension, and a pulsatile abdominal mass.
- The differential diagnosis is broad and is dependent on the presentation of the patient. Possible alternative diagnoses include:
  - Renal colic
  - Diverticulitis
  - Perforated ulcer
  - Pancreatitis
  - Gastrointestinal bleed
  - Myocardial infarction
  - Pulmonary embolism

PATIENT HISTORY AND PHYSICAL FINDINGS

- Patients with AAA are typically asymptomatic and the aneurysm is diagnosed as an incidental finding. A patient of lower body habitus or with a large aneurysm may notice a palpable pulsatile mass.
- Rarely, patients may present with distal limb ischemia related to embolization of thrombus from within the aneurysm.
- Patients with a ruptured aneurysm may present with abdominal or back pain, or pain radiating to the testes, inguinal canal, rectum, or hip. A history of syncope or hypotension in a patient with a tender, pulsatile abdominal mass indicates a possible ruptured aneurysm. Rarely, patients may present with an aortocaval fistula secondary to the ruptured aneurysm and demonstrate symptoms of heart failure, a systolic bruit in the abdomen, and central venous hypertension.
- Risk factors for aneurysmal disease are similar to atherosclerotic disease and include advancing age, male gender, chronic obstructive pulmonary disease, smoking, family history of aneurysms, and connective tissue disorders. A thorough history should be taken from the patient to elicit risk factors for an aneurysm and medical comorbidities. The history and physical exam are important to determine the etiology of the aneurysm and overall health of the patient as this will influence the choice of operative approach.
- Risk factors for rupture include female gender, large initial aneurysm diameter, low forced expiration volume in 1 second, current smoking history, immunomodulation therapy after major organ transplantation, and elevated mean blood pressure.[1]
- An AAA may be identified on physical exam as a palpable pulsatile mass, typically supraumbilical and in the midline; however, the position may vary due to aortic tortuosity. The ability to palpate the aneurysm is affected by the aneurysm size and body habitus of the patient. Given the incidence of concomitant aneurysms, patients should be examined for other aneurysms such as femoral or popliteal aneurysms.

IMAGING AND OTHER DIAGNOSTIC STUDIES

- Multiple randomized controlled trials (RCTs) have demonstrated that a one-time screening for an AAA by ultrasound is effective at reducing aneurysm-related mortality and incidence of aneurysm rupture.[2] The Multicentre Aneurysm Screening Study (MASS) randomized over 67,000 men aged 65 to 74 to ultrasound AAA screening vs no screening, and found that screening led to a 40% reduction in aneurysm-related mortality, and this benefit persisted for over a decade.[3]
- Society for Vascular Surgery (SVS) guidelines recommend a one-time screening ultrasound for men and women aged 65 to 75, or over 75 in good health, with a history of tobacco use, and patients aged 65 to 75, or older than 75 years and in good health, with a first-degree relative with an AAA.[1]
- CT angiogram (CTA) is the current standard modality for operative planning and provides excellent imaging of AAAs, with increased accuracy of diameter measurements compared to ultrasound. CTA allows for three-dimensional reconstruction and includes essential anatomic information such as dimensions, neck angulation, thrombus, calcification, occlusive disease, and assessment of arterial access.

SURGICAL MANAGEMENT

Indications

- The goal of AAA repair is to prevent rupture; therefore the decision to treat is based on the risk of rupture, the risk of treatment, the patient's life expectancy, and patient preference.[2]
- The current recommendation for repair of AAA in low- and average-risk patients is aneurysms >5.5 cm in men and >5 cm in women. There is no long-term benefit of survival of open or endovascular repair in small aneurysms, 4 to 5.5 cm, as demonstrated by multiple RCTs.[4]

- Other indications include rupture, aneurysm growth rate of >1 cm in 1 year, and symptomatic aneurysms.

Preoperative Planning

- Successful EVAR excludes an aneurysm from blood flow through placement of the stent, typically through the common femoral arteries. A stent graft consisting of a metallic stent framework covered with a synthetic fabric material is used. The metal skeleton is made of nitinol or stainless steel. There are multiple aortic stent grafts currently available and the selection of the device should be tailored to the individual anatomic requirements, as each device has different parameters for the IFU.
- Anatomic measurements obtained from a high-quality CTA are essential for a successful EVAR. 3-D reconstruction software programs (eg, TeraRecon) provide precise diameter and path length measurements for operative planning. Graft oversizing of 10% to 20% is typically used in the aortic neck. Length measurements are obtained from the lowest renal artery to the iliac bifurcations and can be repeated intraoperatively with marking catheters.
- The IFU of the device and the patient's anatomy should be carefully scrutinized for suitability for EVAR and device selection. If the patient does not have good anatomy for standard EVAR, they should be considered for fenestrated or branched EVAR or open repair. Other patient characteristics to factor into the decision for operative repair include the age of the patient and durability of repair, and potential for the presence of a connective tissue disorder.
- When EVAR is performed within IFU criteria, the results are excellent, with <1% type 1a endoleaks. However, a large number of patients undergo standard EVAR with anatomy outside IFU. Reduced adherence to IFU is associated with higher rates of aneurysm sac expansion, which ultimately translates into treatment failure, costly reintervention, and possibly late aneurysm rupture.[5] The Ad Hoc Committee of Standardized Reporting Practices for the Society of Vascular Surgery defined a marginal neck as having length <15 mm, diameter >28 mm, angle >60, and presence of significant calcification or thrombus. These guidelines predominantly coincide with the instructions for use for the majority of EVAR devices.[6]
- With the increasing use of EVAR for patients with hostile or short necks, techniques to prevent or treat type 1a endoleaks have become important tools, such as the Heli-FX EndoAnchor System (Medtronic Vascular). This is an adjunctive sealing device that can be placed to treat or prevent type 1a endoleak. It delivers 3.0 × 4.5 mm helical screws to improve the seal between the endograft and the aortic wall (**FIGURE 1**).
- The decreasing profile of endovascular devices is beneficial in not only allowing navigation of tortuous, diseased, or small iliac arteries, it also makes totally percutaneous access for the procedure appealing. This technique uses suture-mediated closure devices, such as Perclose ProGlide or Prostar XL, in a "preclose" technique. The Prostar XL Percutaneous Vascular surgery device (Abbott Vascular) is a suture-mediated arterial closure device. It is a CE Mark-approved closure device for large size femoral artery punctures from 8 to 24 Fr; it is delivered over a 0.038 wire. The ProGlide (Abbott Vascular) is also a suture-mediated arterial closure device that will track over a standard 0.035 wire and accommodates 5- to 21-Fr arteriotomies. In arteriotomies >8 Fr, at least two devices are required to close the arteriotomy. Risk factors for failure include heavy arterial calcification, increased ratio of sheath size to common femoral artery diameter, increased patient age, and female sex.[7] In patients with inadequate access vessels for a percutaneous approach, open femoral exposure may be required. Adjunctive measures for inadequate access include the use of a conduit or endoconduit.

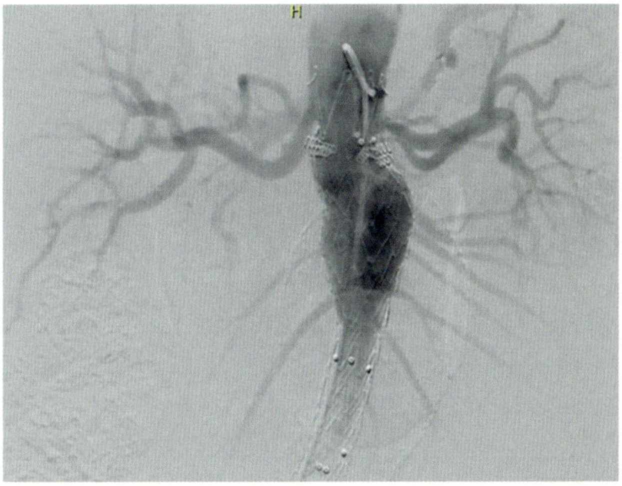

FIGURE 1 • Seven endoanchors inserted in the infrarenal aorta using the Heli-FX EndoAnchor System in an EVAR treating an aneurysm with a short infrarenal neck.

- In patients who do not have ideal anatomy for a standard EVAR with a bifurcated device, an aortouni-iliac endograft may be more appropriate. Some relative indications for aortouni-iliac endograft configuration include a very small (<15 mm) terminal aorta, which would not accommodate a bifurcated device, severe unilateral iliac occlusive disease, or secondary treatment of migration of short body endograft.
- The SMA and celiac arteries should also be examined preoperatively for patency and evidence of severe stenosis or occlusion. If present, the patient should be carefully assessed for symptoms of chronic mesenteric ischemia. In the setting of severe visceral disease, revascularization should be considered prior to EVAR or open repair should be considered given the obligation of covering the IMA during EVAR.

ENDOVASCULAR ANEURYSM REPAIR STANDARD

Percutaneous Access

- After confirming the location of the inguinal ligament, femoral bifurcation, and appropriateness of the artery for percutaneous access, ultrasound guidance is used to puncture the common femoral artery with a 0.018-in micropuncture kit. A 0.035-in starter wire (eg, Bentson, Cook Medical, Bloomington, IN) is advanced into the abdominal aorta and the sheath is exchanged for a 7-Fr sheath.

Preclose Technique

- While the assistant maintains pressure, the 7-Fr sheath is exchanged for a Perclose Proglide (Abbott, Abbott Park, IL) device. This is advanced until the guidewire exit line on the device and the wire is temporarily removed. The device is advanced until pulsatile blood is seen through the pilot tube lumen. The device is turned to the 10-o'clock position and the footplate is activated. Holding back tension on the device, the suture is deployed. The footplate is lowered, and the device removed from the artery until the guidewire is reintroduced. The suture ends are clamped together to avoid premature cinching of the knots (**FIGURE 2**).
- A second Perclose Proglide (Abbott, Abbott Park, IL) device is loaded and deployed at the 2-o'clock position.

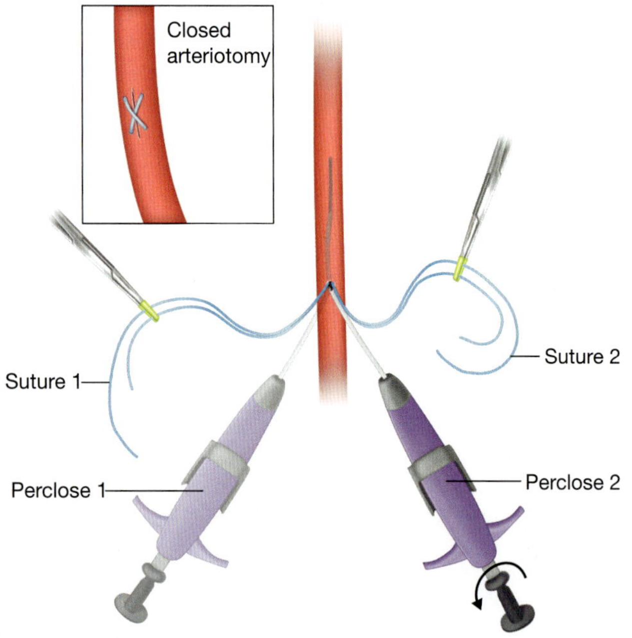

FIGURE 2 • Preclose technique. Two ProGlides are deployed, one at the 10-o'clock position and the other at the 2-o'clock position before beginning serial dilation maneuvers and deployment of delivery catheters. Once the procedure is complete, and large diameter devices are removed, both knots are seated to close the arteriotomy (see inset). Until closure, the free sutures are controlled on suture boots. Once the procedure is complete, both knots are pushed down to close the arteriotomy.

- Once both devices are deployed and the sutures controlled, a 9-Fr sheath may be placed to continue dilation.

Delivery and Deployment of Endograft

- Bilateral straight stiff 260 cm Lunderquist (Cook Medical) or equivalent wires are placed in the proximal descending thoracic aorta. Serial dilation is then performed to place the sheaths required for the chosen device.
- Systemic anticoagulation is established with intravenous unfractionated heparin (100 units/kg) and confirmed with an activated clotting time (ACT) greater than 250 seconds.
- A flush catheter is advanced into the proximal abdominal aorta from the contralateral femoral artery. A catheter with 1 cm markers can be used to concomitantly confirm the length measurements obtained from preoperative imaging.
- The main body endograft is oriented to deploy the contralateral gate anterolaterally, and advanced over the ipsilateral Lunderquist wire (Cook Medical) (**FIGURE 3A**).
- The flush catheter is connected to a power injector and air is flushed from the system. The image intensifier is adjusted cranially to limit parallax in the setting of neck angulation to obtain an orthogonal view to the takeoff of the lowest renal artery, based on the preoperative CT. With the ventilator held to minimize motion artifact, an initial aortogram is obtained to identify the position of the renal arteries.
- The main body endograft is then deployed according to the IFU, with the proximal fabric margin positioned just below the lowest renal artery to obtain maximum seal. Deployment continues until the contralateral gate is open. The flush catheter should be pulled back before deployment of suprarenal fixation to avoid entrapment of the catheter. The suprarenal stents are then deployed (**FIGURE 3B**).

Gate Cannulation

- The flush catheter is retracted to below the contralateral gate, and a combination of hydrophilic wires (such as a Terumo Glidewire guidewire) and direction catheters can be used to cannulate the contralateral gate. Positioning the contralateral sheath within 1 to 2 cm of the gate may assist this (**FIGURE 3C**).
- Once the gate has been cannulated, the flush pigtail catheter is reformed within the limb and presence within the device is confirmed by visualizing the spinning catheter. Cannulation can also be confirmed by using a molding balloon and inflating it across the origin of the limb resulting in a mushroom appearance of the balloon.[8]
- Strategies to obtain gate cannulation include various guidewires, shaped catheters, adjusting the C-arm, or using a snare from the other side. Brachial access can also be used for this same purpose.

Limb extension

- Retrograde iliac angiography is performed through the sheath with the C-arm in the contralateral oblique position to identify the origin of the internal iliac artery. A marker catheter is used to measure the appropriate length limb. For three-piece bifurcated devices, this is completed on both sides. Adequate overlap between stent components and length of seal in the common iliac artery must be considered (**FIGURE 3D**).

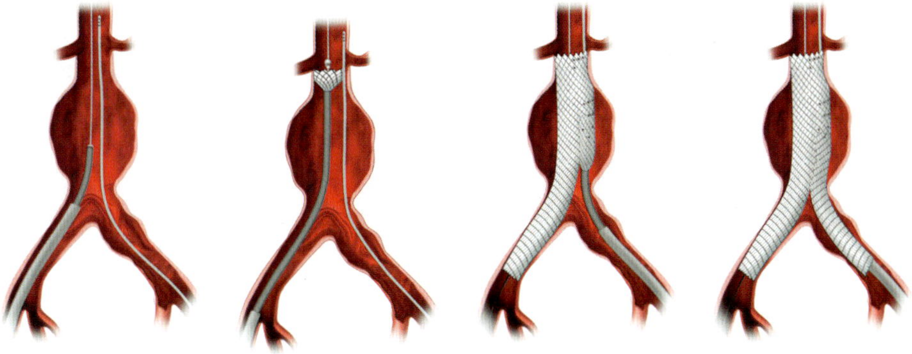

FIGURE 3 • Delivery and deployment of endograft. **A,** The main body is brought up the ipsilateral iliac artery to the level of the renal arteries. An Omni Flush catheter is brought up the contralateral iliac artery and an angiogram is performed. **B,** The main body endograft is deployed under fluoroscopic guidance until the contralateral gate is opened. **C,** The contralateral gate is cannulated. **D,** An extension limb is placed proximal to the iliac bifurcation on the contralateral side and the ipsilateral endograft is finished being deployed (one docking limb systems) or an extension limb is placed (two docking limb systems) to the level of the ipsilateral iliac bifurcation.

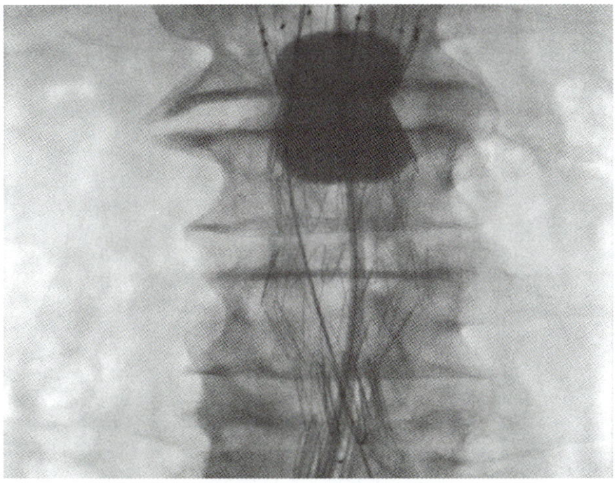

FIGURE 4 • Balloon molding. A semicompliant balloon is inflated at proximal and distal landing zones as well as at all overlapping endografts.

Balloon Molding

- A semicompliant balloon is expanded with diluted contrast solution at all three landing zones, the neck and iliac arteries, areas of overlap, and areas within the gates as appropriate for the specific device. Kissing balloons may be used to treat the presence of a common iliac artery stenosis or narrowing at the aortic bifurcation. Self-expanding bare metal stents may be used in areas of stenosis or at the end of the distal limb into the external iliac artery to prevent kinking (**FIGURE 4**).

Completion Arteriography

- The flush catheter is reintroduced and a completion aortogram is performed with the end of the catheter superior to the stent graft to assess for positioning, stent patency, and the presence of endoleaks (**FIGURE 5A-D**).
- Type I and III endoleaks present as earlier, brisker antegrade filling of the aneurysm sac as opposed to type II endoleaks, which tend to be delayed, slower, retrograde filling of the aneurysm sac.
- All type I and III endoleaks should be addressed prior to completion of the procedure, whereas many type II endoleaks resolve on their own over the first year. If proximal aortic endoanchors are required, they are placed at this time.

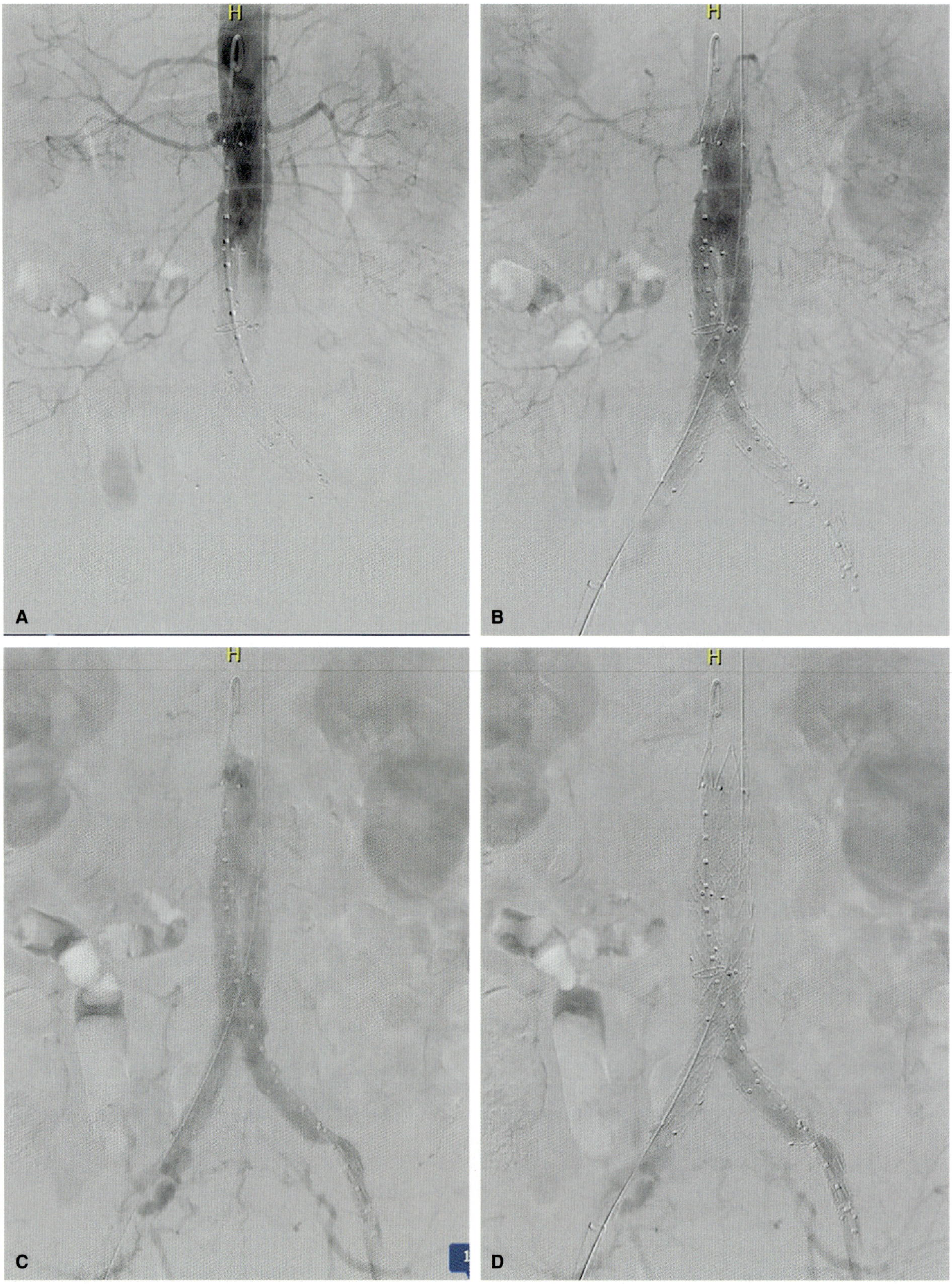

FIGURE 5 • Completion arteriography. Special attention is paid to ensure the renal and iliac arteries are patent, as well as to identify if an endoleak is present. The endograft itself should be scrutinized for any evidence of limb kinking. **A,** Renal artery patency confirmed. **B,** No type 1A endoleak confirmed. **C,** The right external and internal iliac arteries are confirmed to be patient. The left iliac limb extends into the external iliac artery to exclude the left internal iliac aneurysm. The endograft itself should be scrutinized for any evidence of limb kinking. **D,** No type 1B, 2, 3, or 4 endoleak identified with delayed imaging.

ENDOVASCULAR ANEURYSM REPAIR FOR RUPTURED ANEURYSMS OR REVAR

Preoperative Considerations

- Successful treatment of a ruptured AAA with EVAR relies on early diagnosis, rapid completion of a CT scan, and timely transport to the operating room. A standardized protocol developed by the Albany Vascular Group to manage patients with ruptured AAA has shown significant improvements in patient survival.[9]
- In a hybrid OR, the patient is prepped and draped in supine position, including the abdomen for potential conversion to open repair if necessary.

Access

- Access to the common femoral arteries may be performed through a percutaneous approach or open exposure depending on the clinical circumstances, operator experience, and logistics. In hemodynamically unstable patients, access may be obtained under local anesthesia with conversion to general anesthesia once balloon control of the aorta has been obtained if necessary. If time does not permit for the preclose technique, conversion to open femoral closure after the endograft has been fully deployed may be completed.
- After placement of bilateral stiff wires (eg, Lunderquist, Cook Medical), the sheaths are upsized as outlined in the previous section. If an aortic occlusion balloon is to be used due to hemodynamic instability, the sheath on the contralateral side should be advanced into the supraceliac aorta to provide support for the balloon and prevent downward displacement into the aneurysm sac. This also allows for removal of the balloon through the sheath to avoid the balloon getting caught on the barbs of the endograft.
- The use of systemic anticoagulation in the setting of ruptured aortic aneurysm repair is controversial and dependent on the hemodynamic status of the patient, presence of active bleeding, and existing consumptive coagulopathy. Anticoagulation may be withheld until the main body and extension limbs are deployed.

Aortic Balloon Control

- A semicompliant balloon (Coda, Cook Medical) is advanced and positioned in the supraceliac aorta under fluoroscopic guidance (**FIGURE 6**). Once in position, the balloon can be inflated depending on the patient's hemodynamic status.

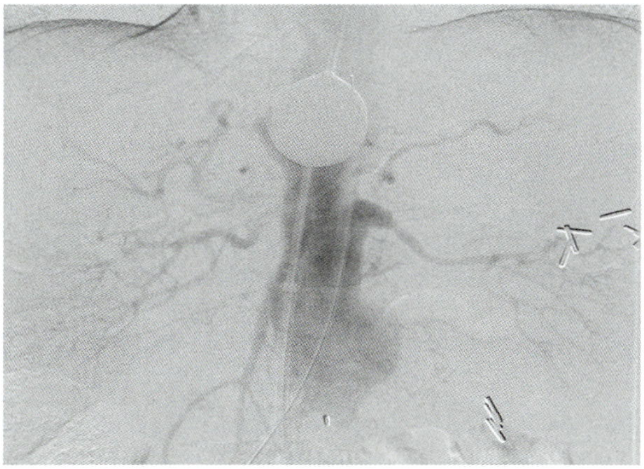

FIGURE 6 • Aortic balloon control for REVAR. A semicompliant balloon is placed up the contralateral iliac artery proximal to the celiac trunk. It can be inflated depending on hemodynamic instability.

Endograft Delivery and Deployment

- Aortography is performed through the contralateral sheath below the balloon to localize the origins of the renal arteries.
- The main body endograft is oriented for anterolateral deployment of the contralateral gate, then placed through the ipsilateral sheath to the level of the renal arteries. A repeat angiogram after adjusting for parallax may be necessary if there is angulation of the aortic neck (**FIGURE 7**).
- If the aortic occlusion balloon is in place without the support of a sheath, it should be deflated and withdrawn to avoid trapping the balloon between the aortic neck and the stent graft. The main body is then deployed just distal to the lowest renal artery, according to the device IFU, and the entirety of the ipsilateral gate is deployed. This allows for a second semicompliant balloon to be advanced up the ipsilateral endograft limb and placed into the main body for inflation depending on hemodynamic instability (**FIGURE 8**).

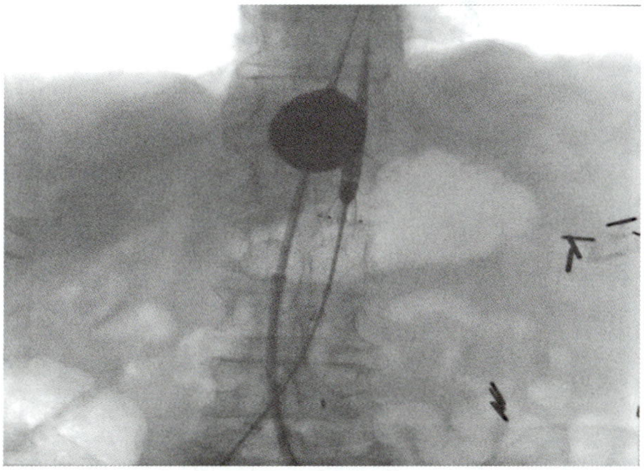

FIGURE 7 • Main body deployment for REVAR. After an angiogram is performed to identify the renal arteries and aortic neck, the main body is deployed up the ipsilateral iliac artery. This can be done with the semicompliant balloon inflated.

Gate Cannulation

- Gate cannulation proceeds in a standard fashion during REVAR. Time awareness is critical to ensure that aneurysm sealing is accomplished in the most expeditious manner possible.

Limb Extension

- Limb extension proceeds in a standard fashion during REVAR.

Balloon Molding

- Balloon molding is performed at all seal zones to optimize hemostasis.

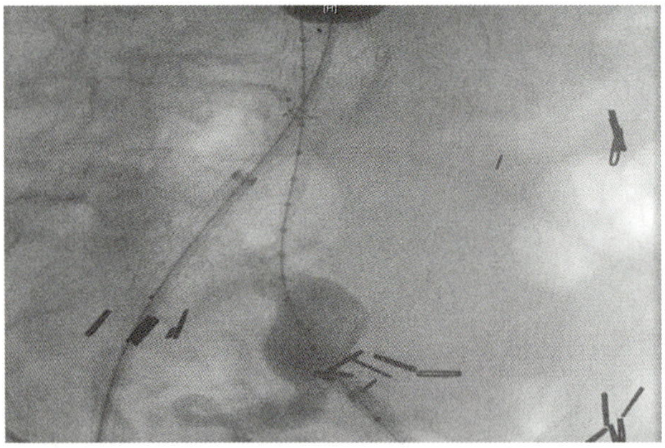

FIGURE 8 • Balloon exchange and gate cannulation for REVAR. The entire ipsilateral gate is deployed prior to contralateral gate cannulation. A second semicompliant balloon is placed up the ipsilateral endograft limb (top of image) and placed into the main body of the endograft. It can be inflated depending on hemodynamic instability. The first semicompliant balloon is removed and the sheath is brought to distal to the contralateral gate to prepare for gate cannulation. Retrograde angiography with a marking catheter is performed through the contralateral sheath to identify the iliac bifurcation and desired limb extension length.

Completion Aortography

- Completion aortography is performed as previously described. Attention should be paid to all the general considerations of presence and nature of endoleaks, kinking of the limbs, and sufficient overlap in the landing zones to meet IFU.

Closure

- Closure proceeds as indicated for standard EVAR.

Abdominal compartment syndrome (ACS)

- Abdominal compartment syndrome occurs in up to 20% of patients after treatment of a ruptured AAA by EVAR, with a high rate of perioperative mortality of 50%.[10]
- The pathophysiology of ACS after EVAR for ruptured AAA is multifactorial and includes the presence of the retroperitoneal hematoma, ongoing bleeding from lumbar arteries and the IMA, and shock associated with rupture, which can induce alterations in microvascular permeability and lead to visceral and soft tissue edema.[9]
- Several variables have been identified as contributing factors to ACS including the use of an aortic occlusion balloon, need for massive blood transfusion, and coagulopathy at the com pletion of the case.

PEARLS AND PITFALLS

Patient selection and preoperative planning	Careful preoperative assessment of the patient and their anatomy is essential to obtaining a good, durable result from EVAR to ensure anatomic suitability and availability of equipment.
Access	Ultrasound guidance is essential to limiting access complications. The needle tip should be visualized entering the anterior artery wall, in an area deemed appropriate for access.
Gate cannulation	In general, the main body should be advanced through the more tortuous of the iliac arteries to all a more "straight shot" for the contralateral gate cannulation. However, in some scenarios this may not be practical if the tortuosity of the iliac precludes main body positioning and deployment altogether. Crossing the iliac limbs of the graft during placement of the main body graft may allow a straighter line for gate access.
Tortuous iliacs	Remove the stiff wires and leave catheters in place for the completion angiogram. This allows the vessels to take their native position and reveal any type 1a endoleak or kinking of the limbs that may not be evident when the graft is straightened out by the stiff wire.
Graft angioplasty	If using one smaller sheath (ie, 12 or 14 Fr) and one larger, place the compliant balloon through the smaller sheath first. Once the balloon is inflated, it is more difficult to pass through a 12-Fr sheath.
Closure	Tie down the sutures of the closure device with the wire in place. If there is still significant bleeding, deploy another closure device or place an occlusive sheath and proceed with open conversion of the femoral artery closure under more controlled circumstances.

POSTOPERATIVE CARE

- After percutaneous EVAR, patients should remain supine for 3 hours and are free to ambulate thereafter. Most elective EVARs are discharged on postoperative day 1, or in some cases as same-day surgery. Given the decreasing size of access sheaths, the preclose technique, and advanced anesthesia techniques, several centers have advocated for the safety and efficacy of outpatient EVAR, with nearly 40% of patients estimated to be candidates.
- As recommended by SVS guidelines, an initial postoperative contrast-enhanced CT is performed at 1 month to assess stability of the aneurysm sac, and for endoleaks and graft position. Patients are then reassessed with CT or color duplex ultrasound at 6 months if there is a type II endoleak or 1 year if there is no endoleak and no aneurysm sac enlargement[1] (**FIGURE 9**).
- EVAR has been shown to have lower perioperative morbidity and mortality compared to OSR. The early survival

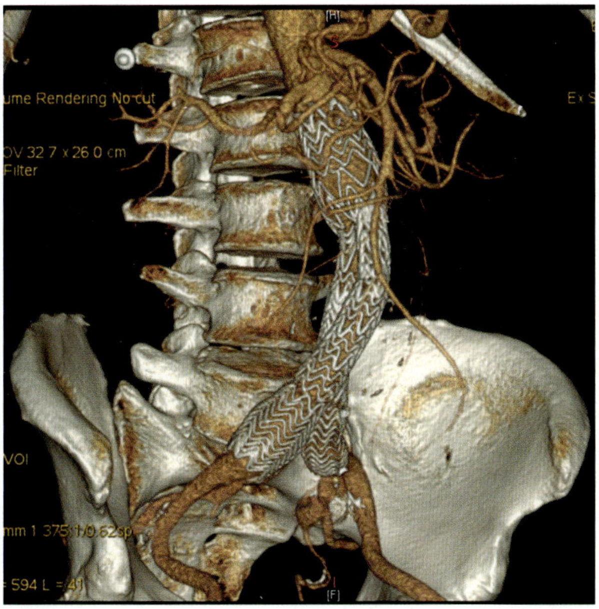

FIGURE 9 • Postoperative imaging. 3-D reconstruction of a CT aortogram in a patient who have undergone successful EVAR at 1-month follow-up.

benefit of EVAR is lost over time; the 15-year results from EVAR-1 showed now difference in survival between EVAR vs OSR.[11] Beyond 8 years, EVAR has been found to have higher all-cause and aneurysm-related mortality, primarily due to aneurysm rupture in the EVAR group.[11]

COMPLICATIONS

- Endoleak and delayed rupture
- Graft limb occlusion
- Thromboembolism
- Migration
- Stent graft infection
- Renal dysfunction
- Renal artery occlusion
- Bowel ischemia
- Pelvic ischemia

REFERENCES

1. Chaikof EL, Dalman RL, Eskandari MK, et al. The Society for Vascular Surgery practice guidelines on the care of patients with an abdominal aortic aneurysm. *J Vasc Surg*. 2018;67(1):2-77.e2. doi:10.1016/j.jvs.2017.10.044
2. Swerdlow NJ, Wu WW, Schermerhorn ML. Open and endovascular management of aortic aneurysms. *Circ Res*. 2019;124(4):647-661. doi:10.1161/CIRCRESAHA.118.313186
3. Ashton HA, Buxton MJ, Day NE, et al. The Multicentre Aneurysm Screening Study (MASS) into the effect of abdominal aortic aneurysm screening on mortality in men: a randomised controlled trial. *Lancet*. 2002;360(9345):1531-1539. doi:10.1016/s0140-6736(02)11522-4
4. Filardo G, Powell JT, Martinez MA, Ballard DJ. Surgery for small asymptomatic abdominal aortic aneurysms. *Cochrane Database Syst Rev*. 2015;2015(2):CD001835. Published 2015 Feb 8. doi:10.1002/14651858.CD001835.pub4
5. Schanzer A, Greenberg RK, Hevelone N, et al. Predictors of abdominal aortic aneurysm sac enlargement after endovascular repair [published correction appears in Circulation. 2012 Jan 17;125(2):e266]. *Circulation*. 2011;123(24):2848-2855. doi:10.1161/CIRCULATIONAHA.110.014902
6. Chaikof EL, Blankensteijn JD, Harris PL, et al. Reporting standards for endovascular aortic aneurysm repair. *J Vasc Surg*. 2002;35(5):1048-1060. doi:10.1067/mva.2002.123763
7. Smeds MR, Charlton-Ouw KM. Infrarenal endovascular aneurysm repair: new developments and decision making in 2016. *Semin Vasc Surg*. 2016;29(1-2):27-34. doi:10.1053/j.semvascsurg.2016.06.001
8. Wilson WRW, Benveniste GL. Confirmation of contralateral limb gate cannulation using a moulding balloon. *Eur J Vasc Endovasc Surg Extra*. 2010;20:25-26.
9. Mehta M. Technical tips for EVAR for ruptured AAA. *Semin Vasc Surg*. 2009;22(3):181-186. doi:10.1053/j.semvascsurg.2009.07.010
10. SÁ P, Oliveira-Pinto J, Mansilha A. Abdominal compartment syndrome after r-EVAR: a systematic review with meta-analysis on incidence and mortality. *Int Angiol*. 2020;39(5):411-421. doi:10.23736/S0392-9590.20.04406-5
11. Patel R, Sweeting MJ, Powell JT, Greenhalgh RM. EVAR trial investigators. Endovascular versus open repair of abdominal aortic aneurysm in 15-years' follow-up of the UK endovascular aneurysm repair trial 1 (EVAR trial 1): a randomised controlled trial. *Lancet*. 2016;388(10058):2366-2374. doi:10.1016/S0140-6736(16)31135-7

Chapter 24

Advanced Aneurysm Management Techniques: Management of Internal Iliac Artery Aneurysm Disease

Olamide Alabi, Erica L. Mitchell, and Laura B. Pride

DEFINITION

- An internal iliac artery aneurysm (IIAA) is defined as a ≥50% increase in the expected diameter. Internal iliac arteries for both men and women measure 0.54 ± 0.15 cm,[1] therefore threshold diameter of 8 mm is used to define IIAA.
- IIAA are exceedingly rare, representing <0.5% of all aortoiliac aneurysms. Ninety percent are unilateral and not associated with abdominal aortic aneurysms (AAA)[2,3] (**FIGURE 1**).
- Patients with IIAA are typically males in their seventh and eighth decade of life in line with their association with atherosclerotic disease.[2,3]
- The natural history of IIAA is not well described as prospective studies are lacking. Retrospective data show that IIAAs are typically slow growing and aneurysms <4 cm rarely rupture.[4,5]

DIFFERENTIAL DIAGNOSIS

- The differential diagnosis of IIAA is primarily limited to atherosclerotic degenerative aneurysms.
- Aneurysmal degeneration of the internal iliac artery may result from infection, trauma, inflammatory or connective tissue disorders, and dissection.[6]

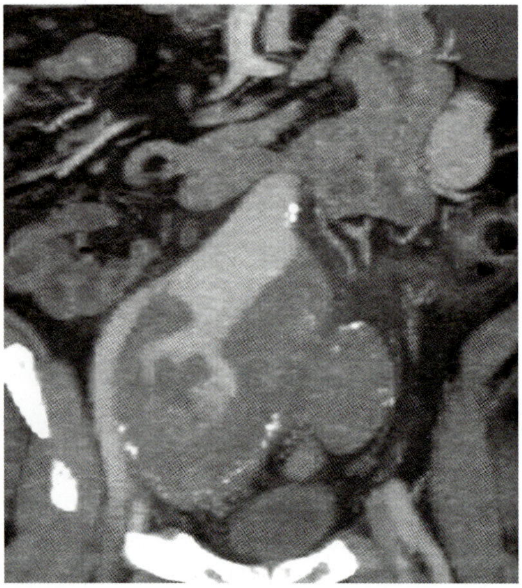

FIGURE 1 • Large right internal iliac artery aneurysm.

PATIENT HISTORY AND PHYSICAL FINDINGS

- IIAAs are difficult to detect on physical examination because they are situated deep in the posteromedial pelvis.
- Most IIAAs are asymptomatic and found incidentally on imaging.
- Symptoms may result from compression of adjacent structures including lumbosacral nerves, pelvic veins, and portions of the urinary or lower gastrointestinal tract and result in lower back, flank, or groin discomfort, as well as urinary changes. The nonspecific nature of these symptoms often delays diagnosis and treatment of IIAA. Less common presentations include renal failure, rectal bleeding from fistulization, constipation, lower extremity swelling, and deep vein thrombosis.[2,6]
- When IIAA present as rupture, mortality rates are high and reported at >30%.[6] Survival for ruptured IIAA is improving with endovascular treatment.[5]
- Data related to rupture risk and threshold for repair are limited to common iliac artery (CIA) aneurysms, with treatment indicated for aneurysms >3 to 3.5 cm in diameter.[4,5,7] This threshold can be extended to IIAA management as well.
- Repair is indicated for all symptomatic IIAA, regardless of size.

IMAGING AND OTHER DIAGNOSTIC STUDIES

- Although plain abdominal x-rays can detect heavily calcified aortoiliac aneurysms, the imaging modalities used to make the diagnosis include duplex ultrasound (DUS), computed tomography angiography (CTA), magnetic resonance imaging (MRI), and magnetic resonance angiography (MRA).
- DUS is an excellent screening and surveillance tool for asymptomatic aortoiliac disease; however, image quality can be limited by bowel gas and increased abdominal girth. Distinguishing common, internal, or external iliac artery (EIA) aneurysmal involvement may be challenging by DUS alone.[6,8,9]
- CTA, with 1-mm cuts, represents the "gold standard" for the diagnosis and anatomic evaluation of abdominal aneurysms and is essential for endovascular case planning. Contrast enhancement allows for comprehensive evaluation of luminal irregularities, relationship to other anatomic structures, and for the identification of impending or overt rupture.[9,10]
- MRI and MRA are highly sensitive and allow for detailed evaluation of aneurysmal disease without the use of ionizing radiation. Their use is limited for operative planning because they are less able to demonstrate aortic wall calcification.
- Digital subtraction angiography (DSA) is invasive and adds little to the identification and analysis of iliac aneurysms.

SURGICAL MANAGEMENT

- The goals of surgical management are to prevent death from rupture and maintain suitable pelvic perfusion.
- The majority of IIAAs are now repaired via endovascular methods[2] as traditional surgical repair can be challenging and fraught with pelvic venous bleeding complications.
- Endovascular repair is associated with lower operative morbidity and mortality rates and shorter inpatient length of stays compared with open repair.[3,4,11]
- Open surgical repair remains a reasonable option with excellent long-term durability for patients with aneurysm anatomy not suitable for endovascular repair, failed endovascular repair, aneurysmal compression of local structures, and/or the presence of an infected endovascular graft.

Preoperative Planning

- High-quality preoperative imaging is essential for precase planning.
- CTA, with multiple phases, is optimal for this purpose. Multiple phases allow for complete evaluation as precontrast phase provides information regarding vessel calcification, contrast images reveal luminal irregularities such as mural thrombus, dissections or ulcerations, and delayed phase images allow for endoleaks to be detected postprocedurally.[12]
- A combination of axial imaging and 3D postprocessing should allow for complete evaluation of the following:
  - IIAA diameter and length of proximal and distal landing zones
  - Iliac artery tortuosity and angulation
  - Presence and severity of associated occlusive disease
  - Ipsilateral and contralateral internal iliac artery patency
  - Status of the ipsilateral deep femoral artery
  - Concomitant CIA, abdominal or thoracic aortic pathology
- Determination of IIAA endovascular repair suitability needs to be answered at the start. Suitability is determined by pelvic perfusion, landing zone, vessel tortuosity, and access.
- The optimal method for endovascular repair of IIAA depends largely on the adequacy of pelvic perfusion. Preservation of at least one internal iliac artery, if feasible, is recommended to prevent future buttock claudication and erectile dysfunction.
- Spinal cord ischemia, colonic ischemia, and buttock necrosis can result from loss of flow to both internal iliac arteries.[2,13,14] If obliteration of perfusion to both internal iliac arteries is planned, a staged approach can minimize ischemic complications.[9]
- In general, landing zones are sited in nonaneurysmal arterial segments that manifest minimal angulation, tortuosity, and/or occlusive disease. The allowable diameter range for treatment may vary, depending on the device deployed. In all circumstances, reference should be made to the "Instructions for Use," or IFU, included in the package insert or available online.
- Device selection is based on the need for durable aneurysm exclusion and endograft fixation, accomplished with the fewest component pieces possible.
- If the patient is not an endovascular candidate, then a decision needs to be made on how best to manage the IIAA via open surgical techniques.
- Options for open repair include total internal iliac artery aneurysm inflow and outflow ligation, endoaneurysmorrhaphy, or aneurysmectomy with interposition grafting. Treatment option will drive operative exposure and extent of IIAA dissection.

Positioning

- Open surgical repair is typically performed under general or spinal anesthesia. The iliac artery can be accessed through a low midline/transperitoneal or a paramedian/retroperitoneal approach. Exposure will depend on the patient's body habitus, extent of the aneurysm, presence of concomitant AAA and/or CIA aneurysm, or if there are bilateral IIAAs.
- Endovascular repair can be performed under general, regional, spinal, or local anesthesia. For this approach, the patient is positioned supine, arms by their side, with both groins and the entire abdomen prepared and draped into the sterile field. The C-arm is typically positioned contralateral to the operative team.

OPEN SURGICAL REPAIR

- Exposure of the Internal Iliac Artery Aneurysm
  - Our preferred approach for open repair of a unilateral IIAA is an ipsilateral lower quadrant retroperitoneal approach.
  - A curvilinear, or "kidney transplant-type," incision is created with dissection through the skin, subcutaneous tissue, external and internal oblique muscles, and transversus abdominis musculature to the retroperitoneal space. Sweep the preperitoneal fat, peritoneum, and contents medially.
  - Note the psoas muscle, the iliac artery lies laterally. The iliac vein is posteromedial to the artery.
  - Utilize a Bookwalter or an OMNI-TRACT retractor system to aid in exposure.
  - Identify the ureter as it crosses over the iliac artery bifurcation. Avoid devascularizing the ureter.
  - Appropriately expose the common and external iliac arteries at the origin while avoiding injury to the underlying iliac veins.
  - If the operative plan includes total internal iliac artery aneurysm inflow and outflow ligation, endoaneurysmorrhaphy, or aneurysmectomy with interposition grafting, dissect medially and caudally to expose the outflow branches of the internal iliac artery.

Options

- Proximal Ligation: One of the simplest options for management of an IIAA is surgical ligation of proximal internal iliac artery. Unfortunately, this procedure is associated with a high recurrence rate with IIAA enlargement resulting from retrograde filling of the aneurysm sac.[15] Continued surveillance is needed for all IIAA treated in this manner.
- Distal Ligation: Distal ligation eliminates retrograde filling of a residual IIAA. The procedure can be technically difficult due to the depth of the dissection deep in the pelvis.
- Endoaneurysmorrhaphy: Involves proximal ligation of the internal iliac artery followed by opening of the aneurysm sac and ligation of the branch vessels from within. Endoaneurysmorrhaphy is used to treat proximal ligation failures.

- Aneurysmectomy: Maintaining perfusion to the distal internal iliac artery can be achieved with aneurysmectomy and interposition bypass. This option is generally applied for concomitant treatment of EIA aneurysms. Jump grafts can arise off of this bypass for EIA perfusion.[14] Transposition of the internal iliac artery to the external iliac artery has also been described.[13]

ENDOVASCULAR REPAIR

- There are various methods to perform endovascular flow interruption or exclusion of the IIAA.
- Proximal Exclusion:
  - In the setting of normal bilateral pelvic perfusion, simple stent graft coverage of the arterial origin of the IIAA is an option. Continued aneurysm growth is inevitable with this approach since the IIAA is still perfused via distal branches. Further IIAA treatment, especially for an enlarging IIAA, can be a challenge with this treatment algorithm.[2] Continued surveillance is needed for all IIAA treated in this manner.
- Proximal Embolization:
  - Coil embolization of the IIAA ostium carries similar risk and outcome as proximal exclusion.
- Distal Embolization with Proximal Exclusion/Embolization:
  - The preferred IIAA obliterative endovascular treatment option involves coil embolization or plug occlusion of the internal iliac artery branch vessels and/or the aneurysm itself. A stent graft is then deployed across the origin of the internal iliac artery (**FIGURE 2**).
  - Outflow vessel embolization with proximal exclusion is chosen in the setting of no adequate proximal landing zone for embolic devices. Proximal embolization is selected for adequate proximal landing zone for embolic devices.
  - Some interventionalists choose to fill the aneurysm sac in addition to outflow vessel embolization to decrease the risk for future endoleak. There are no studies to determine how prevalent or effective this technique is.
- Internal iliac artery preservation: Given the risk of associated ischemic complications with the above-mentioned techniques, several methods have been employed in attempt to preserve pelvic perfusion.
  - Iliac branch endoprosthesis:
    - While outside of the manufacturer's IFU, an iliac branch endoprosthesis (IBE) can be used to treat IIAA while preserving internal iliac artery flow. In these cases, a large internal iliac artery branch vessel is used as the distal landing target[4,16,17] (**FIGURE 3**).
  - Parallel stent grafts
    - For IIAA lacking an adequate proximal landing zone for stent grafting, a "chimney" or "snorkel" type graft can be extended from the internal iliac artery into the EIA or CIA. Alternately, a "sandwich" technique can be used, via simultaneous release of parallel covered stent grafts, to create an iliac artery neo-bifurcation.[2]
  - Hybrid Stent and Embolization
    - In the absence of a distal landing zone, a stent graft can be placed into the largest of the branch vessels after coil embolization of smaller vessels draining the aneurysm.

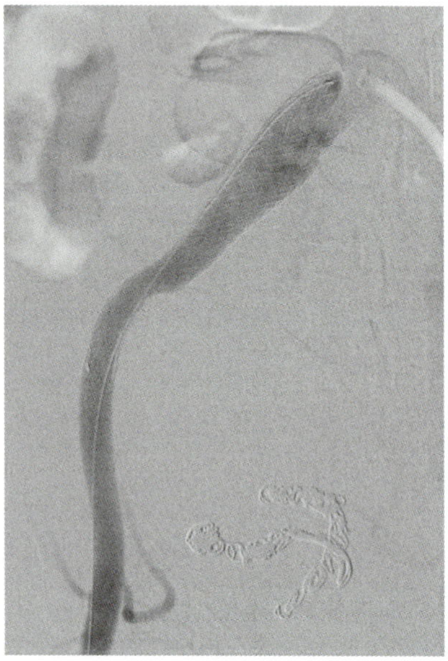

FIGURE 2 • Endovascular exclusion of large internal iliac artery aneurysm with distal coil embolization and proximal exclusion with stent graft.

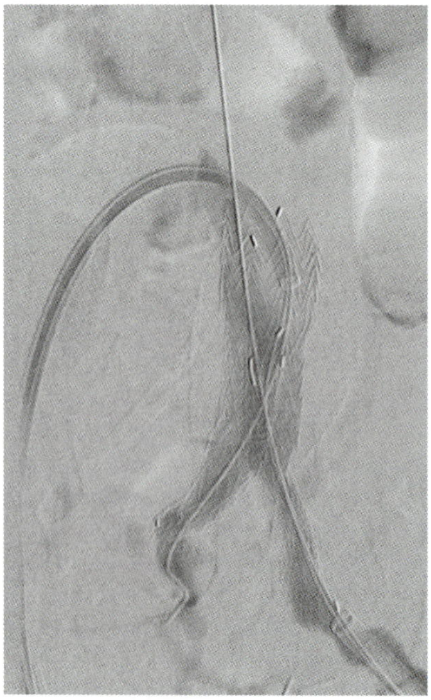

FIGURE 3 • Iliac branch endoprosthesis delivery for exclusion of left internal iliac artery aneurysm.

PEARLS AND PITFALLS

Open vs endovascular management	■ The preferred treatment for IIAAs is endovascular over open repair because endovascular repair is associated with lower operative morbidity and mortality rates and shorter inpatient length of stays compared with open repair.[3,4,11]
Preoperative planning	■ Determination of IIAA endovascular repair suitability needs to be answered at the start. ■ Suitability is determined by pelvic perfusion, landing zone, vessel tortuosity, and access as described above. CTA, with multiple phases, is optimal for this purpose.
Adequate exposure (Open)	■ The iliac artery can be accessed through a low midline/transperitoneal or a paramedian/retroperitoneal approach. Exposure will depend on the patient's body habitus, extent of the aneurysm, presence of concomitant AAA and/or CIA aneurysm, or if there are bilateral IIAAs.
Adequate access	■ Endovascular access requires suitable arterial access. Arterial suitability is driven by arterial diameter, degree of atherosclerotic burden, and vessel tortuosity. These parameters are typically outlined and driven by the device IFU.

POSTOPERATIVE CARE

- For endovascular treatment of the IIAA, postoperative care is similar to a standard endovascular aneurysm repair. Complete blood count and basic metabolic panel may be checked the following morning.
- Groin access should be checked routinely immediately after the procedure, the following morning, and prior to discharge. The duration for strict immobilization is driven by the arterial closure technique of the interventionalist. Oral intake is started immediately, the Foley catheter is removed, and the patient is encouraged to ambulate and discharged on following postoperative day.
- For open surgical treatment, both trans- and retroperitoneal approaches, diet can be advanced, and labs drawn in alignment with institutional protocols. Patients can be discharged when ambulatory, pain is well managed, and bowel function resumes.

COMPLICATIONS

- In general, morbidity and mortality rates are higher for open surgical vs endovascular repair of IIAA.
- Thirty-day mortality rates for both urgent and elective open surgical repair is 4% to 6% compared to 1% to 2% for endovascular repair.
- Hospital length of stay (LOS) is greater for open (5-9 days) vs endovascular (2-3 days) IIAA repair.[11]
- The main complication associated with open IIAA repair is bleeding related to venous injury. Other less common complications include ureteral injury, bowel injury, ipsilateral leg ischemia, and early graft thrombosis.
- Complications related to endovascular treatment include access site injuries, early graft thrombosis, and ischemia related to iliac artery occlusion.
- Graft occlusions to both the external and internal iliac arteries occur at significantly higher frequency with endovascular preservation techniques than with open surgery.[13,16]
- Complications specifically related to internal iliac artery occlusion include buttock claudication (30% unilateral, 40% bilateral),[13,16,18] ischemic colitis or ischemic bowel requiring surgery (0.5% unilateral, 1% bilateral), gluteal necrosis and spinal ischemia (<1%),[18] and erectile dysfunction (10%-15% of cases).[13,18]
- IBE with preservation of at least one internal iliac artery for the management of aortoiliac disease is associated with a notably lower (2%) rate of buttock claudication with 97% technical success, 7% reintervention rate, and <1% 30-day mortality.[16]
- Embolization of the internal iliac artery with vascular plugs vs coil embolization is associated with lower procedural time, total fluoroscopy time, and radiation dose when applied to EVAR (**FIGURE 4**).[19] Unfortunately, in the management of IIAA, it may not be feasible to use plugs alone to sufficiently embolize the distal branch vessels.[18]

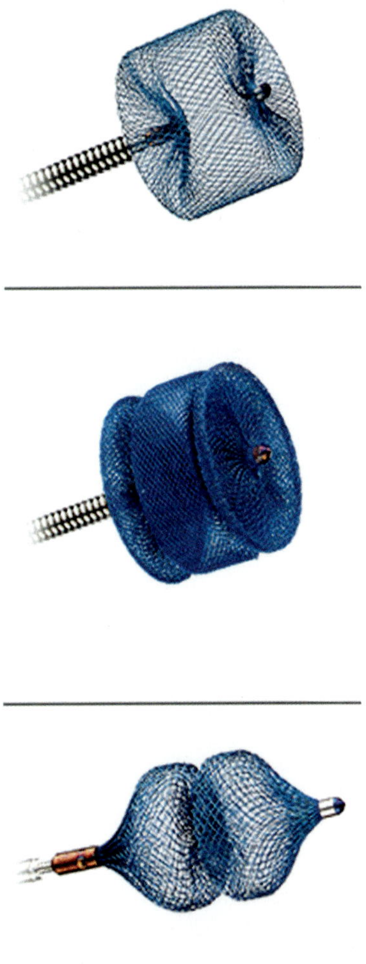

FIGURE 4 • Variety of vascular plugs used for vessel embolization. (Absolute Pro, Amplatzer, and Omnilink Elite are trademarks of Abbott or its related companies. Reproduced with permission of Abbott, © 2022. All rights reserved.)

REFERENCES

1. Johnston KW, Rutherford RB, Tilson MD, Shah DM, Hollier L, Stanley JC. Suggested standards for reporting on arterial aneurysms. Subcommittee on reporting standards for arterial aneurysms, Ad Hoc Committee on reporting standards, Society for vascular surgery and North American Chapter, International Society for Cardiovascular surgery. *J Vasc Surg*. 1991;13(3):452-458.
2. Perini P, Mariani E, Fanelli M, et al. Surgical and endovascular management of isolated internal iliac artery aneurysms: a systematic review and meta-analysis. *Vasc Endovasc Surg*. 2021;55(3):254-264.
3. Antoniou GA, Nassef AH, Antoniou SA, Loh SYY, Turner DR, Beard JD. Endovascular treatment of isolated internal iliac artery aneurysms. *Vascular*. 2011;19(6):291-300.
4. Wanhainen A, Verzini F, Van Herzeele I, et al. Editor's Choice - European Society for Vascular Surgery (ESVS) 2019 Clinical practice guidelines on the management of abdominal Aorto-iliac artery aneurysms. *Eur J Vasc Endovasc Surg*. 2019;57(1):8-93.
5. Laine MT, Björck M, Beiles CB, et al. Few internal iliac artery aneurysms rupture under 4 cm. *J Vasc Surg*. 2017;65(1):76-81.
6. Dix FP, Titi M, Al-Khaffaf H. The isolated internal iliac artery aneurysm—a review. *Eur J Vasc Endovasc Surg*. 2005;30(2):119-129.
7. Santilli SM, Wernsing SE, Lee ES. Expansion rates and outcomes for iliac artery aneurysms. *J Vasc Surg*. 2000;31(1 pt 1):114-121.
8. Freel KA, Nutley WK. Internal iliac artery aneurysm detected by sonography. *J Diagn Med Sonogr*. 2013;29(5):234-237.
9. Chaikof EL, Dalman RL, Eskandari MK, et al. The Society for Vascular Surgery practice guidelines on the care of patients with an abdominal aortic aneurysm. *J Vasc Surg*. 2018;67(1):2-77 e2.
10. Biancari F, Paone R, Venermo M, D'Andrea V, PeräläJ. Diagnostic accuracy of computed tomography in patients with suspected abdominal aortic aneurysm rupture. *Eur J Vasc Endovasc Surg*. 2013;45(3):227-230.
11. Buck DB, Bensley RP, Darling J, et al. The effect of endovascular treatment on isolated iliac artery aneurysm treatment and mortality. *J Vasc Surg*. 2015;62(2):331-335.
12. Lau C, Feldman DN, Girardi LN, Kim LK. Imaging for surveillance and operative management for endovascular aortic aneurysm repairs. *J Thorac Dis*. 2017;9(suppl 4):S309-S316.
13. Kouvelos GN, Katsargyris A, Antoniou GA, Oikonomou K, Verhoeven ELG. Outcome after interruption or preservation of internal iliac artery flow during endovascular repair of abdominal aorto-iliac aneurysms. *Eur J Vasc Endovasc Surg*. 2016;52(5):621-634.
14. Bacharach JM, Slovut DP. State of the art: management of iliac artery aneurysmal disease. *Cathet Cardiovasc Interv*. 2008;71(5):708-714.
15. Wilhelm BJ, Sakharpe A, Ibrahim G, Baccaro LM, Fisher J. The 100-year evolution of the isolated internal iliac artery aneurysm. *Ann Vasc Surg*. 2014;28(4):1070-1077.
16. Giosdekos A, Antonopoulos CN, Sfyroeras GS, et al. The use of iliac branch devices for preservation of flow in internal iliac artery during endovascular aortic aneurysm repair. *J Vasc Surg*. 2020;71(6):2133-2144.
17. Noel-Lamy M, Jaskolka J, Lindsay TF, Oreopoulos GD, Tan KT. Internal iliac aneurysm repair outcomes using a modification of the iliac branch graft. *Eur J Vasc Endovasc Surg*. 2015;50(4):474-479.
18. Bosanquet DC, Wilcox C, Whitehurst L, et al. Systematic review and meta-analysis of the effect of internal iliac artery exclusion for patients undergoing EVAR. *Eur J Vasc Endovasc Surg*. 2017;53(4):534-548.
19. Abbott C *The Amplatzer Family of Vascular Plugs*. 2021 [cited January 9, 2021] https://www.cardiovascular.abbott/int/en/hcp/products/peripheral-intervention/amplatzer-family-vascular-plugs.html.

Chapter 25

Aortoiliac Occlusive Disease: Open Surgical Management

Ashley R. Gutwein and Raghu L. Motaganahalli

DEFINITIONS

- Peripheral artery disease (PAD) is a condition that, due to atherosclerosis and chronic plaque accumulation, leads to arterial occlusion that results in diminished blood supply to distal arterial beds. Patients experience a wide range of symptoms from claudication to rest pain, nonhealing wounds, and gangrene.
- PAD is then further subclassified depending on the anatomical location of the atherosclerotic burden. In general, PAD is classified as aortoiliac, femoral-popliteal, tibial, or multilevel disease.[1,2]
- The Trans-Atlantic Inter-Society Consensus Classification (TASC) historically was used to help classify the anatomic disease patterns and recommend open vs endovascular therapy.[3] TASC has made way for the Global Anatomic Staging System (GLASS).
- GLASS evaluates the arterial occlusive disease of the entire limb as well as the presence of wounds and infections to help determine the chances of success with endovascular vs open treatment[2] (**TABLE 1**).
- When patients have the multilevel disease, treatment is first focused on treating the aortoiliac and femoral occlusive disease (termed inflow disease), followed by the more distal (or outflow) arterial occlusive disease.[1]
- This chapter will focus on open surgical options for aortoiliac occlusive disease.

DIFFERENTIAL DIAGNOSIS

- Several conditions can mimic vascular claudication. It is important to differentiate if the lower extremity pain is due to vascular occlusive disease or due to neurogenic or musculoskeletal etiology. A thorough history, physical examination, x-rays, and continuous-wave Doppler can help differentiate between arterial, venous, neurogenic, or musculoskeletal causes for pain.[4,5]

Table 1: GLASS Classifications of Aortoiliac Occlusive Disease

I. Stenosis of the common and/or external iliac artery, chronic total occlusion of either common or external iliac artery (not both), stenosis of the infrarenal aorta: any combination of these
II. Chronic total occlusion of the aorta; chronic total occlusion of common and external iliac arteries; severe diffuse disease and/or small-caliber (<6 mm) common and external iliac arteries; concomitant aneurysm disease; severe diffuse in-stent restenosis in the AI system
A, no significant CFA disease; B, significant CFA disease (>50% stenosis)

AI, aortoiliac; CFA, common femoral artery.
A simplified staging system for inflow (AI and CFA) disease is suggested. Hemodynamically significant disease (>50% stenosis) of the CFA is considered a key modifier (A/B).
Adapted from Conte MS, Bradbury AW, Kolh P, et al. Global vascular guidelines on the management of chronic limb-threatening ischemia. J Vasc Surg. 2019;69(6S):3S-125S.e40. Copyright © 2019 by the Society for Vascular Surgery and European Society for Vascular Surgery. With permission.

- Patients with aortoiliac occlusive disease may experience gluteal, thigh, or calf muscle pain. Symptoms are reproducible and occur with walking.
- Neurogenic claudication occurs with standing, does not require walking to bring it on, and can be relieved by positional changes. Use of spinal support while walking, such as a shopping cart or wheeled walker, may relieve the pain. Patients with neurogenic claudication may also have vasculogenic claudication complicating the diagnosis. Spinal imaging and ankle-brachial indices (ABIs) can help differentiate between neurogenic and arterial occlusive disease. It is important to understand the patient's symptoms and expectations before proceeding with any form of intervention.
- Venous claudication is described as a bursting type of pain that occurs after walking longer distances and requires a longer rest period with leg elevation. Physical examination findings of swelling and discoloration are often present. Once again, ABIs and duplex examinations can help distinguish the etiology.
- Pain secondary to osteoarthritis can mimic arterial claudication; however, the pain is localized to the joints, exacerbated by activity, and relieved by rest. X-rays and ABIs can help differentiate these two diagnoses.

PATIENT HISTORY AND PHYSICAL FINDINGS

- Patients with aortoiliac disease have up to a 50% risk of concomitant coronary artery disease with the same risk factors of smoking, hypertension, lipid abnormalities, diabetes mellitus, male gender, increased age, and family history.
- The disease burden in the internal and external iliac blood supply leads to a variety of clinical presentations, which is most notable for Leriche syndrome, which comprises the symptoms of buttock claudication, impotence in men, muscle atrophy, and absent or diminished femoral pulses.[6,7] Impotence as an isolated symptom in men should be evaluated for other possible causes. Impotence is only seen in 30% of men with decreased hypogastric perfusion as there are abundant collaterals from the mesenteric, profunda, and lumbar arteries.
- A physical examination will show a decrease or lack of femoral and distal pulses, although at rest the pulses may be present. More severe disease may present with extremity hair loss, coolness, decreased capillary refill, dependent rubor, as well as gangrene.
- ABIs are decreased but not generally below 0.5 to 0.6 unless the patient also has outflow disease.

IMAGING AND OTHER DIAGNOSTIC STUDIES

- Noninvasive vascular laboratories
  - Patients with aortoiliac disease will have decreased ABI with dampened waveforms of the common femoral artery indicating proximal stenosis or occlusion[7] (**FIGURE 1**).

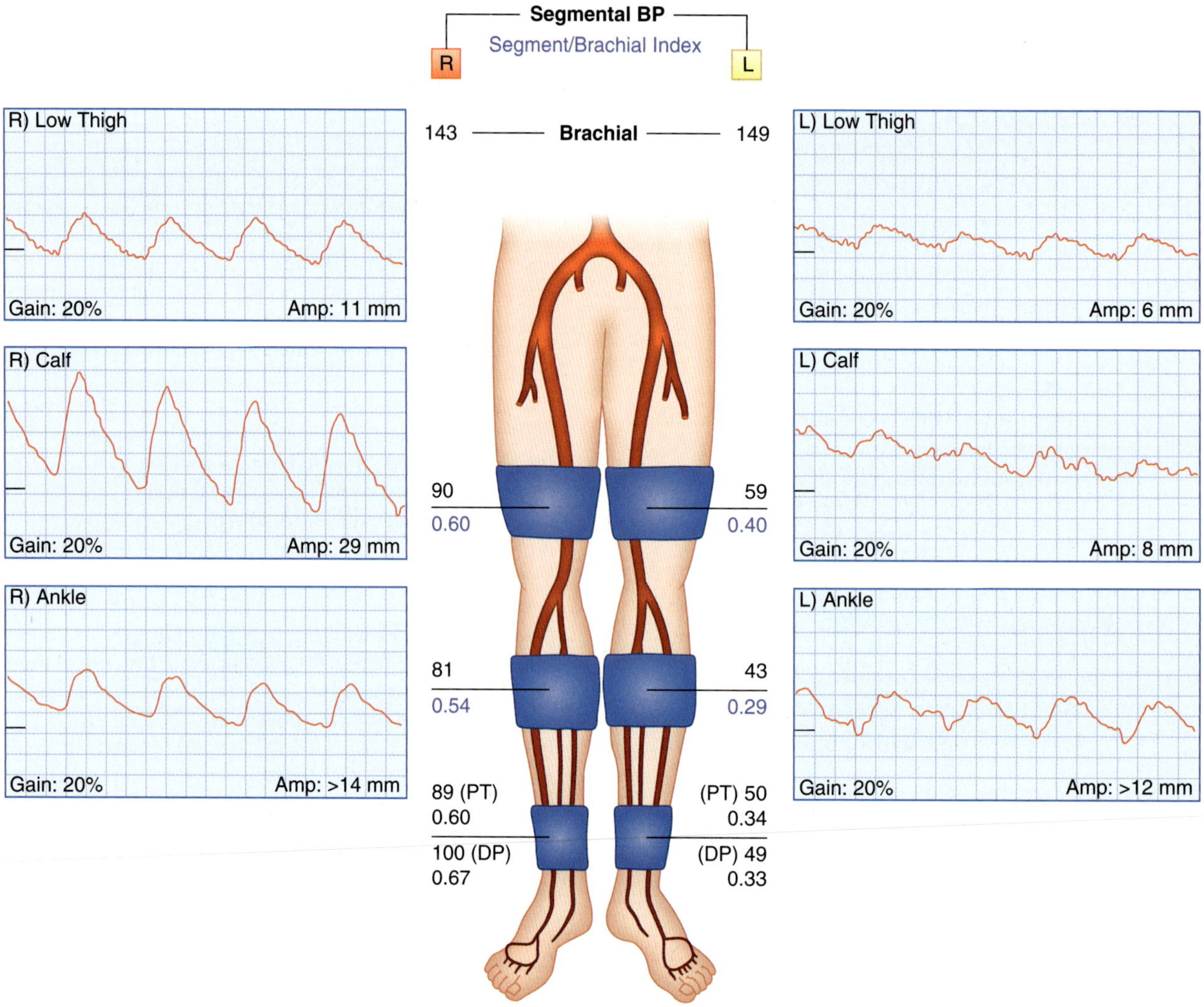

FIGURE 1 • Arterial waveforms showing monophasic waveform in both lower extremities with decreased ABI suggestive of aortoiliac occlusive disease.

    - If the patient has a normal ABI at rest, exercise testing should be completed. A drop by 15% of the ABI from resting value is considered significant and leads to diminished blood flow distal to the point of stenosis or obstruction during exercise.
    - Duplex ultrasound for the aortoiliac system is limited by body habitus and bowel gas.
- Computed tomography angiography (CTA)
    - CTA is excellent at estimating the degree of stenosis as well as the degree of calcification. It is often considered the noninvasive imaging study of choice for preoperative planning. It is important to evaluate the aortoiliac, femoral, popliteal, and tibial vessels.
    - CTA can help in deciding graft size, location of cross-clamping, enlarged collateral pathways to preserve, and operative approach (open, endovascular, or hybrid)[8] (**FIGURE 2**).
- Magnetic resonance angiography (MRA)
    - MRA often can overestimate the degree of stenosis, and the presence of stents and other metallic objects can interfere with imaging. Motion artifacts may limit the quality of the study.
    - MRA can be considered if the patient has a contraindication to CTA, such as contrast allergy.
- Arteriography
    - Iliac occlusion and diseased femoral arteries can make diagnostic angiography complicated and may require using a radial or brachial artery approach.
    - Arteriography does not always show the degree of calcification, which is important in operative planning.
    - CO_2 angiography may be the best option in patients with severe renal insufficiency.

SURGICAL MANAGEMENT

- The decision to proceed with revascularization vs medical therapy is based on the patient's symptoms. Claudication is generally treated medically while rest pain or tissue loss require revascularization.[4]
- Patients should be advised to quit smoking and start statin therapy and aspirin if tolerated.

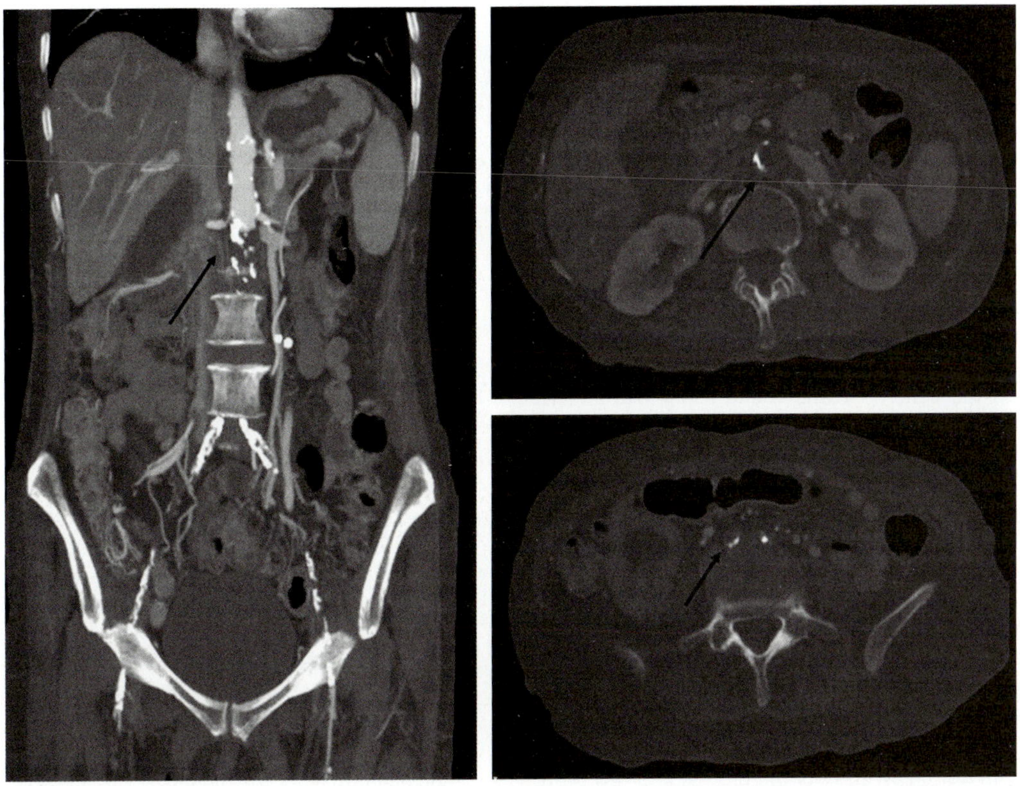

FIGURE 2 • CTA showing juxtarenal aortic occlusion at the level of the renal arteries including calcific plaques in bilateral common iliac arteries (*black arrows*).

- Preoperative anesthesia visits should include inquiries into cardiac, lung, and renal systems to evaluate overall operative risk as patients with PAD are at high risk for coronary artery disease, chronic obstructive pulmonary disease, and chronic kidney disease.[6]
- The decision to proceed with open vs endovascular interventions is multifactorial and depends on the patient's anatomy, comorbidities, and age, as well as the surgeon's experience.
- Patients with aortoiliac occlusive disease can be treated with either an inline direct reconstruction such as aortobifemoral or thoracobifemoral bypass. Extra-anatomic options include an axillofemoral or femoral-to-femoral bypass. In general, aortobifemoral bypass (AFB) is durable with excellent long-term patency, but if the patient is not a candidate due to comorbidities, anatomy, or prior abdominal surgeries, extra-anatomic bypass is a good alternative.

AORTOBIFEMORAL BYPASS

- The patient is prepared from nipples to knees with chlorhexidine preparation and draped with a sterile technique using skin-protective barriers.

Exposure of Femoral Vessels

- Exposure of femoral outflow vessels is the initial step in AFB.
- The inguinal ligament marks the transition point from the external iliac artery to the common femoral artery and is identified by connecting the anterior superior iliac spine to the pubic tubercle. The common femoral artery is located over the medial third of the femoral head and two finger breaths lateral to pubic symphysis but may be difficult to palpate in aortoiliac occlusive disease. Ultrasound can be used to identify the common femoral artery and femoral bifurcation to allow for optimal incision placement.
- There are two options for groin incision: vertical and oblique. A vertical incision over the common femoral artery and bifurcation allows for greater access to the proximal and distal vessels in extensive femoral artery disease that requires common femoral endarterectomy and profundoplasty. These techniques are discussed in Chapter 26. If the patient has no significant common femoral or deep femoral artery disease noted on imaging studies, then an oblique incision is better for cosmesis and wound healing. A transverse incision is made parallel and just caudal to the inguinal ligament.
- The subcutaneous tissue is then dissected with electrocautery with careful attention to ligate superficial crossing vessels to control bleeding and ligating lymphatics to prevent seroma formation. A self-retaining retractor is used to help expose the tissues and is repositioned as the dissection proceeds deeper.
- Once the fascia lata is divided vertically, the femoral sheath is identified. The femoral artery lies lateral to the femoral vein. Dissection is carried out cranially to identify the distal external iliac artery. Circumflex femoral veins cross the femoral artery just beneath the inguinal ligament. It is advisable to

ligate this venous branch to prevent inadvertent injury resulting in bleeding during the tunneling process. Circumferential control is also obtained of the inferior epigastric artery, circumflex femoral artery branches. These branches provide important collateral flow to the lower extremities and pelvis in case of aortoiliac occlusive disease. Progressing caudally, circumferential dissection of the profunda femoral and superficial femoral arteries is performed until a soft healthy portion of the artery is encountered and tagged with a vessel loop or moist umbilical tape using a right angle. All arterial side branches are identified and are controlled with vessel loops or temporary clips. The branches are rarely ligated to help preserve collaterals. The extent of femoral dissection depends on the patient's outflow, and if diseased adjunct endarterectomy may be required.

- Dissecting the femoral arteries before opening the abdomen minimizes the time that the abdomen is open. The groin incision is then packed with an antibacterial saline-soaked gauze to avoid desiccation.

Exposure of the Aorta

- A transperitoneal approach is routinely used to expose the infrarenal aorta, although a retroperitoneal approach may also be used depending on surgeons' preference and associated visceral arterial occlusive disease being addressed.
- For transabdominal exposure, a longitudinal midline incision is made from just below the xiphoid process to a few centimeters below the umbilicus or down to the symphysis pubis when iliac arterial exposure will be required. Subcutaneous tissue is dissected, and the abdomen is entered through linea alba between the rectus muscles.
- In a transabdominal approach, the transverse colon is retracted cephalad, and the small bowel is shifted to the patient's right side and packed in soft, moist lap sponges to the right. The ligament of Treitz is taken down and the duodenum is mobilized to the right. A self-retaining retractor is then placed to sweep the bowel to the right with a moist laparotomy pad. The retroperitoneal tissue overlying the aorta is dissected, and the aorta is exposed superiorly to at least the level of the left renal vein.
- Retroperitoneal aortic exposure offers the advantages of exposing the aorta at or above the level of the renal arteries. The benefits of retroperitoneal exposure include less postop morbidity and decreased pulmonary complications. The disadvantage of retroperitoneal exposure includes difficulty to expose the right femoral artery with difficulties experienced during the tunneling process. The risk of bleeding due to venous injuries also limits the use of this technique for AFB. These limitations could be overcome by limiting the extent to which the patient is positioned in the lateral decubitus position. The incision is made beginning at the tip of the 12th rib and extended toward the umbilicus. The Rectus muscle is not generally divided. Care is taken to prevent inadvertently entering the peritoneal cavity while entering the retroperitoneal space. Blunt dissection ensures that peritoneal contents are swept off the abdominal wall providing additional working space in the retroperitoneum.
- Preoperative CTA can help identify renal arteries anatomy, the position of the left renal vein, inferior mesenteric artery (IMA), and a portion of the aorta that is free of disease for clamping and sewing the proximal anastomosis. Manual palpation is also used to identify a portion of the artery amenable to clamping. Care should be taken to prevent circumferential dissection of the aortic neck in patients with a retro aortic renal vein.
- If there is a juxtarenal occlusion of the aorta, or if there is a need for an aortic endarterectomy at the level of the renal arteries or adjunct aortic endarterectomy is needed, then one should expose a segment of suprarenal aorta. The left renal vein is either ligated between sutures or mobilized by dividing the lumbar and adrenal veins. This will enable mobilization and control of the origins of the renal arteries, which are controlled with doubly passed silastic loops so that they may be occluded during endarterectomy to prevent atheroma embolization. Accessory renal arteries and the IMA should be identified and be evaluated if reimplantation is necessary.

Tunneling and Graft Selection

- Blunt finger dissection under the inguinal ligament and over the aortic bifurcation is used to make the tunnel. It is important to stay directly anterior to the external iliac artery and posterior to the ureter. The crossing vein off the femoral vein beneath the inguinal ligament must be ligated or carefully avoided. Moist umbilical tapes, Penrose drain, or red rubber catheters are fed through to the tunnels using a smooth aortic clamp to mark the tunnels.
- Aortic sizers and preoperative imaging are used to select the appropriately sized graft. Typically, a bifurcated polyester (Dacron) graft is used, although others prefer polytetrafluoroethylene (PTFE). Grafts range from 12 × 6 mm to 22 × 11 mm.

Proximal Anastomosis

- There are two options for proximal aortic anastomosis: end to end and end to side. Both are acceptable and have advantages depending on the patient's anatomy and surgeon preference. End-to-side anastomosis can preserve blood flow to the pelvis and is necessary when there is bilateral external iliac artery occlusion with patent hypogastric arteries and IMA. An end-to-end anastomosis allows an aortic endarterectomy of the proximal aorta as well as the renal arteries to be performed. This configuration has a decreased risk of aortoenteric fistula as it lies flat in the retroperitoneum; however, it does not preserve antegrade flow into the pelvis or IMA. Before aortic clamping, heparin is given intravenously. Typically, 100 units/kg is administered and allowed to circulate for 3 minutes with a goal activated clotting time (ACT) around 250. ACT is checked every 30 minutes and readministered as needed.
- If a patient has juxtarenal aortic occlusion (**FIGURE 3A**), both the renal artery vessel loops are placed on tension to prevent any embolic debris from embolizing into renal arteries at the time of clamping the proximal neck. Suprarenal clamps are placed followed by transecting the aorta leaving a stump to move the clamps down below the renal arteries soon after endarterectomy (**FIGURE 3B**). This will reduce the renal ischemia time and resultant postoperative acute kidney injury.
- If end-to-side anastomosis is planned a side-biting aortic clamp can be used. For the infrarenal aorta it may be difficult to perform an anastomosis using a side-biting clam without

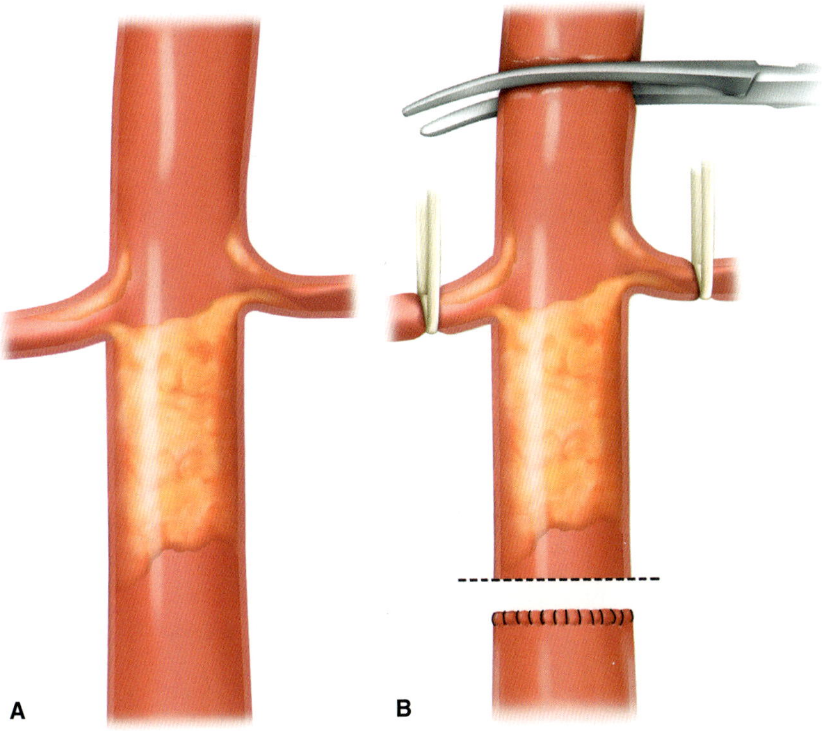

FIGURE 3 • Image showing juxtarenal aortic occlusion with stenosis of both renal arteries **(A)**. Adjunct aortic endarterectomy, renal endarterectomy with brief suprarenal control would be necessary to complete the proximal anastomosis **(B)**.

risking bleeding from the suture line due to the caliber of the aorta and thickness of the aortic wall. Hence the authors prefer using two clamps to occlude the aorta before aortotomy below the level of renal arteries. An appropriately sized graft is chosen; the graft is then trimmed and beveled. The anastomosis is completed using a running 3.0 polypropylene (**FIGURE 4A**). When there is need to preserve the flow into the internal iliac artery, one can also consider doing the distal anastomosis to the common iliac artery or to the internal iliac artery with additional graft limbs to the femoral artery (**FIGURE 4B**).

- If an end-to-end anastomosis is planned: The aorta is transected just distal to the renal arteries leaving sufficient length for anastomosis. If the aorta is heavily calcified, an aortic endarterectomy can be done to facilitate the proximal anastomosis. The graft is trimmed to leave the main body length of 3 to 4 cm, and a running 3.0 polypropylene is used for anastomosis (**FIGURE 6C**). Felt pledged sutures can be used if the aortic wall is thinned due to endarterectomy. If the aortic wall is thin, authors prefer to use interrupted sutures using a 4-0 Prolene to complete the anastomosis. One can also reinforce the proximal suture line with a sleeve of the Dacron especially if the aorta is of poor quality at the suture line. The distal aorta then is oversewn with a 3-0 Prolene. The graft limbs are then clamped, and the proximal clamp is then released to check for suture line bleeding. Repair sutures can be used for any suture line bleeding with 4-0 or 5-0 sutures on a pledget as needed.
- The decision to reimplant the IMA depends on the status of pelvic perfusion and superior mesenteric arterial collaterals. Traditionally, if there is no pulsatile back bleeding from the ostium of the IMA, then a reimplantation is indicated. If the IMA is occluded, then reimplantation is not indicated. However, reimplantation itself cannot prevent colonic ischemia (**FIGURE 5A** and **B**).

Graft Tunneling

- Using the umbilical tape or Penrose drain as a guide, an aortic clamp is then used to tunnel each graft limb from the abdomen into the femoral incision. The graft is then pulled gently through the tunnel above the external iliac vessels and below the ureter. Care must be taken to minimize kinking, twisting, and redundancy in the graft tunnels. Once tunneled the graft limbs are flushed to confirm adequate inflow, reclamped in the abdomen, and flushed with heparinized saline solution.

Distal Anastomosis

- The common femoral, superficial femoral, and profunda arteries are clamped, using the surgeon's preferred clamp, on healthy portions of the artery. Side branches are controlled by placing the vessel loops on tension. A longitudinal arteriotomy is then made with a no. 11 blade followed by Potts scissors. If there is significant common femoral or profunda disease the arteriotomy should be carried onto the profunda, and common femoral endarterectomy or profundoplasty performed if needed as poor outflow is a common cause of late graft occlusion. The graft is then cut on a taper to allow a natural reimplantation angle into the common femoral artery with minimal tension. The anastomosis is then completed as an end-to-side fashion with 5-0 or 6-0 polypropylene sutures in a running fashion (**FIGURE 6**).

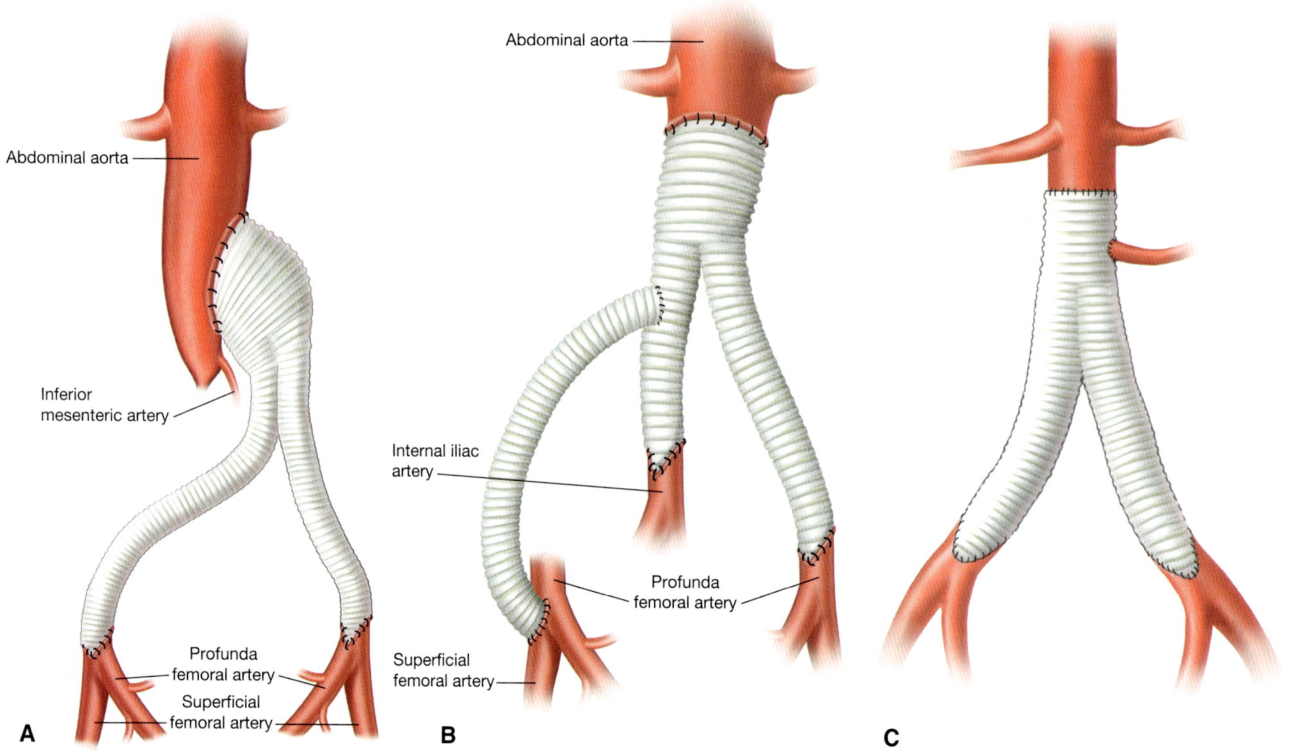

FIGURE 4 • Configurations for aortobifemoral artery bypass. End-to-side aortobifemoral bypass for patients with occluded bilateral external iliac arteries **(A)**. Frame **(B)** shows aorta to common iliac or to internal iliac bypass with an additional graft limb to the femoral artery. Both **(A and B)** techniques are designed to preserve pelvic arterial flow. Frame **(C)** shows aorta to bifemoral bypass with reimplantation of the inferior mesenteric artery.

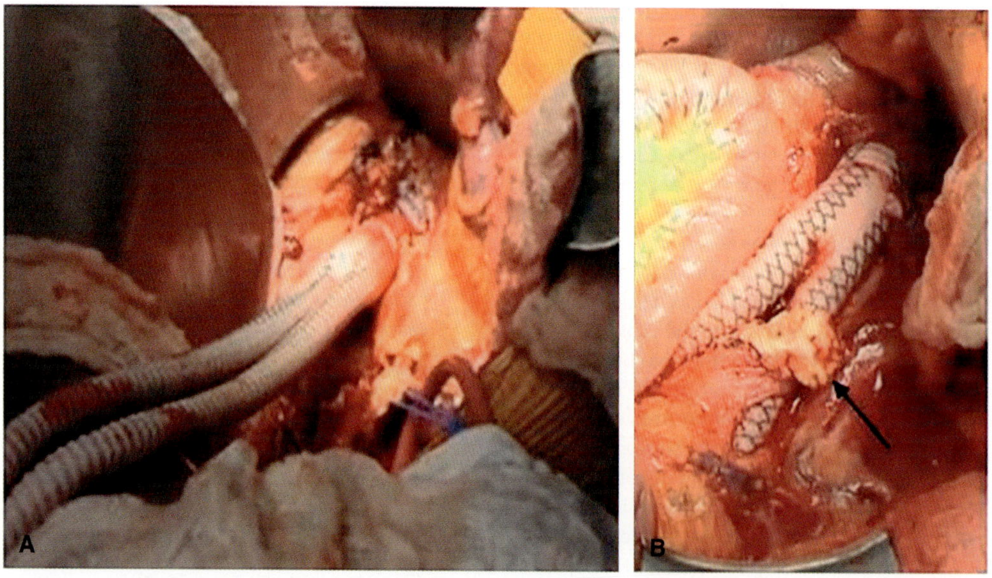

FIGURE 5 • Intraoperative image shows completion of the proximal anastomosis to aorta with end-to-end technique **(A)**. Frame **(B)** shows completion of the aortobifemoral artery bypass. *Black arrow* shows the inferior mesenteric artery patch ready to be reimplanted to the graft limb.

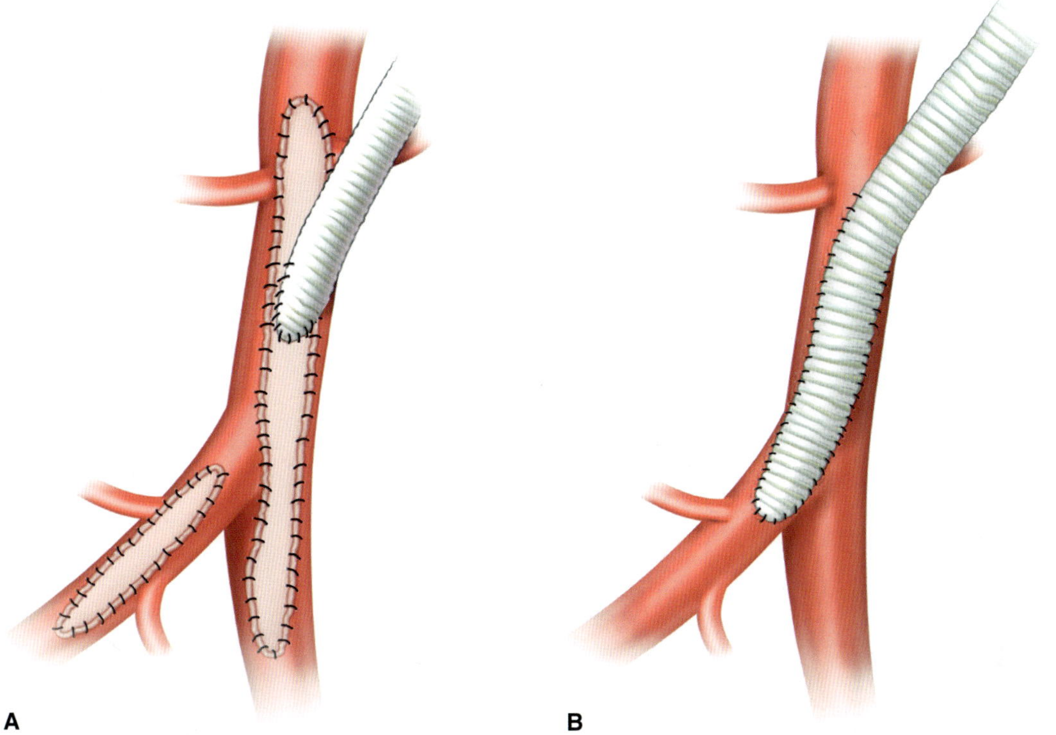

FIGURE 6 • Femoral artery reconstruction configurations. Common femoral endarterectomy with deep femoral endarterectomy, patch angioplasty, and reimplantation of the aortofemoral graft limb onto the patch **(A)**. Femoral endarterectomy with profundoplasty extending the hood of the graft onto deep femoral artery **(B)**.

The same procedure is completed for the contralateral limb. Graft limbs and native vessels are flushed and back bled before completion of the arteriotomy closure.

Closure

- Protamine may be given, depending on the time of the last heparin bolus or according to the intraoperative ACT reading. Approximately 10 mg is given for every 1000 units of heparin given, adjusted for time decay and the heparin half-life or can be estimated of the last ACT measurement. After adequate hemostasis is achieved, the groins are closed in multiple layers and the dead space is closed to prevent seroma formation and minimize groin infections. In the case of redo groin incisions, if tissue is not adequate for closure, a prophylactic muscle flap should be strongly considered. Groin complications can be catastrophic as they can place the graft at risk for infection.
- In the abdomen, the retroperitoneum is closed over the graft to prevent aortoenteric fistulas and the abdominal fascia is closed according to surgeon preference. In situations where the retroperitoneum cannot be approximated with ease, a tongue of omentum is brought into the infracolic compartment through the transverse mesocolon and placed over the graft to keep the bowel and the graft separated.[5,6]

Thoracofemoral Bypass

- If the infrarenal aorta is not suitable for clamping due to heavy calcification, or if there is extensive disease burden in the paravisceral aorta (**FIGURE 7A**), thoracofemoral bypass may be considered. In addition, in a patient with a hostile abdomen, making it difficult to gain access to retroperitoneum without risking injury to peritoneal contents, thoracofemoral bypass may be preferred.
- In general, patients undergoing thoracobifemoral bypass will need a similar preprocedure evaluation as for an AFB. One anticipates that patients can withstand single lung ventilation and recover from a thoracotomy.
- Preparation will include chest wall, abdomen, pelvis, both lower extremities up to the knee with the patient in semidecubitus position to allow access to the right femoral artery. As described earlier for the retroperitoneal exposure, one would anticipate some difficulty with the tunneling process specifically for the right lower extremity if the patient is positioned in true lateral decubitus position.
- The procedure involves the following major components:
  - Bilateral femoral artery exposure as described above.
  - Thoracotomy through the 8th intercostal space to gain access into the left hemithorax. The inferior pulmonary ligament is divided to allow mobilization of the left lung. Single lung ventilation is required at this point to expose the descending thoracic aorta. Care should be taken to prevent injury to the thoracic duct for complications of chylothorax. Once the mediastinal pleura is divided, the distal descending thoracic aorta is exposed.
  - The thoracic aorta is partially occluded with a side biting Satinsky clamp of appropriate configuration.
  - As described above, an end-to-side anastomosis is performed with 3-0/4-0 Prolene sutures. The suture line is examined for any bleeding before proceeding to the infrainguinal reconstruction.

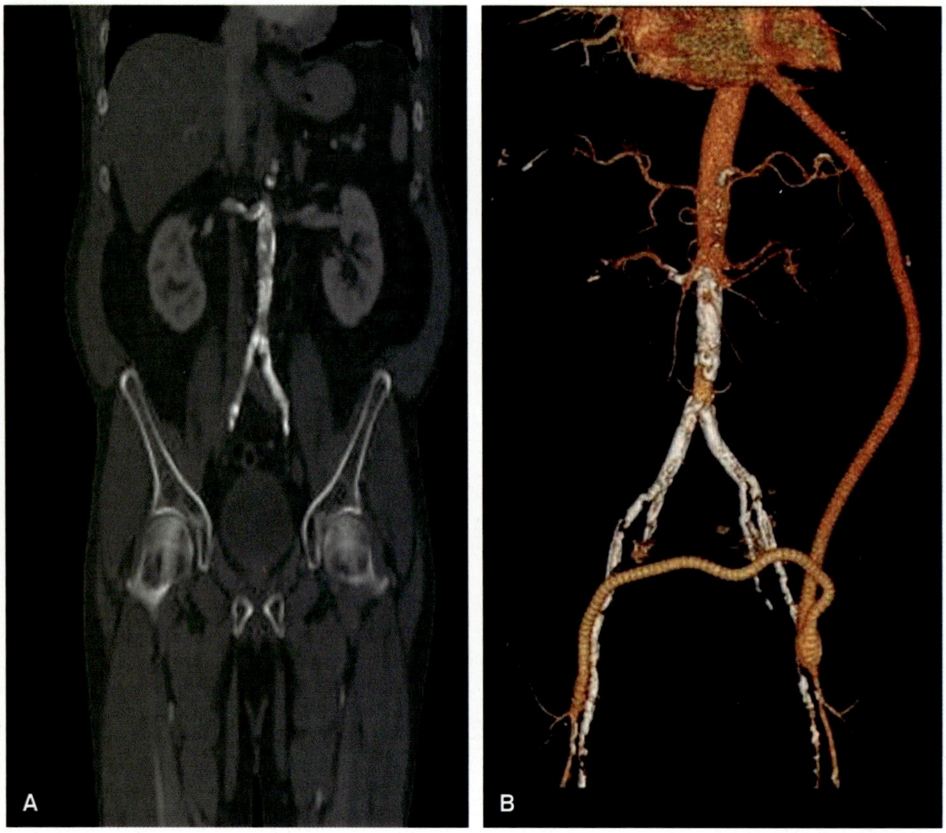

FIGURE 7 • CT Angiographic image shows heavily calcific juxtarenal aorta not suitable for placing a clamp **(A)**. Frame **(B)** shows a completed thoracic aorta to bifemoral bypass.

- The retroperitoneal tunnel lies behind the diaphragm along the posterolateral abdominal wall into the pelvis (**FIGURE 7B**).
- Typically, a 10- to 12-mm straight Dacron tube or an externally supported PTFE is chosen as the conduit. A femoral-to-femoral artery graft is then performed to revascularize the right lower extremity.
- A chest tube is placed in the left hemithorax to allow the drainage and removed at the earliest opportunity after ensuring adequate lung expansion. Wound closure is performed in multiple layers by approximating the anatomical layers with absorbable suture material.[8,9]

EXTRA-ANATOMIC BYPASS

Graft Configuration

- Depending on the extent of the aortoiliac occlusive disease and symptoms a variety of graft configurations may be used: axillofemoral bypass using commercially available PTFE grafts or axillounifemoral bypass using an 8-mm externally supported straight graft along with femoral-to-femoral bypass. **Femoral Exposure**: See section under Aortobifemoral Bypass-Exposure of Femoral Vessels.

Axillary Exposures

- Choosing the donor axillary artery: In general, patients will need an upper extremity arterial Doppler study including blood pressure in both upper extremities to look for pressure gradients before choosing the donor artery. The decision also depends on the presence of other prosthetic material, pacemaker, defibrillator, access port, prior radiation, dialysis access, presence of ostomies and fistulas, and coexisting conditions that would require thoracotomy in the future.
- The patient should be positioned with the arm abducted at 90° with a shoulder roll. The surgical field involves the upper arm, shoulder, chest wall, abdomen, as well as both lower extremities to the knees. A two-team approach is useful to limit the duration of the procedure in these critically ill patients.
- An oblique incision is made a couple of centimeters inferior to the middle third of the clavicle. The deep fascia is opened, and the pectoralis major muscles are split. Pectoralis minor tendon may have to be divided to obtain exposure of the axillary artery. The axillary artery is then dissected. There are often large venous branches that need to be ligated. Several branches of the axillary artery must be controlled to prevent back bleeding during the anastomosis.
- The anastomosis is performed to the first part of the axillary artery, which is medial to the tendon of the pectoralis major muscle. Anastomosis at this location generally prevents anastomotic disruption that may result from hyperabduction of the upper extremity.

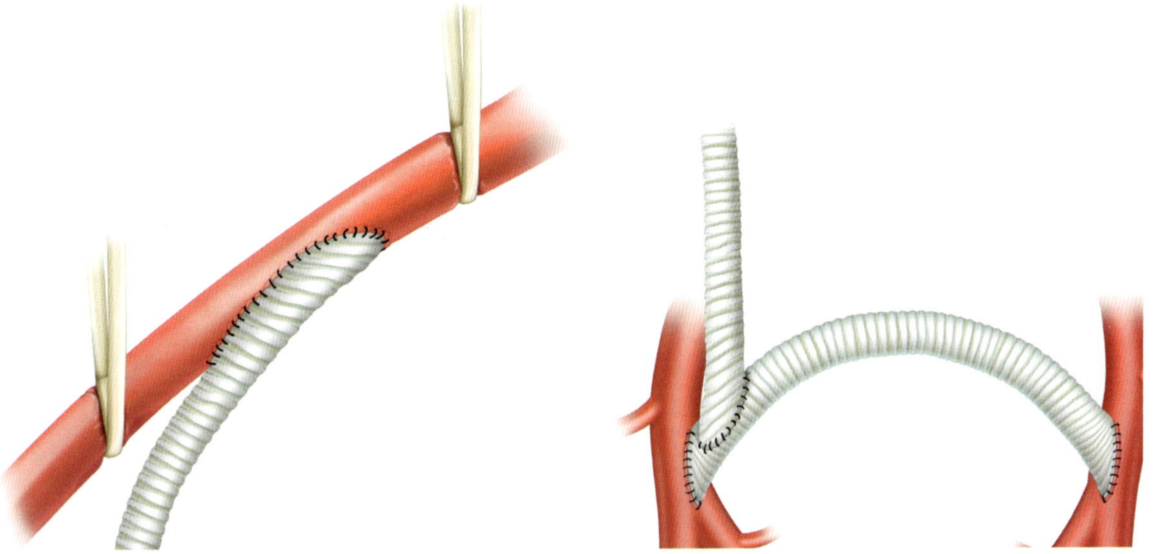

FIGURE 8 • Axillary artery to externally supported PTFE graft. Note configuration of the inflow anastomosis to axially artery **(A)**, axillounifemoral bypass and femoral to femoral bypass **(B)**.

Tunneling and Graft Selection

- For the axillofemoral bypass an 8-mm externally supported PTFE graft is typically used, and 6- to 8-mm externally supported PTFE is used for the femoral-to-femoral bypass. If planning an axillobifemoral bypass, there is a bifurcated externally supported PTFE graft available.
- The tunneling process differs if an axillary unifemoral bypass is planned vs using an off the shelf axillobifemoral bypass graft.
- The axillofemoral tunnel is started using blunt dissection from the axillary incision medial and posterior to the pectoralis minor muscle and groin incision medial to the anterior superior iliac spine. A long metallic tunneler is then passed between the incisions on the anterior lateral aspect of the abdominal and chest wall, anterior to the external oblique aponeurosis. Occasionally one may need a counter incision over the lower chest wall to facilitate the tunneling process.
- The femoral-to-femoral artery bypass tunnel is completed by using blunt dissection just anterior to the inguinal ligament. The tunnel is then completed in the suprapubic region just anterior to the external oblique aponeurosis fascia with a gentle large arc using blunt dissection. A long aortic clamp can be used to pass the graft from one side to the other in the subcutaneous tissue, avoiding entry into the peritoneal cavity.

Axillary Anastomosis

- After heparinizing the patient as previously described, the axillary artery is clamped. The arteriotomy should be made as medial as safely possible to avoid tension on the graft that could result in an axillary artery anastomotic disruption. An 11 blade is used to make the arteriotomy along the inferior wall of the axillary artery and extended using Potts scissors. The graft is spatulated and an end-to-side anastomosis is completed with a running 5-0 or 6-0 polypropylene. A gentle curve is then allowed before the graft takes a vertical course inferiorly (**FIGURE 8A**).
- After completion, the anastomosis is inspected for hemostasis before feeding the graft through the tunnel. Some redundancy should be left in the graft to avoid tension on the axillary artery, which could cause anastomotic disruption.

Femoral Anastomosis

- Similar principles described in the aortobifemoral portion of this chapter are used in the femoral anastomosis of extra-anatomic reconstruction, ensuring adequate outflow with the adjunct endarterectomy or profundaplasty in patients with extensive femoral artery disease.
- If planning an axillobifemoral configuration, an oval graftotomy is made on the hood of the axillounifemoral bypass for the femoral-femoral graft (**FIGURE 8B**). This is an additional anastomosis that is required if one is not using a prefabricated axillobifemoral graft configuration.

Closure:

- Protamine can be administered as described earlier in this chapter. Continuous waveform Doppler is used to evaluate the outflow arteries with the graft open and clamped. The groin incisions are closed in the same fashion as described in the aortobifemoral portion of this chapter. The axillary incision is closed first by approximating the deep fascia followed by soft tissue and skin.[10,11]

PEARLS AND PITFALLS

Aortofemoral reconstruction	▪ Adequate exposure is critical to success. ▪ Localized endarterectomy at both proximal and distal anastomotic sites is generally required. ▪ Tunneling errors can lead to both early and late complications with graft failure. ▪ The hood of the distal anastomosis should be placed onto the deep femoral artery to improve graft patency.
Extra-anatomical reconstruction	▪ Adequate inflow and outflow must be assured for success. ▪ Concomitant femoral endarterectomy should be used freely. ▪ Tunneling and closure errors frequently cause early graft failure. ▪ Axillary anastomosis should be placed as medially as possible to prevent anastomotic disruption.

POSTOPERATIVE CARE

- Patients are admitted to a cardiac monitored floor postoperatively as patients are at high risk for cardiac and respiratory disease.
- High-frequency neurovascular checks are needed to assess early graft thrombosis requiring reintervention or initiation of anticoagulation.
- Patients are encouraged to ambulate at the earliest once they have no bleeding concerns and have adequate pain control.
- When the abdomen is entered, in the case of aortobifemoral grafting, patients are kept NPO until bowel function returns while enhanced recovery protocols suggest early return to feeding.
- The decision to place the patient on antiplatelet and anticoagulation is based on the patient's comorbidities, and prior vascular procedure history.
- Patients should be seen in clinic immediately postoperatively and then 3, 6, and 12 months and then every 6 to 12 months thereafter with an ABI and graft duplex.[12]

COMPLICATIONS

- Early
  - Hemorrhage
  - Early graft thrombosis
  - Infections
  - Colon ischemia
  - Femoral nerve injury
  - Venous thrombosis
  - Abdominal or lower extremity compartment syndrome
  - Postoperative pneumonia
  - Acute kidney injury
- Late
  - Aortoenteric fistula
  - Graft restenosis, thrombosis of graft
  - Anastomotic pseudoaneurysm
  - Graft infection

REFERENCES

1. Bismuth J, Duran C. Bypass surgery in limb salvage: inflow procedures. *Methodist Debakey Cardiovasc J*. 2013;9(2):66-68.
2. Conte MS, Bradbury AW, Kolh P, et al. Global vascular guidelines on the management of chronic limb-threatening ischemia. *J Vasc Surg*. 2019;69(6s):3S-125S.e140.
3. Norgren L, Hiatt WR, Dormandy JA, Nehler MR, Harris KA, Fowkes FG. Inter-Society Consensus for the management of peripheral arterial disease (TASC II). *Journal of vascular surgery*. 2007;45(suppl S):S5-S67.
4. Conte MS, Pomposelli FB, Clair DG, et al. Society for Vascular Surgery practice guidelines for atherosclerotic occlusive disease of the lower extremities: management of asymptomatic disease and claudication. *J Vasc Surg*. 2015;61(3 suppl):2s-41s.
5. Menard M, Shah SK, Belkin M. Aortoiliac disease: direct reconstruction. In: Sidway AN, ed. *Rutherfords Vascular Surgery and Endovascular Therapy*. Vol IV. Elesvier; 2019:1397-1415.
6. Crawford R, Brewster D. *Direct Surgical repair of aortoiliac disease*. In: *Atlas of Vascular Surgery and Endovascular Therapy*. Vol IV. Elsevier; 2014:350-361.
7. Mylankal KJ, Fitridge R. Assessment of chronic limb ischemia. In: Loftus I, Hinchliffe RJ, eds. *Vascular and Endovascular Surgery: A Companion to Specialist Surgical Practice*. Vol. VI. Elseiver; 2019:13-35.
8. Crawford JD, Scali ST, Giles KA, et al. Contemporary outcomes of thoracofemoral bypass. *Journal of vascular surgery*. 2019;69(4):1150-1159.e1151.
9. Kalman PG, Johnston KW, Walker PM. Descending thoracic aortofemoral bypass as an alternative for aortoiliac revascularization. *J Cardiovasc Surg*. 1991;32(4):443-446.
10. Schneide JR. Extraanatomic repair of aortoiliac occlusive disease. In: Chaikof EL, ed. *Atlas of Vascular Surgery and Endovasular Therapy*. Vol IV. Elsever; 2014:362-372.
11. Schneide JR. Aortoiliac disease: open extraanatomic bypass. In: Sidawy AN, ed. *Rutherfords Vascualr Surgery and Endovascular Therapy*. Vol. IV. Elsevier; 2019:1416-1422.
12. Zierler RE, Jordan WD, Lal BK, et al. The Society for Vascular Surgery practice guidelines on follow-up after vascular surgery arterial procedures. *J Vasc Surg*. 2018;68(1):256-284.

Chapter 26

Aortoiliac Occlusive Disease: Endovascular and Hybrid Management

Shernaz S. Dossabhoy and Venita Chandra

DEFINITION

- Multilevel atherosclerotic occlusive disease involving the distal aorta, iliac vessels, and common femoral arteries is a commonly occurring pathology seen often by vascular surgeons. Traditional approaches to this disease process involved open surgical reconstruction with an aortobifemoral bypass or iliofemoral bypass. Over the past 20 years, however, there has been a paradigm shift toward endovascular and hybrid approaches often as first-line therapy. Combining femoral endarterectomy with endovascular iliac stenting is now a common minimally invasive approach to this problem, providing an effective alternative to open strategies with the potential of shorter hospitalizations and decreased morbidity. Compared to iliac stenting alone, proper evaluation of femoral disease and, if indicated, a hybrid approach with concomitant femoral endarterectomy has been associated with increased durability of endovascular aortoiliac interventions.[1]

PATIENT HISTORY AND PHYSICAL FINDINGS

- Aortoiliac and femoral occlusive disease can present, as with all peripheral arterial diseases (PADs), in a variety of ways.
- The typical presentation of aortoiliac occlusive disease includes claudication of the buttock and upper thigh and erectile dysfunction. When multilevel vascular disease occurs, as in the case of combined aortoiliac and femoral occlusive disease, distal lower extremity symptoms such as calf claudication, rest pain, and tissue loss may ensue.
- Typical physical examination includes the absence or diminution of femoral pulses. Other than the peripheral pulse assessment, the physical examination can demonstrate other signs of PAD such as cool digits and active wounds or ulcers, including more subtle findings such as shiny skin and lack of hair over the shins.

IMAGING AND OTHER DIAGNOSTIC STUDIES

- The initial evaluation of a patient with PAD should involve noninvasive evaluation of peripheral blood flow with arterial waveforms and ankle–brachial indices (ABIs) (**FIGURE 1**). These studies provide objective data regarding the extent of occlusive disease; however, they do not provide adequate anatomic data for preoperative planning.
- Once the degree and physiologic impact of the disease are determined by noninvasive testing, high-resolution anatomic imaging via either computed tomographic angiography (CTA) or magnetic resonance angiography (MRA) should be obtained for surgical planning.
- CTAs are currently the gold standard for preoperative planning. They have the advantage of providing information regarding the degree and location of stenosis as well as the anatomy of the arterial wall (including degree of calcification and presence of aneurysms). Three-dimensional reformatting can provide additional valuable information (**FIGURE 2**). CTAs, however, are limited by the fact that they involve the use of contrast as well as radiation exposure. MRAs avoid radiation exposure and contrast often, however, at the risk

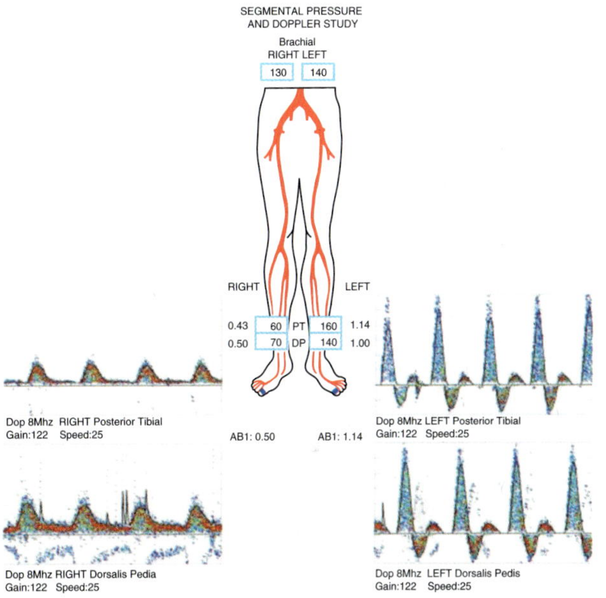

FIGURE 1 • Arterial waveforms and ankle–brachial indices for a patient with aortoiliac disease. Note the monophasic waveforms on the right.

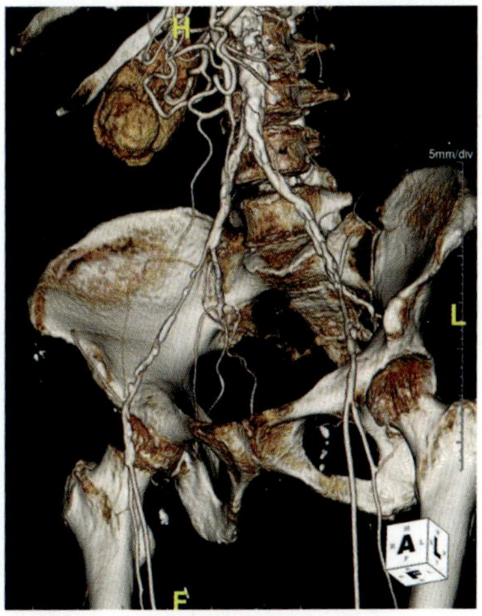

FIGURE 2 • Computed tomographic angiography with 3D reconstruction demonstrating diffuse aortoiliac as well as femoral occlusive disease.

of reduced anatomic precision. Gadolinium magnetic resonance contrast also entails risk of long-term renal dysfunction and nephrogenic systemic fibrosis.

- Catheter-based diagnostic aortography also provides anatomic data; however, it is an invasive procedure with potential complications. In addition, arteriograms only provide an understanding of the luminal anatomy, occasionally obscuring features such as aneurysms, inclusion cysts, or periarterial inflammation. Particularly for aortoiliac-femoral disease, preprocedural CTA identifies significant common femoral disease that may benefit from concomitant open endarterectomy at the time of catheter-based intervention. Alternatively, relying on catheter-based arteriography as the primary diagnostic modality may reduce overall contrast burden, radiation exposure, and need for additional procedures if common femoral level intervention is not required. In general, careful preprocedural physical examination and duplex imaging may suffice to help determine whether the additional cost and potential risks of CTA are justified prior to catheter-based intervention for aortoiliac arterial occlusive disease.

SURGICAL MANAGEMENT

- As with all patients with PAD, initial treatment approach should include comprehensive assessment and management of concomitant cardiovascular disease risk factors. Details regarding maximal medical management of PAD are beyond the scope or purpose of this chapter; at a minimum, however, consideration should be given to beginning statin and antiplatelet therapy prior to intervention, along with consideration of beta blockade and angiotensin receptor blocker or converting enzyme inhibitor therapy in selected patients. Patients should be counseled on risk factor behavior modification including smoking cessation, exercise or walking program such as supervised exercise therapy, and diet modification.
- Regardless of medical or anesthetic risk, however, all patients with critical limb ischemia should be considered candidates for revascularization when faced with potential limb loss. Major limb amputation above or below the knee is not necessarily a "safer" surgical alternative to multilevel hybrid revascularization for these patients. Indications for intervention for intermittent claudication are somewhat more complicated and controversial, however. The risks of a procedure are weighed against the potential gain; typically, only patients with severe lifestyle-limiting claudication who have failed nonoperative strategies are offered surgical revascularization.

Preoperative Planning

- Determining the anatomic distribution of disease is essential to obtaining optimal results. The imperative for precision imaging cannot be emphasized enough—if you cannot appreciate the full extent of disease, you cannot expect to comprehensively address it. As in all aspects of vascular surgery, the biggest disappointments, both during and after the procedure, usually arise from underestimating the extent of underlying disease.
- Historically, the Trans-Atlantic Inter-Society Consensus (TASC) II guidelines have provided a classification scheme based on anatomic patterns of disease (**FIGURE 3**).[2] The recommendations of the TASC II guidelines is an endovascular management for TASC A and B iliac lesions, whereas open surgical reconstruction is recommended for TASC C and D lesions in good-risk patients. Frequently, however, patients with multilevel disease as seen in TASC C and D lesions have more virulent atherosclerotic processes that often make them poorer surgical candidates. In addition, the development of an increasingly sophisticated armamentarium of endovascular tools and strategies is leading more and more vascular surgeons to attempt endovascular revascularization first, even for patients with TASC C or D lesions.
- More recently, the 2019 Global Limb Anatomic Staging System (GLASS) for critical limb threatening ischemia (CLTI) provided a simplified staging system for inflow disease (both aortoiliac and common femoral artery) (**TABLE 1**).[3] These guidelines recommend an endovascular-first approach for the treatment of CLTI patients with moderate to severe (eg, GLASS stage IA) aortoiliac disease.[3]
- Targeted perioperative risk assessment should be undertaken in appropriate patients, particularly in those with reduced exercise tolerance, known or suspected congestive heart failure, clinically significant pulmonary disease, exercise-induced angina, arrhythmias, or recent history of myocardial infarction. The presence of additional relevant comorbidities, including diabetes, reduced glomerular filtration rate, iodinated contrast allergies, thrombophilia or coagulopathic disorders, concomitant bacterial infection, or liver disease, should also be identified and, when present, evaluated.

Positioning

- Patients are generally placed in the supine position, either in a hybrid operating suite with fixed imaging capabilities or on a radiolucent table with a mobile imaging unit (C-arm) in a traditional operating room environment.
- Positioning should be arranged in such a way as to ensure adequate exposure of the entire aortoiliac and femoral vasculature, with room on either side of the patient to rotate the imaging unit to various angles to obtain appropriate oblique images. In angiographic parlance, in many important circumstances (such as identifying and protecting the origin of the ipsilateral internal iliac artery), "one view is no view."

Type A Lesions

- Unilateral or bilateral stenosis of CIA
- Unilateral or bilateral single short (<3 cm) stenosis of EIA

Type B Lesions

- Short (<3 cm) stenosis of infrarenal aorta
- Unilateral CIA occlusion
- Single or multiple stenoses totaling 3-10 cm involving the EIA not extending into the CFA
- Unilateral EIA occlusion not involving the origins of internal iliac of CFA

Type C Lesions

- Bilateral CIA occlusions
- Bilateral EIA stenoses 3-10 cm long not extending into the CFA
- Unilateral EIA stenosis extending into the CFA
- Unilateral EIA occlusion that involves the origins of internal iliac and/or CFA
- Heavily calcified unilateral EIA occlustion with or without involvement of origins of internal iliac and/or CFA

Type D Lesions

- Infrarenal aortoiliac occlusion
- Diffuse disease involving the aorta and both iliac arteries requiring treatment
- Diffuse multiple stenoses involving the unlateral CIA, EIA, and CFA
- Unilateral occlusions of both CIA and EIA
- Bilateral occlusions of EIA
- Iliac stenoses in patients with AAA requiring treatment and not amenable to endograft placement or other lesions requiring open aortic or iliac surgery

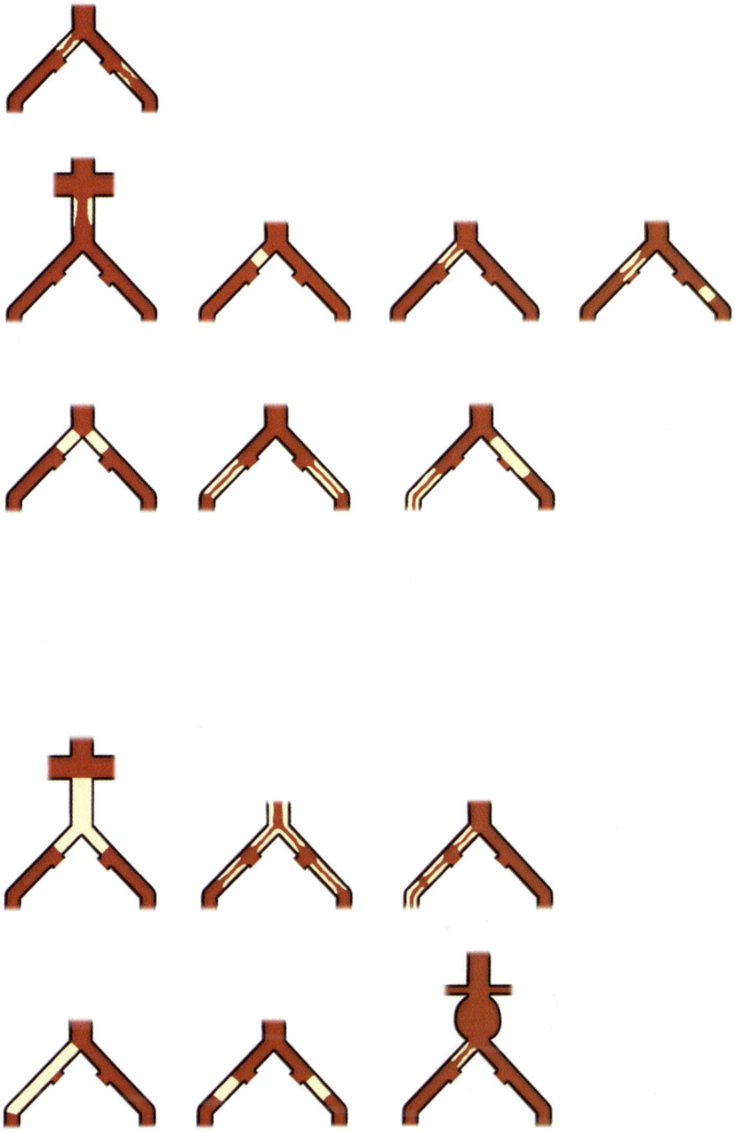

FIGURE 3 • TASC II classification scheme for iliac disease. (Reprinted from Norgren L, Hiatt WR, Dormandy JA, et al. Inter-Society Consensus for the Management of Peripheral Arterial Disease [TASC II]. *J Vasc Surg*. 2007;45(suppl S):S5–S67. Copyright © 2007 The Society for Vascular Surgery. With permission.)

Table 1: Global Anatomic Staging System (GLASS) Simplified Staging System for Aortoiliac Inflow Disease

GLASS stage	Description
I	• Stenosis of common and/or external iliac artery • Chronic total occlusion of common or external iliac artery (not both) • Stenosis of infrarenal aorta, or • Any combination of the above
A	No significant CFA disease
B	Significant CFA disease (>50% stenosis)
II	• Chronic total occlusion of aorta • Chronic total occlusion of common and external iliac arteries • Severe diffuse disease and/or small-caliber (<6 mm) common and external iliac arteries • Concomitant aneurysmal disease • Severe diffuse in-stent restenosis of aortoiliac system
A	No significant CFA disease
B	Significant CFA disease (>50% stenosis)

CFA, common femoral artery.

Adapted from Conte MS, Bradbury AW, Kolh P, et al. Global vascular guidelines on the management of chronic limb-threatening ischemia. J Vasc Surg. 2019;69(6S):3S-125S.e40. Copyright © 2019 by the Society for Vascular Surgery and European Society for Vascular Surgery. With permission.

FEMORAL ENDARTERECTOMY

First Step

- For extended femoral endarterectomy (often requiring exposure of the proximal deep femoral or "profunda" artery as well as the entire length of common femoral artery), optimal exposure is obtained via a longitudinal incision placed directly over the femoral artery (**FIGURE 4**). The inguinal ligament should be identified by palpation of the pubic tubercle and anterior superior iliac spine (an oblique line between these two structures is the typical course of the inguinal ligament) and used as a guide for femoral localization. Typically, the femoral artery is located approximately one-third the distance from the pubic tubercle to anterior superior iliac crest. Even when no pulse is palpable, a firm calcified linear mass can usually be palpated in this area. Alternatively, duplex ultrasound or fluoroscopic imaging may be used to ensure accurate placement of the incision. Failure to incise directly over the common femoral artery may increase risk for chronic lymphatic drainage, delayed or complicated wound healing, and femoral nerve or venous injury. Although oblique femoral incisions have gained in popularity, especially when used to obtain femoral access for proximal aneurysm repair, these often do not provide sufficient exposure as distal external iliac exposure is often required for a complete endarterectomy.
- The subcutaneous tissues are divided, ligating any lymphatic channels that are encountered. The inferior edge of the inguinal ligament is identified, and the common femoral artery is exposed through the femoral sheath as it exits underneath the inguinal ligament.

Second Step

- Full circumferential dissection of the distal external iliac artery (under the inguinal ligament), the common femoral artery, the superficial femoral artery, and the origin of the deep femoral artery and its initial branches are obtained sequentially (**FIGURE 4**).
- The individual arteries should be assessed for areas of calcification and extensive plaque burden. Soft sections with minimal calcification, or plaque limited to the posterior arterial wall, should be identified for consideration of clamp placement as appropriate for the planned procedure.
- The inguinal ligament may be divided for adequate exposure of the distal external iliac artery when necessary to ensure adequate endarterectomy. When considering the relative margin of distal endarterectomy vs proximal stent placement, it is important to avoid stent placement across the inguinal ligament, as this may greatly reduce long-term patency of the procedure as well as complicate stent delivery through an ipsilateral retrograde sheath. In general, operators should err of the side of more extensive proximal endarterectomies as opposed to distal extension of external iliac stents.
- Careful ligation of the circumflex iliac vein as it crosses over the external iliac artery under the inguinal ligament should be considered to prevent accidental tearing of the vessel during clamping.
- External iliac collaterals, like the epigastric artery or circumflex iliac artery, should be preserved during dissection and endarterectomy whenever possible to ensure optimal long-term outcome.

Third Step

- Once exposure is complete, the common femoral artery can be punctured under direct visualization with advancement of a wire under fluoroscopic guidance across the iliac lesion (**FIGURE 5**).

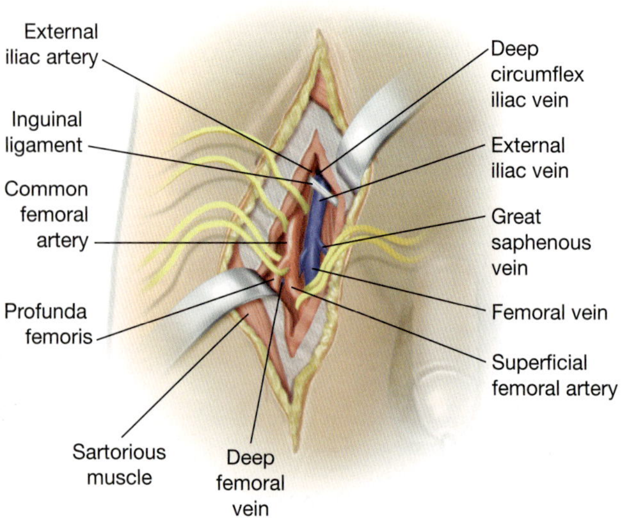

FIGURE 4 • Typical longitudinal femoral artery exposure and anatomy. CFA, common femoral artery; DCIV, deep circumflex iliac vein; EIA, external iliac artery; EIV, external iliac vein; GSV, greater saphenous vein; SFA, superficial femoral artery.

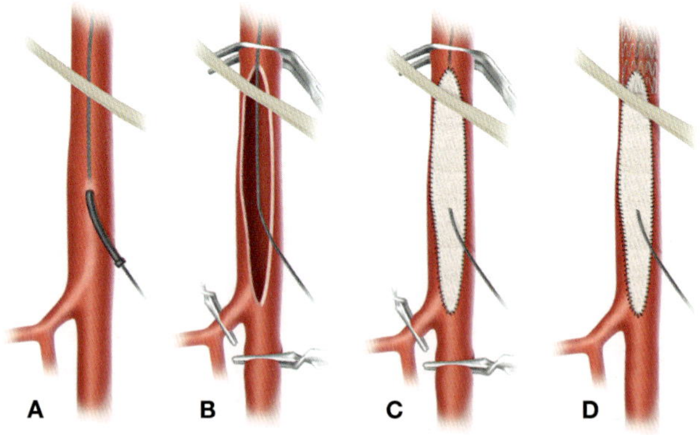

FIGURE 5 • Technique for concurrent femoral endarterectomy and iliac stenting. **A,** Direct puncture of common femoral artery and advancement of wire under fluoroscopic guidance. **B,** With wire across iliac lesion, clamp proximal and distal end proceed with arteriotomy. **C,** After endarterectomy, patch is sewn in. Prior to completion of patch center, the distal portion of the patch is punctured with an 18-gauge needle and the wire is passed through the patch. **D,** After completion of the patch, flow is restored and a sheath can be advanced over the wire and iliac stenting can proceed. For patients with distal external iliac disease, the iliac stents can be carried down into the proximal portion of the endarterectomy and patch.

- This approach eliminates the possibility of creating a retrograde dissection when a wire is passed after the endarterectomy is performed, as well as the need to puncture the endarterectomy patch to gain access.
- If the disease burden is confined to the common iliac artery or only the proximal external iliac artery, then iliac stenting can proceed at this point, prior to proceeding with the endarterectomy. Occasionally, however, the amount of femoral disease burden is so great that the sheath will be occlusive or otherwise impair runoff, which may limit the ability to obtain digital subtraction angiography images during or after stent placement. Therefore, consideration should be given to initial endarterectomy depending on individual anatomic circumstances.
- When retrograde wire passage is not possible due to extensive proximal plaque burden, tortuosity, or other anatomic considerations, antegrade passage from the contralateral iliofemoral system (obtained via either percutaneous or open femoral access) or left axillary or brachial access may be attempted. Importantly, longer sheath/catheter/guidewire combinations will be needed for these procedures and positioning considerations will be affected as well (eg, arm will need to be exposed and prepped on a radiolucent surface). Once antegrade wire access is accomplished, this may be used to deliver treatment devices directly or snared and externalized through the ipsilateral femoral access for retrograde intervention as originally planned.

Fourth Step

- Leaving the wire in place, the patient is systemically heparinized, and proximal and distal femoral control is obtained with vascular clamps. Especially proximally, a padded clamp (eg, Fogarty Hydragrip) should be chosen to allow the external iliac artery to be clamped over the existing wire to prevent or minimize wire-related injury.
- A longitudinal common femoral arteriotomy is performed to expose the full extent of femoral disease that needs to be addressed to ensure adequate runoff from the iliac intervention. A single femoral incision for the femoral endarterectomy is often sufficient to achieve adequate outflow; however, additional distal femoral bypass procedures may be required if extensive forefoot gangrene is present, which is often a consequence of multilevel arterial occlusive disease. Extended deep femoral endarterectomy is highly effective in achieving suitable runoff when few other revascularization options may be available (**FIGURE 4**).
- The arteriotomy can extend onto either the superficial or deep femoral artery. Occasionally, an eversion endarterectomy of the deep femoral artery can be performed when the arteriotomy extends onto the superficial femoral artery. Alternatively, the arteriotomy may be extended down the deep femoral artery when the superficial femoral artery is chronically occluded. Selection of the reconstruction technique is influenced by the occlusive pathology, level of debility, indications for revascularization, and optimal revascularization strategy (**FIGURE 6**).

Fifth Step

- Carefully, an endarterectomy plane is developed between the plaque and remaining mural media or adventitia using a Penfield dissector or Beaver blade. The plane most typically is developed within or exterior to the media, leaving the adventitia intact. Failure to appreciate the appropriate endarterectomy plane may weaken the adventitia, leading to bleeding or postoperative hematoma or pseudoaneurysm formation. Care should be taken to dissect the plaque away from the remaining arterial wall, not vice versa. The endarterectomy plane is developed on each side of the vessel and advanced posteriorly until the planes meet in the midline. Following this maneuver, the plaque is transected flush with

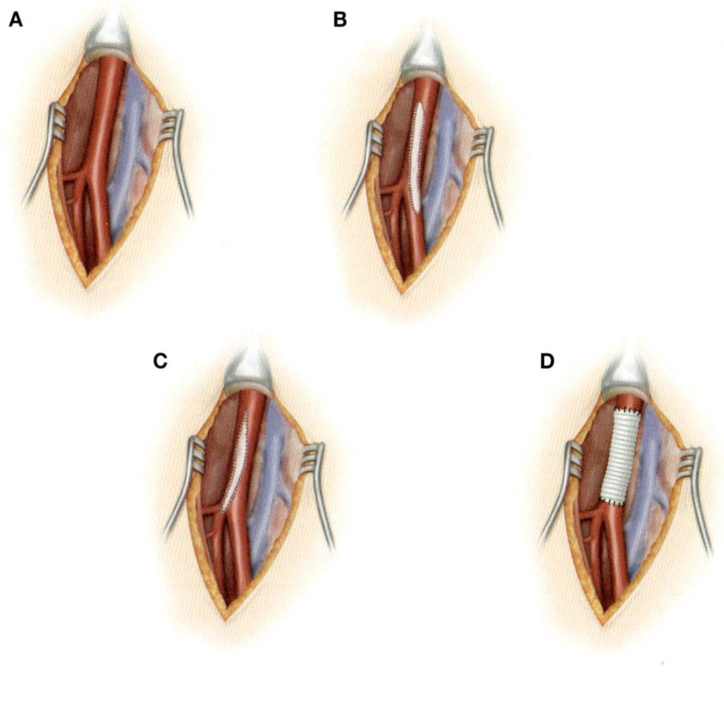

FIGURE 6 • Various femoral endarterectomy closure strategies. **A,** Typical anatomy; occasionally, primary repair, can be considered if common femoral artery is of adequate size. **B,** Arteriotomy and patch extended onto superficial femoral artery; deep femoral artery endarterectomy can be performed using an eversion technique. **C,** Arteriotomy and patch extended onto deep femoral artery. Particularly useful in chronically occluded superficial femoral artery (SFA). **D,** Interposition repair of common femoral artery; can syndactylize deep femoral artery and SFA if needed.

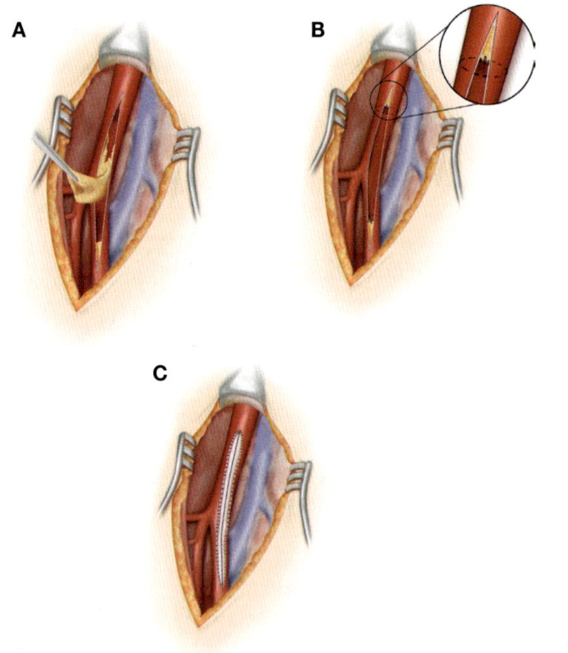

FIGURE 7 • Femoral endarterectomy technique. **A,** Longitudinal arteriotomy and development of endarterectomy plane. **B,** Ensure adequate endpoints on either end. **C,** Patch closure.

the arterial wall. Care should be taken to achieve good quality and minimally diseased endpoints in both the superficial and deep femoral arteries as necessary (**FIGURE 7**). Tacking sutures, as commonly employed during carotid endarterectomy, may also be necessary in the femoral artery to ensure adequate endpoints. Particularly in the case of the deep femoral artery, care should be taken to extend the endarterectomy well past the mass of common femoral artery–related plaque. This may require exposing the deep femoral artery well beyond its initial branches, dividing crossing branches of the deep femoral vein, and avoiding excessively deep placement of self-retaining retractors to limit the possibility of traction injury to femoral nerve branches.

- Often, significant posterior plaque extends proximally into the external iliac arteries. As previously discussed, care should be taken in deciding at which point the endarterectomy should end vs distal extension of iliac stents (**FIGURE 5**).

Sixth Step

- Once the full extent of plaque has been removed and suitable irrigation performed to identify and eliminate remaining mobile fragments of residual media, patch angioplasty should be performed typically using running 5-0 polypropylene suture initiated at both the proximal and distal endpoints and tied in the middle. Bovine pericardium, extruded polytetrafluoroethylene (ePTFE), and polyester or autogenous vein segments all may represent reasonable patch options, depending on individual circumstances. In general, autogenous vein is more resistant to infection, whereas prosthetic patch options are available off the shelf in a variety of configurations. ePTFE patches tend to bleed more through their suture holes following placement, although this tendency may be tempered by use of ePTFE sutures. Currently, our preference is to use bovine pericardial patch as the default choice in the absence of infection or other contraindication (eg, patient objection due to religious reasons) (**FIGURE 6**).
- Rarely, when arterial wall integrity appears compromised following endarterectomy, femoral interposition grafting may be performed in lieu of patch angioplasty. Interposition grafting may also be a good choice when the femoral plaque burden is so great that endarterectomy is impractical; in this case, an interposition graft (ePTFE or knitted polyester) can be placed instead of a patch. This can be configured in any number of ways:
    - Distal anastomosis to distal common femoral artery
    - Distal anastomosis to syndactylized superficial and deep femoral arteries (**FIGURE 6**)
    - Distal anastomosis to superficial femoral artery with reimplantation of the deep femoral artery
    - Distal anastomosis to the deep femoral artery with reimplantation of superficial femoral artery
    - Distal anastomosis to the deep femoral artery only, when the superficial femoral artery is already occluded

Seventh Step

- Before completion of patch closure, the middle or distal portion of the patch is punctured with an 18-gauge needle and the back of the previously placed wire is routed through the needle. Patch closure is then completed and the clamps are removed; at this point, an appropriately sized sheath can be advanced over the wire, through the patch, in preparation for iliac stenting.

COMMON ILIAC STENTING

First Step

- Typically, a 6-Fr or 7-Fr sheath is adequate for iliac stenting. Once the sheath is placed after completion of the patch, appropriate arteriogram images are obtained.
- For distal aorta and proximal common iliac disease, often the best approach is passage of a flush catheter into the aorta and a power-injected aortogram.
- For primarily iliac disease, retrograde arteriography through the femoral sheath is usually sufficient to obtain adequate iliac opacification.
- Contralateral anterior oblique (15°-30°) projections are typically chosen for visualization of the respective iliac systems to ensure identification of the origin of the ipsilateral internal iliac arteries. Also, the full extent of disease burden may be most adequately addressed by multiple obliquities in any circumstance.
- A marking catheter may be used to assist in length measurements and "buddy" wires may also be placed from contralateral femoral access. Every effort should be made to maintain perfusion to the hypogastric arteries.

Second Step

- Selection of the appropriate balloon and stent diameter for the common iliac arteries is crucial. Slight oversizing of 5% to 10% is recommended, except in the case of heavily calcified lesions, where oversizing may increase the risk of arterial rupture.
- Optimal target vessel diameter can be estimated preoperatively from CTA measurements based on the diameter of adjacent or contralateral nondiseased arterial segments and confirmed intraoperatively during the hybrid procedure itself. Common iliac artery target diameters range from 7 to 10 mm while external iliac artery diameters range from 5 to 8 mm with both depending on patient gender, body habitus, and burden of disease.
- Balloon "predilation" may facilitate stent placement and assist with stent sizing.
- Mild pain during dilation is to be anticipated and indicates stretching of the adventitia; excessive or persistent pain, however, may indicate arterial compromise or rupture. In the latter circumstance, consideration should be given to additional placement of a covered stent when contrast extravasation is present on arteriography and not immediately controlled with extended balloon deployment. In the retroperitoneum, unlike the lower extremities, tamponade will not likely limit further bleeding and extended balloon deployment may not be advisable as definitive treatment. When general anesthesia is required for the concomitant endarterectomy, this warning sign may not be present and completion arteriography should be closely examined for indications of iliac artery disruption or contrast extravasation.
- There are numerous commercially available stents, with some specifically indicated for iliac arterial intervention (eg, "on label") (TABLE 2). Appropriate diameter and length stents generally fall into two categories, balloon-expandable or self-expanding, and can be covered or uncovered (eg, with adherent graft material).

Table 2: Various Stent Options for Treating Aortoiliac Disease[a]

	Balloon-expandable	Self-expanding
Covered	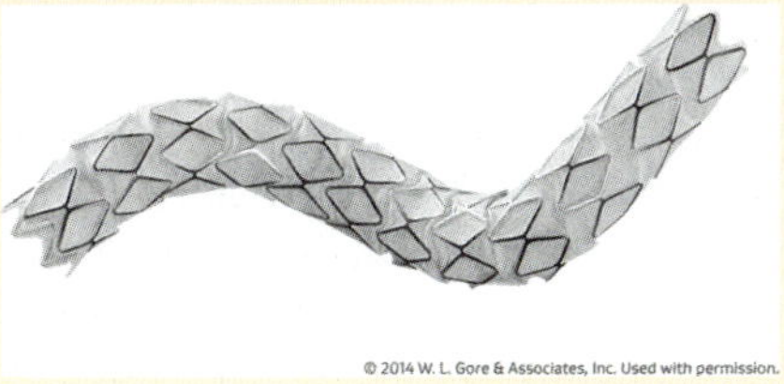 GORE® VIABAHN® VBX Balloon Expandable. See Instructions for Use for complete device information, including approved indications and safety information. (Copyright © 2014 W. L. Gore & Associates, Inc. Used with permission) Lifestream™ Balloon Expandable Vascular Covered Stent (Bard Peripheral Vascular Inc., Tempe, Ariz) iCAST (Atrium Medical, Hudson, NH)[a]	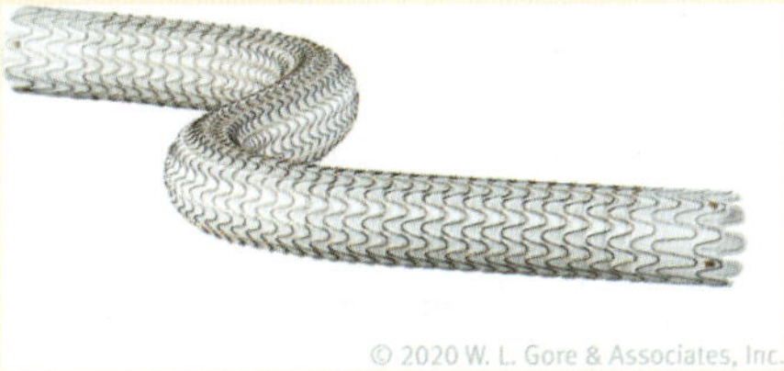 GORE® VIABAHN® Endoprosthesis. See Instructions for Use for complete device information, including approved indications and safety information. (Copyright © 2020 W. L. Gore & Associates, Inc. Used with permission.)

(Continued)

Table 2: Various Stent Options for Treating Aortoiliac Disease[a] (Continued)

	Balloon-expandable	Self-expanding
Uncovered (Bare metal)	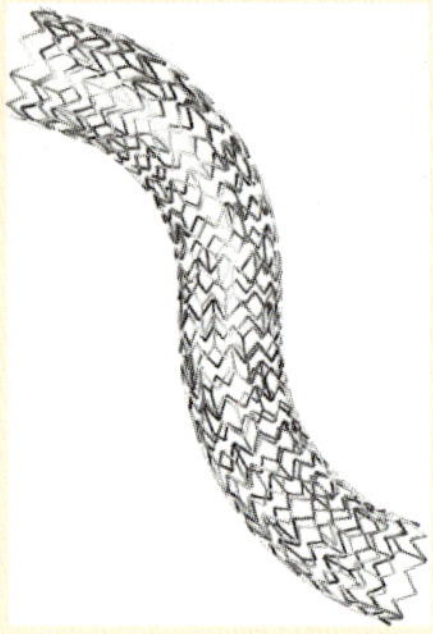 Image provided courtesy of Boston Scientific. Copyright © 2022 Boston Scientific Corporation or its affiliates. All rights reserved.	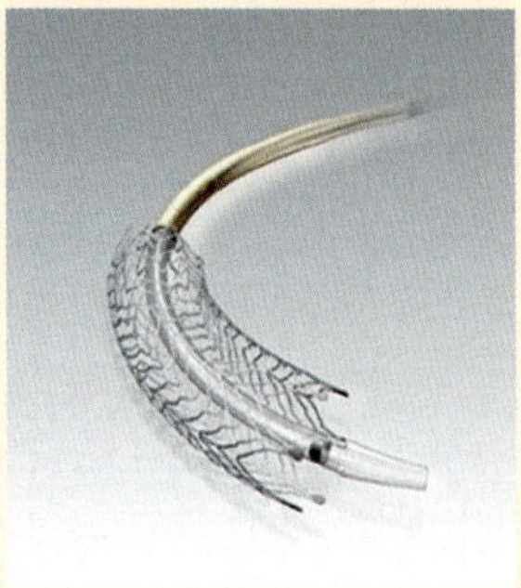 Absolute Pro, Amplatzer, and Omnilink Elite are trademarks of Abbott or its related companies. Reproduced with permission of Abbott, © 2022. All rights reserved.
	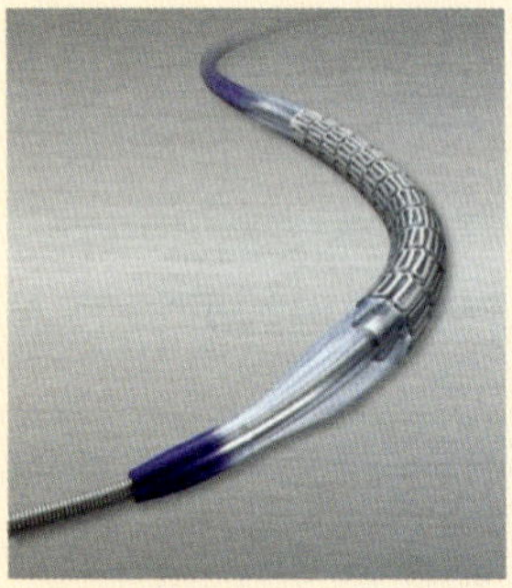 Absolute Pro, Amplatzer, and Omnilink Elite are trademarks of Abbott or its related companies. Reproduced with permission of Abbott, © 2022. All rights reserved.	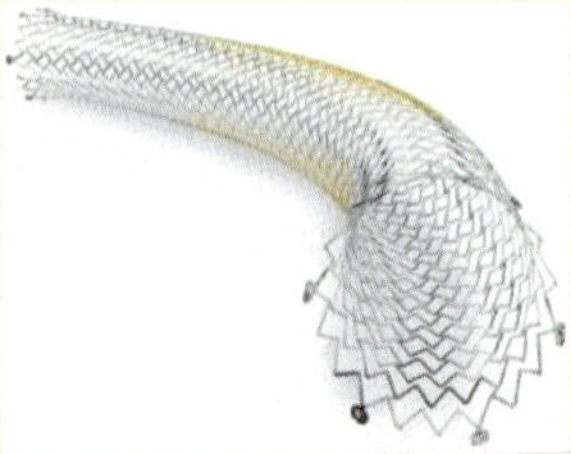 S.M.A.R.T Vascular Stent (Cordis, Miami Lakes, FL)
	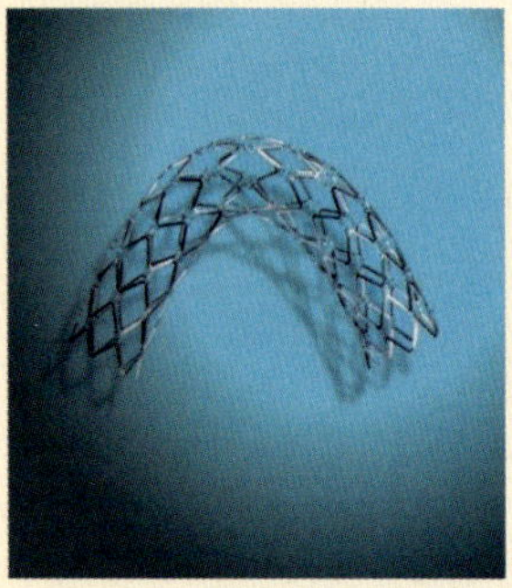 Palmaz Genesis Balloon Expandable Stent (Cordis, Miami Lakes, FL)	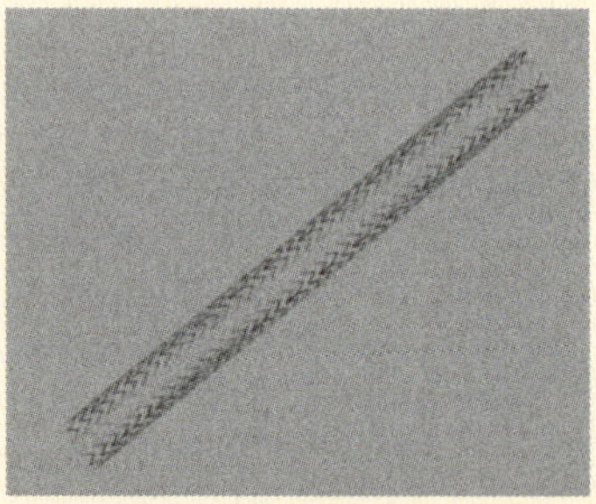 Courtesy of Cook Medical
	Assurant Cobalt Iliac Stent System (Medtronic, Minneapolis, Minn)	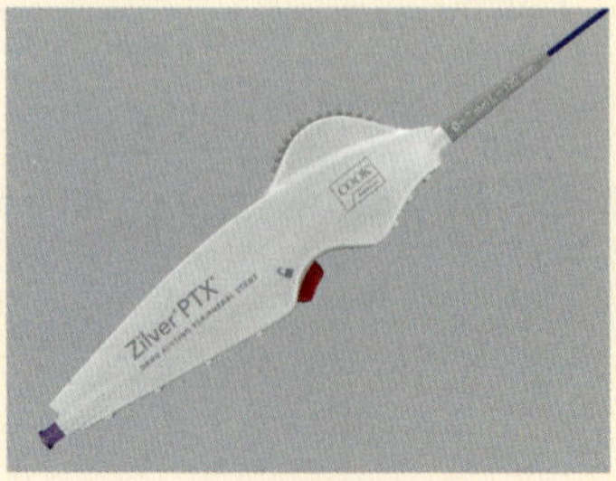 Courtesy of Cook Medical[b]
		LifeStent™ and LifeStent™ XL Vascular Stent System (Bard Peripheral Vascular Inc., Tempe, Ariz)[b]

[a]*The devices listed are approved by the FDA for iliac disease, unless otherwise stated.*
[b]*Off-label use; not FDA-approved for iliac lesions.*

- The length of the balloon or stent should cover the entire length of the diseased area.
- Balloon-expandable stents have the advantage of higher precision of placement and greater radial strength; however, they are less flexible than self-expanding stents. In general, balloon-expandable stents are best suited for common iliac artery lesions where "kissing" stents in the contralateral iliac artery may be needed to deal with excessive plaque burden or calcification, or the aortic bifurcation may need to be "advanced" into the distal aorta to completely ensure adequate luminal recanalization. Alternatively, external iliac lesions are often best treated with self-expanding stents, which are more flexible and compliant with the radius of curvature present in this artery. Exceptions exist for both indications, however, and device placement should be individualized to specific anatomic and clinical requirements.
- In heavily calcified vessels, to better facilitate angioplasty and stenting, plaque modification with intravascular lithotripsy (eg, Shockwave, Shockwave Medical Inc., Santa Clara, CA) can be considered.

Third Step

- In the setting of bilateral or even unilateral proximal common iliac artery disease or distal aortic disease, bilateral aortic bifurcation balloon dilation and stenting should be completed simultaneously to protect the contralateral common iliac artery from dissection, plaque dislodgement, or subsequent embolization. This is generally referred to as "kissing" iliac stents.
- Alternatively, the Covered Endovascular Reconstruction of the Aortic Bifurcation (CERAB) technique can be used when the distal aortic wall is calcified. This involves placing two kissing iliac stents (usually covered) within a covered aortic stent graft to endovascularly reconstruct the aortic bifurcation in a more anatomic and physiologic fashion (**FIGURE 8**).[4]
- Balloon-expandable stents are typically used for these proximal common iliac lesions and may be deployed well into the distal aorta, essentially raising the level of the aortic bifurcation.

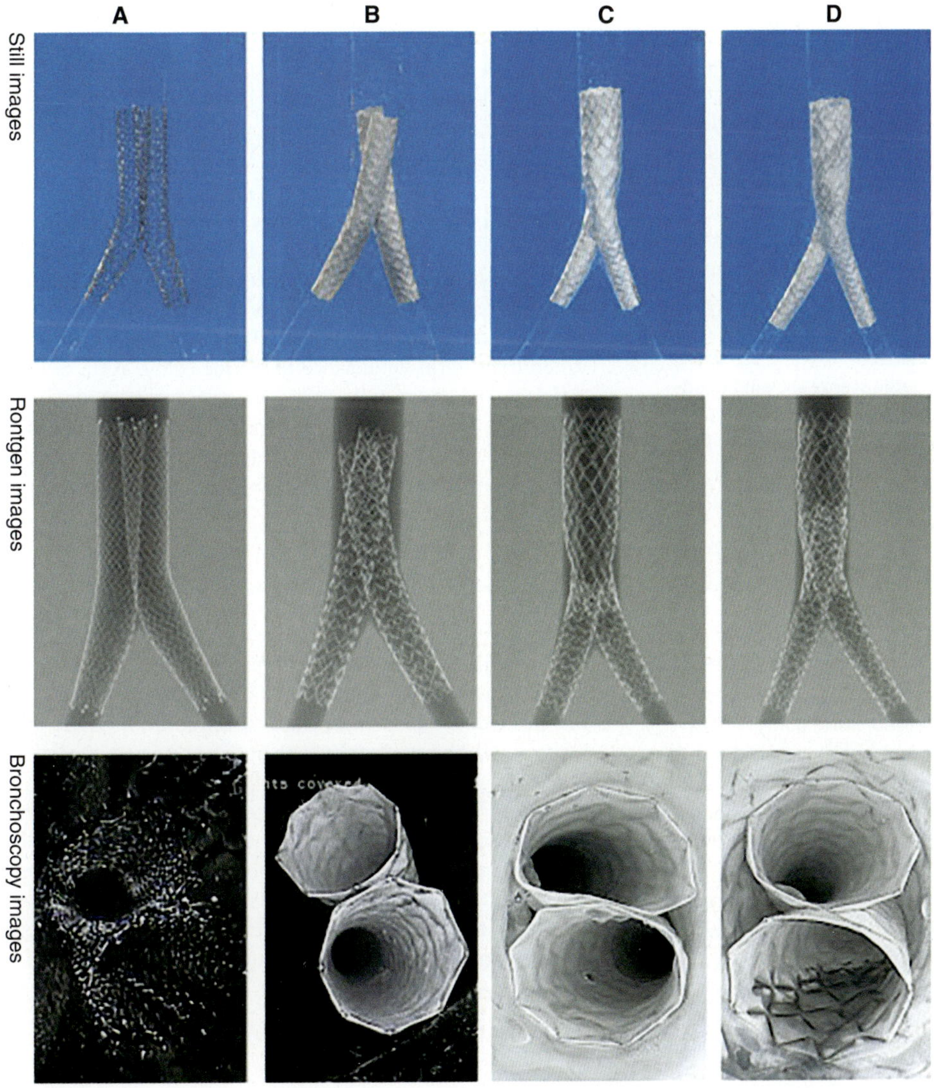

FIGURE 8 • Still, Rontgen, and bronchoscopic images of **(A)** self-expandable nitinol kissing bare metal stents; **(B)** balloon-expandable kissing covered stents; **(C)** Covered Endovascular Reconstruction of the Aortic Bifurcation (CERAB)-1 with limbs starting in the tapered portion of the aortic cuff; **(D)** CERAB-2 with the iliac limbs starting just above the tapered part of the aortic cuff. (Reprinted with permission from Groot Jebbink E, Grimme FA, Goverde PC, et al. Geometrical consequences of kissing stents and the Covered Endovascular Reconstruction of the Aortic Bifurcation configuration in an in vitro model for endovascular reconstruction of aortic bifurcation. *J Vasc Surg.* 2015;61(5):1306-1311.)

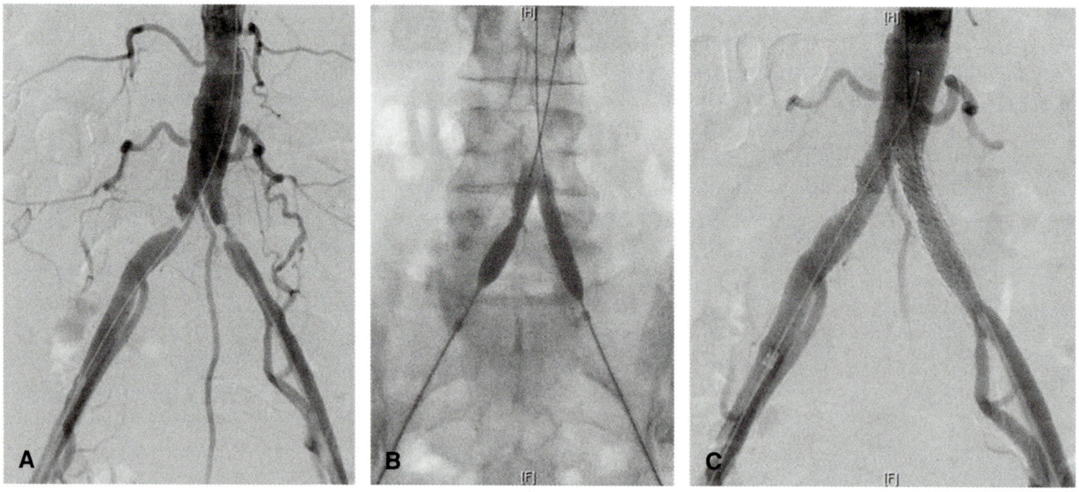

FIGURE 9 • Bilateral common iliac artery stenosis treated with kissing stent technique. **A,** Initial aortogram demonstrating high-grade bilateral proximal common iliac stenosis. **B,** Balloon dilation demonstrating waist in balloon at location of stenosis. **C,** Completion aortogram with bilateral kissing iliac stents, raising the aortic bifurcation by a few centimeters.

Fourth Step

- For common iliac lesions immediately adjacent to the aortic bifurcation, after precise arteriographic localization of the aortic and iliac bifurcations and extent of plaque burden, appropriately sized stents are selected. Unilateral or bilateral sheaths of sufficient diameter for the selected stents are advanced into the distal aorta. When common iliac lesions are not strictly "orificial," concomitant contralateral stenting is generally not required. Again, careful angiographic assessment should be made to determine the extent of plaque burden present at the origin of the common iliac arteries to make this determination.
- Appropriately sized balloon-expandable stents are advanced within the sheaths and positioned across the respective lesions. The sheaths are then pulled back to expose the entire stent; this sequence prevents accidental dislodgement of the stent off the balloon, attempting to cross the lesion, and limits the risk of plaque embolization during stent passage.
- Once both stents are positioned appropriately, they are inflated simultaneously to achieve the kissing configuration (**FIGURE 9**).

Fifth Step

- Completion arteriography, typically through a pressure injection in the distal aorta through "side-hole" or flush catheters, is obtained to confirm stent placement, evaluate degree of residual stenosis, and rule out complications such as dissection or thrombus/embolization.
- When the clinical significance of plaque in the aorta or iliac arteries is unknown, pressure measurement may be required. Pull-back pressures are obtained with the goal of eliminating pressure gradients across the treated lesion at rest or limiting to less than 15 mm Hg following injection of a distal vasodilator such as papaverine.

EXTERNAL ILIAC ARTERY STENTING

First Step

- When the external iliac artery is diseased, particularly the distal segment, self-expanding stents are typically used due to the increased tortuosity of these vessels and the increased flexibility of self-expanding stents as opposed to balloon-expandable stents (as described in *Common Iliac Stenting, Second Step*).
- The same principles exist in terms of sizing, although for self-expanding stents, 10% to 20% oversizing is typically recommended in the respective instructions for use.

Second Step

- Deployment of self-expanding stents does not require advancement of the introducer sheath past the lesion. The self-expanding stents usually are mounted on a carrier and constrained. The stents should be positioned across the lesion and deployed.
- Close fluoroscopic monitoring should occur during deployment, as self-expanding stents tend to be far less precise in positioning in comparison to balloon-expandable stents and typically may advance across the lesion during deployment. Carefully applying negative tension and ensuring slow deployment can help increase accuracy of stent placement.

Third Step

- Predilation and postdilation may be performed as necessary with appropriately sized balloons before and after stent deployment.
- In the setting of very distal external iliac artery disease or incomplete distal external iliac endarterectomy (as described earlier), the distal end of the stent may be carried down to the level of the endarterectomy, again with care to avoid crossing the inguinal ligament as previously described (**FIGURE 5**).

Fourth Step

- Just as in common iliac stenting, completion arteriograms should be performed, and pressure gradients may be obtained as necessary to confirm sufficient resolution of the stenosis.

Fifth Step

- Usually, a single-repair stitch can be used to close the patch sheath access site, regardless of the diameter of the sheath used for stent deployment.
- Once hemostasis is achieved, the sheaths removed, and anticoagulation reversed with protamine injection, the femoral exposure should be closed with a multilayer, anatomic closure with absorbable suture.

PEARLS AND PITFALLS

Occluded iliac artery strategies

Reentry devices	■ When attempting to cross an occluded segment with catheter-guidewire combinations, a subintimal plane may be developed. This subintimal technique is appropriate as long as the true lumen can once again be regained prior to entering the aorta. In some circumstances, this reentry may be challenging. In these situations, reentry devices can be employed. These devices have nitinol cannula that can be advanced through the device and used to puncture into the true lumen; a 0.014-in wire is then advanced. Free passage of the wire indicates true lumen access, which is confirmed by contrast injection. The passage can then be dilated and stented in a conventional manner (**FIGURE 10**). Care should be taken to attempt reentry before the dissection plane is advanced too far proximally into the distal aorta, as this may compromise the ability to properly deploy balloon-expandable stents and/or compromise inferior mesenteric arterial flow. Similarly, reentry systems should be used with caution in the iliac arterial system to avoid perforation and retroperitoneal bleeding.

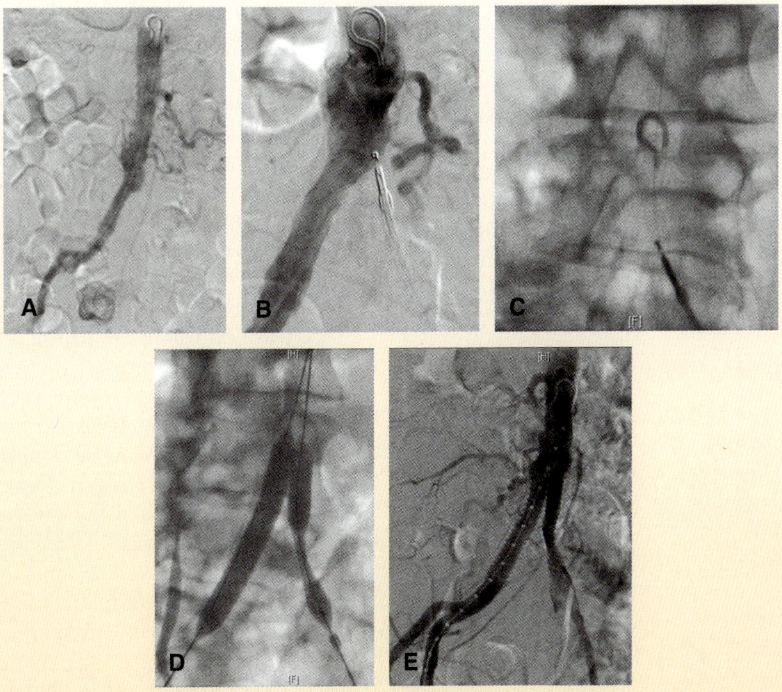

FIGURE 10 ● Use of an Outback reentry catheter in treatment of a chronic total iliac occlusion. **A,** Aortogram showing complete occlusion of the left iliac arterial system. **B,** The majority of the occlusion was crossed; however, reentry into the true aortic lumen was unsuccessful using traditional techniques. The Outback reentry catheter was advanced and positioned. **C,** After advancement of the reentry needle, a 0.014-in wire was able to be passed into the aorta. **D,** Retrograde kissing balloon-expandable stent placement into bilateral common iliac arteries. **E,** Completion aortogram demonstrating reconstitution of flow in left iliac system. (Cordis, Miami Lakes, FL.)

Alternative approach	■ Antegrade approach from either a brachial or contralateral femoral access sometimes provides more "pushability" across recalcitrant lesions and may be more successful at obtaining wire access. This is particularly true when a small invagination is apparent angiographically in the ipsilateral common iliac artery (when totally occluded). Once the occlusion or stenosis is traversed, the wire can be snared from the ipsilateral femoral and an ipsilateral sheath can still be advanced to complete the procedure as previously described from the ipsilateral femoral access. This is generally advisable as compared to attempted stent placement from left brachial access, due to proximity and control issues, as well as the availability of suitably sized stents on long delivery catheters.
Severe calcified disease strategies	■ In patients with significant atherosclerotic burden, care should be taken during the intervention to minimize atheroembolization. Use of covered stent grafts can be considered in these scenarios. Additionally, as an added benefit of the hybrid approach, flushing maneuvers of the patch angioplasty site may be performed to eliminate embolic debris. ■ Prior to angioplasty or stenting, plaque modification with intravascular lithotripsy (eg, Shockwave) can be considered. ■ If the distal aorta is diseased, the Covered Endovascular Reconstruction of the Aortic Bifurcation (CERAB) technique deploys two kissing iliac stents within a covered aortic stent graft to more anatomically and physiologically reconstruct the aortic bifurcation.
Arterial rupture	■ Cover with stent graft. Consider proximal balloon occlusion.
Arterial dissection	■ Extend stent if the dissection is flow limiting.

POSTOPERATIVE CARE

- Following femoral endarterectomy and iliac stenting, patients are usually monitored in the hospital for 1 to 2 days.
- Postoperative antithrombotic management is not well studied in this population; however, most surgeons treat patients with dual antiplatelet therapy such as aspirin and clopidogrel (Plavix), with a loading dose of clopidogrel (ie, 300 mg) followed by a daily dose (ie, 75 mg), for the first 6 weeks following the procedure. Long-term antiplatelet management is usually achieved with acetylsalicylic acid (ASA 81 mg) alone, except in circumstances of aspirin allergy.
- Routine follow-up with arterial duplex and ABIs is important to monitor for continued patency and potential need for secondary intervention. Typical postoperative surveillance includes 1 month, 3 month, 6 months, and annually thereafter. Patients with active wounds should be more closely monitored until healed.

OUTCOMES

- Early and long-term results of concomitant common femoral artery endarterectomy and iliac stenting have been excellent since their first reports in the early 2000s.[5,6] More recent studies continue to report excellent patency results. In a series of 108 patients (127 procedures), 2-year primary, primary-assisted, and secondary patency were 91%, 94%, and 98%, while 5-year patency rates were 87%, 92%, and 98%, respectively.[7]
- There is some evidence that covered stent grafts may have improved patency compared to bare metal stents, particularly in TASC C and D lesions.[6,8] In a study of 61 patients with TASC C and D iliac lesions all treated with the VIABAHN self-expanding PTFE-covered stent graft (W.L. Gore and Associates, Flagstaff, Ariz), primary patency at three years was 95%.[9]
- Iliac artery stenting combined with open femoral endarterectomy also appears to be equally effective as open surgical revascularization with aortobifemoral or iliofemoral bypass. Piazza and colleagues[10] found similar 30-day morbidity and mortality as well as primary patency at 3 years when comparing a 10-year cohort of patients treated in both manners. These similarities were maintained even after stratification for TASC group. In the long-term, endovascular repair with kissing iliac stents (with and without femoral endarterectomy) continues to have comparable outcomes with open aortobifemoral bypass. Dorigo and colleagues studied 210 patients (82 aortobifemoral, 128 iliac stenting) with TASC C and D lesions and found a significantly lower rate of postoperative complications in the stenting group (7% vs 21%, $P < .001$) but no significant difference in 6-year survival, patency (primary, primary-assisted, or secondary), or reintervention.[11]
- Endovascular stenting and/or hybrid therapy has comparable early and late outcomes to open surgical revascularization but is associated with shorter hospital length of stay and lower hospital expense.[12] Therefore, endovascular or hybrid treatment can be considered a first-line therapy option for aortoiliac occlusive disease in appropriate patients.
- Endovascular aortobifemoral bypass or hybrid iliac stenting with femoral endarterectomy is associated with complications (see below) and the need for reinterventions, ranging from approximately 6% to 11%.[9,11] Thus, routine surveillance, often lifelong, is critical for these patients.

COMPLICATIONS

- Contrast nephropathy
- Wound complications, including infection, dehiscence, seroma formation, and nerve entrapment
- Arterial rupture

- Arterial dissection
- Embolization
- Common or external iliac stent stenosis, thrombosis, or occlusion
- Common femoral artery stenosis
- Common femoral artery pseudoaneurysm

REFERENCES

1. Rzucidlo EM, Powell RJ, Zwolak RM, et al. Early results of stent-grafting to treat diffuse aortoiliac occlusive disease. *J Vasc Surg*. 2003;37(6):1175-1180.
2. Norgren L, Hiatt WR, Dormandy JA, Nehler MR, Harris KA, Fowkes FGR. Inter-society Consensus for the management of peripheral arterial disease (TASC II). *J Vasc Surg*. 2007;45:S5-67.
3. Conte MS, Bradbury AW, Kolh P, et al. Global vascular guidelines on the management of chronic limb-threatening ischemia. *J Vasc Surg*. 2019;69(6):3S-125S.e40.
4. Groot Jebbink E, Grimme F, Goverde P, van Oostayen J, Slump C, Reijnen M. Geometrical consequences of kissing stents and the covered endovascular reconstruction of the aortic bifurcation configuration in an in vitro model for endovascular reconstruction of aortic bifurcation. *J Vasc Surg*. 2015;61(5):1306-1311.
5. Nelson PR, Powell RJ, Schermerhorn ML, et al. Early results of external iliac artery stenting combined with common femoral artery endarterectomy. *J Vasc Surg*. 2002;35(6):1107-1113.
6. Chang RW, Goodney PP, Baek JH, Nolan BW, Rzucidlo EM, Powell RJ. Long-term results of combined common femoral endarterectomy and iliac stenting/stent grafting for occlusive disease. *J Vasc Surg*. 2008;48(2):362-367.
7. Maitrias P, Deltombe G, Molin V, Reix T. Iliofemoral endarterectomy associated with systematic iliac stent grafting for the treatment of severe iliofemoral occlusive disease. *J Vasc Surg*. 2017;65(2):406-413.
8. Mwipatayi BP, Thomas S, Wong J, et al. A comparison of covered vs bare expandable stents for the treatment of aortoiliac occlusive disease. *J Vasc Surg*. 2011;54(6):1561-1570.
9. Bracale UM, Giribono AM, Spinelli D, et al. Long-term results of endovascular treatment of TASC C and D aortoiliac occlusive disease with expanded polytetrafluoroethylene stent graft. *Ann Vasc Surg*. 2019;56:254-260.
10. Piazza M, Ricotta JJ, Bower TC, et al. Iliac artery stenting combined with open femoral endarterectomy is as effective as open surgical reconstruction for severe iliac and common femoral occlusive disease. *J Vasc Surg*. 2011;54(2):402-411.
11. Dorigo W, Piffaretti G, Benedetto F, et al. A comparison between aortobifemoral bypass and aortoiliac kissing stents in patients with complex aortoiliac obstructive disease. *J Vasc Surg*. 2017;65(1):99-107.
12. Rocha-Neves J, Ferreira A, Sousa J, et al. Endovascular approach versus aortobifemoral bypass grafting: outcomes in extensive aortoiliac occlusive disease. *Vasc Endovasc Surg*. 2020;54(2):102-110.

SECTION V: Infrainguinal Arterial Disease Management

Chapter 27 Surgical Exposure of the Lower Extremity Arteries

Young Kim and Anahita Dua

DEFINITION

- The primary etiology of chronic lower extremity ischemia is atherosclerosis, although other, rare causes may exist. These include embolic disease, adventitial cystic disease, popliteal artery entrapment, radiation arteritis, and other disease processes. The symptomatic manifestation of chronic lower extremity ischemia is termed peripheral arterial disease (PAD). Atherosclerotic stenosis or occlusion of the peripheral arterial tree results in arterial insufficiency and limb ischemia. PAD is a major contributor to reduced quality of life (QOL) and increased morbidity and mortality among an increasing elderly patient population.

DIFFERENTIAL DIAGNOSIS

- The challenge for the vascular specialist is to determine whether the nature and severity of presenting symptoms correlate with the degree of chronic arterial insufficiency present. Many alternative diagnoses must be considered, including neuropathy (eg, spinal stenosis), inflammation, infection, lymphatic or venous disease, repetitive trauma (eg, diabetic foot ulcers), or peripheral embolism. Definitive diagnosis is derived from a detailed history and physical examination correlated with appropriately directed noninvasive vascular laboratory and adjunctive imaging studies. The vascular specialist must also differentiate chronic limb ischemia from acute limb ischemia, which is quicker-onset (within 14 days) and more likely to require an urgent intervention.

PATIENT HISTORY AND PHYSICAL FINDINGS

- Approximately half of patients with PAD are asymptomatic. Symptoms related to PAD can range from intermittent claudication to chronic limb-threatening ischemia (CLTI), where CLTI includes ischemic rest pain, ulceration, and gangrene. Pulse examination is an integral component of the vascular-focused physical examination. Femoral, popliteal, posterior tibial, and dorsalis pedis pulses should be noted and graded (0 = absent; 1+ = diminished; 2+ = normal; 3+ = enlarged/aneurysmal). If pulses are absent, a handheld Doppler probe may be utilized to localize signals. Additionally, the femoral pulses may be auscultated to listen for bruits, indicating aortoiliac occlusive disease (as opposed to an infrainguinal process). Femoral bruits may be further exacerbated by having the patient perform several squats prior to auscultation.
- Claudication is defined as muscular pain, cramping, aching, or discomfort in the lower limb, reproducibly elicited by exercise and relieved within 10 minutes of cessation. Classically, the muscle group impacted by claudication is one level inferior to the atherosclerotic lesion. For example, aortoiliac lesions present with buttock claudication, and femoropopliteal lesions present with calf claudication. Lesions at multiple levels are responsible for the development of CLTI. CLTI has traditionally been defined as (1) persistent, recurring ischemic rest pain requiring opiate analgesia for longer than 2 weeks and (2) ankle systolic blood pressure (SBP) less than 50 mm Hg or toe pressures less than 30 mm Hg (or absent pedal pulse in patients with diabetes).[1] Ischemic rest pain worsens with leg elevation and is relieved by dependency. In addition to absent pulses, dependent rubor, elevation pallor, and calf muscle atrophy are frequently present among patients with CLTI. CLTI also includes ischemic foot ulceration and gangrene in the setting of ankle SBP less than 50 mm Hg or toe pressures less than 40 mm Hg in patients without diabetes (<50 mm Hg in diabetics).
- Patients with PAD often have multiple medical comorbidities. These include coronary artery disease (CAD), diabetes mellitus, hypertension, hyperlipidemia, chronic kidney disease, chronic obstructive pulmonary disease, and a prolonged smoking history. Frailty is also common among patients with PAD due to older age and limited ambulation. Therefore, all patients with PAD require comprehensive medical management and risk factor modification. Additionally, given that PAD often manifests through pain, patients with PAD should also be questioned regarding use of narcotic and non-narcotic analgesics.
- For patients with intermittent claudication, revascularization is indicated for those with persistent, lifestyle-limiting symptoms, despite adequate risk factor modification, exercise, and optimal medical management. For patients with lifestyle-limiting claudication, the primary goal of intervention is to improve exercise tolerance and thereby QOL. All patients with CLTI, on the other hand, are indicated for surgical revascularization to prevent limb loss. Therefore, revascularization among the CLTI cohort is focused on wound healing and functional limb salvage, in addition to symptomatic relief and QOL improvements.[2,3]

IMAGING AND OTHER DIAGNOSTIC STUDIES

- Adequate preoperative planning depends on a thorough history and detailed physical examination. The vascular specialist must determine the severity of ischemic symptoms, along with any infectious complications, functional status, and anticipated longevity. Once it is decided that revascularization will improve the patient's functional status and QOL, imaging and other diagnostic studies can be utilized to determine the location, extent, and severity of occlusive arterial lesions. These studies can also help determine whether endovascular, open, or hybrid revascularization procedures are indicated.
- The delineation of the relevant arterial anatomy on the index limb is facilitated by high-quality, noninvasive vascular laboratory studies (ankle-brachial index and toe pressure measurements). These are supplemented by arterial color duplex ultrasound imaging. Arterial duplex is extremely accurate in the assessment of iliofemoral and femoropopliteal arterial occlusive disease but less so for infrageniculate lesions. Duplex enables differentiation of stenosis from occlusion and determination of lesion length and degree of calcification.
- Cross-sectional imaging studies, such as computed tomography angiography (CTA) or magnetic resonance arteriography, can also help define arterial anatomy when defining disease extent and severity. CTA is better suited for assessing aortoiliac and femoral disease and suboptimal for infrageniculate arteries. Catheter-based angiography is better suited for assessing infrageniculate disease. Both CTA and conventional angiography utilize intravenous contrast, and the practitioner should be cognizant of contrast-induced nephropathy.

SURGICAL MANAGEMENT

Preoperative Planning

- In terms of cardiovascular health, PAD is considered equivalent to CAD. Therefore, preoperative risk evaluation for overall cardiovascular-related mortality represents an integral component of preoperative planning. For patients with stable or minimally symptomatic CAD, preoperative evaluation is focused on risk-reduction efforts. Frequently, this includes antiplatelet therapy, plaque stabilization via statin therapy, β-blockade, and optimization of hypertension management.
- For an open bypass, the goals of preoperative planning include identification of diseased arterial segment(s), selection of the most appropriate arterial inflow source, selection of the optimal bypass target for maximal outflow and target bed perfusion, and selection of the best available conduit. Conduit availability is almost always the rate-limiting factor because the best quality conduit is a single-segment great saphenous vein (GSV). Alternatives to GSV grafts include prosthetic conduits (eg, polytetrafluoroethylene, Dacron), arm veins, and spliced vein segments.
- The surgical plan should be individualized based on patient's functional status, medical comorbidities, extent of arterial disease, and conduit availability. Infrainguinal bypass may originate from the common femoral artery (CFA), superficial femoral artery (SFA), profunda femoris artery (PFA), or popliteal artery, with a bypass target of the popliteal, tibial, or pedal/plantar arteries. Patient positioning, selection of incisions, and surgical techniques are all dictated by the type of bypass procedure deemed most appropriate under the circumstances.

EXPOSURE OF THE FEMORAL VESSELS

Positioning

- The patient is placed in supine position. Foley catheter should be inserted, as long as the patient is not anuric at baseline. Arms may be tucked to facilitate intraoperative and completion angiography.

Placement of Incision

- The inguinal ligament can be identified as a line between the pubic tubercle and anterior superior iliac spine. The CFA is located along this imaginary line, two fingerbreadths lateral to pubic tubercle. Palpation of the inguinal ligament and femoral pulse, or direct visualization with duplex ultrasound, can localize the CFA bifurcation and help to guide optimal incision placement. Even when pulseless due to excessive calcification or occlusive disease, the CFA may be localized by reliance on anatomic landmarks and direct palpation, recognized as a firm tubular structure positioned within the femoral sheath.
- The vertical groin incision is most commonly employed to provide optimal access to the entire length of the CFA. This should be created coaxially along the artery itself, continued from the inguinal ligament distally, and aimed at the medial aspect of the knee. This incision may be extended cephalad or caudad to increase arterial exposure as necessary (**FIGURE 1**, *incision A*).
- Alternatively, a transverse incision can be placed 1 cm below and parallel to the inguinal ligament to avoid potential skin maceration and wound complications that may accompany vertical incisions in this situation (**FIGURE 1**, *incision B*). This incision is particularly useful in obese patients with substantial abdominal pannus. Although the proximal SFA and PFA may be exposed through a transverse incision, further proximal or distal exposure is prohibited by the incision itself. Therefore, if an extensive common and deep femoral endarterectomy is anticipated to optimize inflow, a vertical incision should be planned.

Dissection and Control of the Common, Superficial, and Proximal Deep Femoral Arteries

- The incision is carried through the subcutaneous tissue and superficial fascia using electrocautery. A self-retaining retractor, such as a Weitlaner or Beckmann, may be placed at this time. Deep to the subcutaneous tissue and superficial fascia, the dissection is extended longitudinally, even when using an oblique incision, to optimize the length of femoral exposure. Self-retaining retractors are carefully repositioned to

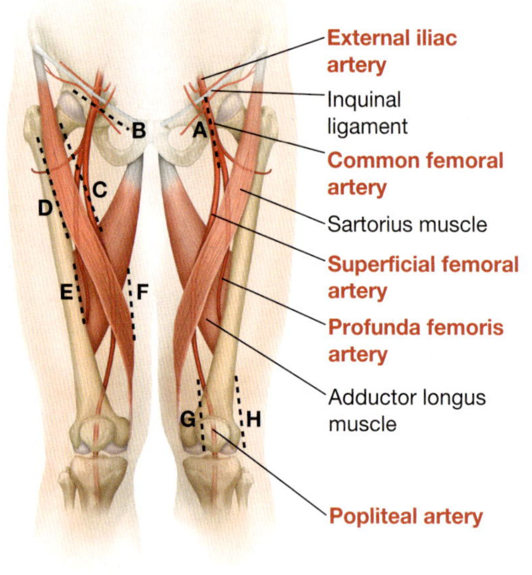

FIGURE 1 • Exposure of the femoral vessels. The proximal femoral vessels may be exposed through a *(A)* longitudinal or *(B)* transverse incision. The mid- and distal superficial femoral and profunda femoris arteries may be exposed through a number of incisions *(C-F)*. The suprageniculate popliteal artery may be exposed through a *(G)* medial or *(H)* lateral approach.

optimize exposure, while avoiding traction injury to femoral nerve branches or the common femoral vein. Sharp dissection through the femoral sheath exposes the anterior surface of the CFA.

- The dissection plane should remain centered directly over the CFA, which can be identified by digital palpation. Encountering venous structures indicates medial deviation from the optimal plane; whereas the iliopsoas muscle, femoral nerve fibers, or lymphatic vessels are indicative of lateral deviation. Incorrectly placed femoral incisions are associated with an increased risk of wound complications, including wound necrosis and separation, lymphatic leaks, femoral neuropraxia, and venous injury.
- Sharp dissection should proceed along the CFA both proximally and distally. The CFA and its branches are circumferentially dissected and individually isolated. Placement of a red rubber catheter or silastic vessel loops around the CFA and its branches aid in retraction, dissection, and mobilization.
- Proximal dissection is continued along the CFA to the inguinal ligament. At this point, the inguinal ligament may be divided if exposure of the external iliac artery is necessary. Caution is necessary in this area, as a prominent femoral vein tributary crosses anteriorly over the CFA in this area, underneath the inguinal ligament, and is prone to injury if not identified, ligated, and divided early in the dissection. Inadvertent injury to this so-called "vein of pain" results in retraction and troublesome bleeding. If the inguinal ligament is divided, it should be repaired prior to the end of the procedure to prevent hernia formation.
- The medial and lateral femoral circumflex arteries, important collaterals in iliofemoral arterial occlusive disease, are identified at level of the inguinal ligament and individually controlled with removable clips or silastic vessel loops. Use of the former reduces clutter in the wound during endarterectomy or creation of the proximal anastomosis. If removable clips are placed, then they should be removed prior to the end of the procedure.
- As the dissection proceeds distally, an abrupt caliber change marks the femoral bifurcation and the origins of the PFA (Latin for *deep femoral artery*) and SFA. The SFA continues distally in the same plane, while the PFA usually courses posteriorly and laterally away from the femoral bifurcation. Occasionally, multiple PFAs may be encountered. The lateral circumflex iliac vein is encountered crossing the anterior surface of the PFA and should preclude any blind dissection in this area. After silastic loops are placed on each vessel, gentle upward traction on the CFA and SFA may help bring the PFA into view (**FIGURE 2A**).
- Medial and distal dissection provides extended exposure of the proximal SFA (**FIGURE 1**, *incision F*). This vessel only occasionally has small branches in its proximal segment. A sensory branch of the femoral nerve may be present crossing the SFA from lateral to medial. Transection may result in pain, numbness, and paresthesia along the medial thigh distribution. Even extended femoral bifurcation dissections rarely require division of femoral nerve branches, which should be avoided to minimize postoperative discomfort.

Exposure of the Profunda Femoris Artery—Middle and Distal Segments

- Exposure of the distal portions of the PFA often enables use of shorter vein conduit in distal leg bypass or may improve outflow from proximal revascularization procedures (eg, iliac angioplasty and stenting, aortobifemoral bypass). These segments can be exposed through either posteromedial or anteromedial approaches (**FIGURE 1**, *incisions C–F*). The approach should be dictated by the surgical indication (inflow sources or outflow target), with additional consideration for native vs reoperative field.
- Incisions are placed along either the medial (**FIGURE 1**, *incisions C and F*) or lateral borders of the sartorius muscle (**FIGURE 1**, *incisions D and E*). The dissection plane is deepened through the subcutaneous tissue and fascia using electrocautery, passing lateral or medial to the sartorius, respectively. The sartorius muscle is then mobilized and retracted laterally or medially, depending on the approach. Dissection is carried posteriorly, passing lateral to the superficial femoral vessels and accompanying nerve, to the space between the adductor longus muscle (medially) and vastus medialis (laterally) (**FIGURE 2B**, *incisions C–E*). The PFA and profunda vein pass directly underneath.
- Dissection between adductor longus and vastus medialis muscle exposes the middle segments of the PFA. Crossing venous tributaries should be ligated and divided as necessary to provide optimal exposure. Distal segments of PFA begin to course posterior to the femur beyond this point and are therefore less useful for bypass planning.
- Alternatively, dissection between the adductor longus (anteriorly) and gracilis muscle (posteriorly) allows for medial exposure of the PFA in the distal thigh (**FIGURE 1**, *incision F*; **FIGURE 2B**, *incision F*).

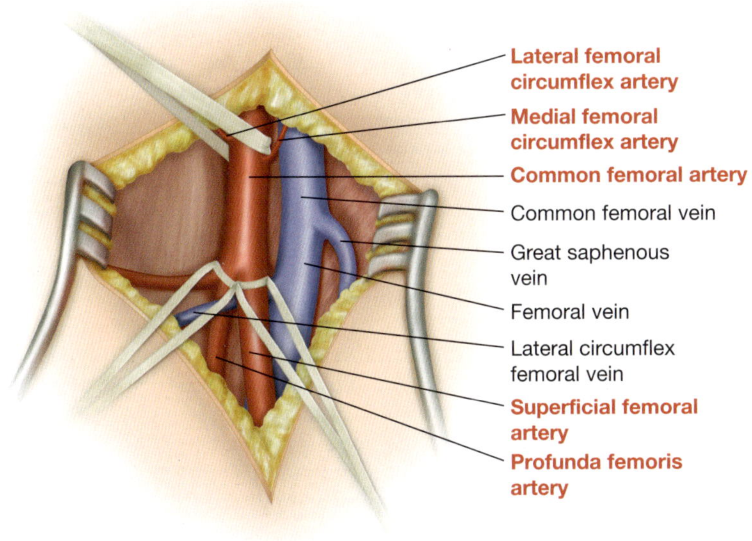

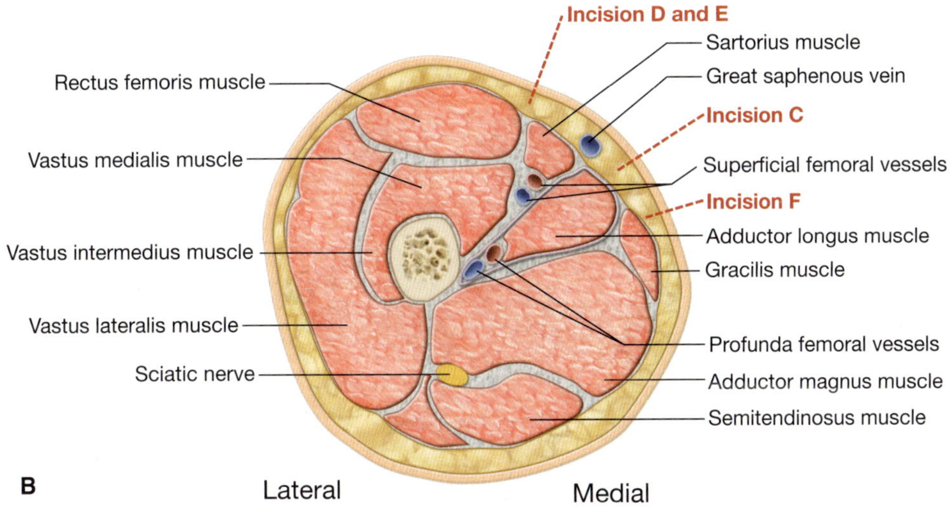

FIGURE 2 • **A,** Exposure of femoral vessels at groin through a longitudinal incision. **B,** Anteromedial and posterolateral approaches to expose middle and distal segments of the superficial and deep femoral arteries. Incisions *(C-F)* correspond to **FIGURE 1**.

EXPOSURE OF THE POPLITEAL ARTERY

Medial Exposure of the Above-Knee Popliteal Artery

- The patient is placed in a supine position. The operative leg is then flexed and rotated laterally. A bump may be placed underneath the knee for stabilization; however, this may hinder the use of gravity to aid in exposure.
- A longitudinal incision is made along the groove formed by the vastus medialis (anteriorly) and the sartorius muscles (posteromedially), measuring approximately 10 to 12 cm (**FIGURE 3A**, *incision A*). The incision is carried through the subcutaneous tissue and fascia using electrocautery. A self-retaining retractor is carefully placed without undue tension, taking care not to injure the GSV or saphenous nerve. At this location, the GSV is likely to be encountered more posteromedially in the subcutaneous tissue. The saphenous nerve may be encountered at distal end of the incision as it joins the GSV near the medial aspect of the knee.
- The deep fascia is then longitudinally incised above the sartorius muscle to enter the above-knee popliteal fossa. The popliteal artery can be palpated against the posterior surface of the femur (**FIGURE 3B**).
- Multiple veins are encountered in the popliteal fossa. The popliteal artery is often surrounded by venae comitantes (Latin for *accompanying veins*), and the popliteal vein is posterolateral to the artery in this location. The popliteal and/or superficial femoral veins may be duplicated throughout the popliteal fossa and distal thigh. Isolation and control of the artery usually requires ligation and division of surrounding collateral veins. A sclerotic popliteal vein can easily be mistaken for the popliteal artery, and care must be taken to distinguish the two vessels.

Lateral Exposure of the Above-Knee Popliteal Artery

- Lateral exposure of the above-knee popliteal artery is useful in select clinical scenarios. For instance, axillopopliteal bypass is logistically easier through a lateral approach. Another instance is when the medial approach has previously been dissected or is complicated by infection or injury.
- The patient is placed in a supine position. The operative leg is then flexed and rotated medially. A bump may be placed underneath the knee for stabilization.
- A longitudinal incision is made between the vastus lateralis and the biceps femoris muscles, measuring approximately 10 to 12 cm (**FIGURE 4A**, *incision A*). The incision is carried through the subcutaneous tissue and fascia using electrocautery. A self-retaining retractor is carefully placed without undue tension. Once the fascia lata has been exposed, a generous cruciate incision ("T-ed") is created at both ends to prevent bypass graft impingement by its dense fibers.
- After self-retaining retractors are placed, the popliteal space is entered. The sciatic nerve and popliteal vein will be encountered first, as they are lateral to the popliteal artery. The sciatic nerve is gently retracted downward. The popliteal vein is then circumferentially dissected and mobilized to expose the above-knee popliteal artery.

Posterior Exposure of the Popliteal Vessels

- Although direct and relatively uncomplicated, posterior access is limited by the medial and lateral heads of the gastrocnemius muscle distally and the hamstrings proximally. Therefore, only limited popliteal artery access is achievable through this incision. Despite its limitations, posterior exposure may be the preferred approach for management of popliteal artery entrapment syndrome, popliteal adventitial cystic disease, focal popliteal artery aneurysms, or arterial injury following traumatic posterior knee dislocation.
- The patient is placed in a prone position, using a pillow to prop up the lower leg and foot.

An S-shaped incision is made, starting medially at the distal thigh. The incision is carried across the posterior crease of the knee joint, ending laterally at the proximal leg. Dissection is then carried anteriorly through the subcutaneous tissue and superficial fascia, entering the popliteal fossa. After placing self-retaining retractors, exposure is maximized by mobilizing the popliteal artery between the two heads of the gastrocnemius muscle inferiorly and between the hamstring muscles (semimembranosus and biceps femoris) superiorly.

- The muscles are gently retracted to expose the entire popliteal fossa. The tibial and common peroneal nerves are

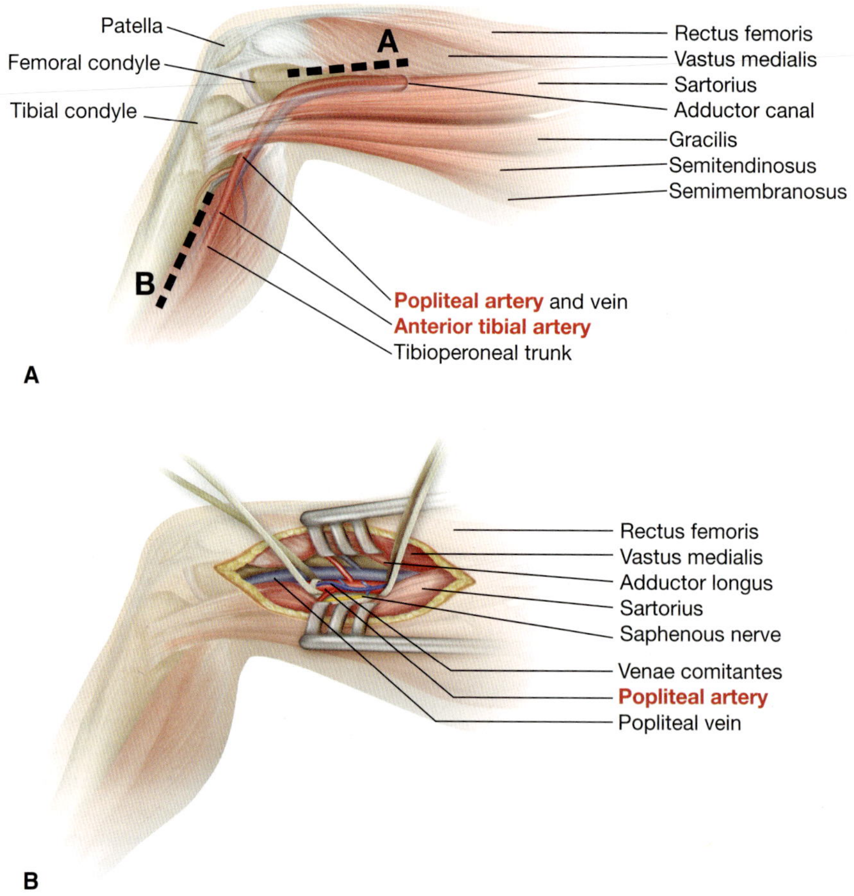

FIGURE 3 • **A,** Medial exposure of the *(A)* suprageniculate and *(B)* infrageniculate popliteal artery. **B,** Exposure of the suprageniculate popliteal artery. **C,** Exposure of the infrageniculate popliteal artery and its trifurcation. **D,** Exposure of the popliteal artery through a posterior approach.

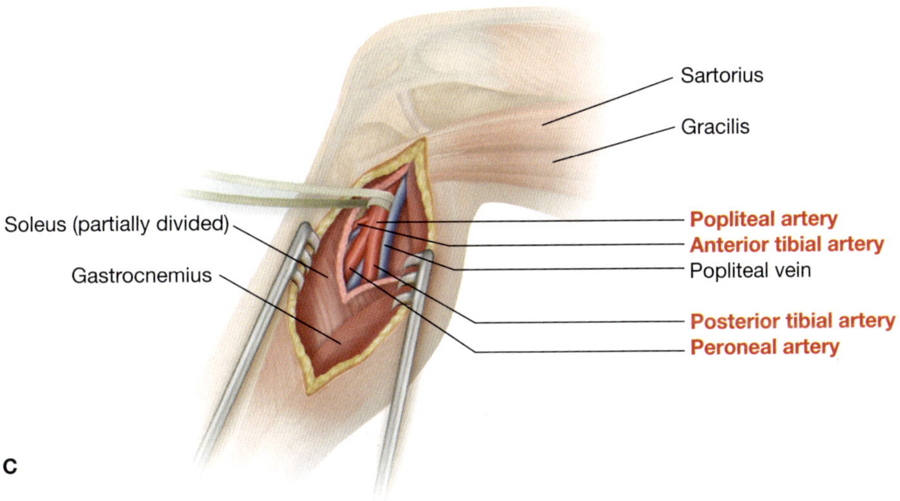

C

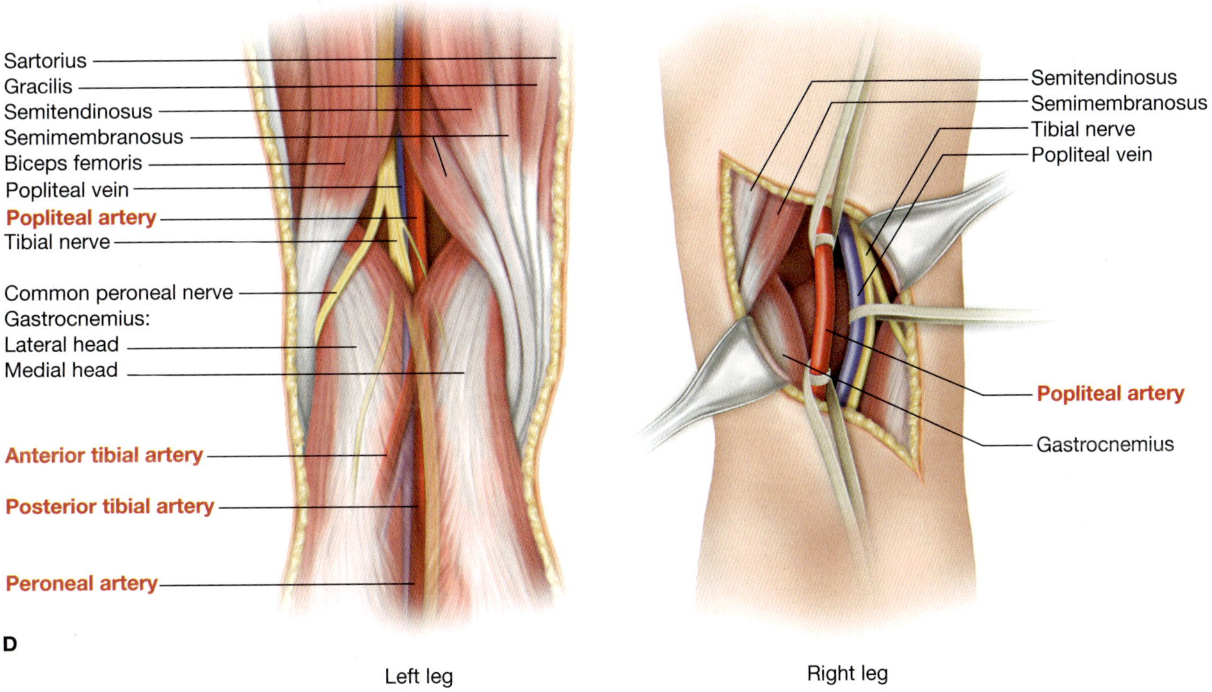

D

FIGURE 3 • Cont'd

encountered superficially in this exposure. The popliteal artery is anterior (deep) to the popliteal vein in the popliteal fossa.

- It may be necessary to mobilize the popliteal vein with ligation and division of popliteal venous tributaries to fully expose the artery. Once the appropriate segment is circumferentially dissected, silastic vessel loops are placed proximally and distally.

Medial Exposure of the Infrageniculate Popliteal Artery

- The medial approach to the below-knee popliteal artery is the most common approach (**FIGURE 3A**).
- The patient is placed in a supine position. The operative leg is then flexed and rotated laterally. A bump may be placed underneath the knee for stabilization; however, this may hinder the use of gravity to aid in exposure.
- A longitudinal incision is made one fingerbreadth below the edge of the tibia, along the course of the GSV (**FIGURE 3A**, *incision B*). The dissection is carried through subcutaneous tissue and fascia into the deep posterior compartment. The infrageniculate popliteal vessels reside in the deep posterior compartment and are partially covered by the origin of the soleus muscle.
- Division of the soleus muscle fibers (**FIGURE 3C**) will facilitate exposure of the tibioperoneal trunk and takeoff of the anterior tibial artery; however, it is not entirely necessary for exposure of the below-knee popliteal artery itself. As previously described, the popliteal artery lies

in close proximity to the popliteal vein and tibial nerve. Mobilization of the popliteal vein from the adjacent artery is imperative to provide adequate exposure of all relevant structures, including the anterior tibial artery, tibioperoneal trunk, and its two branches (posterior tibial and peroneal arteries). It may be necessary to ligate and divide the anterior tibial vein at its confluence with the (often paired) popliteal vein to expose the tibial vessels. Dissection and retraction must proceed deliberately in this location to avoid injury to the neighboring tibial nerve and its distal branches.

Lateral Exposure of the Infrageniculate Popliteal Artery

- The lateral approach to the below-knee popliteal artery is rarely performed, given the need for fibulectomy, but may be beneficial in the setting of active infection or a reoperative surgical field.
- A longitudinal incision is made a fingerbreadth anterior to the fibula, starting 2 cm inferior to the fibular head and extending caudally. Dissection is carried directly onto fibula (**FIGURE 4A**, *incision B*). Note the location of the common peroneal nerve, which courses from posterior to anterior around the neck of the upper fibula just below its head, before it branches into the superficial and deep peroneal nerves. Injury to the common peroneal nerve can result in foot drop and sensory deficits.
- After exposure of the fibula, the periosteum of the fibula is circumferentially dissected. A bone saw is then used to excise the exposed segment of the fibula, while protecting the underlying structures. The popliteal vessels and branches are found directly underneath the fibular periosteum, with the popliteal artery usually located anterior to the popliteal vein and posterior tibial nerve. By extending the dissection distally, the anterior tibial artery takeoff and the tibioperoneal trunk can also be exposed.

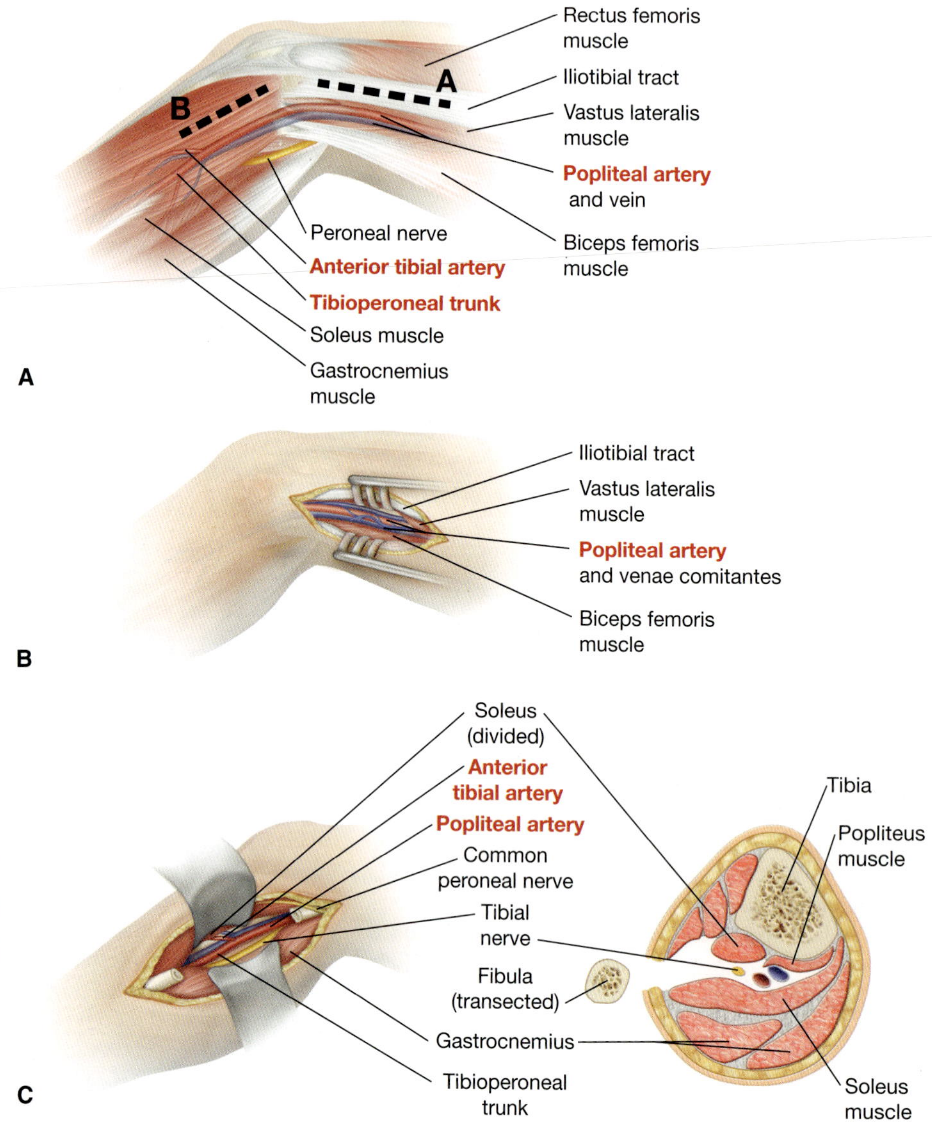

FIGURE 4 • **A,** Lateral exposure of *(A)* supragenicuate and *(B)* infrageniculate popliteal artery. **B,** Exposure of suprageniculate popliteal artery. **C,** Exposure of infrageniculate popliteal artery and its trifurcation.

EXPOSURE OF THE TIBIAL VESSELS

Exposure of the Anterior Tibial Artery—Proximal Segment

- Exposure of the origin of the anterior tibial artery is similar to the technique for medial exposure for the infrageniculate popliteal artery.

Exposure of the Anterior Tibial Artery—Middle Segment

- Exposure of the middle segment of the anterior tibial artery is useful for situations in which there is limited length of autogenous vein graft.
- An axial incision is made in a vertical plane about two fingerbreadths lateral to the anterior edge of the tibia (**FIGURE 5A**). The incision is then deepened between the tibialis anterior and the extensor hallucis longus muscles. The anterior tibial artery is found superficial to the interosseus membrane between the cleft formed by these two muscles.
- Dissecting away the overlying collateral veins allows for exposure and control of the middle segment of the anterior tibial artery. Use of a proximal sterile tourniquet during exposure of all the crural arteries may significantly accelerate the dissection while limiting bleeding from the numerous and redundant collateral veins. Prior to placing the sterile tourniquet, an Esmarch bandage should be used to drain the leg of its venous blood, otherwise venous congestion may result in persistent bleeding from any venous structures.

Exposure of the Posterior Tibial Artery—Proximal Segment

- Exposure of the proximal segment of the posterior tibial artery is similar to the technique for medial exposure for the infrageniculate popliteal artery. The soleus muscle must be dissected free from its tibial attachments for adequate exposure.

Exposure of the Posterior Tibial Artery—Middle Segment

- Exposure of the middle segment of the posterior tibial artery is useful for situations in which there is limited length of autogenous vein graft.
- A longitudinal incision is made just anterior to the soleus muscle. The overlying soleus muscle must be divided to expose the underlying vessels (**FIGURE 5B**). The posterior tibial artery lies anterior to soleus muscle with the peroneal artery located laterally, in the same plane, between the soleus and tibialis posterior muscles.
- Careful dissection is necessary to avoid injury to the tibial nerve, which commonly runs between the posterior tibial and peroneal vessels.

Exposure of the Peroneal Artery—Proximal Segment

- Exposure of the proximal segment of the peroneal artery is similar to the technique for medial exposure for the infrageniculate popliteal artery, extended caudally to expose the tibioperoneal trunk and its branches.

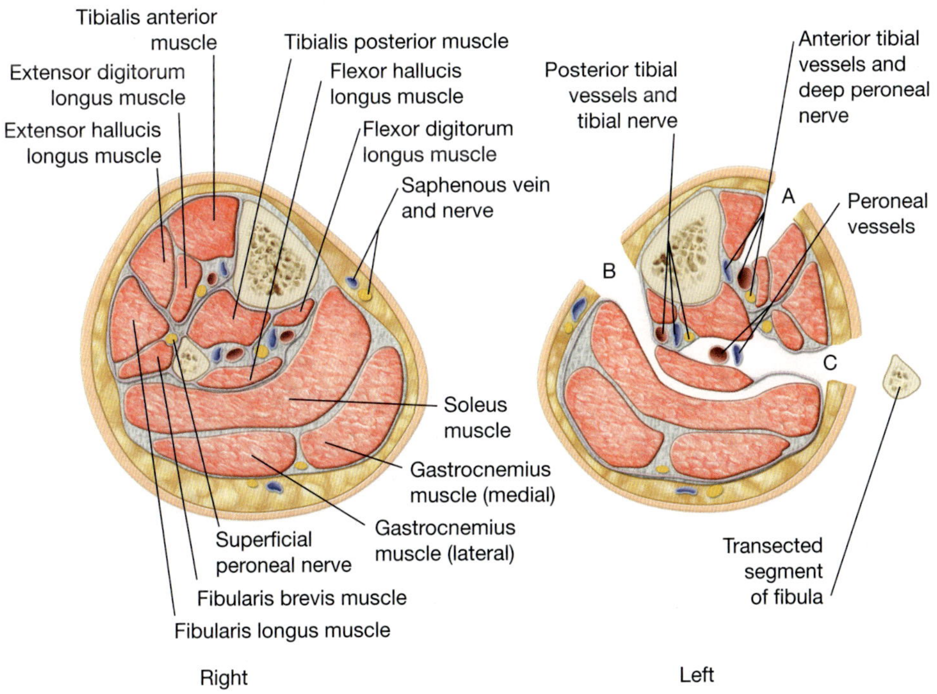

FIGURE 5 • Exposure of anterior tibial, posterior tibial, and peroneal arteries at mid-lower leg.

Exposure of the Peroneal Artery—Middle Segment

- Exposure of the middle segment of the peroneal artery may also be performed from an anterolateral approach. This is rarely performed, given the need for fibulectomy.
- A vertical incision is made over the fibula at the desired level of exposure (**FIGURE 5C**). Dissection is then carried down through the overlying muscle using electrocautery, eventually exposing the fibula. The fibular periosteum is dissected circumferentially. A bone saw is then used to excise the exposed segment of the fibula, while protecting the underlying structures. After incising the inner periosteal membrane, the peroneal vessels are found immediately beneath this structure. The artery usually is anterior to flexor hallucis longus and posterior to the tibialis posterior muscles.
- The peroneal artery is exposed and controlled after mobilization from circumferential collateral veins and the main peroneal vein. Use of a proximal sterile tourniquet and Esmarch bandage is prudent.

EXPOSURE OF PEDAL VESSELS

Exposure of the Inframalleolar Posterior Tibial Artery

- Exposure of the distal segment of the posterior tibial artery enables pedal bypass, which may be useful in patients with tibial disease (eg, diabetic macroangiopathy).
- Intraoperative ultrasound may be used to locate the trajectory of the posterior tibial artery. A longitudinal incision is made through skin and fascia at the midpoint between the medial malleolus and the Achilles tendon. If this exposure is used for an *in situ* bypass procedure, the incision should be deviated anteriorly to accommodate the anterior course of the GSV, as it crosses the medial malleolus.
- The flexor retinaculum is identified as a thick tendon sheath and divided sharply to provide optimal exposure. The posterior tibial vessels are located between the flexor digitorum longus and flexor hallucis longus muscles/tendons. A small Weitlaner self-retaining retractor is placed for exposure. The neurovascular bundle is usually enveloped by fatty tissue underneath the fascia. Within the neurovascular bundle, the posterior tibial artery is usually found anterior to the tibial nerve. There is typically a rich network of venous collaterals present. These may either be mobilized or (more commonly) divided to facilitate distal posterior tibial artery exposure.
- When more distal bypass targets are needed (eg, prohibitive burden of disease in the posterior tibial artery itself), the dissection may be continued distally along the posterior tibial artery to its bifurcation into the medial and lateral plantar arteries. In these cases, however, preoperative angiogram is paramount to immediate and long-term surgical success and only in rare circumstances should the operative plan be changed by unexpected findings at the time of surgery. The presence of luminal calcification alone, without substantial compromise to the target lumen diameter, is not a contraindication to bypass reconstruction. If there is any uncertainty regarding the optimal bypass target, consideration should be given to intraoperative arteriography to guide surgical decision-making. To this end, we perform all open bypass procedures in a hybrid operating room environment with high-quality imaging capabilities to ensure the optimal outcome of all procedures, regardless of the initial operative plan.

Exposure of the Supramalleolar Anterior Tibial Artery

- Exposure of the supramalleolar anterior tibial artery is useful as a distal bypass target, especially in the presence of substantial tibial atherosclerosis. It may also be preferable to bypass to this segment in the presence of a dorsal foot wound.
- Ultrasound may help to localize this artery intraoperatively. A longitudinal incision is placed made between the tibialis anterior (medially) and extensor hallucis longus and the extensor digitorum longus (laterally) (**FIGURE 6A**). The anterior tibial artery and peroneal nerve usually course through the groove between these structures. Dissection and retraction of these tendons will expose the supramalleolar segment of the anterior tibial artery.

Exposure of the Dorsalis Pedis Artery

- The dorsalis pedis artery (Latin for *dorsal artery of foot*) is the extension of the anterior tibial artery as it passes beneath the extensor retinaculum. It can serve as a suitable distal bypass target, especially in patients with diabetes.
- Ultrasound may help to localize this artery intraoperatively, as the location and course of this artery can vary widely between patients. The artery is best exposed beyond the inferior extensor retinaculum. A longitudinal incision is made on the dorsum of the foot, between the first and second metatarsal shafts and distal to the extensor retinaculum (**FIGURE 6B**).
- The dorsalis pedis artery typically resides in the groove between the first and second metatarsal heads, lateral to the extensor hallucis longus tendon, which is readily identified by dorsiflexion of the great toe, and medial to extensor hallucis brevis. Dissection is carried through subcutaneous tissue and the fascial layer must be divided to expose the artery. The dorsalis pedis artery is surrounded by two venous structures which must be carefully identified prior to placement of a sterile tourniquet. Methylene blue dye is useful for marking the artery at this point. After placement of the tourniquet, it can be quite difficult to differentiate the artery from the surrounding veins.

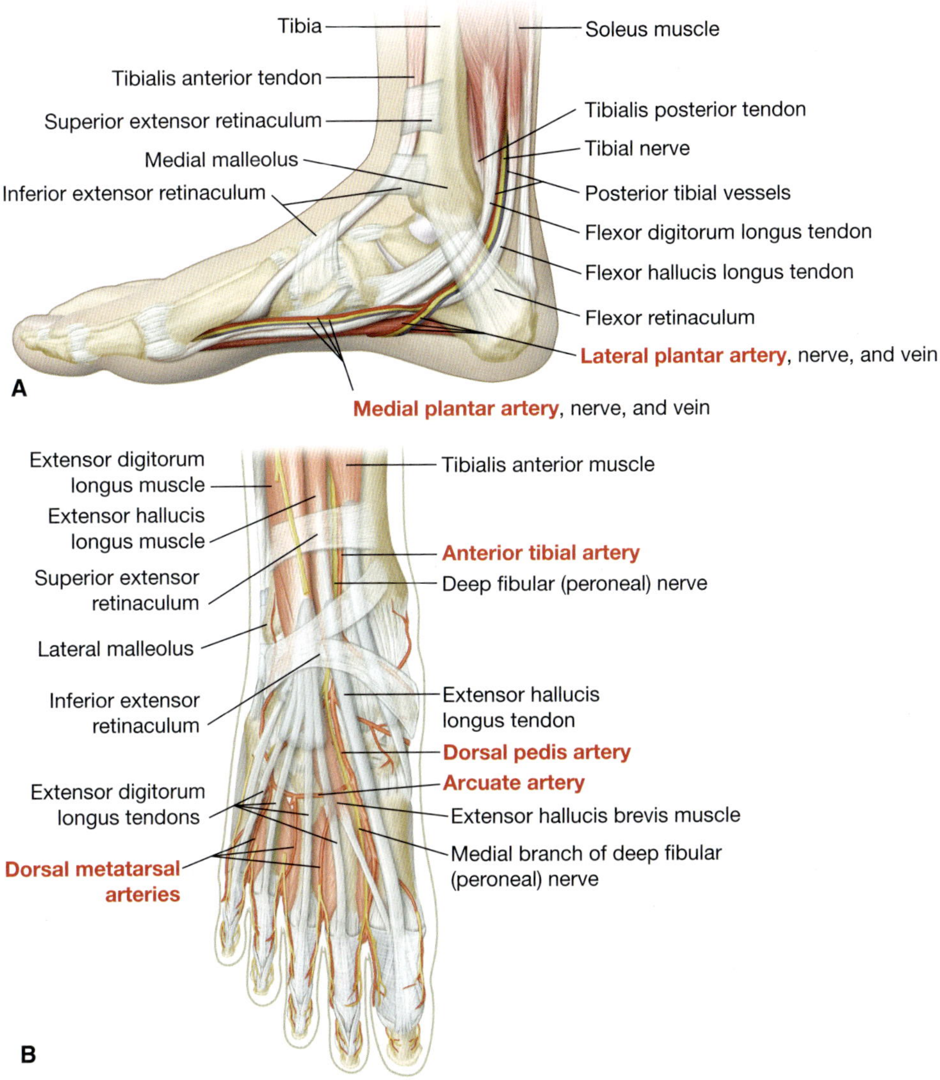

FIGURE 6 • **A,** Exposure of posterior tibial artery. **B,** Exposure of anterior tibial and dorsalis pedis arteries.

PEARLS AND PITFALLS

- Preoperative and intraoperative ultrasound aids the selection and placement of the incision. Dissection can be guided by palpation of the underlying arterial pulse. In many cases, given the burden of atherosclerotic disease, distal pulses are frequently absent or difficult to palpate. Use of an intraoperative Doppler probe can aid in the localization and dissection of target vessel. Nonetheless, knowledge of appropriate anatomic landmarks will greatly facilitate careful and expeditious exposure and avoid inadvertent injury to surrounding structures. In all circumstances, dissection should be directly targeted on and around the artery. This principle is similar in many ways to the orthopedic axiom to "stay on the bone" during dissection—keeping exposure centered on the target artery minimizes venous bleeding and damage to surrounding structures. Placement of an encircling silastic vessel loop will aid in vascular control and further mobilization.
- In the exposures of the thigh arteries, the sartorius muscle serves as an important landmark for the exposure of the common, superficial, and profunda femoris arteries.
- In the setting of reoperation, alternative surgical exposures allow operation in a virgin field that is unscarred by previous operation. Active infection may also preclude certain approaches to a target vessel, and alternative access is prudent in these situations.
- At the end of the procedure, if the inguinal ligament was divided for proximal exposure, it should be reapproximated. Any removable clips placed on the femoral circumflex arteries should be removed. Completion angiography is not always necessary, but may be useful if there is any question regarding the quality of the bypass.

POSTOPERATIVE CARE

- Following bypass, patients should be maintained on a comprehensive medical regimen to optimize their cardiopulmonary status. Lower extremity bypass operations are often performed on patients with diabetes and debilitating symptoms of claudication or CLTI. Postoperative care should also aim to optimize nutritional status, functional status, and maintenance of euglycemia. If the indication for bypass was tissue loss, the patient may develop a worsening infection secondary to increased distal perfusion.
- Most surgeons routinely employ routine antiplatelet and selective anticoagulation therapy to improve graft patency in lower extremity bypass patients. The Dutch Bypass Oral Anticoagulants or Aspirin (BOA) trial suggested that oral anticoagulation improved vein graft patency compared with aspirin, whereas aspirin improved prosthetic graft patency compared with anticoagulation.[10] The antiplatelet and/or anticoagulation regimen must be tailored to each individual patient following bypass with consideration of risk for graft failure vs risk of bleeding.
- We routinely administer aspirin to bypass patients and reserve anticoagulation (warfarin) for high-risk situations (redo bypass, marginal or alternative vein conduits, spliced vein grafts, poor outflow, prior graft thrombosis) due to the increased bleeding risk associated with anticoagulation. If anticoagulation is initiated, we begin with a low-dose heparin infusion after a routine postoperative check and then titrate accordingly if there is no evidence of hematoma or bleeding. The patient is transitioned to an oral anticoagulant following dietary intake and ambulation.
- Considerable efforts on wound care are required to achieve wound healing after lower extremity revascularization in patients with CLTI and tissue loss. Meticulous nursing care and early ambulation are also crucial to prevent decubitus ulcer in the lower extremities and the sacrum, creating new wounds in patients with lower extremity ischemia. Physical therapy consultation is advisable following bypass procedures. We routinely use *Prevalon* boots to protect the affected extremity from developing pressure ulcers against the bedpost.

OUTCOMES

- Outcomes of revascularization should be reported and interpreted through the reporting standards created and updated by the Society for Vascular Surgery.
- In general, autogenous vein conduits are superior to all others for infrainguinal bypass, even for the suprageniculate popliteal insertion site, where vein has proven superior to PTFE beyond 2 to 3 years. Ipsilateral and contralateral GSV conduits exhibit patency rates superior to alternative vein grafts, such as small saphenous vein, arm vein, and spliced veins. Vein graft primary patency rates for femoral-to-infrageniculate popliteal bypasses are approximately 70% to 75% at 5 years, and assisted primary patency can be improved even further by a duplex vein graft surveillance protocol. Infrapopliteal vein graft primary patency rates range from 60% to 70% at 5 years. Multiple randomized trials have shown no benefit of reversed vs in situ vein configurations.
- PTFE grafts have acceptable short-term and intermediate-term patency rates only in the suprageniculate popliteal position and therefore should only be used in limb salvage situations if autologous vein is truly unavailable. When PTFE must be used, an adjunctive venous Miller cuff or Taylor patch may improve results. The primary factors influencing graft patency are indication, conduit type, conduit quality (diameter), and arterial runoff. Poor runoff adversely impacts prosthetic graft patency.
- The reader is further referred to standard textbook sources such as *Rutherford's Vascular Surgery*, 7th edition, Chapter 109, for a more detailed discussion of the expected outcomes after surgical revascularization for infrainguinal disease.[2]

COMPLICATIONS

- Incomplete hemostasis: Satisfactory hemostasis should be achieved prior to skin closure. Full anticoagulation from heparin can be reversed with protamine to reduce the risk of postoperative bleeding. Channel drains may be placed in extensively dissected wounds. Hypertension is also a strong risk factor for postoperative hemorrhage and blood pressure should be strictly controlled during the postoperative phase.
- Vascular injury: Vascular clamps or silastic loops can lift atherosclerotic plaques and create inadvertent dissection planes and arterial injury in the presence of calcified plaques. Vascular clamps should therefore be placed at relatively soft, disease-free segments. Occasionally, this requires lateral positioning of a clamp to provide anterior/posterior rather than lateral compression of a vessel. In the CFA, the accumulation of significant posterior plaque often mandates modification of "atraumatic" clamp placement. In the tibial vessels, care should be taken to obtain control in the least traumatic fashion possible to limit compression of inelastic runoff vessels and the potential for clamp injury and restenosis. Alternative devices (eg, *Pruitt* occlusion catheters, *Fogarty* embolectomy catheters) may provide sufficient control to maintain a hemostatic field during completion of the distal anastomosis without exerting undue tension on the target vessel. As previously mentioned, strategic use of proximal thigh tourniquets and Esmarch bandage, deployed following creation of the proximal anastomosis and graft tunneling, may also be useful in minimizing bleeding and the risk of clamp injury in diseased tibial vessels.
- Distal embolization: Most frequently, periprocedural embolization is due to fragmentation of atherosclerotic plaque fragments or thrombus during dissection or clamping. Full systemic anticoagulation with intravenous heparin prior to clamping the vessel and intraoperative monitoring of activated clotting time will minimize the risk of graft or native vessel thrombosis. Prior to closure of arteriotomy and clamp release, all involved arteries must be meticulously back-bled and flushed to remove residual thrombus or loosen plaque fragments. Attention to this portion of the procedure, as well as to the precise course of graft tunneling, will optimize outcome and eliminate the need for revisions at the end of a long procedure.
- Nerve injury: Nerves and vessels are often intimately associated. Nerve injury can be caused by surgical dissection, a poorly placed self-retaining retractor, aggressive

spreading and clamp placement, and thermal energy from diathermy. These injuries can be prevented via intimate knowledge of appropriate anatomic landmarks, accurate incision placement, and meticulous sharp dissection. Importantly, excessively deep placement of self-retaining retractors during CFA/PFA exposure can result in substantial traction injuries to motor branches of the femoral nerve, significantly limiting the ability of patients to stand or bear weight for weeks following the procedure. As a general rule, retractors should be placed in the most superficial plane possible to obtain sufficient exposure of target vessels. All retractors should be removed as soon as they are no longer needed, or if attention is turned to alternative sites or other portions of the procedure that do not require continuous exposure.

- Lymphatic injury: Lymphatic vessels usually course close to the arteries and veins. Any visible lymphatic vessels should be suture ligated. Cautery may be used to the divided end of lymphatic channels. Careful dissection respecting tissue planes allows layered closure to eliminate dead space and lymphatic accumulation, formation of seroma, or hematoma. Lymph nodes should not be transected. When lymph nodes are inadvertently injured, extra time should be taken to control, ligate, and divide afferent and efferent vessels and remove the node completely.

REFERENCES

1. Norgren L, Hiatt WR, Dormandy JA, et al. Inter-society consensus for the management of peripheral arterial disease (TASC II). *J Vasc Surg*. 2007;45(suppl S):S5-S67.
2. Mills JL. Infrainguinal bypass. In: Cronenwett JL, Johnston KW, Rutherford RB, eds. *Rutherford's Vascular Surgery*. 7th ed. Saunders/Elsevier; 2010:1682-1703.
3. London NJM. Surgical intervention for lower extremity arterial occlusive disease: femoropopliteal and tibial interventions. In: Hallett JW, Mills JL, Earnshaw J, et al, eds. *Comprehensive Vascular and Endovascular Surgery*. 2nd ed. Mosby, Inc; 2009:192-214.
4. Netter FH. *Atlas of Human Anatomy*. 5th ed. Saunders/Elsevier; 2010.
5. Ouriel K, Rutherford RB. *Atlas of Vascular Surgery: Operative Procedures*. Saunders; 1998.
6. Rohen JW, Yokochi C, Lutjen-Drecoli E. *Color Atlas of Anatomy: A Photographic Study of the Human Body*. 7th ed. Lippincott Williams & Wilkins; 2011.
7. Zarins CK, Gewertz BL. *Atlas of Vascular Surgery*. Churchill Livingstone; 1989.
8. Mills JL, ed. *Management of Chronic Lower Limb Ischemia*. Arnold Publishing Inc and Oxford University Press; 2000.
9. Mills JL, Lucas LC. Reversed vein bypass grafts to popliteal, tibial and peroneal arteries. In: Fischer JE, ed. *Mastery of Surgery*. 6th ed. Lippincott Williams & Wilkins; 2012.
10. Efficacy of oral anticoagulants compared with aspirin after infrainguinal bypass surgery (The Dutch Bypass Oral Anticoagulants or Aspirin Study): a randomised trial. *Lancet*. 2000;355(9201):346-351.

Chapter 28 Management of the Infected Femoral Graft

Alyssa Jaesun Pyun and Vincent Lopez Rowe

DEFINITION

- Early prosthetic graft infection: <4 months, often hospital acquired, more virulent, associated with more severe presentation
- Late prosthetic graft infection: >4 months, often low virulence (eg, *Staphylococcus epidermidis*)
- Szilagyi Classification (postoperative wound infection)
  - Grade I: cellulitis
  - Grade II: extend into subcutaneous tissue
  - Grade III: involving vascular prosthesis

PATIENT HISTORY AND PHYSICAL FINDINGS

- The symptoms of an infected femoral graft can vary widely, from a chronically draining wound to sepsis and hemodynamic collapse.
- Symptoms may have been present from hours to weeks.
- Infections are more likely to occur when bypass grafts are implanted emergently or required prolonged operative times.
- Physical examination should include inspection of the surgical wounds and graft tunnels for induration, erythema, tenderness, open wounds, aneurysmal degeneration of the graft or anastomosis, or drainage.

IMAGING AND OTHER DIAGNOSTIC STUDIES

- When possible, causative organisms should be identified prior to surgery to aid in choosing appropriate systemic antibiotics and the optimal surgical approach. Surface culture swabs may result in false negatives, especially for low-virulent organisms with low numbers and slow growth not penetrating the perigraft tissue.
- Positive blood cultures are uncommon and laboratory testing may be normal, especially in late appearing low-virulent perigraft infections.
- Duplex ultrasonography is often the first imaging study obtained as it can be performed quickly, can demonstrate graft patency, and can differentiate anastomotic pseudoaneurysms, hematomas, seromas/fluid collections, and solid tissue masses. Duplex ultrasonography can also help define the tissue planes involved and proximity to the underlying bypass graft.
- Prior to surgery, detailed imaging with computed tomographic angiography (CTA) can provide critical information for developing a cohesive plan for surgical exploration with graft removal and replacement.
- CT can accurately identify anatomic signs of infection including loss of normal tissue planes, soft tissue gas, and presence of fluid collections/abscesses or anastomotic pseudoaneurysms.
- CTA provides high-resolution imaging of the aorta and runoff vessels, which will aid in determining revascularization options, including in situ reconstruction, obturator bypass, or ilioprofunda bypass.
- Radionuclide scans may provide evidence for graft infection when other imaging studies are nondiagnostic; however, this may result in false positives in the early postoperative period due to nonspecific uptake of healing perigraft tissue.

SURGICAL MANAGEMENT

- Aggressive and wide debridement of devitalized or infected tissue must accompany graft excision and replacement in the setting of infection. This may require multiple/staged debridements.
- Partial or complete excision of infected prosthetic grafts is generally required to eliminate the infection.
- Excision of infected autogenous graft infections may be necessary when associated with sepsis caused by *Escherichia coli*, *Pseudomonas*, or *Proteus* spp.
- Graft preservation with local debridement may be considered when low-virulent infections of shorter graft segments do not include the anastomoses and are limited to the immediate perigraft area. We recommend against graft preservation with virulent organisms such as *Pseudomonas*, *Serratia*, *methicillin-resistant Staphylococcus aureus*, and *E. coli*.
- Thrombosed grafts with adequate collateral circulation may tolerate excision without reconstruction.
- Graft excision and extra-anatomic bypass is preferred in the presence of severe sepsis and/or hemorrhage. Examples of extra-anatomic bypasses include axillary-to-femoral bypass (**FIGURE 1**), obturator bypass, or cross-femoral bypass.

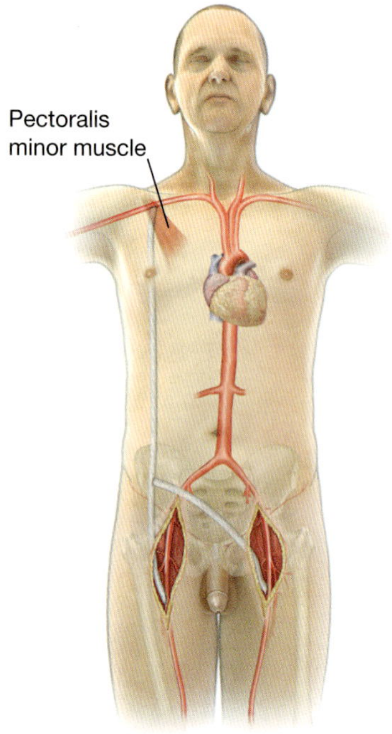

FIGURE 1 • Axillofemoral bypass. Note that the proximal graft is placed behind the pectoralis minor muscle.

- In situ replacement is generally preferred in low-virulent infections without sepsis or invasive infection and in those with distal occlusive disease.
- There continues to be a limited role for endovascular therapy in the setting of femoral graft infections; however, it has been described in rare circumstances.[1]
- Potential options for replacement graft material include autogenous vein (saphenous, cephalic, basilic, or superficial femoral vein [SFV]), cryopreserved tissue (aorto-iliac-femoral artery, femoral vein, saphenous vein),[2] or antibiotic-impregnated prosthetic graft (rifampin-soaked Dacron or polytetrafluoroethylene [PTFE]).
- Debridement of an infected groin wound may result in a large defect that either cannot be covered or closed. Muscle flaps can provide coverage of healthy well-vascularized tissue to protect the repair.
- Small to medium defects can be covered with a sartorius muscle flap, which is divided from its attachment to the anterior superior iliac spine and mobilized medially to cover the wound.
- A pedicled flap from the leg or abdominal wall may be required for larger wounds. These flaps may utilize the rectus femoris, rectus abdominis, tensor fasciae latae, or gracilis.[3-5]
- Negative pressure wound therapy can be considered with adequate tissue coverage over the bypass graft.

GENERAL CONSIDERATIONS

- It is preferable when considering an extra-anatomic reconstruction to revascularize before excising the infected graft. This can be accomplished with a bypass and tunnel performed across clean tissue planes. Once the bypass is completed and wounds closed, the groin can be explored and the infected graft removed. With this approach, the continuity between the superficial femoral and deep femoral arteries should be maintained by either oversewing the distal common femoral artery or anastomosing the profunda femoris artery (PFA) to the superficial femoral artery with proximal ligation (**FIGURE 2**).
- Debridement of the infected site should include removal of infected or necrotic tissue and complete excision of the anastomosis. Dissection may be aided by lack of incorporation of the infected graft but also may prove challenging due to the extensive scarring in the reoperative field. Sharp dissection techniques are critical for minimizing the risk of inadvertent injury to vessels or adjacent structures.
- Other measures such as the use of antibiotic-loaded beads and pulse lavage irrigation can be used as adjunctive measures for wound sterilization.[6,7]
- It is important to send cultures of the perigraft fluid, tissue, and graft.[8] Instructions can be given to the microbiology lab to perform sonication of the graft to separate biofilm from graft and maximize the bacteriology yield.

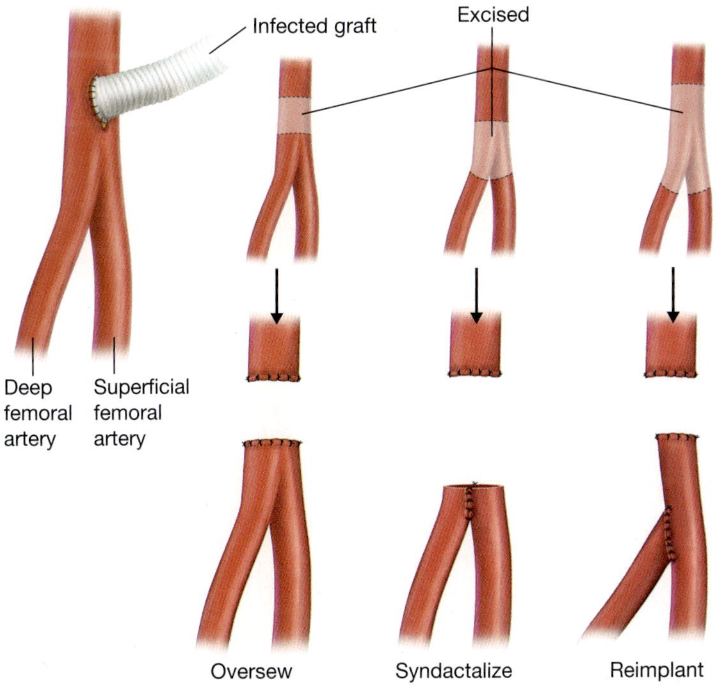

FIGURE 2 • Surgical options for maintaining continuity of arterial flow to the profunda femoris artery after obturator bypass and common femoral artery ligation.

OBTURATOR BYPASS

- Using the obturator foramen may be a useful approach for bypassing an infected groin through a sterile field.[9-11] A reinforced PTFE graft is preferred and can be used if sepsis has been controlled and the bypass can be performed without violating the infected field.
- The proximal anastomosis can be performed to the common iliac artery, external iliac artery (ipsilateral or contralateral), or previous graft if not infected (**FIGURE 3**). Exposure can be obtained through a standard retroperitoneal incision, by dividing the external and internal oblique and transversus abdominis muscles, identifying the preperitoneal space, and retracting the peritoneum medially with blunt dissection techniques. The obturator foramen is just posterior to the anterior ramus of the pelvis, although it may not be easily palpated due to the overlying obturator membrane.
- The distal anastomosis can be performed to the distal superficial femoral artery, the midportion of the PFA (see the following section, lateral approach to the Lateral Profunda Femoris Artery Exposure), or the popliteal artery. During this dissection, the adductor longus and magnus can be identified with the leg abducted and externally rotated. The tunnel will be placed deep to these muscles, which insert on the external surface of the obturator foramen.
- The tunnel should be performed in a cranial direction with a long aortic clamp or tunneling instrument (**FIGURE 4**). The instrument is passed deep to the adductor magnus while a hand is placed over the obturator foramen from the retroperitoneal incision. The instrument can be directed through the obturator foramen. The tunnel should be made through the anteriomedial portion of the obturator foramen to avoid injury to the obturator artery and nerve, which traverses laterally.
- Once the tunnel is made, the graft can be placed and the bypass performed. Once completed, the incisions should be closed and protected before proceeding with excision of the infected graft.

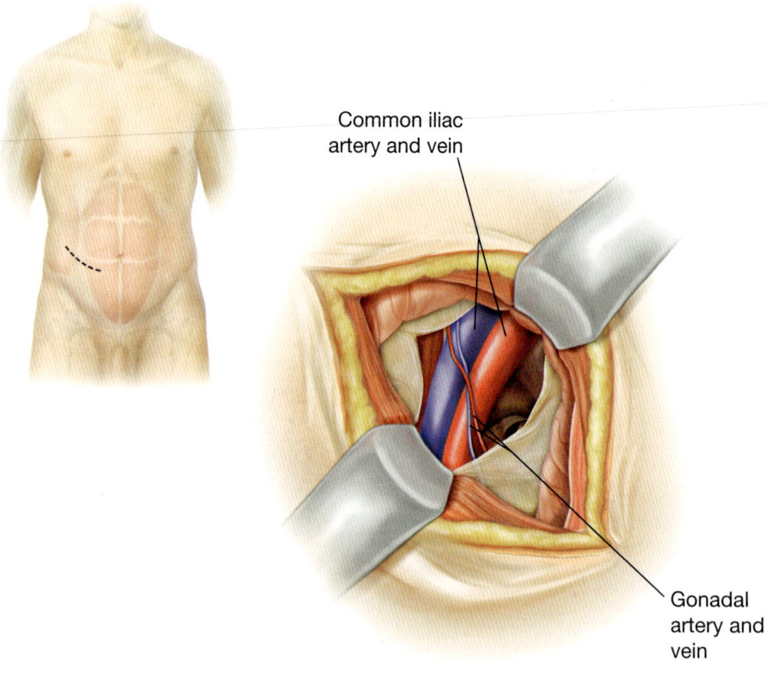

FIGURE 3 • Operative incision for retroperitoneal exposure of the iliac artery. Peritoneum and its contents are retracted medially to aid in exposure.

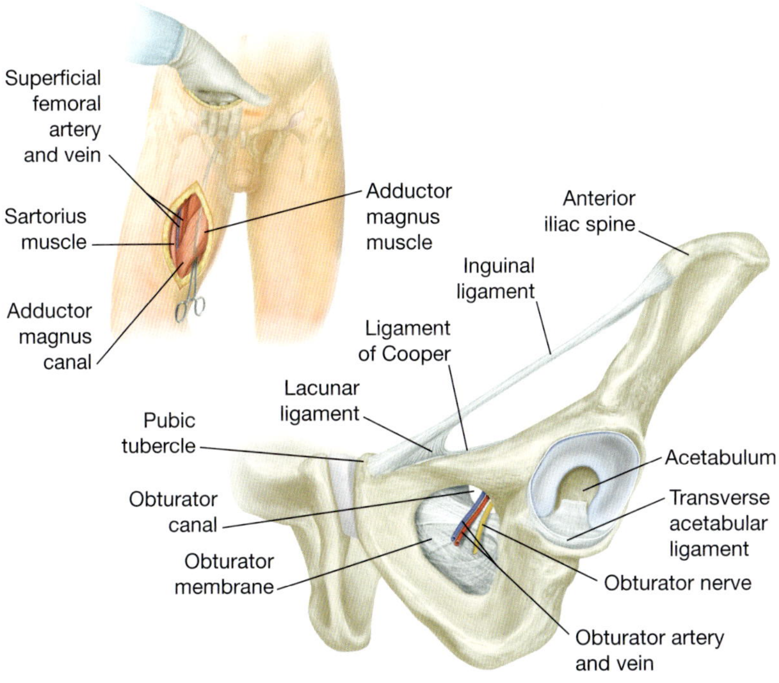

FIGURE 4 • Exposure of the superficial femoral artery and tunneling for an obturator bypass. **Left:** creating the tunnel behind the adductor magnus muscle. **Right:** placement of the tunnel through the obturator membrane.

LATERAL FEMORAL BYPASS

- The lateral femoral bypass allows for tunneling lateral to the infected field.
- A retroperitoneal approach allows for inflow vessel exposure and anastomosis. The graft is then tunneled medial to the anterior iliac spine and under the inguinal ligament through the psoas canal before continuing anterolaterally, coursing lateral to the femoral nerve subcutaneously to the outflow vessel for distal anastomosis.[12]

LATERAL PROFUNDA FEMORIS ARTERY EXPOSURE

- Another option for remote revascularization is to use the second portion of the PFA, exposed through a lateral incision.[13] This approach may be useful if the superficial femoral artery is occluded and the goal is to establish flow from the axillary artery via a tunnel medial to the anterior iliac spine and lateral to the femoral infection.
- The PFA is exposed through an incision placed along the lateral border of the sartorius muscle 4 to 6 cm below the anterior superior iliac spine (**FIGURE 5**). The sartorius and superficial femoral vessels can be retracted medially to expose the adductor longus. Its overlying fascia is divided, and with medial retraction, the PFA is exposed.

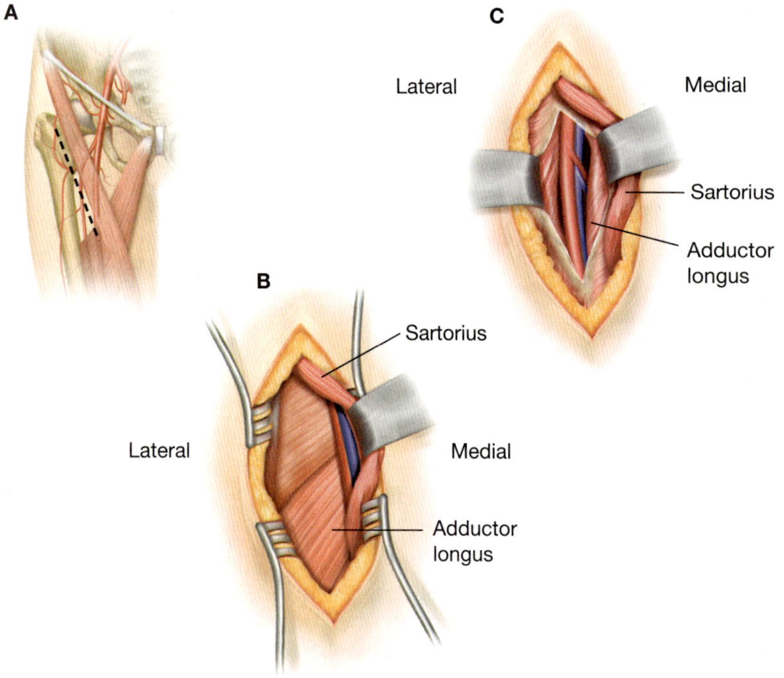

FIGURE 5 • Lateral exposure of the profunda femoris artery. **A,** Incision along the lateral border of the sartorius muscle. **B,** Medial retraction of the superficial femoral artery and vein to expose the adductor longus. **C,** Fascial incision and medial retraction of the adductor longus to expose the profunda femoris vessels.

SUPERFICIAL FEMORAL VEIN HARVEST

- SFV can be a suitable graft for reconstruction, with a low incidence of recurrent or uncontrolled infection.[14] Preoperative evaluation should include duplex imaging of the SFV to exclude deep venous thrombosis and to determine the vessel diameter.
- Dissection can be performed through a standard anteromedial leg incision or placed over the lateral border of the sartorius (**FIGURE 6**). The vein should be dissected from its confluence with the profunda femoris vein distally to obtain sufficient length for reconstruction. Care should be taken to preserve the profunda femoris vein and the common femoral vein. The dissection can be continued distally through the adductor canal if an extensive segment of vein is required for reconstruction.
- Once harvested, branches of the SFV should be doubly ligated or suture ligated a distance 2 mm from their junction with the SFV to prevent slippage of the ligature once the conduit is pressurized.

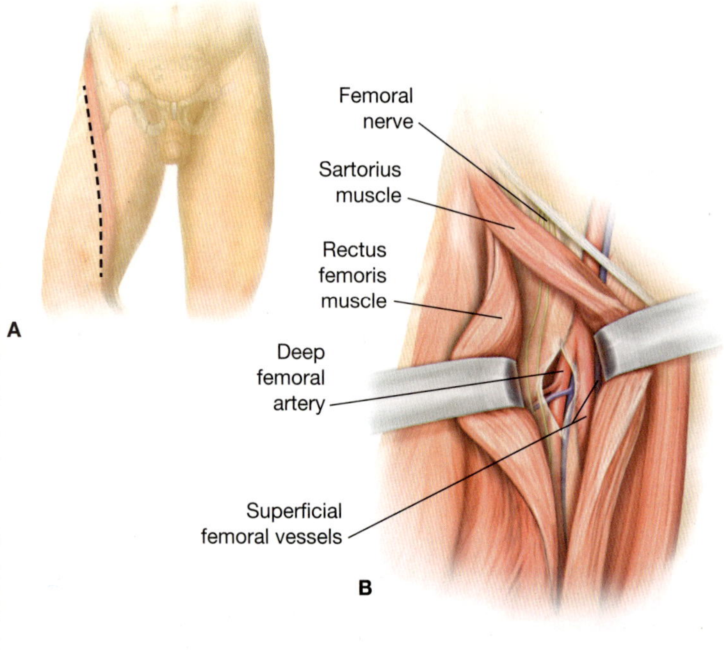

FIGURE 6 • Exposure of the superficial femoral vein. **A,** Incision along the sartorius muscle. **B,** medial retraction of the sartorius to expose the superficial femoral vein.

CRYOPRESERVED GRAFTS

- Some studies have shown favorable results for cryopreserved allografts with regard to limb loss, recurrent infection, and survival compared with other in situ replacements.[15]
- When considering an allograft, greater than 24 hours may be required to locate suitable graft material and length if there is no on-site inventory.
- Grafts should be prepared immediately before implantation. The thaw-and-rinse process takes approximately 45 minutes.
- Ligated branches should be tested for hemostasis and suture ligatures placed if necessary. Antibiotic-impregnated fibrin glue may be considered at suture lines. If using an aortoiliac homograft, it is easier to confirm hemostasis if the graft is placed with the lumbar branches facing anterior.
- Graft length should allow for a tension-free anastomosis. When possible, avoid allograft-to-allograft anastomoses.

PROFUNDA TO SUPERFICIAL FEMORAL ARTERY TRANSPOSITION

- Alternatively, in scenarios of significant common femoral artery interruption with gross infection and no suitable conduits available, a profunda to superficial femoral artery transposition can be done.
- Femoral artery exposure with common femoral, profunda, and superficial femoral artery control should be obtained, followed by sufficient profunda and superficial femoral artery mobilization to minimize tension while avoiding redundancy/kinking. After suture ligation of the common femoral artery, an end-to-side or end-to-end anastomosis of the profunda and superficial femoral artery can be done to maintain distal perfusion (**FIGURE 2**). In theory, by maintaining the continuity of the femoral bifurcation, the collaterals from the profunda femoral artery are allowed back into the axial circulation earlier, as opposed to through the small collateral networks around the knee.

PEARLS AND PITFALLS

Preoperative considerations	■ When possible, consideration should be made prior to surgery for the best option(s) of graft material, allowing time to obtain it if required. For autogenous vein, preoperative duplex is essential to determine the size and quality of the proposed conduit.
Proximal and distal vessel control	■ When possible, proximal and distal vessel control should be obtained through extension of the original incision or through separate incisions before dissecting the infected vessels. Remote bypass with subsequent removal of infected material may be preferable to in situ repair.
Intraoperative cultures	■ It is important to obtain Gram stain, aerobic, and anaerobic cultures of the perigraft fluid, perigraft tissue, and graft. The yield of the graft will be increased if sonication of the graft is performed in the microbiology lab prior to incubation.
Tunnels	■ Tunnels, when possible, should be placed in sterile fields.
Systemic antibiotic treatment	■ Broad-spectrum antibiotics should be initially considered for patients with severe sepsis. For those without sepsis, blood and wound cultures should be performed prior to starting antibiotics. Initial antibiotics should include coverage for methicillin-resistant *Staphylococcus aureus* (MRSA). After surgery, parenteral antibiotics should be considered for 2-6 weeks, especially for invasive infections or in situ repair.

POSTOPERATIVE CARE

- Antibiotics should be continued for at least 2 to 6 weeks, depending on the type of organism, and should be chosen based on antimicrobial sensitivity when available.
- Patients should be inspected daily for signs of infection, which may include fever, leukocytosis, erythema or drainage from the wound, or wound breakdown. Persistent infection should trigger consideration of wound exploration and reevaluation of the antibiotic regimen.
- Drains, if placed, should be removed as soon as possible, based on quantity and appearance of fluid. Ongoing purulent drainage or continued fever and leukocytosis may indicate lack of source control, which may require wound exploration and washout.
- Arterial surveillance should be performed prior to discharge to confirm the integrity of the repair and establish a baseline for future surveillance examinations.

COMPLICATIONS

- Bleeding from the wound should raise immediate concern for arterial disruption from persistent infection leading to tissue destruction. If present, patients should undergo arterial duplex and be considered for re-exploration. Under these circumstances, complete evaluation of the arterial reconstruction (even if remote) is advisable as vascular resection and reconstruction may be required. At times, arterial ligation may be the only option for local control of sepsis.

- If not already performed, patients requiring re-exploration and debridement for persistent infection will most often benefit from muscle flap coverage of the defect.

REFERENCES

1. Naddaf A, Hasanadka R, Hood D, Hodgson K. Repair of an anastomotic pseudoaneurysm with a novel hybrid technique. *Ann Vasc Surg*. 2020;63:439-442.
2. Furlough CL, Jain AK, Ho KJ, Rodriguez HE, Tomita TM, Eskandari MK. Peripheral artery reconstructions using cryopreserved arterial allografts in infected fields. *J Vasc Surg*. 2019;70(2):562-568.
3. Ryer EJ, Garvin RP, Kapadia RN, et al. Outcome of rectus femoris muscle flaps performed by vascular surgeons for the management of complex groin wounds after femoral artery reconstructions. *J Vasc Surg*. 2020;71(3):905-911.
4. Ali AT, Rueda M, Desikan S, et al. Outcomes after retroflexed gracilis muscle flap for vascular infections in the groin. *J Vasc Surg*. 2016;64(2):452-457.
5. Dua A, Rothenberg KA, Lavingia K, Ho VT, Rao C, Desai SS. Outcomes of gracilis muscle flaps in the management of groin complications after arterial bypass with prosthetic graft. *Ann Vasc Surg*. 2018;51:113-118.
6. Stone PA, Armstrong PA, Bandyk DF, et al. Use of antibiotic-loaded polymethylmethacrylate beads for the treatment of extracavitary prosthetic vascular graft infections. *J Vasc Surg*. 2006;44(4):757-761.
7. Mote GA, Malay DS. Efficacy of power-pulsed lavage in lower extremity wound infections: a prospective observational study. *J Foot Ankle Surg*. 2010;49(2):135-142.
8. Bandyk DF, Bergamini TM, Kinney EV, et al. In situ replacement of vascular prostheses infected by bacterial biofilms. *J Vasc Surg*. 1991;13(5):575-583.
9. Pearce WH, Ricco JB, Yao JS, et al. Modified technique of obturator bypass in failed or infected grafts. *Ann Surg*. 1983;197(3):344-347.
10. Bath J, Rahimi M, Long B, Avgerinos E, Giglia J. Clinical outcomes of obturator canal bypass. *J Vasc Surg*. 2017;66(1):160-166.
11. Dunphy KM, Hassey J, Vallabjaneni R, et al. Results of obturator foramen bypass in patients with groin infection and arterial involvement. *Ann Vasc Surg*. 2021;S0890-5096(21):00202-00208.
12. Madden NJ, Calligaro KD, Dougherty MJ, Zheng H, Troutman DA. Lateral femoral bypass for prosthetic arterial graft infections in the groin. *J Vasc Surg*. 2019;69(4):1129-1136.
13. Bridges R, Gewertz BL. Lateral incision for exposure of femoral vessels. *Surg Gynecol Obstet*. 1980;150(5):732-733.
14. Smith ST, Clagett GP. Femoral vein harvest for vascular reconstructions: pitfalls and tips for success. *Semin Vasc Surg*. 2008;21(1):35-40.
15. Kieffer E, Gomes D, Chiche L, et al. Allograft replacement for infrarenal aortic graft infection: early and late results in 179 patients. *J Vasc Surg*. 2004;39(5):1009-1017.

Chapter 29 Femoral Pseudoaneurysm Management: Open and Endovascular

Joseph Patrick Hart

DEFINITION

- Common femoral aneurysms are either true aneurysms or pseudoaneurysms and are usually chronic. True aneurysms are typically either degenerative or due to familial or genetic disease. Pseudoaneurysms differ in that not all the arterial wall layers are typically involved, and they are most often acute. The name pseudoaneurysm indicates an aneurysm wall consisting only of connective tissue histologically similar to the adventitia.
- Femoral pseudoaneurysms are a common reason for urgent or emergent vascular surgery inpatient consultation that usually arise from transfemoral vascular access with or without iatrogenic procedural and periprocedural mishaps. Active pseudoaneurysms contain a nonthrombosed or partially thrombosed area of extravascular flow. This chapter focuses on the treatment of pseudoaneurysms of the femoral artery and bifurcation.
- Consultation for femoral pseudoaneurysms (PSAs) remains common due to increasing utilization of endovascular access as well as the use of larger devices. Closure devices have become routine and have led to earlier discharge and mobilization times; however, closure devices can cause their own set of possible complications, including concomitant dissection, back wall to front wall closure, vessel occlusion, distal embolization, and infection. These concerns should inform the approach to any patient with PSA after closure device use.

DIFFERENTIAL DIAGNOSIS

- If concern for femoral PSA arises, a mass may be present anterior to the femoral artery, which may or may not be pulsatile. It is generally considered most appropriate to obtain an early directed vascular ultrasound whenever suspicion arises.
- The differential diagnosis includes:
  - Periprocedural hematoma without pseudoaneurysm
  - Femoral arterial to venous fistula
  - Lymphadenopathy
  - Seroma
  - Abscess
- An isolated iatrogenic arteriovenous fistula (AVF) will often have a palpable thrill or audible bruit and may present with limb swelling. This can coexist with a femoral PSA. A firm groin mass can be either a hematoma or thrombosed pseudoaneurysm or could represent groin lymphadenopathy from a variety of causes. An abscess or seroma typically presents with a softer mass in the groin, with or without overlying cellulitis. Simple duplex ultrasound can often confirm the diagnosis when a groin mass is discovered on physical examination.

PATIENT HISTORY AND PHYSICAL FINDINGS

- Patients with femoral PSA often present with history of recent cardiac catheterization, peripheral angiography or intervention, endovascular graft placement, intracardiac device placement, extracorporeal life support (ECMO) use, or any other procedure via a transfemoral arterial access.
- Closure device use is an essential historical point to elucidate as the presence of a closure device may change the spectrum of anticipated concomitant findings and proposed repair.
- Many patients who develop PSA after arterial access are on aggressive perioperative antiplatelet and anticoagulation regimens, which increase their risk for PSA formation. These may not be able to be discontinued, depending on the procedure performed or devices placed (eg, drug-eluting devices).
- Multiple femoral accesses, previous open common femoral surgery, prosthetic patch graft or adjacent stent deployments, radiation, or other historical factors are important details to determine in the patient's history.
- Morbid obesity is an important risk factor, history element, and potentially complicating perioperative/-interventional factor.
- Some patients report a sudden popping sensation preceding groin mass formation. Not infrequently, an episode of straining or lifting just precedes complaints of PSA formation.
- Physical examination of PSA can vary from obvious and quite striking to relatively benign and occult. Tenderness anterior to the common femoral artery on the side of access is common, and concomitant ecchymosis and hematoma is often noted. A pulsatile mass on the side of the access is often appreciated if the femoral artery pseudoaneurysm is patent. A bruit may be audible and may be due to PSA, or concomitant AVF, stenosis, or dissection.
- The ipsilateral limb should be examined carefully for distal perfusion, and pulse examination should be documented. The contralateral limb distal vascular examination is also important as the status of distal perfusion is critical. If pulses are not palpable, the status of Doppler signals should be assessed and documented bilaterally.
- Skin viability over the PSA should be assessed. If the pseudoaneurysm or pseudoaneurysm and hematoma in combination have led to so-called shiny skin or otherwise evident compromised skin perfusion, expeditious and most likely open surgical management will be necessary.
- Hemoglobin concentration may be decreased, especially if there is a concomitant large groin or retroperitoneal hematoma.
- Patients with hemodynamic instability or requiring ongoing transfusion should undergo rapid assessment with stabilization and may then require expedited treatment.

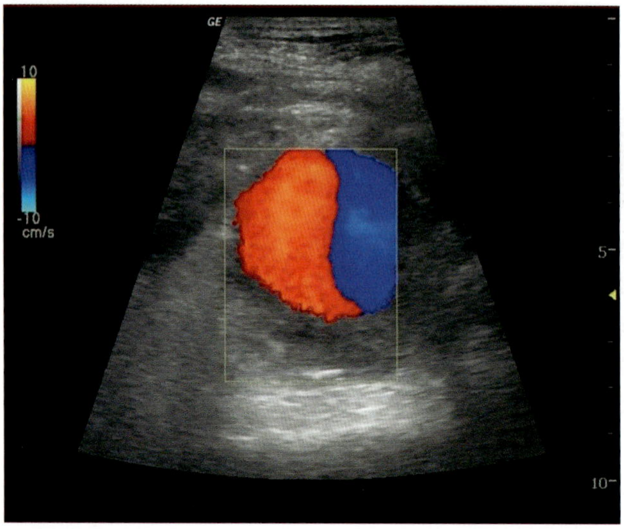

FIGURE 1 • Duplex ultrasound of CFA with pathognomonic finding of arterial pseudoaneurysm.

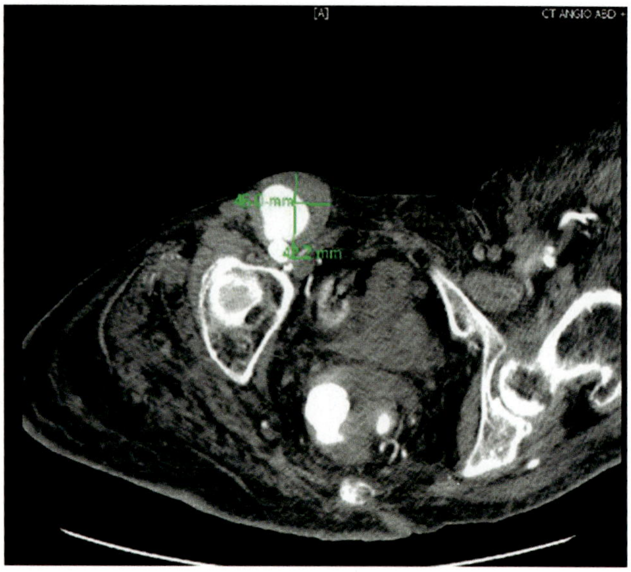

FIGURE 2 • CT angiography of pelvis with finding of arterial pseudoaneurysm.

IMAGING AND OTHER DIAGNOSTIC STUDIES

- Imaging to confirm or exclude groin PSA is usually initiated by a screening duplex ultrasound (**FIGURE 1**). This will often confirm the diagnosis and may be all the imaging necessary prior to attempting repair. Typical and pathognomonic bicolor signal within the pseudoaneurysm cavity makes the diagnosis. In addition, ultrasound can provide confirmation of the length and dimensions of the pseudoaneurysm neck, which is critical to confirming suitability for thrombin injection to treat noninvasively.
- Other potential findings on ultrasound can include AVF, femoral or common femoral deep venous thrombosis, additional technical problems within the common femoral artery (CFA) lumen, existing occlusive disease, arterial thrombosis, hematoma, seroma, or other problems.
- CT angiography (CTA), contrasted or even noncontrast CT, magnetic resonance angiography all may detect a groin pseudoaneurysm in various clinical scenarios. If malperfusion is detected on physical examination, CTA is indicated to confirm or exclude distal embolization, femoral artery bifurcation or other related vessel thromboses, chronic occlusive disease, and/or steal (**FIGURE 2**).
- While CTA can be omitted from the workup in many cases, it may be helpful to establish the runoff status below the pseudoaneurysm, as well provide information regarding inflow and surrounding anatomy.
- Catheter angiography may be a useful adjunct to either thrombin injection or, in some cases, even operative repair.

NONOPERATIVE MANAGEMENT

- Importantly, under a certain threshold size, PSAs are likely to thrombose spontaneously. Observation with serial weekly ultrasound follow-up is indicated in those patients with PSAs under 2 cm, with no associated skin compromise or infection.[1] Repeat ultrasound often will demonstrate occlusion of the PSA after 1 to 2 weeks, obviating any need for intervention. If the patient is maintained on anticoagulation the PSA is less likely to occlude without assistance.
- Ultrasound-guided compression is a potentially successful, although tedious, approach that accelerates otherwise spontaneous closure in some patients. This approach is undertaken by the ultrasound tech. The femoral vessels and the PSA neck is visualized. Ultrasound-guided compression is held to occlude flow through the neck but allow flow through the femoral vessels. This is held for 15 to 30 minutes, and the flow in the PSA is evaluated. Repeat pressure can be applied if partial occlusion is observed. This technique can be very uncomfortable for the patient and may require sedation. If the patient is maintained on anticoagulation, this technique is not likely to be successful, and this technique is generally reserved for those PSAs that are smaller. We typically reserve ultrasound-guided compression for those PSAs that are less than 2 cm but are not candidates for observation only.[1]

ENDOVASCULAR APPROACH

- Endovascular management is the most common approach to femoral PSA today. With its less invasive approach without the need for a formal open incision, thrombin injection remains the workhorse of femoral PSA treatment.
- After a femoral PSA is identified by duplex ultrasound, neck length and width must be evaluated carefully and confirmed to be greater than or equal to 10 mm long and less than 5 mm wide.[2]
- In PSAs that do not have otherwise acceptable necks, some can still be salvaged for endovascular management by use of endoluminal angioplasty balloon protection, usually from a contralateral approach to protect against distal embolization of thrombin, when a neck of more conventional dimensions for unprotected thrombin injection is not present.

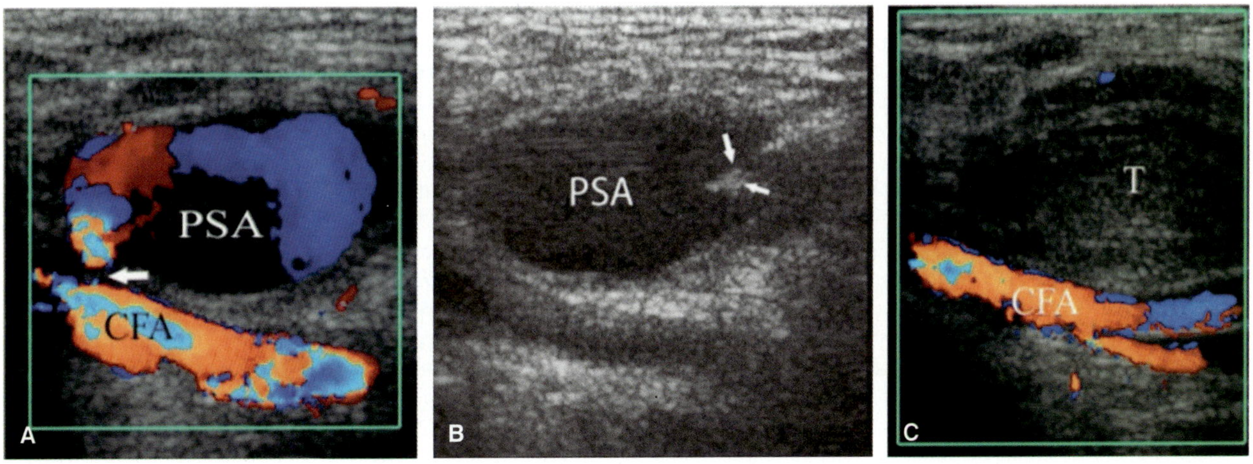

FIGURE 3 • Duplex ultrasound of CFA with **(A)** arterial pseudoaneurysm (arrow indicates PSA neck), **(B)** needle tip for thrombin injection (arrow indicates needle tip), and **(C)** thrombotic pseudoaneurysm occlusion with preservation of native vessel luminal flow.

- Following prep and drape and a time out, an appropriately prepped and draped ultrasound probe is used to confirm the presence of the pseudoaneurysm again and that spontaneous thrombosis has not occurred. Neck length and width are quickly generally confirmed.
- A micropuncture needle on an injection system using extension tubing and a three-way stopcock is placed under ultrasound guidance into the PSA sac. Agitated saline without thrombin is then injected to confirm luminal access to the PSA (**FIGURE 3**). (Alternatively, an etched EchoTip micropuncture needle can also provide direct evidence of correct needle position.)
- After this is confirmed by a swirling pattern on grayscale duplex (or etched tip needle use), thrombin can be injected while maintaining meticulous attention to awareness of needle tip position. An initial injection of as little as 0.1 mL of a 1000 U/mL thrombin solution is used, and ultrasound visualization of the PSA is maintained.[3] Use of a total dose greater than 1.0 mL of such a solution should not be necessary in most moderate-sized PSAs. Thrombosis of the PSA is visualized, usually almost immediately, upon thrombin injection. Continuous duplex monitoring is used during extremely slow and measured injection to look for increased echogenicity and/or loss of color flow indicating PSA thrombosis.
- Avoiding overinjection and treatment beyond the PSA or its neck into the CFA is most critical and necessitates excellent on-field ultrasound imaging guidance and highly coordinated, stable injection technique.
- Ultrasound is then used to confirm complete thrombosis during the index procedure. Visualization of appropriate thrombosis of the pseudoaneurysm lumen by grayscale as well as elimination of color flow within the pseudoaneurysm with preservation of flow within the arterial lumen are confirmed and documented.
- Critically, those attempting thrombin injection should be prepared to perform rescue thrombus aspiration or other catheter-directed intervention should there be distal thrombin embolization.
- Most vascular surgeons perform a follow-up duplex ultrasound to confirm pseudoaneurysm thrombosis and exclude the need for retreatment or further observation at 24 to 48 hours post procedure.

SURGICAL MANAGEMENT

- Surgical management first mandates orderly control of inflow and outflow. PSA having surgical repair will usually be larger, present with one of the other complications outlined above, and occur in patients who have failed, or were not a candidate for, ultrasound-guided compression or thrombin injection.
- The first step is to obtain proximal control. Given the common femoral PSA proximity to the inguinal ligament in many cases, this raises specific challenges with regards to proximal control. In patients with adequate distance above the pseudoaneurysm, relatively high exposure of the common femoral from the groin can be accomplished. In this case, a longitudinal incision is made over the femoral vessels and, in the most proximal aspect, carried down to the femoral artery at the level of the inguinal ligament. Care must be taken to avoid entrance into the pseudoaneurysm itself. Circumferential control is obtained, and a vessel loop is placed around the vessel. Extensive mobilization of the inguinal ligament to allow high external iliac control through the groin is critical if working to do the whole repair from the groin only.
- If there is not enough room proximal to the pseudoaneurysm to facilitate operative exposure of the common femoral artery, there are two choices. A separate curvilinear incision can be made above the inguinal ligament, and the retroperitoneal space can be entered after dividing the abdominal musculature and dissecting the retroperitoneal space. The distal external iliac artery can be circumferentially controlled above the inguinal ligament via this approach, which provides excellent proximal control.
- Alternatively, endovascular balloon control can be obtained from the contralateral groin or, if necessary, the arm or the ipsilateral superficial femoral artery (SFA). However, this provides another arterial access site at risk for PSA or other

complication; therefore, careful planning and execution of this access must be taken (**FIGURE 4**).

- The second step is to obtain distal control of the femoral bifurcation. This is generally done by dissecting distal from the PSA sac and getting circumferential control of both the SFA and the profunda.
- Once proximal control is obtained, distal control of the femoral bifurcation is also required.
- The third step is then to clamp both proximally and distally, typically after heparin is administered, and then directly enter the PSA sac. Further dissection of the common femoral artery is done at this point, and the arterial defect should be clearly seen. Often, the defect is small and can be repaired with one or two interrupted Prolene sutures. If the defect is large, or the edges require resection due to friable tissue, a patch angioplasty should be undertaken. In our practice, this is typically completed with bovine pericardium (**FIGURE 5**).
- However, in the setting of infection, a section of saphenous vein should be used. In the presence of a known chronically occluded SFA (and absent chronic limb threatening ischemia), the occluded SFA may be harvested (caudally away from the bifurcation) and endarterectomized to create autologous conduit with which to form a patch.
- Occasionally, despite all intentions, the PSA sac is entered directly prior to control being obtained. While clearly a secondary strategy, in this situation more formal proximal control can be obtained by one operator while another operator applies direct digital hemostasis at the femoral arteriotomy site.
- Once the arterial repair is complete, evacuation of large communicating hematomas either within the groin and thigh or retroperitoneum should be completed as necessary. Any necrotic skin should be resected. Wide drainage, careful and meticulous incision

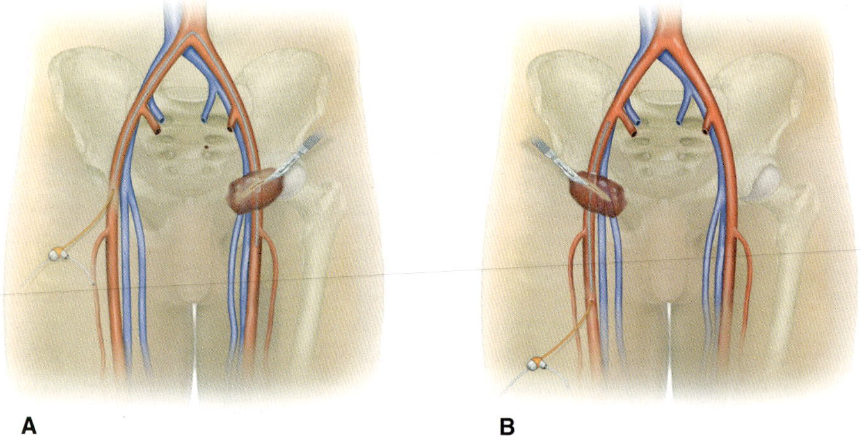

FIGURE 4 • Strategies (contralateral CFA and ipsilateral SFA) for endovascular external iliac artery control to facilitate dissection.

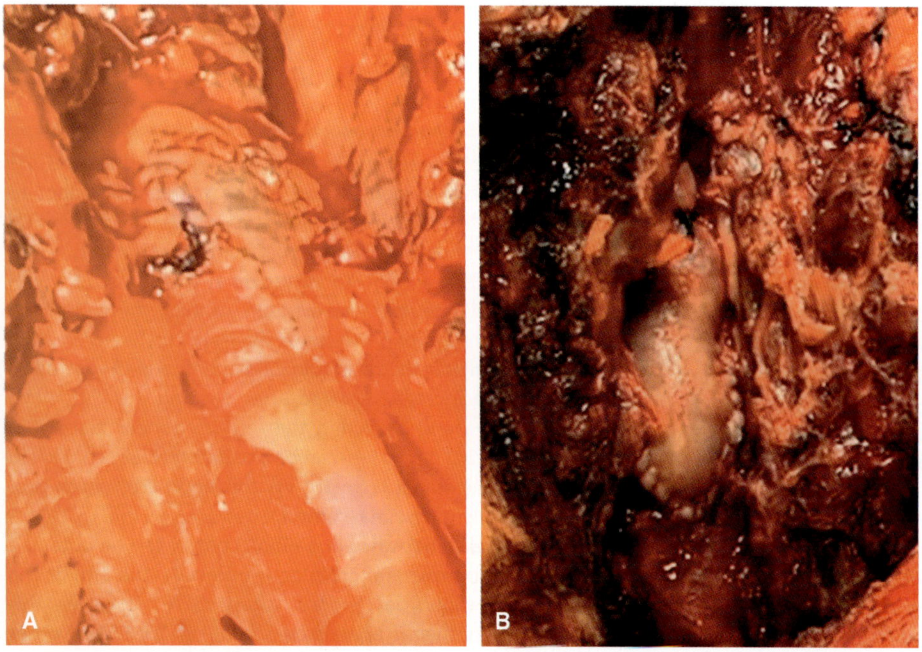

FIGURE 5 • If primary repair is not an option, **(A)** bovine patch angioplasty and **(B)** vein patch angioplasty are options. Dacron (with Rifampin) or PTFE interposition grafting can also be considered in more severe cases.

management, delayed primary closure techniques (with a planned return to the operating room for definitive closure once infection clearance is achieved), vacuum assisted closure dressings with specialized sponges for atraumatic dressing near or directly on vascular structures, temporary antibiotic bone cement bead placement, and other steps may be considered.

- It is usually feasible to do a multilayer primary closure. However, in the event of a large soft tissue defect, it may be necessary to perform a sartorial or other muscle flap, and plastic surgery assistance for formal muscle flap or other composite closure may be necessary to achieve a satisfactory outcome.
- If primary closure is feasible, it is our practice to place drains into these wounds to prevent seroma formation. Often it is necessary to get some tissue closure over the vessels and use the vacuum-assisted closure device for the skin, when there is a skin defect due to necrosis.

PEARLS AND PITFALLS

Duplex ultrasound	▪ The workhorse of femoral artery PSA diagnosis is color duplex ultrasound with a stereotypical two-color flow pattern within the PSA.
Management	▪ The mainstay of active management of the iatrogenic common femoral PSA, beyond observation or ultrasound-guided compression, is thrombin injection. ▪ Clinicians performing thrombin injection must be familiar with limits regarding the neck geometry, balloon protection techniques, and operative or endovascular techniques to treat luminal displacement of thrombin as needed or should distal thrombosis occur.
Operative approach	▪ In the case of operative approaches, the extent of proximal control concomitant with the overall clinical situation balancing patient body habitus, adjacent disease, previous procedures, and comorbidities vs security of proximal artery inflow control is critical.
Endovascular adjuncts	▪ Endovascular adjuncts to inflow control may be critical as a hybrid approach to open repair. Likewise, definitive open control of the external iliac artery either by extensive mobilization of the inguinal ligament for more proximal control or formal counter incision to access the iliac arteries in the pelvis will be needed in a subset of cases.
Open repair	▪ In the case of open repair, successful operative management or even staged operative management with delayed closure is only the beginning of successful treatment. Careful management of this incision with close monitoring of skin closure both prior to discharge and follow-up as an outpatient is critical. Reoperation, management of seromas, and a need for secondary plastics coverage will be frequent in the open management group.

POSTOPERATIVE CARE

- Operative repairs, especially those in the case of infection or extensive hematoma creating dead space and or increasing risk of seroma, will require meticulous postoperative care and frequent reintervention. Re-exploration, seroma evacuation, adjuncts to achieve primary closure, and early plastic surgery consultation will be the cornerstone of successful management of wound problems.
- Finding a way to at once be both hopeful and reassuring—yet clear—with patients and families that these are risks in these cases is important from a patient satisfaction and medical-legal standpoint in this author's estimate.
- Duplex follow-up even of operative repairs is helpful to exclude seroma, technical defects, thrombosis, and other problems. If an occlusive process component was of concern, follow-up ankle brachial indexes may also be valuable.
- In most cases anticoagulation regimen will not be impacted by a successful minimal direct primary pseudoaneurysm repair. In the event of a more complex repair, antiplatelet or other medication recommendations may need tailoring to the specific patient scenario.
- Patients treated with thrombin injection or ultrasound-guided compression should be kept on strict bed rest for a minimum of 6 hours with close observation immediately following the procedure and then general bed rest with minimal necessary activity overnight. Duplex ultrasound confirmation of satisfactory thrombosis without local complication should be performed at 24 to 48 hours post injection.

COMPLICATIONS

- Complications of open repair of femoral pseudoaneurysm align closely with those of any open procedure involving the common femoral artery or its bifurcation.
- Groin wound infection, incisional dehiscence, seroma, infection, anastomotic suture line or patch dehiscence, neuropathic pain or injury, venous thrombosis or bleeding, postoperative

thrombosis or hemorrhage, chronic wound formation, biologic or prosthetic implant infection with need for removal, and other typical perioperative problems may arise.

- Multiple complicating comorbid conditions may combine to leave a given patient at significant risk of extensive and complex local wound problems.
- In complex cardiac patients, volume overload, renal failure, pulmonary compromise, further cardiac issues, or related problems may serve to undermine an otherwise technically successful operative repair.
- For local wound complications, prolonged serial washouts and VAC dressing placements to support delayed reclosure or formal plastic surgery operative coverage with muscle flap or other pedicled coverage for ultimate definitive closure may be necessary.
- Thrombin injection has potential complications of immune reaction, incomplete thrombosis, failure, distal embolization of thrombin with distal leg ischemia, recurrence, or other similar problems.
- Recurrent or persistent pseudoaneurysms can be treated with further thrombin injection if it is felt a safe neck still exists or (if small) with expectant management and observation/reimaging for further complete pseudoaneurysm thrombosis and resolution.

REFERENCES

1. Fellmeth BD, Roberts AC, Bookstein JJ, et al. Postangiographic femoral artery injuries: nonsurgical repair with US-guided compression. *Radiology*. 1991;178(3):671-675. doi:10.1148/radiology.178.3.1994400
2. Saad NE, Saad WE, Davies MG, Waldman DL, Fultz PJ, Rubens DJ. Pseudoaneurysms and the role of minimally invasive techniques in their management. *Radiographics*. 2005;25(suppl 1):S173-S189. doi:10.1148/rg.25si055503
3. Stone PA, Campbell JE, AbuRahma AF. Femoral pseudoaneurysms after percutaneous access. *J Vasc Surg*. 2014;60(5):1359-1366. doi:10.1016/j.jvs.2014.07.035

SUGGESTED READINGS

1. Altin RS, Flicker S, Naidech HJ. Pseudoaneurysm and arteriovenous fistula after femoral artery catheterization: association with low femoral punctures. *AJR Am J Roentgenol*. 1989;152(3):629-631. doi:10.2214/ajr.152.3.629
2. Dzijan-Horn M, Langwieser N, Groha P, et al. Safety and efficacy of a potential treatment algorithm by using manual compression repair and ultrasound-guided thrombin injection for the management of iatrogenic femoral artery pseudoaneurysm in a large patient cohort. *Circ Cardiovasc Interv*. 2014;7(2):207-215. doi:10.1161/CIRCINTERVENTIONS.113.000836
3. Gorecka J, Chen JF, Shah S, Dardik A, Guzman RJ, Nassiri N. A hybrid approach for vascular control and repair of an expanding iatrogenic femoral artery pseudoaneurysm. *J Vasc Surg Cases Innov Tech*. 2020;6(3):460-463. doi:10.1016/j.jvscit.2020.07.010
4. Hayakawa N, Kodera S, Miyauchi A, et al. Effective treatment of iatrogenic femoral pseudoaneurysms by combined endovascular balloon inflation and percutaneous thrombin injection. *Cardiovasc Interv Ther*. 2021;37(1):158-166. doi:10.1007/s12928-021-00764-9
5. Kalapatapu VR, Shelton KR, Ali AT, Moursi MM, Eidt JF. Pseudoaneurysm: a review. *Curr Treat Options Cardiovasc Med*. 2008;10(2):173-183. doi:10.1007/s11936-008-0019-8
6. Kang SS, Labropoulos N, Mansour MA, et al. Expanded indications for ultrasound-guided thrombin injection of pseudoaneurysms. *J Vasc Surg*. 2000;31(2):289-298. doi:10.1016/s0741-5214(00)90160-5
7. La Perna L, Olin JW, Goines D, Childs MB, Ouriel K. Ultrasound-guided thrombin injection for the treatment of postcatheterization pseudoaneurysms. *Circulation*. 2000;102(19):2391-2395. doi:10.1161/01.cir.102.19.2391
8. Liau CS, Ho FM, Chen MF, Lee YT. Treatment of iatrogenic femoral artery pseudoaneurysm with percutaneous thrombin injection. *J Vasc Surg*. 1997;26(1):18-23. doi:10.1016/s0741-5214(97)70141-1
9. Madia C. Management trends for postcatheterization femoral artery pseudoaneurysms. *JAAPA*. 2019;32(6):15-18. doi:10.1097/01.JAA.0000558236.60240.02
10. Schahab N, Kavsur R, Mahn T, et al. Endovascular management of femoral access-site and access-related vascular complications following percutaneous coronary interventions (PCI). *PLoS One*. 2020;15(3):e0230535. doi:10.1371/journal.pone.0230535
11. Stone PA, AbuRahma AF, Flaherty SK, Bates MC. Femoral pseudoaneurysms. *Vasc Endovasc Surg*. 2006;40(2):109-117. doi:10.1177/153857440604000204
12. Yang EY, Tabbara MM, Sanchez PG, et al. Comparison of ultrasound-guided thrombin injection of iatrogenic pseudoaneurysms based on neck dimension. *Ann Vasc Surg*. 2018;47:121-127. doi:10.1016/j.avsg.2017.07.029

Chapter 30

Infrainguinal Embolectomy Techniques

Kathryn Marie Swanson and Malachi G. Sheahan

DEFINITION

- Acute limb ischemia is defined as the sudden loss of blood flow to an extremity resulting in acute ischemia. If the ischemia persists untreated, it can lead to muscle death, limb loss, and possibly death. To be considered acute limb ischemia, the onset must be within 2 weeks of presentation. The condition is often associated with embolic events secondary to atrial fibrillation or aortic mural thrombus. In addition, acute limb ischemia can be thrombotic in nature secondary to preexisting atherosclerotic disease or trauma. Occlusions can occur at the aortic, iliac, femoral, popliteal or tibial levels. Based on the anatomy and etiology of ischemia, a broad range of techniques exist, both open and endovascular, which can be used to restore blood flow to an acutely ischemic extremity. In this chapter, we will focus on the technique for infrainguinal embolectomy.

DIFFERENTIAL DIAGNOSIS

- The diagnosis of acute limb ischemia can be attributed to an embolic source or a thrombotic state (**TABLE 1**). Sources of embolism can be cardiac or noncardiac. Examples of a thrombotic state include atherosclerotic obstruction, arterial bypass thrombosis, hypercoagulable state, vasospasm, and aortic dissection.

PATIENT HISTORY AND PHYSICAL FINDINGS

- Acute limb ischemia can occur secondary to an embolic or thrombotic event.
- Embolic events can be cardiac or noncardiac in origin. Cardiogenic embolism usually arises from a thrombus that forms in the heart due to an arrhythmia or from wall motion abnormality after a myocardial infarction. Noncardiac sources of emboli are usually due to aortic mural thrombus secondary to trauma or underlying atherosclerotic lesions.
- Thrombotic events can be precipitated by vessel dissection, hypercoagulable state, lower extremity bypass thrombosis, or trauma.
- Acute limb ischemia usually presents with severe pain to the affected extremity. This can progress to motor and/or sensory loss depending on the duration of ischemia time.
- Acute limb ischemia can be classified according to the Rutherford classification (**TABLE 2**).
- In the setting of acute on chronic limb ischemia, the sudden onset of worsening pain with motor/sensory loss is usually preceded by a history of claudication and/or rest pain.
- The presentation of acute limb ischemia differs from chronic limb ischemia due to the development of collateral vessels surrounding the chronic occlusion. Chronic occlusions can lead to progressive claudication symptoms and occasionally pain at rest. This progression happens over months to years, rather than hours, as is seen in acute limb ischemia.
- Physical examination findings include tenderness to palpation in the affected limb, pallor, decreased or absent pulses, and motor and sensory loss. If the acute limb ischemia is advanced, the extremity will appear mottled with absent pulses and total loss of motor and sensory function.
- In the setting of acute on chronic limb ischemia, the presence of chronic limb ischemia signs may be present as well. These signs include hair loss, hypertrophic toenails, dependent rubor, and chronic wounds.

IMAGING AND OTHER DIAGNOSTIC STUDIES

- Historically, catheter-based angiography is the gold standard for evaluating acute limb ischemia as it allows simultaneous diagnosis and treatment of the occlusion. In addition, contralateral femoral or brachial access will allow you to obtain inflow images of the aortoiliac segments. Angiography is limited, however, by the availability of an angiography suite, potentially poor visualization of the outflow vessels, and the

Table 1: Etiology of Acute Limb Ischemia

Embolic	Thrombotic	Miscellaneous
Cardiac embolism secondary to atrial fibrillation or myocardial infarction, cardiac mural thrombus, aortic mural thrombus, thrombus from more proximal aneurysm	Acute thrombosis of preexisting atherosclerotic lesion, trauma with resulting vessel thrombosis, aneurysm thrombosis, hypercoagulable states, dissection	Dynamic flap from aortic dissection, access site complication

Table 2: Rutherford Classification of Acute Limb Ischemia

Rutherford class	Prognosis	Arterial signal	Venous signal	Sensory loss	Motor loss
I	Viable	+	+	−	−
IIa	Threatened	−	+	+	−
IIb	Threatened	−	+	+	+
III	Nonviable	−	−	+	+

calcium burden in the affected vessels, which might inhibit imaging.

- Computed tomography angiogram (CTA) has become the test of choice due to widespread availability and high speed when diagnosing acute limb ischemia. However, the use of CTA is limited by the risk of contrast-induced nephropathy, especially in patients with preexisting renal dysfunction. CTAs allow the physician to view relevant anatomy and pathology, including aortoiliac disease, as well as calcification along the vessels in the affected extremity. In addition, CTA may allow for better visualization of distal runoff when compared with catheter-based angiography.
- Duplex ultrasonography is also available to evaluate blood flow in an ischemic extremity. This modality has the advantage of being low cost and easy to access. However, it is operator dependent and can be limited by body habitus. In addition, duplex ultrasonography does not provide images of the aortoiliac segment.

SURGICAL MANAGEMENT

Preoperative Planning

- Surgical management of acute limb ischemia is largely guided by the Rutherford ischemia classification (**TABLE 2**). All patients with acute limb ischemia should be placed on a heparin drip upon presentation to prevent thrombus propagation unless a contraindication exists. In the setting of Rutherford class 1 ischemia, the patient may be managed conservatively with anticoagulation alone. Rutherford class IIa or IIb warrants revascularization. Endovascular revascularization can be attempted with Rutherford class IIa ischemia. Rutherford class IIb ischemia requires immediate open surgical revascularization such as open embolectomy. Rutherford class III ischemia is nonviable, and primary amputation should be considered to avoid sequelae of systemic reperfusion injury. In the event that there is a role for endovascular or hybrid intervention or a completion angiogram, most cases should be performed in a hybrid suite with both operative and angiographic capabilities.

Positioning

- The patient should be positioned supine on the table. The sterile prep should include the abdomen along with the affected lower extremity and the contralateral groin and thigh. In certain circumstances, the antecubital fossa should be prepared for brachial access and the entire contralateral lower extremity may be prepped for saphenous vein harvest. The entire involved extremity should always be included in the sterile field in case an embolectomy is not possible and a bypass procedure is required. In addition, depending on ischemia time, concurrent four-compartment fasciotomy may be necessary.

TECHNIQUES

- Prior to revascularization, four-compartment fasciotomies should be performed in the lower extremity if the ischemic time is greater than 6 hours or if any concern for compartment syndrome exists. For further information, please see the corresponding chapter in this text.
- A longitudinal skin incision is made overlying the femoral artery in the groin of the affected limb. The landmark halfway between the pubic symphysis and the anterior superior iliac spine can be used to guide incision placement as the femoral pulse will frequently be absent (**FIGURE 1**).

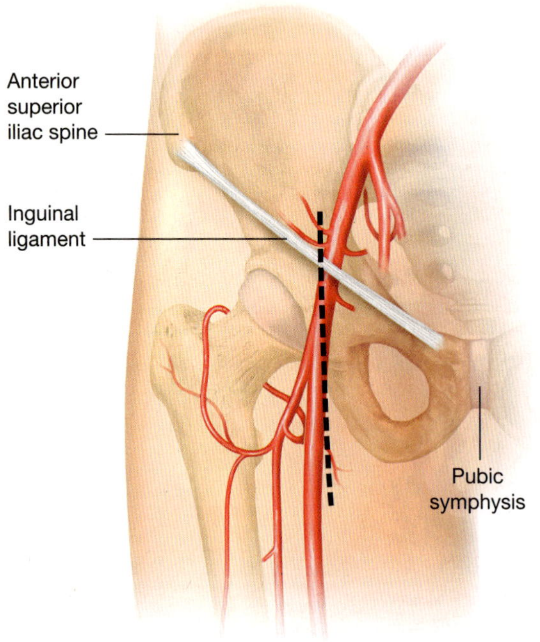

FIGURE 1 • The halfway point between the anterior superior iliac spine and public symphysis is the anatomic landmark used to guide incision placement for common femoral artery exposure.

- Dissection is then carried down to the level of the common femoral artery with Bovie electrocautery and Metzenbaum scissors, taking care to ligate or cauterize any exposed lymphatics to avoid postoperative groin seroma. Care should be taken not to injure any of the other contents of the femoral triangle including the femoral nerve and femoral vein (**FIGURE 2**).
- As there are rarely anterior branches of the femoral artery, the vessel is safely approached from this direction.
- The distal external iliac artery and proximal profunda femoris and superficial femoral arteries are encircled with Silastic vessel loops. Any side branches are controlled with vessel loops or ligated with silk suture or surgical clips (**FIGURE 3**).

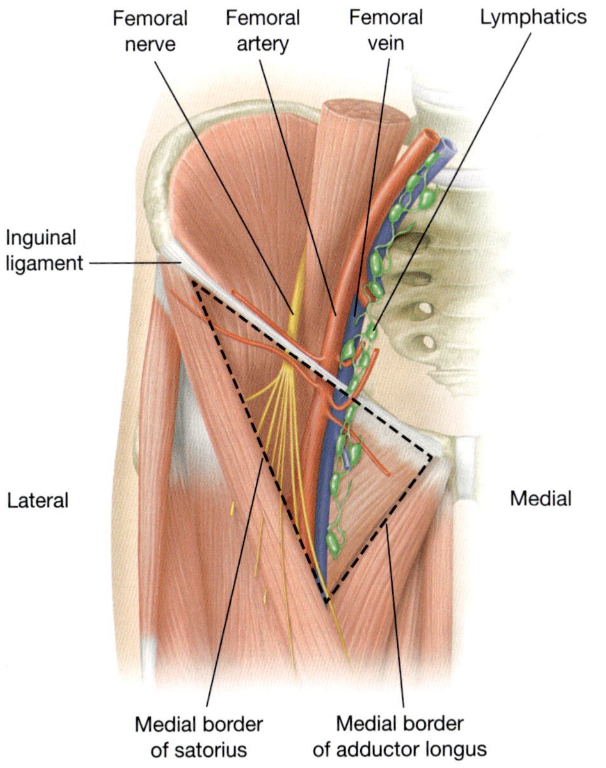

FIGURE 2 • The femoral triangle is bound by the inguinal ligament, medial border of the sartorius muscle, and border of the adductor longus muscle. The femoral triangle contains, from lateral to medial, the femoral nerve, femoral artery, femoral vein, and inguinal lymphatics.

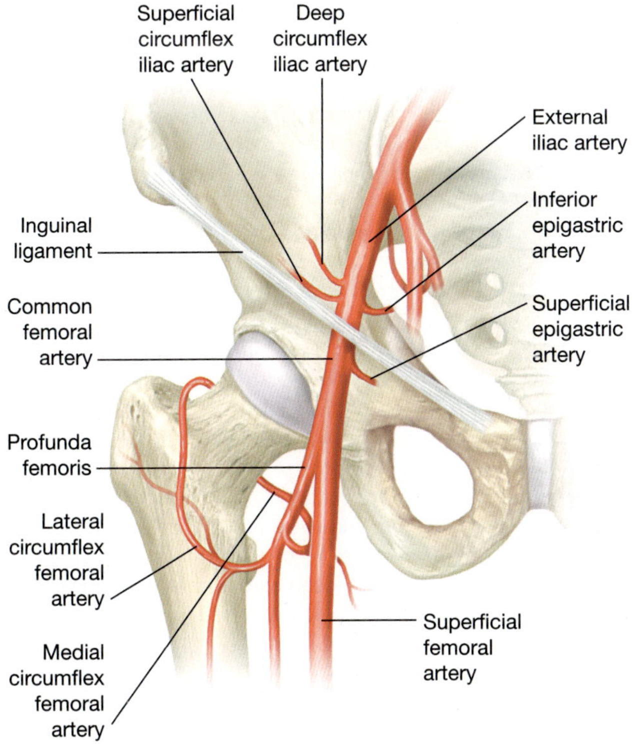

FIGURE 3 • Branches of the common femoral artery.

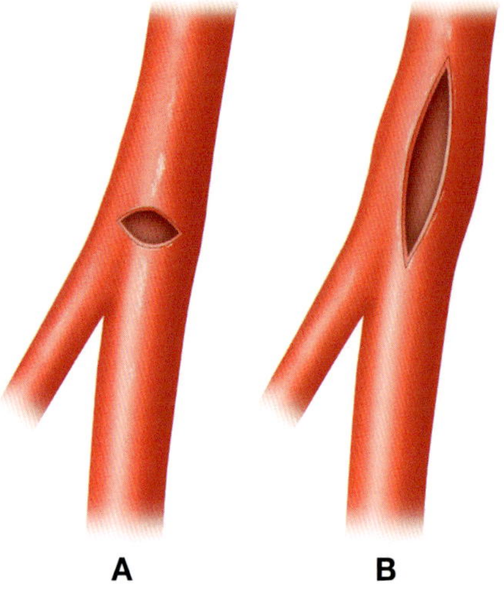

FIGURE 4 • Transverse **(A)** vs longitudinal **(B)** arteriotomy.

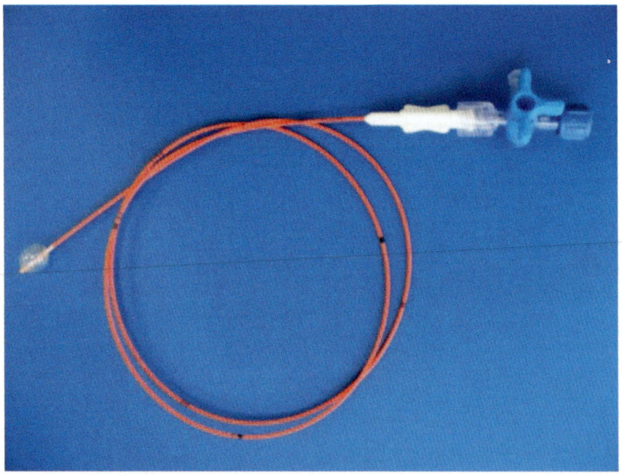

FIGURE 5 • Fogarty embolectomy catheter.

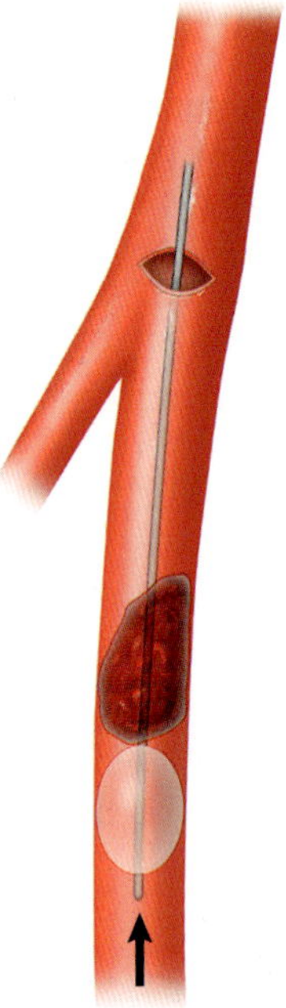

FIGURE 6 • The Fogarty embolectomy catheter is advanced down the artery past the point of thrombus. The balloon is gently inflated and then pulled back so as to remove any thrombus in the artery.

- If they are not already on a heparin drip, the patient is systemically heparinized to obtain an activated clotting time (ACT) greater than 250 seconds. The heparin should be redosed as needed every 30 minutes throughout the case to maintain an ACT >250 seconds.
- If thrombus is suspected in the common femoral artery, clamping in this region should be avoided so as not to transect any preexisting clot.
- An arteriotomy is made in the common femoral artery with a #11 blade scalpel and extended with Potts scissors. A transverse vs longitudinal arteriotomy is chosen based on the presence or absence of chronic disease in the femoral artery (**FIGURE 4**) (see pearls and pitfalls for more information).
- Any thrombus initially encountered can be removed with DeBakey forceps and sent to pathology as a specimen.
- A Fogarty balloon embolectomy catheter (**FIGURE 5**) is then advanced down the superficial artery into the popliteal artery. The authors usually start with a 3 French catheter. The balloon is inflated with saline as indicated and withdrawn from the artery in order to remove any thrombus from the vessel (**FIGURE 6**). As the balloon is withdrawn the control of the superficial femoral artery is released to allow concurrent back-bleeding. Multiple passes are made with the Fogarty catheter until there is adequate back-bleeding and no return of thrombus. If there is concern for thrombus in the profunda femoris artery, Fogarty embolectomy is again performed down the profunda until good back-bleeding is encountered and there is no further return of thrombus.
- Distal control is then obtained by placing tension on the Silastic vessel loops.
- Attention is then turned toward the inflow. Fogarty embolectomy is performed of the inflow until there is strong pulsatile inflow bleeding and no return of thrombus. Proximal control is then reestablished with a vascular clamp or a Silastic vessel loop.
- At this point, the foot should be checked for pulses or Doppler signals. If signals are present and adequate in the ipsilateral foot, the arteriotomy can be closed. If the arteriotomy was made in transverse fashion, arterial closure is performed by primary repair of the arteriotomy using 5-0 Prolene suture with a C1 needle in an interrupted fashion. If a longitudinal arteriotomy was performed, it is prudent

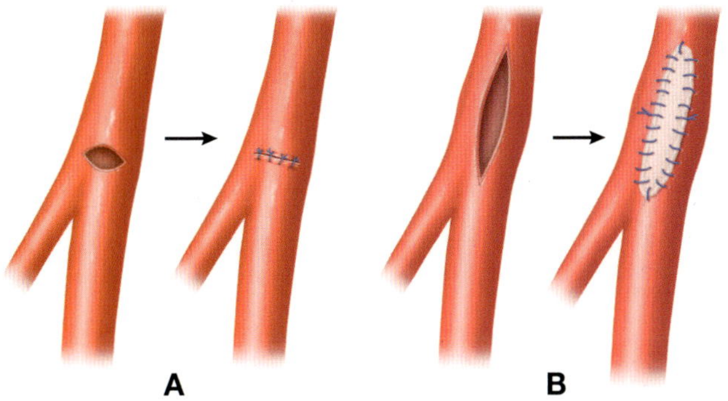

FIGURE 7 • Arterial closure techniques. Transverse arteriotomy should be closed primarily with interrupted Prolene suture **(A)**. Longitudinal arteriotomy should be closed with bovine pericardial or autologous vein patch angioplasty **(B)**.

to proceed with patch angioplasty with bovine pericardial patch vs autologous vein so as not to cause stenosis of the vessel (**FIGURE 7**).

- If palpable pulses are not obtained in the foot, an angiogram should be performed. This will help guide further decision making. If there are no fluoroscopic capabilities, the above-knee vs below-knee popliteal artery should be exposed.
- The above-knee popliteal artery is exposed through a distal medial thigh incision. With the leg externally rotated and knee flexed, an incision is made along the anterior border of the sartorius muscle in the distal third of the thigh (**FIGURE 8**). The sartorius muscle is then retracted posteriorly, and the vastus medialis muscle is identified and retracted anteriorly. This will expose the popliteal vessels. The sheath enveloping the popliteal artery and vein is incised. The artery should immediately be encountered as it lies medial to the vein (**FIGURE 9**).
- Proximal and distal control of the artery should be obtained with Silastic vessel loops. A longitudinal arteriotomy is made with a #11 blade scalpel and Fogarty embolectomy is again performed both distally and proximally.
- At this point, if there are adequate distal signals or pulses, the arteriotomy should be closed as described above.
- If there are not adequate signals or pulses in the foot at this point, the below-knee popliteal artery should be exposed. This is usually performed via a medial calf incision with the leg externally rotated and flexed at the knee. The incision is made 1 cm posterior to the tibial border in the proximal third of the calf (**FIGURE 10**). Care should be taken not to injure the great saphenous vein.
- Dissection is carried down to the level of the gastrocnemius, which is retracted posteriorly to expose the neurovascular sheath (**FIGURE 11**). The popliteal vein will be encountered first in the neurovascular bundle. This should be encircled with a Silastic vessel loop and retracted to expose the popliteal artery laterally. The tibial nerve lies posterior to the artery. Care should be taken not to injure the tibial nerve during this dissection.
- For more distal exposure, the soleus can be divided and retracted posteriorly (**FIGURE 11**). This will allow further dissection of the popliteal artery to identify the tibioperoneal trunk as well as anterior tibial arteries. These should be encircled with Silastic vessel loops, so as to allow for selective Fogarty catheterization of each tibial vessel.
- For more proximal exposure, the tendons of the semitendinosus, gracilus, and sartorius can be divided (**FIGURE 11**). These should be reapproximated at the time of closure.

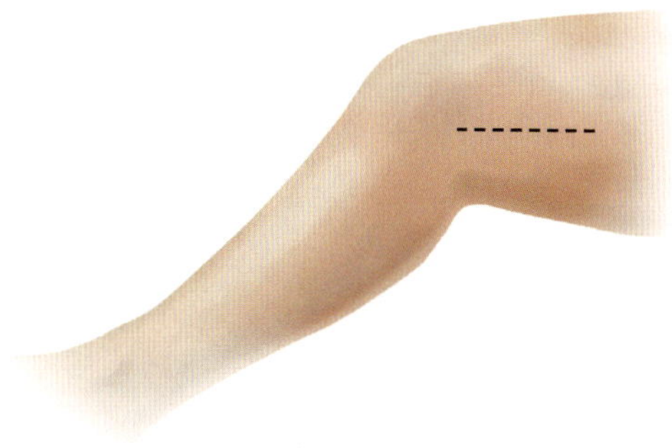

FIGURE 8 • The skin incision for suprageniculate popliteal exposure is made along the anterior border of the sartorius in the distal third of the thigh.

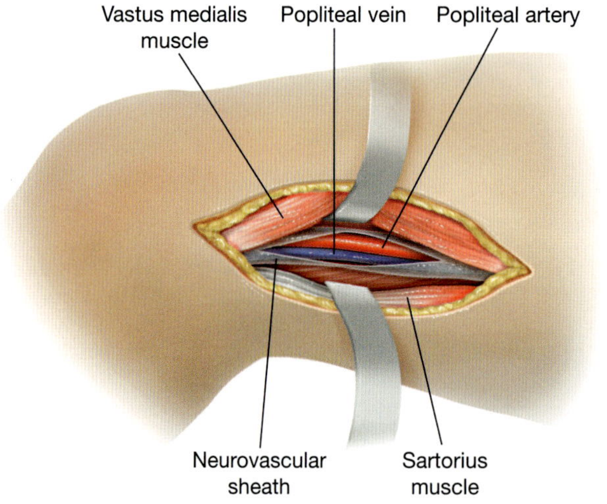

FIGURE 9 ● The supragenicualte popliteal artery is exposed by retracting the sartorius muscle posteriorly and the vastus medialis muscle anteriorly. This will expose the neurovascular bundle containing the popliteal artery.

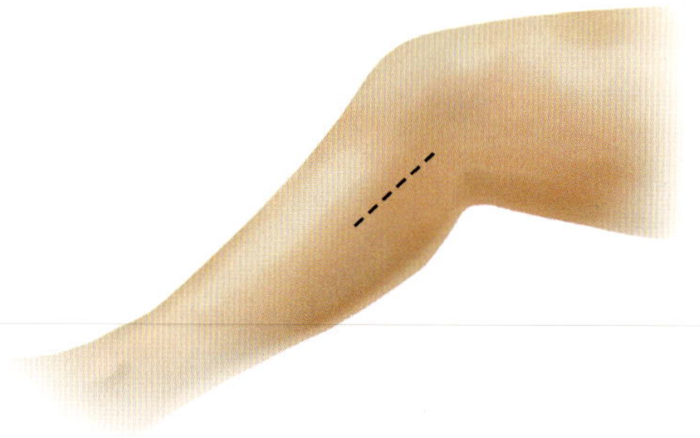

FIGURE 10 ● Skin incision for infrageniculate popliteal exposure is made 1 cm posterior to the tibial border in the proximal third of the calf.

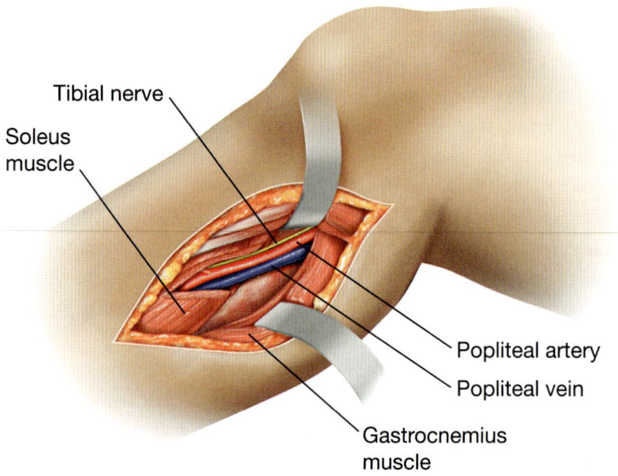

FIGURE 11 ● The infrageniculate popliteal artery is exposed by retracting the gastrocnemius posteriorly. Division of the soleus may be necessary to further expose the distal infrageniculate popliteal artery and tibial arteries.

- A longitudinal arteriotomy is then made with a #11 blade scalpel and extended with Potts scissors. Fogarty embolectomy is then performed of all three tibial vessels. For Fogarty embolectomy technique, see above.
- At this point, the below-knee popliteal artery should be closed with bovine pericardial patch angioplasty or autologous vein patch angioplasty.
- The groin incision is closed in *multiple* layers including the femoral sheath, deep dermal layer, and skin. If incisions from distal arterial exposures were made, a layered closure of these should be performed as well.

PEARLS AND PITFALLS

Common femoral embolectomy	■ For common femoral embolectomy, transverse arteriotomy is sufficient as long as the artery is free of significant atherosclerosis. In the setting of moderate to substantial calcium and plaque burden, it is prudent to perform a longitudinal arteriotomy with endarterectomy and patch angioplasty. ■ In the event of a common femoral embolectomy, it is important to make the arteriotomy sufficiently close to the bifurcation of the superficial femoral and profunda femoris arteries. This will allow the catheter to be directed into either lumen for embolectomy.
Popliteal embolectomy	■ For above-knee popliteal embolectomy, it is advised to perform a longitudinal arteriotomy with patch angioplasty with bovine pericardium or autologous vein patch. ■ Below-knee popliteal embolectomy should always be performed with longitudinal arteriotomy and patch angioplasty closure so as not to narrow the lumen of the vessel significantly.
Complications	■ In the event that the embolectomy catheter cannot be passed due to chronic disease or a dissection, a bypass may be necessary to reestablish inline flow.
Fasciotomy	■ Concurrent fasciotomy should be performed for ischemia time greater than 6 hours, or if the patient develops signs of compartment syndrome. The threshold for fasciotomy should be low as a missed compartment syndrome has devastating long-term effects.

POSTOPERATIVE CARE

- Postoperatively, the patient should be admitted to a hospital unit capable of performing cardiac monitoring and hourly neurovascular checks.
- The patient will require embolic workup including CTA chest/abdomen/pelvis with runoff and echocardiogram. If those studies do not reveal an embolic source, the patient will need a hypercoagulability workup. This can be done as an outpatient.
- In most cases, the patient should be anticoagulated postoperatively on a heparin drip with transition to an appropriate oral agent upon discharge.

COMPLICATIONS

- Postoperative cardiac events: As is true of most vascular surgery procedures, myocardial infarction remains a leading cause of morbidity and mortality after this procedure secondary to the prevalence of preexisting cardiac vascular disease and the increased stress on the body caused by acute limb ischemia. In addition, arrhythmias are a common cause of emboli and may be encountered postoperatively. All patients should be monitored on telemetry in the postoperative period.
- Renal failure: Circulating myoglobin, a by-product of muscle death, is associated with prolonged periods of limb ischemia. Elevated myoglobinemia can lead to toxic nephropathy. This, combined with contrast load from preoperative imaging or on-table angiography, puts the patient at risk for acute renal failure.
- Infection: Groin wounds should be closely monitored for signs of infection. Suspected infections should be treated promptly with antibiotics to avoid involvement of any underlying prosthetic material, such as bovine pericardial patch used for angioplasty. Groin wounds have high rates of infections.
- Lymphocele: Groin lymphoceles are a possible sequela of inadequately ligated lymphatic channels. These can be observed if they are small. However, if they persist or cause compressive symptoms, the lymphocele should be surgically excised and closed in multiple layers. Groin muscle flaps can also prove helpful in preventing lymphocele recurrence.
- Arterial complications: Dissection can occur during Fogarty embolectomy if the catheter is advanced into a subintimal plane. If the entry flap is easy to identify, the intimal flap should be tacked down with interrupted Prolene suture. If the dissection flap occurs proximally or distally in the artery, endovascular intervention with balloon or stent placement may be required. In addition, postoperative pseudoaneurysm can develop at the arteriotomy site if there is not an adequate seal on the arteriotomy after repair. This will usually require reexploration and open repair.
- Distal embolization: Distal embolization may occur following angiography or after advancing the Fogarty catheter through the thrombus in the artery.
- Compartment syndrome: Compartment syndrome can develop secondary to ischemia-reperfusion phenomenon. This results in muscle death and worsening interstitial edema. It is associated with ischemia times greater than 6 hours. Generally speaking, the threshold to perform fasciotomy at the time of reperfusion is low as missed compartment syndrome has devastating consequences including permanent motor/sensory deficits and limb loss.
- Limb loss: Rates of limb loss despite revascularization remain high as many patients have underlying vascular disease prior to their acute ischemic event. In addition, patients who present with higher Rutherford acute limb ischemia scores are found to have decreased rates of limb salvage.

SUGGESTED READING

1. Creager M, Kaufman J, Conte M. Acute limb ischemia. *N Engl J Med*. 2012;366:2198-2206.
2. Hemingway J, Emanuels D, Aarabi S, et al. Safety of transfer, type of procedure, and factors predictive of limb salvage in a modern series of acute limb ischemia. *J Vasc Surg*. 2019;69(4):1174-1179.
3. Kempe K, Starr B, Stafford J, et al. Results of surgical management of acute thromboembolic lower extremity ischemia. *J Vasc Surg*. 2014;60(3):702-707.
4. Suggested standards for reports dealing with lower extremity ischemia. Prepared by the Ad Hoc Committee on Reporting Standards, Society for Vascular Surgery/North American Chapter, International Society for Cardiovascular Surgery. [published correction appears in J Vasc Surg. 1986;4(4):350]. *J Vasc Surg*. 1986;4(1):80-94.
5. Tawes R, Harris E, Brown W, et al. Acute limb ischemia: thromboembolism. Symposium: Nontraumatic Vascular Emergencies. *J Vasc Surg*. 1987;5(6):901-903.
6. Wang J, Kim A, Kashyap V. Open Surgical or endovascular revascularization for acute limb ischemia. *J Vasc Surg*. 2016;63(1):270-278.

Chapter 31

Percutaneous Femoral-Popliteal Reconstruction Techniques: Antegrade Approaches

Kellie R. Brown

DEFINITION

- Femoral-popliteal revascularization for indications of limb salvage or claudication is performed using open, endovascular, or hybrid approaches. Advanced open surgical techniques are detailed elsewhere.
- Basic procedural goals: Improve functional status, quality of life, and, in the setting of ischemic tissue loss, augment wound healing and limb preservation.
- Challenges influencing long-term clinical success: (1) superficial femoral and popliteal artery movement during activities of daily living, including flexion, compression, torsion, and stretching; (2) compromised runoff; (3) the generally diffuse nature of femoral-popliteal disease, requiring angioplasty of long segments of diseased and stiffened artery; and (4) complex pathology, including ostial lesions, luminal thrombus accumulation, and mural calcification.
- Indications for intervention:
  - Rutherford class 1, 2, and 3 ischemia—exercise therapy and medical management are pursued as primary intervention.[1]
  - Rutherford class 4, 5, and 6 ischemia—rest pain, ischemic ulcer, and gangrene warrant revascularization as initial therapy.
- Guidewire-catheter combinations are particularly effective and widely used to cross femoral-popliteal stenoses or occlusions. Once across, reconstructions are performed with any combination of angioplasty, stenting, stent grafting, or atherectomy.
- Reentry devices facilitate true lumen reentry after subintimal recanalization for endovascular treatment of complex lesion morphologies and occlusions in the femoral-popliteal segment.
- Subintimal recanalization and reconstruction of the femoral and popliteal arteries have diminished reliance upon femoral-popliteal bypass. Reentry into the true lumen can be challenging and is often the rate-limiting factor for the success of this procedure. Improved wires, support catheters, and reentry devices have been developed for crossing chronic total occlusions (CTOs).
- Tools for managing CTOs are listed in **TABLE 1** CTO support catheters may be used to support the guidewire that is being used to cross the occlusion. These typically have lubricious surface and a stiff tip. Distal access may be used to recanalize infrainguinal occlusions from a retrograde direction. Reentry catheters may be used to reenter the true lumen.

Table 1: Tools for Managing Chronic Total Occlusions in the Lower Extremity

Tool for managing CTO	Purpose	Examples
CTO support catheters	Support during wire crossing	CXI (Cook Medical) Quick-Cross (Spectranetics) TrailBlazer (Covidien) Gopher (Vascular Solutions) Seeker (BD)
Distal access	Access for bidirectional approach	Retrograde puncture of SFA–popliteal Tibial-pedal
Reentry catheters	Enter true lumen from subintimal space	Outback (Cordis) Pioneer (Medtronic) Enteer (Covidien) OffRoad (Boston Scientific)
CTO crossing devices	True lumen crossing	Crosser (Bard) Frontrunner (Cordis) Laser (Spectranetics) TruePath (Boston Scientific) Wildcat (Avinger) Viance (Covidien)

CTO, chronic total occlusion; SFA, superficial femoral artery.

PATIENT HISTORY AND PHYSICAL FINDINGS

- History includes a detailed description of ischemic symptoms pertaining to claudication, rest pain, or tissue loss. The progression of symptoms and timeframe are helpful in determining the urgency of therapy.
- The presence and severity of cardiovascular disease risk factors should be assessed and managed to ensure optimal perioperative and long-term clinical results, including tobacco use, diabetes, hypertension, hyperlipidemia, renal dysfunction, and sedentary lifestyle.
- Previous vascular or endovascular procedures should be reviewed in detail, including obtaining operative notes, prior imaging and surveillance studies, and prior physiologic testing results whenever possible.
- For claudicants, the potential presence and contribution of nonvascular causes of leg pain with exercise should be considered; for example, neurologic claudication secondary to lumbar radiculopathy and other degenerative spine diseases.[2]
- Physical examination should document peripheral pulses at all levels, both lower extremities, including the strength and quality of femoral pulses and skin integrity at potential access sites.
- The severity and extent of ischemia, degree of existing tissue damage, and presence of infection are documented prior to initiating intervention.

IMAGING AND OTHER DIAGNOSTIC STUDIES

- Physiologic vascular testing provides objective determination of the location and severity of disease, assists in procedural planning, and provides documentation of baseline conditions.
  - Ankle-brachial index (ABI): ratio of the continuous wave Doppler–determined blood pressure in the anterior or posterior tibial arteries (whichever is higher) to the

blood pressure in the brachial artery (>0.9 = normal; 0.5-0.9 = usually consistent with mild to severe claudication; <0.5 = present in patients with very short distance claudication, rest pain, or tissue loss).

- Toe pressures: The ABI may be artifactually elevated in diabetic patients with calcified tibial arteries. Toe pressures may provide more reliable assessment of pedal and forefoot perfusion when the ABI is greater than 1.2. Hallux pressure less than 50 mm Hg may predict delayed or inadequate wound resolution, 50 to 80 mm Hg is indeterminant, and greater than 80 mm Hg is generally sufficient to promote healing.
- Duplex arterial imaging: Direct insonation provides insight into the location and severity of disease. The ratio of the peak systolic velocities (PSV) obtained from the most compromised location divided by PSV from the most adjacent, proximal noninvolved segment provides additional guidance regarding the severity of disease; greater than or equal to 2.5:1 usually identifies a stenosis greater than 50% (**FIGURE 1**).
- Computed tomographic arteriography (CTA): CTA has assumed an increasing role in guiding peripheral vascular intervention, particularly in regard to choosing appropriate devices and optimal interventional approach (eg, ipsilateral antegrade vs contralateral retrograde). Patients who might benefit from subintimal recanalization and reentry typically have complex lesion morphology, such as arterial occlusion, that may be managed by creating a new channel outside of the potential space offered by the subintimal area. Imaging studies that define the anatomy and lesion morphology are

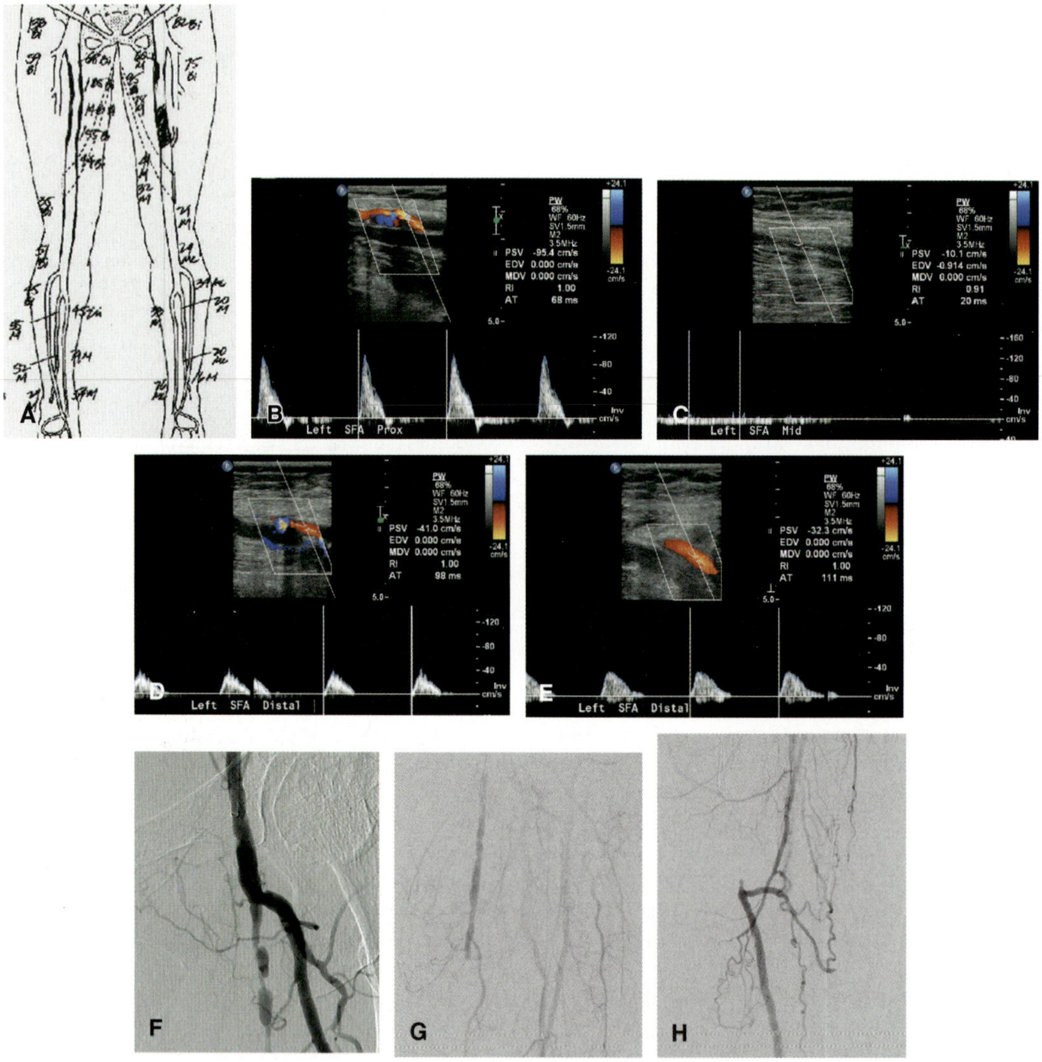

FIGURE 1 • Duplex evaluation of lower extremity arteries. **A,** Duplex mapping was performed on a patient with very severe left lower extremity claudication. There is a left SFA occlusion with reconstitution of the distal SFA. **B,** Duplex image of proximal left SFA shows some plaque formation and a peak velocity of 95 cm per second. **C,** This duplex image demonstrates no flow in the occluded segment of the SFA. **D,** The left distal SFA duplex image shows the point of reconstitution of the artery with a patent distal artery and low velocity flow. **E,** The more distal SFA is a healthier artery with a reasonable lumen, but it has a low peak velocity of 32 cm per second. **F,** The arteriogram performed on the left lower extremity of this patient at the time of intervention showed a patent but diseased proximal SFA. The CFA and profunda femoris artery do not have significant occlusive disease. **G,** There is a mid-SFA occlusion as demonstrated by duplex evaluation. **H,** There is reconstitution of the left distal SFA as indicated by duplex mapping.

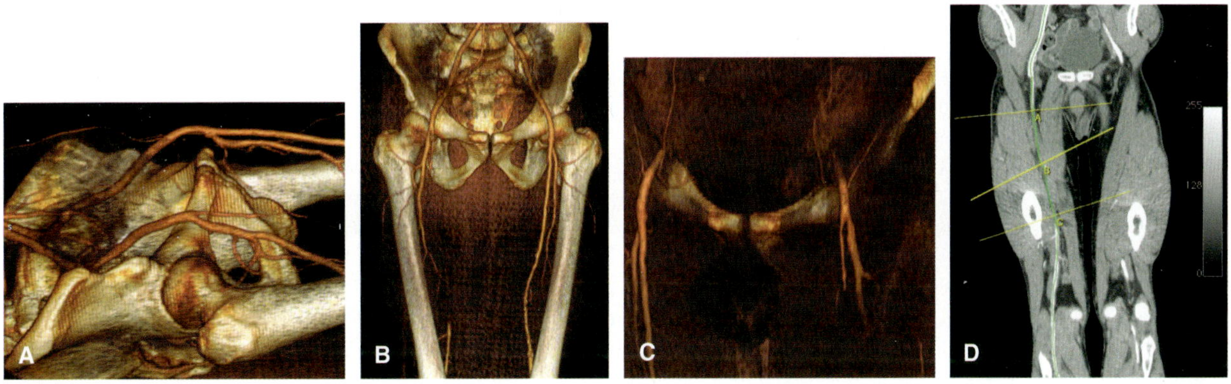

FIGURE 2 • CT angiography for infrainguinal occlusive disease. Volume rendering technique. Preoperative study of puncture zones in the CFA in a patient with a long right SFA occlusion. **A,** Evaluation of iliac artery inflow. **B,** Long right SFA occlusion with reconstitution of the above-the-knee popliteal artery. **C,** CT evaluation of the CFAs and femoral bifurcations prior to access. **D,** Centerline measurements performed to measure diameters and plan for stent graft placement in the right SFA.

useful prior to revascularization. This additional guidance, however, comes at the cost of substantially more iodinated contrast and radiation exposure than that provided by catheter-directed, intra-arterial contrast arteriography, augmented by direct ultrasonic visualization and physiologic testing (**FIGURE 2**).

- Magnetic resonance arteriography (MRA): MRA may also assist preoperative planning. Although MRA does not expose patients to ionizing radiation, artifactual overestimation of disease severity is common in low-flow conditions. Also, gadolinium contrast administration is contraindicated in patients with a glomerular filtration rate of less than 30 mL per minute due to risk of contrast-associated glomerulosclerosis (**FIGURE 3**).

SURGICAL MANAGEMENT

- Overview—Success in percutaneous management of femoral-popliteal occlusive disease requires detailed preoperative planning, thoughtful choice of access site and closure techniques, and familiarity and facility with a wide range of complementary intraluminal wire-guided devices.

Preoperative Planning

- The operative plan includes access site selection, planned method of crossing, and options for arterial reconstruction.
- Endovascular inventory: An essential element of endovascular success is a robust and redundant device inventory. In contrast to open reconstruction techniques, where similar instruments will suffice for all lower extremity bypass configurations regardless of routing, a unique and task-specific repertoire is required for almost every endovascular approach. Procedural success requires that the necessary devices, including guidewires, sheaths, catheters, angioplasty balloons, stents, reentry devices, stent grafts, and atherectomy catheters are identified and available before intervention is attempted.
- Appropriate radiation protection must be available for all individuals involved in interventional procedures. All team members must conscientiously wear a radiation dosimeter, submitted monthly for aggregate exposure documentation. Leadership ensures that all team members adhere to basic radiation safety tenants, including limiting the length and intensity of exposure to the minimum required for precision imaging and intervention (the "as low as reasonably achievable" [ALARA] principle). Safety principles, including distance from the radiation source, appropriate shielding and optimal table height, and source-image intensifier distance, must be understood and applied during every procedure.
- Antibiotic prophylaxis is administered prior to the initiation of the procedure, whenever permanent implants are considered.
- Percutaneous procedures are performed under local anesthesia with appropriate sedation. Care should be taken to avoid

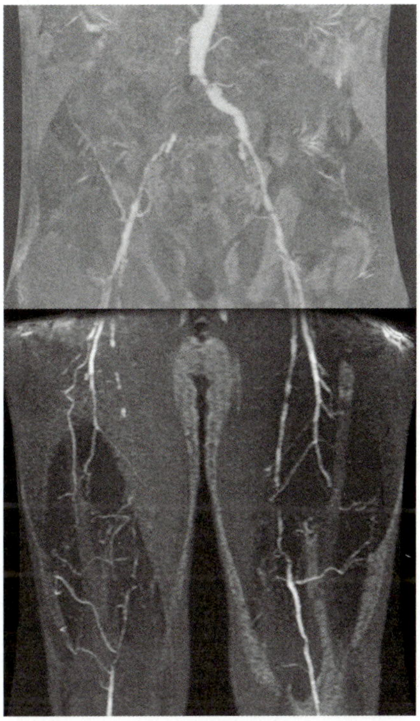

FIGURE 3 • Magnetic resonance angiography as preoperative assessment of lesion location and severity. This patient has extensive iliac and femoral artery occlusive disease. Both femoral artery puncture sites are compromised. There are long lesions in both superficial femoral arteries.

oversedation to ensure that patients can cooperate with instructions and imaging requirements during the procedure. When hybrid open endovascular procedures are contemplated, general anesthesia may facilitate more rapid and accurate device deployment, with reciprocally less radiation exposure for the patient, catheterization laboratory team, and operator.

- An important initial consideration is the approach and optimal puncture site. The common femoral artery (CFA) is the most frequent access site. The approach is typically either up and over the aortic bifurcation from the contralateral femoral artery or ipsilateral antegrade femoral puncture. The transbrachial, transthoracic approach may also provide optimal antegrade access under certain circumstances.
- Subintimal recanalization of the femoral-popliteal segment may be performed using an up and over approach from the contralateral common femoral artery or using an antegrade approach from the ipsilateral common femoral artery. A reentry catheter may be used through either of these access choices. Preoperative noninvasive imaging is very helpful in making this plan for approach.
- The location of lesion helps determine access site and approach. Many patients with superficial femoral artery (SFA) and/or popliteal artery disease are treated with an up and over approach. If the patient has inflow iliac artery disease or has an SFA lesion that begins near the origin of the SFA, an up and over approach is warranted. Reentry devices require placement of a 6-French (Fr) sheath. If an up and over approach is anticipated, the aortic bifurcation should also be assessed to make sure that the reentry device can be passed.
- Patients with extensive disease below the knee and without iliac or proximal SFA disease and who are not obese can be treated using an antegrade approach.

Positioning

- Surgeon position should provide forehand access, whenever possible (**FIGURE 4**).
- Retrograde femoral puncture: This is the most common type of access for all endovascular procedures, including femoral-popliteal revascularization (**FIGURE 5**). The needle is placed in the CFA and the guidewire is advanced retrograde into the iliac artery.

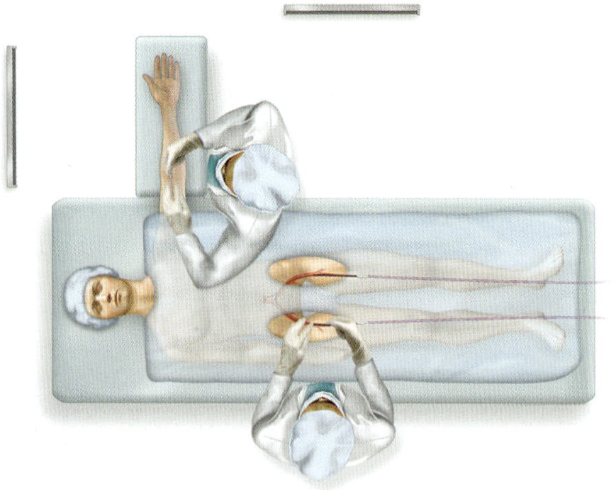

FIGURE 4 • Patient positioning. The operator works forehand when possible. The right-handed operator stands on the patient's right side for a retrograde femoral puncture of either groin. The right-handed operator stands at the inferior aspect of the left arm when performing a left brachial puncture. The monitors are placed so that they can be comfortably observed by the operator.

- The femoral area is examined prior to puncture of the artery. The inguinal ligament extends from the anterior superior iliac spine to the pubic tubercle. The best puncture site is inferior to the inguinal ligament and at least a centimeter superior to the femoral bifurcation. Ultrasound provides useful guidance for arterial puncture and is used routinely in the authors practice (**FIGURE 6**). Following needle insertion, spot fluoroscopy from an ipsilateral oblique angle is obtained to confirm position. If arterial insertion is determined to be proximal to the femoral head, the access attempt is aborted before larger devices are inserted to minimize the risk of retroperitoneal hematoma formation due to inadequate compression or control following the procedure. Common femoral access also enables closure devices to be employed with confidence when necessary.
- Closure devices: recommended for retrograde femoral access site management following insertion of greater than or equal to 6-Fr sheaths. Sheath puncture less than 6 Fr is best managed by compression for 10 to 15 minutes, with or without adjuncts such as a thrombin-impregnated dressing (eg, D-stat patch).
- When pulses are not palpable at the desired access site, ultrasound or fluoroscopic guidance (assisted by mural femoral artery calcification) may provide valuable assistance. Under these circumstances, bilateral femoral access and ipsilateral iliac intervention may be required for procedural success. Ideally, this eventuality is anticipated based on the results of preprocedural examination and physiologic testing. Fortunately, the pulseless femoral artery is often palpable based on mural calcification alone. Patience and spot fluoroscopic images to confirm needle and artery position following failed needle passes often ensures ultimate success.
- Secondary puncture of the postoperative groin presents special challenges. Whenever possible, scar tissue and anastomoses should be avoided. Access in native artery is preferable to prosthetic or autogenous grafts. Considerable force may be required for needle and micropuncture set access; consideration should be given to using "stiff" 0.018-in wires and micropuncture sets specifically manufactured to facilitate difficult groin access.
- Antegrade femoral puncture: The femoral pulse and inguinal ligament are carefully marked (**FIGURE 7**). Needle placement is directed proximal to the femoral artery bifurcation under real-time ultrasound guidance.
- Guidewire placement into the superficial femoral artery (SFA) requires patience and practice. Ultrasound imaging in a longitudinal view may facilitate SFA wire intubation. When using a micropuncture set with a "steerable" 0.018-in wire (eg, one with a slight curve placed at the tip), fluoroscopic control may also be employed. If repeated attempts result in deep femoral artery placement, the micropuncture set should be exchanged for an 11-cm 4- or 5-Fr sheath over a standard multipurpose (eg, Bentsen) wire. Once safe antegrade deep femoral access is obtained, the 5-Fr sheath may be gradually withdrawn with sequential fluoroscopic contrast "puffs" of 1 mL or less performed until the femoral bifurcation is imaged (but while the sheath tip is still in the CFA). At this juncture, roadmapping or last-image-hold digital subtraction

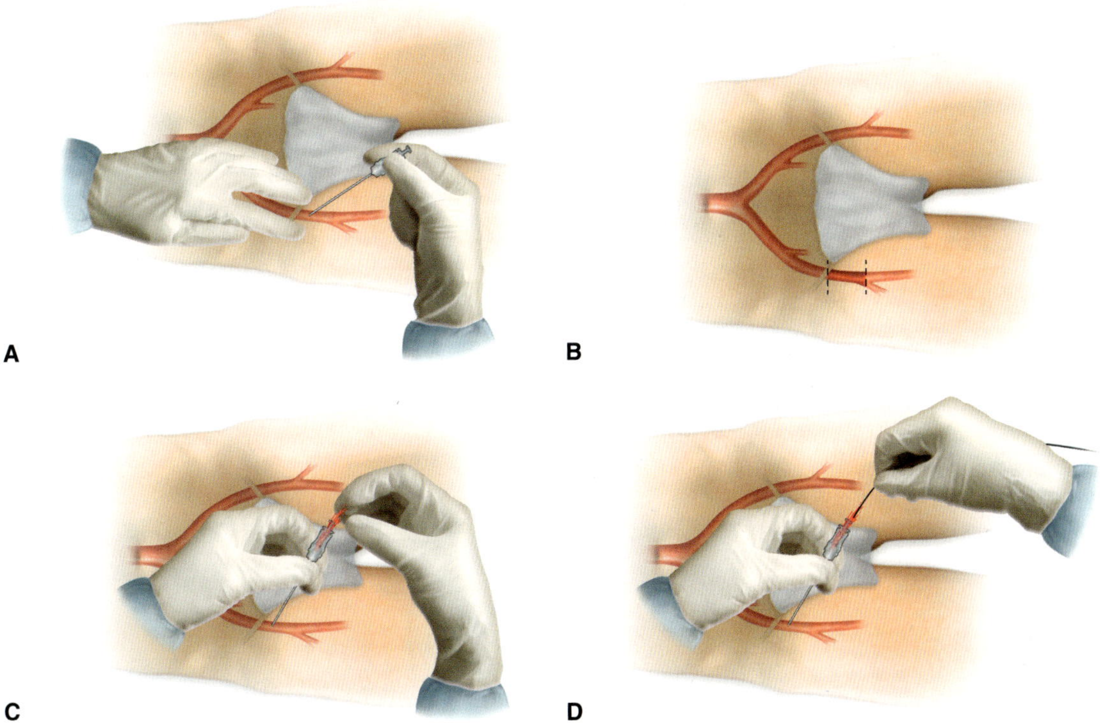

FIGURE 5 • Retrograde femoral puncture. **A,** The anatomic relationships are evaluated. The left hand may be used to help guide the needle. **B,** The access needle is placed in the CFA inferior to the inguinal ligament and superior to the femoral bifurcation. **C,** The needle is advanced into the CFA until arterial blood return is apparent. **D,** In the image a prolongation of the guide inside the retrograde femoral should be included, in order to understand that with this approach and these needle angulation the guide should never go to the SFA, or profunda artery.

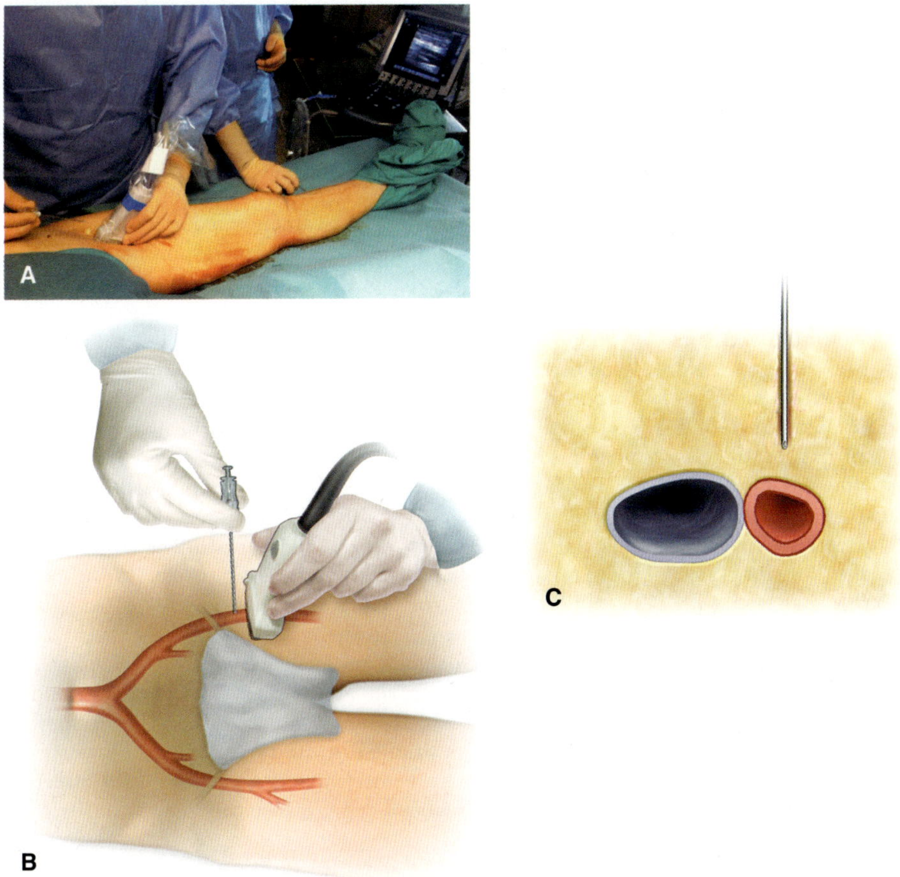

FIGURE 6 • Ultrasound-guided puncture. **A,** In this case, the operator is evaluating the left CFA using the ultrasound probe with a longitudinal orientation. The monitor is placed in a location where the operator can visualize the arterial puncture real time. **B,** In the drawing, the operator is preparing for an antegrade femoral puncture with ultrasound guidance. **C,** In this rendering of an ultrasound image that is seen during common femoral arterial puncture, the common femoral vein is typically much larger in diameter, lies side by side to the artery, and the vein is typically easily compressible. The entry needle can be visualized as it enters the artery to ensure the correct location of the puncture.

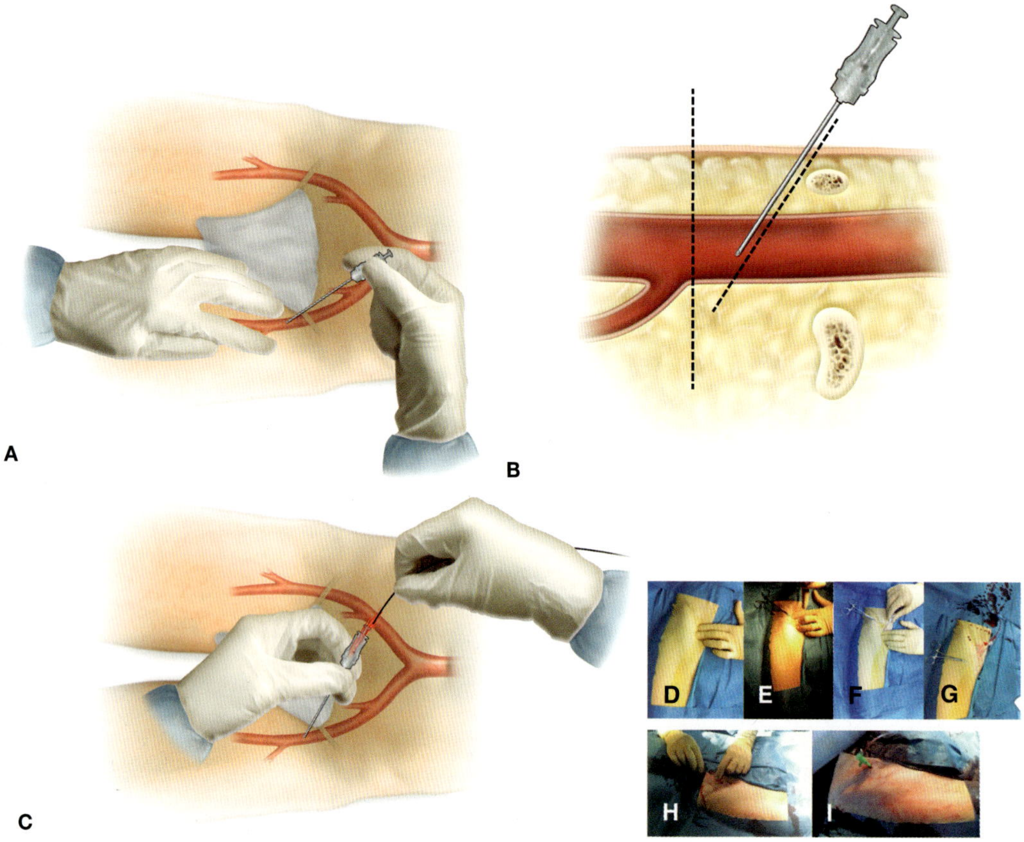

FIGURE 7 • Antegrade puncture. **A,** The needle punctures the skin at the level of the inguinal ligament or just superior to that level. The angle of trajectory of the needle will permit the artery puncture to be proximal to the femoral bifurcation. **B,** The further proximal to the femoral bifurcation the artery puncture is located, the easier it is to steer the wire into the SFA. The best location for needle placement is inferior to the inguinal ligament but well proximal to the femoral bifurcation. **C,** The needle enters the CFA, and when arterial return is achieved, the floppy-tip guidewire is advanced into the artery. **D,** The artery and the anatomic boundaries are palpated. **E,** A clamp is used to assist with fluoroscopic identification of the desired puncture location. **F,** The needle is placed. **G,** Arterial return is achieved. **H,** A guidewire is placed. **I,** A sheath is advanced.

angiography from an ipsilateral oblique angle is performed to outline femoral bifurcation anatomy, after which a steerable hydrophilic guidewire and, ultimately, the 5-Fr sheath is directed under fluoroscopic imaging into the SFA.

- Antegrade femoral access should be avoided in the obese, in patients with a short CFA, or in patients with extreme proximal or orificial SFA disease. Although antegrade access improves "pushability" across total occlusions and enables usage of a wider inventory of guidewire-catheter combinations, there is no option for inflow disease management using this approach.
- Brachial puncture and transaortic sheath placement may provide an alternative option for "antegrade" femoral access. Upper extremity arteries are smaller, less forgiving, more prone to spasm, and less predictably managed with compression following access. Notoriously, small amounts of arterial extravasation may catalyze debilitating and permanent neurapraxia, even when brachial access is obtained well distal to the axillary fossa. Debilitating nerve injury from "axillary" sheath hematomas may occur at any location proximal to the antecubitum. Open exposure effectively minimizes this risk, and exposure is easily obtained with local anesthetic in most patients.
- The longer guidewires and catheters required to access the femoral and popliteal arteries are less responsive to surgeon manipulation from a brachial approach and also limit the available inventory of appropriate devices for femoral or popliteal intervention.
- When brachial access is required, the level of access is determined by the diameter of the largest sheath required to complete the procedure. For 6- or 7-Fr sheaths, the segment immediately proximal to the antecubital fossa is sufficient. For larger sheaths, access should be obtained in the distal axillary artery, proximal to the bifurcation of the deep brachial artery. The left arm should be used whenever possible to minimize risk for embolic iatrogenic stroke. During micropuncture access, even under direct vision, back-bleeding may not be pulsatile due to the smaller caliber of the brachial artery. Sheaths should be managed with frequent flushing with 100 U/mL heparin, as well as systemic anticoagulation once definitive interventional sheaths (6-7 Fr, 55-90 cm from the arm) are positioned in the target artery, or whenever sheaths appear to be occlusive. Intra-arterial nitroglycerine injection may reduce arterial vasospasm to the distal extremity when necessary.

- Percutaneous femoral-popliteal revascularization techniques include balloon angioplasty alone, or self-expanding stent graft implantation as an adjunct to angioplasty. These techniques require placement of interventional-grade sheaths, braided when required to cross the aortic arch or bifurcation to prevent kinking as well as sufficient length to reach the treatment site without limiting device selection. Sheath access also permits serial angiographic imaging to guide device positioning, deployment, and confirm procedural success.

SHEATH PLACEMENT

- Ensure that the appropriate sheath is selected and that alternatives are available should plans or needs change.
- Decide on optimal sheath positioning. Usually, placement immediately adjacent to the target lesion maximizes the ability to cross the lesion, control the procedure, and minimize contrast usage. In many circumstances, it may not be possible or practical to advance the sheath past the femoral bifurcation when approaching from the contralateral femoral artery.
- Heparin is typically administered, 50 to 100 U/kg, following sheath placement and prior to intervention.

Up and Over Approach

- Crossing the aortic bifurcation (**FIGURE 8**): Through a contralateral retrograde puncture, an infrarenal aortogram is performed to evaluate aortic bifurcation anatomy and location. Usually located at the level of the iliac crest, vascular calcifications may outline the bifurcation and guide positioning. The aortic bifurcation must be free of occlusive or aneurysmal disease to ensure safe sheath passage. Occasionally, iliac artery lesions must be treated prior to femoral intervention to ensure optimal outcome.
- Selective catheterization of the aortic bifurcation is performed, followed by antegrade catheterization of the contralateral iliac artery system, either with the flush or pigtail catheter used for the aortogram or an exchange catheter advanced at least to the femoral bifurcation.
- The sheath tip is placed somewhere between mid-iliac artery and the mid- to distal SFA, depending on lesion location and interventional intention. A 6-Fr sheath may be adequate for this purpose, but 7 Fr may be required for many devices (read the package insert). The angioplasty catheter length for proximal SFA lesions is 75 to 80 cm; for more distal lesions, 90 to 110 cm.
- Access to the deep femoral artery may be required to safely advance the "up and over" sheath over a stiff exchange wire (eg, Rosen). After flushing and dilator placement, ensure that the sheath sidearm stopcock is turned to the "off" position. The skin incision may need to be enlarged to facilitate placement. Consider serial dilator exchanges when upsizing a sheath by two or more French sizes. Occasionally, depending on the angle of the aortic bifurcation, sheath placement may be facilitated by passage over a stiff, exchange length hydrophilic wire. When using hydrophilic wires for this purpose, care should always be taken to keep the tip of the wire in the image screen field to prevent inadvertent arterial puncture and extravasation from wire injury. Similarly, when confronted by extreme tortuosity in the iliac arterial system, interval advancement of the sheath into the internal iliac artery may be required to gain access to the contralateral iliac artery with a second or "buddy" wire, following which, standard catheter and guidewire techniques may be used to advance the sheath to its ultimate desired location.
- Regardless of procedure or access approach, it is always advisable to keep the wire tip in the imaging field whenever sheaths are exchanged or advanced—arterial perforation and extravasation may limit procedural options, or the ability to initiate systemic anticoagulation, and may increase compartment pressures to the point of requiring surgical release if not recognized and managed promptly.

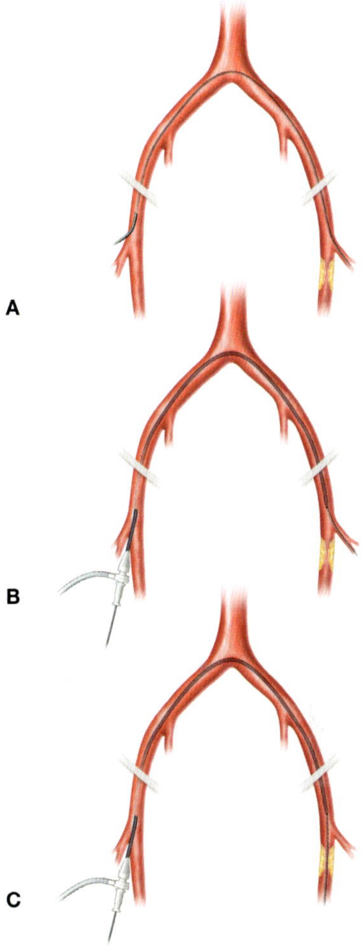

FIGURE 8 • Sheath access. **A,** An exchange guidewire is placed over the aortic bifurcation. The tip of the guidewire is placed in a large, safe branch. In this example, the profunda femoris artery is used to anchor the wire. **B,** The sheath is advanced over the stiff guidewire. The advancement of the sheath is observed under fluoroscopic control to ensure that it is being passed safely. **C,** After sheath placement over the aortic bifurcation, the stiff wire is removed and the directional wire is advanced across the lesion in preparation for treatment.

TECHNIQUES

Table 2: Approach: Up and Over or Ipsilateral Antegrade

Approach	Antegrade	Up and over	Brachial
Puncture	More challenging	Simple retrograde femoral	Retrograde brachial
Catheterization	Proximal femoral puncture and selective catheters	Challenging with tortuous arteries, diseased bifurcation Easy to catheterize SFA	Challenging, long distance, diseased aorta
Catheter control	Excellent	Fair	Fair
Catheter inventory	Minimal	More supplies, long catheters Up and over sheaths	Specific material, long sheaths, catheters
Indications	Infrapopliteal, femoropopliteal disease	Proximal SFA disease	Proximal SFA, femoropopliteal disease
Limitations	Obesity, CFA disease, proximal SFA disease	Contralateral disease, bifurcation disease	Aortic disease, infrapopliteal disease

CFA, common femoral artery; SFA, superficial femoral artery.

Ipsilateral Approach

- See prior recommendations for securing access (**TABLE 2**). Obesity and excessive abdominal pannus may significantly limit the use of this approach. Before initiating treatment, obtain angiographic documentation of existing ipsilateral anatomy, including infrapopliteal runoff.
- Shorter guidewires and devices improve the efficiency of the ipsilateral antegrade approach.
- If balloon angioplasty alone is planned, 4- or 5-Fr sheath can be used to treat ipsilateral SFA lesions. More complex reconstructions require 6-Fr and occasionally 7-Fr sheaths.

CROSSING OCCLUSIVE LESIONS

- Guidewire-catheter skills form the basis of all endovascular procedures. Successful guidewire positioning requires familiarity with a range of devices and guidewire-catheter pairings. The guidewire required for crossing the lesion could not be adequate for working or deploying a stent or a stent graft. Familiarity with and access to a wide selection of wires (depending on length, diameter, tip pressure, and hydrophilic qualities) is essential for success (**FIGURE 9**).
- Guidewire features to be considered:
  - Length: Must be adequate to cover the cumulative distance, both inside and outside the patient, to perform the procedure and support the catheter.

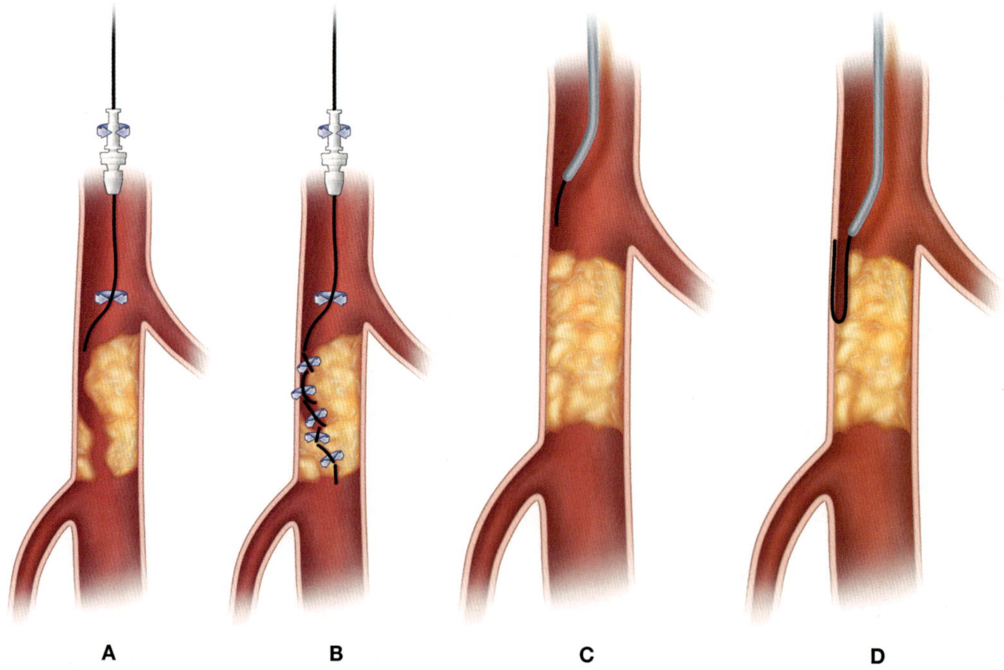

FIGURE 9 • Crossing the lesion. **A,** In this case, a critical stenosis is crossed. The image intensifier is angulated to get the best view of the pathway through the lesion. **B,** Typically, a hydrophilic wire with a directional tip is used and the wire tip is steered through the lesion. **C,** In this case, an occlusion is crossed using subintimal technique. The guidewire is advanced and is supported by a catheter with an angled tip. **D,** The guidewire is pointed toward the arterial wall at the beginning of the lesion and is pointed away from the collateral that fills the segment and is near the location where the lesion begins. The wire is pushed until an elbow forms and enters the subintimal space. **E,** The loop is advanced. The loop is maintained in a narrow configuration by supporting it closely with the catheter. **F,** After the loop pops into the patent distal segment, the catheter is advanced. The wire is removed and contrast is administered to confirm the location of the catheter tip in the true lumen.

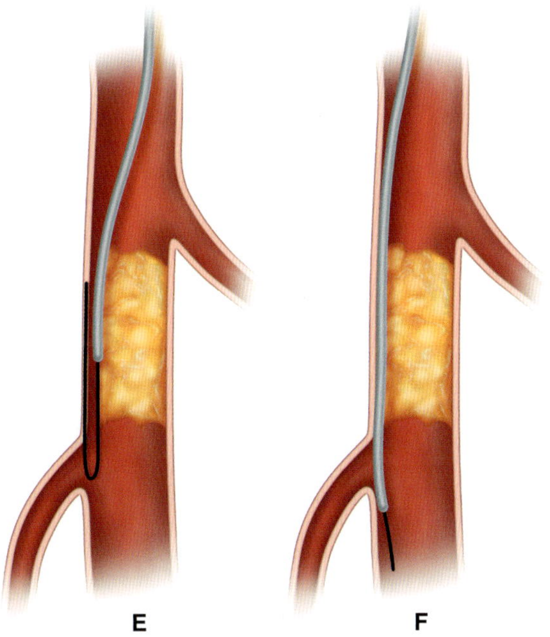

FIGURE 9 • Continued

Guidewire lengths vary from 145 to 300 cm. For an ipsilateral antegrade approach, 145- to 180-cm guidewires are adequate, but for contralateral or brachial access 260- to 300-cm lengths are necessary.

As a general rule of thumb, guidewire length must be at least twice that of the coaxial device to be positioned over the wire.

- Diameter: Most femoral-popliteal procedures are performed with 0.035-in guidewires, but smaller-caliber angioplasty is generally performed with 0.018-in or 0.014-in guidewires.
- Stiffness: An inner steel core confers different magnitudes of stiffness on the shaft of the wire. A stiffer wire may help to cross a calcified lesion, but it is also easier to injure the vessels. In wires specifically designed to cross femoral-popliteal lesions, tip pressure may also vary across wires with similar stiffness along the majority of their length.
- Coating: Hydrophilic guidewires may reduce the coefficient of friction. Typically, they are passed in conjunction with purpose-specific crossing catheters.

- Crossing catheters support guidewire passage and, depending on design, confer varying degrees of support and directionality. After the guidewire is used to cross the lesion, the catheter may be advanced so that the choice working wire may be placed. Crossing catheter technology has advanced considerably in the last 5 to 10 years. Options abound for torsionality (braided or unbraided), tip taper, tip shape, length, and diameter. Examples include the Quick-Cross and CTX catheter families. Some experience is required to learn how to use these catheters optimally in most situations.

RECANALIZATION STRATEGY IN CHRONIC TOTAL OCCLUSIONS

- With most complex lesions of the femoral and popliteal arteries, it is quite common to recanalize the true lumen. Stenosis can almost always be crossed transluminally using a wire supported by a catheter. A steerable, hydrophilic, low-profile wire is best. Long lesions, particularly if completely occluded, may not be able to be crossed in the true lumen. In this case, subintimal recanalization and reentry is the best option.
- Strategy is based on selection of a reentry site where the artery has an acceptable lumen, collaterals can be preserved, calcification is avoided, and potential bypass sites remain intact. Staying in the true lumen offers the shortest reconstruction and preservation of the most collaterals. When subintimal passage is required, reentry should be accomplished as close to the distal true lumen reconstitution as possible. The most common method of subintimal recanalization is using a loop of hydrophilic wire to dissect the subintimal space reenter the true lumen.
- There is typically a large incoming collateral feeding the reconstituted segment. If the reentry site is calcified, the success rate for loop passage is lower and use of a reentry catheter is more likely to be needed.
- If there is a substantial plaque at the intended reentry site, consider a site more distal than the initial reconstitution site. If there is another lesion distal to but near the reentry site, this can pose a challenge for passing the guidewire distally after it has popped into the true lumen.
- The operator must decide in this case whether to reenter distal to all the lesions, given that it might negatively affect bypass options. If reentry fails and the patient needs a bypass, target sites for distal anastomosis should be anticipated, although failed reentry usually does not result in thrombosis of that segment.

TREATMENT PLATFORM

Sheath Placement

- Place the sheath tip close to the origin of the occlusion. Contrast administered through the sheath fills the distal reconstitution site through collaterals. For an SFA occlusion, the tip of the sheath is usually positioned near the femoral bifurcation and the distal artery is visualized with contrast flowing through profunda collaterals. Use a sheath that is one size larger than that used for angioplasty and stenting, usually 7 Fr. This permits contrast administration even if a reentry device is being positioned (**FIGURE 10**).

- Heparin is typically administered, 50 to 100 U/kg following sheath placement and prior to intervention.

Entering the Subintimal Space

- Place an angled-tip catheter pointing toward the artery wall at the origin of the occlusion. Point it opposite the location where the largest runoff collateral is located. Advance a Glidewire into the wall. Push it and the tip will catch and a loop will form (**FIGURE 11**).

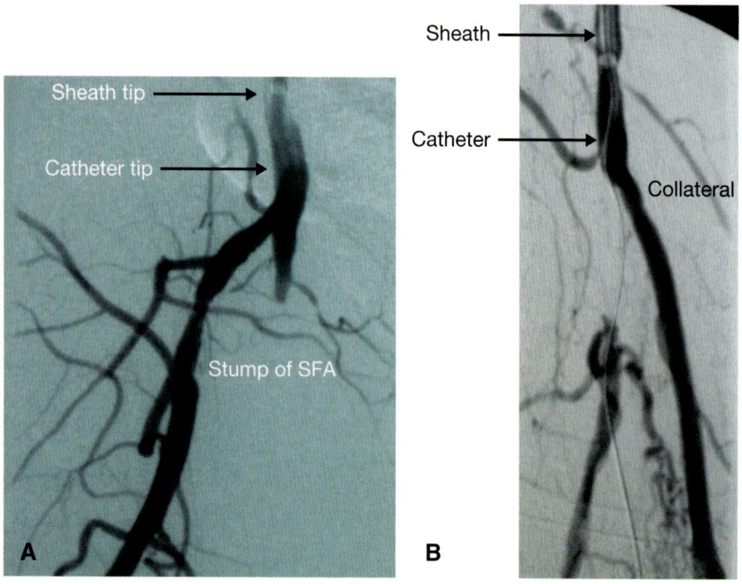

FIGURE 10 • Sheath placement. **A,** There is a stump of proximal SFA that is patent. The sheath was placed up and over the aortic bifurcation. The tip of the sheath is in the common femoral artery and can be recognized by a radiopaque tip. The catheter is used to direct the guidewire into the blind sac of the occluded proximal SFA. **B,** This arteriogram shows a short popliteal artery occlusion. The tip of the sheath is placed directly into the proximal popliteal artery to support the recanalization. There is a large perigenicular collateral that originates from the popliteal artery at the location where the artery occludes. Typically, the subintimal space is entered by directing the catheter tip and the guidewire to the arterial wall on the side opposite the origin of the large collateral.

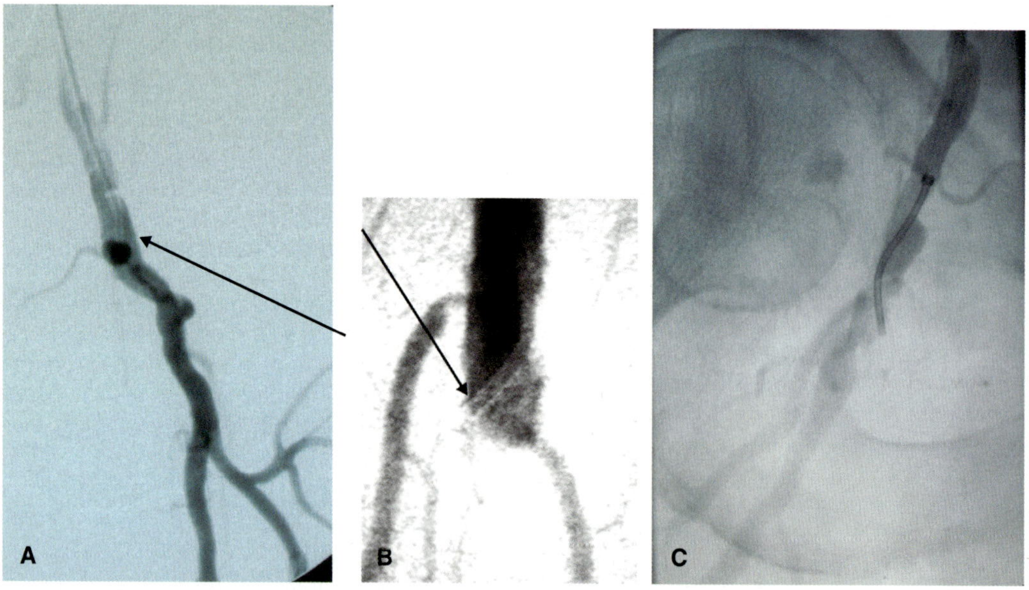

FIGURE 11 • Enter the subintimal space. **A,** After sheath tip placement near the origin of the occlusion and where the administered contrast will opacify the location where the artery reconstitutes. An angled-tip catheter is used (*arrow*) to direct the wire toward the superficial femoral artery origin. **B,** In the popliteal artery, the catheter is pointed to the interface between the artery and the occlusion on the side opposite the largest exiting collateral (*arrow*). **C,** The tip of the catheter is pointed against the artery wall at the location where the occlusion starts. **D,** The hydrophilic guidewire is pushed into the wall until the tip of the wire catches and a loop forms. The loop usually forms at the transition zone along the wire between the soft, floppy tip of the hydrophilic wire and the stiffer shaft of the wire. **E,** After the wire loop is embedded within the occlusion, the supporting catheter is advanced.

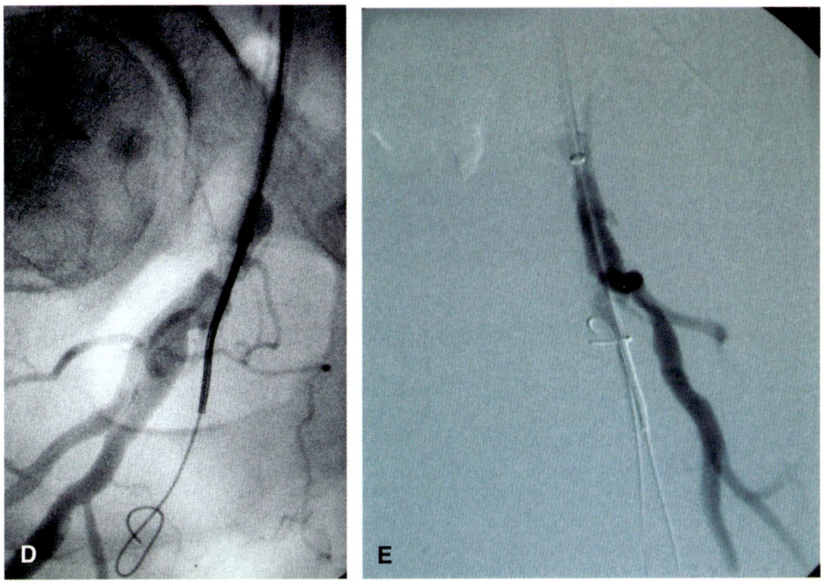

FIGURE 11 • Continued

LOOP MANAGEMENT

Loop Advancement

- Visualization, loop management, and assessment of the reentry site are the maneuvers that enhance success. The looped hydrophilic wire is advanced past the lesion (**FIGURE 12**). The loop is kept narrow and is optimal if less than the diameter of the artery lumen. This is done by closely following the loop with a supporting catheter. Because the loop is in the subintimal space, keeping the loop narrow keeps the subintimal space tight. This helps to direct the wire in a straighter trajectory toward its target and makes the knuckle of the wire loop a more effective tool for piercing tissue to get into the true lumen.
- The standard Glidewire (Terumo) has a directional tip with a soft shaft. If subintimal passage is being performed past a heavily calcified lesion, the artery wall may be more adherent to the calcified segment, making wire passage alone more difficult. Catheter support is required, and sometimes a low-profile balloon must be used to create space in the

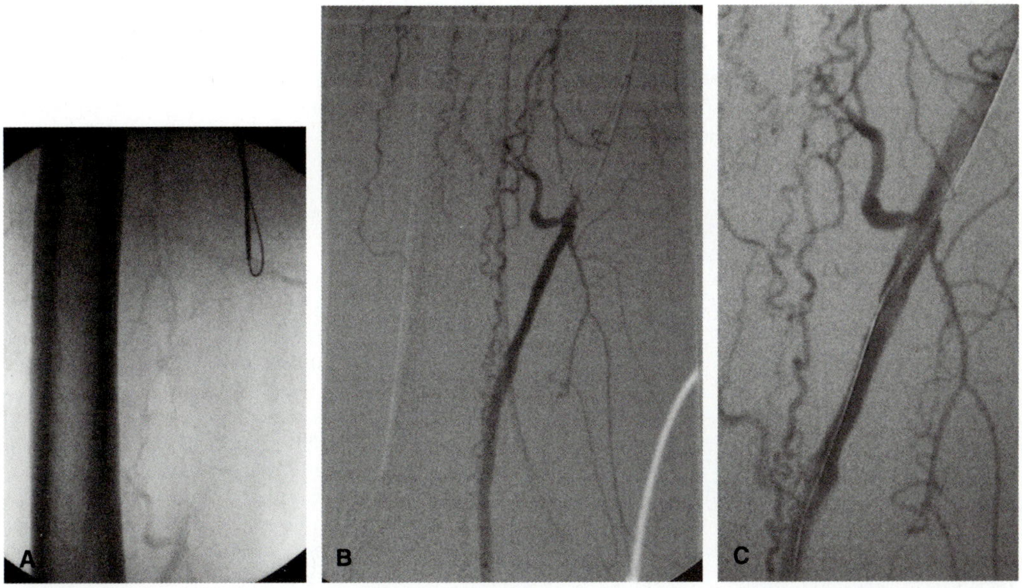

FIGURE 12 • Loop advancement. **A,** After entering the subintimal space, the loop is advanced with the support of the catheter. The loop works best when it is maintained in a narrow configuration. This is enhanced by closely following the loop with the supporting catheter. If the loop encounters a heavily calcified segment, it tends to widen or to spiral around the calcific segment. **B,** The loop is advanced to the arterial segment where the true lumen is reconstituted. Quite commonly, the loop of wire will pass into the true lumen. The location where the artery reconstitutes is visualized by administering contrast into the sheath. **C,** After the loop passes into the true lumen, advance the catheter into the true lumen. Always confirm location in the true lumen before starting reconstruction. This is usually done by removing the wire and administering contrast into the catheter. The guidewire of choice for use during treatment can then be placed.

subintimal plane. Typically, a standard Glidewire is used, but when passing a very calcified lesion, a stiff Glidewire should be considered. A nylon catheter, 4 or 5 Fr, with an angled tip and a hydrophilic coating is best.

- CTO support catheters, such as the Quick-Cross (Spectranetics) or the CXI (Cook Medical), offer more support and low profile than a standard catheter and are generally helpful in crossing CTOs. The loop usually seeks the weakest point in the tissue and breaks across the membrane from subintimal potential space to true lumen more than 70% of the time in our experience. Orthogonal views are helpful in assessing the trajectory of the loop and whether it is progressing toward the reentry site.
- Even if the reentry site is calcified, a wire loop or a stiff wire with catheter support may reenter the true lumen, and it is worth an attempt. If this approach is unsuccessful, a reentry catheter is used as the next step, both to save time and to maintain the integrity of the reentry before too much manipulation has taken place.

REENTRY DEVICE

Reentry Device Placement

- The subintimal wire is exchanged for a stiff 0.014-in guidewire.
- The reentry device is advanced.
    - If the proximal part of the subintimal space is too tight to allow passage of a 6-Fr reentry catheter (approximately 2 mm), a long, low-caliber balloon may be used to slightly enlarge the subintimal space. Do not dilate the area intended for reentry. If the subintimal space at the reentry site is enlarged, it prevents the reentry needle from having adequate support to puncture the true lumen.

REENTRY INTO TRUE LUMEN

- After the catheter is in place, a needle in the tip of the catheter is advanced into the true lumen.
- A 0.014-in guidewire is advanced from the reentry catheter into the true lumen.
    - The direction of the needle is oriented using fluoroscopy.
    - Orthogonal views are obtained to locate the juxtaposition of the true and false lumens.
    - The image intensifier is positioned so that the catheter and an acceptable target vessel segment are viewed side by side.
- Rotate the catheter until the "L" shape appears at the tip.
- Advance the needle into the true lumen.
    - Multiple needle passes may be required. The risk of a needle pass is low.
    - The needle may only require a partial advancement to get into the true lumen. A full advancement may go through the true lumen and into the wall on the opposite side.
    - Multiple small adjustments are often required before the true lumen is reentered, especially if the reentry site is diseased.
- The needle throw is oriented with intravascular ultrasound (IVUS) when using the Pioneer catheter (Medtronic). The needle is at the 12-o'clock position on the IVUS image, and the catheter is rotated to face the true lumen. Using color ultrasound, the true and false lumens can be distinguished and the wire passed into the true lumen.
- After passing the wire, the needle is retracted and the reentry catheter is removed over the wire.
- Some commercially available reentry catheters are listed in **TABLE 1**. Reentry catheters may be guided by fluoroscopy or IVUS, and reentry is achieved by passage of a needle, stiff wire tip, or drill. Orthogonal views are obtained to locate the juxtaposition of the true and false lumens, and the image intensifier is positioned so that the catheter and an acceptable target vessel segment are viewed side by side (**FIGURE 13**).

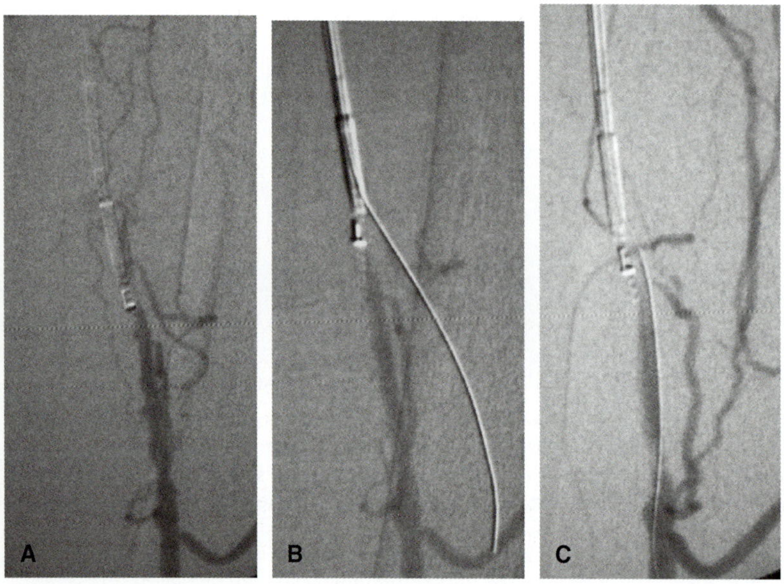

FIGURE 13 • Use of a reentry catheter. **A,** If the wire loop does not pass into the true lumen, consider a reentry device. In this example, the Outback (Cordis) device is used. This is a 6-Fr catheter that is advanced in the subintimal space, along the same course where the channel was created by the catheter and guidewire. The reentry catheter is oriented side by side with the true lumen. The catheter is rotated so that the "L" shape at the tip of the reentry catheter is pointing toward the true lumen. **B,** The needle is advanced. In this case, the tip of the needle had passed beyond the true lumen and the wire is outside the artery. **C,** The needle is passed again, this time not quite so deeply, and the wire passes into the true lumen. After each throw of the needle, if it appears to be going in the correct direction into the true lumen, the wire is passed to explore and see if the tip progresses into the correct location in the true lumen.

ALTERNATIVE REENTRY OPTIONS

Reentry Device Cannot Be Used

- Use a catheter with a stiff tip to bluntly push on the reentry site or use a low-profile balloon angioplasty to break up the tissue membrane in hopes of achieving a fenestration as shown by active blood return.
- This approach is sometimes successful, but it enlarges and occasionally perforates the subintimal space at the reentry site and will render the reentry catheters less efficacious because they rely on a tight subintimal space to provide leverage for the needle passage into the true lumen.
- Another option is to consider a straight 0.035-in Glidewire or a straight 0.014-in or 0.018-in CTO wire to push on the reentry site to see if it can be drilled into place.

Retrograde Approach

- Retrograde puncture can be performed on a distal artery, such as a tibial or pedal artery. Retrograde passage of a wire is often possible, even when antegrade passage across the same lesion was not. This is especially the case for occlusions of the popliteal and proximal tibial level where there are collaterals that an antegrade wire tends to follow blindly along and where reentry devices are not as applicable.
  - Contrast is administered through the proximal access to obtain a roadmap of the distal puncture site, or ultrasound is used to guide the access.
  - A 4-cm 21-gauge micropuncture needle is used.
- A V18 wire (Boston Scientific) is introduced.
  - Sheath placement is avoided if possible to keep the arteriotomy small.
  - If the retrograde wire cannot break into the true lumen, a coronary balloon catheter is passed over it.
- A balloon introduced from the antegrade direction and the balloon introduced retrograde are juxtaposed and inflated and are usually able to split the dissection flap to open the true lumen (**FIGURE 14**).

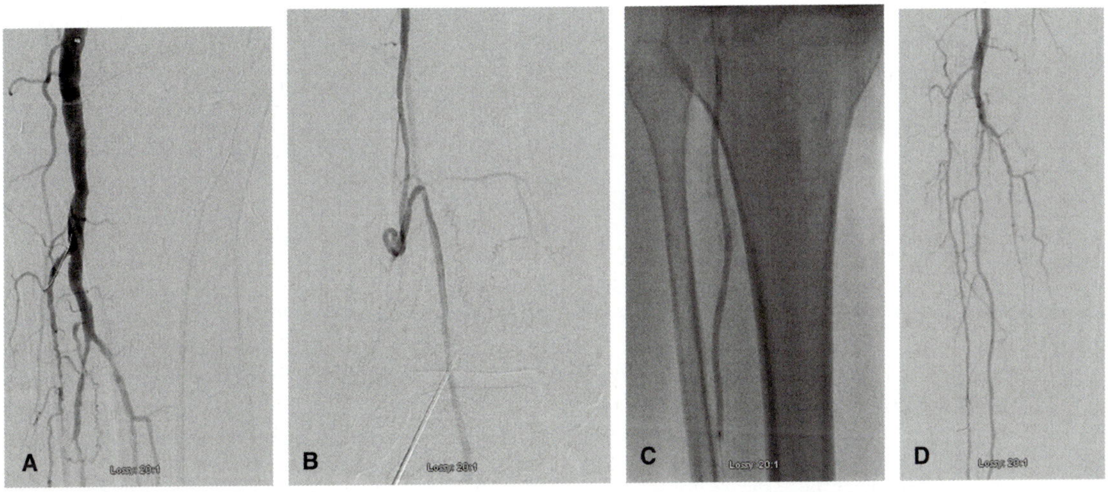

FIGURE 14 • Retrograde puncture using pedal access. **A,** This patient has a pedal gangrene in an angiosome that is perfused by the anterior tibial artery. Revascularization of the anterior tibial artery using a traditional antegrade approach was not successful. **B,** A roadmap of the distal anterior tibial artery was performed. The arterial access needle is advanced into the distal anterior tibial artery under roadmapping. **C,** After retrograde access, the guidewire is passed into the antegrade sheath. The angioplasty balloon is then introduced through the antegrade sheath. **D,** After angioplasty, the anterior tibial artery is patent.

BALLOON ANGIOPLASTY

- Once wire access is obtained across the lesion, angioplasty is undertaken. The angioplasty process enlarges the lumen by compressing and rupturing the plaque, as well as stretching and, in some cases, damaging the media and adventitia (**FIGURE 15**).
- The balloon length and diameter are typically selected to treat the entire lesion, with minimal proximal or distal overlap, to restore the original diameter as determined by proximal or distal measurement. The balloon catheter is positioned over the guidewire and inflated to nominal pressure to achieve the specified diameter. Occasionally, higher pressures may be required to reduce lesion "waisting."
- Inflate slowly. Balloon inflation is maintained for 2 minutes.
- Deflate slowly, and ensure full deflation fluoroscopically before withdrawal.
- The balloon angioplasty catheter may be used repeatedly during the same procedure; however, its capacity to recover the predeployment diameter following deflation degrades with sequential use.
- Balloon diameters range from 4 to 7 mm for the SFA and 3 to 6 mm in the popliteal artery.
- Conventional angioplasty is limited somewhat by target artery dissection. Not all dissections need further treatment. In general, only flow-limiting dissections as judged by sequential contrast injections through the interventional sheath need additional treatment. Dissections may be managed by prolonged periods of inflation followed by gradual deflation to "tack" the plaque up to the arterial wall. Persistent flow obstruction following angioplasty is the most common indication for subsequent secondary stenting.

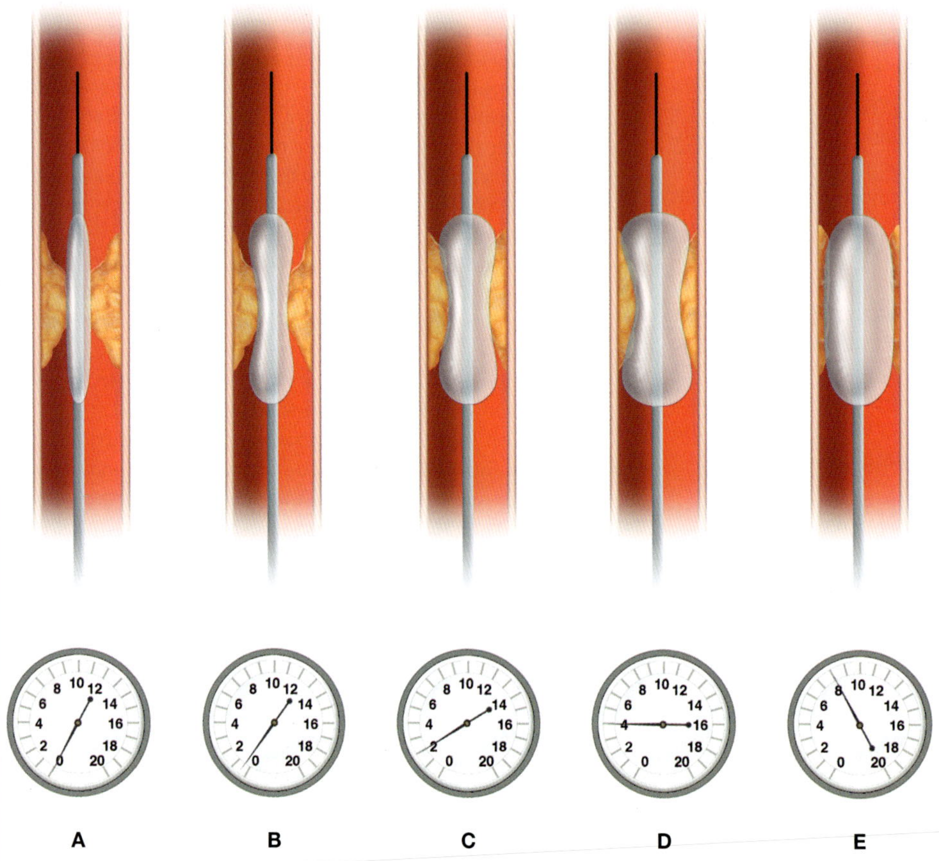

FIGURE 15 • Balloon angioplasty. **A,** The balloon catheter is advanced over the guidewire and into the lesion. If possible, an angioplasty balloon is selected that is able to treat the whole lesion length with a single inflation. **B,** The balloon is inflated, and this is observed using fluoroscopy. At very low pressure, the balloon will inflate freely in the locations where there is minimal or no impingement of the lesion on the balloon. **C,** Usually with 2 atm of pressure, the waist on the balloon becomes apparent and the lesion begins to yield to the outward force exerted by the balloon. **D,** The balloon is inflated gradually. This helps to avoid delivering more pressure to the artery than is required. This also allows the lesion to gradually give way. At higher pressure, the waist becomes smaller. **E,** Pressure in the balloon is gradually increased until the balloon reaches its full diameter. The balloon is typically inflated for 2 to 3 minutes in situations where the operator is hoping to use angioplasty as stand-alone therapy.

STENTS

- Although all vascular-compatible, size-appropriate, self-expanding (nitinol) stents may be deployed in the superficial femoral or popliteal arteries as clinically indicated, select devices have obtained specific indications for this application from the US Food and Drug Administration. The operator is encouraged to familiarize themselves with this designation and to use application-approved devices whenever appropriate to ensure optimal outcome.
- Material and characteristics of peripheral stents have evolved in recent years. Self-expanding nitinol stents are most appropriate for SFA and popliteal applications. The ideal stent should have the ability to adapt to the vessel with a precise deployment and without kinking, collapsing, or fracturing as well as limit long-term arterial injury and restenosis. More recently, drug-eluting stents have been developed and are approved for use in the United States to limit chronic restenosis of the stent arterial segment following deployment. The potential clinical benefits derived from these devices are offset to a significant degree by their substantial increase in cost over "bare metal" stents.
- Femoral-popliteal stents may be placed routinely or selectively. Selective stent placement may be considered for significant postangioplasty dissection, long lesions (>15 cm), residual stenosis postangioplasty, pressure gradient (>10 mm Hg) after angioplasty, recurrent stenosis, occlusion, or to prevent or limit postangioplasty embolization of plaque.
- Localization: A stent is typically deployed to span the distance between the relatively healthy artery proximal and distal to the target lesion. "Healthy" is a relative term in this sense, and care should be taken to limit stent coverage to the minimal distance required to achieve an optimal result. Long lesions in the SFA are most commonly stented, but be aware that stents in the distal superficial femoral and popliteal arteries may be damaged by stress from knee flexion (**FIGURE 16**). Excessive stent coverage may accelerate long-term restenosis and luminal compromise, regardless of the degree of initial success or the type or size of deployed stent.
- Sheath size: Most stents for infrainguinal deployment require a 6- or 7-Fr sheath. Refer to the individual instructions for use for each individual device.
- Deployment: Most infrainguinal nitinol stents are deployed using a pin and pull maneuver that retracts the cover from the constrained stent and the underlying mandrel. A ratcheting mechanism may also be integrated into the deployment process. Typically, these may be removed for basic pin/pull deployment if the ratchet becomes jammed or disabled. After deployment, completion angioplasty is performed to bring the stent to profile.
- Complications of stent deployment:
  - Acute: arterial dissection, occlusion, rupture, stent migration or embolization, embolization of atherosclerotic material, thrombosis
  - Chronic: intimal hyperplasia, recurrent stenosis, infection, stent damage, thrombosis

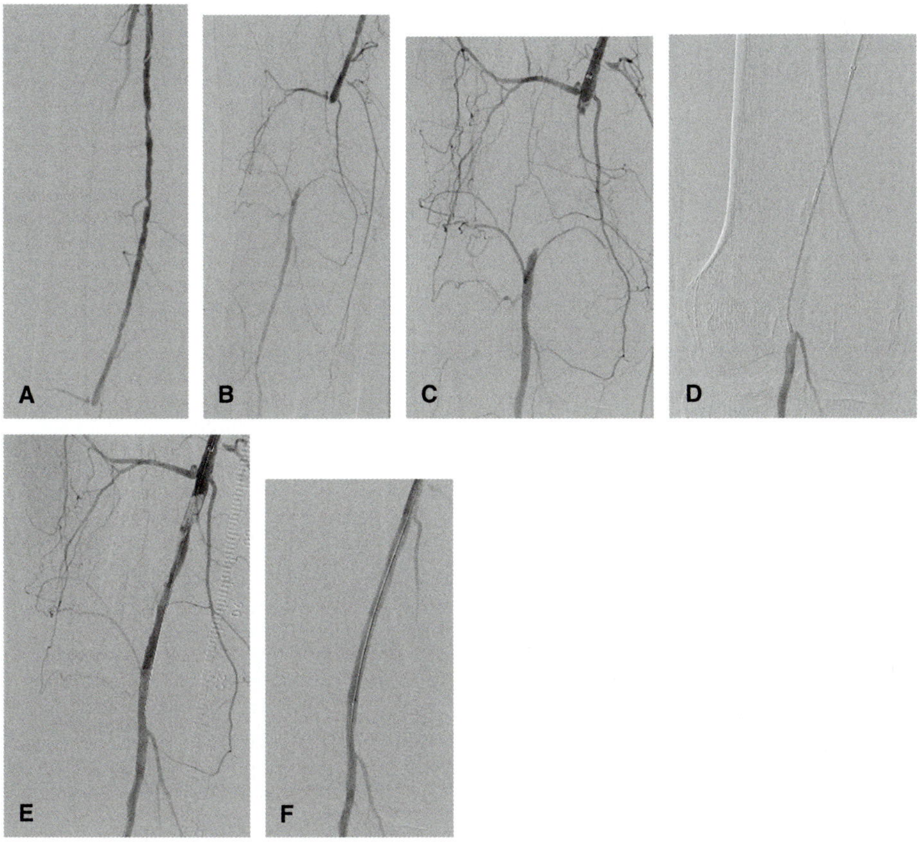

FIGURE 16 • Stent placement. **A,** The patient represented by these arteriograms presented with a right foot Rutherford 5 gangrene. Arteriography demonstrated several mid-SFA stenoses. **B,** The distal SFA and proximal to mid-popliteal arteries were occluded. **C,** The SFA stenoses were treated with balloon angioplasty and the sheath was advanced distally so that its tip was close to the occlusion. **D,** A chronic total occlusion (CTO) catheter is used to support the guidewire in crossing the lesion and the location in the true lumen is confirmed. **E,** After balloon angioplasty, there was a significant dissection and residual stenosis. **F,** A self-expanding nitinol stent was placed for mechanical support of the arterial wall and to enhance immediate patency of the reconstruction.

STENT GRAFTS

- Nitinol-based, flexible stent grafts may be deployed over long and calcified SFA lesions as an alternative to bare metal or drug-eluting stents. In general, the longer and more complex the target lesion(s) and length of required coverage, the more suitable the indication for covered stent placement.
- Stent grafting may require exchange of a 0.035-in wire system for smaller guidewires (eg, 0.025 in or 0.018 in); the operator is again cautioned to refer to the instructions for use for each device considered for placement. Stent grafts must be deployed over the specific guidewire adequate for the stent graft. Sheath upsizing may also be required, depending on the diameter selected. Choosing a larger sheath at the outset will minimize the need for awkward or inefficient sheath exchange after the procedure is well underway. Aggressive predilatation is also often necessary in order to create sufficient space for bulkier covered stent to pass the lesion prior to deployment. Similar to bare metal stents, covered stent deployment is usually followed by completion angioplasty to bring the covered lumen to profile (**FIGURE 17**).
- Relative advantages of stent grafts compared with bare metal stents include the ability to create an entirely new lining for a disease arterial segment. This coverage obviates the possibility of in-stent stenosis within the graft. However, experience has shown that unlike surgically placed prosthetic bypass grafts, covered stents in the superficial femoral and popliteal arteries tend to incite restenosis at the proximal end. Thus, placement usually requires coverage up to the origin of the SFA. Any uncovered artery in this region is likely to develop critical restenosis. Disadvantages include the necessary coverage of all collateral vessels encompassed in the covered segment, as well as the increased risk for graft infection inherent in fabric-covered metal stents. Also, although some stent grafts are heparin bonded, the thrombogenicity of covered stents varies directly with the length of segment covered, such that complete SFA coverage from the origin to the adductor canal necessitates long-term oral anticoagulation therapy in patients treated in our practice. Anticoagulation in this circumstance is designed to limit thrombus extension following future graft occlusion rather than increasing long-term graft patency. Anticoagulation does not typically extend prosthetic graft patency in the lower extremity, regardless of open or endovascular placement.

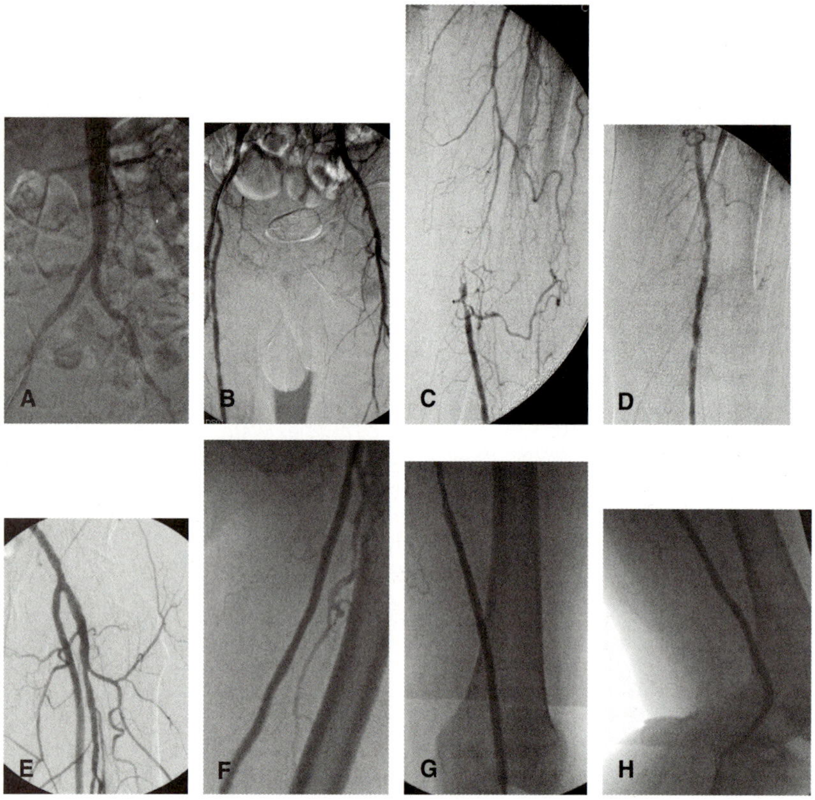

FIGURE 17 • Stent graft. **A,** This patient has a long SFA occlusion that was relined with Viabahn stent graft. An aortoiliac arteriogram was performed using contralateral access. **B,** The left SFA is occluded. There is a patent proximal stump of SFA. **C,** The point of reconstitution is the above-the-knee popliteal artery. **D,** The proximal popliteal artery, extending to the knee, is diffusely diseased. **E and F,** After recanalization and aggressive balloon angioplasty, the artery is reconstructed with Viabahn stent graft placement. **G and H,** The distal end of the graft is fully dilated and without flow limitation in the straight leg and bent knee positions.

PEARLS AND PITFALLS

Artery puncture	■ The puncture is planned prior to the procedure. Access site issues are the most common type of complication. A well-performed access will set the procedure up for success.
Specific material	■ In planning the procedure, check to make sure that all the necessary inventory is available prior to the procedure.
Crossing the lesion	■ Do not force the wire across the lesion. If staying within the true lumen is not successful, utilize subintimal passage or try a retrograde approach.
Subintimal passage	■ The subintimal space often can be converted to a smooth, large-diameter conduit. ■ Entry and reentry sites usually require extra angioplasty or mechanical support from implants.
Optimal reentry site	■ Minimal calcifications. ■ Healthy true lumen. ■ Shortest subintimal channel.
Collaterals	■ Reenter as close to distal reconstitution as possible. ■ Typically, a large incoming collateral feeds the reconstituted segment. ■ The subintimal space has collaterals and can fail suddenly. Consider anticoagulation or dual antiplatelet therapy post procedure to maintain patency.
Follow-up	■ The patient is evaluated after the procedure at 1 week and 1 month and then 6-month intervals after that. We typically obtain some assessment of perfusion (ABI). Duplex mapping may also be performed for surveillance.

POSTOPERATIVE CARE

- The patient should remain at bedrest for at least 6 hours after the procedure. After use of a closure device, usually 2 hours of bedrest is required.
- Puncture site management: Obtaining hemostasis is made safer and simpler when the arteriotomy site is carefully managed during the procedure. Ensure the patient is comfortable prior to removing the sheath.
- Holding pressure: After ipsilateral antegrade puncture, use two hands to hold pressure. One is placed proximal to the inguinal ligament to apply pressure over distal external iliac artery to decrease the pressure flowing through the puncture. The other hand applies pressure over the area of arterial puncture just distal to the inguinal ligament. There are no approved closure devices for antegrade puncture. Following a retrograde puncture, digital pressure is held at the location of arteriotomy, proximal to the skin puncture site.
- Closure devices: Closure devices are used whenever possible to reduce risk of access site complications and limit patient immobility following the procedure.
- The patient is seen in clinic 1 week post procedure for an access site check and at 1 month where a new baseline ABI and duplex ultrasound of the treated segment is obtained. In our practice we then follow these patients with ABI and duplex every 6 months. This surveillance program is modified as necessary for high-risk patients, who are sometimes seen at closer intervals.
- True lumen recanalizations have collaterals, whereas subintimal passages do not. Patients with subintimal recanalization should be monitored with duplex because they may fail suddenly in a manner similar to a bypass. We typically perform duplex surveillance every 6 months.
- The patient should be encouraged to:
  - Avoid smoking
  - Walk daily
  - Follow best medical treatment
  - Follow-up with the vascular clinic

OUTCOMES

- Patients with peripheral artery disease and critical limb ischemia (CLI) have a shorter life expectancy than the general population. The most effective method of revascularization with the shortest recovery time and the least amount of surgical risk is considered ideal. In this regard, most centers have adopted a percutaneous-first approach to lower extremity revascularization, when intervention is indicated.[3]
- Successful percutaneous revascularization is considered equivalent to traditional open bypass surgery in providing freedom from major and minor amputation in patients with severe limb ischemia up to 2 years following revascularization. To date, the Bypass vs Angioplasty in Severe Ischemia of the Leg (BASIL) trial remains the only randomized prospective trial comparing the success of open surgical bypass vs endovascular therapy for CLI. When life expectancy extends beyond 2 years, bypass patency is superior.[4] With recent advances in technology, the patency of the endovascular procedures may approach that which can be achieved with autogenous vein bypass.[5]
- Others studies have reported that, despite the reduced primary patency, limb salvage rates remain comparable with surgical bypass and range from 74% at 5 years to 84.7% at 8 years.[6]
- On a population level, an endovascular approach has been shown to be associated with improved amputation-free survival as compared with open bypass in a study of propensity matched Medicare beneficiaries. Patients undergoing endovascular repair had improved amputation-free survival compared with open repair at 30 days (92.6 vs 91.1%, $P = .002$) and at 4 years (51 vs 46%, $P < .001$).[7]
- Lower limb revascularization of diabetic patients affected by intermittent claudication, in addition to improved walking performance, is associated with a reduction in the incidence of future major cardiovascular events when accompanied by increased physical exercise and improved glucose management and weight control.[8]
- Loop reentry using standard technique is successful in about 70% to 80% of cases.[9]
- In patients who failed loop reentry, reentry catheters are successful approximately 80% of the time.[9]
- Reentry success was 90% successful in a study using the Outback (Cordis) reentry catheter for all-comers.[10]

COMPLICATIONS

- Artery puncture: hematoma, occlusion, dissection, pseudoaneurysm, arteriovenous fistula
- Failure of recanalization: intimal dissection, branch occlusion, thrombosis, embolization, vessel rupture, remote hemorrhage
- Stent/stent graft complications: stent embolization, stent will not expand lesion, stent kink, stent thrombosis
- Infection

ACKNOWLEDGMENT

We gratefully acknowledge the contributions of F. Gallardo Pedrajas and Peter A. Schneider as portions of their chapter were retained in this revision.

REFERENCES

1. Hirsch AT, Haskal ZJ, Hertzer NR, et al. ACC/AHA 2005 guidelines for the management of patients with peripheral arterial disease (lower extremity, renal, mesenteric, and abdominal aortic): executive summary a collaborative report from the American Association for Vascular Surgery/Society for Vascular Surgery, Society for Cardiovascular Angiography and Interventions, Society for Vascular Medicine and Biology, Society of Interventional Radiology, and the ACC/AHA Task Force on Practice Guidelines (Writing Committee to Develop Guidelines for the Management of Patients With Peripheral Arterial Disease) endorsed by the American Association of Cardiovascular and Pulmonary Rehabilitation; National Heart, Lung, and Blood Institute; Society for Vascular Nursing; TransAtlantic Inter-Society Consensus; and Vascular Disease Foundation. *J Am Coll Cardiol*. 2006;47:1239-1312.
2. Issack PS, Cunningham ME, Pumberger M, et al. Degenerative lumbar spinal stenosis: evaluation and management. *J Am Acad Orthop Surg*. 2012;20(8):527-535.
3. Giugliano G, Perrino C, Schiano V, et al. Endovascular treatment of lower extremity arteries is associated with an improved outcome in diabetic patients affected by intermittent claudication. *BMC Surg*. 2012;12(suppl 1):S19.
4. Adam DJ, Beard JD, Cleveland T. Bypass versus angioplasty in severe ischaemia of the leg (BASIL): multicentre, randomised controlled trial. *Lancet*. 2005;366:1925-1934.

5. Almasri J, Adusumalli J, Asi N, et al. A systematic review and meta-analysis of revascularization outcomes of infrainguinal chronic limb-threatening ischemia. *J Vasc Surg*. 2018;68:624-633. doi:10.1016/j.jvs.2018.01.066
6. Houbballah R, Raux M, LaMuraglia G. Trans-Atlantic debate: lower extremity bypass versus endovascular therapy for young patients with symptomatic peripheral arterial disease. Part two—against the motion. Endovascular therapy is the preferred treatment for patients <65 years old with symptomatic infrainguinal arterial disease. *Eur J Vasc Endovasc Surg*. 2012;44:116-119.
7. Wiseman JT, Fernandes-Taylor S, Saha S, et al. Endovascular versus open revascularization for peripheral arterial disease. *Ann Surg*. 2017;265(2):424-430. doi:10.1097/SLA.0000000000001676 PMID: 28059972; PMCID: PMC6174695.
8. Conrad MF, Crawford RS, Hackney LA, et al. Endovascular management of patients with critical limb ischemia. *J Vasc Surg*. 2011;53:1020-1025.
9. Setacci C, Chisci E, de Donato G, et al. Subintimal angioplasty with the aid of a re-entry device for TASC C and D lesions of the SFA. *Eur J Vasc Endovasc Surg*. 2009;38(1):76-87.
10. Bausback Y, Botsios S, Flux J, et al. Outback catheter for femoropopliteal occlusions: immediate and long-term results. *J Endovasc Ther*. 2011;18(1):13-21.

Chapter 32

Tibial Interventions: Tibial-Specific Angioplasty Considerations and Retrograde Approaches

Georges E. Al Khoury, Adham N. Abou Ali, and Rabih A. Chaer

DEFINITION

- Endovascular tibial intervention is a minimally invasive, endoluminal revascularization of the infrapopliteal vessels. It is an accepted treatment of critical limb ischemia (CLI) in patients with tibial occlusive disease. It is usually performed from a transfemoral access (antegrade approach) and, in selected cases, from transpedal or tibial access (retrograde approach).
- Therapeutic interventions performed in tibial arteries include plain or drug-eluting balloon angioplasty, atherectomy, or bare metal or drug-eluting stents.
- Procedures are typically performed under local anesthesia with moderate conscious sedation in a fixed-imaging hybrid operating room or in the interventional angiography suite. Portable imaging systems may also provide sufficient resolution for precise, image-guided intervention depending on circumstances.

DIFFERENTIAL DIAGNOSIS

The differential diagnosis for peripheral arterial disease includes, and is not limited to, the following:

- Diabetic neuropathy pain is described as a burning or aching sensation that commonly occurs at night associated with numbness or hypoesthesia. The symptom complex of diabetic neuropathy may be confused with ischemic rest pain or metatarsalgia, given the similar dermatomal distribution and overlapping risk factors.
- Venous ulcers are associated with skin pigmentation, induration from chronic venous hypertension, and inflammation. They develop primarily in the perimalleolar region of the ankle and usually do not involve the forefoot.
- Musculoskeletal pain resulting from mechanical etiology, stress fracture, arthritis, and plantar fasciitis.
- Soft tissue infection and malperforans ulcers in diabetic patients with advanced sensory neuropathy and/or Charcot deformity of the foot.
- Chronic, nondiabetic peripheral neuropathies such as dorsal foot paresthesias and dysesthesias following long saphenous vein harvest.

PATIENT HISTORY AND PHYSICAL FINDINGS

- Patients with infrainguinal occlusive disease present with symptoms of claudication (Rutherford ischemia classification categories 1, 2, and 3), ischemic rest pain, or tissue loss (Rutherford ischemia categories 4, 5, and 6). When the atherosclerotic disease is limited to the infrapopliteal arterial segments, pain is mainly located in the forefoot. Advanced arterial insufficiency can also lead to ischemic ulceration, gangrenous changes, and nonhealing wounds. This constellation of symptoms represents chronic limb-threatening ischemia and typically occurs when the ankle pressure is less than 50 mm Hg, the ankle-brachial index is less than 0.4, and the great toe pressure is less than 30 mm Hg (**FIGURE 1A** and **B**).

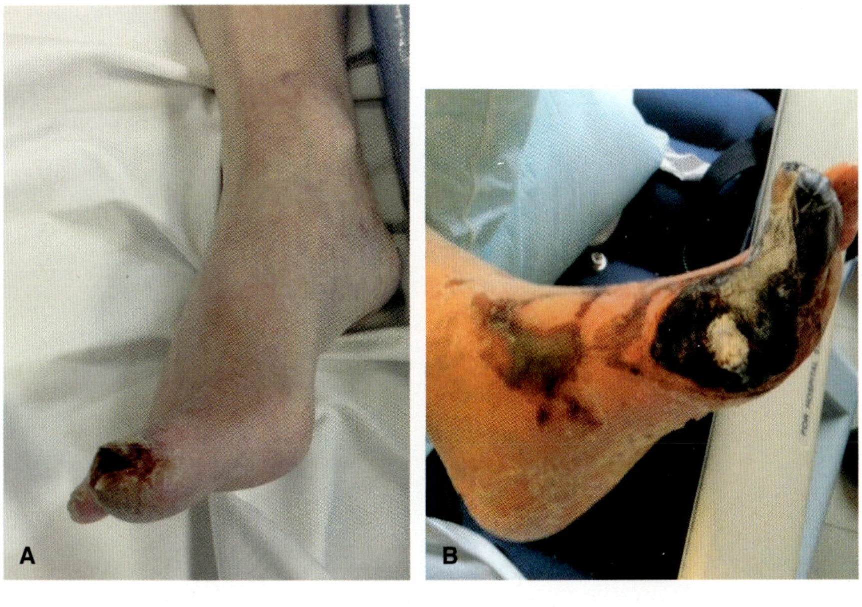

FIGURE 1 • **A,** Patient with tibial occlusive disease and ischemic right first toe ulceration. Rutherford class 5. **B,** Patient with severe multilevel occlusive disease with gangrene of the left first toe and ulcerations on the dorsum of the foot. Rutherford class 6.

- CLI with tissue loss often occurs not only in the setting of multilevel arterial occlusive disease but also with isolated diabetic tibial occlusive disease. In that setting, femoral, and frequently popliteal, pulses remain palpable. In either circumstance, limb-threatening ischemia may ensue. In the latter circumstance, multilevel approaches to complete revascularization, either staged or simultaneous, should be pursued.
- Neurovascular examination, with particular focus on the wound location and the extent of tissue loss, should be evaluated and documented. Probably, the most deterministic variable is the extent of tissue loss—Wagner wound classification, the presence and severity of osteomyelitis, exposure or involvement of the calcaneus bone, residual intact skin on either the dorsal or plantar foot.
- The Society of Vascular Surgery Lower Extremity Threatened Limb (SVS WIfI) classification system categorizes critical limb ischemia based on wound, ischemia, and foot infection grades. The resulting score and clinical stage correlate with the amputation risk for each limb.[1] Wound grading depends on the size, depth, and severity of the wound. Ischemia grading depends on the ankle-brachial index, ankle pressures, and transcutaneous oxygen pressure levels. Foot infection grading depends on local and/or systemic signs of infection.
- These conditions all impact decision making and clinical outcomes. Patient's functional capacity also plays an important role in the intensity of the therapeutic strategy. Options and outcome goals vary substantially between ambulatory and nonambulatory patients.

IMAGING AND OTHER DIAGNOSTIC STUDIES

- Pulse volume recordings (PVRs) and toe pressure measurements when possible (**FIGURE 2**).
- Duplex (**FIGURE 3**).
- Computed tomography and magnetic resonance angiograms have limited diagnostic utility in the infrapopliteal vessels. This is usually due to inaccurate contrast bolus timing with distal extremity cross-sectional imaging techniques, heavy vessel wall calcification, and the diminutive size of reconstituted target arteries.
- Intra-arterial angiography remains the gold standard imaging study for tibial occlusive disease for both diagnostic and therapeutic purposes (**FIGURE 4**).

SURGICAL MANAGEMENT

- Technical skills, careful planning, and knowledge of the relevant arterial anatomy determine tibial revascularization strategies for limb salvage. Current controversies include the potential value of restoring patency in more than one tibial vessel to optimize blood flow and maximize the chances of wound healing. Proponents of this approach reference the "angiosome" concept of the foot or the idea that specific skin regions derive primary perfusion from end arterioles arising primarily from either the dorsal pedal or posterior tibial arteries as they cross the ankle. This practice is pursued in marked contradistinction to the open surgical imperative to restore in-line flow to the foot in the single largest, most continuous crural artery. The many advantages of endovascular reconstruction techniques in tibial reconstruction include restoring partial flow in multiple target arteries as compared with a single artery following surgical bypass, as well as opportunities to repeat procedures with relatively simple outpatient interventions as needed, to maintain patency and skin integrity. Treatment decisions regarding revascularization strategy in individual circumstances should be guided by patient-specific comorbidities and anatomic considerations, arterial runoff into the foot, patient habitus and ambulatory status as well as patency and feasibility considerations related to either open or endovascular options.
- Currently available endovascular technology facilitates successful treatment of complex occlusive lesions at and below the malleolar level. Limitations remain and include limited durability and patency, as well as technical limitations highlighted by risks of arterial perforation (**FIGURE 5**), difficulty in true lumen reentry in complete occlusions (**FIGURE 6**), procedure-related distal arterial embolization, and limited pedal vessel outflow in certain circumstances.

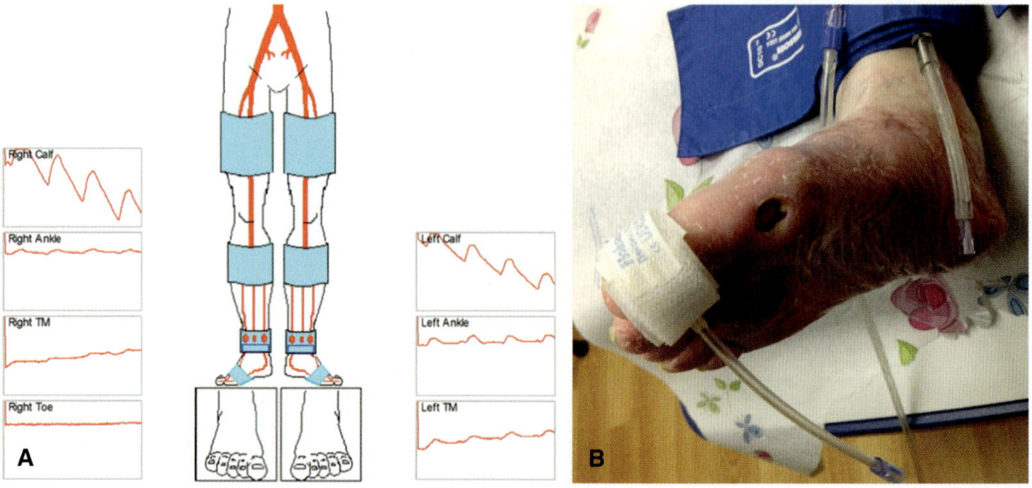

FIGURE 2 • PVR on a patient with severe right tibial occlusive disease and nonhealing toe ulcer. The tracings are pulsatile at the calf level consistent with adequate femoropopliteal flow; however, the waveforms are flat, distally suggestive of tibial occlusive disease.

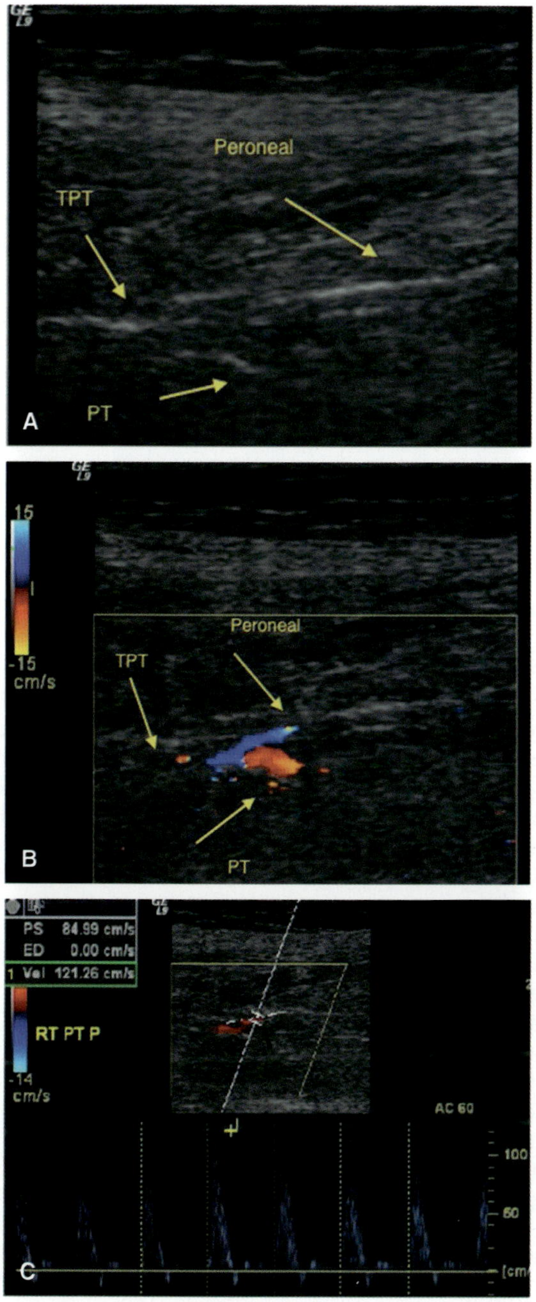

FIGURE 3 ● **A,** Duplex B-mode image shows the calcified tibioperoneal trunk bifurcation into the posterior tibial artery and peroneal artery. **B,** Duplex of the tibioperoneal trunk bifurcation shows flow into the posterior tibial artery. **C,** Duplex of the proximal posterior tibial artery shows normal triphasic Doppler waveform.

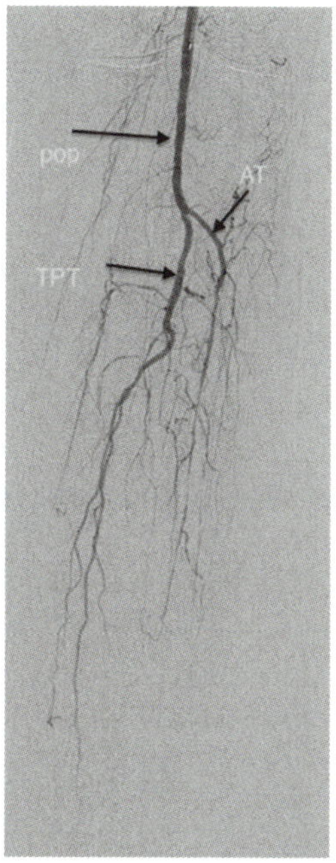

FIGURE 4 ● Selective left leg angiogram shows patent popliteal artery, patent tibioperoneal trunk, complete occlusion of the anterior tibial artery, and complete occlusion of the peroneal artery.

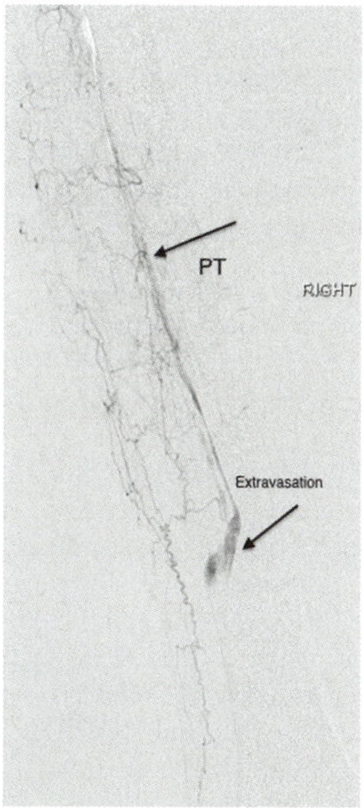

FIGURE 5 ● Angiogram shows extravasation from distal posterior tibial artery in an attempt to cross a total occlusion with a catheter and wire.

- The retrograde or SAFARI (Subintimal Flossing with Antegrade-Retrograde Intervention) tibial intervention technique may improve technical results in challenging lesions, particularly those resistant to ipsilateral antegrade access, including flush occlusions at the origin of the target artery or with large collateral arteries adjacent to the occluded origin. In nearly every circumstance, even chronic and recalcitrant occlusions may be crossed more easily from the retrograde rather than antegrade approach; this is true regardless of the chronicity of the lesion in question, degree of calcification, or length of occlusion.
- The pedal loop technique has been proposed in certain clinical situations requiring significant improvement in blood flow via the restoration of flow through both the anterior tibial and posterior tibial arteries (through the plantar arteries and their

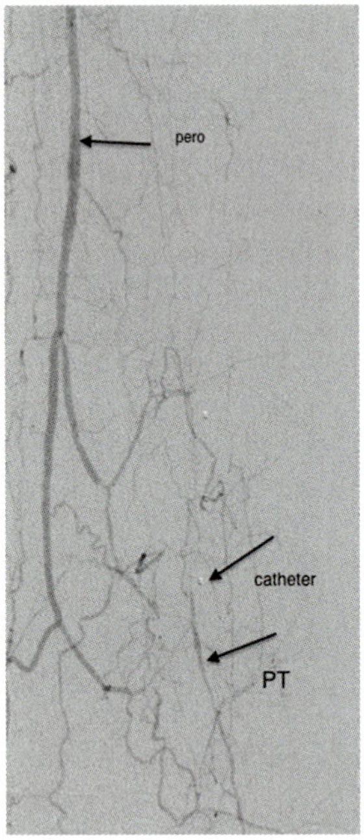

FIGURE 6 • Angiogram from sheath shows the catheter in the subintimal plane after recanalization of posterior tibial (PT) with reconstitution of distal PT away from the catheter.

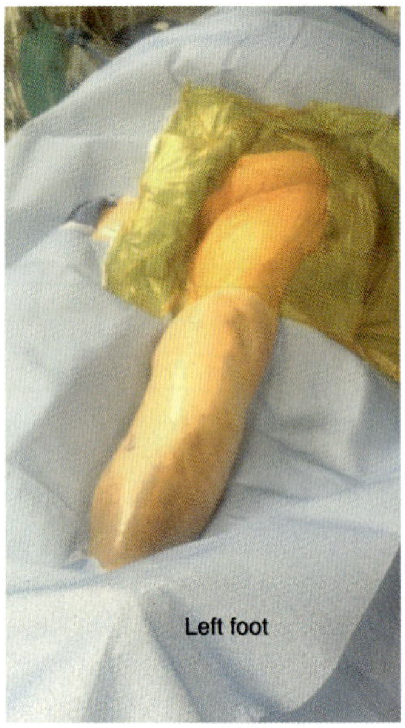

FIGURE 7 • Patient is placed in the supine position on the angiographic table; the groins and lower extremity are prepped and draped in anticipation of antegrade and retrograde approaches.

anatomical anastomoses). It entails one of two approaches: A. Antegrade recanalization of the anterior tibial artery (ATA) and the dorsalis pedis (DP) and then retrograde recanalization of the plantar artery and then the posterior tibial artery. B. Antegrade recanalization of the posterior tibial artery and the plantar artery and then retrograde recanalization of the DP and then the ATA. Very low-profile balloon catheters are recommended particularly while navigating the tortuous vessels of the foot.

Preoperative Planning

- Preoperative vein mapping prior to the diagnostic angiogram is helpful in handicapping potential surgical alternatives and determining the extent to which interventional alternatives are to be pursued.
- Patients should be medically optimized prior to their procedure: preventive strategies are advised to reduce the risk of kidney injury in patients at risk for contrast nephropathy; smoking cessation is encouraged as well as antiplatelet and statin therapy. Carbon dioxide angiography is a useful tool in aortoiliac and femoral (inflow) evaluation; however, its utility in tibial angiography is limited.
- Tibial interventions can entail significant radiation exposure. Protective shields, lead glasses, and judicious use of fluoroscopy are recommended to protect all participants in the procedure. Ultrasound-guided access can minimize radiation exposure, particularly for pedal access; needle extenders allow the operator to puncture remotely and minimize hand exposure.
- Micropuncture and pedal access kits are useful access tools.
- Sheaths: 5- and 6-Fr, braided, 90 cm or 110 cm from contralateral femoral access; 45- to 55-cm sheath from the ipsilateral transfemoral access; 4- and 5-Fr Slender Glidesheaths (Terumo) with the ultrathin wall technology have been suggested for diagnostic angiograms from the transradial access; 120- to 150-cm (Sublime) length sheaths are currently available for intervention.
- Wires: 300-cm, 0.014-in, or 0.018-in wires; 260-cm, 0.035-in floppy Glidewire.
- Catheters: 150- to 170-cm catheters and balloons.
- Medications: heparin (or other anticoagulant), clopidogrel, nitroglycerin, papaverine, alteplase, and calcium channel blockers.

Positioning

- The patient is placed supine on the angiographic table with both groins prepped and draped. Consider preparing the foot and the leg in anticipation for retrograde approach if needed (**FIGURE 7**).

TECHNIQUES

ANTEGRADE TIBIAL REVASCULARIZATION

First Step: A. Femoral Access and Anticoagulation

- Contralateral femoral access with standard up and over technique is our routine approach for diagnostic arteriograms and most tibial interventions.
- Antegrade femoral approach has distinct advantages for tibial or pedal interventions, especially in the setting of a hostile and narrow aortic bifurcation. Antegrade access generally provides easier pushability and reduced radiation to the patient and procedural team. Therefore, it is our preferred approach in the treatment of recurrent disease or known distal disease.
- Ultrasound-guided access may minimize risk for access site complications.
- Diagnostic arteriogram to image the inflow is performed.

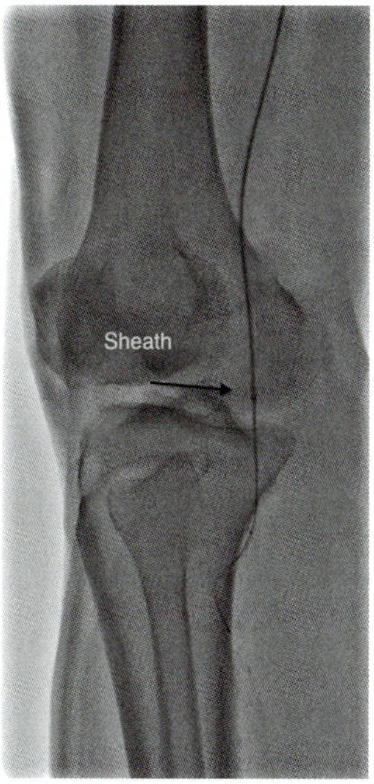

FIGURE 8 • After obtaining femoral access, the sheath is advanced to the popliteal artery for the intervention. It allows better visualization of the tibial vessels and facilitates the pushability and the ability to cross total occlusions.

- A 5- or 6-Fr sheath is advanced over a stiff wire to the popliteal artery, positioned as close as possible to the tibial trifurcation (Sheath: 90-110 cm from the contralateral femoral access and 45 to 55 cm from the ipsilateral femoral access) (**FIGURE 8**).
- Sheath tip positioning close to the target vessel maximizes pushability across total occlusions. Also, improved visualization of tibial vessels is achieved with reduced contrast volumes.
- Anticoagulation is established using unfractionated heparin or other alternatives to achieve an activated clotting time (ACT) of more than 250 seconds.

B. Transradial Access

- The improved safety and patient convenience profile for transradial compared with transfemoral access has made this approach attractive to interventionalists with lower access site complication rates and shorter ambulation times.
- Patient selection is of paramount importance given the greater distance that needs to be traversed compared with transfemoral access. Typical distances to tibial arteries are 200 to 250 cm.
- Left radial access is typically preferred (to right radial access) given the shorter working distance and avoiding the need to cross the aortic arch and compromising the cerebral vessels.
- It is helpful to have the working table parallel to the abducted left arm and to have the imaging monitor to the left of the patient's head (if accessing from the left radial artery) for improved working flow.
- Ultrasound-guided access is also encouraged to minimize access site complications.
- Slender Glidesheaths (Terumo), 4 and 5 Fr, with the ultrathin wall technology have been suggested for diagnostic angiograms through the transradial access.
- An antispasmodic cocktail of vasodilators (a calcium channel blocker and nitroglycerin with a heparinized saline solution) is subsequently administered.
- An angled catheter (Kumpe, Angled Glidecath) can be used to traverse the arch into the descending thoracic aorta with the image intensifier in a left anterior oblique view. An upper extremity angiogram may be helpful if the operator encounters difficulties crossing the subclavian artery.
- Selective lower extremity diagnostic angiograms can be performed utilizing a 5-Fr 125-cm-long pigtail catheter.
- The relatively recent Terumo R2P Destination Slender sheath available in 149 cm lengths allows for placing the sheath tip as close as possible to the target lesion to allow for better pushability.
- Similarly, anticoagulation is established using unfractionated heparin to achieve an ACT of more than 250 seconds.

Second Step: Selective Angiogram

- Imaging of the tibial outflow is obtained from sheath injections or through diagnostic catheters (5- to 10-mL power or hand injection). To reduce contrast load, contrast may be diluted 50% for all but the most distal arterial beds.
- Anteroposterior or ipsilateral anterior oblique projections are obtained to visualize the popliteal "trifurcation" and separate the tibia and fibula. True lateral oblique projections are obtained to visualize pedal outflow.
- Arteriographic images must be carefully examined to optimize outcome; multiple projections may be required to sufficiently opacify tibial and pedal vascular anatomy, especially distal to extended or serial occlusions. Delayed views (prolonged digital subtraction angiography [DSA] time) may improve opacification of patent tibial or pedal vessels distal to occluded segments (**FIGURE 9**). Withdrawing the sheath to the femoral bifurcation may uncover reconstitution of distal tibial artery segments through extended deep femoral artery collateral pathways.

Third Step: Crossing the Occlusion

- Angled catheters and guidewires are typically used to select the respective tibial arteries.
- The catheter/guidewire combination is advanced into the target tibial artery proximal to the occlusion or stenosis.
- Anatomy is confirmed with magnified arteriographic views.
- "Road mapping" may improve guidance across occlusions. The wire leads through the occlusion, followed by the crossing catheter (eg, Quick-Cross or Cook CXI or TrailBlazer, 0.014 in or 0.018 in) (**FIGURE 10**).
- Transluminal passage is preferred to subintimal access because reentry into the true lumen may be unpredictable and challenging.
- Soft-tipped hydrophilic guidewires are used to negotiate and traverse tibial stenosis with the support of crossing catheters under magnified road map guidance.
- Heavier weighted tip, chronic total occlusion (CTO) guidewires (either 0.014-in or 0.018-in platforms) are designed to provide improved performance and penetration across total occlusions.
- For longer occlusions, leading with a 2-mm percutaneous transluminal angioplasty (PTA) balloon as an alternative to low-profile crossing catheters (eg, Quick-Cross or CXI) can

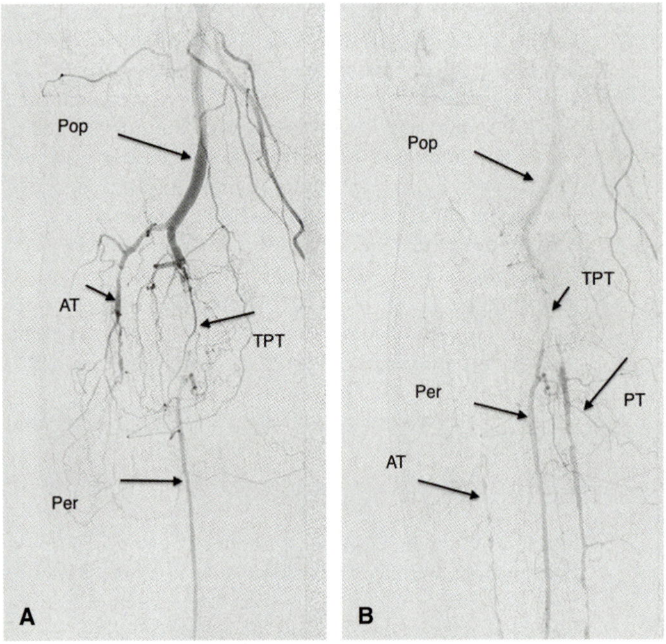

FIGURE 9 • **A,** Diagnostic angiogram from the popliteal sheath demonstrates patent right popliteal artery, occluded anterior tibial artery, and occluded distal tibioperoneal trunk with reconstitution of peroneal artery. The posterior tibial artery appears to be occluded. **B,** Angiogram with delayed DSA time identifies a patent diseased posterior tibial artery distal to the occluded tibioperoneal trunk and patent peroneal artery.

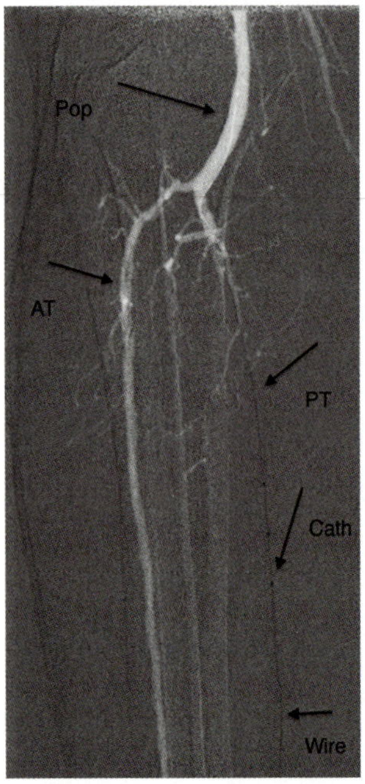

FIGURE 10 • Recanalization of occluded PT. Under road map guidance, the PT was selected, and using a wire and support catheter, the occlusion was crossed.

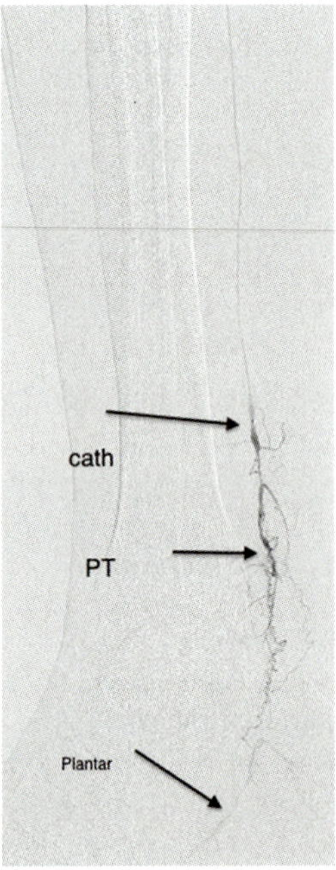

FIGURE 11 • Angiogram from catheter in PT during recanalization of occluded PT.

improve access by extending or reestablishing the recanalization plane during transit.

Fourth Step: Reentry Into the True Lumen

- Reenter into the true lumen under road map guidance (**FIGURE 11**).
- Advance the catheter over the wire into the true lumen beyond the target lesion and remove the wire.
- Check for back-bleeding and subsequently perform a selective angiogram through the catheter to confirm the proper intraluminal position (**FIGURE 12**).
- Advance a stiff wire with long, soft tip into the target vessel as distal as possible (**FIGURE 13**).
- Remove the catheter carefully under fluoroscopic guidance while maintaining wire access into the distal patent artery.
- Reentry devices can be used to select the true lumen from a dissection plane. Alternatively, if failure to reenter the true lumen persists despite the use of reentry devices or balloon angioplasty to disrupt the dissection membrane, retrograde access into the distal true lumen can be attempted at the time or in a staged future setting.

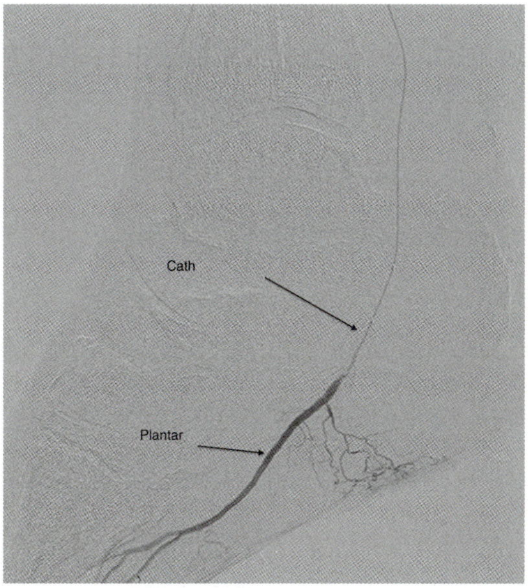

FIGURE 12 • Angiogram from catheter in the plantar artery to confirm the proper intraluminal position after recanalization of PT.

Fifth Step: Treatment With Balloon Angioplasty

- The proximal and distal ends of the lesion are demarcated by a repeat contrast injection through the sheath. The use of radiopaque adhesive rulers applied on the affected leg may help with measurement and device selection.
- Deliver the appropriate size balloon (typically 2-3.5 mm in diameter) to the target lesion and perform the balloon angioplasty for 2- to 3-minute inflation time (**FIGURE 14**).
- Single inflation using a long balloon decreases the procedural time and reduces the risk of postangioplasty dissection requiring reintervention (**FIGURE 15**). Tapered balloons can help treat lesions across vessels of variable size.

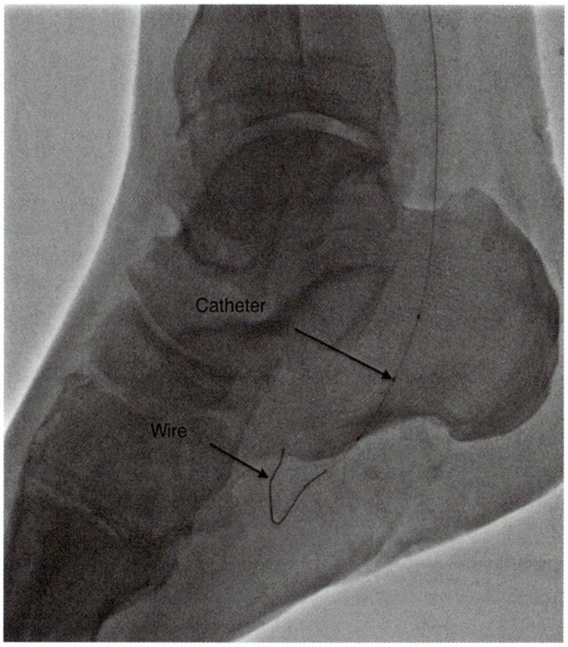

FIGURE 13 • Placement of wire into the plantar artery prior to angioplasty of the occluded PT.

- Heparin flush, continuous or intermittent, through the sheath is recommended during balloon inflation and throughout the procedure.
- Selective injection of intra-arterial nitroglycerin through the sheath will minimize the effects of spasm at or distal to the intervention.

Sixth Step: Angiogram Post Balloon Angioplasty

- The treatment balloon is retracted back over the wire to the popliteal artery level.
- The completion arteriogram is performed from a sheath injection to assess the angioplasty outcome and pedal runoff (**FIGURE 16**).

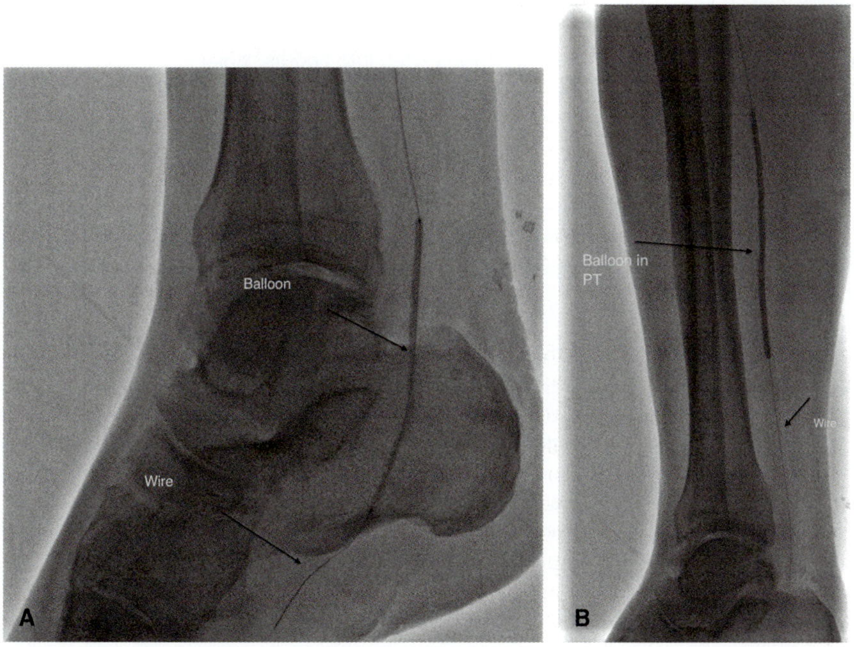

FIGURE 14 • **A,** Balloon angioplasty of distal PT with 2-mm balloon for 2-minute inflation time. **B,** Balloon angioplasty of PT with 3-mm balloon for 2-minute inflation time.

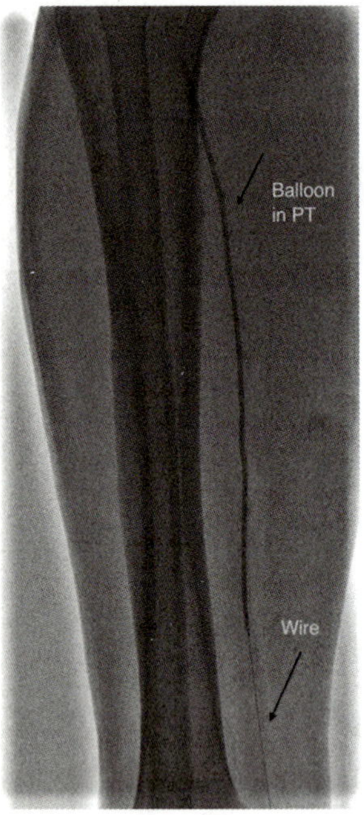

FIGURE 15 • Angioplasty of PT with long balloon.

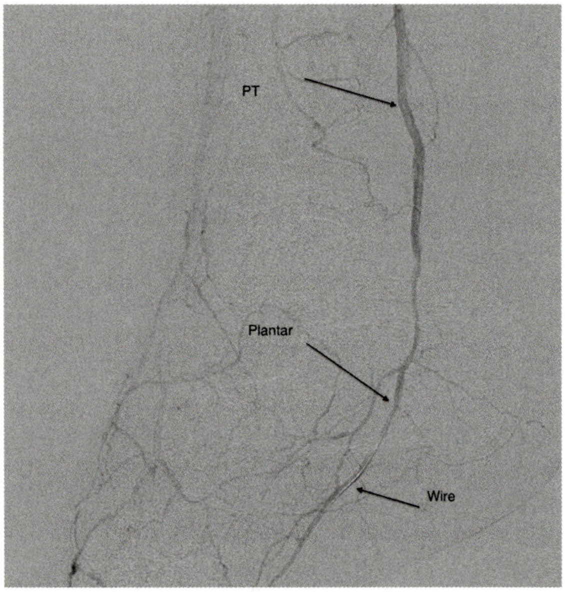

FIGURE 16 • Angiogram from sheath postrecanalization and angioplasty of PT shows good flow without any flow-limiting dissection.

- Recoil or dissections are treated with sustained reinflation of the balloon for 3 to 5 minutes or by upsizing the balloon, followed by more gradual deflation.
- Flow-limiting dissections in the proximal tibioperoneal trunk and proximal tibial arteries may be resolved with stent or tack placement when necessary.
- Distal embolization can be managed by aspiration through the existing catheter or aspiration with a purpose-specific catheter such as the Export. Catheter-directed thrombolysis may be attempted in select cases.
- Other modalities may be useful in restoring patency, such as atherectomy devices and can be used as stand-alone therapy or as adjuncts to balloon angioplasty.
- The routine use of tibial stenting is not advocated at this stage. Although there is some evidence to suggest that drug-eluting stents may result in improved durability, these are subject to cost restrictions, regulatory approvals, and availability depending on the country of practice. Ongoing trials on bioabsorbable drug eluting tibial scaffolds may add to the device armamentarium.

Seventh Step: Treatment With Atherectomy

- Treatment with atherectomy devices necessitates crossing the occlusive lesion with a wire prior to device use. In our practice it is reserved to heavily calcified lesions that cannot be crossed with a catheter or a balloon over the wire (**FIGURE 17**).
- Different atherectomy devices have different technical considerations. Operator familiarity with the respective device is important for the technical success of the procedure.
- After crossing the lesion as described in step 3 above, the existing wire is exchanged for a 0.014-in wire.
- The atherectomy device is typically introduced over its respective 0.014-in wire. Atherectomy is performed following device-specific instructions for use.
- Postatherectomy balloon angioplasty is subsequently performed as mentioned in the fifth step above (**FIGURE 17**).
- Distal embolic protection devices are frequently employed during atherectomy of femoropopliteal lesions due to the concern for embolization. These devices are rarely employed with atherectomy of tibial vessels.

Eighth Step: Revascularization of Another Tibial Vessel

- The ultimate goal is to reestablish direct, in-line arterial flow to the ischemic part of the foot. A secondary goal is to optimize flow by reconstructing more than one occluded tibial artery, when possible.
- The wire is redirected into another tibial vessel, and recanalization is performed as described earlier (**FIGURE 18**).
- When the peroneal artery is the sole outflow vessel, revascularization to the level of the peroneal collaterals at ankle is needed.
- Ostial lesions at the bifurcation of anterior tibial artery and tibioperoneal trunk can be treated with kissing balloon technique to prevent plaque shifting.

Ninth Step: Completion Angiogram and Hemostasis

- If the completion angiography is satisfactory (**FIGURE 19**), the sheath is pulled back to the common femoral artery and injection from that level is recommended to rule out any complications in the femoropopliteal segment related to sheath position.
- The sheath is removed, and hemostasis is obtained at the access site either by using closure device or manual compression without heparin reversal unless necessary.

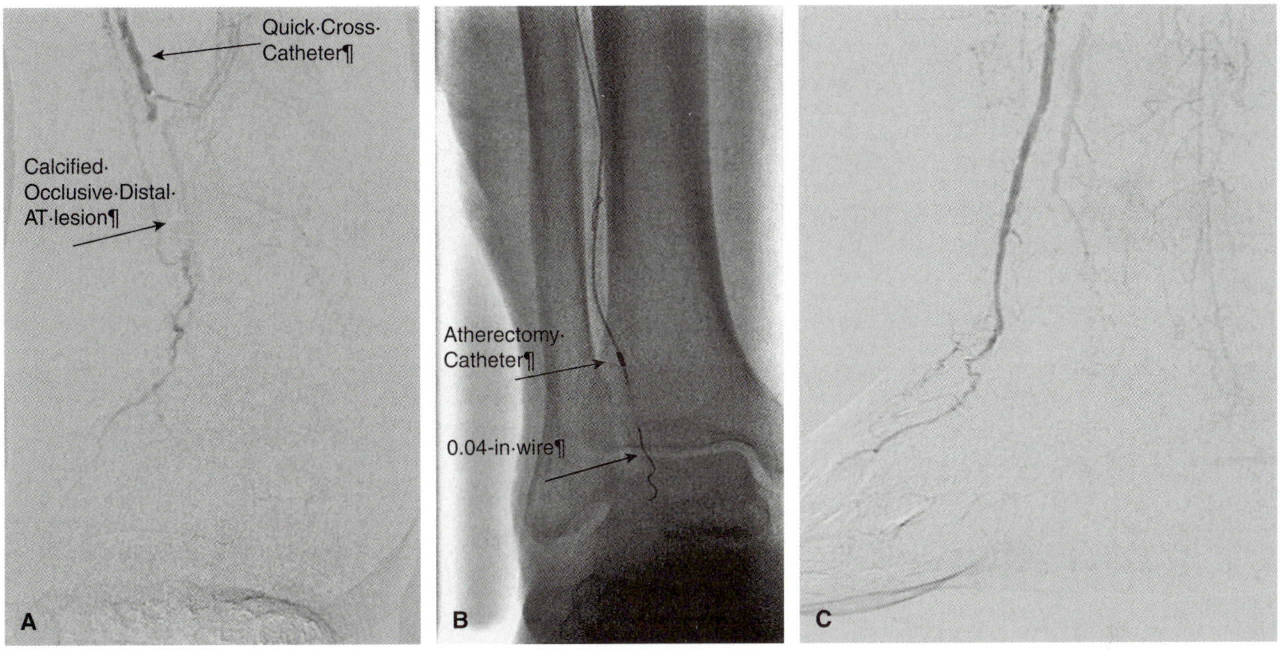

FIGURE 17 • **A,** Occluded distal anterior tibial (AT) artery lesion **(B)**. Rotational atherectomy CSI catheter in the distal anterior tibial artery over a 0.014-in wire. **C,** Postatherectomy and standard balloon angioplasty completion angiogram.

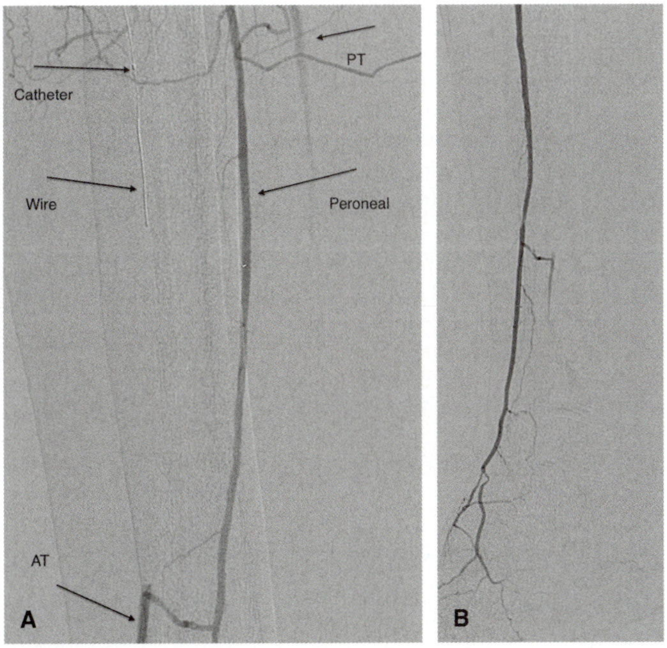

FIGURE 18 • **A,** Angiogram from the sheath at the time of recanalization of anterior tibial (AT) artery with a wire and catheter. The peroneal artery is patent and reconstitutes a distal anterior tibial artery. **B,** Angiogram from the sheath postangioplasty of the AT with 3-mm balloon shows patent AT without any dissection or flow-limiting stenosis.

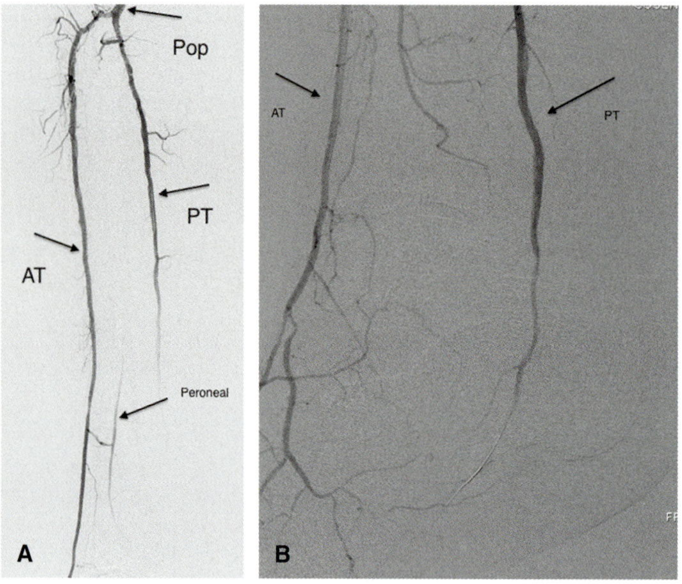

FIGURE 19 • **A,** Completion angiogram from the sheath postrecanalization of occluded AT and PT shows patent vessels with good flow mainly in the AT without any significant dissection. The peroneal artery reconstituted in a retrograde fashion from the AT. **B,** Patent distal AT and PT runoff into the foot.

RETROGRADE TIBIAL RECANALIZATION

First Step: Retrograde Access

- Antegrade access is obtained first as described earlier. This is used for initial imaging and delivery of treatment devices.
- Administration of vasodilators through the antegrade sheath can facilitate tibial access and minimize vasospasm.
- Retrograde tibial arterial access is performed under ultrasound or fluoroscopic guidance using a micropuncture 21-gauge needle; a 300-cm, 0.018-in or 0.014-in wire; and balloon or support catheter. An introducer dilator, although potentially useful, is not essential.
- Sedation should be managed to minimize movement when road mapping is used to identify target arteries; excess sedation will worsen patient cooperation as they will not be able to follow the physician's instructions.
- Local anesthesia is infiltrated at the intended puncture site; excess anesthetic volume may deepen the vessel and make cannulation more difficult.
- Access to the posterior tibial artery is obtained in the region of the medial malleolus. Dorsiflexion and/or eversion of the foot may facilitate access.
- Access to the anterior tibial artery is obtained on the dorsum of the foot or the distal aspect of the leg anteriorly, where the target artery may be larger. Dorsalis pedis access is facilitated by plantar flexion of the foot.
- The peroneal artery should be approached laterally through the interosseous membrane.
- More proximal access to the posterior or anterior tibial arteries may be obtained with road map guidance when necessary. The use of intra-arterial vasodilators will help with vessel visualization and subsequent access.
- Inadvertent venous puncture may occur during attempts at retrograde access, and when it does, consider leaving the wire in place to help guide further attempts at arterial access.
- Ultrasound-assisted retrograde access, as an adjunct to road map guidance alone, may help to define the three-dimensional orientation of the needle in relation to the target artery (**FIGURE 20**).
- Image quality is optimized by incorporating a sufficient delay following contrast injection to maximize opacification of the target artery. Selective use of intra-arterial vasodilators through the antegrade sheath may reduce the severity of access-related vasospasm, when present, distally.
- The C-arm is adjusted to best align the needle to the target vessel, typically using an ipsilateral oblique projection.
- Surgical exposure may become necessary to ensure adequate access for retrograde tibial reconstruction. Retrograde access may also be obtained concomitant with planned

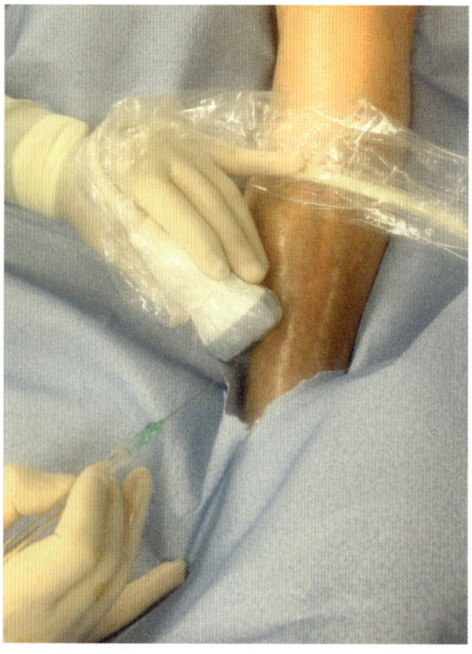

FIGURE 20 • Retrograde approach: access to PT under ultrasound guidance.

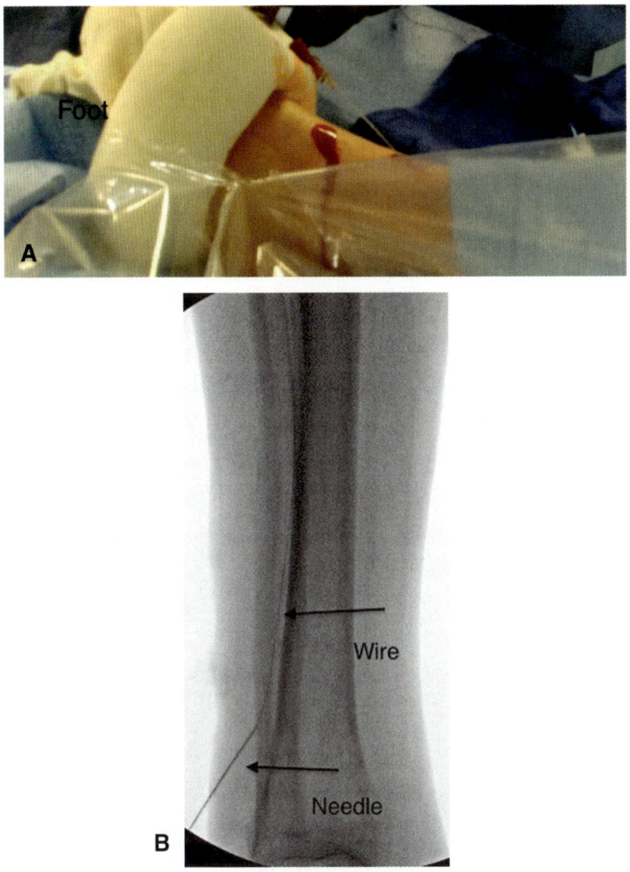

FIGURE 21 ● **A,** Retrograde access to AT with adequate arterial back-bleeding from the micropuncture needle. **B,** Needle in AT and wire advanced proximally under fluoroscopic guidance.

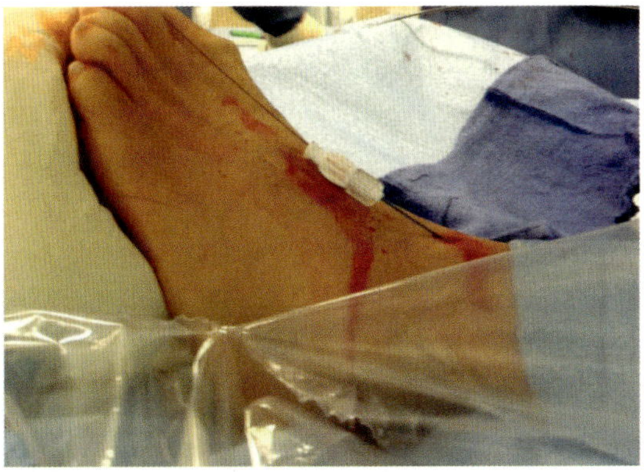

FIGURE 22 ● Retrograde access: wire and inner dilator of the microsheath.

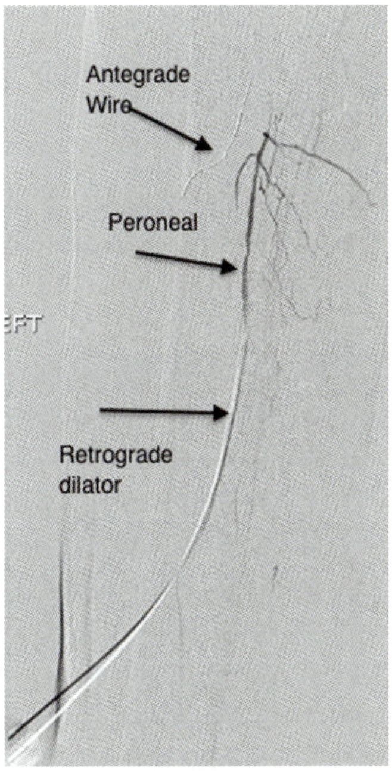

FIGURE 23 ● Retrograde access of the peroneal artery angiogram from the introducer confirms the intraluminal position.

transmetatarsal amputation by identifying and cannulating the open end of transected distal dorsal pedal artery.

Second Step: Retrograde Angiogram

- Once back-bleeding is seen, the micropuncture 0.018-in access wire is advanced under fluoroscopic guidance (**FIGURE 21**), followed by an appropriately sized support catheter, balloon, or the inner dilator of the 4-Fr microsheath.
- In most cases, retrograde sheaths are generally *not* deployed to minimize trauma to the puncture site and distal target artery (**FIGURE 22**). When sheaths are required, use of a radial access sheath will facilitate atraumatic access.
- Intraluminal position is confirmed by retrograde angiography through the catheter or dilator (**FIGURE 23**).

Third Step: Recanalization of Tibial Occlusion

- Antegrade sheath arteriography is used to delineate the extent of the target lesion.
- The occlusion is crossed using 0.018-in or 0.014-in wires, supported by a crossing catheter or low-profile angioplasty balloon (**FIGURE 24**). The 0.014-in wire may lack the necessary support to allow retrograde crossing of tibial lesions, and therefore, the 0.018-in wire can be utilized.
- The wire and crossing catheter combination is advanced from distal to proximal and into the popliteal artery if possible. The wire is removed.
- Following aspiration to confirm luminal position, a selective arteriogram is performed from the retrograde catheter.

Fourth Step: Exteriorization of the Wire From the Femoral Access Site

- Next, an attempt is made to advance the guidewire into the antegrade sheath or catheter (**FIGURE 25**).
- When this proves difficult on its own, a snare is deployed through the antegrade sheath to capture and externalize the distal retrograde wire (**FIGURE 26**).
- Following successful externalization of the retrograde wire, through and through "wire access" is available from both ends.
- A crossing catheter is then advanced from the antegrade access site over the wire to the patent tibial vessel distal to the occlusion.
- Distal intraluminal position is confirmed with arteriography through the crossing catheter.

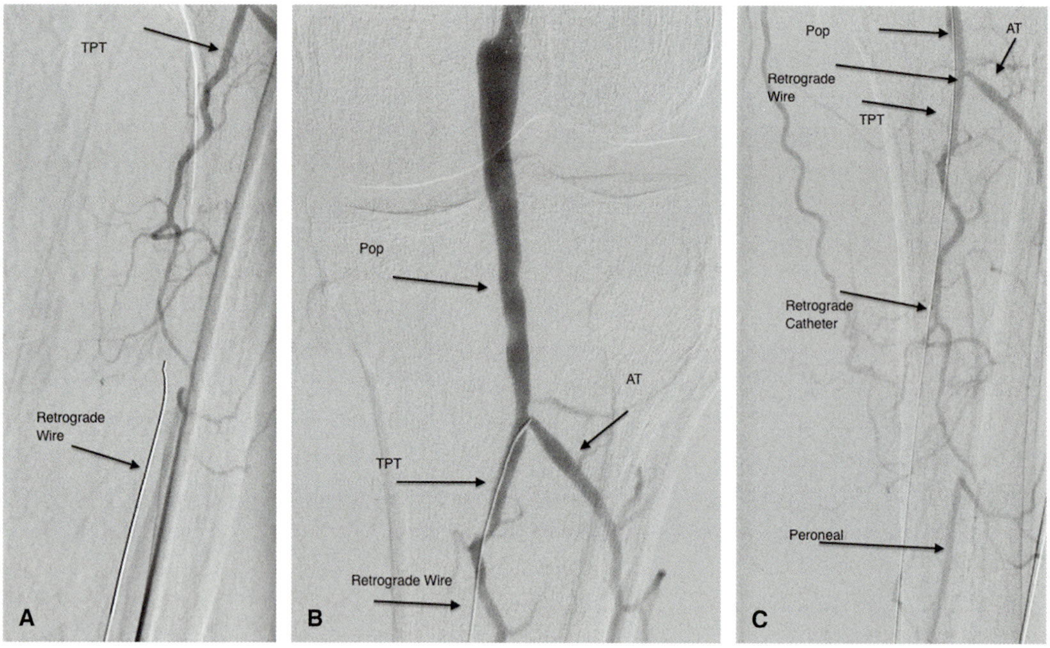

FIGURE 24 • **A,** Angiogram from antegrade sheath. Wire crossing the occluded PT. **B,** Angiogram confirming entry of the wire into the tibioperoneal trunk (TPT). **C,** Angiogram shows the retrograde wire and catheter across the occlusion into the popliteal artery proximally.

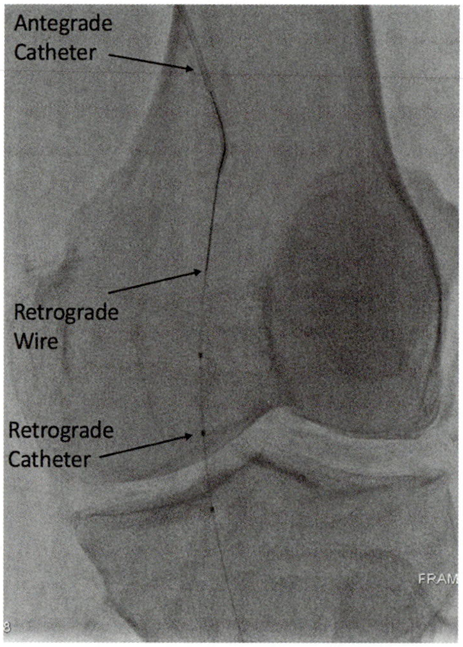

FIGURE 25 • Retrograde wire is advanced into the antegrade catheter to establish "wire access" from both antegrade and retrograde access sites.

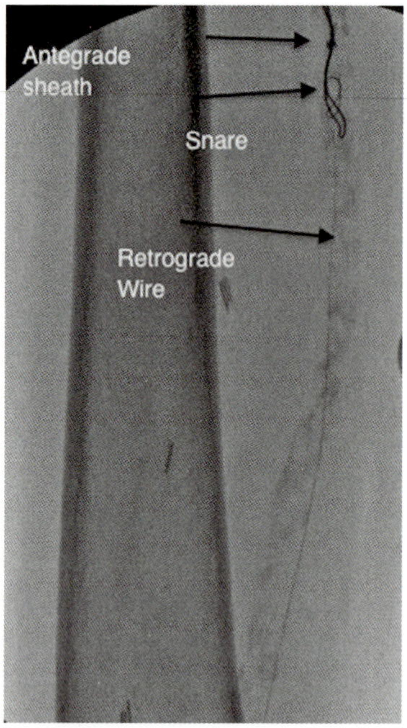

FIGURE 26 • Snaring the retrograde wire into the proximal sheath.

- Next, the through and through wire is removed from the antegrade sheath, leaving the crossing catheter across the lesion. The wire is exchanged for a 300-cm 0.014-in working wire, advanced distally through the antegrade crossing catheter.
- The retrograde access catheter or micropuncture 4-Fr access dilator is subsequently removed from the distal target artery.

Hemostasis is obtained and maintained by manual pressure at the access site (**FIGURE 27**), the application of a blood pressure cuff across the site (**FIGURE 28**), or a radial compression device (Dstat Radial Hemostat Band). Vasospasm at the retrograde access sites can be addressed with intra-arterial vasodilator administration.

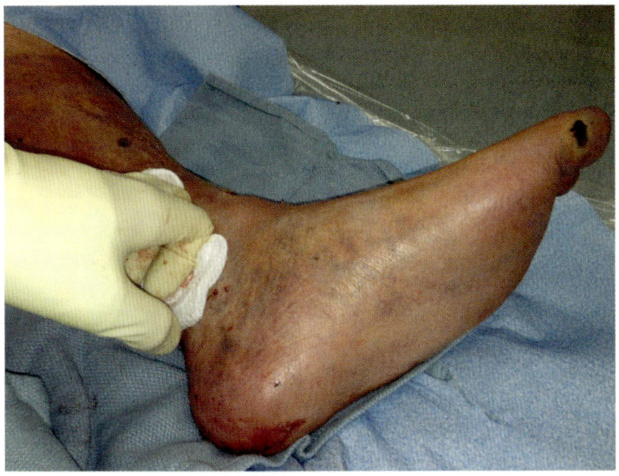

FIGURE 27 • Hemostasis with manual compression postretrograde PT access.

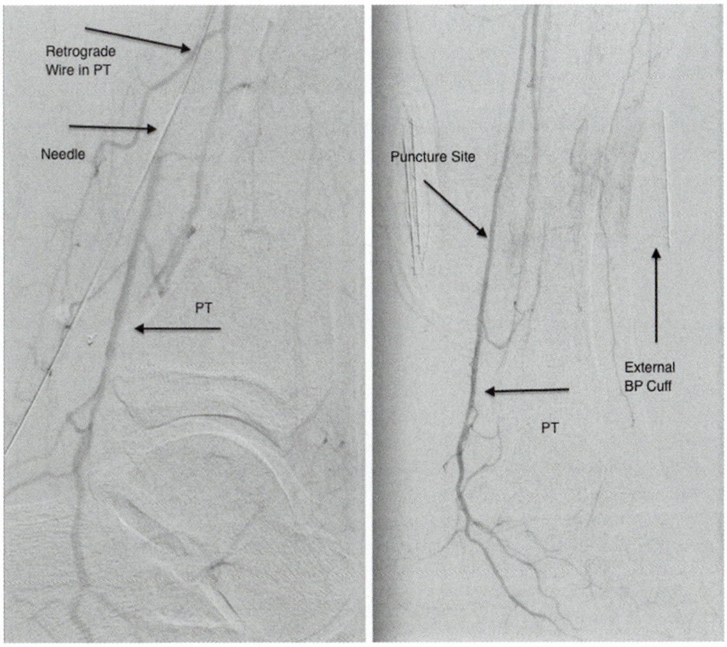

FIGURE 28 • Angiogram of PT access site with blood pressure cuff used for hemostasis (image on the right of the screen).

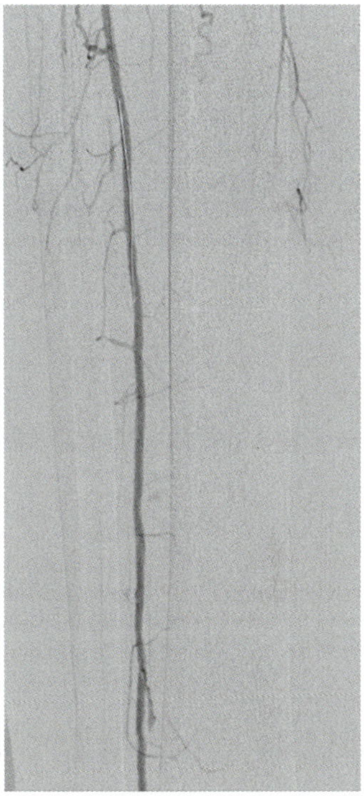

FIGURE 29 • Angiogram shows extravasation from retrograde peroneal access site postrecanalization of TPT.

- Removing all devices from the retrograde access site as quickly as possible reduces instrumentation time and potential for arterial injury and distal thrombosis.
- Inflating a balloon advanced from the antegrade access sheath across the retrograde access site (**FIGURE 29**) not only may affect hemostasis but can also increase traumatic injury and access site bleeding and is rarely needed.

Fifth Step: Treatment With Balloon Angioplasty

- The intervention is then performed in the standard fashion from the antegrade approach (**FIGURE 30**).

Antegrade-Retrograde Approach

- If the retrograde wire is not able to cross the lesion and regain access to the true lumen, an antegrade-retrograde approach may be used to create adjacent subintimal planes in opposing directions (CART technique or controlled antegrade and retrograde subintimal tracking) (**FIGURE 31**).
- The dissection flap separating the adjacent subintimal spaces may be disrupted by simultaneous inflation in both directions.
- This allows visualization and recanalization of true lumen from either or both directions. The two PTA balloons selected for this maneuver should be sized appropriately to minimize risk for target arterial rupture.

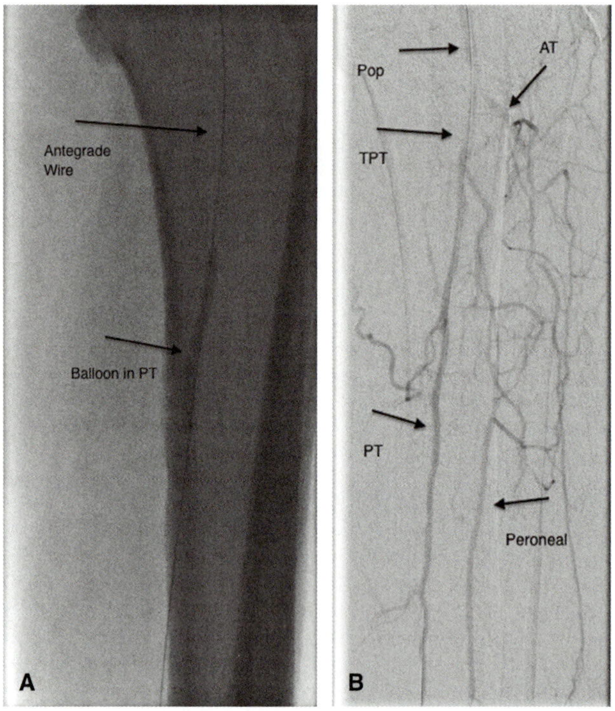

FIGURE 30 • **A,** Balloon angioplasty of the occluded PT postretrograde recanalization and exteriorization of the wire from the antegrade sheath. **B,** Completion angiogram shows good flow into the PT without any dissection.

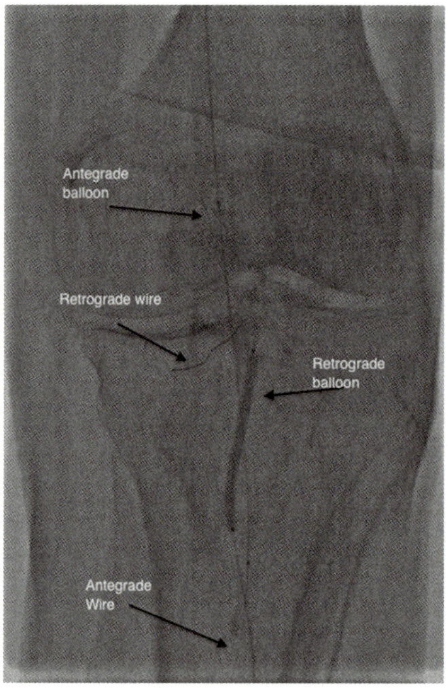

FIGURE 31 • Retrograde/antegrade PTA to disrupt the membrane between two subintimal planes.

PEARLS AND PITFALLS

Goals for percutaneous tibial revascularization	■ Achieve direct in-line flow to the ischemic foot and, when possible, optimize pedal perfusion by recanalizing more than one occluded tibial artery.
Contralateral or antegrade femoral access	■ Choice based on inflow anatomy and target lesion. Advancement of the antegrade sheath tip into the popliteal artery is key for support and successful tibial revascularization.
Ultrasound-guided access	■ Can help access the anterior wall of the vessel in a relatively disease-free spot and minimize access site complications. It is recommended in antegrade femoral access and retrograde pedal access.
Retrograde approach	■ Should not be regarded as the first option for tibial interventions. It is selectively considered after failed attempts at antegrade access and in the setting of flush occlusions of the antegrade artery with large, adjacent collaterals.
Sheathless retrograde technique	■ Is preferred to minimize tibial artery access complications such as dissection and thrombosis. Recanalization is achieved with a wire and support catheter. Hemostasis with manual compression is usually sufficient.
Crossing total occlusions	■ The intraluminal plane is attempted first with a stiff wire and crossing catheter. The proper catheter position should be confirmed with a selective arteriography prior to definitive angioplasty.
Balloon-assisted recanalization	■ Inflation of a 2-mm balloon may assist with the recanalization of long calcified occlusions.
Kissing balloon technique	■ Is sometimes needed to treat the ostial lesions at the origin of the anterior tibial or posterior tibial artery, depending on the amount of plaque in the adjacent peroneal artery or tibioperoneal trunk.
Anticoagulation	■ Maintain an ACT of greater than 250 seconds throughout the intervention. Continuous or intermittent flushing of the popliteal sheath with heparinized solution is recommended.
Vasodilators	■ Are used from the antegrade sheath and at the pedal access site to prevent vasospasm and to allow better visualization of tibial vessels distal to the occlusion. Heparin, verapamil, and nitroglycerin is a frequently used "cocktail" through the pedal access to address vasospasm.

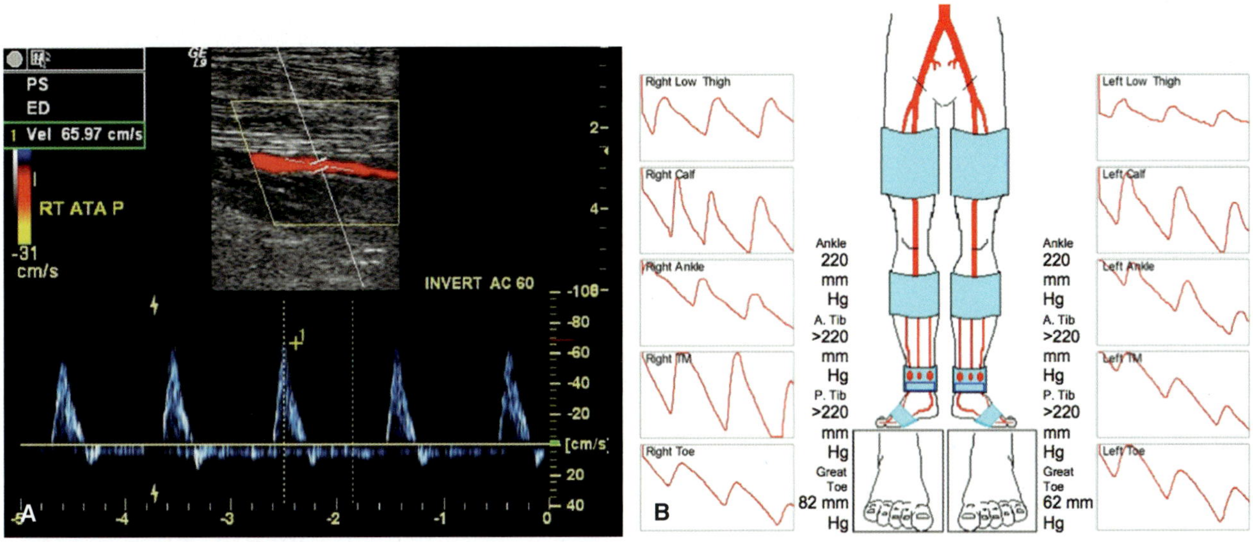

FIGURE 32 ● **A,** Duplex of the anterior tibial artery postrecanalization and angioplasty shows patent vessel with relatively normal Doppler flow. **B,** Follow-up PVRs postrecanalization and angioplasty of the right anterior tibial artery and right posterior tibial artery demonstrate normal PVR waveforms in the foot with adequate toe pressure.

POSTOPERATIVE CARE

- Following the procedure, the patient is observed in the recovery unit with serial neurovascular examinations and intravenous and oral hydration.
- A clopidogrel loading dose (usually 300 mg) is administered when the patient is not already on dual antiplatelet therapy. Dual antiplatelet therapy is recommended for at least 3 months, longer when stents are used.
- Clinical follow-up is obtained 2 to 4 weeks after the procedure is performed, including vascular laboratory studies (usually PVRs, segmental pressures, and Duplex arterial insonation) (**FIGURE 32**).
- Close follow-up is essential to ensure optimal symptom resolution and limb salvage.

OUTCOMES

- Tibial balloon angioplasty carries a relatively low primary patency rate but can greatly augment long-term limb salvage rates. The minimally invasive nature of the procedure is especially advantageous in high-medical-risk patients. One-year primary patency rates in experienced hands range from 30% to 40%; secondary patency rates approach 60%, with ultimate limb salvage greater than 70%.[2,3]
- Retrograde interventions do not impact the patency rates of tibial interventions compared with antegrade transfemoral access. Access site thrombosis appears to be an uncommon complication.[4,5]
- Literature results remain inconsistent regarding drug-eluting balloons for tibial lesions. Results from the randomized IN.PACT DEEP trial comparing drug-coated balloons vs standard angioplasty for the treatment of infrapopliteal lesions revealed no significant differences in amputation rates between the two groups.[6]
- Primary stenting does not appear to offer any advantage over tibial angioplasty alone. A Cochrane review of randomized clinical trials revealed no differences in primary patency, secondary patency, or major amputations between angioplasty alone vs angioplasty and stenting.[7,8] There may be some patency advantage associated with drug eluting, as compared with bare metal stents.[9] Nonetheless, stenting under all circumstances should be considered as a "bailout," used to improve suboptimal results of angioplasty alone.[10]
- Tibial atherectomy does not offer an added benefit compared with plain balloon angioplasty with comparable patency and limb salvage rates.[11]
- Patients with significant tissue loss and gangrene should be followed very closely after successful tibial angioplasty. Lesion restenosis rates trend higher in patients at increased risk for limb loss.[12]
- Multilevel interventions, when necessary, are associated with improved limb salvage rate and wound healing compared with isolated tibial interventions.[3]
- Postangioplasty arterial restenosis may portend less clinical significance once healing is achieved in the distal limb or forefoot. The temporary increase in blood flow following angioplasty is often sufficient to heal small ulcerations.[13]
- There is some evidence of improved patency with drug-eluting stents and drug-eluting balloons.[9,14]
- The LIFE BTK trial is currently enrolling patients in the prospective trial evaluating the safety and effectiveness of the new Everolimus Eluting Resorbable Scaffold system in the tibial vessels.

COMPLICATIONS

- Access site complications (hematoma, bleeding, pseudoaneurysm) are more common with the ipsilateral antegrade femoral approach.
- Contrast-induced nephropathy can be avoided by sufficient preoperative, intraoperative, and postoperative hydration as well as judicious use of contrast.
- Vessel thrombosis can be avoided by maintaining a therapeutic anticoagulation level throughout the procedure. The use of nitroglycerin can help prevent vasospasm and a

low-flow state. Dual antiplatelet therapy is recommended to avoid early postprocedural target artery thrombosis.

- Outflow embolization may be successfully treated with catheter aspiration or thrombolysis if needed.
- Retrograde access site bleeding, dissection, and vessel thrombosis are described after the retrograde pedal access. Using ultrasound-guided access, sheathless technique and the use of local vasodilators may minimize the risk of retrograde access site complications.
- Compartment syndrome may develop either from reperfusion injury following successful intervention or, more commonly, perforation of tibial arteries in the deep compartments of the leg.
- Limb loss may result from failed intervention, iatrogenic vessel thrombosis, distal arterial occlusion following embolization, and compartment syndrome.

REFERENCES

1. Mills JL, Sr., Conte MS, Armstrong DG, et al. The Society for Vascular Surgery Lower Extremity Threatened Limb Classification System: risk stratification based on wound, ischemia, and foot infection (WIfI). *J Vasc Surg* 2014;59:220-234.e1-2.
2. Fernandez N, McEnaney R, Marone LK, et al. Predictors of failure and success of tibial interventions for critical limb ischemia. *J Vasc Surg*. 2010;52:834-842.
3. Fernandez N, McEnaney R, Marone LK, et al. Multilevel versus isolated endovascular tibial interventions for critical limb ischemia. *J Vasc Surg*. 2011;54:722-729.
4. Taha AG, Abou Ali AN, Al-Khoury G, et al. Outcomes of infrageniculate retrograde versus transfemoral access for endovascular intervention for chronic lower extremity ischemia. *J Vasc Surg*. 2018;68:1088-1095.
5. Lai SH, Fenlon J, Roush BB, et al. Analysis of the retrograde tibial artery approach in lower extremity revascularization in an office endovascular center. *J Vasc Surg*. 2019;70:157-165.
6. Zeller T, Micari A, Scheinert D, et al. The IN.PACT DEEP clinical drug-coated balloon trial: 5-year outcomes. *JACC Cardiovasc Interv*. 2020;13:431-443.
7. Hsu CC, Kwan GN, Singh D, Rophael JA, Anthony C, van Driel ML. Angioplasty versus stenting for infrapopliteal arterial lesions in chronic limb-threatening ischaemia. *Cochrane Database Syst Rev*. 2018;12:Cd009195.
8. Randon C, Jacobs B, De Ryck F, Vermassen F. Angioplasty or primary stenting for infrapopliteal lesions: results of a prospective randomized trial. *Cardiovasc Intervent Radiol*. 2010;33:260-269.
9. Bosiers M, Scheinert D, Peeters P, et al. Randomized comparison of everolimus-eluting versus bare-metal stents in patients with critical limb ischemia and infrapopliteal arterial occlusive disease. *J Vasc Surg*. 2012;55:390-398.
10. Donas KP, Torsello G, Schwindt A, Schönefeld E, Boldt O, Pitoulias GA. Below knee bare nitinol stent placement in high-risk patients with critical limb ischemia is still durable after 24 months of follow-up. *J Vasc Surg*. 2010;52:356-361.
11. Todd KE Jr, Ahanchi SS, Maurer CA, Kim JH, Chipman CR, Panneton JM. Atherectomy offers no benefits over balloon angioplasty in tibial interventions for critical limb ischemia. *J Vasc Surg*. 2013;58:941-948.
12. Saqib NU, Domenick N, Cho JS, et al. Predictors and outcomes of restenosis following tibial artery endovascular interventions for critical limb ischemia. *J Vasc Surg*. 2013;57:692-699.
13. Schmidt A, Ulrich M, Winkler B, et al. Angiographic patency and clinical outcome after balloon-angioplasty for extensive infrapopliteal arterial disease. *Cathet Cardiovasc Interv*. 2010;76:1047-1054.
14. Schmidt A, Piorkowski M, Werner M, et al. First experience with drug-eluting balloons in infrapopliteal arteries: restenosis rate and clinical outcome. *J Am Coll Cardiol*. 2011;58:1105-1109.

Chapter 33 Open Infrainguinal Reconstruction Techniques

Gregory J. Landry

DEFINITION

- Lower extremity bypasses are named by the corresponding inflow and outflow arteries. The most common inflow source is the femoral artery (common, superficial, profunda). For disease that is more distal the popliteal or tibial arteries can also be used for inflow. Common sources of outflow include the popliteal (above and below knee), tibial (anterior tibial, posterior tibial, peroneal), and pedal (dorsalis pedis, posterior tibial, medial and lateral plantar) arteries.
- Autogenous conduit is preferred for all lower extremity bypasses when available. The greater saphenous vein (GSV) is the most frequently used conduit. Other options for native conduit include the short saphenous vein, arm vein (basilic, cephalic, brachial), and femoral vein.
- If suitable autogenous conduit is not available, alternate conduit options include prosthetic (polytetrafluoroethylene, polyester) or cryopreserved cadaver grafts.

DIFFERENTIAL DIAGNOSIS

- The majority of patients for whom lower extremity bypass is necessary will have atherosclerotic peripheral arterial disease (PAD).
- Other conditions for which lower extremity bypass may be necessary include aneurysms (eg, femoral, popliteal), trauma, and vasculitis.

PATIENT HISTORY AND PHYSICAL FINDINGS

- PAD can be asymptomatic; however, revascularization is rarely performed in the absence of symptoms. The most frequent symptomatic presentation of PAD is intermittent claudication (leg pain with walking relieved by rest). More severe PAD presents with chronic limb threatening ischemia (CLTI), including rest pain, ulcers, and gangrene.
- A history of cardiovascular risk factors should be elicited in all patients undergoing lower extremity bypass, including history of smoking, cardiac disease, cerebrovascular disease, diabetes, chronic kidney disease, hyperlipidemia, and chronic obstructive pulmonary disease.
- Upper and lower extremity pulse examination should be performed. Because atherosclerosis is a systemic disorder, the following pulses should be assessed bilaterally: carotid, brachial, radial, femoral, popliteal, dorsalis pedis, and posterior tibial. Both the presence and strength of pulses should be recorded.
- If lower extremity pulses are absent, which is usually the case in patients undergoing surgery for peripheral arterial disease, ankle-brachial indices (ABIs) should be measured. The highest ankle pressure is divided by the highest brachial pressure.
- A history of prior vein use or removal should be elicited. Veins may have previously been used for prior lower extremity or coronary artery bypass. Patients with varicose veins may have undergone prior vein stripping or ablation. Patients with chronic kidney disease may have had prior upper extremity arteriovenous fistula placement. In dialysis-dependent patients, upper extremity veins should be used judiciously as they may be necessary for future arteriovenous access.

IMAGING AND OTHER DIAGNOSTIC STUDIES

- ABIs should be calculated in all patients considered for lower extremity bypass. A normal ABI is between 0.9 and 1.3. While there is some overlap, in general, an ABI 0.5 to 0.9 is consistent with intermittent claudication and <0.5 is consistent with CLTI. An ABI >1.3 is likely falsely elevated due to arterial calcification and may or may not be associated with significant arterial occlusive disease.
- Arterial duplex ultrasonography can be performed to determine sites of arterial stenosis and occlusion. In some centers, ultrasonography is the only diagnostic test performed before revascularization; however, in most centers, additional imaging is performed.
- Patients considered for lower extremity bypass should undergo arteriography to define the proximal (inflow) and distal (outflow) targets.
  - Digital subtraction angiography remains the gold standard and provides the greatest anatomic detail for operative planning.
  - Alternative imaging modalities include computed tomography and magnetic resonance angiography or duplex ultrasonography.
- Duplex ultrasonography should be used for preoperative vein mapping to identify suitable autogenous conduit (**FIGURE 1**). If the patient has good-quality GSV, no further

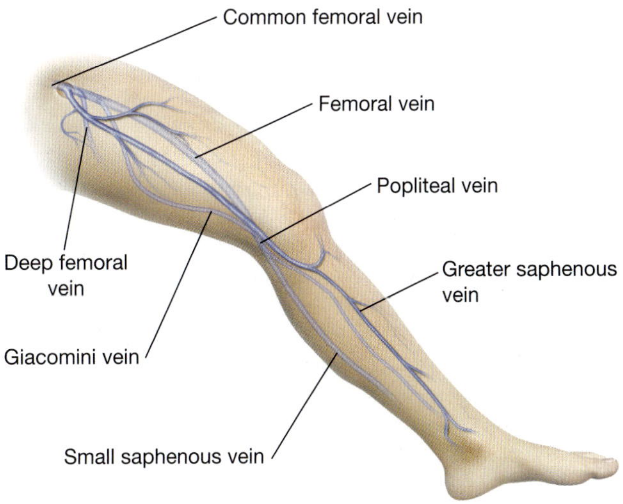

FIGURE 1 • Lower extremity venous anatomy.

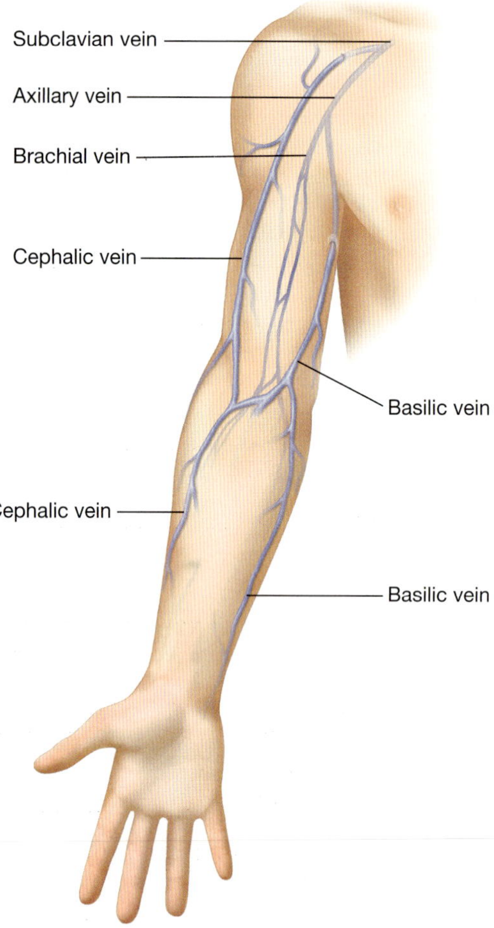

FIGURE 2 • Upper extremity venous anatomy.

vein mapping is typically necessary. If the GSV is of poor quality or absent, small saphenous vein and arm vein should be mapped (**FIGURE 2**).

- Ideal conduit diameter is 3.5 mm or greater.
- The vein should be easily compressible. A thick-walled or noncompressible vein may indicate prior superficial venous thrombosis, and the vein is likely not suitable for bypass.
- Mapping should ideally immediately precede surgery with vein course marked with an indelible marker on the skin.

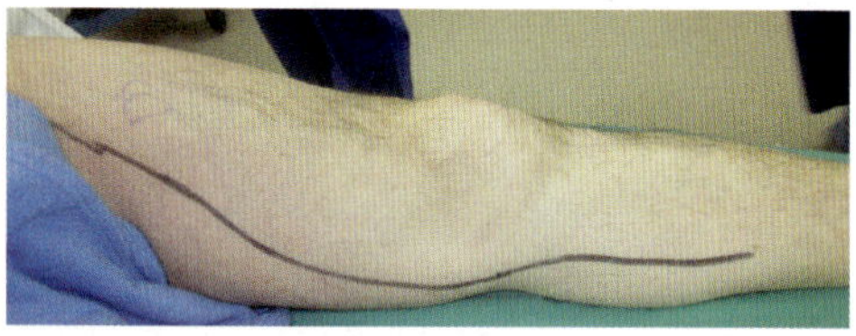

FIGURE 3 • Lower extremity vein mapping with marking of GSV.

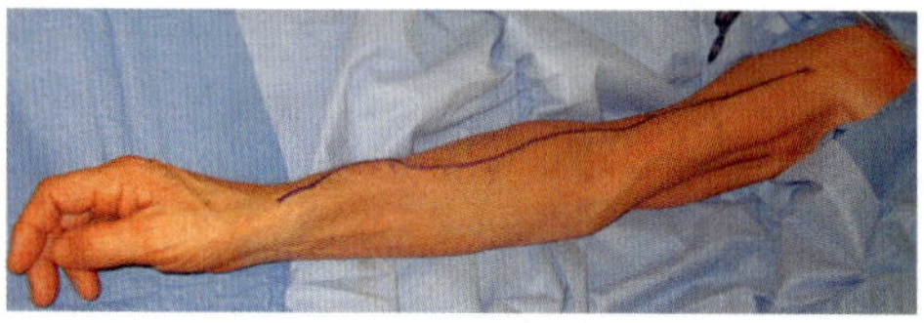

FIGURE 4 • Upper extremity vein mapping with marking of the cephalic and basilic veins.

This allows precise placement of incisions, which avoids the creation of skin and tissue flaps that might impede wound healing.

SURGICAL MANAGEMENT

- Preoperative planning
  - If not previously marked or if marks have faded, it is useful to re-mark the intended venous conduit with ultrasound guidance prior to surgery (**FIGURES 3** and **4**).
  - Open foot lesions or gangrene should be covered with sterile adhesive to prevent contamination of sterile incisions.
  - Prophylactic intravenous antibiotics should be administered to reduce risk of perioperative infection.
  - If arm vein is to be harvested, it is important to avoid blood draws or intravenous lines in the intended arm(s). If veins from both arms are necessary, central venous access may be necessary.
- Positioning
  - The majority of the procedures are performed with the patient supine. If small saphenous vein is the intended conduit, it is often easier to perform this part of the procedure with the patient prone and then to reprepare and drape with the patient supine.
  - If arm vein is to be harvested, the arms should be abducted and placed on arm boards.

TECHNIQUES

- Arterial exposure (for additional details see Chapter 27):
  - The common, superficial, and profunda femoral arteries are exposed through a proximal groin incision. This incision can be either longitudinal or oblique per surgeon preference. The femoral vessels are located in the femoral triangle bordered medially by the adductor longus muscle, laterally by the sartorius muscle, and superiorly by the inguinal ligament.
  - The above-knee popliteal artery is exposed through a medial above-knee incision. The sartorius muscle is reflected posteriorly and the popliteal space entered. The popliteal artery and vein are closely apposed and dissected free from each other.
  - The below-knee popliteal artery is exposed through a medial below-knee incision. The fascia is opened and the popliteal space entered. The gastrocnemius muscle is reflected posteriorly and the popliteal artery identified cephalad to the soleus muscle.
  - Division of the proximal soleus muscle allows dissection of the proximal anterior tibial artery, tibioperoneal trunk, and proximal posterior tibial and peroneal arteries.
  - The mid and distal anterior tibial artery is exposed through a lateral calf incision. The anterior compartment is entered and the tibialis anterior and extensor hallucis longus muscle are separated, with the artery found at the base of the compartment between these two muscles.

  - The mid and distal posterior tibial and peroneal arteries are exposed through a medial calf incision. The fascia is opened to enter the superficial posterior compartment. The soleus muscle is divided to enter the deep posterior compartment. Upon entering the deep posterior compartment, the first vessels encountered are the posterior tibial artery and veins. Tibial veins are often paired with branches over the artery. In the same plane, further lateral dissection is needed to expose the peroneal artery, which is adjacent to the fibula.
  - This distal peroneal artery can be exposed through a lateral calf incision with removal of the distal fibula. The common peroneal nerve should be protected. The lateral malleolus should be preserved to maintain joint stability. Muscle attachments to the fibula should be disconnected with a periosteal elevator or similar device and the fibular segment resected using a saw or bone cutters. Great care should be taken on the medial aspect of the fibula as the peroneal vessels lie immediately underneath.
  - Inframalleolar arteries can be exposed on the foot for pedal bypass. The dorsalis pedis artery is typically located between the first and second metatarsal. The distal posterior tibial and proximal medial and lateral plantar arteries are posterior to the medial malleolus and extend onto the plantar surface of the foot.
- Open vein harvest: GSV
  - A longitudinal incision is made directly over the marked vein. Either a single incision or multiple skip incisions can be used, with some evidence of fewer wound infections with the latter approach (**FIGURE 5**).
  - The necessary length of vein is unroofed. Using blunt and sharp dissection with Metzenbaum scissors, the vein is freed from surrounding structures. Side branches are ligated and divided with silk ligatures and hemoclips.
  - The GSV is divided proximally at the saphenofemoral junction (**FIGURE 6**), distally according to the length of vein needed, once both proximal and distal anastomosis sites have been dissected.
  - It is helpful distally to identify a branch point in the vein that can subsequently be used for the proximal anastomosis if the graft is placed in reversed configuration (**FIGURE 7A** and **B**).
- Open vein harvest: small saphenous vein
  - The same technique is used as for the GSV, except typically with the patient prone.
  - Proximally, the vein is typically divided at the saphenopopliteal junction. Some patients will have continuation of the small saphenous vein in the thigh (Giacomini vein), which allows harvesting additional length of vein in the thigh.
- Open vein harvest: arm vein
  - Both the cephalic and basilic veins can be harvested through longitudinal arm incisions. The same technique is used as for leg vein; however, care must be taken, as the arm veins tend to be more thin walled and fragile than leg vein.
  - The cephalic vein can frequently be harvested as a single conduit from the wrist to the deltopectoral groove (**FIGURE 8A-C**). A single segment is frequently adequate for a femoral-popliteal or femoral to proximal tibial bypass.
  - The basilic vein tends to be larger in diameter than the cephalic vein, although often, only a short segment in the upper arm is available. The basilic vein is well suited for use as an extension graft when revision of a previously placed bypass is necessary. When used as a new bypass, a composite graft composed of two or more vein segments is frequently necessary.
  - The basilic vein often has large branches that communicate medially with the brachial vein. These branches are often broad based and are better ligated with a running monofilament suture than simple ligation.
  - The median antebrachial cutaneous nerve frequently interdigitates with the basilic vein. With meticulous dissection, this nerve can be preserved (**FIGURE 9**).
  - The brachial vein is intimately associated with both the brachial artery and median nerve. This vein can also be

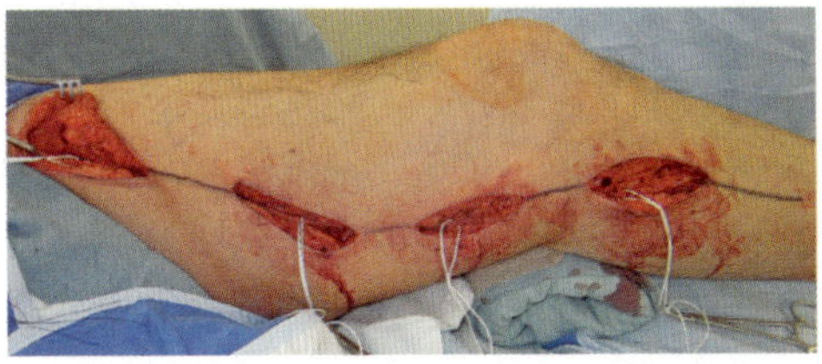

FIGURE 5 ● Open GSV harvest through skip incisions. The vein is encircled with silastic vessel loops.

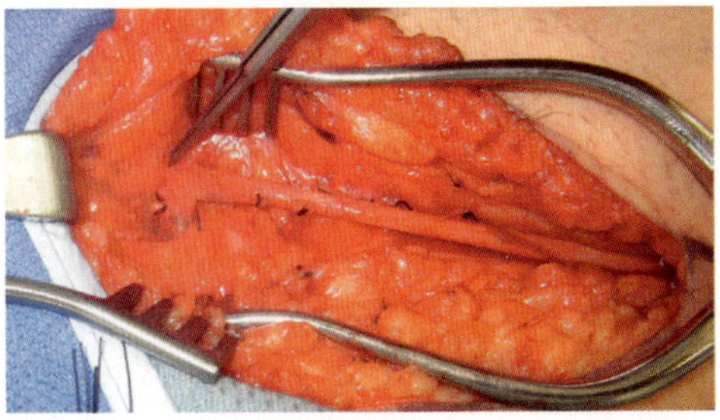

FIGURE 6 ● GSV mobilized proximally to saphenofemoral junction. Side branches ligated with silk ligatures.

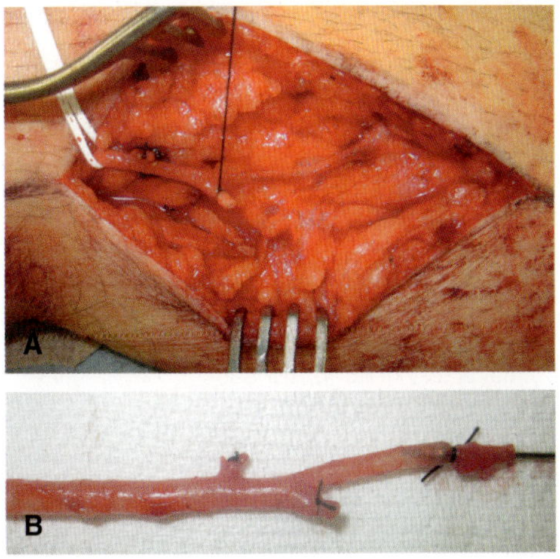

FIGURE 7 ● **A and B,** Distal GSV divided at branch point to provide starting spot for proximal anastomosis of reversed vein graft.

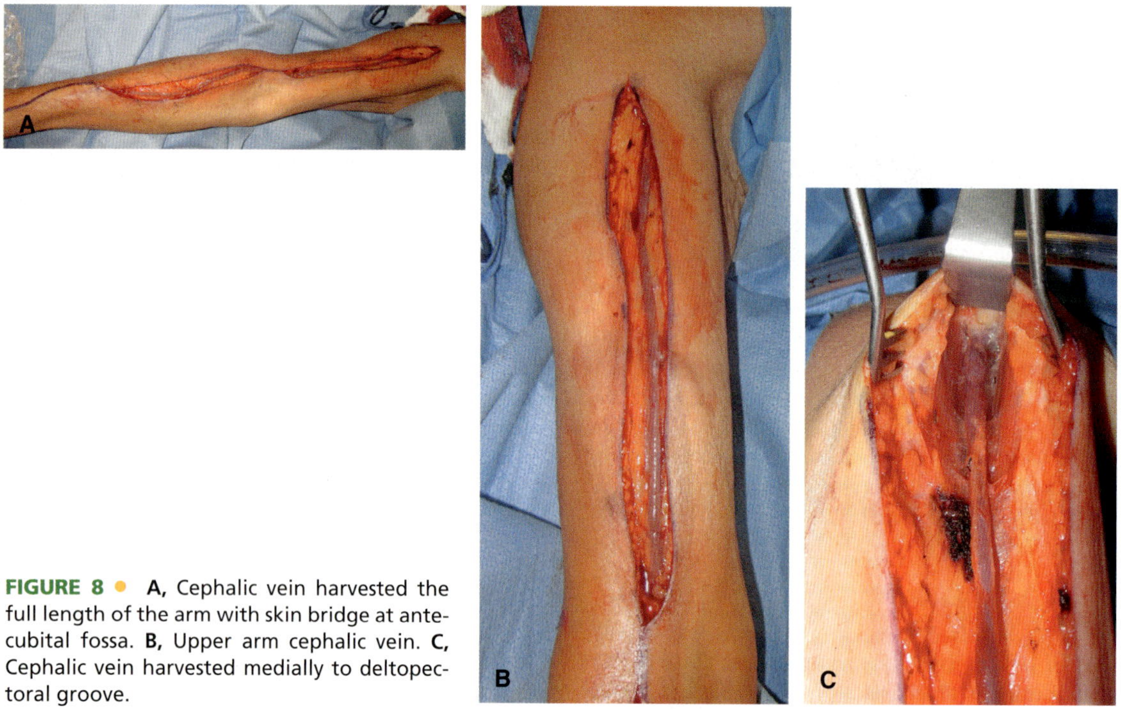

FIGURE 8 • **A,** Cephalic vein harvested the full length of the arm with skin bridge at antecubital fossa. **B,** Upper arm cephalic vein. **C,** Cephalic vein harvested medially to deltopectoral groove.

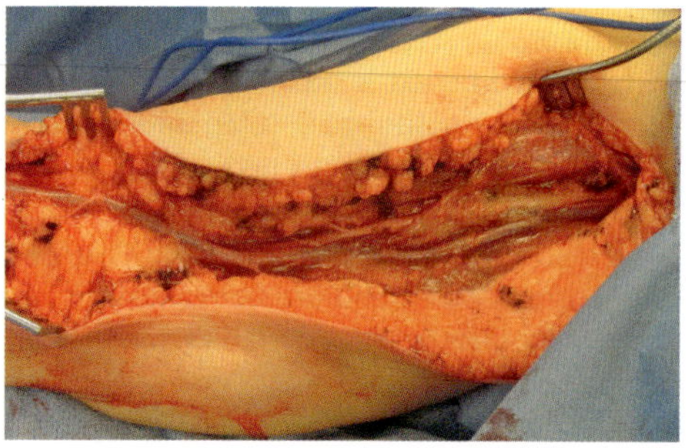

FIGURE 9 • Basilic vein harvested in upper arm. Median antebrachial cutaneous nerve adjacent to and interdigitating with vein.

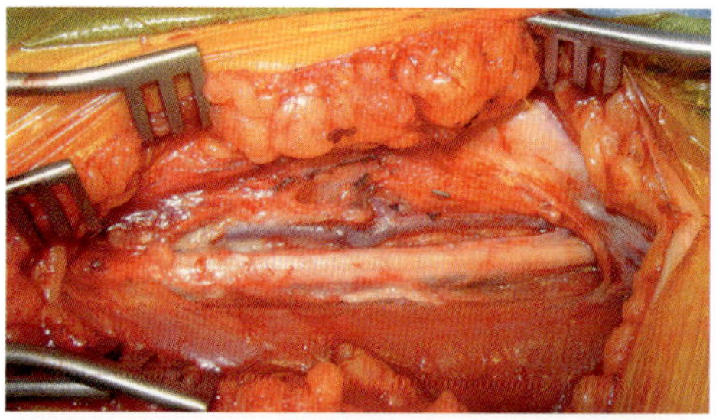

FIGURE 10 • Brachial vein harvest with vein adjacent to median nerve. Brachial artery deep to nerve.

  harvested as conduit, but great care needs to be taken to avoid injury to adjacent structures (**FIGURE 10**).
- Open harvest: femoral vein
  - Although typically used for larger vessel reconstruction, the femoral vein can be used for autogenous lower extremity bypass if necessary.
  - The proximal femoral vein is harvested medial to sartorius muscle. The vein is adjacent to the superficial femoral artery. The vein can be harvested proximally up to the profunda femoral vein.
  - Distally, the femoral vein is easier to harvest with the sartorius muscle reflected posteriorly. The vein can easily be harvested as far as the adductor canal.
  - If a longer segment is needed, the vein can be further harvested caudal to the adductor tendon into the popliteal fossa.
- Endoscopic harvest: GSV
  - Endoscopic harvest works best for veins within the saphenous fascial envelope (**FIGURE 11A**). It is technically more difficult in cases where the vein leaves this fascial envelope and is situated more superficially or in the subcutaneous fatty tissue (**FIGURE 11B**).
  - Available harvesting systems are described in **TABLE 1**.
  - A 2-cm incision is made at the level of the knee and the GSV dissected free at this site and encircled with a silastic vessel loop (**FIGURE 12**).
  - The vein is dissected from the knee to the saphenofemoral junction using a conical dissecting tip (**FIGURE 13**). CO_2 insufflation is performed through an inflatable trocar.
  - The vein is held in place with the C-ring or V-lock mechanism, and side branches are divided with bipolar electrocautery or harmonic scissors depending on the manufacturer (**FIGURE 14**).
  - Harvesting can also be performed in the calf; however, this is more technically challenging due to multiple geniculate venous branches, subcutaneous position of vein, and close approximation with saphenous nerve.
  - If an incision in the groin is going to be made for the proximal anastomosis of the graft, the incision can be

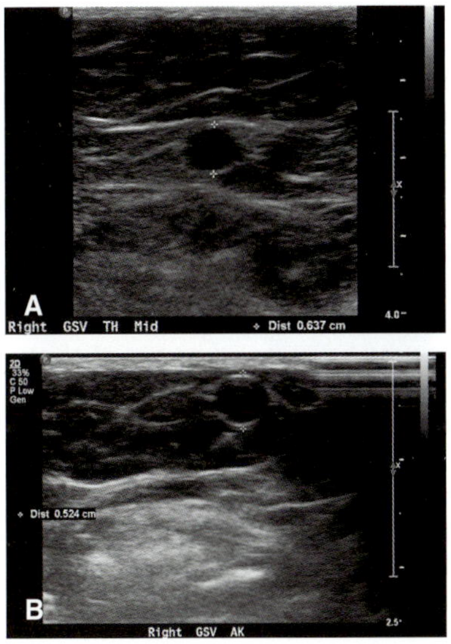

FIGURE 11 ● **A,** GSV (marked by *cursors*) within the saphenous fascial envelope suitable for endoscopic vein harvest. **B,** Subcutaneous GSV outside of saphenous fascial envelope, less suitable for endoscopic harvest.

Table 1: Endoscopic Vein Harvesting Systems

Manufacturer	Device	Dissecting tool	Vein securing	Side branch ligation
Maquet	Vasoview	Conical tip	C-ring	Bipolar ligating forceps
Maquet	Vasoview Hemopro	Conical tip	C-ring	Thermostatic cut and seal
Terumo	VirtuoSaph	Conical tip	V-lock	Bipolar cut and coagulation

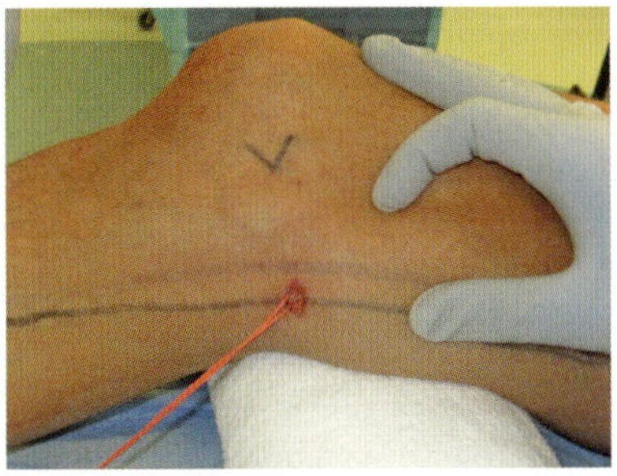

FIGURE 12 ● A 2-cm incision at the level of the knee through which GSV (encircled with silastic loop) dissected for endoscopic harvest.

made at this point to complete the proximal harvest. If an incision is not going to be made in the groin, a stab incision is made in the groin and the vein grasped under direct vision with a tonsil clamp. The vein is then pulled through the incision and ligated and divided with silk ligatures.

- After proximal division, the vein can be pulled out of the tunnel through the knee incision.

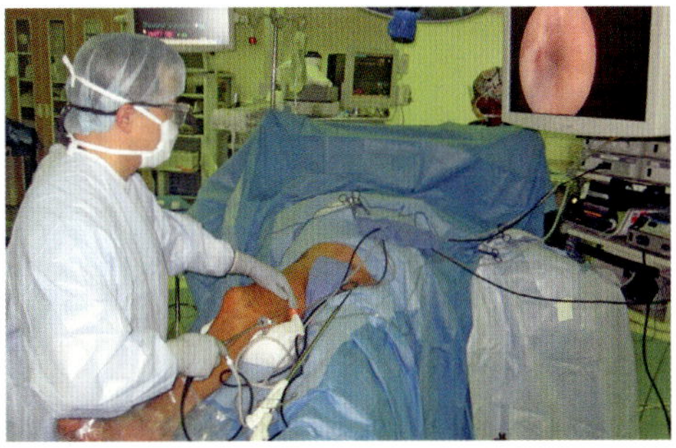

FIGURE 13 ● Conical dissecting tool mounted on camera used to isolate GSV. Operator standing opposite screen depicting endoscopic image.

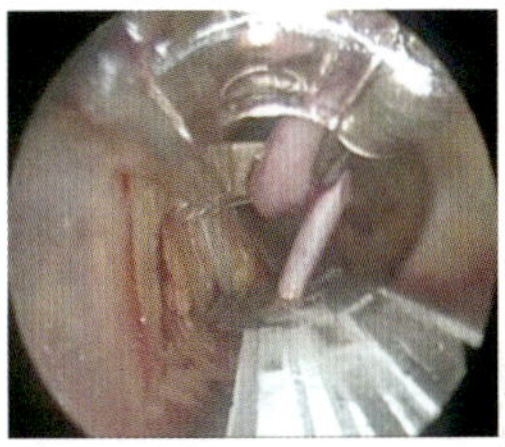

FIGURE 14 ● GSV held in plastic cradle while side branch ligated and divided with bipolar electrocautery.

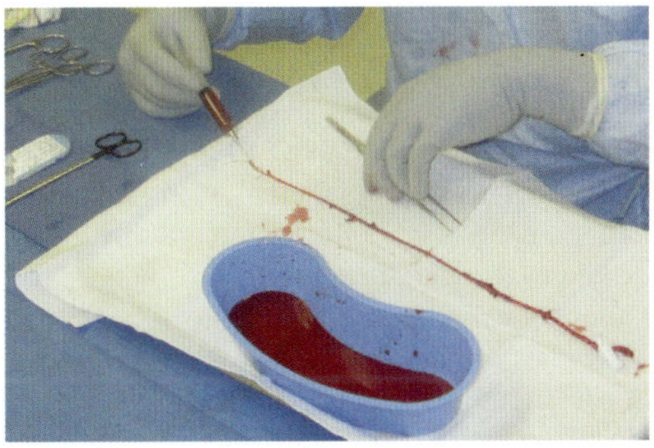

FIGURE 15 ● Back-table preparation of harvested vein.

  - A below-knee incision can be made to harvest the distal vein if this incision is already intended for the distal anastomotic site.
- Back-table vein preparation
  - Harvested veins are prepared on a back table (**FIGURE 15**). Veins are distended with the surgeon's solution of choice. The author prefers using chilled, heparinized autologous blood, although heparinized saline is also sufficient.
  - Any side branches not ligated during the initial harvest are ligated with silk ligatures or, if too small or short, with 7-0 polypropylene suture.
  - For endoscopically harvested veins, because the side branches are not ligated during the initial harvest, they are ligated at a back table with silk ligatures or 7-0 polypropylene suture after vein removal.
- Composite graft creation
  - A venovenostomy can be performed with two (or more) venous segments to create a single conduit of adequate length. The vein of larger diameter should be

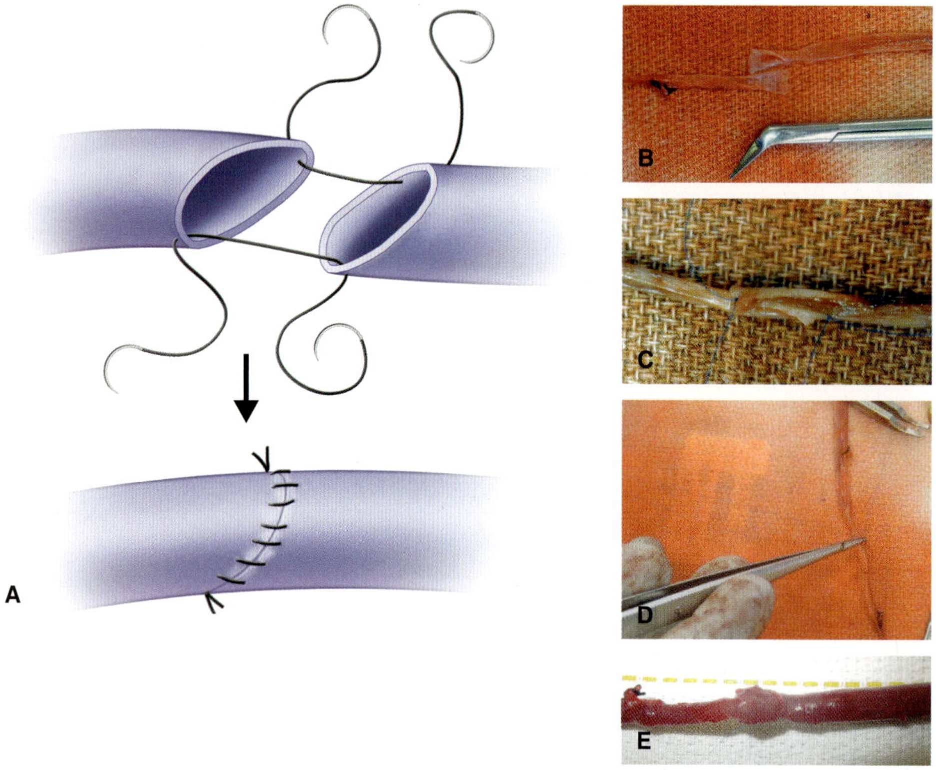

FIGURE 16 • **A,** Diagram depicting vein splicing. **B,** Splicing of arm veins to create single conduit. Veins spatulated with Potts scissors. **C,** A 7-0 polypropylene suture placed to approximate the heel and toe of the two veins. **D,** Venovenostomy performed with running suture. **E,** Final spatulated venovenostomy.

placed proximally. The veins are spatulated and sewn end to end with running 7-0 polypropylene suture (**FIGURE 16A-E**). Additional vein segments can be added as necessary with the same technique to create a conduit of adequate length.

- Nonautogenous conduit
  - The most commonly used prosthetic bypasses are externally supported polytetrafluoroethylene or polyester. Typical diameters are 6 or 8 mm depending on the size of the arteries. No special preparation for these grafts is required.
  - Cryopreserved greater saphenous vein is the most frequently used cryopreserved conduit. Cryopreserved femoral artery and vein can also be used. These conduits are frozen and must be thawed and prepared according to manufacturer specifications.
- Graft tunneling
  - Grafts are best tunneled using a hollow tube tunneler, such as a Scanlan tunneler, in order to avoid unnecessary tension on the vein as it is pulled through the subcutaneous tissue. This is particularly important in a composite graft where suture line disruption can potentially occur. The same tunnelers can be used for prosthetic conduits.
  - Tunneling performed after the proximal anastomosis allows the graft to be passed under pressure, which lessens the likelihood of twisting or kinking during tunneling.
  - In a first-time bypass, tunneling anatomically through the popliteal fossa for below-knee targets provides the most direct route to minimize vein length (**FIGURE 17**). In redo procedures in which previous grafts were tunneled through the popliteal fossa, a subcutaneously tunneled graft may be necessary.

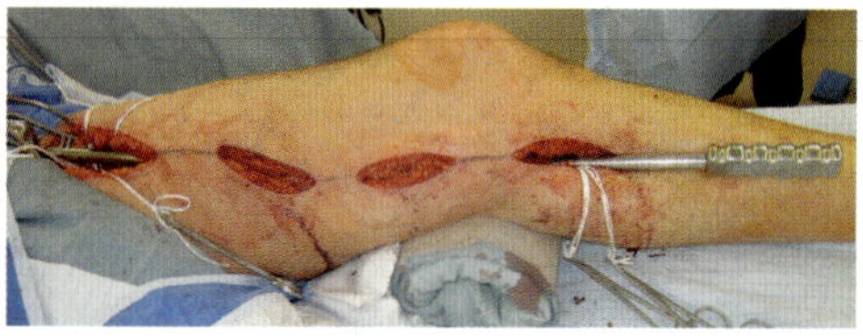

FIGURE 17 • Anatomic tunnel through popliteal fossa for femoral to below-knee popliteal artery bypass.

  - Two options exist for grafts tunneled to the anterior tibial artery. For grafts based on the common femoral artery, a lateral, subcutaneously tunneled graft is the most straightforward. For grafts based further distally on the superficial femoral or profunda femoral arteries, an anatomic tunnel through the popliteal fossa and interosseous membrane is more direct and minimizes vein length. The interosseous membrane should be directly visualized and a cruciate incision made to prevent graft stricture. Grafts to the posterior tibial or peroneal artery are tunneled either through the popliteal fossa or medially and subcutaneously (**FIGURE 18**).
  - Vein grafts can either be placed reversed or nonreversed depending on the size match at the proximal and distal anastomotic site. Reversed grafts require no further treatment. Nonreversed grafts require valve lysis with a valvulotome. This is best performed with the vein pressurized, so is typically performed after placement of the proximal anastomosis prior to tunneling so that lysis occurs under direct vision.

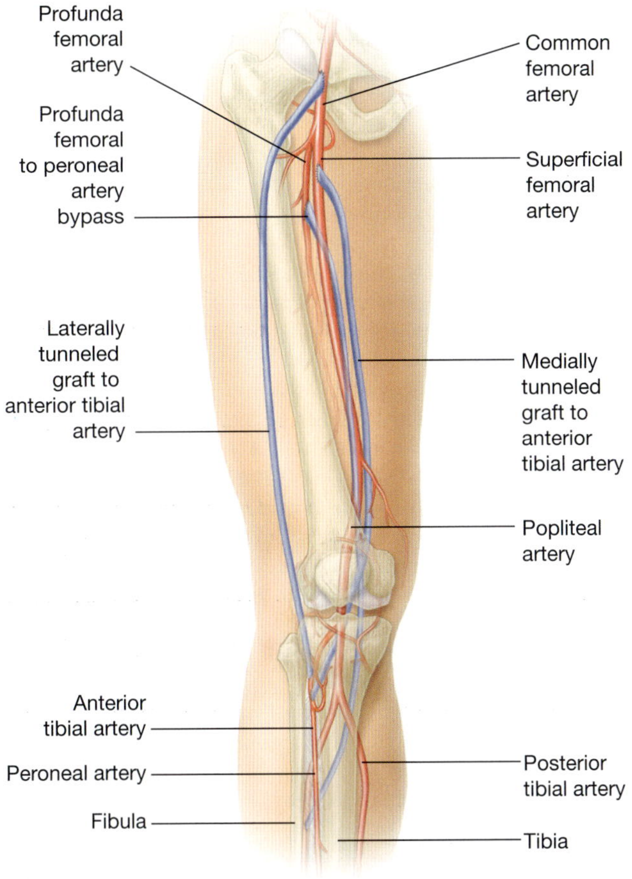

FIGURE 18 ● Diagram depicting tunneling options for tibial grafts.

- Choice of proximal anastomotic site
  - The choice of proximal anastomotic site depends on the anatomy, available vein length, and quality.
    - If adequate vein length is present, an anastomosis to the common femoral artery is generally preferred.
    - If vein length is insufficient, the graft can be based on either the superficial or the profunda femoral artery. For patients with atherosclerotic lower extremity arterial occlusive disease, the profunda femoral artery is more likely to be better preserved than the superficial femoral artery, which is more likely to be affected by atherosclerosis (**FIGURE 19A** and **B**).
    - In the presence of common femoral or proximal profunda femoral artery stenosis, a common and/or profunda femoral endarterectomy with placement of a vein or prosthetic patch (Linton patch) can provide adequate inflow for the graft, with the proximal anastomosis to the distal end of the patch (**FIGURE 20**).
    - In patients with patent superficial femoral arteries and more distal tibial artery disease, as is often seen in patients with diabetes, grafts may be based on either the above- or below-knee popliteal artery.
    - For patients requiring tibial or pedal bypasses with insufficient vein length, the superficial femoral

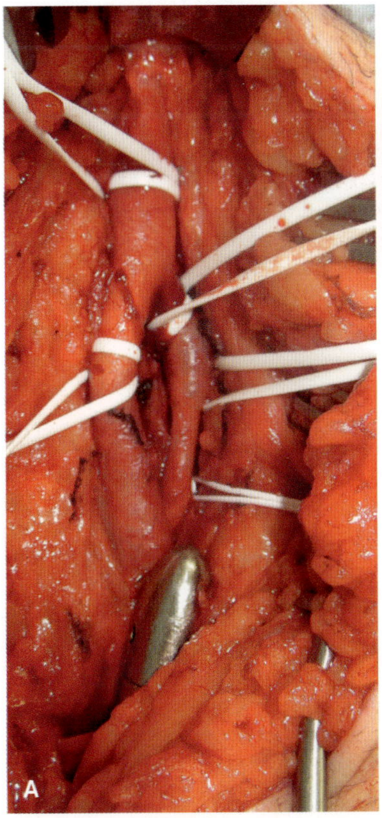

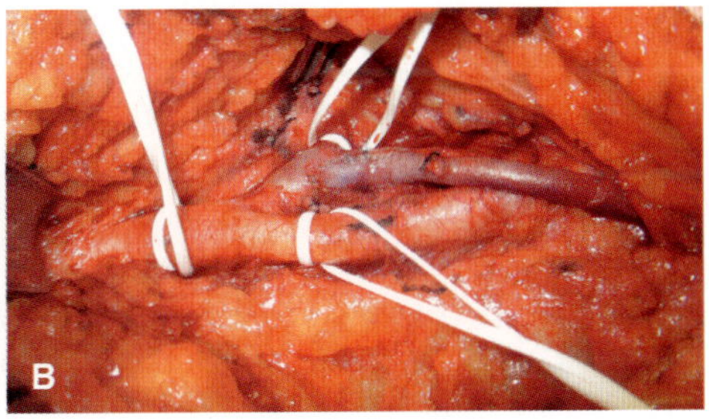

FIGURE 19 ● **A,** Common, superficial, and profunda femoral arteries dissected for proximal anastomosis. Vessels encircled with silastic loops. **B,** Proximal anastomosis to profunda femoral artery in patient with inadequate vein length to base graft on common femoral artery. Note tunneling device in subsartorial position.

artery can be treated with angioplasty with or without stenting to provide inflow for a graft based on the above- or below-knee popliteal artery. This is ideally performed either in a hybrid operating room (OR) suite or in a standard OR with C-arm fluoroscopy.

- Choice of distal anastomotic site
  - In general, the shortest bypass configuration that provides adequate distal flow is chosen.
    - If direct runoff to the foot can be achieved through a bypass to the popliteal artery, this is preferred.

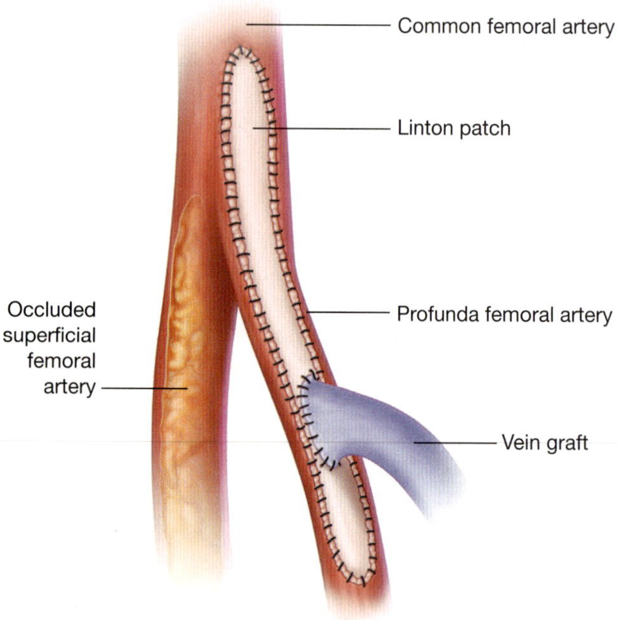

FIGURE 20 • Diagram of Linton patch on common and profunda femoral arteries from which proximal anastomosis of bypass is based.

    - If the popliteal artery is occluded and a tibial artery serves as the distal target, a direct angiosome revascularization should be chosen if possible in cases of foot ulcers or ischemia. For rest pain or claudication, the dominant tibial vessel should be chosen.
- Proximal anastomosis
  - Proximal and distal arterial control is obtained with atraumatic vascular clamps, silastic loops, or Fogarty catheters as needed and per surgeon's choice.
  - The anastomotic arteriotomy is made with a no. 11 scalpel and extended with Potts scissors. The arteriotomy length should be about 1.5 to 2 times the diameter of the vein.
  - The proximal anastomosis is ideally performed using a vein branch as the heel in order to avoid heel stricture (**FIGURE 21**). The vein is spatulated through the heel (**FIGURE 22A-C**).
  - The anastomosis is performed with running polypropylene rule. As a rule of thumb, suture diameter is 4-0 in the iliac artery, 5-0 femoral, 6-0 popliteal, and 7-0 tibial (**FIGURE 23**).
- Distal anastomosis
  - This is performed in similar fashion to the proximal anastomosis, although spatulation through a side branch is generally not possible and less necessary as for the proximal anastomosis, because the graft toe geometry is more important for patency than the heel geometry in the outflow (**FIGURE 24**).
  - Some surgeons prefer using a tourniquet inflated to 250 mm Hg for distal control below the knee. This requires less dissection than control with vascular clamps or silastic loops. In patients with extensive arterial calcification, however, tourniquet control may not be adequate.
  - When prosthetic grafts are used, especially if placed in an infrageniculate position, it is common to use a vein patch or cuff at the distal anastomosis. Since most stenoses occur at the distal outflow

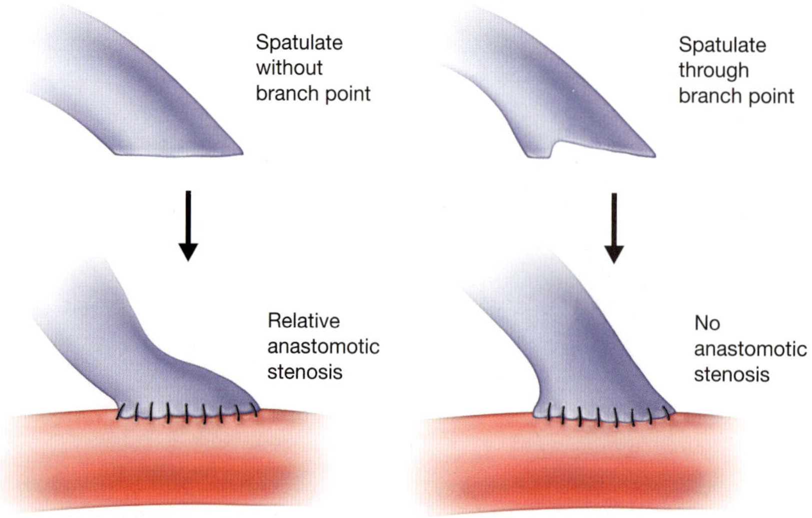

FIGURE 21 • The vein is spatulated through a branch point to avoid a stricture at the heel of the proximal anastomosis, which can occur if a side branch is not used.

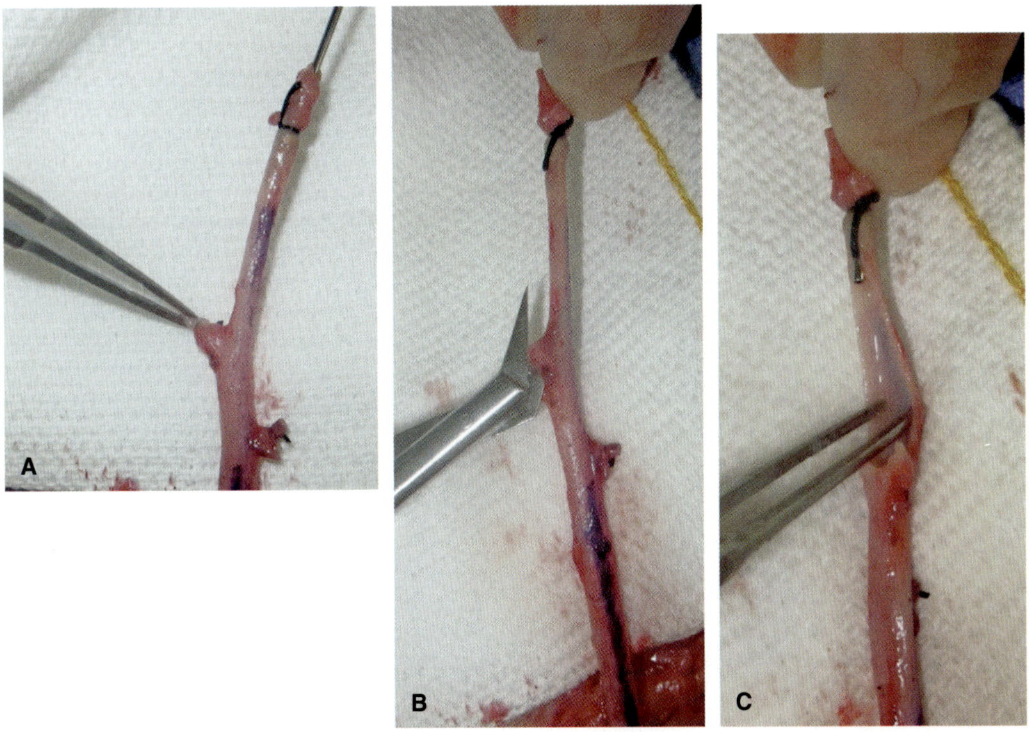

FIGURE 22 • **A,** Preparation of vein for proximal anastomosis. If possible, side branch is chosen for heel of proximal anastomosis to prevent anastomotic stricture. **B,** Vein spatulated with Potts scissors through branch point. **C,** Spatulated vein prepared for proximal anastomosis.

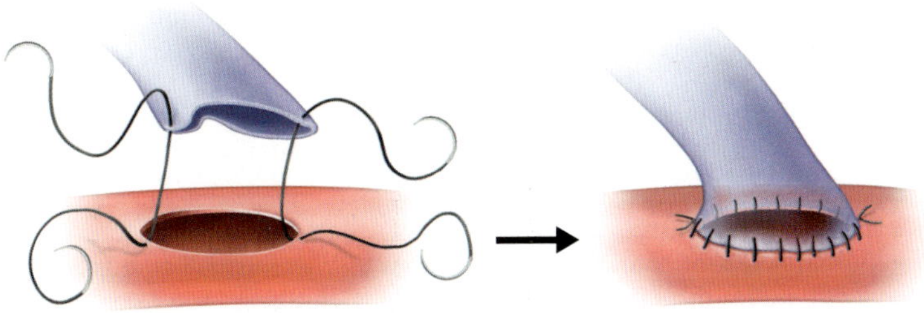

FIGURE 23 • Diagram demonstrating proximal graft anastomosis.

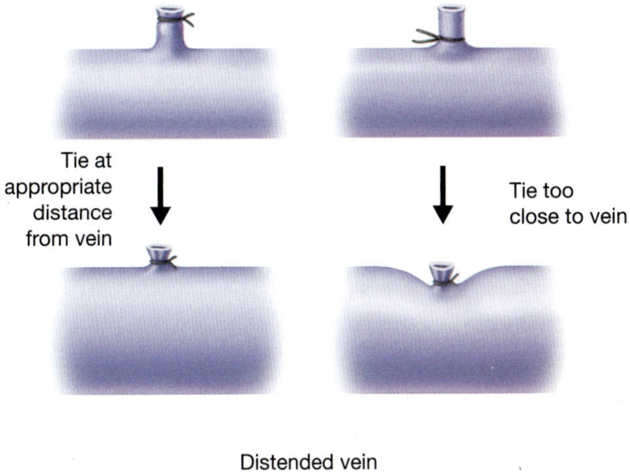

FIGURE 25 • "Dimpling" can occur with graft distention if side branch tie is too close to vein.

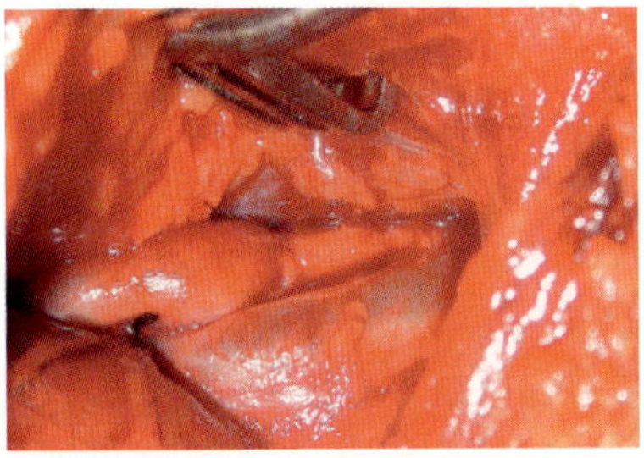

FIGURE 24 • Distal anastomosis to below-knee popliteal artery.

due to the formation of intimal hyperplasia, a vein patch or cuff can help to mitigate intimal hyperplasia formation. Commonly used techniques include the Taylor patch, Linton patch, or Miller cuff.

- In situ bypass:
  - An alternative bypass method utilizing the greater saphenous vein is an in situ bypass. In these bypasses the greater saphenous vein is not harvested, rather, it is left in place. The same graft configurations as a reversed or nonreversed saphenous vein graft can be performed, with the proximal greater saphenous vein and inflow artery exposed in the proximal incision and the distal greater saphenous vein and outflow artery exposed in the distal incision. The greater saphenous vein is ligated and divided at the saphenofemoral junction and the most cephalad vein valve manually lysed. The vein is then anastomosed to the inflow artery in standard fashion. The saphenous vein is then ligated and divided distally, and the valves are lysed with a valvulotome. This is best accomplished with the vein pressurized and can typically be achieved with one or two passages of the valvulotome. The distal anastomosis is then performed in standard fashion.
  - After completing the proximal and distal anastomosis, greater saphenous vein branches must be ligated. This can be done through a continuous or staggered incision. Branches can be identified with intraoperative duplex ultrasound or angiography.
- Adjunctive techniques:
  - In distal tibial or pedal bypasses, if the arterial outflow is deemed suboptimal, an adjunctive arteriovenous fistula can be created. An adjacent tibial or pedal vein is mobilized and the proximal end anastomosed to the bypass graft. This creates a low resistance outflow bed for the graft that may assist in maintaining graft patency in situations where the arterial outflow has high resistance.
- Intraoperative assessment:
  - Augmentation of Doppler signals at the ankle with the graft open compared with the graft occluded generally indicates graft patency with improved arterial perfusion. Intraoperative duplex or arteriography should also be considered to rule out technical problems with the graft.

PEARLS AND PITFALLS

Open vein harvest	■ Preoperative vein mapping is important to localize the site of the incision to avoid tissue flaps that can lead to poor wound healing. ■ Vein branches should not be ligated flush with the vein as "dimpling" can occur when the vein is distended. It is good to ligate the vein branch at least 1 mm away from the vein to allow proper vein expansion (**FIGURE 25**). ■ Arm veins tend to be more fragile than leg veins, requiring gentler handling during harvest.
Endoscopic vein harvest	■ Avoid harvesting veins that are subcutaneous or not enclosed within a fascial envelope as these are technically more difficult to harvest and therefore more prone to injury.
Vein preparation	■ Avoid overdistending the vein during preparation. A good technique is to inject a small amount of fluid into the vein and then manually distending the vein in segments rather than trying to inflate the vein with the syringe.
Graft tunneling	■ Passing the graft while distended reduces the risk of twisting or kinking. ■ Using a sterile marking pen, a line can be drawn on the anterior surface of the vein to help orient the graft distally and prevent twisting.
Anastomotic placement	■ Severely diseased vessels tend to delaminate when handled. Great care must be taken to include all layers in the anastomosis to prevent dissection. ■ In severely calcified vessels, vessel loops may not provide adequate control and vascular clamps may cause a crush injury. In these cases, Fogarty balloons may be needed for arterial control. A thigh tourniquet can also be used to facilitate arterial control.

POSTOPERATIVE CARE

- Patients should be monitored postoperatively in either an intensive care unit or a surgical ward. Hourly vascular checks should be performed with continuous wave Doppler.
- Early ambulation, generally on the first postoperative day, is encouraged, particularly in patients with claudication or rest pain. Patients with ulcers or gangrene may require a longer period of non–weight-bearing if lesions are on a weight-bearing surface.

OUTCOMES

- Anticipated 3-year primary patency rates for reversed saphenous vein grafts are 70% to 80% for femoral-popliteal and 60% to 75% for femoral-tibial. Comparable patency rates for arm vein bypasses are 60% to 70% and 50% to 60%, respectively, and for prosthetic grafts, 45% to 65% and 20% to 30%, respectively. Anticipated 5-year limb salvage in patients with critical limb ischemia is 80% to 90%, with 5-year survival in 40% to 70%.[1-5]

- Reversed and in situ vein grafts have been shown to have comparable patency rates in multiple studies.[6]
- Ambulatory function and independent living status is preserved in the majority of patients who undergo successful revascularization.
- Quality of life measures are improved in the majority of patients who undergo successful revascularization.[7]
- About 20% to 30% of patients will develop vein graft stenoses requiring either open or endovascular revision during follow-up.[8,9]
- Data on patency rates of open vs endoscopically harvested vein grafts are mixed, making definitive recommendations on the preferred approach difficult.[10,11]

COMPLICATIONS

- Wound infection
- Seroma
- Hematoma
- Graft occlusion
- Myocardial infarction

REFERENCES

1. Chew DK, Owens CD, Belkin M, et al. Bypass in the absence of ipsilateral greater saphenous vein: safety and superiority of the contralateral greater saphenous vein. *J Vasc Surg*. 2002;35(6):1085-1092.
2. Curi MA, Skelly CL, Woo DH, et al. Long-term results of infrageniculate bypass grafting using all-autogenous composite vein. *Ann Vasc Surg*. 2002;16(5):618-623.
3. Faries PL, Arora S, Pomposelli FB, et al. The use of arm vein in lower-extremity revascularization: results of 520 procedures performed in eight years. *J Vasc Surg*. 2000;31(1):50-59.
4. Gentile AT, Lee RW, Moneta GL, et al. Results of bypass to the popliteal and tibial arteries with alternative sources of autogenous vein. *J Vasc Surg*. 1996;23(2):272-279.
5. Taylor LM Jr, Edwards JM, Porter JM. Present status of reversed vein bypass: five-year results of a modern series. *J Vasc Surg*. 1990;11(2):193-206.
6. Harris PL, Veith FJ, Shanik GD, et al. Prospective randomized comparison of in situ and reversed infrapopliteal vein grafts. *Br J Surg*. 1993;80(2):173-176.
7. Nguyen LL, Moneta GL, Conte MS, et al. Prospective multicenter study of quality of life before and after lower extremity vein bypass in 1404 patients with critical limb ischemia. *J Vasc Surg*. 2006;44(5):977-983.
8. Idu MM, Buth J, Hop WCJ, et al. Factors influencing the development of vein-graft stenosis and their significance for clinical management. *Eur J Vasc Endovasc Surg*. 1999;17:15-21.
9. Conte MS, Bandyk DF, Clowes AW, et al. Results of PREVENT III: a multicenter randomized trial of edifoligide for the prevention of vein graft failure in lower extremity bypass surgery. *J Vasc Surg*. 2006;43(4):742-751.
10. Kronick M, Liem TK, Jung E, et al. Experienced operators achieve superior patency and wound complication rates with endoscopic great saphenous vein bypass compared with open harvest in lower extremity bypass. *J Vasc Surg*. 2019;70:1534-1542.
11. Guo Q, Huang B, Zhao J. Systematic review and meta-analysis of saphenous vein harvesting and grafting for lower extremity arterial bypass. *J Vasc Surg*. 2021;73(3):1075-1086.

Chapter 34

Perimalleolar Bypass and Hybrid Techniques

Robin B. Osofsky and Erika R. Ketteler

DEFINITION

- Perimalleolar bypasses are defined by the anatomic location of the distal target outflow vessel and refer to any revascularization in which the distal target vessel is the posterior tibialis, anterior tibialis, or peroneal arteries in the distal lower leg and usually referring to the level just above the ankle malleoli. The pedal vessels (dorsalis pedis, posterior tibialis, and lateral or medial plantar artery) can also be target vessels, but by definition these bypasses should be identified as pedal as there are different patency expectations as compared with perimalleolar targets.
- Infrapopliteal (perimalleolar and pedal) bypasses are generally performed in patients with advanced critical limb threatening ischemia (CLTI), which includes tissue loss and/or ischemic rest pain. Surgical management of distal tibial disease can be performed with open surgical bypass, endovascular therapy (EVT), or a hybrid approach. To the date of this chapter publication, no randomized control trials exist that clarify whether EVT or surgical bypass is better in patients with distal tibial disease. Regardless of technique, the specific therapy is tailored to an individual's clinical picture, functional status, and correlating anatomic limitations.

DIFFERENTIAL DIAGNOSIS

- The three major etiologies of lower extremity ulceration include ischemic, neuropathic, and venous stasis disease. Although all of these can have poor perfusion as a primary contributing factor, the diagnostic workup and management is different. Arterial ulcerations typically have a punched-out dry appearance and occur on the distal forefoot and toes, whereas neuropathic ulcerations often occur due to pressure at callus points. Venous stasis ulcerations are typically located on the medial malleolus ("gaiter") location and have associated edema, skin changes, and brawny induration and possible serous drainage.

PATIENT HISTORY AND PHYSICAL FINDINGS

- Peripheral arterial occlusive disease (PAOD) is the chronic atherosclerotic disease of the lower extremities. It is a spectrum of disease that ranges from asymptomatic to intermittent claudication (IC) and finally critical limb threatening ischemia (CLTI). Patients with CLTI will present with one or both of the following factors: rest pain or tissue necrosis (gangrene or nonhealing ulceration). Ischemic rest pain is characterized specifically by burning pain localized primarily to the distal forefoot and is associated with dependent rubor and elevation pallor.
- It should be noted that the natural history of PAOD and IC differ drastically from that of patients with CLTI. Rates of limb loss for patients with IC is <1% per year of life, whereas patients with CLTI have rates of 22% (2%-42%) at 1 year.[1]
- In general, the demographics for patients with PAOD, IC, and CLTI are similar and can differentiate into modifiable and nonmodifiable risk factors. Modifiable risks factors include smoking, hypertension, hyperlipemia, and diabetes, with smoking being the risk offering most opportunities for physician input. Nonmodifiable risk factors include age, gender, African American ethnicity, and family history of atherosclerosis. Of note, patients with CLTI have a higher prevalence of renal disease and diabetes. In addition, many of such patients do have the classic history of IC but rather present initially with tissue loss (embolic or caused by minor trauma). This fact is especially pertinent in diabetic patients who may not have any pain as a symptom of the critical limb ischemia.
- Due to significant comorbid conditions, it is critical to perform risk stratification when deciding between different revascularization modalities. In addition, managing and optimizing risk factors are keys to a successful outcome following lower extremity revascularization, regardless of the technique used. As such, optimizing lipid profile, glycemic control, smoking cessation, minimizing renal dysfunction, and managing hypercoagulable states are all essential components to the perioperative medical management, in addition to managing any concomitant coronary disease. Many patients may already be followed by a team of physicians for their co-morbidities and it is imperative that consultants remain actively involved in the perioperative period to optimize both the short-term quality of life and long-term limb salvage and overall survival.
- Included in surgical decision making is understanding that, although operative procedures may be technically and anatomically feasible, palliative expectant wound care may be more appropriate. This is important especially if the patient has small, limited wounds without pain or infection in a high-risk surgical patient who may be nonambulatory.
- Primary amputation may sometimes best meet patient expectations and goals of care rather than revascularization, especially if there is limited life-expectancy, nonambulatory status, or an imminent dying trajectory.
- Physical examination should include a thorough peripheral vascular examination, including assessment of the potential presence of a palpable aortic aneurysm on abdominal examination as a source of emboli causing the limb ischemic changes. The quality and symmetry of pulses and/or handheld Doppler signals at the femoral, popliteal, and pedal levels will assist in determining the anatomic level of disease. Wound documentation, when present, should note location, depth, presence of infection, bone exposure, and extent of soft tissue defects. Neuropathic deformities of the foot should also be taken into careful consideration for offloading purposes. If there is gross purulence or systemic signs of infection, a debridement of the affected area is usually required prior to revascularization for sepsis control.

- Classically, scoring systems for CLTI such as the Fontaine and Rutherford systems have been utilized to determine the likelihood of amputation and need for revascularization. However, in the past decade, such systems have been replaced with the Society for Vascular Surgery Lower Extremity Threatened Limb Classification System. The system stratifies limb risk by three factors: Wound, Ischemia, and foot Infection (WIfI) score. This system is similar to the "TMN" score for malignancy and grades each of the three main criteria on a four-point severity scale (0,1,2,3), which altogether yield a total of 64 distinct combinations. These 64 combinations are then assigned to one of four stages of clinical severity that are expected to correlate with amputation risk at 1 year. Clinical stage 1 is "very low risk" with 1 year rate of major amputations 0.75%, whereas stage 5 corresponds to an unsalvageable limb (**FIGURE 1**).[2]

IMAGING AND DIAGNOSTIC STUDIES

- The initial diagnostic workup of patients with ischemic ulcerations, rest pain, or significant claudication involves noninvasive vascular testing. This involves calculation of ankle-brachial indices (ABIs) and pulsed volume recordings in addition to duplex imaging of the extremity. An ABI of less than 0.4 is typically seen in patients with CLTI (**FIGURE 2**). Toe pressures of less than 40 mm Hg suggest inadequate microvascular perfusion for wound healing even with normal macrovascular arterial perfusion (eg, palpable dorsalis pedis [DP] and posterior tibial [PT] pulses). In cases of severely calcified vessels, it is important to obtain associated pulsed volume recordings or segmental waveforms along with toe pressures because ABIs can be falsely elevated due to vessel incompressibility generating an ABI >1.4. Transcutaneous oxygen tension ($TcPO_2$) measurement can also be used to determine the severity of ischemia and probability of wound healing (**FIGURE 3**).
- Computed tomography arteriography (CTA) is the preferred imaging modality for aortoiliac and femoropopliteal disease. However, CTA is limited in assessment of the tibial vessels often due to calcification or concomitant proximal stenosis, which ultimately limits distal contrast opacification. Magnetic resonance angiography has some use in CLTI but in general infrapopliteal disease tends to be overestimated by this modality and the injection of heavy metal gadolinium is not without concern for patients with concomitant renal insufficiency. Thus, digital subtraction angiography (DSA) remains the gold standard for diagnosis of infrapopliteal disease especially as the treatment of arterial stenoses/occlusions could occur in the same setting in an endovascular approach. Prior to obtaining either CTA or DSA, the surgeon must consider to optimize renal function to decrease the risk for contrast-induced nephropathy.

TREATMENT STRATEGY

- The goal of therapy in patients with CLTI should be to relieve pain, heal wounds, preserve functional status, and avoid major amputation. Pulsatile flow at the level of the tissue loss is the general goal; however, sometimes a pulse is not achievable and global improvement of perfusion to the

Assessment of the risk of amputation: the WIfI classification (for further details see Mills et al[317])

Component	Score	Description		
W (Wound)	0	No ulcer (Ischaemic rest pain)		
	1	Small, shallow ulcer on distal leg or foot without gangrene		
	2	Deeper ulcer with exposed bone, joint or tendon ± gangrenous changes limited to toes		
	3	Extensive deep ulcer, full thickness heel ulcer ± calcaneal involvement ± extensive gangrene		
I (Ischaemia)		ABI	Ankle pressure (mmHg)	Toe pressure or $TcPO_2$
	0	≥0.80	> 100	≥60
	1	0.60–0.79	70–100	40–59
	2	0.40–0.59	50–70	30–39
	3	<0.40	<50	<30
fI (foot Infection)	0	No symptoms/signs of infection		
	1	Local infection involving only skin and subcutaneous tissue		
	2	Local infection involving deeper than skin/subcutaneous tissue		
	3	Systemic inflammatory response syndrome		

Example: A 65-year-old male diabetic patient with gangrene of the big toe and a <2 cm rim of cellulitis at the base of the toe, without any clinical/biological sign of general infection/inflammation, whose toe pressure is at 30 mmHg would be classified as Wound 2, Ischaemia 2, foot infection 1 (WIfI 2-2-1). The clinical stage would be 4 (high risk of amputation). The benefit of revascularization (if feasible) is high, also depending on infection control.

ABI = ankle-brachial index, $TcPO_2$ = transcutaneous oxygen pressure.

FIGURE 1 • Society for Vascular Surgery Lower Extremity Threatened Limb Classification. (System: Risk stratification based on Wound, Ischemia, and foot Infection [WifI].) (Reprinted from Mills JL, Conte MS, Armstrong DG, et al. The Society for Vascular Surgery Lower Extremity Threatened Limb Classification System: risk stratification based on wound, ischemia, and foot infection (WIfI). *J Vasc Surg*. 2014;59(1):220-234.e1-2. Copyright © 2014 The Authors. With permission.)

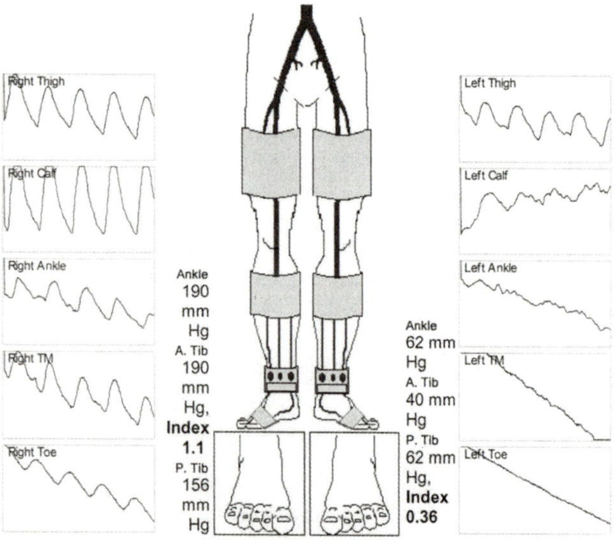

FIGURE 2 • Severely reduced ABI and flattened distal pulsed volume recordings.

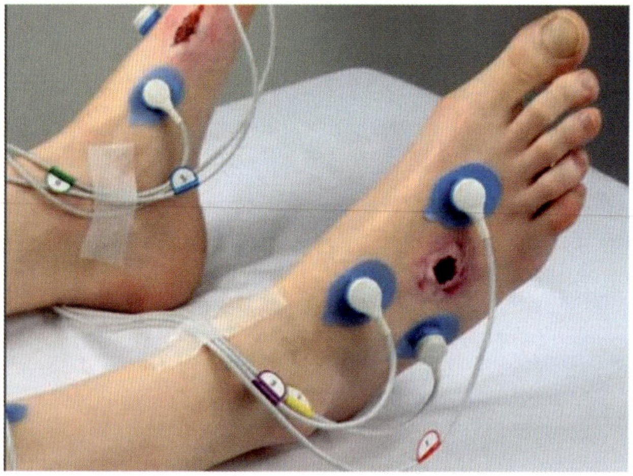

FIGURE 3 • Transcutaneous oxygen tension ($TcPO_2$).

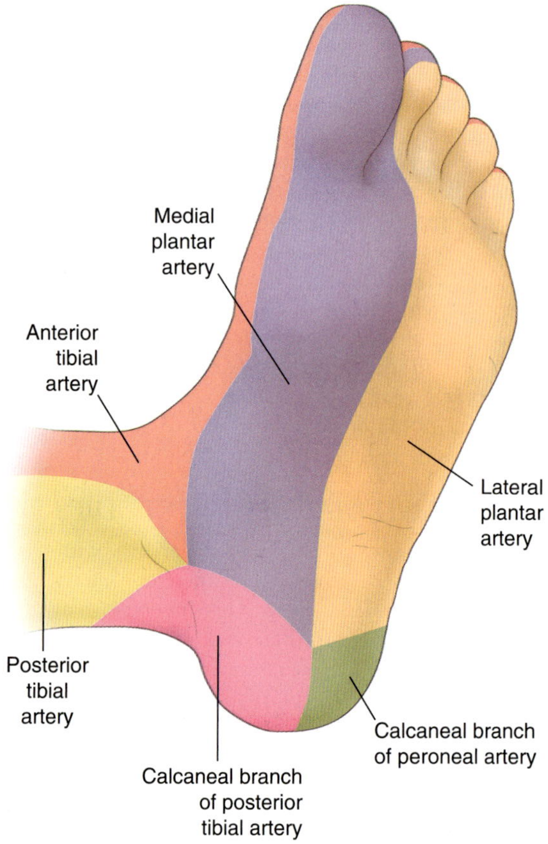

FIGURE 4 • Angiosome concept.

ischemic area is the objective. Historically, angiosome revascularization (**FIGURE 4**) was implemented to guide the choice of distal anastomosis, based on the feeding vessel for the vascular territory of interest.[3] Attempts at distal revascularization should only proceed when adequate arterial inflow is present. Hence, proximal revascularization of the aorta and iliac and femoral arteries may need to be performed prior to or concomitantly with perimalleolar revascularization.

- Treatment strategy regarding choice of EVT vs open surgical bypass remains complex. The Trans-Atlantic Inter-Society Consensus (TASC) classification system does assist in such decision-making. In 2007, the TASC II classifications were published, which classified disease pattern involvement from types A through D for both aortoiliac and femoropopliteal segments. The group advocated for endovascular treatment for TASC type A and open surgical treatment for TASC type D. For TASC type B and C lesions, the authors stated there was insufficient evidence for recommending one modality over another (**FIGURE 5**). As mentioned in the introduction, there are no trials that ideally compare tibial EVT to surgical bypass and at the time of this publication, the ongoing BEST CLI and BASIL2 trials remain open to try to answer such questions.
- The decision to proceed with open perimalleolar bypass is made in the context of the patient's overall clinical functional status, cardiopulmonary and renal comorbidities, presence of autogenous saphenous vein conduit, and options for endovascular revascularization. Preoperative autogenous conduit assessment is best performed by detailed duplex imaging along the length of the vein. Preference is always given to a single segment of the great saphenous vein (GSV) from the ipsilateral leg that is at least 2.5 to 3 mm in diameter, compressible, and free of thrombus throughout. Assessment of the contralateral GSV is useful in cases that ipsilateral vein is found to be of poor quality during operative exploration. Small saphenous vein or arm vein is rarely used, but both are options realizing that the quality and frequency of valves is less ideal for long conduits. Combining multiple segments of veins may be necessary for adequate length with each anastomosis being a future site of stenosis impacting long-term patency. Composite bypass with vein and prosthetic, or full prosthetic bypass, is least ideal due to patency and infection risks but may be necessary if autogenous vein is not available. Composite bypasses do have limited long-term patency but may be appropriate if patency is only needed for wound healing and/or pain control in unique patient scenarios.
- Inflow artery selection for perimalleolar bypass is usually based on the length of available conduit and extent of proximal disease. The common, superficial, or deep femoral arteries or the popliteal artery may all serve as suitable inflow. Pulse by examination of such vessels is usually adequate

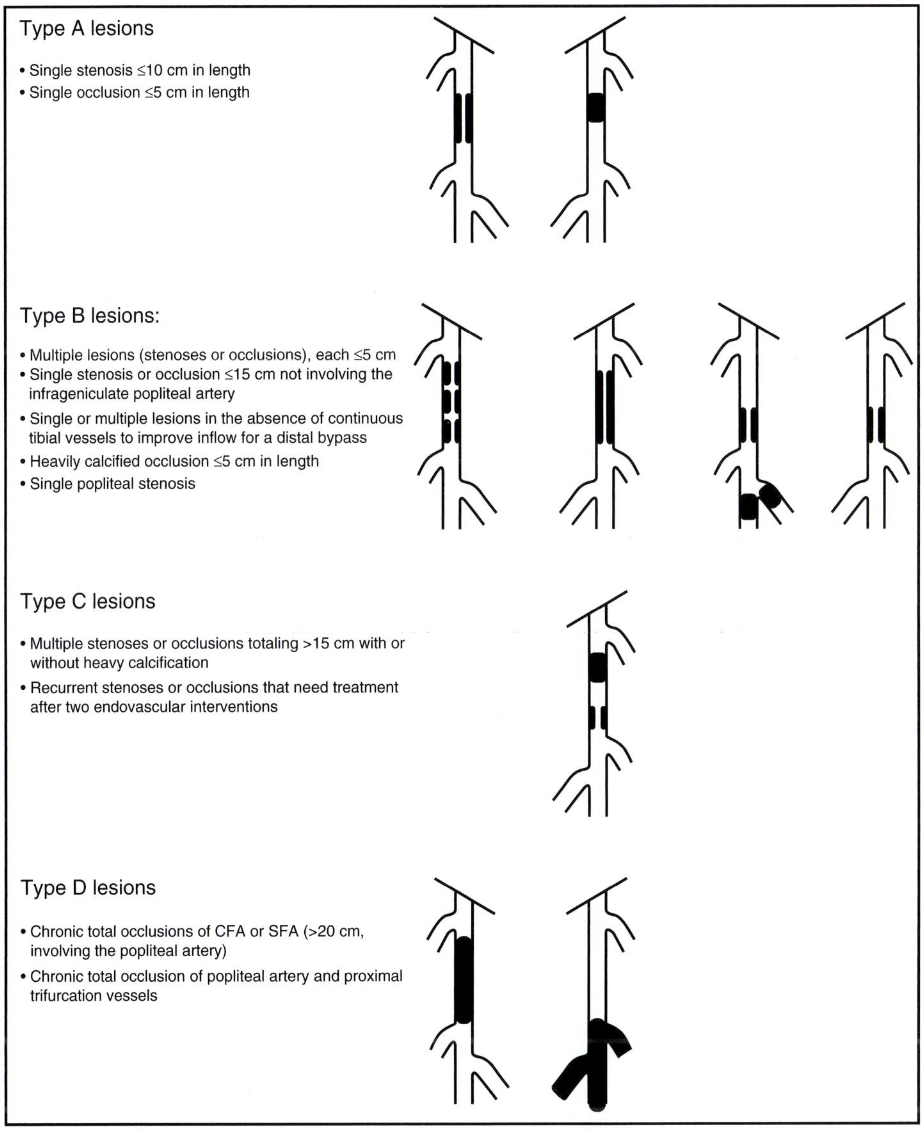
Type A lesions
• Single stenosis ≤10 cm in length
• Single occlusion ≤5 cm in length
Type B lesions:
• Multiple lesions (stenoses or occlusions), each ≤5 cm
• Single stenosis or occlusion ≤15 cm not involving the infrageniculate popliteal artery
• Single or multiple lesions in the absence of continuous tibial vessels to improve inflow for a distal bypass
• Heavily calcified occlusion ≤5 cm in length
• Single popliteal stenosis
Type C lesions
• Multiple stenoses or occlusions totaling >15 cm with or without heavy calcification
• Recurrent stenoses or occlusions that need treatment after two endovascular interventions
Type D lesions
• Chronic total occlusions of CFA or SFA (>20 cm, involving the popliteal artery)
• Chronic total occlusion of popliteal artery and proximal trifurcation vessels

FIGURE 5 • Trans-Atlantic Inter-Society Consensus (TASC) classification for femoropopliteal disease. (Reprinted from Kukkonen T, Korhonen M, Halmesmäki K, Lehti L, Tiitola M, Aho P, Lepäntalo M, Venermo M. Poor inter-observer agreement on the TASC II classification of femoropopliteal lesions. *Eur J Vasc Endovasc Surg*. 2010;39(2):220-224. Copyright © 2010 European Society for Vascular Surgery. With permission.)

but can be supplemented by duplex imaging or even with diagnostic angiography. The need for concomitant endarterectomy should also be evaluated at this time and may be needed to ensure inflow is adequate to service the revascularization method by vein, prosthetic, or endovascular recanalization.

SURGICAL MANAGEMENT

Preoperative Planning

- The type of anesthesia is determined by the type of cardiopulmonary comorbidities and the anatomic level of arterial occlusive disease. Preoperative consultation with anesthesiology and cardiology can be utilized in the CLTI patient population to gauge the appropriate amount of surgical risk vs a nonoperative approach. Generally, limb threat with tissue loss does not require preoperative cardiac testing as time to allow cardiac revascularization is not appropriate. Cardiac disease optimization with medical management should be continued or initiated with antiplatelet, anti-inflammatory statin therapy and blood pressure and diabetic control to assist in prevention of perioperative complications. General anesthesia, peripheral nerve block, and spinal anesthesia are all potential options for bypass procedures. Intraoperative fluid administration should be used judiciously, and preoperative preparation should include blood type determination and crossmatching as necessary. Therapeutic anticoagulation may be held prior to the revascularization procedure, but most patients remain on antiplatelet agents without cessation.

Positioning

- Any lower extremity bypass might require intraoperative angiography and, as such, procedures should be performed on a fluoroscopy-appropriate table. The patient is positioned supine, with the leg slightly abducted and externally rotated to provide optimal exposure of the ipsilateral GSV harvest site. It is our practice to localize the GSV by ultrasound to assist in incision planning and try to access the conduit vein in discontinuous incisions to provide for better healing with less disruption of the lymphatics to avoid excessive edema. Intraoperative vein mapping also helps determine whether the contralateral leg should also be prepped as an alternative site for vein harvesting.

- Other items that should be available in the room include a sterile pneumatic tourniquet and a surgical bump constructed of towels to allow elevation of the knee for best anatomic exposure and dissection. A sterile on-table tourniquet can be useful to avoid clamp injury to target distal artery. Open forefoot wounds should be excluded from the operative field with adhesive drapes prior to limb preparation.

TECHNIQUES

OPEN BYPASS

Perimalleolar Bypass to the Distal Posterior Tibialis Artery

First Step: Exposure of the Posterior Tibialis Artery at the Ankle

- The distal incision is marked by palpating posterior to the medial malleolus, taking care to avoid injury to adjacent GSV (**FIGURE 6**). Dissection is carried sharply through skin and subcutaneous tissues and through the flexor retinaculum. The tendons of the flexor digitorum longus muscle and flexor hallucis longus pass anteriorly and posteriorly, respectively, to the neurovascular bundle at this level. Careful attention to finding perforating collaterals can guide the dissection to the main artery of interest especially as a pulse is generally not present to assist. The paired tibial veins are often seen first as overlying the artery. The tibial nerve travels posterior to the artery and may not be seen clearly during this exposure. The tibial artery does not need to be dissected circumferentially if a pneumatic tourniquet is deployed for proximal control. For plantar bypass/exposure of the medial and lateral plantar arteries, the same incision can be carried further distally onto the medial aspect of the foot. Avoidance of circumferential occlusion of the target artery is recommended, and often only single vessel loop retraction can occlude any arterial flow to allow visualization for anastomosis creation.

Second Step: Exposure of the Inflow Artery

- Concurrent dissection of the arterial inflow can be performed with a second surgical team if available while the tibial target is being exposed to assist in limiting operative time in high-risk patients with CLTI. If the common femoral artery is chosen, then a longitudinal vertical incision just below the inguinal ligament will allow for simultaneous exposure of both the femoral bifurcation and the saphenofemoral confluence for dissection of the GSV. If femoral bifurcation disease is not suspected by prior imaging, then a transverse groin incision localized over the femoral artery erring medially toward the GSV is also a useful exposure as it is more anatomic with less tension to provide for decreased risks of wound separation and lymph leak (**FIGURE 7**). If the deep femoral artery is to be used as inflow, then division of the lateral femoral circumflex vein may be helpful in controlling the first-order branches past the origin. If the deep femoral origin is more posterior, the muscle bellies of the adductor longus and vastus medialis can be divided to limit the angle from which the graft originates from the arterial anastomosis. Another approach to the deep femoral artery for inflow is a lateral sartorius approach (**FIGURE 8**).
- If the below-knee popliteal artery is to be used as the inflow, which might be the case in diabetic patients with severe tibial disease not amenable to endovascular revascularization, this exposure is best obtained through a medial calf incision 1 cm posterior to the tibia (**FIGURE 9**). Utilizing the surgical bump under the distal thigh to allow the calf muscles to be tension-free, the infrageniculate popliteal artery is found by dividing the skin and avoiding the GSV. The crural fascia is incised again 1 cm posterior to the tibia with the incision extended to the border of the semitendinosus tendon to allow retraction of the gastrocnemius muscle (and sometimes also the deeper soleus muscle) posterior to enter the

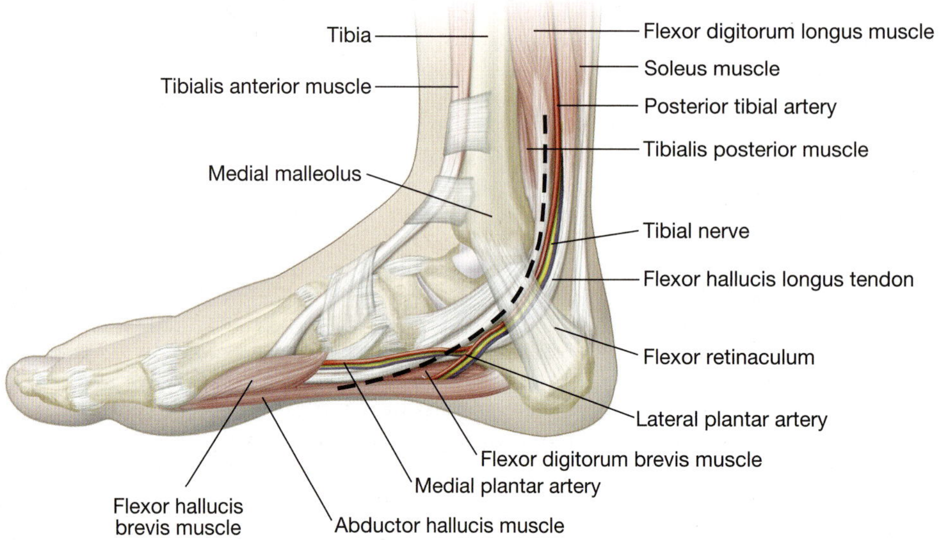

FIGURE 6 • Incision for exposure of the posterior tibialis artery at the medial malleolus.

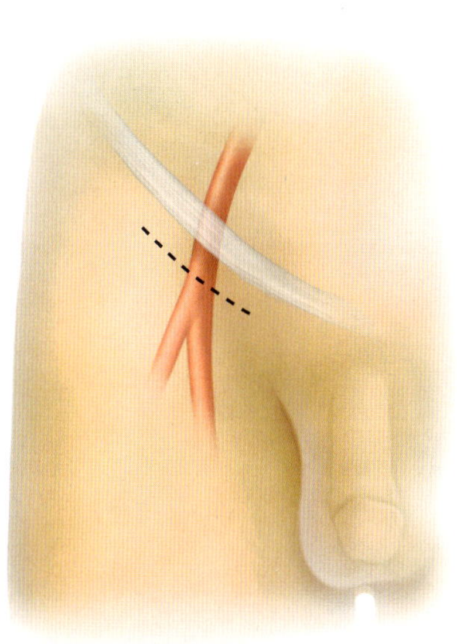

FIGURE 7 • Transverse groin incision for femoral artery exposure.

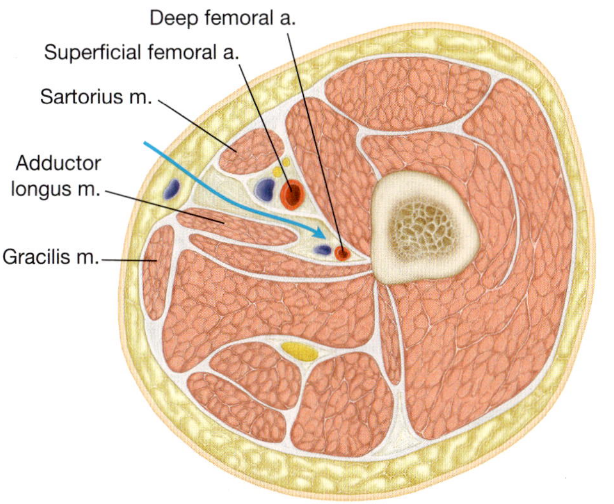

FIGURE 8 • Deep femoral artery exposure via lateral sartorius approach (*solid blue arrow*).

fascia of an avascular plane to find the neurovascular popliteal bundle proximal and deep along the tibia (**FIGURE 10**).

Third Step: Harvest and Preparation of Autogenous Vein

- The course of the GSV is marked on the skin prior to prepping. The shortest segment of suitable caliber and quality GSV is harvested. Incision placement is partially determined by the location of the arterial access incisions. Care should be taken to avoid creating skin flaps during vein exposure. Harvesting vein through skip incisions may help to minimize wound complications but is not necessary for a good result. Minimal vein manipulations, with care being taken to accurately ligate side branches with permanent suture without crimping the main vein lumen is important. Minimal dissection of the vein is typically required when in situ bypass is planned, as the vein can be left in its bed with only limited dissection of the anastomotic segments. Skip incisions provide access to ligate larger side venous branches.

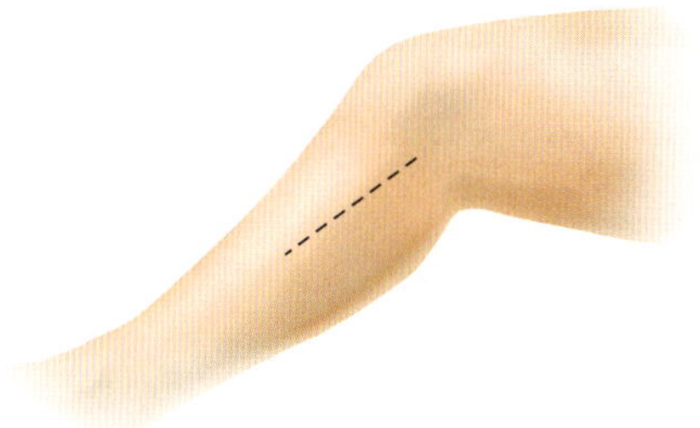

FIGURE 9 • Incision for below-knee popliteal exposure.

- After an adequate length of saphenous is exposed, it is prepared for use. If a reversed bypass is being planned, the vein is removed from its bed and reversed for bypass placement. The saphenofemoral confluence is oversewn or suture ligated. If an in situ bypass is planned, the saphenous vein is transected at the saphenofemoral confluence, and the proximal vein is transposed to the femoral bifurcation and the anastomosis is constructed. Value lysis is performed after proximal anastomosis creation to allow dilation of the vein for ease in using the valvulotome. A third option, nonreversed translocated, is used when the size mismatch is too great to use the reversed technique but the vein needs to be tunneled under the muscle or across the leg (as in a distal anterior tibial bypass). In situ and translocated vein conduits are useful, but there is a technical learning curve with needed ability to troubleshoot patent branches especially if skip incisions were created (**FIGURE 11**).
- When using reversed vein, we generally try to use the largest overall diameter segment for the bypass conduit. The vein is distended gently with heparinized saline, any branches that are not ligated well are repaired using 7-0 polypropylene suture, and small holes are oversewn in a longitudinal fashion taking care not to narrow the vein. Depending on institutional expertise, endoscopic vein harvest is an alternative method to minimize incisional length and potential wound complications, but it has a steep learning curve. There is evidence to suggest that endoscopic vein harvest may decrease the infection risks but this benefit may be outweighed by long-term patency concerns.[4]
- After systemic anticoagulation is achieved with intravenous heparin, the proximal anastomosis is performed after controlling the inflow artery with vessel loops or vascular clamps. The loops or clamps are released, and the anastomosis is confirmed to be hemostatic. If significant atherosclerotic disease in the inflow artery is present, a separate arterial patch repair may be needed with our preference in using bovine pericardium on the host artery with the vein conduit anastomosed to such. Other patch options can be a separate segment of vein or even prosthetic such as Dacron or PTFE (**FIGURE 12**).
- If valve lysis is required, it is done after proximal anastomosis creation. Once complete, the vein is distended with blood. The vein is then marked for orientation with marker to avoid twisting and it is passed through the tunneler to exit the distal incision and clamped proximally with an atraumatic bulldog clamp or Yasargil clip. The length of vein needed is determined after the vein has already been tunneled and distended, with the leg in a maximally extended position.

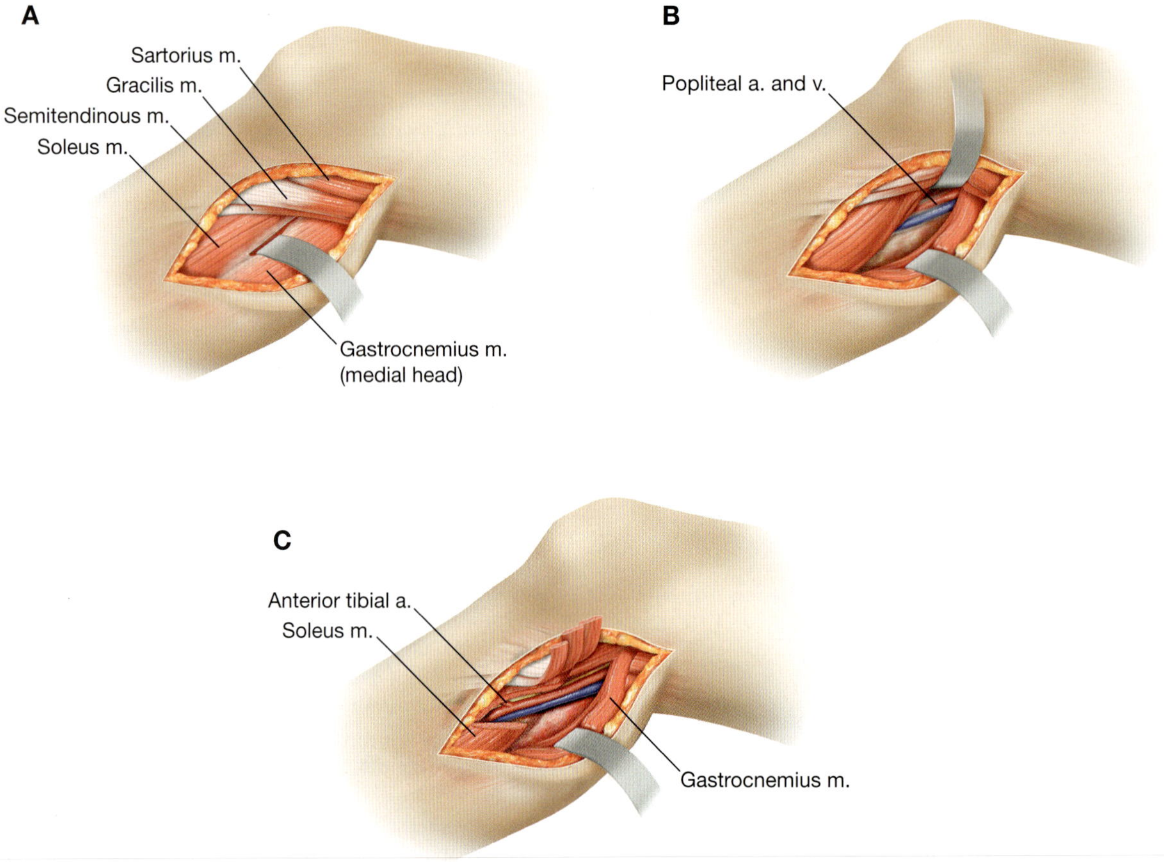

FIGURE 10 • **A-C,** Dissection for below-knee popliteal exposure.

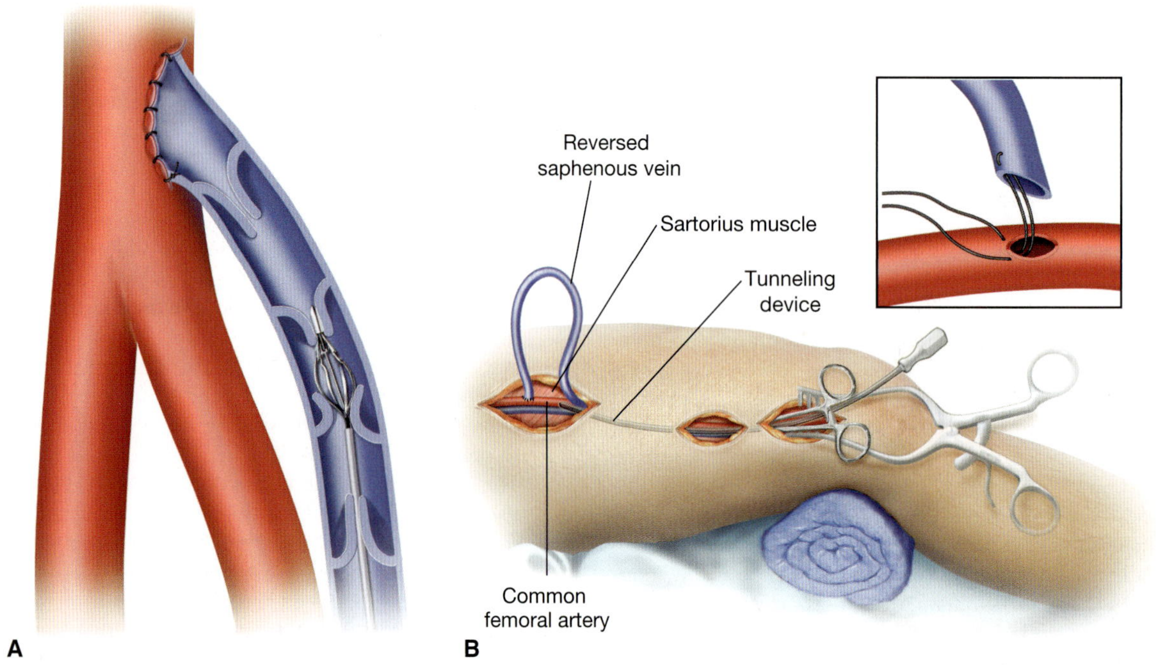

FIGURE 11 • **A,** A valvulotome being used to lyse valves in a nonreversed vein under distension. **B,** Tunneling with hollow tunneling device through the subcutaneous tissues away from saphenectomy site.

The leg can be manipulated in various positions with knee flexion to make sure any excess or redundant vein is appropriately trimmed prior to embarking on the distal anastomosis.

- Tunneling is generally performed using a hollow tunneler (eg, Gore, Scanlan, Jenkner) with a blunt appropriately sized tip (6 mm at least) in a subcutaneous plane away from the saphenectomy incision, if possible, to avoid wound complications. The vein is carefully inspected at the entry and exit site of the tunnel to ensure it is not constrained by fascial or muscular bands. Of note, unique vein tunneling may be required as situations arise in a more anatomic approach (such as through the tibial/fibular space when going from medial inflow artery to ATA).

Fourth Step: Distal Anastomosis Creation

- If a tourniquet is to be used for distal control, then the lower leg is exsanguinated using an Esmarch bandage. The tourniquet is placed around the thigh if the inflow is at the level of the common femoral, profunda femoris, or proximal superficial femoral arteries. It is inflated to 250 to 300 mm Hg. The target is then identified. Care is taken to identify the artery instead of the vein because they can appear deceptively similar when exsanguinated under tourniquet hemostasis. The distal anastomosis is created using a 6-0, 7-0, or 8-0 polypropylene suture depending on the size of the target artery. Loupe magnification is helpful and generally mandatory in this setting. The first assistant should sit beside the operating surgeon to maintain suture tension around the anastomosis and suction away blood and debris from the operative field.
- Tourniquet, intra-arterial balloon occlusion, occlusion without circumferential occlusion, or cautious atraumatic clamps are all options for hemostatic control. If the tourniquet fails to maintain sufficient hemostasis due to medial calcification in the larger proximal arteries, other options for hemostasis include vessel loops and vascular clamps for tibial control, use of vessel stoppers, or use of a carbon dioxide (CO_2) blower suction device. Circumferential tibial artery dissection must be done with care to avoid injury to the adjacent paired tibial veins, or venae comitantes, that give off several crossing branches above and below the target artery.
- Prior to completion of the anastomosis, the tourniquet is deflated and flushed. The proximal graft clamp or bulldog is released, and the anastomosis is thoroughly flushed prior to tying down and completing the anastomosis. Cautious limited probing of the outflow artery with coronary dilators can ensure no concerns of the anastomosis but should be judiciously utilized as dissection or injury to the artery can occur even with proper technique. Topical agents such as thrombin/Gelfoam, Surgicel, or Floseal may be helpful in obtaining hemostasis following reversal of anticoagulation with protamine. Wound closure is covered later in the chapter.

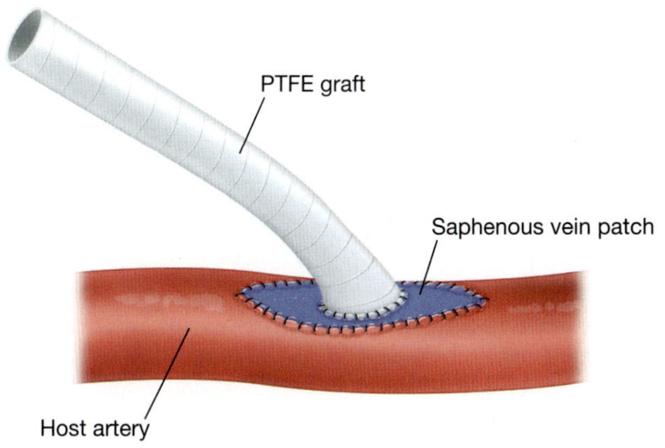

FIGURE 12 • Schematic for Linton patch anastomosis.

Perimalleolar Bypass to the Distal Anterior Tibialis Artery

First Step: Exposure of the Anterior Tibialis Artery at the Ankle

- Simultaneous dissection of the vein and proximal inflow artery should occur while the distal bypass target is identified and controlled as described earlier. The distal exposure of the anterior tibial above the ankle is performed by identifying the tendon of the extensor hallucis longus and creating an incision just lateral to this and medial to the tibialis anterior tendon. Plantar flexing the ankle and palpating the space that opens between the two tendons often easily identify this groove in which the artery runs. The extensor retinaculum is divided at the malleolus and the vascular bundle should be easily identified at this level lying along the anterior surface of the tibia (**FIGURE 13**).

Second Step: Tunneling the Vein to the Anterior Tibialis Artery

- The GSV is harvested and either reversed or used in a nonreversed fashion depending on factors described earlier. The tunnel from the inflow artery to the anterior tibial can be maintained in a subcutaneous plane across the anterior surface of the tibia medial to the exposure site, but this is difficult due to thin skin and limited subcutaneous tissue in most patients. A counterincision may be needed at the ankle to allow for a gentler curvature of the vein graft toward the dorsum of the foot. If there is concern about potential compression of the vein graft in this region because of its superficial nature, the alternative is to tunnel through the interosseus membrane. This tunnel is created higher in the calf between the deep posterior and anterior compartments (**FIGURE 14**). Because the GSV harvest incision is already on the medial calf, the dissection can be extended deeper by retracting the gastrocnemius muscles posteriorly and partially dividing the soleus to reach the posterior tibial vessels. These are protected and gently retracted posteriorly while the fibers of the tibialis posterior muscle are separated and the tunneler is bluntly passed through the interosseus membrane here. Once the vein graft is in the anterior compartment, it can be tunneled in a subcutaneous or subfascial plane to reach the exposed anterior tibialis artery just above the ankle. Another path for the vein conduit if there is enough length is to tunnel across the anterior thigh to the lateral calf, taking care in the subcutaneous space of the lateral knee, which should be kept lateral/posterior to avoid the fibular head where nerve injury can occur.

Third Step: Exposure of the Dorsalis Pedis Artery

- If the dorsal pedal artery is the target vessel, then the exposure distally is on the dorsum of the foot and the tunneling

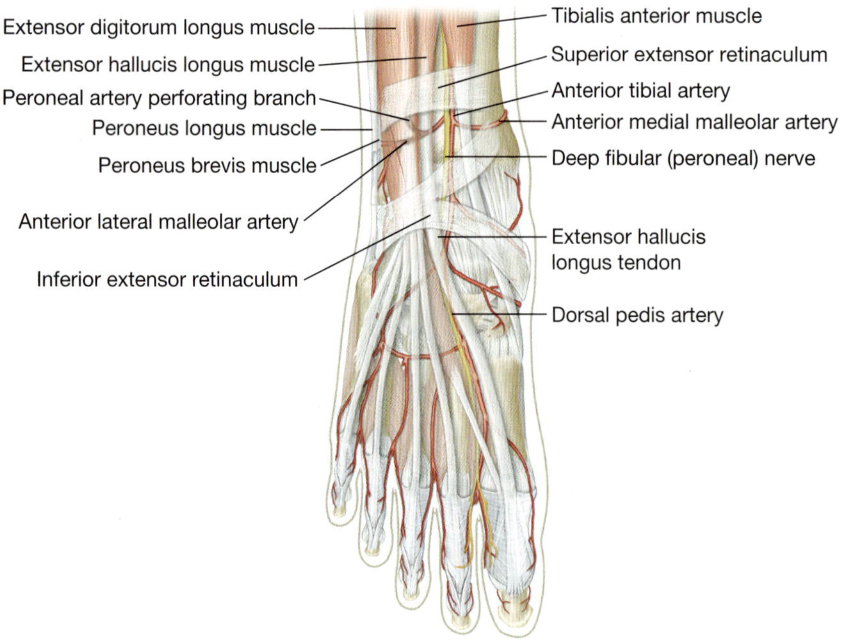

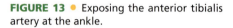

FIGURE 13 • Exposing the anterior tibialis artery at the ankle.

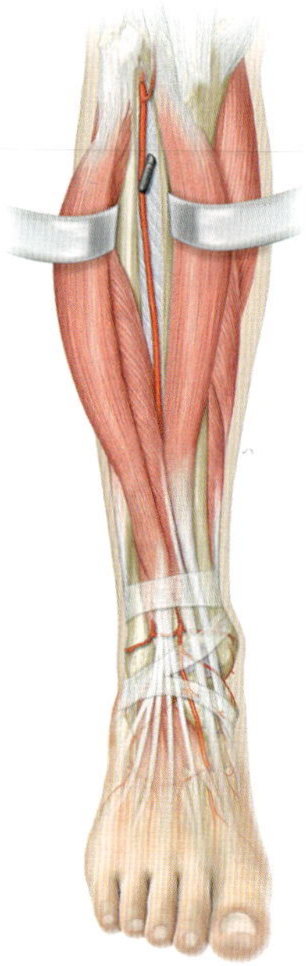

FIGURE 14 • Tunneling through the interosseous membrane at the midcalf.

techniques remain similar to what is outlined earlier for the anterior tibial artery at the ankle. An incision is created on the dorsum of the foot just lateral to the extensor hallucis longus tendon and carried down through the fascia. The dorsal pedal artery lies lateral to the deep peroneal nerve here (**FIGURE 15**).

- Care should be taken to not leave self-retaining retractors in for too long in these smaller distal incisions to avoid tension on the wound edges and potential skin necrosis.

Exposure of the Peroneal Artery at the Ankle

First Step: Peroneal Artery Anatomy

- The peroneal artery comes off the tibioperoneal trunk at the upper calf and then distally branches into two perforating branches at the ankle joint, termed anterior and posterior perforating peroneal arteries, which supply the anterior and lateral compartments and communicate with the anterior tibial artery and some tarsal branches.

Second Step: Exposure of the Distal Third of the Peroneal Artery

- The proximal segment of the peroneal artery can be accessed easily from a medial approach similar to the posterior tibial artery exposure just dissection more laterally toward the fibula. Using Doppler signal can ensure proper trajectory. The perimalleolar or distal third of the peroneal artery needs to be approached laterally and requires resection of a portion of the fibula. An incision is created along the lateral border of the fibula, and dissection is carried down through the fascia to the fibula after which the periosteum is cleared proximally and distally (**FIGURE 16**). The peroneal artery is near the fibula medially, and care should be taken to avoid injury to the vascular bundle when clearing the bone (**FIGURE 17**). The bone can then be excised, and the peroneal artery is identified behind the interosseus membrane. The bone can be transected using a Gigli saw or oscillating power saw. The advantage of either a traditional bone cutter or power saw is that the bone does not necessarily have to be circumferentially dissected.
- The peroneal artery can also be exposed posteriorly, but this is somewhat challenging to do when the patient is supine. An incision just above the ankle posterolaterally between the tendons of the flexor hallucis longus and the flexor digitorum longus reveals the artery in its most distal segment

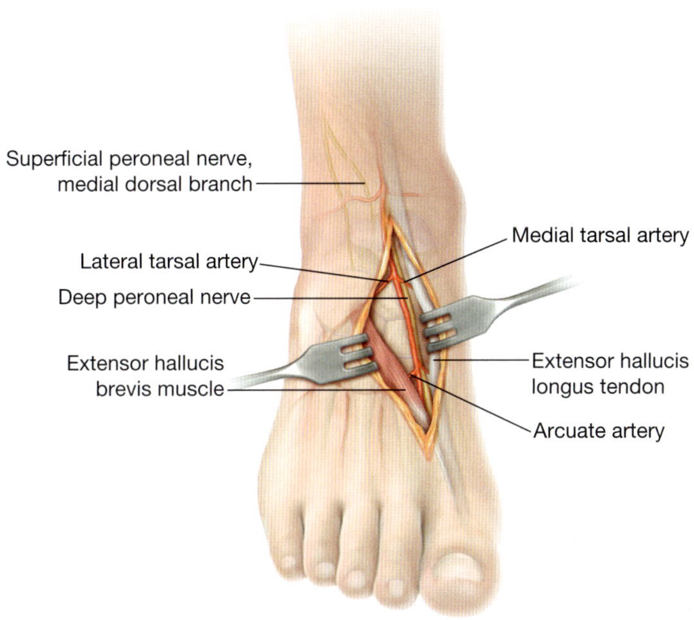

FIGURE 15 • Exposure of the dorsalis pedis artery.

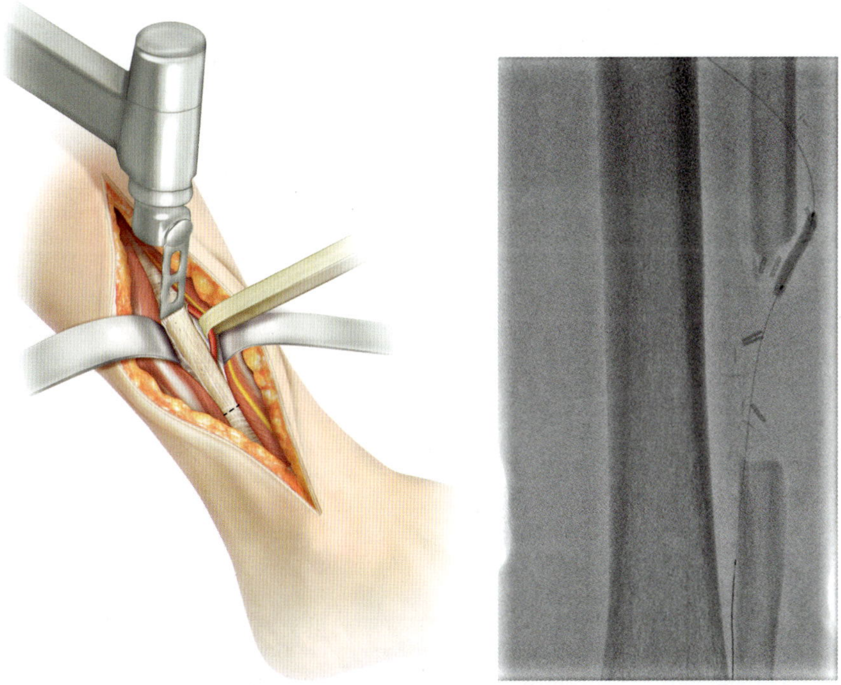

FIGURE 16 • Clearing the fibula and resection for exposure of the distal peroneal artery.

(**FIGURE 18**). This approach is favored when the small saphenous vein will also be harvested for the graft conduit.

Additional Considerations

Alternative Conduits

- Despite careful preoperative planning and efforts to fully interrogate adequate conduit, the great saphenous vein may prove to be unsuitable for the intended purpose once exposed. If length of vein is a concern, then careful consideration should be given to either moving the inflow anastomosis more distally or moving the target artery more proximally. An additional alternative is to create a shorter tunnel, harvest the great saphenous vein from the contralateral leg, or harvest arm vein when other options are not available or advisable.
- Occasionally, if no suitable autogenous vein conduit exists (especially in the case of redo bypasses), consideration may

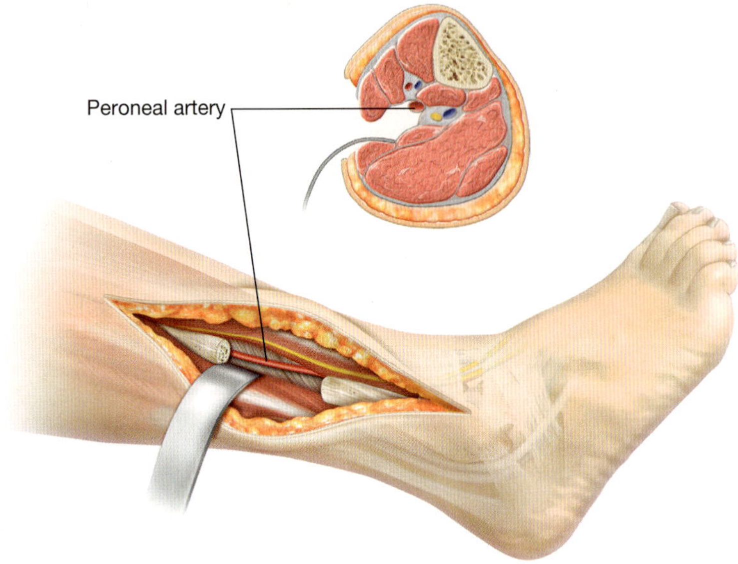

FIGURE 17 • Exposure of the distal third of the peroneal artery.

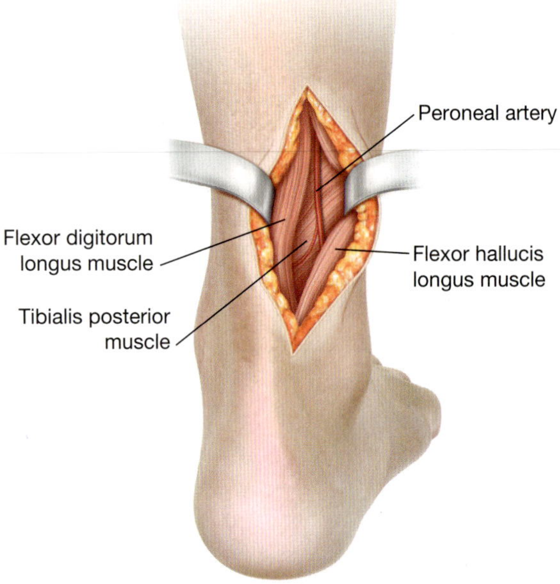

FIGURE 18 • Posterior approach to the distal third of the peroneal artery.

be given to cadaveric cryopreserved vein or prosthetic bypass with vein cuffs or patches or creation of arteriovenous fistulae distally. The limitations of these nonautogenous options must be weighed against the known patency limitations of spliced vein or arm vein grafts. In addition, composite vein/PTFE remains a viable option, but patency and infection limitations must also be considered.

Bypass Evaluation

- Following open, endovascular, or hybrid procedures the authors advocate for thorough evaluation of the intervention performed. The patency of the bypass is assessed intraoperatively by multiple potential methods. Feeling a strong bypass pulse in the tunnel and in the target vessel distal to the anastomosis is reassuring but could suggest nonideal outflow (obstructive at or distal to anastomosis). Listening with a handheld Doppler to assess the quality of the Doppler signal of the artery distal to the distal anastomosis is also helpful. A multiphasic strong Doppler signal that augments significantly when the graft is first compressed and then released is suggestive of a patent bypass. In the absence of strong clinical signs of graft patency (eg, palpable distal pulse), an intraoperative color flow duplex scan may be used to identify potential flow limiting defects, such as retained valves in the bypass if in situ or transposed or focal velocity elevations or low flow in the graft itself due to twisting or vein injury.
- Completion arteriography provides useful detail regarding potential technical problems, including the status of the anastomoses, tunneling issues, and the presence of retained valves, if any. Angiography is performed using a small-caliber needle in the most proximal artery or vein bypass with runoff views through the venous conduit into the outflow arterial tree. Some degree of spasm may be seen at the site of clamp placement or vessel loop manipulation but should be considered thrombus or stenosis until proven otherwise. Reimaging, treatment of spasm with intra-arterial papaverine, or exploration of the concerning area of vein or artery is required if angiography reveals concerns. When tunneling concerns arise, dynamic arteriography with the leg flexed and extended in various positions can be helpful to prevent kinking of the bypass in the early postoperative period.

Wound Closure

- Wound closure is a key component of the operation and should not be minimized or relegated to inexperienced team members as much of the morbidity from bypass procedures arises from wound complications. These patients have significant postoperative edema related to vein harvesting as well as the arterial reperfusion of the ischemic limb. The vein harvest bed should be irrigated, inspected for hemostasis, and closed in multiple layers of running or interrupted absorbable suture and/or staples. Generally, suture multilayer closure is preferably for any areas where a nonanatomic bypass is present. Care is taken to avoid injury to the saphenous nerve. At the ankle and around points of flexion, such as the knee, it is useful to use mattress nylon sutures. It is also important to close the ankle incision first before reperfusion edema makes tension-free closure challenging. It is often difficult to get more than one layer of subcutaneous tissue over the bypass and distal anastomosis at the perimalleolar level (**FIGURE 19**). Wound closure should be planned for while making the initial incisions with other closure options including use of vacuum-assisted device or even a bedside or return to operating room for secondary closure; both of these closure management options are generally rare events but are useful to consider if needed in some scenarios.

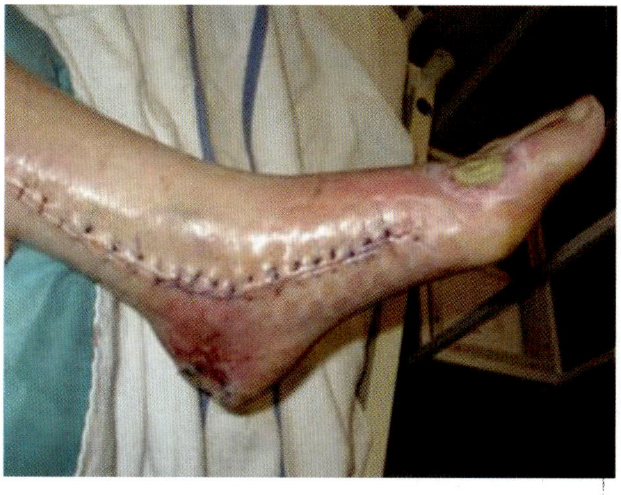

FIGURE 19 • Perimalleolar wound closure.

ENDOVASCULAR TECHNIQUES

Endovascular and Hybrid Approaches

- For completeness in presentation of the perimalleolar revascularization topic, a discussion must occur regarding endovascular interventions. In the past few decades, there have been numerous advances in endovascular techniques pertaining to lower extremity arterial disease. These endovascular approaches provide many advantages and generally are associated with less morbidity in the patient with CLTI with many comorbidities because endovascular interventions can be performed under local sedation without needing general or regional anesthesia as is needed for open bypass. Nonetheless endovascular revascularization techniques have their own limitations and disadvantages. Hence, it is of paramount importance to first identify appropriate anatomic stenoses and/or occlusions amenable to EVT as discussed above in TASC II guidelines. In addition, it is essential to identify the patient is an appropriate candidate for EVT from the clinical presentation, functional status and comorbidities, and anatomic pattern of disease. Surgical calculators can be helpful to decide if endovascular approaches offer the patient less risk than open bypass revascularization.
- As mentioned, PAOD can present in a variety of permutations with regards to disease pattern. Often, EVT may need to be offered in a hybrid approach with an open bypass. As an example, a patient with a short segment proximal stenosis may be treated with angioplasty and stent to augment inflow while the patient's distal long segment stenosis/occlusion may be managed with open vein bypass. The contrast is true as well, as many patients undergo proximal bypasses and completion management with distal endovascular interventions especially with venous conduit limitations. The ideal hybrid approach must be customized to the patient's anatomy and disease distribution. Endovascular therapy has greatly expanded the toolbox for interventions in the management of lower extremity revascularization.

Endovascular Arterial Access

Endovascular access approaches and outcomes are topics that need to be discussed in greater detail than this chapter covers. In general, the percutaneous Seldinger technique is utilized to gain arterial access via a retrograde or anterograde approach. Once access is obtained with a micropuncture (4Fr) system, an appropriately sized working sheath is inserted to guide wires and catheters to cross and treat the angiographic stenoses and occlusions that are imaged (**FIGURE 20**).

- Retrograde access via the contralateral common femoral artery is commonly utilized for lower extremity revascularization. Once a working sheath is situated, the treatment limb is accessed by fluoroscopical guidance of wires and catheters up and over the aortic bifurcation. The retrograde technique offers advantages given ease of access and less risk of the development of dissection flaps.
- Alternatively, retrograde access can be accomplished in the ipsilateral limb distal to the target lesion for intervention. For example, the dorsalis pedis artery can be used allowing for direct access below a tibial arterial target lesion. Nonetheless, this technique is limited by sheath size as well as the quality of distal access and is technically challenging with a learning curve.
- Finally, anterograde access via the ipsilateral common femoral and superficial femoral with the patient supine or the popliteal artery with the patient prone. Each technique has advantages and disadvantages based on target vessel intervention goals, but in general an antegrade approach provides shorter distance for maneuvers and allows for greater ease in push ability and maneuverability of wires and catheters. With that said, anterograde access carries a risk for the development of anterograde dissection flap, which can result in acute limb ischemia and need for emergent open repair. Furthermore, anterograde access can be technically difficult in obese patients especially for common femoral artery access through a large pannus.

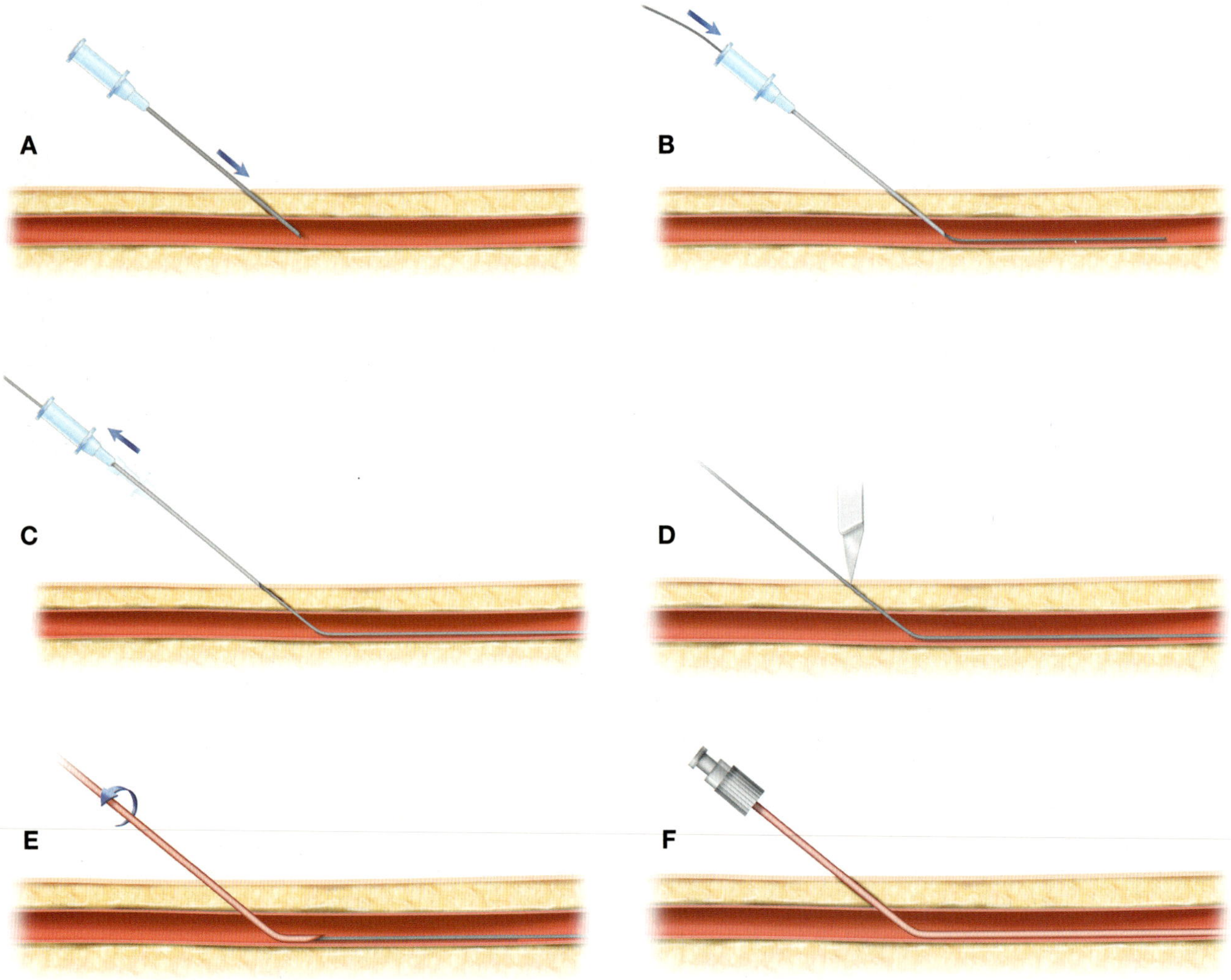

FIGURE 20 • Seldinger technique. **A,** Hollow needle introduction into artery. **B,** Passage of guidewire into artery via hollow needle. **C,** Removal of needle over the wire. **D,** Incision of skin along wire. **E,** Placement of dilator over the wire into the artery and then removal of dilator. **F,** Placement of the sheath over the wire into the artery and removal of the wire.

Image Acquisition

- Equipment and room setup are essential components for successful endovascular revascularization procedures. The surgeon must ensure they have access to a procedure room with fluoroscopy imaging on an appropriate table. Preoperatively the patient's renal function should be assessed, and if needed, preoperative hydration should be provided. In addition, surgeons should have appropriate radiation safety equipment available. Contrast agents can ultimately be injected via syringe or with power injector. Finally, digital subtraction angiography should be utilized to optimally interpret the fluoroscopic images.

Treatment

- The rate-limiting step of endovascular revascularization procedures is the ability to cross or traverse the target lesion or lesions. This process often requires an ability to modify the operative plan based on the patient's anatomy, therapeutic goals, and comorbidities. The intervention performed will ultimately be determined by the quality of the lesion (eg, calcific) and total length of the stenosis or occlusion. Various treatment modalities available include percutaneous balloon angioplasty (PTA) with or without stent placement, cryotherapy, and atherectomy. The rationale and details of such techniques is complex and beyond the scope of this chapter, but each endovascular technique is deployed based on the goal of the procedure related to the desired clinical outcome and the time for patency of the intervention. These outcomes are weighed with the expense of both the endovascular supplies and the degree of patient and staff radiation and the contrast dye requirements for a patient especially if there is underlying renal insufficiency. Perimalleolar endovascular revascularization procedures should be performed by providers with experience and training to allow appropriate technical skills combined with clinical judgments to obtain optimal outcomes with least risk and most benefit.

Closure

- Access site closure is a broad topic with goal to avoid hematomas or arterial injury. In general, manual pressure can be employed for sheath sizes less than 8 French, but this method requires movement restrictions for a period to prevent pseudoaneurysm or bleeding. Thus, to expedite time and patient comfort, numerous percutaneous closure devices exist on the market that include a variety of physical, chemical, and combination of such to close the percutaneous access site without complications of bleeding, thrombosis, or arterial injury and stenosis. Postoperative anticoagulation also is a consideration when selecting a closure method. If hemostasis is not satisfactorily achieved following removal of access sheath and appropriate manual pressure, a deferral to an open repair is required with resultant risks and benefits.

PEARLS AND PITFALLS

	Open bypass perimalleolar procedures
Preoperative planning	▪ The bypass target is chosen to provide the best option for direct in-line perfusion to area of tissue loss on the forefoot. Autogenous vein bypass is preferred over prosthetic for both patency and limb-salvage outcomes.
Placement of incision	▪ Using ultrasound in the operating room to identify the GSV in relation to the proximal and distal incisions can help avoid raising flaps or creating postoperative wound complications. ▪ Use of a tourniquet above the knee can assist in avoiding unnecessary manipulation and potential injury to distal tibial vessels.
Tunneling	▪ Tunneling the bypass away from the vein harvest incision can help protect the bypass from exposure and infection in case of wound complications and wound dehiscence postoperatively.
Intraoperative assessment of bypass	▪ Manipulating the leg in slightly different positions can assist with evaluating the course of the vein bypass in the tunnel during intraoperative assessment with on-table angiography.
Wound closure	▪ Avoid leaving self-retaining retractors in distal incisions for prolonged periods to avoid skin edge necrosis. ▪ Closure of distal wounds is best accomplished with nylon suture in a mattress fashion to avoid tension on the wound. Wounds over the dorsum of the foot can be closed with mattress sutures. Alternatively, deep-dermal Vicryl sutures and subcuticular Monocryl sutures can be employed and dressed with Dermabond. Occasionally, a counter incision may be necessary to provide adequate coverage over the exposed artery at the ankle. Rare cases may need secondary wound closure after reperfusion edema and/or utilization of vacuum-assisted devices.
Postoperative care	▪ A gently placed soft cast can prevent significant lower leg edema and subsequent wound breakdown in the immediate postoperative period. ▪ Predischarge duplex assessment of the graft is important if intraoperative assessment of the bypass was not performed with angiography or duplex.

POSTOPERATIVE CARE

Open Bypass

- Because of the length and location of the vein harvested for conduit, the patient will undoubtedly have significant edema postoperatively throughout the affected leg. Drains (eg, flat 10Fr Jackson-Pratt to bulb) can be placed in the vein harvest sites especially with deep harvest sites and if the patient requires postoperative anticoagulation; key is to exit the drain proximal to the drain placement in a separate skin incision to avoid creating any more distal wounds that could leak or weep. Tape should be avoided on all skin in the lower leg especially as postoperative edema can cause blisters and infection in compromised skin. The authors do not routinely wrap the leg for at least 48 hours to prevent conduit compression and thrombosis. Limb elevation must be employed in the postoperative setting such that the ankle is above the knee and the knee is above the hip. When the patient is ready for compression wrappings, the foot, ankle, and lower leg may be wrapped in a soft cast consisting of an inner layer of Webril and outer layer of gently compressive Ace wrap or Coban. Care needs to be taken to minimize external compression on the vein graft itself, especially in the areas around the ankle. The patient can ambulate starting on postoperative day 1, but the leg should be elevated when the patient is sitting or in bed.
- The authors will universally put the bypass patient on single or dual antiplatelet therapy in the perioperative setting. Depending on the clinical scenario and the surgeon's assessment of the conduit and runoff quality, a short course of

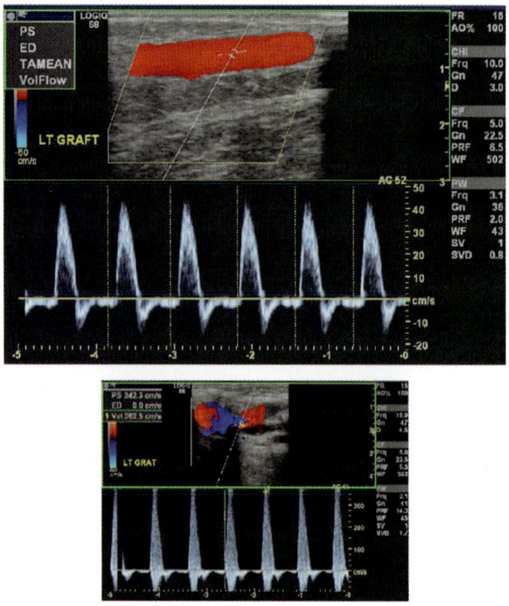

FIGURE 21 • Surveillance duplex of vein bypass.

therapeutic anticoagulation may be employed; however, this must be balanced against the risk of bleeding in individual patients. In addition, the patient should remain on a statin, ensure adequate glucose control, and remain normotensive.

- For perimalleolar bypass patients who did not get an intraoperative assessment of their bypass with an on-table angiography, a predischarge duplex is performed to document patency and pedal perfusion. If a significant abnormality is identified on duplex (significantly low flows in the bypass or focally high velocities), then this should be addressed prior to discharge with angiography or exploration of the area with appropriate intervention.
- Once discharged, patients either return weekly for a change of their soft cast until their edema has sufficiently resolved or follow up at the 1-month interval for formal duplex interrogation of the bypass. Certainly, more frequent visits may be warranted in patients with wound concerns.
- Surveillance duplex of vein bypasses is obtained at the 3-month, 6-month, and 12-month postoperative time points and then every 6 or 12 months with both ABI and graft duplex (**FIGURE 21**). After the 1-year time point with no previous abnormalities on postoperative imaging, the surveillance can be moved to once a year. Occasionally, the surveillance interval is shortened for high-risk bypasses or prosthetic tibial bypasses and especially if the patient is still using tobacco.

COMPLICATIONS

- Early complications of distal bypasses include bleeding, wound infection/breakdown, and graft occlusion. Early graft occlusion in the first 24 to 48 hours must be considered technical errors and require urgent operative re-exploration.

Late complications include graft stenosis, limb swelling, graft occlusion, and aneurysmal degeneration of the vein bypass. Most patients with CLTI have concomitant coronary disease, and the rate of perioperative myocardial infarction can be as high as 5%. It is very important to maintain patients on their cardiac medications in the perioperative period and manage fluids judiciously to avoid precipitating coronary events.

OUTCOMES

Perimalleolar Bypass Revascularization

- In a systemic review and meta-analysis in 2018 for bypass surgery to any infrainguinal target, the incidence rate of major amputation within 1 year was 0.11 with great saphenous vein graft, 0.24 with nonautogenous graft, and 0.16 with ectopic vein or spliced arm vein graft. Primary patency of the bypass at 1 year was 0.77 in nonautogenous grafts, 0.64 in great saphenous vein grafts, and 0.45 in ectopic vein or spliced arm vein graft. At 2 years and beyond, superior patency (primary and secondary) and limb salvage rates for great saphenous vein over nonautogenous and ectopic vein conduits were evident and increasingly amplified. Mortality was similar for the three types of bypass grafts. Data for major adverse cardiovascular events, reintervention/readmission, amputation-free survival, reintervention and amputation-free survival, quality of life, and wound healing were limited.[5]

Perimalleolar Endovascular Revascularization

- In a systemic review and meta-analysis in 2018, in patients with infrapopliteal artery lesions, primary patency at 1 year was as follows: bare-metal stent (BMS): 0.50, drug-eluting stent (DES): 0.73, atherectomy 0.78, and balloon angioplasty 0.66. At 3 years, in patients with infrapopliteal artery lesions, primary patency of DES was 0.49 and that of BMS was 0.10 with no data available for PTA. Data on major amputation and mortality in patients with infrapopliteal disease were not significantly different for various endovascular techniques at 1 and 3 years of follow-up.[5]

REFERENCES

1. Anton N. Sidawy BAP. *Rutherford's Vascular Surgery and Endovascular Therapy*. 9th ed. Russell Gabbedy; 2014.
2. Aboyans V, Ricco JB, Bartelink MLEL, et al. 2017 ESC Guidelines on the Diagnosis and Treatment of Peripheral Arterial Diseases, in collaboration with the European Society for Vascular Surgery (ESVS): document covering atherosclerotic disease of extracranial carotid and vertebral, mesenteric, renal. *Eur Heart J*. 2018;39(9):763-816. doi:10.1093/eurheartj/ehx095
3. Fujii M, Terashi H. Angiosome and tissue healing. *Ann Vasc Dis*. 2019;12(2):147-150. doi:10.3400/avd.ra.19-00036
4. Zhao AH, Kwok CHR, Jansen SJ. How to prevent surgical site infection in vascular surgery: a review of the evidence. *Ann Vasc Surg*. 2022;78:336-361. doi:10.1016/j.avsg.2021.06.0455
5. Almasri J, Adusumalli J, Asi N, et al. A systematic review and meta-analysis of revascularization outcomes of infrainguinal chronic limb-threatening ischemia. *J Vasc Surg*. 2018;68:2 PMID: 29804736 doi:10.1016/j.jvs.2018.01.066

Chapter 35 Popliteal Aneurysm Management: Open and Endovascular Repair

Lindsey Marie Korepta and Bernadette Aulivola

DEFINITION

- Popliteal artery aneurysms (PAAs) are the most frequently encountered peripheral arterial aneurysm, accounting for 70% of aneurysms in the peripheral vasculature. In general, an artery is considered aneurysmal when it measures 1.5 times the diameter of the normal adjacent segment. Normal popliteal artery diameter varies depending on body habitus but is typically between 5 and 9 mm and can be up to 1 to 2 mm larger in men than in women.[1,2]
- In characterizing PAAs for indications for repair, not only the maximal diameter but also the presence or absence of intraluminal thrombus and the symptomatic status are important.
- Clinical practice guidelines advocate for repair of any PAA measuring greater than 2 cm in diameter, although smaller aneurysms may have an indication for repair if they are symptomatic or if there is evidence of thromboembolism. The diameter of the popliteal artery is typically larger proximally, at its transition from the superficial femoral artery as it emerges from the adductor hiatus, than in the more distal portion. Aneurysms are more common in the proximal or mid portions of the popliteal artery and may extend to involve the superficial femoral artery proximally or tibial vessels distally.[3]

DIFFERENTIAL DIAGNOSIS

- The asymptomatic PAA may present with a palpable pulsatile mass or fullness in the popliteal fossa on physical examination. The differential diagnosis for a popliteal fossa mass includes PAA, Baker cyst, deep venous thrombosis, and neoplasms such as rhabdomyosarcoma. In the symptomatic patient with ischemia, the differential diagnosis includes other etiologies of acute or chronic ischemia, including popliteal entrapment syndrome, cystic adventitial disease, atherosclerotic peripheral artery disease (PAD), and thromboembolism.

PATIENT HISTORY AND PHYSICAL FINDINGS

- When evaluating any patient, it is important to consider risk factors for aneurysm disease in general, including advanced age, male sex, smoking history, personal history of PAD or atherosclerosis in other vascular beds, and family history of aneurysm disease or connective tissue disorder. Most patients with PAAs are male, accounting for approximately 95% of those affected.[1] Additional risk factors for atherosclerotic disease include hypertension and hyperlipidemia. Diabetes, while a risk factor for atherosclerotic peripheral artery disease, is protective against the development of aneurysm disease.
- In patients with a diagnosis of abdominal aortic aneurysm (AAA), a thorough physical examination should be performed to rule out the presence of concomitant peripheral aneurysms including PAAs, which are present in over 10% of these patients. Palpation of the popliteal pulse is best performed using a technique where the examiner encircles both hands around the knee with thumbs positioned anteriorly over the patella and all other fingertips of both hands pressed against the popliteal fossa. If palpation reveals evidence of a widened popliteal pulse or pulsatile mass, or if the examination is equivocal, duplex ultrasound should be performed to evaluate further for the presence of a popliteal artery aneurysm.
- In patients with PAA, bilateral involvement is present in over 60%, emphasizing the importance of evaluating the contralateral extremity in patients diagnosed with PAA. In addition, approximately 40% of patients with PAA will also have an AAA; therefore, aortic imaging is indicated in all patients with PAA.[4] While femoral artery aneurysms are less common, they may be seen with increased frequency in patients with other extremity aneurysms or AAA; therefore, femoral pulse palpation and/or imaging is recommended as well.
- While PAAs may be diagnosed when small and asymptomatic, patients may present with symptoms of acute or chronic ischemia due to thromboembolism, mass effect on surrounding structures, or rupture, the latter of which is quite rare. Popliteal artery aneurysms, in contrast to AAAs, more commonly present with ischemic symptoms when symptomatic rather than rupture. PAAs can develop intraluminal thrombus, which may embolize to distal vessels. Distal embolization may, in fact, be asymptomatic. Most patients presenting with acute limb ischemia (ALI) related to PAA do so given popliteal artery thrombosis; therefore, PAA should be in the differential diagnosis of any patient presenting with ALI.
- It is important to remember that digital subtraction angiography (DSA) alone may not identify PAA in the patient presenting with ALI; therefore, duplex ultrasound or axial imaging such as computed tomography angiography (CTA) or magnetic resonance angiography (MRA) is essential to identify the presence of PAA and characterize the maximal diameter of the artery.
- Distal embolization due to intraluminal thrombus may present in the asymptomatic state or with intermittent claudication, ischemic rest pain, or tissue loss with distal ulceration or gangrene.
- While uncommon, patients with large PAAs may present with compressive symptoms related to mass effect on the surrounding structures. This may result in complaints of popliteal fossa fullness, discomfort or pain, or lower extremity swelling from popliteal vein compression, which may result in deep venous thrombosis. Compression of the common peroneal nerve by the PAA may present with neurologic symptoms such as foot drop.[5]
- Significant risk of limb loss exists in the patient presenting with signs and symptoms of ALI associated with PAA thromboembolism (36%).[4] This emphasizes the importance of diagnosis of the PAA at an early stage such that proper surveillance

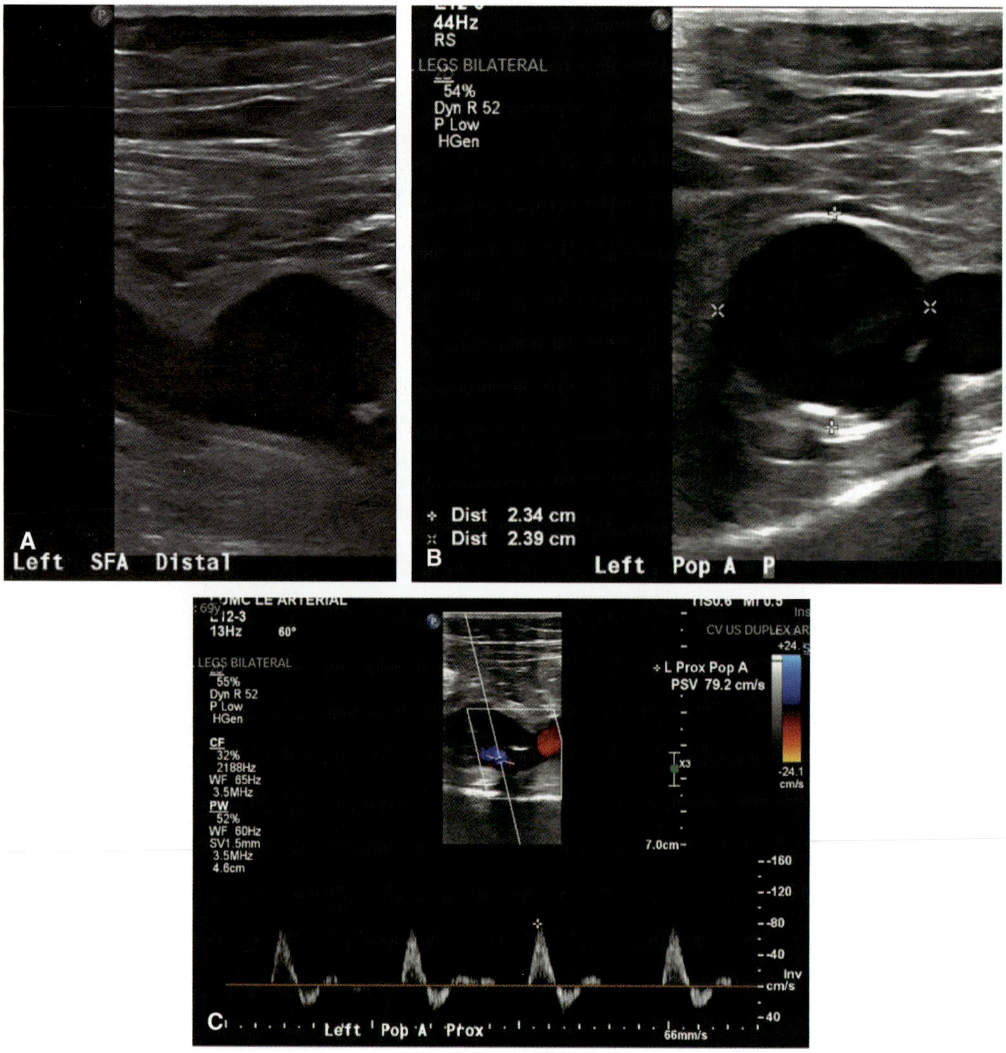

FIGURE 1 • Popliteal artery aneurysm imaging using duplex ultrasound, depicted in **(A)** b-mode longitudinal view, **(B)** b-mode transverse view and **(C)** color flow longitudinal view.

and elective intervention may be performed when indicated. Of PAAs that are identified when asymptomatic, 14% to 24% will become symptomatic within 1 to 2 years and 31% to 68% will become symptomatic within their lifetime.[4,6]

IMAGING AND OTHER DIAGNOSTIC STUDIES

- As previously mentioned, given the high rate of bilateral PAAs and concomitant AAA, bilateral lower extremity arterial duplex ultrasound (US) and abdominal aortic US should be performed whenever a popliteal artery aneurysm is identified. Screening duplex US has been demonstrated to have a nearly 100% accuracy in detection of PAAs and thus is recommended by the Society for Vascular Surgery clinical practice guidelines to be the first step in diagnosis.[1] As demonstrated in **FIGURE 1**, duplex US is able to determine PAA diameter and can detect color Doppler flow through the aneurysm lumen and presence of intraluminal thrombus.
- When repair is indicated for a PAA, CTA (**FIGURE 2**), MRA, or DSA can be used to further characterize the size and extent of the PAA and the runoff vasculature beyond the aneurysm.

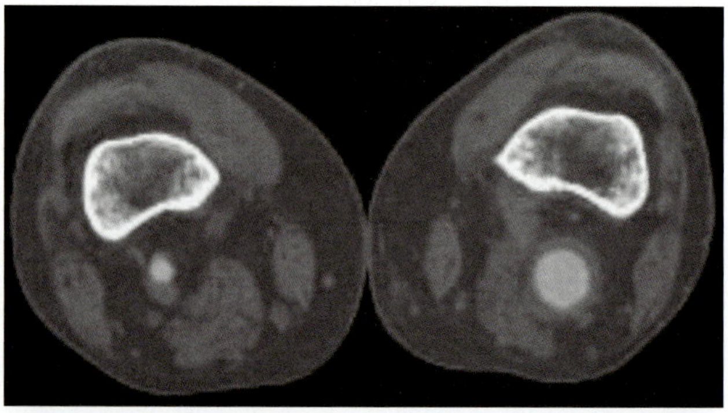

FIGURE 2 • Axial slices of computed tomography angiogram (CTA) imaging demonstrating a left popliteal aneurysm with contrast enhancement of the lumen and presence of a rim of intraluminal thrombus.

It is important to note that DSA demonstrates only the flow lumen and therefore is not an accurate technique to determine aneurysm diameter and may not detect aneurysm at all in cases of PAA thrombosis.

SURGICAL MANAGEMENT

Preoperative Planning

- Workup may vary significantly in the asymptomatic vs the acutely symptomatic patient. Ideally, if the PAA is identified in the asymptomatic state, surveillance may be performed with duplex US and elective repair may be planned once the aneurysm meets size criteria for repair. Asymptomatic PAAs should be considered for elective repair if they measure >2 cm in maximal diameter, or smaller if there is evidence of intraluminal thrombus and runoff vessel occlusion, a possible result of distal embolization. In all cases of elective aneurysm repair, the risk–benefit ratio is assessed prior to recommending intervention. The size of the aneurysm, evidence of distal embolization, and the patient's overall health and medical comorbidities should be taken into consideration. Risks of intervention vary based upon whether the aneurysm is repaired using open surgical or endovascular means. Planning prior to operative repair typically includes venous mapping to identify the suitability of autogenous conduit. Cardiac risk stratification and optimization is essential, as in all elective vascular procedures.
- In the elective setting, lower extremity runoff CTA is the ideal imaging study to provide anatomic detail for intervention planning. This imaging modality provides an adequate assessment of thrombus burden within the aneurysm and runoff to the foot. If the aneurysm is large, contrast enhancement of the aneurysm sac and runoff may be slow, requiring a delayed phase of imaging to properly assess the distal runoff vessels (**FIGURE 3**). During an on-table angiogram, the catheter can be advanced into and beyond the aneurysm to better identify the runoff vessels. Either technique will be able to identify the anatomy of the patent arteries including any large geniculate arteries in the vicinity of the aneurysm, which can be helpful when determining appropriate operative management. Both endovascular and open techniques are used to treat PAAs.
- Endovascular stent placement is a reasonable treatment option for PAA, but patency outcomes are improved in patients with better distal runoff. In our practice, to be considered a candidate for endovascular therapy the patient must have more than one tibial artery vessel runoff to the foot and an adequate sealing zone proximal and distal to the aneurysmal segment. The proximal and distal landing zones must measure between 4 and 12 mm in diameter, as currently available self-expanding covered stents for use in the peripheral vasculature range between 5 and 13 mm in diameter (Viabahn, W. L. Gore & Associates, Flagstaff, AZ). Geniculate vessel anatomy should be assessed preoperatively, as there is potential for retrograde flow via these vessels into the aneurysm sac after stent graft placement (type 2 endoleak), which may lead to progressive aneurysm growth. Preoperative side branch embolization with coils or plugs may be considered if such branches are present and the patient is not a candidate for open repair.

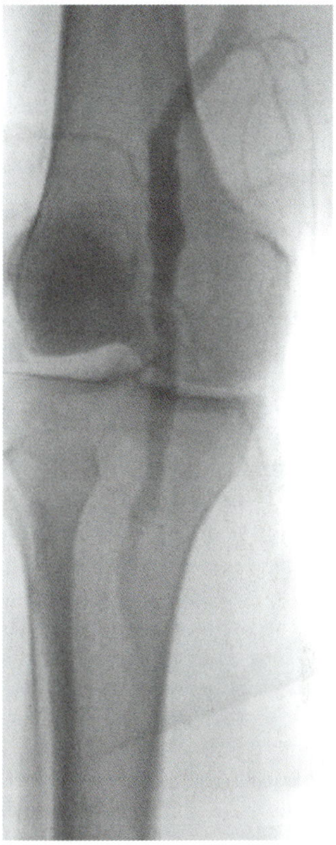

FIGURE 3 • Preintervention angiography with catheter positioned in the distal superficial femoral artery.

- In general, open repair of PAAs is preferred if the patient is deemed to be reasonable operative risk with life expectancy >2 years, especially if the patient is at a young age at intervention, if compressive symptoms are present, or if the aneurysm crosses the knee joint, which is often the case. Techniques for open repair include posterior approach to the popliteal artery with interposition grafting or medial approach with ligation of the artery proximal and distal to the aneurysm and surgical bypass around the aneurysmal segment. Infrequently in the patient presenting with ALI due to acute PAA thrombosis, primary amputation may be considered if the limb is deemed to be nonviable or if the patient is nonambulatory.

POSITIONING AND TECHNIQUE

Endovascular Technique

First Step: Thrombolytic Therapy

- If the patient presents with acute thrombosis of a PAA and endovascular PAA repair is being considered, a patent flow lumen must be restored and runoff artery flow must be optimized prior to stent graft deployment. Typically, on initial diagnosis with ALI, a therapeutic heparin bolus (80 U/kg intravenous [IV]) is given and IV infusion (18 U/kg/h) is instituted.
- Restoration of flow of the occluded popliteal artery is performed typically via a contralateral retrograde femoral artery ultrasound-guided access. The access site must be assessed for the presence of an aneurysm, and it is helpful to know if AAA is also present since puncture site and catheter navigation may be affected by this knowledge. A sheath is placed

up and over the aortic bifurcation with its tip positioned within the external iliac or femoral artery of the affected lower extremity.

- If ischemic symptoms are mild, thrombolytic agent may be infused over a course of hours to dissolve thrombus in the artery. This typically commits the patient to a 12- to 24-hour course of thrombolysis, sometimes longer. For catheter-directed thrombolysis, a multi-side hole catheter is positioned through the thrombosed segment over a guidewire. The location of the tip of the catheter must be confirmed within a patent artery distally prior to infusion. Tissue plasminogen activator (TPA) is then infused at a rate of 1 mg/h through the catheter, which instills the medication throughout the length of the thrombus through multiple side-holes of the catheter. The sheath side-arm is flushed continuously with a low-dose heparin infusion, typically 500 U/h. This is intended to assure patency of the sheath, rather than as a therapeutic dose of anticoagulation. The patient undergoing drip thrombolytic therapy requires close observation, often in the intensive care unit, with Q1 hour neurovascular checks and access site inspection for bleeding complications. Laboratory values including CBC, PT, PTT, and fibrinogen should be checked every 6 hours looking for signs of bleeding or coagulopathy that may alter plans for ongoing thrombolytic therapy. The administration of thrombolytic agents is associated with a risk of bleeding, so patients should be appropriately screened for bleeding risks prior to instituting therapy.
- Often, the degree of ischemia in the patient presenting with a thrombosed PAA does not lend itself to pharmacologic thrombolysis, as described above, given the risk of ongoing nerve, muscle and soft tissue damage from prolonged ischemia during the treatment time. In that case, more rapid thrombolysis results may be seen with the use of pharmacomechanical thrombectomy techniques. There are several commercially available mechanical thrombectomy devices available. In our practice, we pulse-spray 10 mg of TPA (diluted in 100 mL of normal saline) into the thrombus, let it dwell within the thrombus for 20 minutes, then perform thrombus removal using suction thrombectomy. If persistent residual thrombus is seen, a lytic catheter may be left in place for 12 to 24 hours as described above for more complete thrombolysis. After lysis, the patient can be considered for endovascular or open repair. The use of thrombolytic therapy in general requires that the degree of ischemia present would allow for time for thrombolysis, which is generally faster when using mechanical adjunctions to pharmacologic therapy. Open operative thrombectomy should always be a consideration if the degree of ischemia is advanced and rapid flow resolution is warranted.

Second Step: Endovascular Stent Graft Repair

- If endovascular PAA repair is planned, whether in the setting of elective PAA repair or in the symptomatic patient after thrombolysis, the patient is placed on a radiolucent table in the supine position. The sheaths required for delivery of large covered self-expanding stents can be as large as 10 French. In our practice, an up and over technique is used from a contralateral groin approach if there is a favorable access site and aortic bifurcation anatomy. Otherwise an open cut-down on the ipsilateral groin with antegrade access of the common femoral artery may be performed.
- A preintervention DSA run is performed, and the proximal and distal landing zones are identified. A marker catheter can be used to guide stent graft length selection (**FIGURE 4**). Large geniculate branches may be coil embolized prior to stent graft placement. The patient is systemically heparinized (80 U/kg), with a goal activated clotting time (ACT) >200 seconds. The stent is selected based upon seal zone vessel diameter, typically upsizing the stent graft 1 mm from the size of the artery.
- The stent graft is then deployed across the aneurysm, and postdeployment angioplasty may be performed with the appropriate-sized balloon at the seal zones to assure adequate graft expansion and seal. Completion DSA is performed to evaluate the stented segment and runoff arteries. This will assess for artery patency as well as presence of endoleaks (**FIGURES 5** and **6**). Runoff DSA images to the foot are then obtained to document outflow to the foot.

Third Step: Closure of Access

- If endovascular access from the contralateral groin has been carried out, we use PerClose ProGlide closure (Abbot Laboratories, Abbott Park, IL). If open arterial exposure has been performed, the sheath is removed and the artery is closed in a transverse arteriotomy technique with running 6-0 Prolene suture, flushing the artery antegrade and retrograde before completion of the closure down. The femoral exposure is then closed in a standard layered technique.

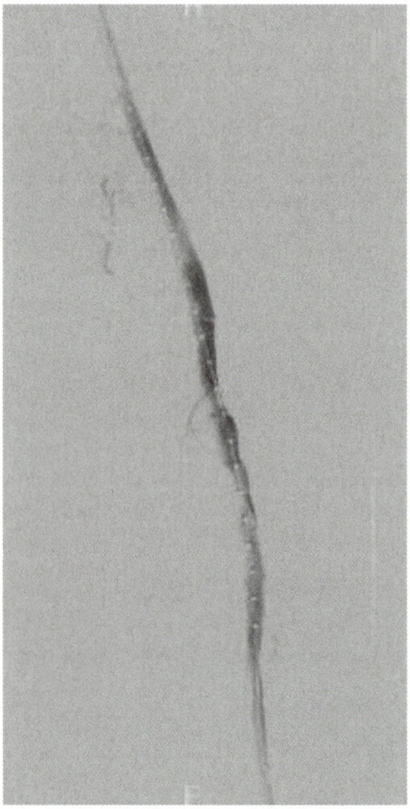

FIGURE 4 • Marker catheter in place to assist with choosing stent length during endovascular repair of PAA.

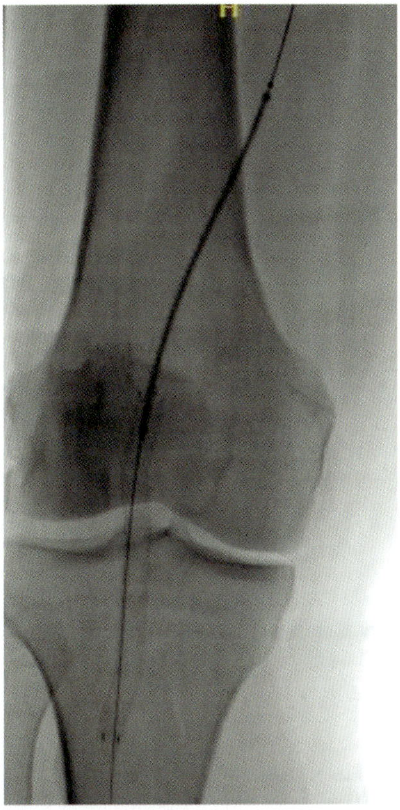

FIGURE 5 • Intraoperative angiogram depicting two covered stent deployment with one stent deployed and adequate overlap with second stent about to be deployed.

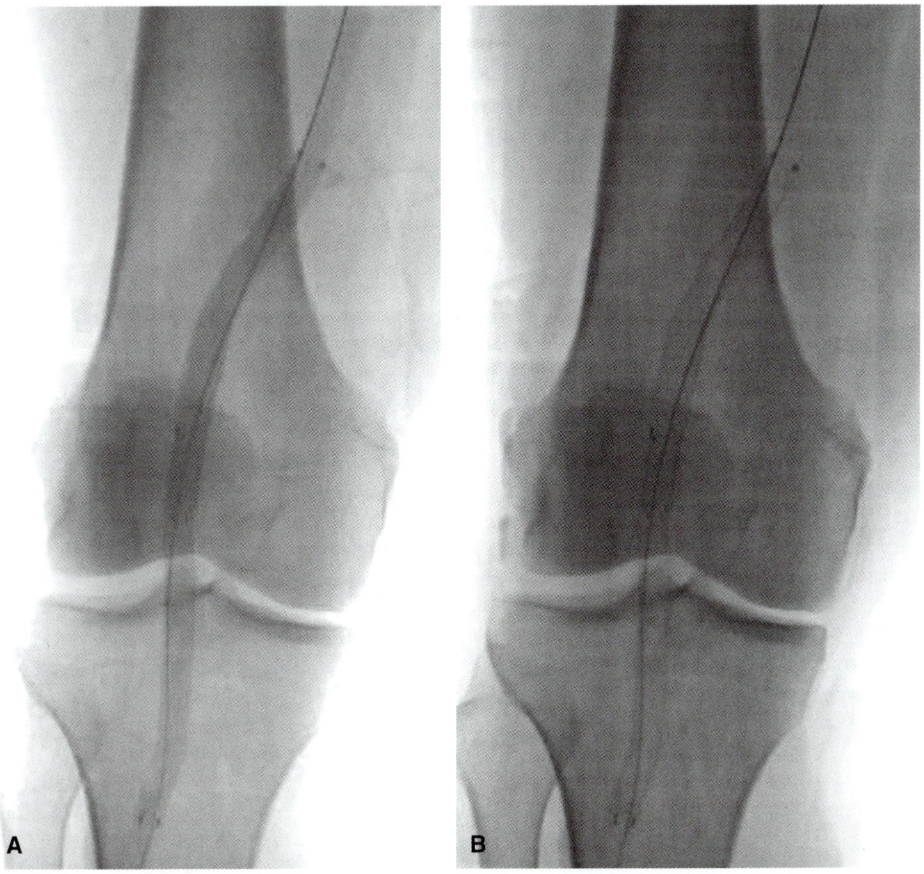

FIGURE 6 • Completion angiogram after covered stent deployment in endovascular repair technique with **(A)** and without **(B)** contrast.

OPEN OPERATIVE TECHNIQUE

- Depending on the size and location of the aneurysm, there are two standard approaches to open popliteal artery aneurysm repair.

Medial Approach (Ligation and Bypass)

First Step: Harvest of Autogenous Conduit

- Preoperatively, the patient should undergo venous mapping with ultrasound. Ipsilateral great saphenous vein (GSV) is the conduit of choice. Before prepping and draping the patient, ultrasound may be performed, marking the course of the GSV with a skin marker on the surface. If autogenous vein is not available, prosthetic graft may be used, typically 6 mm or 8 mm ringed polytetrafluoroethylene (PTFE). The patient is positioned supine, and the extremity is then prepped and draped in the standard sterile fashion. Before or after proximal and distal arterial exposure, the GSV is harvested from one incision to the other, assuming that the size of the vein at this location is adequate. If better conduit quality is present more proximally, then separate GSV harvest incisions may be made. The goal is to use the highest-quality segment of the GSV for bypass.

Second step: Exposure of the Proximal Popliteal Artery

- Assuming the PAA does not extend proximally into the distal superficial femoral artery, proximal exposure is achieved with a longitudinal incision above the knee, taking care to identify and preserve the GSV. A bump is placed just below the knee, facilitating exposure of the above-knee popliteal artery. The artery is exposed by retracting the sartorius muscle posteriorly and entering the popliteal space. The popliteal vein is usually encountered first, and the popliteal artery is located just lateral to this. The artery is dissected free of the neighboring veins and surrounding tissue sufficiently to allow for passage of a vessel loop proximal and distal to the planned proximal anastomosis site. There should be enough space distal to this to ligate the popliteal artery proximal to the aneurysm.

Third Step: Exposure of the Distal Popliteal Artery

- Depending on the extent of the aneurysm, the distal anastomosis of the bypass graft may be the above-knee popliteal artery for very focal aneurysms, but more commonly is located at the distal popliteal artery and approached from a medial incision below the knee. The bump is repositioned under the distal thigh. A longitudinal incision is made below the knee on the medial aspect of the proximal calf. Again, care is taken to avoid injury to the GSV. The fascia of the superficial posterior compartment of the calf is opened longitudinally and the popliteal space is entered. As with the proximal exposure, the vein is encountered first and retracted posteriorly to dissect the artery and place a proximal and distal vessel loop for control. Care should be taken to avoid traction on the nearby tibial nerve. Since the inflow and the outflow to the PAA will be ligated during the operation, one may choose to place a 0-silk tie around the popliteal artery at the proximal aspect of the exposed artery here for ligation rather than a vessel loop in order to tie off the vessel later. If the popliteal artery is aneurysmal throughout its length, the exposure may be extended distally to identify and control a tibial artery target for bypass. The posterior tibial or peroneal arteries can be easily accessed from a medial approach. If the anterior tibial artery or mid to distal peroneal arteries are chosen as the distal bypass target, a separate lateral incision is needed.

Fourth Step: Tunneling

- The bypass conduit can be tunneled anatomically between the heads of the gastrocnemius along the course of the native popliteal artery; however, if the aneurysm is large this may not be feasible due to risk of compression of the bypass graft or risk of rupture/bleeding during tunneling. In this case a "bucket handle" bypass may be performed with subcutaneous tunneling of the bypass instead. Once the tunnel is created with a vascular clamp or tunneling device, the patient is systemically heparinized with 80 U/kg of IV heparin and an ACT is checked to assure therapeutic anticoagulation with a goal ACT of 200 to 250 s.

Fifth Step: Conduit Preparation

- Assuming adequate GSV conduit is available for use, it is harvested assuring adequate length, ligating all branches with 3-0 or 4-0 silk ties and tying it off proximally and distally using 2-0 silk ties. The GSV is stored in an isotonic solution (500 cc of Plasmalyte or Normosol with 60 mg papaverine and 5000 U heparin) in an effort to reduce vasospasm. The GSV conduit may be used in the reversed or nonreversed orientation. This is typically based on surgeon preference as there is no significant impact of vein orientation on bypass patency rates. If the plan is to position it nonreversed, then standard preparation with valve lysis should be performed. If GSV is not available, the bypass may be performed with ringed PTFE, and if so, a distal target artery vein or bovine pericardium patch may be performed prior distal anastomosis at the target site.

Sixth Step: Arterial Bypass

- Arterial bypass is performed in standard fashion with either proximal end-to-side or end-to-end anastomosis. End to side is usually easier from a technical standpoint given size discrepancy with the artery larger than the conduit. The proximal anastomosis is performed first, then the bypass conduit is allowed to inflate with pulsatile inflow and inspected for hemostasis prior to tunneling to the distal anastomosis site. The distal anastomosis is then performed. The inflow and outflow arteries to the aneurysm sac should be ligated as close to the aneurysm sac as possible to ensure aneurysm thrombosis and to decrease the risk of further growth. Completion arteriography can be performed if there is a question about the status of the bypass based on Doppler signal and pulse examination at the end of the case, but it is not our routine to perform completion arteriography.

- When possible, the medial approach is our preferred method of bypass given the ability to harvest the entire length of the GSV, the familiarity of the exposure, and the ability to reach the tibial vessels, if needed for the distal bypass target.

Posterior Approach (Interposition Grafting)

First Step: Harvest of Autogenous Conduit

- If the aneurysm is located directly behind the knee or demonstrates significant compressive symptoms requiring decompression, the posterior approach is preferable. If GSV is to be harvested from the groin of proximal thigh, this is performed supine, then the patient is turned prone. The distal GSV may be harvested in the prone position. The patient is then placed in prone position, assuring proper padding with axillary rolls, a pillow beneath the hips, soft padding underneath the knees, and a roll beneath the ankles. If the small saphenous vein is of adequate size, it can be used as the bypass conduit and harvested via the same incision as outlined below. The popliteal artery is exposed from a posterior approach and aneurysmorrhapy with aneurysm sac decompression can be performed at the same time.

Second step: Exposure of the Proximal Popliteal Artery

- A lazy S-shaped incision is used with the proximal incision positioned on the medial aspect of the posterior distal thigh and the distal part of the incision on the lateral aspect of the posterior calf (**FIGURE 7**). The proximal popliteal artery is identified distal to the adductor canal and exposed by separating the semimembranous and semitendinosus muscles medially from the long head of the biceps femoris, which lies laterally.

Third Step: Exposure of the Distal Popliteal Artery

- Dissection is then carried along the course of the popliteal artery distally to gain distal control of the artery beyond the aneurysm. Care should be taken to gently retract the tibial nerve to gain visualization of the popliteal artery along its course if needed. As there is no tunneling required, the patient is then systemically anticoagulated with heparin as previously described.

Fourth Step: Arterial Bypass

- Vascular clamps are placed distally and proximally for arterial control. The aneurysm sac is opened longitudinally and any intraluminal thrombus is removed. Back bleeding geniculate arteries are oversewn with silk figure-of-eight sutures. End-to-end interposition bypass is then performed in a method similar to that used for open repair of aortic aneurysms (**FIGURE 8**). Alternatively, an end-to-side proximal and distal anastomosis can be carried out, which may be preferable if there is a significant size discrepancy between the bypass conduit and the native artery. An alternative is to use appropriately sized prosthetic conduit, either Dacron or PTFE, to assure a better size match. Often, posterior approach repair may be performed with a short interposition graft. Wound closure is performed with two deep layers and a subcuticular stitch.

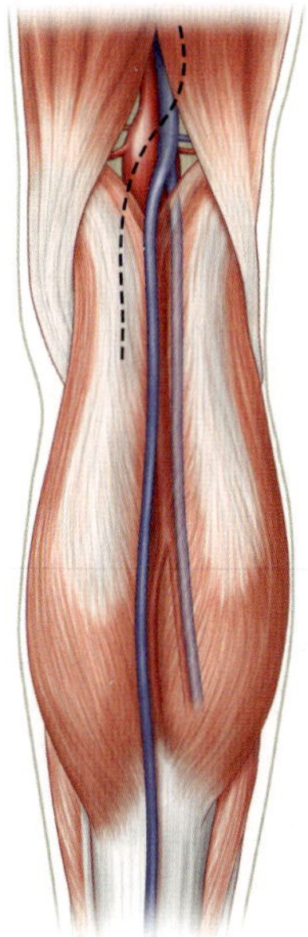

FIGURE 7 Posterior approach to the popliteal artery depicting the lazy-S incision with the incision medial on the thigh and lateral on the calf.

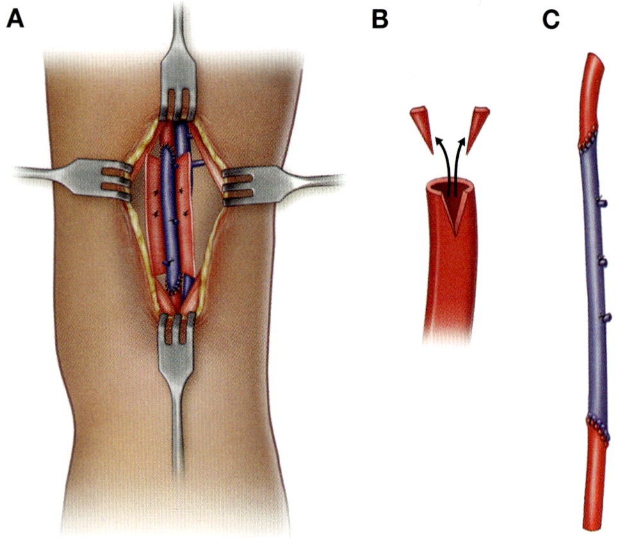

FIGURE 8 • End-to-end bypass technique with saphenous vein conduit using a splicing technique of the proximal and distal arteries and veins to prevent stenosis at the anastomoses.

PEARLS AND PITFALLS

Popliteal artery aneurysm thrombosis	■ As with any acute limb ischemia case, the potential to develop compartment syndrome after revascularization should be taken into consideration and calf four-compartment fasciotomies should be performed when the risk of this is deemed to be significant. If calf fasciotomies are required, we often apply a vessel loop with staples in a "Roman sandal" configuration across the fasciotomy site. This allows for the vessel loop to be tightened at the bedside day by day, and eventually bedside wound closure may be performed without a return trip to the operating room. ■ If open intervention is planned in a patient with PAA thrombosis and there is an adequate runoff artery, bypass may and should be performed without efforts at thrombolysis as long as the runoff artery is deemed to be adequate.
Endovascular technique considerations	■ When planning an endovascular approach to repair of a PAA, we try to use as few stents as possible to decrease the risk of stent migration or thrombosis. We ensure adequate proximal and distal seal into healthy artery to prevent the development of endoleaks in the future. We often perform an open cutdown onto the proximal superficial femoral artery (SFA) or distal common femoral for safe delivery of larger sheaths (typically greater than 8 French in diameter or a steep aortic bifurcation).
Open surgery technique considerations	■ Size mismatch between the artery and the bypass conduit can be considerable. For larger arteries or arteriomegaly, a PTFE bypass conduit that can be chosen closer to the size of the artery should be considered. Studies have demonstrated acceptable patency rates with prosthetic conduit.[7]

POSTOPERATIVE CARE

- With either technique, the popliteal aneurysm can continue to grow if patent geniculate arteries are left unaddressed. Careful postoperative duplex ultrasound (DUS) surveillance should be carried out to assure the best chance of long-term patency. Clinical practice guidelines recommend DUS surveillance be performed at 30 days, 3 months, 6 months, 12 months, and then yearly if the aneurysm does not grow during this interval.[1]
- We place all patients treated with endovascular repair on dual antiplatelet therapy with aspirin 81 mg/d and clopidogrel 75 mg/d for at least 90 days. For vein bypasses, we place

all patients on aspirin 81 mg daily indefinitely. For patients with prosthetic bypass conduits or compromised tibial runoff, we consider dual antiplatelet therapy. For patients presenting with ALI and PAA thrombosis, we often treat with therapeutic anticoagulation in addition to antiplatelet therapy for at least 1 to 3 months.

- The posterior approach incision may be compromised if significant edema is present, therefore we apply compression wraps to the lower extremity for at least a few weeks or until edema is under control.

COMPLICATIONS

- Stent thrombosis has been noted with single vessel runoff, stent coverage below the knee, and large aneurysm size.[1] Stent thrombosis can be detected on DUS surveillance (**FIGURE 9**), CT angiography, or digital subtraction angiography. These stents can often be reopened with pharmacomechanical thrombolysis using the same technique as referenced above. If an underlying lesion is noted as a cause of the stent thrombosis, it may undergo angioplasty or stenting as needed (**FIGURE 10**). In patients with only single vessel runoff, open bypass should be considered given the elevated risk of stent graft thrombosis.
- In order to prevent stent and bypass thrombosis, initiation of postoperative anticoagulation and/or antiplatelet therapy is very important.
- Poor tibial artery runoff is associated with worse outcomes for both open and endovascular interventions.[8] In a patient with poor tibial runoff after open bypass we often will add low-dose rivaroxaban 2.5 mg BID to aspirin 81 mg. We ensure that all stented patients are on dual antiplatelet therapy for at least 90 days and occasionally lifelong if they are noted to have poor tibial runoff.
- Wound complications are increased in open repair over endovascular repair.[1,8] We make every effort to ensure that our patients are medically optimized before surgery. This includes initiation of antihypertensive and statin medications as indicated as well as nutritional support.

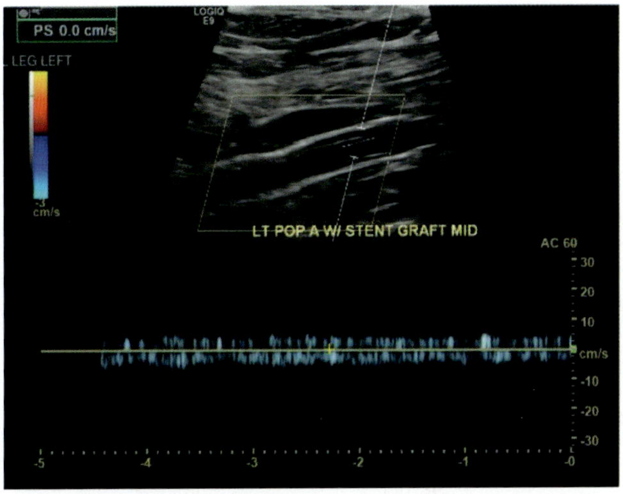

FIGURE 9 • Duplex US demonstrated stent occlusion.

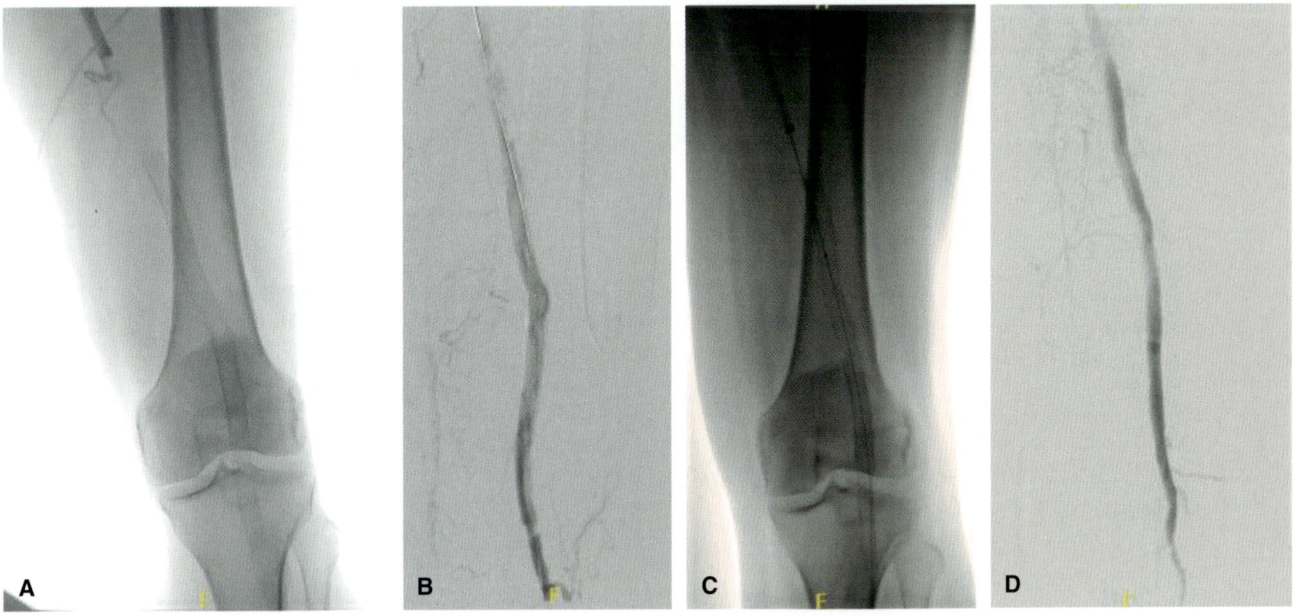

FIGURE 10 • Digital subtraction angiography depicting an occluded stent **(A)**, which was able to be reopened with AngioJet thrombectomy **(B)**, and an area of stenosis just distal to the existing stents **(C)** was treated with an additional stent **(C)** with good result **(D)**.

REFERENCES

1. Farber A, Angle N, Averginos E, et al. The Society for Vascular Surgery clinical practice guidelines on popliteal artery aneurysms. *J Vasc Surg*. 2022;75(1S):109S-120S.
2. Johnston KW, Rutherford RB, Tilson MD, et al. Suggested standards for reporting on arterial aneurysms, Ad Hoc Committee on Reporting Standards, Society of Vascular Surgery and North American chapter, International Society for Cardiovascular Surgery. *J Vasc Surg*. 1991;13(3):452-458.
3. Pomposelli F, Hamdan A. Rutherford's vascular surgery, chapter 136: Lower extremity aneurysms. In: Cronenwett JL, Johnston KW, Rutherford BS, eds. *Rutherford's Vascular Surgery*. 7th ed. Saunders/Elsevier; 2010.
4. Vermilion BD, Kimmins SA, Pace WG, Evans WE. A review of one hundred forty-seven popliteal aneurysms with long-term follow-up. *Surgery*. 1981;90(6):1009-1014.
5. Dawson I, Sie R, van Baalen JM, et al. Asymptomatic popliteal aneurysm: elective operation versus conservative follow-up. *Br J Surg*. 1994;81(10):1504-1507.
6. Dawson I, Sie RB, van Bockel JH. Atherosclerotic popliteal aneurysm. *Br J Surg*. 1997;84(3):293-299.
7. Beseth BD, Moore WS. The posterior approach for repair of popliteal artery aneurysms. *J Vasc Surg*. 2006;43(5):940-944; discussion 944-5.
8. Leake AE, Segal MA, Chaer RA, et al. Meta-analysis of open and endovascular repair of popliteal artery aneurysms. *J Vasc Surg*. 2017;65:246-256.

SECTION VI: Surgical Management of Venous Disease

Chapter 36 Acute Iliofemoral Deep Vein Thrombosis and May-Thurner Syndrome: Surgical and Interventional Management

Sharon C. Kiang and Brian G. DeRubertis

DEFINITION

- Acute iliofemoral occlusion is defined as complete or partial thrombosis of any part of the iliac vein and/or the common femoral vein (CFV), with or without associated femoropopliteal thrombosis, in which symptoms have been present for 14 days or less or for which imaging indicates that thrombosis has occurred within the past 14 days or less.[1] Acute iliofemoral occlusion may occur de novo following unprovoked deep vein thrombosis (DVT) or may occur (or reoccur) in the setting of prior ipsilateral DVT or external compression (May-Thurner syndrome or neoplasia). Treatment options include (1) systemic anticoagulation alone, (2) open surgical venous thrombectomy, or (3) percutaneous intervention, including catheter-directed thrombolysis, pharmacomechanical thrombectomy, and stenting of intrinsic or extrinsic obstructive lesions or masses.

DIFFERENTIAL DIAGNOSIS

- Iliofemoral DVT most commonly presents with unilateral leg swelling and pain. Although patient history and simple diagnostic testing can generally distinguish from other causes, differential diagnoses include cellulitis or worsening of chronic conditions such as venous insufficiency or lymphedema.

PATIENT HISTORY AND PHYSICAL FINDINGS

- There are three objectives in the treatment of iliofemoral thrombotic occlusion: (1) prevent propagation of DVT and subsequent pulmonary embolism (PE), (2) provide symptomatic relief for the patient, and (3) prevent the development of postthrombotic syndrome (PTS).
- A thorough history must be obtained prior to treatment because decisions regarding choice of treatment modality are impacted by severity of symptoms as well as the patient's overall functional status.
- Specific risk factors that merit individualized questioning include history of trauma, current or past episodes of DVT or PE, history of thrombophilia, history or current diagnosis of cancer, and a history of tobacco or substance use. Family history of DVT or PE is important to ascertain. A thorough investigation of current medications should be undertaken, making note of any contraceptive therapy, hormone replacement therapy, or use of anticoagulation (ie, warfarin, enoxaparin).
- Symptoms of iliofemoral occlusion can range from nondescript mild symptoms to severe disabling symptoms, and manifestations of symptoms can vary widely. Commonly reported symptoms of iliofemoral occlusion include limb edema, heaviness, pain, lifestyle-limiting venous claudication, stasis dermatitis, and, in advanced cases, venous ulcerations.[2] Duration of symptoms and consideration of inciting events at the time of symptom development will help differentiate acute occlusion from exacerbation of chronic disease.
- Symptom severity is an important differentiating variable in the management rubric of acute iliofemoral occlusion; severe and persistent symptoms, especially those continuing following the initiation of therapeutic anticoagulation, increase the likelihood of long-term disabling sequelae. The more severe and persistent the symptoms, the more justified the indication for aggressive thrombus removal.
- A detailed physical examination is essential. Conditions that produce symptoms mimicking those associated with iliofemoral occlusion should be excluded. A thorough abdominal and lower extremity pulse examination, with noninvasive physiologic testing, if necessary, will exclude possibility of arterial insufficiency. Comprehensive assessment of peripheral motor and sensory nerve function and of the spine and lower limb joints can rule out these confounding etiologies.
- The affected limb(s) should be examined for evidence of chronic venous insufficiency and/or stasis dermatitis, as well as signs and symptoms of acute DVT. Signs of acute iliofemoral occlusion may include pain, swelling, and bluish discoloration. Extensive thrombus propagation throughout the ipsilateral venous system may lead to phlegmasia alba dolens, characterized by profound painful swelling and a pale, milk-like skin hue. Further thrombus propagation from the deep to the superficial venous system increases outflow obstruction to the point of impeding arterial inflow, precipitating phlegmasia cerulea dolens, limb threat, and tissue loss.
- In patients with either acute or chronic venous disease, objective evaluation and prognostic stratification is best accomplished by using the CEAP (Clinical, Etiology, Anatomy, Pathophysiology) system and venous clinical severity score (VCSS).[3,4]
- Because multiple interventions may be required to optimize outcome in acute iliofemoral disease, patients' expectations

should be managed accordingly. In addition, iliac and femoral venous intervention commonly requires extended periods of postoperative anticoagulation (warfarin and/or low-molecular-weight heparin) to ensure long-term procedural success. The likelihood of patient compliance thus represents an additional important prognostic indicator.

- Long-term functional outcomes are discouraging for patients who refuse interventional management of acute iliofemoral occlusive disease. Forty-four percent of patients treated with medical therapy alone will experience venous claudication, and up to 60% will develop PTS within 2 years.[5-7]

IMAGING AND OTHER DIAGNOSTIC STUDIES

- Imaging provides important prognostic and interventional guidance to surgical management of acute iliofemoral occlusive disease. Current modalities include duplex ultrasonography; catheter-based contrast phlebography; and reconstructed, cross-sectional, contrast-based whole body (computed tomography [CT] and magnetic resonance [MR]) imaging.

Duplex Ultrasonography

- In experienced hands, duplex ultrasonography (US) provides extremely sensitive and specific information regarding the chronicity and extent of infrainguinal venous obstruction. Diagnostic accuracy in the iliocaval venous system is less predictable due to the presence of overlying bowel gas and abdominal adiposity.
- Duplex-derived criteria for acute venous occlusion include incompressibility under direct vision, partial luminal obstruction within the normally echo-free lumen, and absent or abnormal venous flow characteristics with respiration or following a Valsalva maneuver or distal compression.[8]
- The primary advantages of duplex imaging include its noninvasive nature, avoidance of ionizing radiation or nephrotoxic contrast agents, easy reproducibility, portability, and accessibility in the outpatient setting. In addition, substantial cost savings are realized compared with other imaging modalities. Other advantages include the ability of duplex scanning to differentiate hematomas, lymphatic system obstruction, superficial thrombophlebitis, and other soft tissue abnormalities from deep venous obstruction. Thus, duplex scanning is the initial imaging modality of choice in all patients with suspected iliofemoral DVT. When sufficient imaging parameters are met, definitive therapeutic intervention may be safely performed based on duplex-derived anatomic and diagnostic imaging alone.

Computed Tomography Venography

- CT phlebography is frequently ordered for assessment of limb swelling in the inpatient setting. Advantages of this modality include nearly universal availability day or night, less reliance on skill and experience of the technical staff performing the procedure, outstanding spatial resolution, reproducibility and sensitivity throughout the entire venous system, the simultaneous ability to image pulmonary arterial flow and lung perfusion, freedom from limb pain induced by direct probe compression during ultrasound examinations, and the ability to incidentally diagnose concurrent conditions (such as solid organ neoplasia) that may influence thrombogenicity or suitability for treatment with open vs endovascular techniques.
- The modern helical CT phlebogram provides a diagnostic sensitivity and a specificity of nearly 100% per year and was found to detect previously unsuspected venous thrombosis at a prevalence of 1.1%.[9,10]
- CT phlebography also provides useful information regarding thrombus density (and thus chronicity), the presence of residual luminal patency in obstructed veins, and the nature and severity of extrinsic iliac vein compression when present.
- The applicability of CT phlebography to the diagnosis of venous obstruction is limited by the volume of iodinated intravenous contrast required to obtain optimal spatial resolution in target vessels, as well as considerable whole-body radiation exposure inherent in CT imaging. On average, the radiation dosage delivered by diagnostic CT phlebography is equivalent to that of over 1200 chest x-rays or over 10 years environmental exposure at sea level (dosage equivalents courtesy of Radiation Physics Department, Stanford Hospital & Clinics). This is particularly true in patients with reduced creatinine clearance, women of childbearing age who may be pregnant, or in children. For many reasons, including the considerable expense associated with the study, CT phlebography should not be considered a first-line study but rather reserved for patients in whom duplex scanning does not provide sufficient anatomic guidance or where additional diagnoses (eg, pulmonary embolization, solid organ malignancy, or external iliac vein compression) merit evaluation or exclusion.

Magnetic Resonance Venography

- MR phlebography shares many of the advantages and disadvantages of CT-derived cross-sectional imaging, including the ability to obtain high-quality, high-resolution images of surrounding soft tissues and delineate the extent of accompanying lymphadenopathy, soft tissue sarcomas, venous aneurysms, malformations, and compression syndromes that may influence treatment and long-term management considerations. MR phlebography also provides a sensitivity and specificity of nearly 100%, respectively, in the diagnosis of acute iliofemoral venous occlusion.[11]
- However, unlike computed tomography venography, magnetic resonance venography can be used during pregnancy and provide reduced risk of nephrotoxicity in patients with reduced creatinine clearance (although gadolinium is contraindicated in patients with an estimated glomerular filtration rate [eGFR] of more than 60 mL/min).
- Contraindications for MR-based venous imaging include the presence of implantable pacemakers/defibrillators/infusion systems or other ferromagnetic devices and surgical clips/endografts, as well as claustrophobia in affected patients. MR studies are also expensive compared with duplex US, and dedicated personnel and equipment are less widely available than are modern, multirow-detector CT imaging capabilities. Thus, MR phlebography is considered most appropriate as a secondary examination in the absence of suitable duplex imaging or in the presence of contraindications to CT phlebography. MR phlebography may be particularly useful in the evaluation of coexisting or complicating ipsilateral or central venous vascular malformations.

Catheter-Based Contrast Phlebography

- Despite continuing improvements in the quality and widespread availability of noninvasive imaging, catheter-based contrast phlebography remains the gold standard for iliofemoral venous evaluation. Sensitivity and specificity are also nearly 100%, and in addition to anatomic information, physiologic venous pressure and flow information are also provided throughout the iliocaval system when accessed in a retrograde fashion from the CFV.
- Typical fluoroscopic findings include abrupt vessel cutoff in the case of total occlusion or visualization of a filling defect with residual luminal flow around the margins, a phenomenon known as "tram tracking."
- An obvious limitation is the relatively high degree of operator dependency, both in terms of physician and facility capabilities. Catheter-based contrast phlebography may be nondiagnostic in up to 18% of cases due to misinterpretations, artifacts, or superimposition of overlying structures.[12] Thus, experience and suitable infrastructure are necessary to ensure accuracy and precision.
- Other major drawbacks include the inherent invasiveness of the procedure and attendant procedural risk, radiation and contrast exposure (although significantly less than that required for CT imaging), and cost. Thus, contrast phlebography is also inappropriate as the initial diagnostic modality for most patients and best employed in conjunction with planned interventions directed at active thrombus removal.

Intravascular Ultrasound

- Intravascular ultrasound (IVUS) with the 9F Volcano IVUS catheter (Volcano Corporation, San Diego, CA) provides direct intraluminal visualization during catheter-based phlebographic assessment and intervention.
- IVUS-based imaging allows for precise measurement of cross-sectional area and maximum and minimum lumen diameter. Flow within the residual lumen may be determined, as well as precise analysis of residual luminal irregularities. The superior two-dimensional imaging characteristics of IVUS compared with contrast phlebography make this modality the measurement instrument of choice when assessing extrinsic iliac vein compression from tumors or overlying iliac arteries (eg, May-Thurner syndrome).

INTERVENTIONAL AND SURGICAL MANAGEMENT

Preoperative Planning

- Serologic and hematologic evaluation should include the basic metabolic panel (to assess renal function and concomitant electrolyte abnormalities), complete blood count, and a coagulation profile. It is also important to ascertain the status of antiplatelet or anticoagulation therapies when present (eg, dose, dosing frequency, prior complications).
- Prior to operative intervention, the index treatment limb should be marked as required for World Health Organization's preoperative checklist and "time-out" requirements and extent and severity of edema "baselined" for future comparison.
- When appropriate access requires multiple sites (eg, bilateral femoral and/or internal jugular vein approaches), those should be marked and initialed as well.

Positioning

- Patients can be placed supine or prone depending on the site necessary for access. On the operating table, the patient should be placed supine, with their arms secured at the side to facilitate ancillary access from the groin or neck. When popliteal access is required, prone positioning is required.

TECHNIQUES

PERCUTANEOUS MANAGEMENT OF ILIOFEMORAL DEEP VEIN THROMBOSIS (± VENOUS COMPRESSION SYNDROMES)

Duplex-Guided Femoral Vein Access

- Access site is chosen based on duplex US findings, proximal (peripheral) to the site of thrombotic occlusion. This may be the CFV in patients with isolated iliac DVT or the popliteal or tibial veins in patients with iliofemoral DVT.
- Under ultrasound guidance, a 0.018-in micropuncture set is used to access the target vein. In the setting of proximal obstruction, the vein is typically large and easily identified. Wire and catheter exchange is performed to upsize to a 5-Fr interventional sheath.

Baseline Phlebography

- The initial phlebogram is performed either through the interventional sheath or through a diagnostic catheter advanced to the suspected site of occlusion. When using digital subtraction angiography, a mixture of 50% Visipaque and 50% saline provides adequate volume and visualization while minimizing contrast load.
- The ease with which guidewire passage is accomplished, as well as historical information regarding duration of symptoms, informs interventional decision making. Patients with symptoms of less than 7 days duration are frequently conclusively treated with single-session pharmacomechanical thrombectomy, whereas patients with longer duration will more frequently require pretreatment with multiday courses of catheter-directed thrombolytic therapy. The initial phlebogram is instrumental in determining the course of therapy in this regard. Regardless of approach, the goal of therapy is to achieve rapid thrombus removal, minimize venous obstruction, reduce the likelihood of venous valvular damage, uncover underlying venous compression syndromes, and at least theoretically, reduce the likelihood of symptomatic recurrence.

Catheter-Directed Thrombolysis

- Until recently, catheter-directed thrombolysis has been the mainstay of interventional management for iliofemoral

DVT. Following guidewire traversal of thrombus, treatment length is determined via insertion of a marker catheter. Subsequently, an appropriately sized side-hole infusion catheter is positioned over the occluding thrombus. Infusion catheters come with infusion (perforated segment lengths) ranging from 5 to 50 cm or longer, and infusion segment length should be selected to direct infusate specifically into luminal thrombus only—for example, not into patent luminal segments where it will be rapidly dissipated into the venous and systemic circulation. Prior to initiating infusion, the multipurpose guidewire used to position the catheter is exchanged for a purpose and catheter-specific end-occlusion wire, which typically forces the infusate to exit through the side holes rather than leak out coaxially along the guidewire lumen.

- Once proper positioning is obtained, a continuous infusion of tissue plasminogen activator (tPA or alteplase, Genentech, San Francisco, CA) is initiated at the rate of 0.25 to 1.0 mg/h, depending on the extent of thrombus burden and perceived chronicity. A concurrent, coaxial heparin infusion (400-700 U/h) is administered through the sheath to prevent thrombus accumulation around the infusion system.
- Monitoring in a step-down or intensive care environment is an essential safety requirement during extended periods of catheter-directed intravenous thrombolysis outside of the catheterization laboratory. Fibrinogen levels, coagulation profile, and hematocrit are assessed every 4 to 6 hours. Typically, tPA infusion is halted if/when fibrinogen levels drop below 200 mg/dL or evidence of bleeding is present. Repeat phlebography is performed every 12 to 24 hours to assess therapeutic progress and residual thrombus load. As thrombus burden recedes, replacement catheters with shorter infusion segments are typically chosen to concentrate drug delivery within the remaining clot. Infusion rarely continues beyond 48 hours regardless of progress, as experience has demonstrated that complication rates vary directly with total tPA dosage and length of infusion. Also, infusion rates may be reduced when significant progress is noted during periodic phlebographic assessment, again to reduce risks of dosage-related bleeding complications while still pursuing complete dissolution of clot.
- Ultrasound-assisted thrombolysis using the EKOS infusion catheter (EKOS Corporation, Bothell, WA) may reduce the duration of infusion and total tPA dose. This 6-Fr catheter is also available in multiple infusion lengths and contains a core wire producing ultrasound energy that may disrupt fibrin bonds and increase tPA diffusion within thrombus. Clinical studies have demonstrated equivalent clinical outcomes with reduced infusion times using the EKOS system.

Pharmacomechanical Thrombectomy

- Pharmacomechanical thrombectomy (PMT) uses mechanical forces to assist tPA dispersion within the thrombus, typically during a single treatment session. Concurrent aspiration capabilities help remove thrombus fragments during treatment sessions. Devices currently used for this purpose in the venous system include the AngioJet catheter (MEDRAD, Warrendale, PA) and Trellis (Covidien, Mansfield, MA) infusion systems.
- The AngioJet systems comprise an infusion catheter and dedicated reusable drive unit. Radially oriented infusion ports generate high-pressure jets to disperse heparinized saline, with or without tPA, into the thrombus and an adjacent aspiration port to export fragments and debris.
- The AngioJet catheter is most commonly used in acute iliofemoral occlusion in the "power pulse" mode; in this setting, the aspiration function of the catheter is temporarily disabled, whereas tPA pulsation is delivered directly into the thrombus. Typically, 6 to 8 mg of tPA is delivered in this fashion at the beginning of a treatment session. With power pulse activated, the catheter is repeatedly advanced and withdrawn through the thrombus over the guidewire (**FIGURE 1**). After allowing the tPA to dwell for 10 to 15 minutes, the aspiration function is activated and thrombus removed to the greatest extent possible.

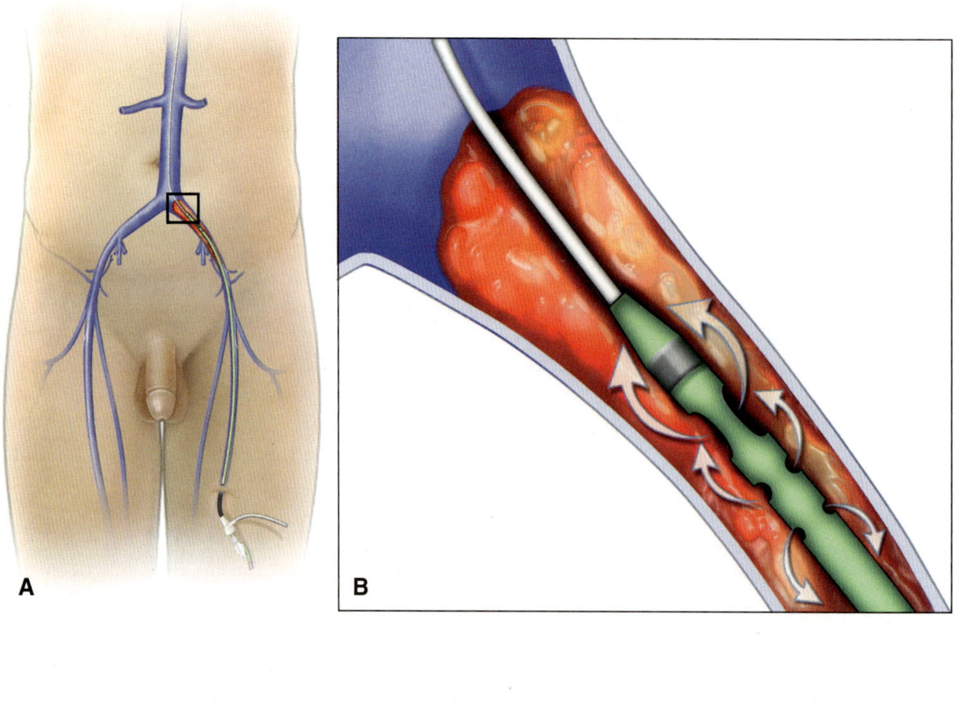

FIGURE 1 • **A,** The 6-Fr AngioJet thrombectomy catheter is useful in the treatment of DVT. This catheter is advanced through a sheath situated in the popliteal or femoral vein over a 0.035-in guidewire. The catheter has radially oriented infusion side holes that deliver saline and tPA directly into the thrombus **B,** and aspiration ports that remove dissolved thrombus and debris.

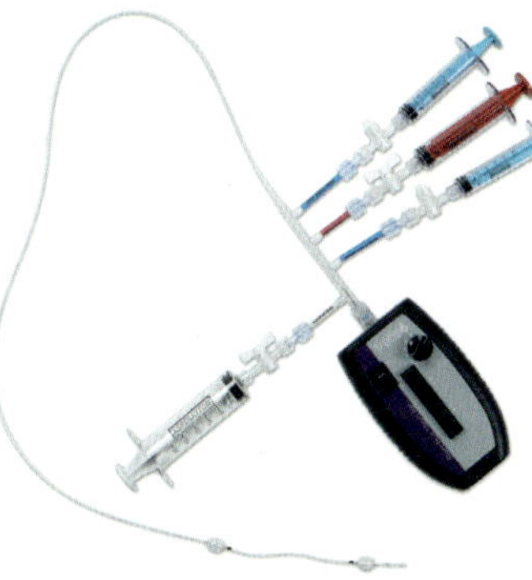

FIGURE 2 • The Trellis peripheral infusion system is an 8-Fr catheter with a single-use disposable drive unit. The catheter has compliant occlusion balloons that are inflated on either side of the treatment zone after advancing the catheter over the guidewire through the thrombus. The treatment zone of the catheter (either 15 or 30 cm length) contains both infusion side holes and aspiration ports. (©2022 Medtronic. All rights reserved. Used with the permission of Medtronic.)

- The Trellis system is composed of an infusion catheter of either 15- or 30-cm infusion length, with compliant occlusion balloons at either end of the infusion ports (FIGURE 2). Following placement over the guidewire, the end occlusion balloons are inflated in order to isolate the area of planned pharmacomechanical thrombolysis (FIGURE 3). A sinusoidal dispersion wire is then advanced through the core of the catheter and attached to a disposable drive unit, which when activated uses mechanical forces to disperse the tPA through the thrombus. After an infusion of 6 mg of tPA over the span of 10 minutes, aspiration of thrombus and debris is performed from the treated segment. The occlusion balloons concentrate tPA within the treatment segment, enabling multiple infusion and dispersal sessions during the same procedure with minimal systemic delivery of thrombolytic agent (FIGURE 4).

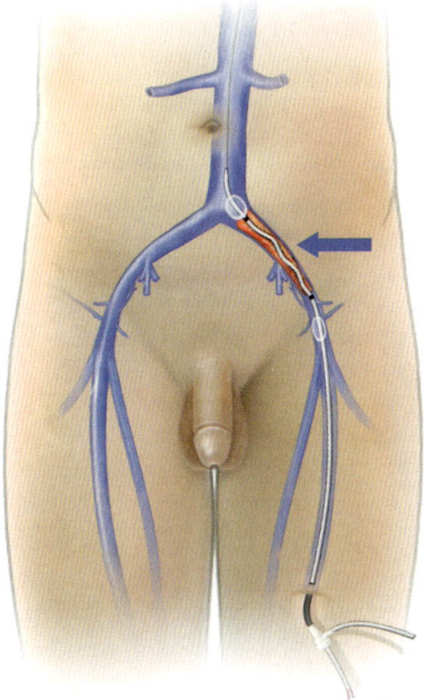

FIGURE 3 • Once the Trellis catheter is in position, the guidewire is replaced by the mechanical dispersion wire, which is attached to the drive unit and enables the treatment portion of the catheter to oscillate back and forth (*arrow*) to facilitate tPA dispersion. During the 10-minute treatment time, tPA is infused through the infusion port at a rate of 1 mg (1 mL) per minute, and following treatment, the dissolved thrombus and remaining tPA is aspirated through the aspiration port.

Stenting of Underlying Venous Stenoses or Venous Compression Syndromes

- Following clearance of acute thrombus from the iliofemoral system, underlying venous lesions that provoked DVT formation or focal external compression may become apparent on completion phlebography. These lesions should be addressed during the same treatment session to minimize the risk of recurrence. IVUS may be particularly useful in this regard.
- Although fixed stenoses may occur throughout the venous system, the most common location for extrinsic compression occurs at the point where the left common iliac vein passes beneath the overlying right common iliac artery (RCIA) (FIGURE 5). After recognizing this compression and successful removal of thrombus proximal or distal to this lesion, the stenosis may be safely resolved with stenting (FIGURE 6). This is best performed by upsizing the interventional sheath to at least 10 Fr followed by deployment of a self-expanding, braided, stainless steel Wallstent (Boston Scientific, Watertown, MA). In conjunction with completion venography, IVUS is then used to quantify the extent of residual compression.

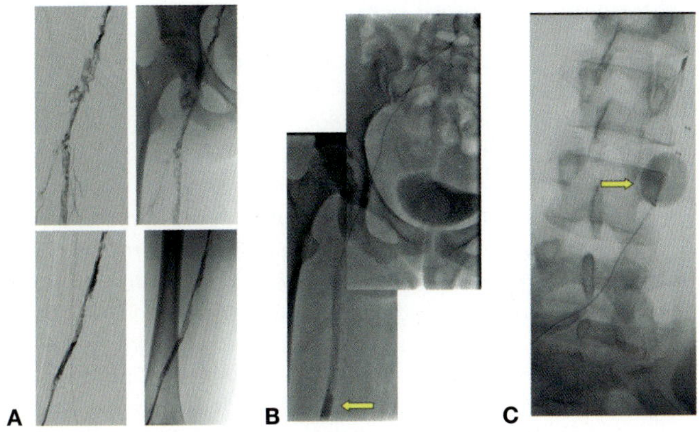

FIGURE 4 • Patient with left iliofemoral venous thrombosis secondary to May-Thurner syndrome. Note the extensive thrombus within the iliac and femoral veins **(A)**. **B and C,** The patient is being treated in the prone position through popliteal vein access. The Trellis catheter has been inserted and advanced through the thrombus, and the occlusion balloons are inflated on either side of the treatment zone (*arrows*). Note the oscillating dispersion wire that improves tPA delivery during infusion.

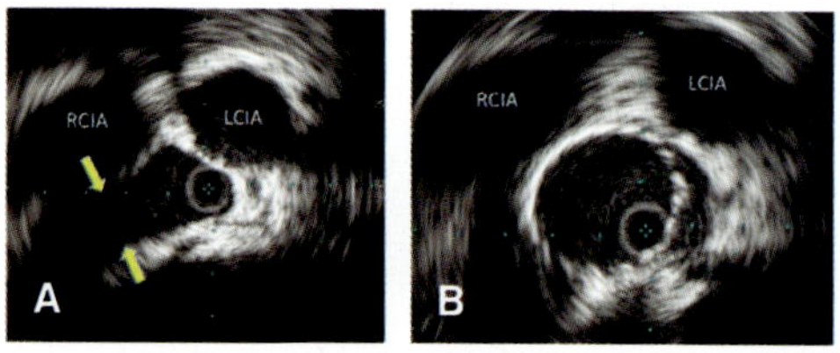

FIGURE 5 • Intravascular ultrasound is the most sensitive assessment tool for detecting May-Thurner compression of the left common iliac vein. **A,** The RCIA is lying directly over and compressing the left common iliac vein (between *yellow arrows*). **B,** Following stenting of the left common iliac vein, there is complete resolution of the compression by the RCIA.

- Stent diameter is chosen based on IVUS-obtained measurements, but diameters commonly chosen for common iliac vein placement in May-Thurner patients range from 16 to 20 mm. In this application, it is important to choose longer stents that provide additional surface apposition in the common or even external iliac veins to present stent dislodgement and migration. Wallstents are particularly appropriate in this regard as they will shorten or extend in proportion to the ultimate treatment diameter and feature exposed wires at either end to optimize vein wall engagement.
- Once appropriately sited and deployed, poststent dilation is necessary to ensure optimal deployment and migration resistance. Some discomfort will be experienced by the "awake" patient during these procedures, and stenting molding should be guided by patient tolerance under these circumstances.

Completion Imaging

- Completion phlebography documents resolution of target stenosis and reciprocal reduction in collateral venous flow.

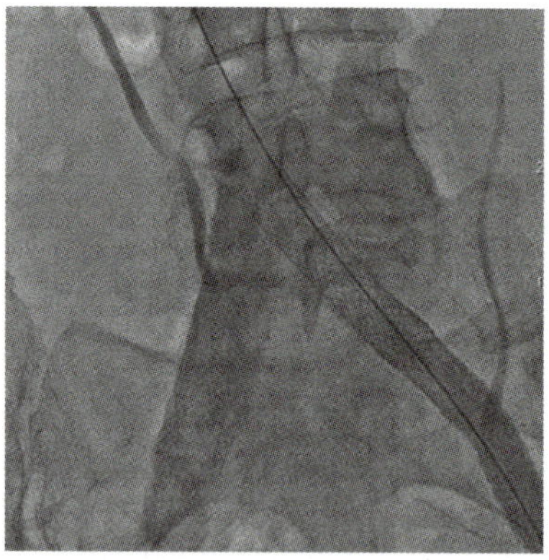

FIGURE 6 • Stenting of the left common iliac vein for May-Thurner syndrome is performed with a braided self-expanding stainless steel stent, usually in diameters ranging from 16 to 20 mm.

- The presence of persistent collaterals suggests residual venous stenosis or compression; IVUS should be reperformed in this circumstance to confirm wall apposition and stent expansion. Repeat balloon dilation may be necessary in these circumstances until sufficient expansion is achieved.

Closure of the Femoral Vein Access

- Following sheath removal, manual pressure is held over the venous puncture site. Closure devices are not appropriate or indicated for management of venous access.
- Patients need to remain supine for at least 1 hour following sheath removal.
- Therapeutic intravenous anticoagulation with unfractionated heparin is initiated at the completion of the procedure. Maintenance of full anticoagulation without interruption throughout the early postoperative period is imperative to procedural success.

OPERATIVE MANAGEMENT OF ILIOFEMORAL DEEP VEIN THROMBOSIS

Iliac Venous Thrombectomy

- For most clinical scenarios, open venous thrombectomy has largely been supplanted by the interventional, image-guided techniques described in the preceding sections. In patients with limb-threatening phlegmasia cerulean dolens or those with contraindications to lytic therapy or contrast administration, open surgical thrombectomy remains an effective and necessary treatment modality.
- Whenever possible, surgical thrombectomy is performed under general anesthesia with positive pressure ventilation to reduce the risk of intraoperative PE.
- A vertical inguinal incision is made to allow exposure and control of the CFV, femoral vein, saphenofemoral junction, and the profunda femoris vein. Once these venous structures have been exposed, the patient is systemically anticoagulated with 100 U/kg of intravenous heparin.
- A longitudinal venotomy is made in the CFV, and a no. 8 or no. 10 venous thrombectomy catheter is then passed up to the level of the common iliac vein and thrombectomy is performed. Attempts are made to clear the majority of the iliac thrombus before passing the thrombectomy catheter into the vena cava in order to reduce the likelihood of pulmonary embolization.
- Back-bleeding may not be present due to competent iliac vein valves, or back-bleeding can occur from the hypogastric vein even without clearance of the thrombus within the common iliac vein. Therefore, back-bleeding should not be used as an indicator of effective thrombus clearance and venography should be performed as a routine after completion of iliac and infrainguinal thrombectomy.

Infrainguinal Femoral Venous Thrombectomy

- Following iliac venous thrombectomy, heparinized saline should be used to flush the iliac vein, the proximal external iliac vein (or distal CFV) should be clamped, and then any thrombus at the proximal (peripheral) aspect of the venotomy should be extracted with forceps.
- Infrainguinal thrombus can then be removed by manual massage or by exsanguinating the leg with an Esmarch bandage, sequentially applied from the foot to the groin, with sufficient overlap to provide continuous compression (**FIGURE 7**). Clot is delivered through the venotomy at the groin.
- Balloon thrombectomy can be performed using a no. 3 thrombectomy catheter passed from the venotomy in the CFV in a retrograde fashion down toward the popliteal

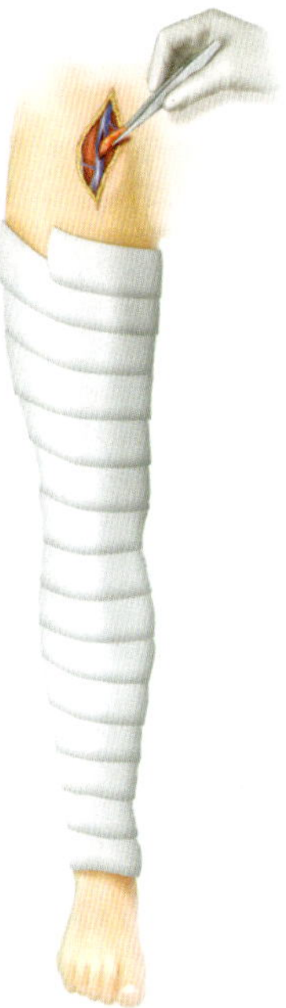

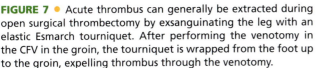

FIGURE 7 • Acute thrombus can generally be extracted during open surgical thrombectomy by exsanguinating the leg with an elastic Esmarch tourniquet. After performing the venotomy in the CFV in the groin, the tourniquet is wrapped from the foot up to the groin, expelling thrombus through the venotomy.

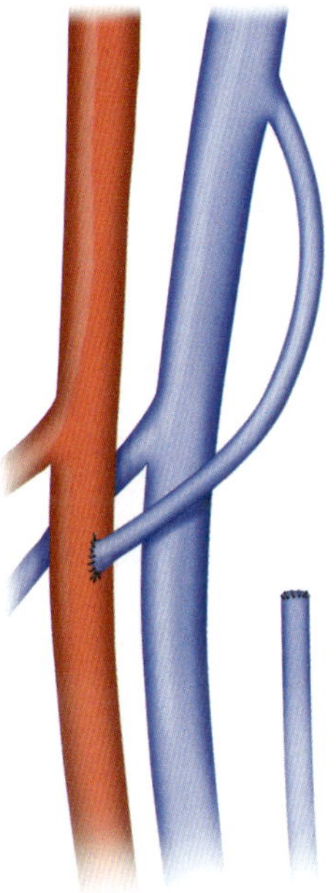

FIGURE 8 • Patency rate following open surgical thrombectomy is significantly improved by creation of an AVF. Following thrombectomy of the iliac and femoral veins, the venotomy is closed with running monofilament suture and an end-to-side anastomosis is created between the saphenous vein and superficial femoral artery.

and tibial veins. Following thrombectomy, the infrainguinal venous circulation should be flushed vigorously with heparinized saline before closure of the venotomy.

- If infrainguinal thrombus persists after thrombectomy, additional techniques for thrombus removal include on-table tPA administration. For on-table tPA administration, 6 mg of alteplase in 200 mL saline is infused retrograde into the femoral vein through the venotomy in the CFV, then the vein is clamped and the solution is allowed to dwell for 10 to 30 minutes.
- If the infrainguinal venous thrombectomy is not successful due to chronic thrombus in the femoral vein, the femoral vein is then ligated below the profunda, and balloon thrombectomy is then performed on the profunda vein and its branches.
- After open thrombectomy is complete, the venotomy is closed with running continuous monofilament suture, avoiding postclosure stricture of the CFV by precision suture placement. If narrowing is apparent, vein or bovine pericardial patch angioplasty may be performed as necessary to restore luminal diameter.

Adjunct Arteriovenous Fistula Creation

- Rates of rethrombosis following surgical thrombectomy can be as high as 80%. Creation of an arteriovenous fistula (AVF) may significantly reduce this risk and is incorporated in the procedure by most surgeons.
- The same groin incision may be employed for AVF creation, transposing the proximal segment of the ipsilateral greater saphenous vein to the superficial femoral artery (**FIGURE 8**).
- Surgical ligation or interventional occlusion of the AVF is ultimately required for optimal long-term outcome, usually employed within 6 weeks following the procedure. Documented patency of the venous system should be demonstrated on follow-up duplex imaging. Failure to close this fistula may result in significant long-term limb and cardiovascular complications, and follow-up is essential to ensure that this part of the procedure is completed.
- Open thrombectomy procedures by their nature are associated with significant blood loss from the central venous system, and preparations should be made both to crossmatch and bank sufficient packed red blood cells, as well as employ operative scavenging systems to recycle and reinfuse lost blood to ensure that appropriate hemodynamic conditions may be maintained throughout the procedure.

Completion Imaging

- Completion venography of the iliac venous system should be performed following open surgical thrombectomy to assess the adequacy of the thrombectomy.
- Following closure of the venotomy and reestablishment of venous flow through the iliofemoral venous system, an 18-gauge access needle and guidewire can be used to puncture the CFV and place a 5-Fr sheath. Contrast injection directly through this sheath is performed to evaluate the iliac veins and assess for residual thrombus. Following venography, the sheath is removed, and a single monofilament stitch can be used to close the puncture site.

Wound Closure

- A careful search for any transected lymphatics should be conducted prior to wound closure.
- A closed suction drain should be placed in the groin wound to prevent seroma formation.
- The wound is then closed with multilayered running absorb able sutures for hemostatic and lymphostatic closure.

POSTOPERATIVE CARE

- Following open surgical thrombectomy, full therapeutic anticoagulation is imperative to prevent rethrombosis. An intravenous heparin infusion is immediately initiated and maintained for 24 to 48 hours before the patient is transitioned to oral anticoagulation with a low-molecular-weight heparin bridge prior to discharge.
- Ambulation should begin on the first postoperative day. Patients may usually be discharged within 48 to 72 hours following thrombectomy.
- On discharge, the patient should be placed in elastic compression stockings (30- to 40-mm Hg ankle gradient), and the importance of compression should be stressed to the patient in the discharge instructions.

OUTCOMES

Endovascular Intervention

- Pharmacomechanical venous thrombectomy provides clinical success rates of 70% to 100% and may reduce the incidence of the PTS, although this latter conclusion remains controversial.
- Following successful procedures, long-term venous patency is reported at 84% in 5 years.
- Valvular competence is preserved at 80% in 5 years and 56% in 10 years in recent series.

Surgical Thrombectomy

- Surgical thrombectomy provides long-term iliac venous patency, with rates approaching 80% when combined with inclusion of a temporary AVF.
- At 5 years, over one-third of patients can be expected to be symptom free and have retained valvular competence.

REFERENCES

1. Vedantham S, Grassi CJ, Ferral H, et al. Reporting standards for endovascular treatment of lower extremity deep vein thrombosis. *J Vasc Intervent Radiol.* 2005;17:417-434.
2. Kahn SR, Ginsberg JS. Relationship between deep venous thrombosis and the postthrombotic syndrome. *Arch Intern Med.* 2004;164:17-26.
3. Porter JM, Moneta GL. Reporting standards in venous disease: an update. International consensus committee on chronic venous disease. *J Vasc Surg.* 1995;21:635-645.
4. Rutherford RB, Padberg FT, Comerota AJ, et al. Venous severity scoring: an adjunct to venous outcome assessment. *J Vasc Surg.* 2000;31:1307-1312.
5. Prandoni P, Lensing AW, Prins MH, et al. Below-knee elastic compression stockings to prevent the postthrombotic syndrome. *Ann Intern Med.* 2004;141:249-256.
6. Brandjes DP, Buller HR, Heijboer H, et al. Randomized trial of effect of compression stockings in patients with symptomatic proximal-vein thrombosis. *Lancet.* 1997;349:759-762.
7. Delis KT, Bountouroglou D, Mansfield AO. Venous claudication in iliofemoral thrombosis: long-term effects on venous hemodynamics, clinical status, and quality of life. *Ann Surg.* 2004;239:118-126.
8. Kearon C, Ginsberg JS, Hirsh J. The role of venous ultrasonography in the diagnosis of suspected deep venous thrombosis and pulmonary embolism. *Ann Intern Med.* 1998;129:1044-1049.
9. Weinmann EE, Salzman EW. Deep-vein thrombosis. *N Engl J Med.* 1994;15:1630-1641.
10. Zontsich T, Turetschek K, Baldt M. CT-phlebography. A new method for the diagnosis of venous thrombosis of the upper and lower extremities. *Radiology.* 1998;38:586-590.
11. Burke B, Sostman HD, Carroll BA, et al. The diagnostic approach to deep venous thrombosis. Which technique? *Clin Chest Med.* 1995;16:253-268.
12. Allie DE, Hebert CJ, Lirtzman MD, et al. Novel simultaneous combination chemical thrombolysis/rheolytic thrombectomy therapy for acute limb ischemia: the power pulse spray technique. *Catheter Cardiovasc Interv.* 2004;63(4):512-522.

Chapter 37

Vena Cava Filter Placement and Removal

Courtney M. Morgan and John E. Rectenwald

DEFINITION

- An inferior vena cava (IVC) filter is a device designed to filter venous blood returning to the right-sided heart and prevent large venous thrombi from the lower extremities and vena cava below the IVC filter from reaching the pulmonary arteries. Venous thrombus reaching the pulmonary arteries (pulmonary embolus, PE) can inhibit oxygenation of blood in the pulmonary capillaries and venous return to the left-sided heart resulting in a decreased arterial oxygen saturation. In addition, pulmonary emboli increase pulmonary artery pressures resulting in pulmonary hypertension and right heart strain or failure. The combination of these two phenomena may result in significant morbidity and mortality in those in which it occurs.
- Inferior vena cava filters are made from various metal alloys including iron, chromium and nickel (stainless steel), nickel and titanium (Nitinol), or cobalt chromium alloy (Elgiloy). They are generally designed in a classic conical design (**FIGURE 1**) although alternative variations exist. The conical design is very efficient and allows up to 70% of the cone volume to be occupied with thrombus with only a 50% obstruction of cross-sectional area of the IVC. In addition, it allows captured thrombus to be centered within the vena cava, thus allowing venous flow around the clot to facilitate thrombolysis.[1] IVC filters are all designed to be placed within the vena cava through a transvenous route primarily by the internal jugular or common femoral venous route. IVC filters are generally designed to be oversized compared to the IVC at rest and are therefore held in place in the IVC by a combination of the radial force and the presence of hooks at the ends of the filter struts that penetrate the wall of the vena cava.

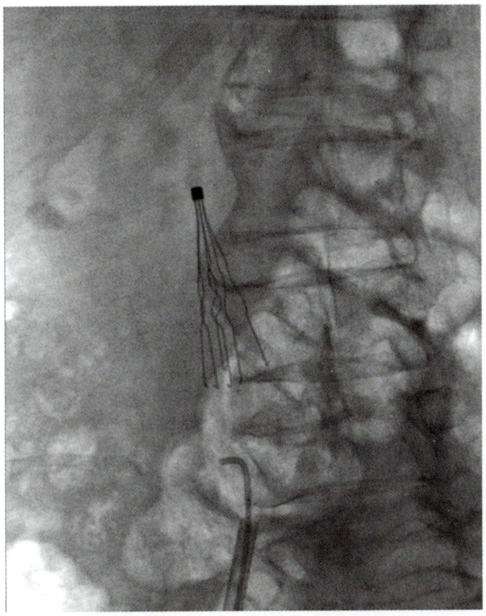

FIGURE 1 • A Greenfield Stainless Steel over-the-wire inferior vena cava filter demonstrating the classic conical design structure. This design allows maximal capture of thrombus while retaining IVC patency as well as promoting venous blood flow around the thrombus to facilitate thrombolysis.

Types of IVC Filters

- Permanent filters, as the name implies, originally developed in the 1960s to 1970s, are intended to be placed in patients indefinitely and are designed to provide life-long filtration, with features that allow maximal fixation to the vena cava intimal surface and promote tissue ingrowth. Permanent IVC filters include the Greenfield Stainless Steel filter (Boston Scientific, MA. USA), the VenaTech LP filter (B. Braun, PA, USA), the TrapEase filter (Cordis, FL, USA), the Simon Nitinol filter (B. Braun, PA, USA), and the Bird's Nest filter (Cook Medical, IN, USA) (**FIGURE 2**).
- Retrievable IVC filters, developed in the early 2000s, are filters that are intentionally designed for removal once the patient no longer needs IVC filtration for the prevention of PE. They are specifically designed to be reconstrained and removed and frequently have hooks incorporated into their designs to facilitate loop ensnarement of the filter and subsequent retrieval. As detailed below, these design features are thought to contribute to the increased complication rates associated with retrievable filters. Examples of currently available retrievable IVC filters include the Günther Tulip and Celect filters (Cook Medical, IN, USA), OptEase filter (Cordis FL, USA), the Option ELITE filter (Argon Medical, TX, USA), the Denali Filter (Bard Medical, NJ, USA) (**FIGURE 3**), and ALN filter (KM Medical, MA, USA).
- Convertible IVC filters are a relatively new concept the first of which only being released in the last few years. This category of IVC filters are intended to be placed permanently but only provide temporary IVC filtration. They convert from an IVC filter to what is essentially a caval stent by means of an absorbable suture or cap that can be removed percutaneously. Examples of this category of IVC filters includes the Sentry Bioconvertible filter (Boston Scientific, MA, USA) and the VenaTech Convertible filter (B. Braun, PA, USA) (**FIGURE 4**). All retrievable and convertible IVC filters are approved by the US Food and Drug Administration for permanent use.

IVC Filter Retrieval

- The rationale for removal of IVC filters has evolved over time. In 1998, PREPIC, a prospective, randomized study that compared patients with IVC filters in place to anticoagulation concluded that patients with filters were at lower risk for symptomatic PE but elevated risk of recurrent deep

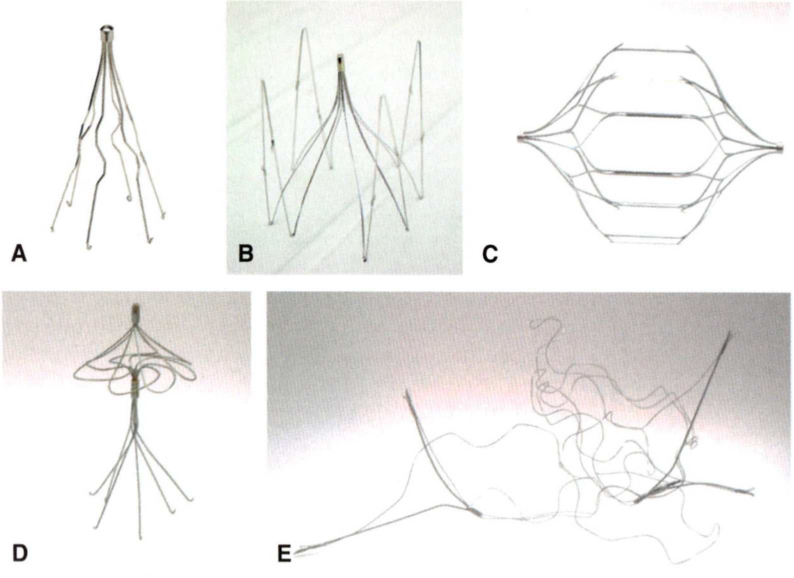

FIGURE 2 • FDA-approved Permanent IVC filters. From left to right: **A,** Boston Scientific Greenfield Stainless Steel over-the-wire filter **B,** B. Braun Vena Tech LP filter; **C,** Cordis Trapease Filter; **D,** BD Interventional Systems, Simon Nitinol Filter; and **E,** Cook Medical Cook Medical Gianturco-Roehm Bird Nest filter. (A, Image provided courtesy of Boston Scientific. Copyright © 2022 Boston Scientific Corporation or its affiliates. All rights reserved. B, © Aesculap AG. C, Cordis, Miami Lakes, FL. D and E, Courtesy of Cook Medical.)

vein thrombosis (DVT).[2] This finding, combined with the data suggesting that risk of death from venous thromboembolism (VTE) is highest in the first 2 weeks after occurrence,[3] spurred the development of IVC filters that could be retrieved to allow for protection from PE when at risk early in the course of VTE and then removed to decrease the risk of recurrent DVT. While this was the intent of retrievable IVC filter, in practicality very few (as low as 5%) of these retrievable filters were actually retrieved.[4-6]

- Recently, the FDA published two safety communications regarding retrievable IVC filters based on analysis of the poor long-term performance of retrievable filters observed in the FDA's Manufacturer and User Facility Device Experience database.[7] Retrievable filters appeared to have significantly higher rates of complications when compared to traditional, permanent IVC filters. The first of these communications, published in August of 2010, recommended that "implanting physicians and clinicians responsible for the ongoing care of

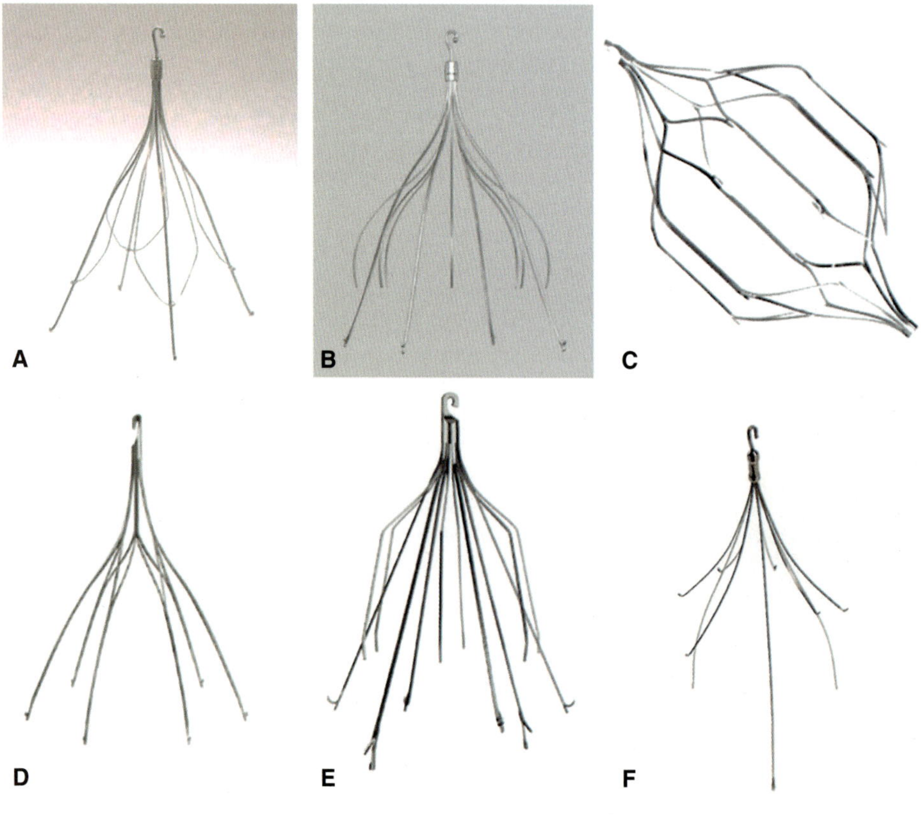

FIGURE 3 • FDA-approved Retrievable IVC filters. From left to right. **A,** Cook Medical Günther Tulip filter; **B,** Cook Medical Celect Platinum filter; **C,** Cordis Optease Filter; **D,** Argon Medical Devices Option ELITE filter; **E,** BD Interventional Systems Denali filter; and **F,** ALN Optional Filter with hook. (A and B, Courtesy of Cook Medical. C, Cordis, Miami Lakes, FL. D, Argon Medical. E, Courtesy and © Becton, Dickinson and Company. F, Used with permission from ALN.)

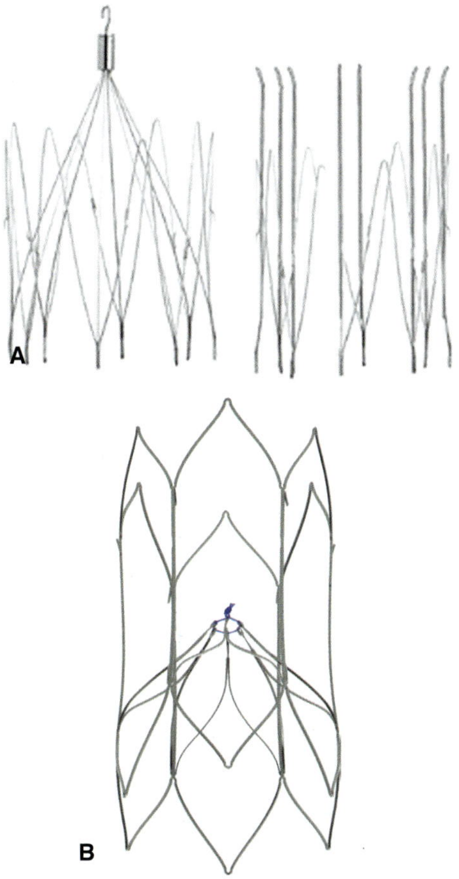

FIGURE 4 • FDA-approved Convertible IVC filters. **A,** B. Braun Vena Tech Convertible filter, and **B,** Boston Scientific Sentry Bioconvertible filter. (A, © Aesculap AG. B, Image provided courtesy of Boston Scientific. Copyright © 2022 Boston Scientific Corporation or its affiliates. All rights reserved.)

patients with retrievable IVC filters consider removing the filter as soon as protection from PE is no longer needed." In May of 2014, the second FDA safety alert letter was published regarding its own decision-analysis regarding IVC filter removal in patients without pulmonary embolism. Based on this analysis, this alert recommends that if the retrievable filter is no longer needed it should be removed between 29 and 54 days after implantation. Based on the FDA's model, the risks of the presence of an IVC filter outweigh the benefits after this time interval.[8]

DIFFERENTIAL DIAGNOSIS

- Patients who are candidates for IVC filters generally present with the signs and symptoms of VTE. These may include unilateral extremity swelling and pain or bilateral lower extremity edema in the case of extensive iliofemoral DVT.
- Patients who suffer PE frequently experience sudden pleuritic chest pain associated with shortness of breath, hypoxia, and signs of right-sided heart failure.
- The diagnosis of VTE can be readily established by assessing for risk factors of VTE and ruling out other potential causes such as lymphedema, chronic venous insufficiency, or cellulitis in the case of extremity DVT and pneumonia, myocardial infarction, pericarditis, and others in the case of pulmonary embolus.

PATIENT HISTORY AND PHYSICAL FINDINGS

- In the United States, DVT occurs in approximately 1 per 1000 people each year. Nearly one-third of patients with symptomatic untreated DVT present with PE.[9] Anticoagulation is the treatment of choice for most cases of VTE, with evidence-based guidelines supporting the use of a vena cava filter when anticoagulation is not possible due to contraindications to anticoagulation or hemorrhagic complications, recurrent PE despite therapeutic anticoagulation, or an inability to achieve therapeutic anticoagulation.[10]
- Expanded indications for prophylactic use of IVC filters are based on clinical factors that place a patient at high risk for both PE and bleeding, making the use of prophylactic anticoagulation for prevention of VTE prohibitive.[11]
- Likewise, relative indications for filter placement include poor compliance with anticoagulation, free-floating iliocaval thrombus, renal cell carcinoma with extension into the renal vein and vena cava, thrombolysis or thromboembolectomy of the iliofemoral veins or IVC, and risk of recurrent PE with pre-existing pulmonary hypertension or limited cardiopulmonary reserve.
- Filter placement may also be considered after DVT in patients with cancer, burns, and pregnancy or for prophylaxis in multitrauma patients, including those with severe closed head injury (Glasgow Coma Scale score <8), spinal cord injury, complex pelvic or multiple long-bone fractures, intra-abdominal injury, pelvic or retroperitoneal hematoma, and ocular trauma.
- Contraindications to vena cava filter placement are few and include chronic occlusion or significant compression of the vena cava and agenesis of the vena cava.
- Upper extremity DVT is becoming more common with the increasing use of central venous lines (particularly peripherally inserted central catheters or P.I.C.C. lines), pacemakers, and implantable defibrillators, with an estimated risk of PE approaching 9% in some series.[12] Standard treatment involves anticoagulation, but with contraindications or complications arising from anticoagulation, superior vena cava (SVC) filter placement can be considered.
    - Since there are no filters specifically designed for placement in the SVC, an adaptation of current IVC filter and available techniques is required. A conical filter with a filter leg hook attachment is most appropriate that these are placed at the confluence of the innominate veins. Filter length should be considered to prevent protrusion into the right atrium. Filter placement is not recommended within an SVC with a diameter >28 to 30 mm.

IMAGING AND OTHER DIAGNOSTIC STUDIES

- In general, there are no required imaging studies prior to placing an IVC filter. This is due to the fact that an IVC venogram is performed at the time of IVC filter placement.

Despite this, the vast majority of patients in which IVC filters are being considered have already had computed tomography (CT) scans or other imaging previously. These studies can be reviewed with special attention paid to the appearance of the common femoral and iliac veins as well as that of the inferior vena cava. Noting the location of the lowest renal vein in relation to the adjacent vertebral bodies can also be a helpful maneuver.

- In patients with renal insufficiency or severe iodinated contrast allergy, alternative contrast agents such as carbon dioxide (CO_2)[13-15] and even gadolinium[13,16] can be used to define and evaluate the IVC and other structures immediately prior to IVC filter placement (**FIGURE 5**). These alternatives to iodinate contrast agents allow for evaluation of IVC patency, presence and location of thrombus, caval anatomy, and location of the renal veins.
- The use of both intravenous[17,18] and transabdominal ultrasound[19,20] for IVC filter placement has become more mainstream. These techniques allow for filter placement without the use of x-ray or contrast agents and are especially well suited for intensive care patients who cannot be easily transported to the fluoroscopy suite for the procedure.[18,21]

SURGICAL MANAGEMENT

Preoperative Planning

- The patient is examined and a thorough history is completed. A review of the indications for filter placement should be conducted prior to filter placement. Based on the clinical scenario, either a permanent or a retrievable filter should be selected for use.

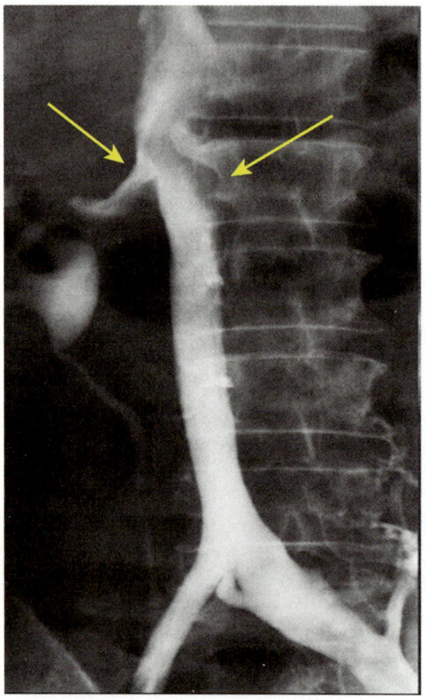

FIGURE 5 • An example of the use of alternative contrast agent for real-time imaging of the vena cava for IVC filter placement. This carbon dioxide (CO_2) inferior vena cavagram well demonstrates the bilateral iliac veins, the inferior vena cava, and the bilateral renal veins (*yellow arrows*).

- Central venous catheters that may be present at the proposed site of access or that extend across the intended location for filter deployment should be removed.
- Coagulopathy or other hematologic issues should be assessed. Discontinuation of anticoagulation before the procedure should be considered based on clinical indication and hemorrhagic risk profile.
- Preoperative imaging studies such as duplex ultrasound or available computed tomography (CT) images, if available, should be reviewed to identify anatomic vena cava variants or other venous anomalies that could potentially alter the treatment plan. During filter placement, selective venography may also help to identify venous anomalies. In this regard, accessory renal veins, retroaortic, and circumferential left renal vein anomalies (5%-7%) are the most common anatomic variation but do not affect filter position. Transposition of the vena cava to the left side with drainage into the left renal vein is rare (0.2%-0.5%) but necessitates accurate anatomic definition. Duplication of the vena cava is also rare (0.2%-0.3%), with the right-sided IVC draining the right iliac vein and right renal vein, whereas the left-sided IVC drains the left iliac veins and joins the left renal vein where it crosses over into the right-sided vena cava. Undiagnosed duplication of the IVC may leave the duplicated vena cava unprotected against PE and would require either separate filters in each vena cava or a suprarenal filter placed above the junction of the left renal vein and the right-sided vena cava. Agenesis of the vena cava is extremely rare, but when present, filter insertion should be avoided, although filter placement into an enlarged azygous segment has been described.[22]
- A preprocedure duplex ultrasound should be obtained to evaluate the presence of venous thrombosis at the intended percutaneous access site or extending into iliofemoral or vena cava. Jugular venous access may be needed if femoral vein access is not possible. A vena cavagram should be performed just before positioning and deployment of a filter to assess the presence and location of any thrombus within the vena cava. The presence of thrombus in the infrarenal IVC may necessitate suprarenal filter placement.
- Ultrasound-guided percutaneous access is generally recommended to allow for direct visualization of the access vein and real-time image guidance for venous cannulation, as well as to avoid concomitant arterial injury.
- The diameter of the IVC, including major and minor axes, should be measured either from venography, transabdominal duplex ultrasound, intravascular ultrasound (IVUS), or a preprocedure CT scan to assist in appropriate filter selection. Vena cava diameter measurements can vary depending on intravascular fluid status and respiratory variation. Vena cava geometry can also range from circular to elliptical.[18] Major and minor axes both should be measured. Nearly all current FDA-approved filters are indicated for vena cava diameters of less than 28 to 30 mm. In patients with a "megacava" defined as a vena cava with diameters larger than 30 mm, a Bird Nest IVC filter can be used within the enlarged IVC. If a Bird Nest IVC filter is not immediately available, either bilateral iliac vein IVC filters or placement for a filter within the suprarenal vena cava (if <30 mm in diameter) can be considered.

- Accurate identification of both renal and common iliac veins is important before filter deployment. The tip of the filter should be positioned at, or below, the lowest renal vein after confirmation of adequate clearance of the filter base above the iliac vein confluence.

Positioning

- The patient is brought to the endovascular suite and placed supine on a radiolucent table.
- If the procedure is being done in the operating room, the patient should be positioned on the radiolucent operating table such that the portable C-arm can be maneuvered over the patient's groin and abdomen for sufficient fluoroscopic visualization of the femoral and iliac vessels as well as the inferior vena cava.
- The patient's arms are placed at their sides and secured to facilitate imaging of the upper abdomen for filter placement.
- If the IVC filter is being delivered via the internal jugular vein, a shoulder roll should be placed beneath the patient's scapulae and the neck extended. In addition, the patient's head should be rotated to the contralateral side. These manipulations better position the internal jugular vein for access.
- In an obese patient, retraction of the abdominal pannus from the groin onto the abdomen can facilitate access of the common femoral vein.

INFERIOR VENA CAVA FILTER PLACEMENT FROM THE GROIN

- The site of puncture is first surveyed with duplex ultrasound to identify the access vessel, nearby structures and assure patency of the vein. The site is then prepped and surgically draped appropriately.
- Local anesthesia is obtained with 1% lidocaine injection over the site of puncture and into the subcutaneous tissues. Conscious sedation can also be utilized if appropriate.
- The right common femoral vein is access with either a 21-gauge micropuncture set or a 19-gauge single-wall puncture needle. The left common femoral vein can also be used for filter placement, however, this approach is less of a straight shot to the IVC and can result in a deployed IVC filter with significantly more tilt.
- After successful access of the common femoral vein, a 0.035 inch "J" or Bentson wire is then advanced through the micropuncture sheath or single-wall puncture needle into the vein and advanced into the inferior vena cava.
- Once the guidewire is in position, a 6-Fr sheath is placed over the wire to secure hemostatic venous access. A 5-Fr marker flush catheter is then advanced over the wire and positioned in the cephalad portion right iliac vein just below the confluence of the inferior vena cava. Many IVC filter manufacturers have designed their IVC filter delivery catheters/sheaths such that the inner dilator functions as a flush catheter and recommend placement of the sheath directly thus skipping this step. The authors choose not to do this as the use of a 6-Fr sheath and flush catheter avoids the risk of unnecessarily opening the IVC filter packaging in the event that an IVC filter cannot be placed such as an occluded IVC for thrombus in the vena cava where the filter is to be positioned.
- An initial contrast venography is performed through a flush catheter or filter delivery sheath to define anatomy and confirm absence of thrombus. A marker or calibrated catheter is positioned at or just below the confluence of the IVC and iliac veins, and a power injection of 20 mL/sec of contrast for 2 seconds for a total of 40 mL ("20 for 40") should confirm normal vena cava and iliac vein relationships. Performance of a breath hold or vagal maneuver will augment filling of the cava. The marker flush catheter facilitates accurate measurement of the diameter of the IVC.
- The inferior vena cava venogram is then carefully reviewed. Special note is made of any thrombus within the vena cava and its location. The contralateral common iliac vein is visualized to confirm normal caval anatomy. The diameter of the IVC is measured with the marker flush catheter to assure that the diameter is not greater than 28 to 30 mm. Finally, the renal veins are identified either directly by contrast refluxed into the vessels or indirectly but the mixing of uncontrasted blood from the renal veins with contrasted blood from the blood within the IVC. The level of the lowest renal vein is then related to a bony anatomic landmark, usually an endplate of a lumbar vertebral body or a vertebral disc space.
- Selection of an IVC filter oriented to the specific approach is essential. In this case, a *femoral*-oriented IVC filter should be selected. Use of a *jugular*-oriented IVC filter from the femoral approach will result in a maldeployed or "up-side down" filter. Review of the device instructions for use is essential. Depending on the specific filter device used, the deployment sequence and technique can vary. Understanding sheath and delivery catheter interactions is essential for successful and accurate deployment of each filter type.
- In general, however, once the IVC filter package is opened and the IVC filter and delivery catheter is flushed, the 5-Fr flush catheter is removed over a stiff 0.035 wire (such as an Amplatz). The skin incision and venotomy are then serially dilated to the size of the delivery sheath. This ranges from 7 to 9 Fr for most devices. The IVC filter delivery sheath is advanced over the wire and positioned appropriately.
- The wire and inner dilator for the filter delivery sheath is removed and the IVC filter with its delivery catheter is advanced into and secured to the filter delivery sheath.
- The authors prefer to have the filter delivery sheath advanced above the level of filter deployment so that the filter can be advanced to the level of deployment within the delivery sheath. The delivery sheath can then be retracted exposing the filter for deployment. This method avoids retracting or worse advancing the exposed IVC filter. Advancing the exposed IVC filter without the benefit of wire guidance risks perforation of the IVC and maldeployment of the IVC filter (**FIGURE 6**).

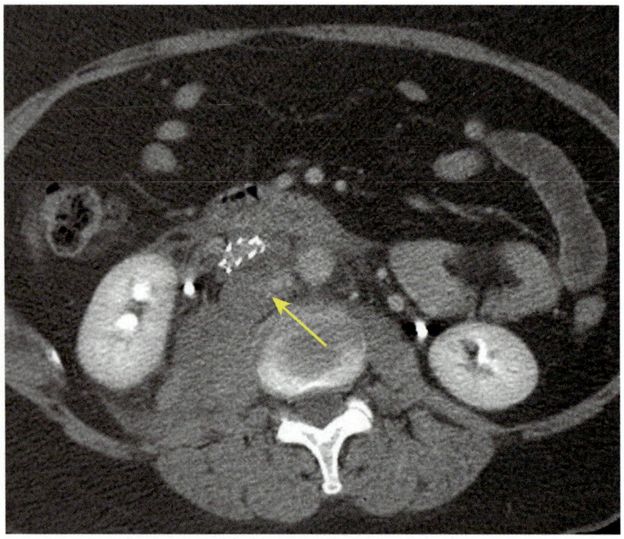

FIGURE 6 • A computed tomographic venogram demonstrating inferior vena cava perforation and surrounding hematoma (*yellow arrow*) after infrarenal IVC filter placement. The filter and IVC are patent but compressed by the resulting retroperitoneal hematoma.

- Once the filter is in the correct position based upon landmarks established on review of the IVC venogram, the filter is deployed according to the manufacturer's instruction for use. Actual deployment of the filter can be accomplished by simple retraction of the deployment sheath over the IVC filter or exposure of the IVC filter and then deployment via a "pin and pull" technique.
- Once the IVC filter has been successfully deployed and is in position, the delivery sheath and catheter are retracted caudally and magnified anterior-posterior and orthogonal single shot x-ray images are obtained. These images are carefully reviewed to assure that the IVC filter has been fully and correctly deployed without crossing of the filter tines or significant tilting with in the vena cava.
- Following successful deployment of an IVC filter, all wires and catheters are removed and pressure is held at the femoral venotomy site until hemostasis is achieved. A sterile dressing is placed and the patient is taken back to the postoperative care unit and remains flat for 4 hours. The patient is then taken back to their inpatient unit or allowed to ambulate and then discharged home.

INFERIOR VENA CAVA FILTER PLACEMENT FROM THE NECK

For the sake of brevity, identical steps in placement of an IVC filter from the internal jugular vein that are identical to placement from the common femoral vein are omitted or truncated.

- As previously mentioned, a shoulder roll is placed beneath the patient scapulae and the neck extended. The patient's head is then rotated toward the opposite side of the site of access.
- The site of puncture is first surveyed with duplex ultrasound to identify the access vessel, nearby structures and assure patency of the vein. The site is then prepped and surgically draped appropriately.
- The right jugular vein is access with either a 21-gauge micropuncture set or a 19 gauge single-wall puncture needle after the area is anesthetized. A 0.035 inch "J" or Bentson wire is then advanced through the micropuncture sheath or needle into the vein and advanced into the inferior vena cava. This may require fluoroscopic guidance and the use of an angled catheter to guide the wire and traverse the right atrium, avoid the right-heart and gain access to the IVC. If catheter guidance is require for traversal of the right heart, then the 6 Fr. sheath is placed at this time with the guide wire within the right atrium or ventricle. Care is taken to monitor the patient's cardiac telemetry and retract the guide wire or catheter if cardiac arrhythmias are observed.
- Once the guidewire is in position and a sheath is in place, the marker flush catheter is advanced into the right or left iliac vein just below the confluence of the inferior vena cava. Again, the IVC filter delivery sheath with the specially designed flush inner dilator can be used instead.
- A power injection of 20 mL/sec of contrast for 2 seconds for a total of 40 mL ("20 for 40") is injected for the vena cavagram prior to IVC filter placement.
- The inferior vena cava venogram is then carefully reviewed as previously detailed and the level of the lowest renal vein is identified and referenced to a boney anatomic landmark.
- Again, selection of a correctly oriented IVC filter delivery device is essential. In this case, a *jugular*-oriented IVC filter should be selected. Use of a *femoral*-oriented IVC filter from the femoral approach will result in a maldeployed filter. Review of the devices instruction for use is essential.
- The IVC filter package is opened and the IVC filter and delivery catheter is flushed, the 5-Fr flush catheter is removed over a stiff 0.035 wire. The skin incision and venotomy are serially dilated. The IVC filter delivery sheath is advanced over the wire and positioned appropriately.
- The wire and inner dilator for the filter delivery sheath is removed and the IVC filter with its delivery catheter is advanced into and secured to the filter delivery sheath.
- Once the filter is in the correct position based upon landmarks established on review of the IVC venogram, the filter is deployed according to the manufacturer's instruction for use. Actual deployment of the filter can be accomplished by simple retraction of the deployment sheath via a "pin and pull" technique.
- Once the IVC filter has been successfully deployed and is in position, the delivery sheath and catheter is retracted cranially and AP and orthogonal single-shot x-rays are obtained to confirm proper filter deployment.
- All wires and catheters are removed and pressure is held at the femoral venotomy site until hemostasis is achieved. For the internal jugular approach, the authors make a point of always placing an occlusive sterile dressing in order to decrease the risk of potential air embolus. The patient allowed to sit upright and is taken back to the postoperative unit. Unlike the femoral approach, there is no need for the patient to remain flat for any period of time. The patient is then taken back to their inpatient unit or allowed to ambulate and then discharged home.

SUPERIOR VENA CAVA FILTER PLACEMENT

Practitioners should consult the applicable Instructions For Use for device indications and contraindications.

A SVC filter can be placed from the common femoral, the internal jugular, and even the subclavian veins depending on circumstances. The femoral approach to placement may be limited by the length of IVC filter delivery devices and patient height. In general, the internal jugular approach is preferred.

- The patient is positioned as previously described for an IVC filter placement placed from the right internal jugular vein approach with the head extended and the neck rotated to the patient's left.
- The skin in anesthetized and the internal jugular vein is punctured and cannulated with a wire under real-time ultrasound guidance.
- A 0.035 guidewire is advanced into and ideally through the right heart and into the perihepatic IVC. A 6-Fr sheath is placed over the wire to secure access.
- A marker pigtail catheter is placed and a venogram is obtained to identify the innominate vein and SVC confluence and unexpected anatomic venous anomalies. Duplication of the SVC occurs in 0.1% to 0.3%. The presence of occlusion, stenosis, or thrombus in the SVC precludes filter placement.
- The IVC filter is then deployed within the SVC using the previously described methods.
- Correct orientation of the filter requires use of a *jugular* filter kit from the *femoral* position or a *femoral* filter set deployed from the *jugular* or *subclavian* position. The filter is deployed so that leg hooks attach at the confluence of the innominate veins and the tip extends into the SVC (see **FIGURE 7**). Care must be taken to avoid filter intrusion in to the right atrium as this may predispose the patient to cardiac arrhythmias and filter migration.
- A chest radiograph is obtained to confirm filter position following placement.

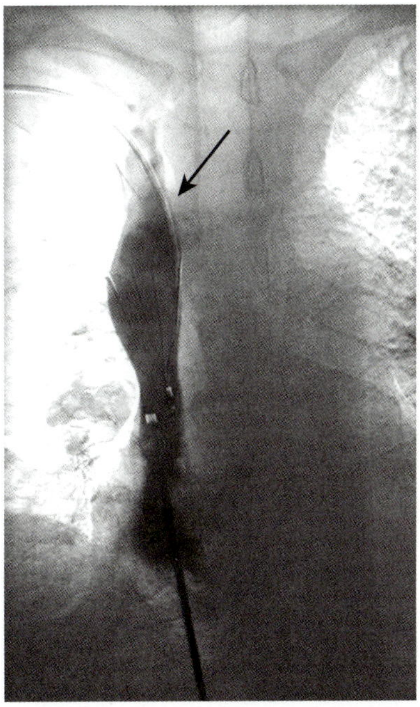

FIGURE 7 • A superior vena cavagram with SVC filter in place. The superior vena cava filter is positioned with the filter base just central to the confluence of the innominate veins (*black arrow*) and the tip proximal to the right atrium.

INFERIOR VENA CAVA FILTER RETRIEVAL

- Prior to an attempt at IVC filter retrieval, the filter should be evaluated radiologically to detect potential technical problems that may complicate or prohibit removal.
- Removal is contraindicated if conventional or CT venography or duplex ultrasound demonstrates thrombus in the filter (**FIGURE 8**).
- Imaging that suggests filter migration, severe tilt, fracture, or other mechanical failure may suggest the need for use of more advanced techniques for IVC filter retrieval.
- Nearly all current retrievable IVC filters require removal from a neck approach due to the conical design of most filters at present.
- For IVC filter retrieval, the patient is positioned and prepped as if undergoing IVC filter from the right internal jugular approach. The skin is anesthetized and the internal jugular vein accessed using real-time ultrasound guidance. Conscious sedation is frequently employed.
- A straight 0.035 guide wire is advanced through the SVC, right atrium of the heart, and into the IVC and a 6-Fr sheath is placed. A 5-Fr straight flush catheter is advanced over the wire. It is the author's preference to avoid recurved wire and catheters for retrieval to avoid the possibility of ensnarement of these instruments with the IVC filter.

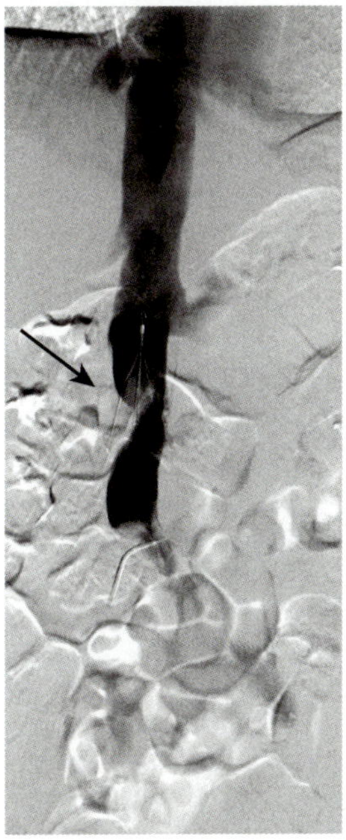

FIGURE 8 • Visualized thrombus (*black arrow*) within an IVC filter on vena cavagram obtained prior to a planned retrieval attempt.

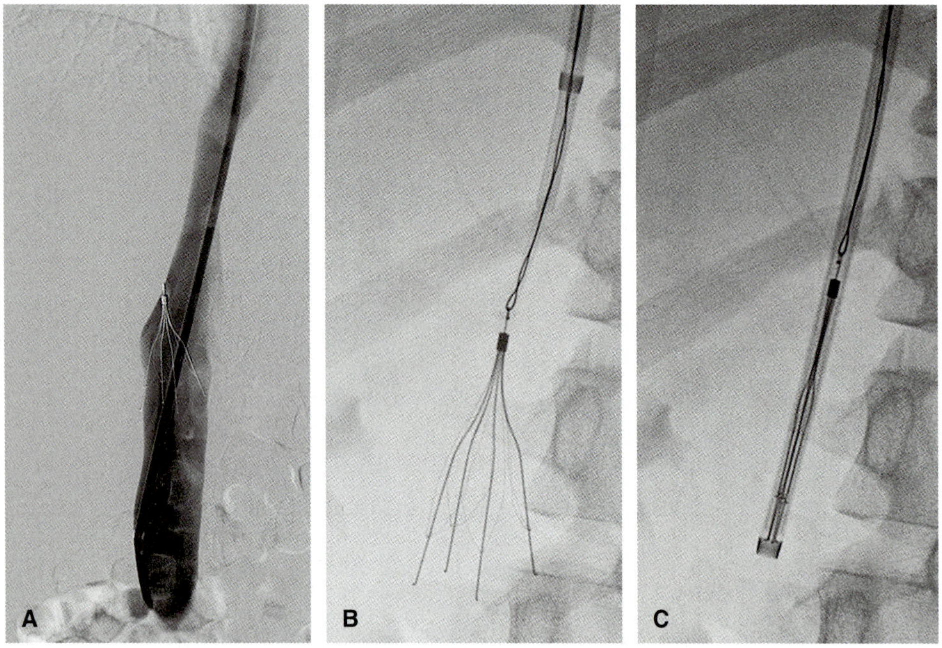

FIGURE 9 • Steps involved in the uncomplicated removal of a Günther tulip retrievable IVC filter. An IVC venogram is first obtained demonstrating patency of the IVC and the absence of thrombus within the filter and visualized cava **(A)**. The tip of the retrieval IVC is then ensnared with snare or conical grappling device **(B)**. The 12-Fr sheath is then advanced over the hooks of IVC filter fully disengaging it from the caval wall and the filter is removed **(C)**.

- The flush catheter is positioned proximally into one of the common iliac veins and an inferior vena cavagram is performed by power injection of 20 mL/sec of contrast over 2 seconds. The venogram is carefully reviewed for the presence of thrombus within the visualized iliac veins, vena cava, and IVC filter (**FIGURE 9A**). If there is significant thrombus present within the filter, the retrieval should be aborted and the filter left in place. The patient can be restudied in 4 to 8 weeks and the IVC filter is removed at that time if imaging demonstrates resolution of the filter thrombus.
- Many manufacturers of IVC filter offer packaged retrieval systems that contain dilators, coaxial retrieval sheaths, and snares that can be used for removal. These are convenient but not necessary.
- The 5-Fr flush catheter is removed over a stiff 0.035 straight-tip Amplatz wire. The 6-Fr sheath is removed and the venotomy site serially dilated to 12 Fr. and a 55 cm 12-Fr sheath is placed over the wire and positioned just at or above the IVC filter.
- A 20 to 30 mm goose neck for multiloop endovascular snare catheter is advanced over the Amplatz wire and the wire is removed and replaced with the snare itself. The snare is used to capture the apex of the filter or apical hook if present (**FIGURE 9B**).
- Once the filter is engaged, the 12-Fr sheath is advanced over the snared filter. The filter legs should release from the vena cava wall allowing the ensnared filter to be retracted into the sheath and removed from the patient (**FIGURE 9C**). It is important to maintain tension on the filter with the snare, but not to retract it into the sheath, rather advance the sheath over the filter.
- If significant resistance is met while attempting to remove the IVC filter, retrieval should be aborted with a plan to consider an additional retrieval attempt utilizing advanced retrieval techniques.
- Once the IVC filter is removed from the patient, it should be carefully inspected to assure that it is intact and without unexpected missing component. Given the current medicolegal environment around IVC filters, the authors routinely photograph the removed IVC filters and upload the images into the patient's medical record.
- A guidewire is replaced into the vena cava and the flush catheter is replaced in the proximal iliac vein. A completion cavagram is performed and carefully reviewed for possible contrast extravasation that might indicate a caval injury or vena cava thrombosis.
- All instruments are removed and the venotomy managed as previously described.

TROUBLESHOOTING IVC/SVC FILTER PLACEMENT AND RETRIEVALS

- A filter deployed with crossed tines can frequently be corrected with simple IVC filter manipulation. This can be as simple as placement of a stiff wire within the vena cava and across the IVC filter or manipulation of the filter with a catheter.
- If the filter is retrievable, then crossed limbs or significant filter tilt can be dealt with by capture, reconstraint, and redeployment of the IVC filter. Complete removal of the filter and replacement should be considered if attempts at correction are not successful.
- A filter that is deployed and exhibits significant tilt >15° can frequently be adjusted and tilt improved by use of stiff wires

and catheters from below the IVC filter. If this should fail, the removable filters can be captured, reconstrained and redeployed to correct tilt.

- IVC filters that are significantly tilted and whose apices abut the wall of the vena cava can make standard retrieval extremely difficult. A simple maneuver such as placement of a stiff wire across the filter to displace it can be used to center the apex and facilitate ensnarement. If this is unsuccessful, after establishing additional venous access, an 8 to 12 mm angioplasty balloon can placed across the filter and inflated. This maneuver frequently displaces the apex of the filter and allows ensnarement and removal. Both of these techniques are simple, frequently successful,[23] and generally within the capabilities of most surgeons placing IVC filters.

PEARLS AND PITFALLS

Vena cava anatomy	▪ Before filter placement, it is best to define the vena cava diameter, the location of the iliac vein confluence and renal veins, as well as the presence of vena cava and renal vein anomalies or thrombus in the vena cava.
Access site complications	▪ Ultrasonography-guided access can evaluate whether there is thrombus at the access site before puncture and also help to avoid concomitant arterial and/or venous injury.
Limitations of imaging	▪ Although the third lumbar vertebral body (or L1/L2 disc space) has been used as a landmark for filter deployment, bony lumbar vertebral anatomy alone is not adequate for proper filter placement as the renal veins and the iliac vein confluence may be found at this level in 5% to 10% of patients.[24] Whether venography, transabdominal duplex ultrasound, or IVUS is used for placement, understanding the limitations of each modality is critical for accurate filter placement.
Filter deployment problems	▪ Filter tilt, crossing of filter legs, entrapment of the filter device inside the filter delivery catheter, filter migration, maldeployment, and vena cava perforation can occur during filter deployment. A thorough understanding of catheter-based techniques, imaging, and *specific filter delivery systems* is required.
The pregnant patient	▪ Indications for filter placement in the pregnant patient include DVT with contraindication to anticoagulation. A suprarenal filter is preferred because of compression of the infrarenal portion of the IVC by the gravid uterus. Jugular access should be considered as well as limiting radiation exposure through use of IVUS if possible. Imaging at the time of placement should confirm the level of the renal veins and the hepatic vein confluence as distal and proximal landmarks. Measurements of the suprarenal IVC should confirm a diameter less than 28 to 30 mm. The filter should be deployed so that the leg attachment point is just above the highest renal vein and below the hepatic vein confluence. This usually positions the filter between the T11 and the L1 vertebral bodies.

Practitioners should consult the applicable Instructions For Use for device indications and contraindications.

POSTOPERATIVE CARE

- *Access site*: Initial postoperative care dictates removal of the sheath from the accessed vein and manual pressure over the puncture site for approximately 15 minutes. A pressure dressing is applied for a few hours, and then the access site is reinspected. If a femoral access is used for filter placement, the patient is keep flat and immobile for 2 to 4 hours. Swelling, hematoma, or bruit would indicate the need for a groin ultrasound to rule out a pseudoaneurysm or arteriovenous fistula.
- *Postprocedural imaging*: An abdominal radiograph is obtained after filter placement to document the position of the filter. The tip should reside between the L1 and the L2 vertebral bodies, but bony vertebral level can vary in relation to renal vein position. Filter tilt should be less than 15°. Tilt greater than 15° suggests filter malpositioning in the iliac vein or migration of the filter tip into a renal or gonadal vein.

COMPLICATIONS

- **Overview on IVC filter-related complications.** Reported technical success rates for a properly positioned filter range between 98% and 100%. Early complications involve access site hematoma, ecchymosis, arteriovenous fistulae, or maldeployment of the filter. Late complications include vena cava thrombosis, pulmonary embolus, access site thrombosis, migration, tilt, and leg penetration through the wall of the vena cava.[25,26] Although most filter types are roughly equivalent in prevention of PE, there is some variation in complication rates among devices.[27-29]
- **Vena cava thrombosis.** Filter design and shape may have some impact on propensity for vena cava thrombosis and rates of vena cava thrombosis varies between 6% and 30%.[30] Conical filter designs seem to have less flow impedance compared with nonconical designs. In a conical design, filling of the filter with thrombus occurs centrally while blood flows peripherally, which may help to maintain vena cava patency.
- **Venous access site thrombosis.** Complications from vascular access for IVC filter placement is reported at a rate of 4% to 11%[31] and similar to that of central line catheter insertion. The two most common access site complications are bleeding at the site of access (6%-15%)[32] and insertion site thrombosis (2%-35%)[33] more common in patient with hypercoagulable states. Factors contributing to access site thrombosis may include larger filter delivery catheter and

sheath size, multiple venous access attempts, extended post-procedure puncture site pressure, and clotting tendency.

- **Filter malpositioning and misplacement.** Filter tilt exceeding 15° may decrease filtration efficiency and lead to pulmonary emboli or vena cava occlusion. Rates of significant tilt vary in the literature between 0% to 39% and may be dependent on the particular filter being used.[34] Filter malpositioning and misplacement occurs at a rate of approximately 1% to 10%.[31] Inadvertent misplacement of the filter in the suprarenal vena cava can lead to renal vein thrombosis, and deployment in the iliac vein can contribute to iliofemoral venous thrombosis. Special care should be taken to delineate vena cava anatomy when using internal jugular access for IVC filter placement. The jugular approach to IVC filter is associated with a higher incidence of nontarget vessel malposition with misdeployment of the IVC filter in the gonadal, paraspinal, and renal veins.[35]
- **Filter leg or hook penetration.** Filter leg or hook penetration through the vena cava wall is fairly common (9%-24%)[36] and is usually asymptomatic. Filter design features such as recurved hooks, thickened J-hooks, and longitudinal filter struts have decreased but not eliminated the risk of penetration. Occasional erosion into the aorta, duodenum, small bowel, colon, ureter, and adjacent vertebral body has been described and, if associated with pseudoaneurysm or infection, may necessitate operative filter removal.
- **Filter migration.** Filters can migrate to a more central vena cava segment or to the heart and can be associated with severe cardiopulmonary compromise and death. Migration occurs in approximately 2% to 5% of cases[37] and is usually the result of inappropriate sizing, deployment over a thrombus with inadequate attachment to the wall of the vena cava, or dislodgement when catheters or guidewires becoming entangled within the filter struts.
- **Filter fracture.** Rates of IVC filter fracture are directly related to design, with variable fracture rates for each individual filter. Retrievable IVC filter fracture rates appear to increase over time and can reach rates of up to 16%.[30,38] Fortunately, overall filter fracture is a relatively rare event occurring in less than 1% of all IVC filters. Filters made from nitinol tend to be more prone to material fatigue and fracture, with an attendant risk of migration.
- **Guidewire entrapment.** Entrapment of guidewires, central venous catheters, or other intravascular devices has been reported and is less than 1%.[39]
- **PE and death.** Nonfatal PE (2%-5%), fatal PE (0.7%), and deaths linked to filter insertion (0.12%) are rare.[32]

REFERENCES

1. Greenfield LJ, Proctor MC. Suprarenal filter placement. *J Vasc Surg*. 1998;28(3):432-438; discussion 438. doi:10.1016/s0741-5214(98)70128-4
2. Decousus H, Leizorovicz A, Parent F, et al. A clinical trial of vena caval filters in the prevention of pulmonary embolism in patients with proximal deep-vein thrombosis. Prévention du Risque d'Embolie Pulmonaire par Interruption Cave Study Group. *N Engl J Med*. 1998;338(7):409-415. doi:10.1056/NEJM199802123380701
3. Carson JL, Kelley MA, Duff A, et al. The clinical course of pulmonary embolism. *N Engl J Med*. 1992;326(19):1240-1245. doi:10.1056/NEJM199205073261902
4. Duszak R, Parker L, Levin DC, Rao VM. Placement and removal of inferior vena cava filters: national trends in the medicare population. *J Am Coll Radiol JACR*. 2011;8(7):483-489. doi:10.1016/j.jacr.2010.12.021
5. Dixon A, Stavropoulos SW. Improving retrieval rates for retrievable inferior vena cava filters. *Expet Rev Med Dev*. 2013;10(1):135-141. doi:10.1586/erd.12.65
6. Guez D, Hansberry DR, Eschelman DJ, et al. Inferior vena cava filter placement and retrieval rates among radiologists and nonradiologists. *J Vasc Interv Radiol JVIR*. 2018;29(4):482-485. doi:10.1016/j.jvir.2017.11.008
7. Andreoli JM, Lewandowski RJ, Vogelzang RL, Ryu RK. Comparison of complication rates associated with permanent and retrievable inferior vena cava filters: a review of the MAUDE database. *J Vasc Interv Radiol JVIR*. 2014;25(8):1181-1185. doi:10.1016/j.jvir.2014.04.016
8. Morales JP, Li X, Irony TZ, Ibrahim NG, Moynahan M, Cavanaugh KJ. Decision analysis of retrievable inferior vena cava filters in patients without pulmonary embolism. *J Vasc Surg Venous Lymphat Disord*. 2013;1(4):376-384. doi:10.1016/j.jvsv.2013.04.005
9. Office of the Surgeon General (US), National Heart, Lung, and Blood Institute (US). *The Surgeon General's Call to Action to Prevent Deep Vein Thrombosis and Pulmonary Embolism*. Office of the Surgeon General (US); 2008. Accessed February 27, 2022. http://www.ncbi.nlm.nih.gov/books/NBK44178/
10. Kearon C, Kahn SR, Agnelli G, Goldhaber S, Raskob GE, Comerota AJ. Antithrombotic therapy for venous thromboembolic disease: American College of Chest Physicians Evidence-Based Clinical Practice Guidelines (8th Edition). *Chest*. 2008;133(6 Suppl):454S-545S. doi:10.1378/chest.08-0658.
11. Rogers FB, Cipolle MD, Velmahos G, Rozycki G, Luchette FA. Practice management guidelines for the prevention of venous thromboembolism in trauma patients: the EAST practice management guidelines work group. *J Trauma*. 2002;53(1):142-164. doi:10.1097/00005373-200207000-00032
12. Muñoz FJ, Mismetti P, Poggio R, et al. Clinical outcome of patients with upper-extremity deep vein thrombosis: results from the RIETE Registry. *Chest*. 2008;133(1):143-148. doi:10.1378/chest.07-1432
13. Brown DB, Pappas JA, Vedantham S, Pilgram TK, Olsen RV, Duncan JR. Gadolinium, carbon dioxide, and iodinated contrast material for planning inferior vena cava filter placement: a prospective trial. *J Vasc Interv Radiol JVIR*. 2003;14(8):1017-1022. doi:10.1097/01.rvi.0000082865.05622.ad
14. Boyd-Kranis R, Sullivan KL, Eschelman DJ, Bonn J, Gardiner GA. Accuracy and safety of carbon dioxide inferior vena cavography. *J Vasc Interv Radiol JVIR*. 1999;10(9):1183-1189. doi:10.1016/s1051-0443(99)70218-6
15. Dewald CL, Jensen CC, Park YH, et al. Vena cavography with CO(2) versus with iodinated contrast material for inferior vena cava filter placement: a prospective evaluation. *Radiology*. 2000;216(3):752-757. doi:10.1148/radiology.216.3.r00au15752
16. Spinosa DJ, Angle JF, Hartwell GD, Hagspiel KD, Leung DA, Matsumoto AH. Gadolinium-based contrast agents in angiography and interventional radiology. *Radiol Clin North Am*. 2002;40(4):693-710. doi:10.1016/s0033-8389(02)00022-2
17. Gunn AJ, Iqbal SI, Kalva SP, et al. Intravascular ultrasound-guided inferior vena cava filter placement using a single-puncture technique in 99 patients. *Vasc Endovascular Surg*. 2013;47(2):97-101. doi:10.1177/1538574412473186
18. Killingsworth CD, Taylor SM, Patterson MA, et al. Prospective implementation of an algorithm for bedside intravascular ultrasound-guided filter placement in critically ill patients. *J Vasc Surg*. 2010;51(5):1215-1221. doi:10.1016/j.jvs.2009.12.041
19. Corriere MA, Passman MA, Guzman RJ, Dattilo JB, Naslund TC. Comparison of bedside transabdominal duplex ultrasound versus contrast venography for inferior vena cava filter placement: what is the best imaging modality?. *Ann Vasc Surg*. 2005;19(2):229-234. doi:10.1007/s10016-004-0163-x
20. Garrett JV, Passman MA, Guzman RJ, Dattilo JB, Naslund TC. Expanding options for bedside placement of inferior vena cava filters with intravascular ultrasound when transabdominal duplex ultrasound imaging is inadequate. *Ann Vasc Surg*. 2004;18(3):329-334. doi:10.1007/s10016-004-0029-2

21. Wellons ED, Matsuura JH, Shuler FW, Franklin JS, Rosenthal D. Bedside intravascular ultrasound-guided vena cava filter placement. *J Vasc Surg*. 2003;38(3):455-457; discussion 457-458. doi:10.1016/s0741-5214(03)00471-3
22. Tanju S, Düşünceli E, Sancak T. Placement of an inferior vena cava filter in a patient with azygos continuation complicated by pulmonary embolism. *Cardiovasc Intervent Radiol*. 2006;29(4):681-684. doi:10.1007/s00270-005-0112-2
23. Brahmandam A, Skrip L, Mojibian H, et al. Costs and complications of endovascular inferior vena cava filter retrieval. *J Vasc Surg Venous Lymphat Disord*. 2019;7(5):653-659.e1. doi:10.1016/j.jvsv.2019.02.017
24. Danetz JS, McLafferty RB, Ayerdi J, Gruneiro LA, Ramsey DE, Hodgson KJ. Selective venography versus nonselective venography before vena cava filter placement: evidence for more, not less. *J Vasc Surg*. 2003;38(5):928-934. doi:10.1016/s0741-5214(03)00911-x
25. Ballew KA, Philbrick JT, Becker DM. Vena cava filter devices. *Clin Chest Med*. 1995;16(2):295-305.
26. Ray CE, Kaufman JA. Complications of inferior vena cava filters. *Abdom Imaging*. 1996;21(4):368-374. doi:10.1007/s002619900084
27. Vena Caval Filter Consensus Conference. Recommended reporting standards for vena caval filter placement and patient follow-up. *J Vasc Surg*. 1999;30(3):573-579.
28. Streiff MB. Vena caval filters: a comprehensive review. *Blood*. 2000;95(12):3669-3677.
29. Hann CL, Streiff MB. The role of vena caval filters in the management of venous thromboembolism. *Blood Rev*. 2005;19(4):179-202. doi:10.1016/j.blre.2004.08.002
30. Wang SL, Siddiqui A, Rosenthal E. Long-term complications of inferior vena cava filters. *J Vasc Surg Venous Lymphat Disord*. 2017;5(1):33-41. doi:10.1016/j.jvsv.2016.07.002
31. Kinney TB. Update on inferior vena cava filters. *J Vasc Interv Radiol JVIR*. 2003;14(4):425-440. doi:10.1097/01.rvi.0000064860.87207.77
32. Joels CS, Sing RF, Heniford BT. Complications of inferior vena cava filters. *Am Surg*. 2003;69(8):654-659.
33. Martin MJ, Blair KS, Curry TK, Singh N. Vena cava filters: current concepts and controversies for the surgeon. *Curr Probl Surg*. 2010;47(7):524-618. doi:10.1067/j.cpsurg.2010.03.004
34. Bae JH, Lee SY. Filter tilting and retrievability of the Celect and Denali inferior vena cava filters using propensity score-matching analysis. *Eur J Radiol Open*. 2018;5:153-158. doi:10.1016/j.ejro.2018.09.001
35. Yun JH, Khanna V, Ahuja RS, Natarajan B. Not so fast with the filter! Is it really in the inferior vena cava? *Am J Interv Radiol*. 2020;4:20. doi:10.25259/AJIR_29_2020
36. Kesselman A, Oo TH, Johnson M, Stecker MS, Kaufman J, Trost D. Current controversies in inferior vena cava filter placement: AJR expert panel narrative review. *AJR Am J Roentgenol*. 2021;216(3):563-569. doi:10.2214/AJR.20.24817
37. Bélénotti P, Sarlon-Bartoli G, Bartoli MA, et al. Vena cava filter migration: an unappreciated complication. About four cases and review of the literature. *Ann Vasc Surg*. 2011;25(8):1141.e9-14. doi:10.1016/j.avsg.2011.03.016
38. Geerts W, Selby R. Inferior vena cava filter use and patient safety: legacy or science?. *Hematol Am Soc Hematol Educ Program*. 2017;2017(1):686-692. doi:10.1182/asheducation-2017.1.686
39. Almestady R, Spain J, Bayona-Molano MDP, Wang W. Iatrogenic migration of VenaTech LP IVC filter to superior vena cava secondary to guidewire entrapment: case report and review of literature. *Vasc Endovascular Surg*. 2013;47(1):48-50. doi:10.1177/1538574412467861

Chapter 38

Superficial Venous Disease Management: Ablation, Phlebectomy, and Sclerotherapy

Meryl Simon Logan and Ruth L. Bush

DEFINITION

- Many consider varicose veins to be a cosmetic concern, yet they can often be a source of pain, distress, and debility.
- Varicose vein symptomatology ranges from asymptomatic to a contributor of nonhealing venous ulcers.
- The diagnosis and management of superficial venous disease has rapidly expanded in recent years, making what was once a surgery performed in the operating room with significant blood loss, now an outpatient in-office procedure with minimal down time.
- In the USA, superficial venous disease, including varicose veins, are common conditions affecting 30% of women and 15% of men. Up to 25% of the Western population is affected by lower extremity venous disease.[1]

Basic Anatomy of the Superficial Venous System

- Superficial veins are located between the skin and deep fascia.
- The main lower limb superficial veins are the great saphenous vein (GSV) and small saphenous vein (SSV).
- The GSV runs from the dorsum of the foot to the proximal thigh, where it empties into the common femoral vein at the saphenofemoral junction. The GSV lies within its own fascial compartment, the "saphenous fascia," and is accompanied by the saphenous nerve, which typically joins at or just below the knee.
- There are *anterior and posterior accessory saphenous veins* throughout the leg. These tributaries lie within the same tissue plane as the GSV.[2]
- There can also be a *duplicated saphenous vein*: a second vein that lies in the same plane as the GSV, has a similar diameter, and drains common cutaneous territories. A duplicated GSV can also be a source of recurrent varicosities after main GSV ablation.[3]
- Varicose veins are dilated subcutaneous veins measuring >3 mm in diameter in the standing position.[4] Of note, most insurance companies will not cover ablation of a GSV measuring <5 mm diameter.
- Pathophysiologic reflux of the superficial veins is defined as reflux lasting >500 ms.

DIFFERENTIAL DIAGNOSIS

- Not all visible veins are varicosities or due to reflux. Leg edema itself has a wide differential, including systemic causes which often lead to bilateral leg swelling (cardiac, renal, liver diseases), lymphedema (which can be primary or secondary), lipedema, as well as rare congenital syndromes such as Klippel-Trenaunay.
- Klippel-Trenaunay is a disorder classically described by a triad of varicosities, cutaneous vascular malformations, and soft tissue or bone overgrowth. This disorder can be associated with absence of the deep venous system. Ablation of superficial veins in a patient with an absent deep system could be catastrophic, highlighting the critical importance of both an appropriate H&P and venous imaging studies preoperatively.[5]
- Symptoms of deep venous disease are similar to those of superficial disease. One must evaluate both deep and superficial venous systems prior to any superficial venous intervention.

PATIENT HISTORY AND PHYSICAL FINDINGS

- Symptoms of venous insufficiency include heaviness, swelling, pain, itching, cramping, and throbbing. Patients can have bleeding from varicosities, or the varicosities can thrombose resulting in thrombophlebitis. Venous ulcer formation can be a result of longstanding venous hypertension due to superficial venous insufficiency.
- Important aspects of the history include prior deep vein thromboses (DVTs), prior venous treatment, hypercoagulable state, smoking, prior surgeries, prior trauma, family history, pregnancy history, and compression use.
- Physical exam should be done in the standing position. The presence/absence of varicosities, palpable cords, tenderness, pulsatility, thrills, or bruits should be noted. Skin changes, including brown discoloration due to hemosiderin staining, fibrotic changes, and thinning of the skin in the distal calf are evidence of more advanced disease and should be noted.
- A full pulse exam should be obtained, including femoral, popliteal, and pedal pulses.
- A standard way of documenting disease severity is using the CEAP classification, which stands for class, etiology, anatomy, pathophysiology. This is an internationally accepted standard for describing chronic venous disease.[6]
- Use of the Venous Clinical Severity Score (VCSS)[7] or other validated scoring tool to document the severity of chronic venous insufficiency is also recommended.

IMAGING AND OTHER DIAGNOSTIC STUDIES

- Venous duplex is the imaging test of choice. This allows DVT to be ruled out, and can evaluate for reflux in both the deep and superficial venous systems. Reflux in the deep system is defined as reflux lasting >1000 milliseconds (ms). Reflux in the superficial system is defined as lasting >500 ms. Perforator reflux is pathologic when it is >500 ms and the perforator measures >3.5 mm in diameter or more.
- A complete venous duplex is typically all that is needed to plan treatment for superficial varicosities. However, abnormal waveforms in the common femoral vein may hint at iliac venous disease, necessitating either CT venogram or catheter-based venogram to evaluate.

SURGICAL MANAGEMENT

General Considerations

- It is important to note that first-line treatment is conservative management, which includes compression therapy, leg elevation, weight loss, and over-the-counter pain medications.
- Compression stockings come in a variety of options (grade, size, length), and are useful in reducing swelling and thus providing symptomatic relief.[1]
- It is important to know the contraindications to surgery, which can include the absence or occlusion of the deep venous system, pregnancy, and the presence of an arteriovenous fistula.

Ablation

- Minimally invasive treatment options have generally supplanted the now mostly historical high ligation and stripping.
- There are multiple options for endovenous ablation including the use of radiofrequency, laser, and glues or sclerosants. All have the common goal of addressing the venous reflux by eliminating the veins that have reflux (**TABLE 1**).

Preoperative Planning

- Most GSV/SSV incompetence can be considered for treatment. The 2020 Appropriate Use Criteria for Chronic Lower Extremity Venous Disease can give further guidance on when to treat.[8]
- These procedures are usually performed in the clinic or minor procedure room. Rarely is an operating room necessary.
- The patient can take an oral benzodiazepine 1 hour preoperatively to handle anxiety, if necessary.
- It is useful to keep the room warm to reduce vasospasm. In addition, the environment should be calming, and often music is chosen to assist in patient relaxation and comfort.

Table 1: Various Endovenous Ablation Options for Axial Vein Reflux

Closure treatment	Thermal?	Tumescent use?	FDA-approved medication
Radiofrequency ablation (RFA)	yes	Yes	N/A
Laser	yes	Yes	N/A
Tissue adhesive "glue"	no	No	VenaSeal
Sclerosant	no	No	ClariVein
Polidocanol Injectable foam	no	No	Varithena

STEP 1. POSITIONING

- The veins are marked in the preoperative area in the *standing position* (**FIGURE 1**).
- The patient is placed supine for GSV treatment and prone for SSV treatment (**FIGURE 2**). If both veins are to be treated at the same setting, we typically start with the GSV and have the patient turn on their side or stomach once this is complete to facilitate access to the SSV.
- The leg is prepped circumferentially and externally rotated into a frog-leg position. The table can be placed into reverse Trendelenburg to increase venous pressure and distend the vein to facilitate access.

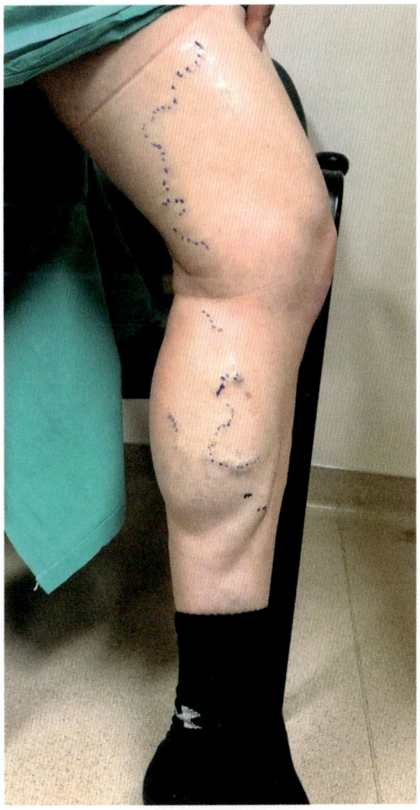

FIGURE 1 • The great saphenous vein and varicosities have been marked in the standing position.

TECHNIQUES

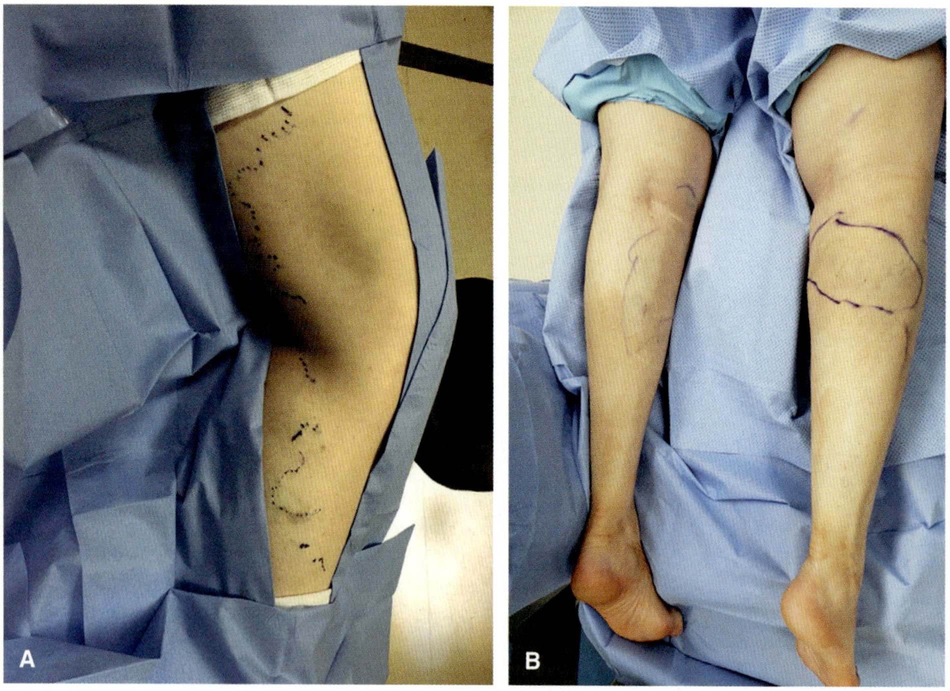

FIGURE 2 • **A,** supine frog-leg position for GSV treatment. **B,** Prone positioning for SSV treatment.

STEP 2. REPEAT THE ULTRASOUND AND CHOOSE AN ACCESS SITE LOCATION

- The ideal access site is as distal on the leg as possible; however, below the knee ablation risks injury to the accompanying saphenous nerve (**FIGURE 3**).

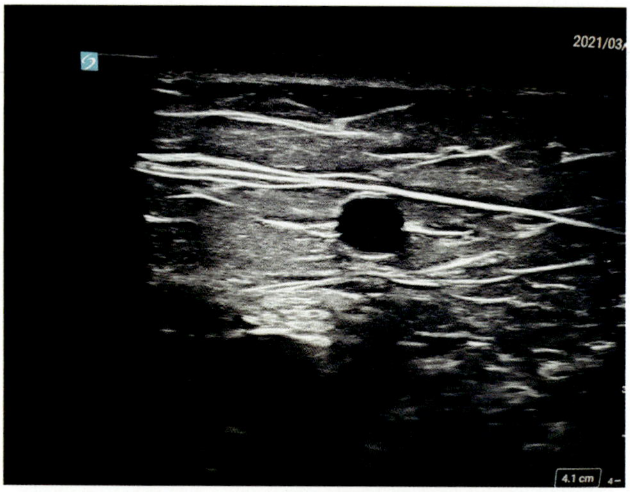

FIGURE 3 • The GSV is seen on B mode ultrasound within the saphenous fascia.

STEP 3 ULTRASOUND-GUIDED ACCESS

- After local anesthetic is placed at the intended access site, using ultrasound guidance a micropuncture needle is placed into the vein, followed by advancement of a .018-inch wire (**FIGURE 4**). The wire is advanced to the SJF (or SPJ) under ultrasound guidance (**FIGURE 5**).
- The micropuncture sheath is exchanged for an appropriately sized sheath for the ablative device.

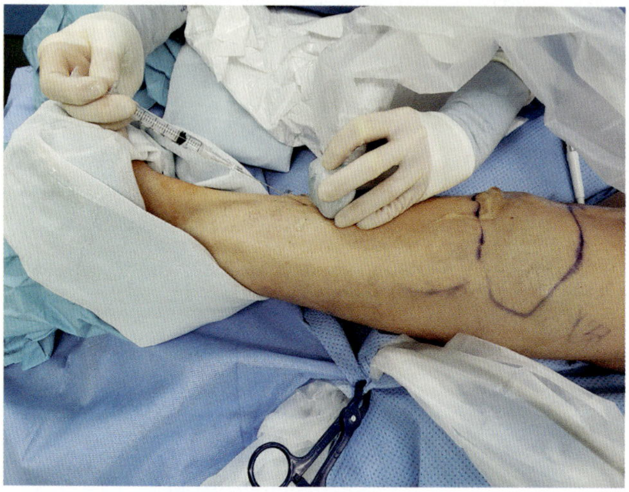

FIGURE 4 • The vein (SSV in this image) is accessed under ultrasound guidance.

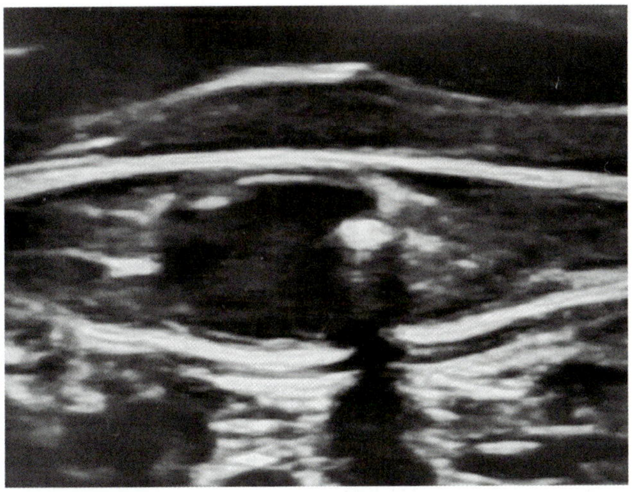

FIGURE 5 ● This B mode ultrasound image shows the radiopaque wire within the GSV lumen. Again, note the saphenous fascia surrounding the vein.

STEP 4

Thermal Ablation

- The tip of the laser or RFA catheter should be 2 to 2.5 cm distal to the SFJ or SPJ or distal to superficial epigastric veins.
- Administer tumescent fluid (approximately 10 mL/cm vein): saline, lidocaine, epinephrine mixture (**FIGURE 6**) to circumferentially surround the vein.
- Treat the vein per device instruction.

Nonthermal Ablation

Includes VenaSeal (n-butyl cyanoacrylate glue) or ultrasound-guided foam sclerotherapy.

- Inject cyanoacrylate glue per instructions for use; Screen patients for adhesive allergic reaction.
- Important to have constant compression at SFJ or SPJ to avoid embolism of glue or sclerosing agent.

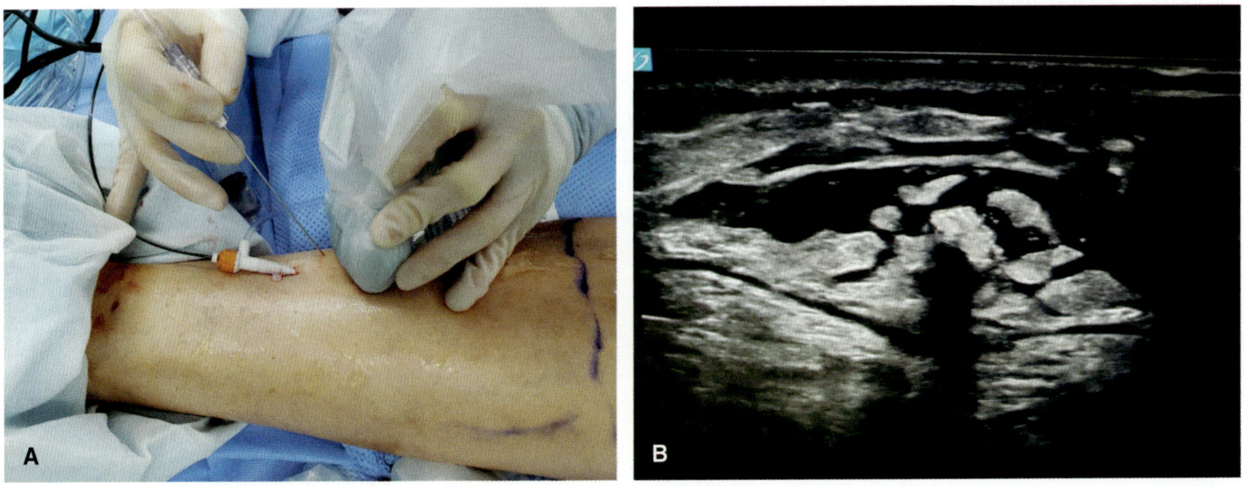

FIGURE 6 ● **A,** The ablation device sheath is in place. The tumescent anesthetic is placed with ultrasound guidance. **B,** Tumescent is seen on B mode ultrasound surrounding the vein, separating the soft tissue off the vein.

STEP 5. REMOVE SHEATH

- Remove sheath, hold light pressure × 5 minutes.

STEP 6. ELEVATE AND WRAP THE LEG

- We use bandage rolls (ie, Kerlix) and elastic wraps (ie, ACE) from foot to proximal thigh. If using cyanoacrylate glue, compression/wraps are not necessary.

TECHNIQUES

PHLEBECTOMY AND SCLEROTHERAPY

- Phlebectomy and sclerotherapy are adjunctive procedures that can be utilized for additional varicosities and spider veins.
- This can be done simultaneously with ablation, or at a later date.
- Preoperative assessment and positioning are as noted in the *Surgical Management* section.

Phlebectomy

- Small "stabs" are made over the varicosities to be excised.
- This is often performed with an 11 blade, followed by a phlebectomy hooks or small hemostats to find, and grab the vein—this is a blind procedure!
- Once grasped, the vein is then gently pulled in a back and forth motion to remove as much vein as possible without tearing (**FIGURE 7**).
- Closure of the stabs can be accomplished with Dermabond or Steri-Strips.
- Compression is then applied as above.

Sclerotherapy

- FDA-approved agents include sodium tetradecyl sulfate (Sotradecol) & polidocanol (Asclera)
- Tools needed-small syringes ideally 3 mL, small needle sizes (such as a 27 or 32 gauge)
    - Use of loupes or a vein light is an option to assist with small vein visualization, but is an added expense
    - It is important to let patients know that the treated areas will initially disappear, but then immediately return and may look red or "angry"—this is temporary
- Compression therapy is applied after sclerotherapy as well to improve outcomes[9]

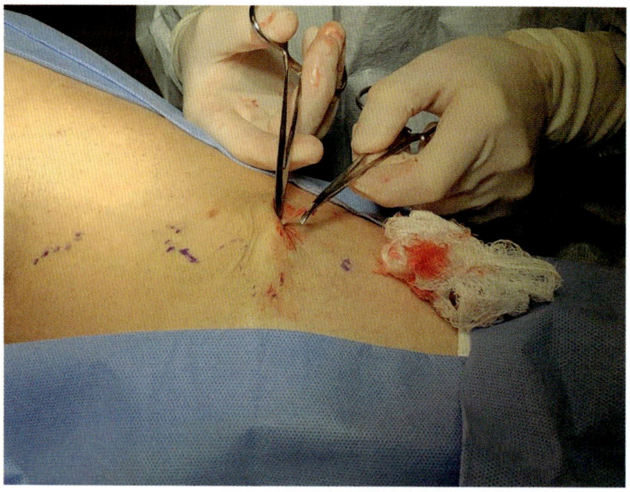

FIGURE 7 • Through a stab incision, a varicose vein has been grasped and is being gently pulled during phlebectomy.

PEARLS AND PITFALLS

Appropriate patient selection is key	▪ Make sure you under promise and over deliver on expectations. No treatment will be perfect in relieving symptoms or providing cosmesis.
Venous insufficiency is a chronic disease	▪ Recurrence is the rule rather than the exception. ▪ Repeated procedures are often necessary in the patient's lifetime.
Pearl	▪ Make sure there is appropriate distance between the end of the catheter and the SFJ or SPJ. Maintaining 2 cm distance for thermal ablation and 5 cm for cyanoacrylate is critical to avoiding femoral vein thrombus.
Postoperative care	▪ Make sure patient is up and ambulating immediately after the procedure, if possible. This will decrease the incidence of post procedure DVT.

POSTOPERATIVE CARE

- Patients are instructed to remove compression wrapping after 48 hours, then transition to their compression stockings.
    - 2 weeks minimum use, recommend continued routine wear
- Acetaminophen or ibuprofen for post-procedure discomfort.
- Ambulation is encouraged immediately.
- Patients are brought back to clinic for a follow-up duplex in 3 to 7 days to confirm saphenous vein ablation and rule out endothermal heat-induced thrombosis (EHIT).

COMPLICATIONS

- Bruising/hematoma
- Superficial thrombophlebitis
- EHIT
    - Classification and treatment recommendations can be found elsewhere. We recommend those provided by the American Venous Forum and Society for Vascular Surgery (https://www.jvsvenous.org/article/S2213-333X(20)30343-7/fulltext)
- Skin reactions/thermal injury/pigmentation

- Saphenous nerve injury and paresthesia
- Recanalization/incomplete ablation
- Neovascularization (less common with ablation then seen with open ligation)

REFERENCES

1. Zhan HT, Bush RL. A review of the current management and treatment options for superficial venous insufficiency. *World J Surg.* 2014;38:2580-2588.
2. Schul MW, Vauvegula S. The clinical relevance of anterior accessory great saphenous vein reflux. *J Vasc Surg Venous Lymphat Disord.* 2020;8:1014-1020.
3. Kockaert M, De Ross KP, Dijk LV, Nijsten T, Neumann M. Duplication of the great saphenous vein: a definition problem and implications for therapy. *Dermatol Surg.* 2012;38:77-82.
4. Gloviczki P, Comerota AJ, Dalsing MC, et al. The care of patients with varicose veins and associated chronic venous diseases: clinical practice guidelines of the Society for Vascular Surgery and the American Venous Forum. *J Vasc Surg.* 2011;53:2S-48S.
5. Wang SK, Drucker NA, Gupta AK, Mashalleck FE, Dalsing MC. Diagnosis and management of the venous malformations of Klippel-Trénaunay syndrome. *J Vasc Surg Venous Lymphat Disord.* 2017;5:587-595.
6. Lurie F, Passman M, Meisner M, et al. The 2020 update of the CEAP classification system reporting standards. *J Vasc Surg Venous Lymphat Disord.* 2020;8:342-352.
7. Passman MA, McLafferty RB, Lentz MF, et al. Validation of Venous Clinical Severity Score (VCSS) with other venous severity assessment tools from the American Venous Forum, National Venous Screening Program. *J Vasc Surg.* 2011;54(6 Suppl):2s-9s.
8. Masuda E, Ozsvath K, Vossler J, et al. The 2020 appropriate use criteria for chronic lower extremity Venous disease of the American Venous Forum, the Society for Vascular Surgery, the American Vein and Lymphatic Society, and the Society of Interventional Radiology. *J Vasc Surg Venous Lymphat Disord.* 2020;8:505-525.
9. Lurie F, Lal BK, Antignani PL, et al. Compression therapy after invasive treatment of superficial veins of the lower extremities: clinical practice guidelines of the American Venous Forum, Society for Vascular Surgery, American College of Phlebology, Society for Vascular Medicine, and International Union of Phlebology. *J Vasc Surg Venous Lymphat Disord.* 2019;7:17-28.

Chapter **39**

Thoracic Vascular Injury—Venous: Brachiocephalic Vein, Subclavian Vein

Michael A. Vella, Michael J. Nabozny, Adam Joseph Doyle, and Nicole A. Stassen

DEFINITION

- Injuries to the brachiocephalic vein (BCV) and subclavian vein (SCV) result most commonly from penetrating mechanisms. Blunt injuries can occur and are often related to hyperextension/traction, shearing, and compression, which ultimately lead to wall disruption, avulsion, and/or occlusion.[1]
- Mortality and need for blood transfusion appear to be higher for venous injuries, likely related to absence of vasospasm, high flow rates, and risk of air embolism.[2-4]
- Injuries to the BCV/SCV are associated with other significant thoracic and extrathoracic trauma, including injuries to the other thoracic great vessels and brachial plexus, depending on mechanism.[1]
- The American Association for the Surgery of Trauma (AAST) classifies injuries to the BCV/SCV as grade II vascular injuries.[5]

DIFFERENTIAL DIAGNOSIS

- Differential diagnosis of suspected BCV/SCV injuries should include injuries to the heart and vasculature of the chest, neck, and proximal upper extremities.

PATIENT HISTORY AND PHYSICAL FINDINGS

- Initial evaluation of any trauma patient, including those with suspected BCV/SCV injuries, should follow ATLS principles of primary and secondary surveys along with adjuncts.[6]
- It is important to understand that history and physical examination findings may be subtle in patients with BCV/SCV injuries, especially in the absence of a concomitant arterial injury.[7]
- Patients with SCV/BCV injuries who are able to communicate may complain of chest, shoulder, or arm pain depending on associated injuries. Neurologic complains (weakness, numbness) in the ipsilateral upper extremity may suggest a brachial plexus injury, which is associated with injuries to the adjacent subclavian vessels.
- Physical examination may reveal penetrating wounds to the chest, neck, axilla, or proximal upper extremity. There may be bruising and/or crepitus over the sternum or clavicle indicating a potential fracture.
- Hemodynamic instability or "hard signs" of vascular injury (expanding hematoma or active bleeding from the retroclavicular area) suggest a major vascular injury. Pulse discrepancy may suggest a subclavian artery injury.
- Neurologic deficits may indicate an associated brachial plexus injury. We find that having a patient perform "rock, paper, scissors" easily evaluates the radial, median, and ulnar nerves, respectively.

IMAGING AND OTHER DIAGNOSTIC STUDIES

- Initial imaging evaluation of a hypotensive blunt trauma patient should include a FAST examination and plain films of the chest and pelvis.
- For patients with penetrating injuries, a thorough physical examination evaluating for ballistic wounds will determine what imaging evaluation is needed for trajectory analysis. Wounds should be marked with radiopaque markers. Plain films of the chest, abdomen, pelvis, head/neck, and extremities are obtained as clinically appropriate in order to identify wound trajectories. A cardiac ultrasound is used to evaluate for pericardial fluid in patients with penetrating anterior or posterior thoracic injuries as well as those with injuries to the epigastrium and thoracoabdominal regions.
- Findings on chest radiograph that suggest a possible BCV/SCV injury include widened mediastinum, hemothorax, and/or apical cap (**FIGURE 1**).
- In general, injuries to the BCV/SCV will not result in hemopericardium on ultrasound unless there is an associated injury to the heart or intrapericardial great vessels.
- Patients who are hemodynamically normal without another indication for urgent operative intervention should undergo computed tomography (CT) angiography of the chest. If a venous injury is suspected, a concomitant CT venogram can be helpful, although most venous injuries will be identified on arterial phase imaging.[7] It is vital that intravenous access is obtained and contrast is administered via the contralateral arm (away from site of potential injury) to avoid contrast artifact.

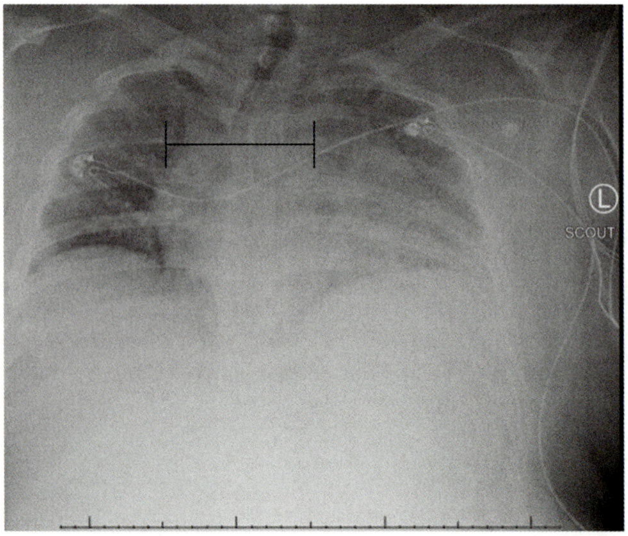

FIGURE 1 • Chest X-ray showing widened mediastinum, which can be seen in thoracic vascular injury.

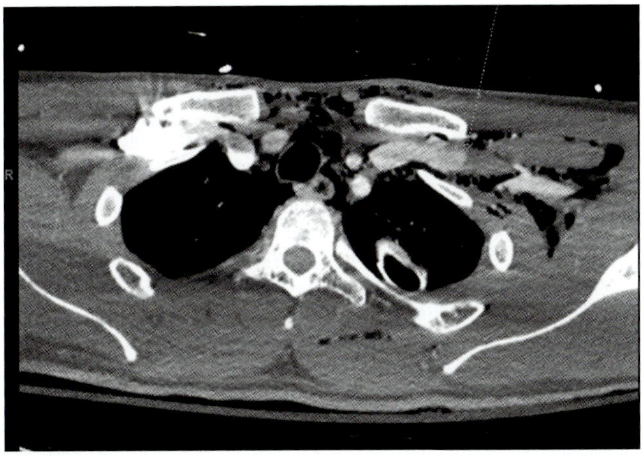

FIGURE 2 ● *Arrow* indicating injury to left subclavian vein as a result of blunt trauma. Contrast was injected in contralateral arm.

- Direct signs of injury on CT include thrombosis/occlusion, avulsion/complete tear, rupture, active extravasation, and pseudoaneurysm. Indirect signs include perivascular hematoma, fat stranding, and vessel wall irregularities[7] (**FIGURE 2**).
- Arterial pressure indices can be obtained if there is concern for arterial injury.

SURGICAL MANAGEMENT

General Considerations

- Nonoperative management of BCV/SCV injuries in hemodynamically normal patients with no other indication for operative exploration is feasible and should occur in a monitored setting.[8] However, the data to guide this practice are limited.
- Overall management of BCV/SCV injuries is based on patient hemodynamics, injury mechanism, concomitant injuries, surgeon experience, and local resources.

Preoperative Planning

- The preoperative management of those with suspected or confirmed BCV/SCV injury should follow the principles of the ATLS primary and secondary surveys.[6]
- Intubation should be considered in patients with immediate airway compromise and in those who are not breathing or are hypoxemic. Intubation in the emergency department should be avoided in penetrating trauma patients with a palpable pulse who are spontaneously breathing and maintaining an appropriate oxygen saturation in order to avoid cardiovascular collapse. Consideration should be given to intubating these patients after surgical prepping and draping is complete. A single-lumen tube is sufficient in most cases.
- Thoracostomy tubes should be placed in patients with suspected or confirmed pneumothorax/hemothorax.
- External junctional hemorrhage related to SCV injury may be temporarily controlled with hemostatic gauze packing. Foley balloon tamponade has also been described for retroclavicular bleeding.[3]
- A brief neurological examination should be performed along with complete exposure of the patient.
- Avoidance of crystalloid in favor of balanced (1:1:1 ratio of packed red blood cells:plasma:platelets) or whole blood resuscitation along with activation of a massive transfusion protocol is recommended. Consideration should be given to the administration of tranexamic acid depending on local practice.
- Preoperative antibiotics and tetanus should be administered.

Positioning/Equipment

- In general, patients should be supine with arms outstretched at 30° if there is concern for SCV injury.
- Prep should include the neck, entire chest, abdomen, and bilateral groins as well as proximal upper extremities.
- Equipment should include thoracotomy/sternotomy and vascular instruments as well as a sternal saw and appropriate lighting. Intraoperative blood salvage equipment should be readily available.

Procedure Descriptions

General Exposure

- The appropriate incision is primarily based on hemodynamic status and location of wounds in penetrating trauma.
- Moribund patients and those in cardiac arrest should undergo left anterolateral thoracotomy with or without extension to a right anterolateral thoracotomy ("clamshell") if presenting signs of life within 15 minutes in penetrating thoracic trauma or witnessed loss of pulses in blunt trauma.[9] This incision may also be of benefit in patients with lateral thoracic penetrating wounds with concern for lung injury.

BRACHIOCEPHALIC VEIN

Incision

- Exposure to the BCV is most often achieved through a median sternotomy.
- A skin incision is made from the suprasternal notch to the xiphoid process (**FIGURE 3**). Dissection is carried down through the presternal fascia, taking care to stay in the midline.
- The interclavicular ligament at the superior aspect of the incision is divided with cautery and blunt dissection and the posterior aspect of the sternum is cleared at the suprasternal notch and under the xiphoid. Respirations are held and a sternal saw (or Lebsche knife) is used to divide the sternum using a steady upward pressure, taking care to stay in the midline. This exposes the underlying pericardium.
- A Finochietto retractor is placed in the upper aspect of the incision with handle directed away from any area that requires additional exposure (ie, direct away from the abdomen if the abdomen may require exploration).

Identification of the Left Brachiocephalic Vein

- The pericardium is entered sharply and incised in the cranial and caudal direction. The remnant thymus tissue/fat is identified in the superior mediastinum anterior to the BCV.
- The crossing left BCV is identified and bluntly separated from surrounding tissue (**FIGURE 4A**).

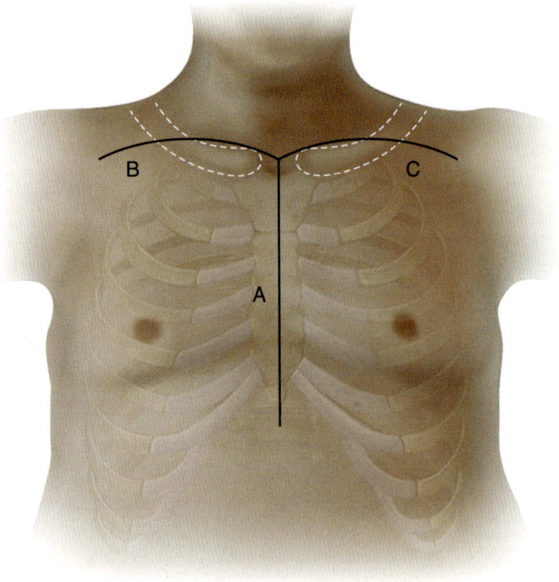

FIGURE 3 • Recommended incisions for exposure of the thoracic vessels. **(A)** Median sternotomy for exposure of the brachiocephalic veins and **(B** and **C)** clavicular incisions for exposure of the bilateral subclavian veins. Median sternotomy and clavicular incisions can be combined for exposure of the proximal subclavian veins. Dotted lines indicate position of clavicles.

- At this point bleeding can be controlled with silastic vessel loops or vascular clamps (**FIGURE 4B**).

Brachiocephalic Vein Injury Management

- Data from the cardiac literature suggest that ligation of the left BCV is well tolerated without significant long-term morbidity due to the presence of venous collaterals.[10-14] Ligation has historically been the most common method of injury management; outcomes are similar between ligation and repair for venous injuries in general[12,14,15] (**FIGURE 4C**).
- We advise ligation in patients who are hemodynamically unstable, require repair beyond simple venorrhaphy, and/or require interventions in multiple cavities. Otherwise, repair (lateral venorrhaphy) can be achieved using fine monofilament suture (5-0 polypropylene) as long as this results in <50% vessel stenosis.

Incision Closure

- Bleeding from the sternal edge is controlled with cautery and bone wax as needed.
- A mediastinal tube is placed. Thoracostomy tubes should be placed if the pleura was entered.
- The sternum is closed with wires (we prefer two in the manubrium and five to close the sternum).
- The presternal fascia and subcutaneous tissues are closed in layers and the skin is closed with staples or running absorbable monofilament suture.

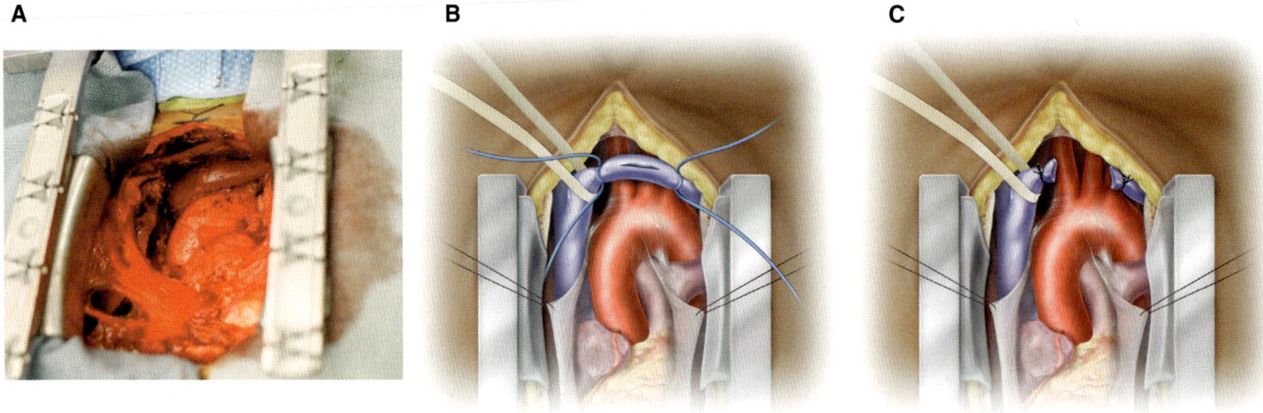

FIGURE 4 • **A,** Median sternotomy has been performed, pericardium opened, and remnant thymic tissue cleared from the brachiocephalic vein, which is seen crossing the aortic arch at the cranial aspect of the wound. **B,** The left brachiocephalic vein has been identified and injury controlled with silastic vessel loops. **C,** The injured brachiocephalic vein injury is suture ligated. (B and C, Reprinted with permission from Lee WA, Kulik A. Arch and great vessel reconstruction with debranching techniques. In: Mulholland MW, Hawn MT, Hughes SJ, et al, eds. *Operative Techniques in Surgery*. Wolters Kluwer; 2015:1804-1809. Figure 2.)

SUBCLAVIAN VEIN

Incision

- The SCV can be accessed through a variety of incisions. We prefer a clavicular incision (with clavicular transection) with extension to a median sternotomy if required. The clavicular incision allows for excellent exposure of the mid and distal SCV with median sternotomy allowing for more proximal access on either side. The incision starts at the sternal notch, is carried over the clavicle, and is extended into the deltopectoral groove (**FIGURE 3**).
- Dissection is carried down through the subcutaneous tissue and platysma muscle until the clavicle is encountered.

Exposure of Subclavian Vein

- The proximal aspect of the clavicle is cleared of all muscular attachments.
- The clavicle is divided near the sternoclavicular junction and distal aspect retracted superiorly. Alternatively, the clavicle

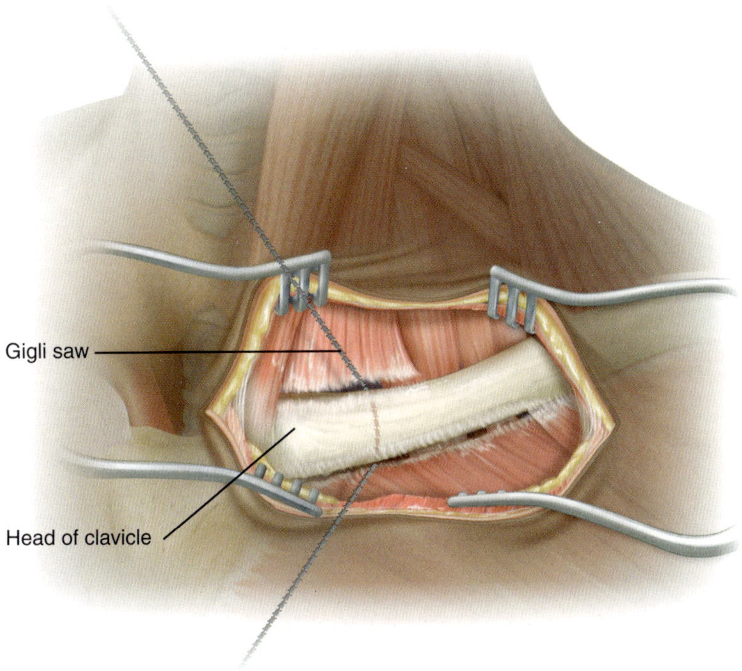

FIGURE 5 • The skin, subcutaneous tissue, and platysma have been divided and clavicle cleared of muscular attachments. A Gigli saw is used to transect the clavicle. Alternatively, a segment of clavicle can be excised.

can be retracted without division, although the exposure is not as good with this approach. A medial claviculectomy (resection of the medial 2/3 of the clavicle) can also be performed and does not require bone reconstruction (**FIGURE 5**).

- The SCV is the first vessel encountered as it is anterior to the artery and anterior scalene muscle. Note that the phrenic nerve courses posterior to the SCV in the medial aspect of this exposure (**FIGURE 6A** and **B**).

Management of Subclavian Vein Injury

- The vein can be encircled with silastic vessel loops or bleeding controlled with vascular clamps.
- Management is similar to that of BCV injuries. Ligation is well tolerated and should be performed in patients who are critically ill or have other management priorities. Lateral venorrhaphy with fine monofilament suture (5-0 polypropylene) can be performed if repair results in less than 50% stenosis. Complex repairs as well as venous shunting should generally be avoided in our opinion[3,4,14,15] (**FIGURE 7A-D**).

Incision Closure

- If the clavicle was divided, it can be reapproximated with wire or plate (**FIGURE 8**).
- The platysma muscle and subcutaneous tissues are closed in layers with absorbable suture. The skin is closed with staples or monofilament suture.
- Median sternotomy, if performed, is closed as previously described.

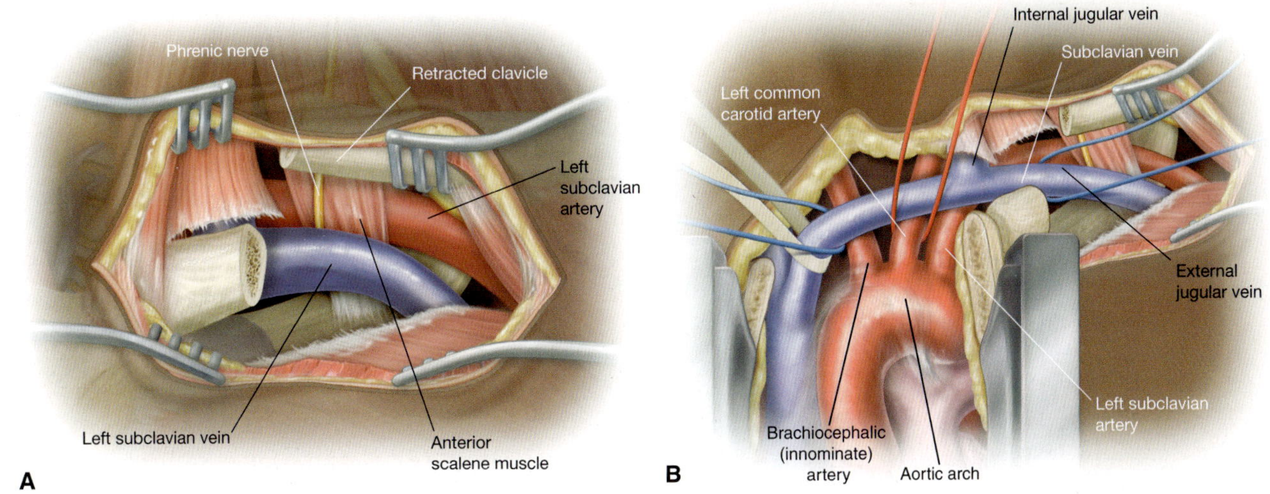

FIGURE 6 • **A,** The clavicle has been transected and retracted upward. The subclavian vein, artery, and phrenic nerve are seen. **B,** Exposure of the proximal left subclavian vein after combined median sternotomy and left clavicular incision.

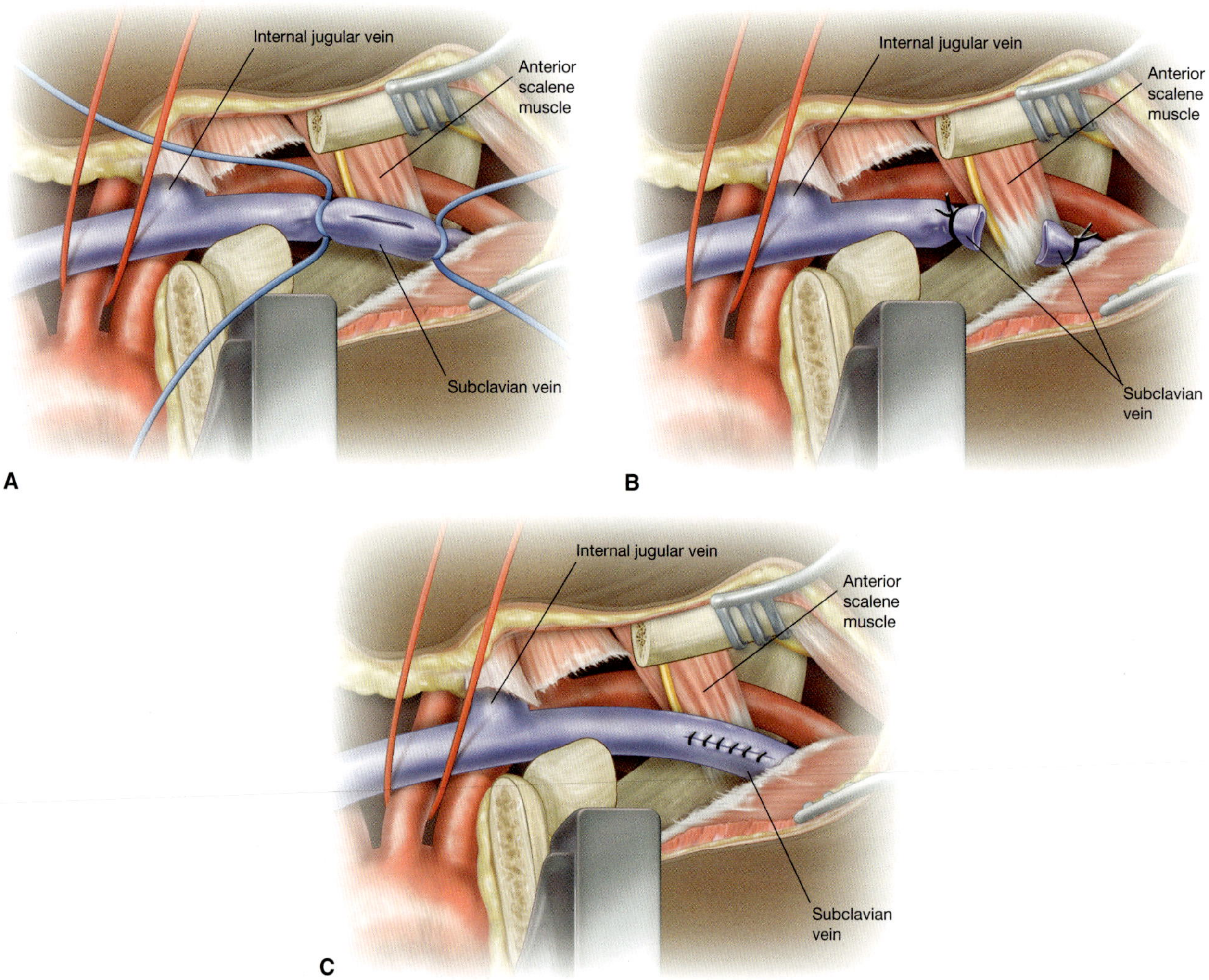

FIGURE 7 • **A,** Subclavian vein injury controlled with silastic vessel loops. **B,** Subclavian vein injury managed with suture ligation. **C,** Subclavian vein injury managed with venorrhaphy.

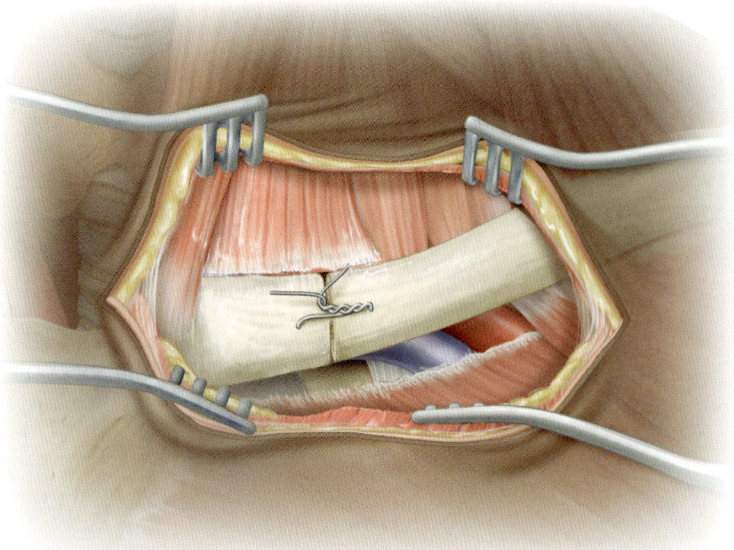

FIGURE 8 • Reapproximation of the transected clavicle with wire.

ROLE OF ENDOVASCULAR MANAGEMENT

- Endovascular management should have a limited role in the treatment of these injuries. Those without active bleeding can typically be managed nonoperatively, and those that are bleeding are usually treated with ligation/or primary repair via appropriate exposure.
- There is limited literature to support the use of covered stents in traumatic venous injuries. Stents are more typically used in the setting of iatrogenic trauma (ruptured central vein during venoplasty in the treatment of central venous stenosis for example) with good effect.

DAMAGE CONTROL

- Patients with severe physiology derangement (acidosis, coagulopathy, hypothermia, hypocalcemia, shock) and/or injuries in multiple cavities may benefit from an abbreviated damage control procedure.
- BCV/SCV injuries can be ligated and the sternotomy/thoracotomy and/or clavicular incisions packed open for delayed return to the operating room following physiologic restoration.
- For temporary chest closure (sternotomy or thoracotomy), we employ a surgical towel covered on one side with a transparent iodine-impregnated dressing to cover the thoracic viscera following placement of thoracostomy tubes (**FIGURE 9**). A transparent dressing can then be used to cover the wound.

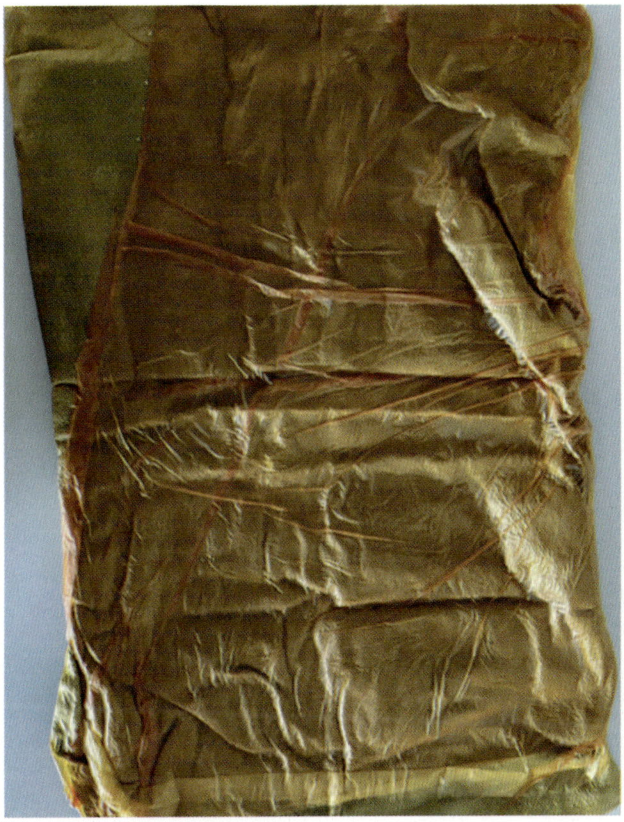

FIGURE 9 • Surgical towel wrapped on one side with iodine-impregnated dressing, which is used to cover the intrathoracic viscera following damage control operation.

PEARLS AND PITTFALLS

Initial evaluation	■ Failure to recognize subtle signs of BCV/SCV injury ■ Failure to recognize associated injuries
Initial airway management	■ Recognize that intubation can lead to cardiovascular collapse in patients with thoracic venous injuries
Operative management	■ Understand the various utility incisions and how these can be extended to achieve additional exposure ■ Avoid complex BCV/SCV repairs, especially in critically ill patients
Postoperative care	■ Failure to start venous thromboembolism (VTE) prophylaxis

POSTOPERATIVE CARE

- Patients with BCV/SVC injuries are generally admitted to the intensive care unit postoperatively.
- The ipsilateral extremity should be elevated over several days to mitigate edema. Most upper extremity edema appears to be transient.[3]
- Serial upper extremity examinations should be performed to monitor for compartment syndrome (tense compartments, pain out of proportion to examination, paresthesia, etc.).
- Chemical VTE prophylaxis should be started immediately if there is no contraindication (ie, traumatic brain injury), as there appears to be an association between venous injury and VTE regardless of method of repair or ligation. In addition, withholding postoperative prophylaxis following venous injury repair has been shown to correlate with increased risk of VTE.[16]
- The need for full anticoagulation following nonoperative and operative repair of venous injuries as well as the role of screening venous duplex ultrasounds require further investigation.

COMPLICATIONS

- Air embolism
- Injury to the phrenic nerve or brachial plexus
- Upper extremity edema
- Upper extremity compartment syndrome
- VTE
- Malunion/osteomyelitis following clavicular division
- Sternal wound infection

REFERENCES

1. O'Connor JV, Byrne C, Scalea TM, Griffith BP, Neschis DG. Vascular injuries after blunt chest trauma: diagnosis and management. *Scand J Trauma Resusc Emerg Med*. 2009;17:42.
2. Demetriades D, Chahwan S, Gomez H, et al. Penetrating injuries to the subclavian and axillary vessels. *J Am Coll Surg*. 1999;188(3):290-295.
3. Sciarretta JD, Asensio JA, Vu T, et al. Subclavian vessel injuries: difficult anatomy and difficult territory. *Eur J Trauma Emerg Surg*. 2011;37(5):439.
4. Iscan S, Etli M, Gursu O, Eker E, El Kilic H. Isolated subclavian vein injury: a rare and high mortality case. *Case Rep Vasc Med*. 2013;2013:152762.
5. Moore EE, Malangoni MA, Cogbill TH, et al. Organ injury scaling. IV: thoracic vascular, lung, cardiac, and diaphragm. *J Trauma*. 1994;36(3):299-300.
6. American College of Surgeons. *Advanced Trauma Life Support Student Course Manual*. 10th ed. 2018.
7. Holly BP, Steenburg SD. Multidetector CT of blunt traumatic venous injuries in the chest, abdomen, and pelvis. *Radiographics*. 2011;31(5):1415-1424.
8. Madsen AS, Bruce JL, Oosthuizen GV, Bekker W, Laing GL, Clarke DL. The selective non-operative management of penetrating cervical venous trauma is safe and effective. *World J Surg*. 2018;42(10):3202-3209.
9. Seamon MJ, Haut ER, Van Arendonk K, et al. An evidence-based approach to patient selection for emergency department thoracotomy: a practice management guideline from the Eastern Association for the Surgery of Trauma. *J Trauma Acute Care Surg*. 2015;79(1):159-173.
10. Sai Sudhakar CB, Elefteriades JA. Safety of left innominate vein division during aortic arch surgery. *Ann Thorac Surg*. 2000;70(3):856-858.
11. McPhee A, Shaikhrezai K, Berg G. Is it safe to divide and ligate the left innominate vein in complex cardiothoracic surgeries? *Interact Cardiovasc Thorac Surg*. 2013;17(3):560-563.
12. Quan RW, Adams ED, Cox MW, et al. The management of trauma venous injury: civilian and wartime experiences. *Perspect Vasc Surg Endovasc Ther*. 2006;18(2):149-156.
13. Feliciano DV. Pitfalls in the management of peripheral vascular injuries. *Trauma Surg Acute Care Open*. 2017;2(1):e000110.
14. Nair R, Robbs JV, Muckart DJ. Management of penetrating cervicomediastinal venous trauma. *Eur J Vasc Endovasc Surg*. 2000;19(1):65-69.
15. O'Connor JV, Scalea TM. Penetrating thoracic great vessel injury: impact of admission hemodynamics and preoperative imaging. *J Trauma*. 2010;68(4):834-837.
16. Frank B, Maher Z, Hazelton JP, et al. Venous thromboembolism after major venous injuries: competing priorities. *J Trauma Acute Care Surg*. 2017;83(6):1095-1101.

Chapter 40 Vascular Injury—Neck: Internal Jugular Vein

Jennifer E. Reid and Deborah M. Stein

DEFINITION

- Traumatic injury to the internal jugular vein (IJV) is most commonly the result of penetrating trauma to the neck and rarely the result of blunt injury.

DIFFERENTIAL DIAGNOSIS

- When a patient presents with a projectile or stab wound injury to the neck, rapid evaluation of the patient's hemodynamic and neurovascular status and knowledge of the complex anatomy of the neck is important to determine the next steps in management.
- Zone I injuries are located between the clavicle and the cricoid cartilage. Important structures contained within this zone include the thoracic outlet vessels, the proximal common carotid arteries, IJVs, vertebral vessels, subclavian vessels, and the trachea.[1]
- Zone II injuries lie between the cricoid cartilage and the angle of the mandible. This zone includes the internal and external carotid arteries, jugular veins, trachea, esophagus, and the recurrent laryngeal nerves.[1]
- Zone III injuries are located between the angle of the mandible and base of the skull and contain the distal portions of the extracranial internal carotid and vertebral arteries, the most superior portions of the jugular veins, and cranial nerves[1] (**FIGURE 1**).
- As you can imagine, the next steps in management will be different for a zone I injury with concern for damage to the thoracic outlet vessels vs an anterior zone II injury with concern for tracheal injury, for example. Also, one should be particularly aware, if an injury crosses midline an aerodigestive injury becomes more likely. Therefore, physical examination becomes extremely important in neck injuries.

PATIENT HISTORY AND PHYSICAL FINDINGS

- In a patient presenting with a traumatic injury to the neck, physical examination is extremely important, as delay in management can result in not only hemorrhagic shock but also rapid airway compromise or neurologic deficits.
- As with any patient presenting with traumatic injuries, these patients should first be assessed using the standard "airway, breathing, circulation" method to determine hemodynamic stability and establish the next steps required for intervention.
- Airway management is of utmost importance in patients with neck injury.
- "Hard signs" of vascular injury within the neck, meaning those that are highly suggestive of vascular injury, include active hemorrhage, pulsatile or expanding hematoma, hematemesis/hemoptysis, audible bruit, palpable thrill, or neurologic deficits.[2]
- However, with isolated jugular venous injuries, the vessel usually tamponades or occludes without any hard signs ever being present since it is a low-pressure venous system.[2] Therefore, most isolated injuries can go unrecognized and can progress without any clinical significance.
- However, given the close proximity to other structures within the neck, damage to which usually warrants surgical intervention, IJV injuries are usually diagnosed during exploration for an arterial injury that presents with hard signs of vascular injury or aerodigestive injury.

IMAGING AND OTHER DIAGNOSTIC STUDIES

- Traditionally, management of penetrating injuries to the neck would have been dictated based on zone. However, these practices have evolved to include selective use of imaging,

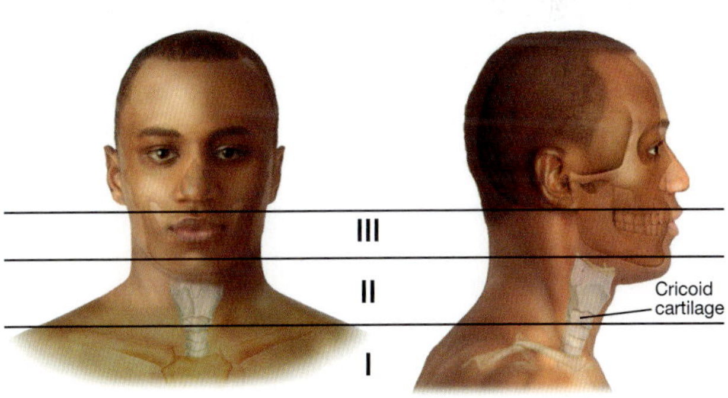

FIGURE 1 • Entry zones for penetrating injury to the neck.

observation, and endoscopy in patients without hard signs of vascular injury dictating emergent surgical exploration for injuries to all three zones.[3]

- Duplex ultrasonography can be performed rapidly at the bedside and is very useful in settings where computed tomographic imaging is not readily available. When color flow duplex and spectral waveform analysis are combined, ultrasound can provide critical information. However, use and interpretation of ultrasound images require sufficient training, and hematoma or soft tissue or bony injuries may obscure vascular injuries; therefore, its use may be limited in the acute setting for penetrating injury to the neck.[4]
- Computed tomographic angiography should be used routinely in patients without any other clear indications for surgical exploration including hard signs of cerebrovascular injury or signs of injury to the aerodigestive tract including stridor or clinically apparent air leak. This use of imaging has resulted in more frequent identification of isolated internal jugular injury, which would have likely otherwise gone undiagnosed.[3]

SURGICAL MANAGEMENT

Selective Nonoperative Management

- In patients with isolated IJV injury diagnosed on imaging, who are hemodynamically stable, nonoperative management is considered safe.[3] Neck exploration is necessary if nonoperative management fails or when other cervical injuries are suspected based on physical examination or diagnostic imaging.

Preoperative Planning

- The patient should undergo the necessary active resuscitation dictated by their clinical status while the operating room is being prepared.
- If available, the surgeon may consider performing the exploration in an operating room that has angiographic capabilities as to have the option for endovascular exploration should the trajectory of injury travel into zone III of the neck and become surgically inaccessible.

Positioning

- Prepare and position the patient in standard fashion with the patient prepped and draped sterilely from chin to knees. In the presence of isolated neck injury, it may be preferable to keep the arms tucked at the patient's sides. Although the injury is to the neck, the surgeon must be prepared if the saphenous vein is required for arterial reconstruction of an arterial injury (discussed elsewhere in this text) discovered during exploration. In addition, the surgeon must be prepared if the trajectory of the projectile dives down into the chest requiring sternotomy.
- The patient's head should be turned away from the side of the injury.

TECHNIQUES

SETUP

- In general, the surgeon should be prepared with the necessary equipment to explore all three zones of the neck, as projectile trajectory is often unpredictable, even if preoperative imaging was obtained.
- Therefore, operative setup for a neck exploration should include vascular instruments, as well as a sternal saw, should proximal control of the great vessels become necessary.
- Bronchoscopy and endoscopy equipment should also be available should there be concern for an occult airway or esophageal injury that cannot be visualized during operative exploration.

INCISION

- Exploration for a presumed IJV injury should begin with an incision at the anterior border of the sternocleidomastoid muscle.
- This anterolateral neck incision can be extended down to the sternal notch or up to the ear if necessary for improved exposure[1] (**FIGURE 2**).
- The incision is carried through the subcutaneous tissue, and the platysma is divided to expose the underlying vessels.

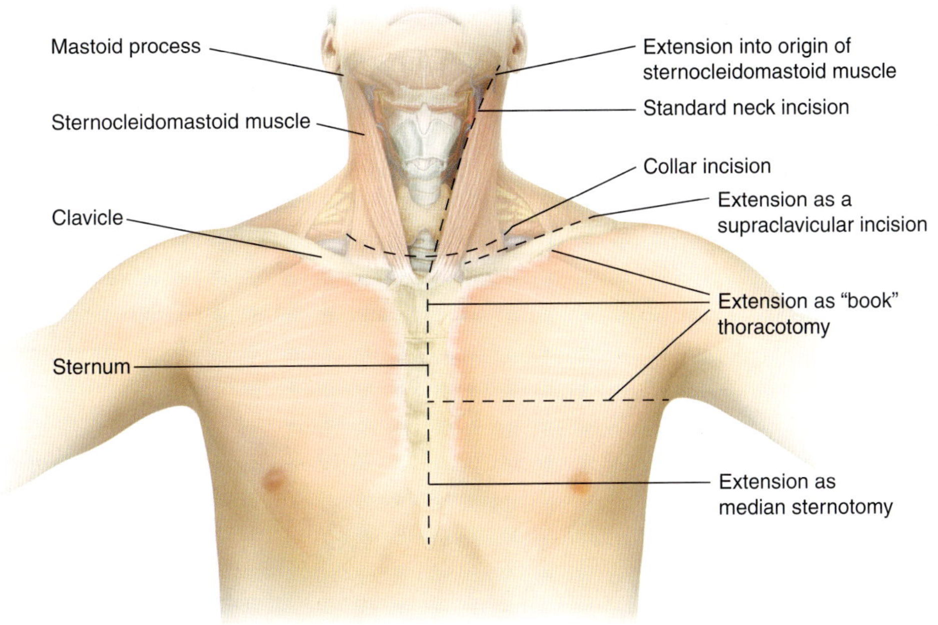

FIGURE 2 • Incisions for exposure of penetrating neck injuries. (Reprinted with permission from Fischer J. *Fischer's Mastery of Surgery*. 7th ed. Wolters Kluwer; 2019. Figure 35.5.)

EXPLORATION

- After making incision and dividing the platysma, there is usually a significant hematoma that distorts the anatomy, especially if there is concomitant carotid or vertebral artery injury.
- Evacuate the hematoma to gain adequate visualization of the trajectory of the injury and to identify structures that lie within the tract.
- Dissect along the plane between the IJV and the carotid to gain full visualization of the area. Use vessel loops if needed for gentle retraction of the vessels.
- Identify the trachea and the esophagus and explore for injury. Further discussion regarding injury to the aerodigestive tract is discussed elsewhere (**FIGURE 3**).
- Once an IJV injury is identified the next steps are determined based on the extent of the injury and the clinical status of the patient.

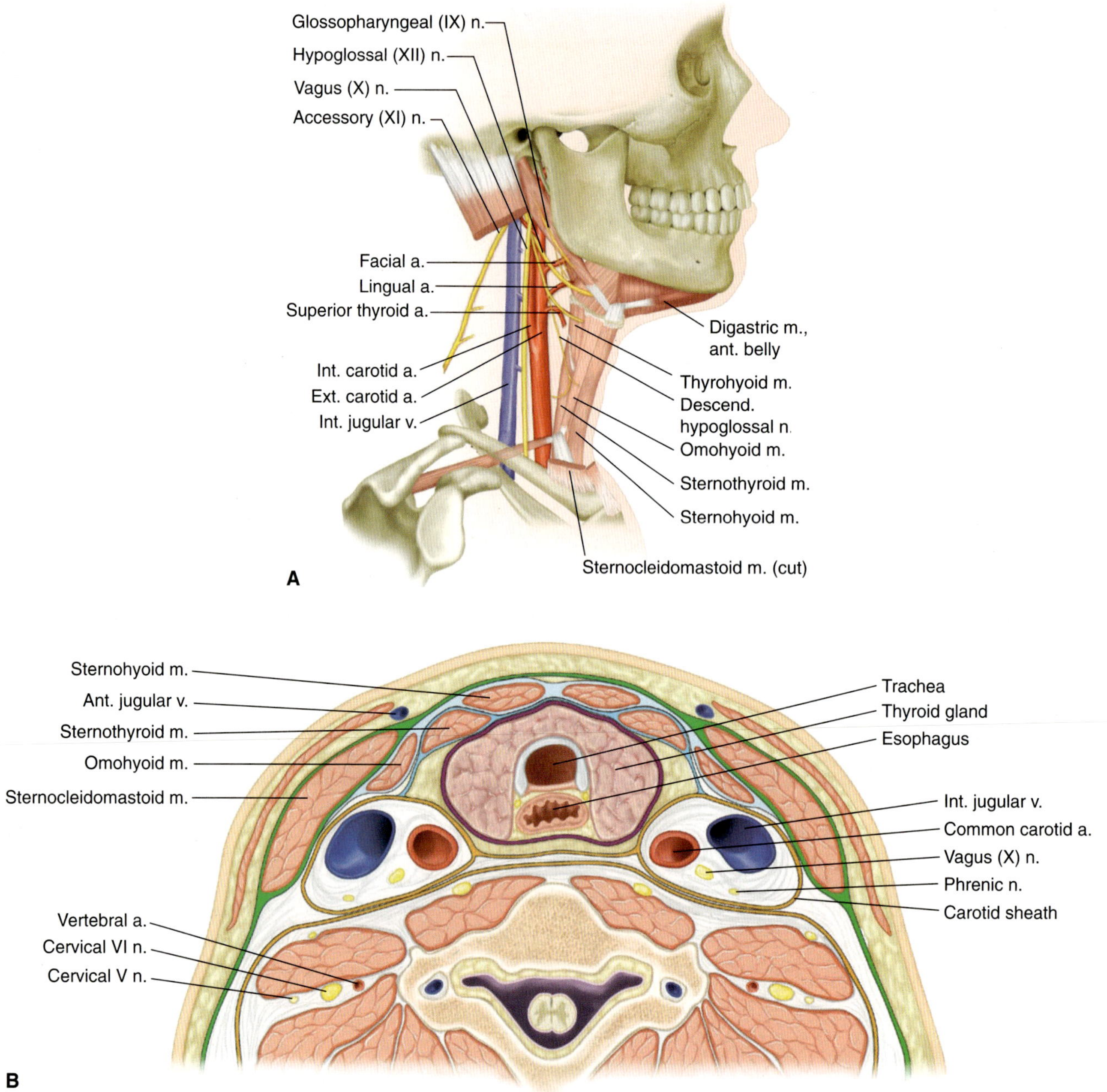

FIGURE 3 • **A,** Anatomy of the neck demonstrating the important structures in the neck exploration. **B,** The cross section shows the carotid sheath and its contents and the anatomy of the trachea and esophagus. (Reprinted with permission from Britt LD, Peitzman AB, Barie PS, et al. *Acute Care Surgery*. 2nd ed. Wolters Kluwer; 2019. Figure 11.2.)

LIGATION

- Ligation of a unilateral IJV is acceptable if repair is difficult or would result in significant stenosis, or if the patient is hemodynamically unstable, or if there are concomitant life-threatening injuries that need to be addressed (**FIGURE 4**).
- Ligation can be performed simply by using a nonabsorbable tie or suture ligation technique.

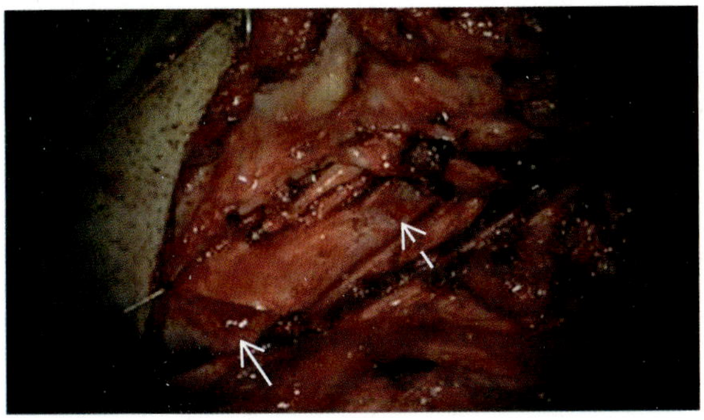

FIGURE 4 • Neck dissection—the carotid artery and the ligated IJV (*arrows*). (Reprinted with permission from Roland, JT Jr. *Master Techniques in Otolaryngology – Head and Neck Surgery*. Wolters Kluwer; 2019. Figure 27.5.)

REPAIR

- At least one IJV should be repaired when there are bilateral injuries to the veins. This is due to a concern that bilateral ligation can result in cerebral venous congestion, which is associated with high mortality.[4]
- Primary repair with lateral venorrhaphy for lateral wall defects to the IJV can be performed using nonabsorbable, monofilament suture in a running fashion with care to not narrow the vessel.
- Vein patches can also be used to repair large defects. The saphenous vein is a good choice for patch repair.

COMPLETION OF THE PROCEDURE

- The procedure is completed once all of the injuries have been addressed and hemostasis has been achieved.
- A muscle flap, most commonly the strap muscles, should be mobilized and placed between the artery and vein in cases of concomitant vein and artery repair as to prevent arteriovenous fistula formation.
- The platysma can be reapproximated and the incision can be closed in layers.
- The placement of a drain can be done at the discretion of the surgeon.

PEARLS AND PITFALLS

Ligation	■ The IJV can typically be ligated without consequence.
Repair	■ Repair of the IJV is associated with a high rate of thrombosis, which leaves the patient at risk of pulmonary emboli.
Nonoperative management	■ When proceeding with nonoperative management, missed aerodigestive injury is a concern, and therefore, endoscopic/bronchoscopic evaluation or exploration may be considered.
High IJV injury	■ Bleeding from the IJV at the base of the skull is best managed by direct pressure.
Concomitant carotid injury	■ The IJV can be used as a patch for arterial reconstruction.

POSTOPERATIVE CARE

- Postoperative care is guided by severity of other injuries and the stability of the patient.
- Most patients with penetrating neck trauma will likely require care in a monitored setting.
- These patients may need to stay intubated to monitor for swelling or hematoma development depending on the extent of injury and other related cervical structure injuries. For example, if a patient had a repair of a destructive airway injury, they may need to stay intubated to allow for healing of the repair.

COMPLICATIONS

- Air embolism
- Vagus nerve or other cranial nerve injury
- Arteriovenous fistula
- Stenosis leading to cerebral venous congestion

REFERENCES

1. Le Roux D, Veller M, Grant I. Carotid, jugular and vertebral blood vessel injuries. In: Velmahos GC, Degiannis E, Doll D, eds. *Penetrating Trauma*. Springer; 2017:257-264. doi:10.1007/978-3-662-49859-0_33
2. Rowe VL, Petrone P, García-Núñez LM, Asensio JA. Carotid, vertebral artery, and jugular venous injuries. In: Petrone P, García-Núñez LM, Asensio JA eds. *Current Therapy of Trauma and Surgical Critical Care*. Mosby; 2008:203-206.
3. Inaba K, Munera F, McKenney MG, et al. The nonoperative management of penetrating internal jugular vein injury. *J Vasc Surg*. 2006;43(1):77-80.
4. Teixeira PGR, DuBose J. Surgical management of vascular trauma. *Surg Clin N Am*. 2017;97:1133-1155.

SECTION VII: Dialysis Access

Chapter 41 Hemodialysis: Open Access Construction

Thomas S. Huber and Salvatore T. Scali

DEFINITION

- The simplistic concept of hemodialysis is that blood is removed from the circulation, filtered through the dialysis machine and then returned. Effective hemodialysis requires a high-flow, low-resistance circuit such that a sufficient quantity of blood can be withdrawn for filtration and then returned. Therefore, the ideal hemodialysis access would be easy to cannulate, sustain sufficient blood flow, maintain patency, have minimal long-term complications, and be cost-effective while remaining acceptable to patients from both an ease of cannulation and cosmetic appearance standpoint.
- The currently available hemodialysis access options include nontunneled and tunneled dialysis catheters (TDCs), usually for more temporary use, and autogenous arteriovenous fistulas (AVFs) and prosthetic arteriovenous grafts (AVGs) for more permanent use. Unfortunately, none of the currently available access options fulfill all criteria for an ideal access and, therefore, they should be viewed as complementary.
- It is generally accepted that a *mature* AVF is the optimal access, although it has been recognized that AVFs are not universally appropriate and that the increased emphasis on their creation has resulted in a higher rate of nonmaturation.[1] In contrast, the potential advantages of AVGs include an unlimited supply of conduit, greater ease of cannulation, a larger surface area for cannulation, and the potential for immediate use.
- The recommendations for permanent hemodialysis access have evolved from a strong emphasis on AVFs, stemming from the original Dialysis Outcome Quality Initiative Guidelines (DOQI)[1] and the Fistula First Breakthrough Initiative (FFBI)[2] to the concept of a "functional access," as summarized by the concept of the "right access, right time, right patient, right reason," that is advocated in the most recent KDOQI Guidelines.[3] The guidelines recommend that each patient should have an ESKD (end-stage kidney disease) Life Plan that is updated on a regular basis and identifies the next dialysis access alternative in the event of failure. Furthermore, the guidelines make recommendations about the role of TDCs for both short-and long-term use (Guideline 2) along with permanent vascular access type and location (Guideline 3). Notably, the guidelines state that AVFs and AVGs are preferred over TDCs, although the choice between AVFs and AVGs should be deferred to the provider, emphasizing that a *usable* AVF is preferred over an AVG if possible.

DIFFERENTIAL DIAGNOSIS

- Patients with ESKD need some type of renal replacement therapy to survive. Although the focus of the chapter is on the open surgical techniques for hemodialysis access, it is important to emphasize that transplantation and peritoneal dialysis are both excellent renal replacement therapies that should be addressed with patients as part of the discussion about their ongoing ESKD Life Plan.
- The traditional choices for permanent upper extremity hemodialysis access are listed in **TABLE 1**. The generic recommendations about the access choice includes AVF > AVG, upper extremity > lower extremity, nondominant extremity > dominant extremity, and forearm > proximal upper arm. However, the optimal choice should be individualized understanding that most access configurations will inevitably fail, further underscoring the importance of the ESKD Life Plan and the need for a remedial access solution. The key determinants that inform the hemodialysis access choice include comorbidities, anatomy, life expectancy, anticipated duration of dialysis, and patient preference.

PATIENT HISTORY AND PHYSICAL FINDINGS

- All patients undergoing evaluation for a permanent hemodialysis access should receive a complete history and physical examination, similar to any major surgical procedure. The physical examination should include assessment of the arterial inflow/venous outflow to the extremity with a focus on any findings such as arm edema, facial swelling, or prominent veins on the chest or shoulder that would suggest central venous obstruction.

Table 1: Traditional Upper Extremity Hemodialysis Access Configurations

Arteriovenous fistula (AVF)
Radial-cephalic (radial artery—wrist)
Radial-basilic (radial artery—wrist)
Radial-cephalic (radial artery—proximal forearm)
Brachial-cephalic (brachial artery—antecubital fossa)
Brachial-basilic (brachial artery—antecubital fossa, distal upper arm)
Arteriovenous graft (AVG)
Brachial-antecubital vein (forearm loop, brachial artery—antecubital fossa, antecubital vein—cephalic, basilic, median antecubital, brachial)
Brachial-axillary (brachial artery—distal upper arm)
Brachial-axillary (brachial artery—proximal upper arm)

- It is important to document all prior access procedures, including any central venous catheters, along with any access-related complications (eg, hand ischemia).
- Notably, pacer and defibrillators with central venous wires are particularly problematic since they can induce an intense fibrotic response that can result in central stenoses or occlusions.

IMAGING AND OTHER DIAGNOSTIC STUDIES

- The noninvasive imaging in the vascular laboratory complements the physical examination.[4] The goals of the duplex ultrasound imaging are to identify all possible artery and vein combinations that can be used for a permanent access. The preoperative imaging includes measurement of the brachial and radial artery diameters, pressures, and velocity waveforms. In addition, an Allen test is performed to determine the dominant blood flow to the hand. The basilic and cephalic vein patency and diameters are measured, and any sign of thickening, scarring, or previous thrombosis is noted. Visualization of the central veins is attempted, although this is limited given the bony thoracic cavity. The potential access configurations can then be determined based upon the history, physical examination, and the noninvasive studies.
- The criteria for a suitable artery include a diameter of ≥2 mm, no evidence of an inflow stenosis, and the ability to vasodilate such that the inflow circuit can sustain adequate blood flow for dialysis. Assessment of vasodilation ability is difficult, but caution should be exercised in patients with severely calcified arteries, as commonly observed in older diabetic patients. The criteria for a suitable vein include a diameter of ≥3 mm, an adequate length for cannulation (in the case of AVFs), and no evidence of venous outflow obstruction.
- Additional imaging with either computed tomography– or catheter-based arteriography/venography can be obtained if necessary. This additional imaging is helpful in patients with presumed arterial inflow problems based upon a history of diabetes mellitus, peripheral artery disease, access-related hand ischemia (ie, steal), abnormal arterial segmental pressures, and/or those individuals undergoing complex access procedures. Similarly, it can be helpful for patients with presumed venous outflow lesions based upon a history of central venous catheters, pacer/defibrillators, arm edema, and/or those undergoing complex procedures.

SURGICAL MANAGEMENT

- The KDOQI Guidelines recommend that the choice of access procedure be dictated by the planned duration of dialysis, after consideration of their ESKD Life Plan (Guideline 3). Specifically, they recommend a forearm AVF, followed by a forearm AVG or a brachial-cephalic AVF, followed by an upper arm AVG or brachial-basilic AVF in patients who are anticipated to be on long-term hemodialysis. In contrast, they recommend a forearm AVG or brachial-cephalic AVF, followed by an upper arm AVG for those with predicted short-term dialysis duration. The Guidelines endorse consideration of early cannulation AVGs for individuals starting dialysis urgently (eg, renal failure without predialysis care) and provide recommendations for patients with complex access needs related to multiple prior failures, although the latter is outside the scope of the current chapter.
- The timing of access creation is dictated by the patient's renal function (ie, chronic kidney disease [CKD] vs ESKD) and the proposed access configuration (ie, AVF vs AVG). The KDOQI Guidelines recommend that patients with CKD with an estimated glomerular filtration rate (eGFR) ≤ 30 mL/min/1.73 m^2 be educated about the various renal replacement therapies while those with an eGFR 15 to 20 mL/min/1.73 m^2 should be referred for access creation. Given the requisite period for AVF maturation, it is ideal to operate on patients with CKD well in advance of their projected dialysis start date, hoping that their access will be suitable for cannulation when needed and obviate the need for TDC placement. Unfortunately, this scenario occurs less than 20% of the time and most individuals start dialysis with a catheter. If an AVG is the only permanent access option for patients with CKD, we prefer to wait until they initiate dialysis before access construction given the uncertainty of predicting when individuals will actually start dialysis, attempting to avoid the scenario that some of the usable lifespan of the AVG is expended before it is actually needed.
- It is imperative that strategies to preserve all potential access options are implemented preoperatively. Central venous catheters should be avoided to prevent the development of stenoses and/or occlusions, particularly subclavian vein catheters and percutaneously inserted central catheters. Similarly, leadless pacers should be used to prevent any fibrotic response from the leads in the central venous system. The cephalic and basilic veins should be spared from blood draws, intravenous catheters, and use as arterial conduits (for example, for lower extremity bypass with arm vein).

Preoperative Preparation

- The preoperative preparation for patients undergoing permanent access should be comparable with any major surgical procedure. It is important to emphasize that patients with CKD and ESKD typically have multiple active medical problems and that these should be optimized, despite that fact that access procedures are generally considered "minor." All infections should be completely treated (ie, catheter-related infection), particularly for those patients in which an AVG is planned. It may be helpful to consult the patient's nephrologist and dialysis center to optimize their preparation. In addition, we prefer to operate on individuals between their dialysis days when possible.

Choice of Anesthesia

- The intraoperative conduct of the various upper extremity permanent access procedures is similar, regardless of whether an AVF or AVG is being created. The options for anesthesia include local, regional, or general with the choice contingent upon the proposed configuration, as well as patient and provider preference. Although regional anesthesia has been purported to provide beneficial vasodilatory effects, the KDOQI Guidelines defer the choice to the provider's discretion (Guideline 8). It is our preference to use regional anesthesia for access procedures based in the antecubital fossa and distally on the forearm while general anesthesia is used for more proximal procedures that extend to the axilla. Importantly, we request that the anesthesiologist use shorter-acting regional agents so that it is possible to perform a neurologic examination of the hand in the recovery room. Intraoperative ultrasound, particularly after the induction of anesthesia, can be particularly helpful to identify the location and size of the outflow veins.

Positioning

- The selected upper extremity is positioned on an arm board or hand table with the shoulder abducted at 90°. The extent of the operative field and skin preparation is dictated by the procedure, typically extending from the hand to the axilla and shoulder. The KDOQI Guidelines failed to identify any intraoperative adjuncts (ie, anastomotic technique, suture type, topical agents) that improved outcome (Guideline 8). Similarly, they did not support the use of one specific graft material, deferring the choice to the operator's discretion (Guideline 4). Although not specifically addressed in the Guidelines, we prefer a fixed dose of heparin (ie, 5000 U intravenously) prior to arterial cross-clamp application in contrast to our more conventional dose for nondialysis-based arterial reconstructions (ie, 100 U/kg), given the intrinsic platelet dysfunction associated with renal failure. It has been our anecdotal impression that there is wide variation in the dosing of heparin across the country with a large percentage of surgeons not using it at all during hemodialysis access procedures.

FOREARM AVF

Radial-Cephalic AVF (FIGURE 1)

- A 3-cm longitudinal incision is made at the midpoint between the radial artery and the cephalic vein and extended distally to the wrist crease. Skin flaps are elevated both medially and laterally to facilitate exposure of the underlying vein and artery, and this can be facilitated with small spring retractors.
- The cephalic vein is dissected and a sufficient length is mobilized to facilitate transposing it to the adjacent artery; this may require ligating any small branches that tether the main vein.
- The vein is then transected proximally (ie, proximal on the vein, distal on the wrist) and the residual segment is suture ligated.
- The mobilized vein is then gently dilated with sterile heparinized saline and marked to prevent any inadvertent twisting during transposition.
- The radial artery is mobilized for approximately 2 to 3 cm, a sufficient length to allow placement of the vascular clamps and create the arteriotomy.
- Patients are administered a fixed heparin dose, the vessels are clamped, and a 1-cm longitudinal arteriotomy is created using an 11-blade scalpel and fine scissors.
- The vein is spatulated and an end of vein to side of artery anastomosis is completed using a running 6-0 monofilament suture under loupe magnification.

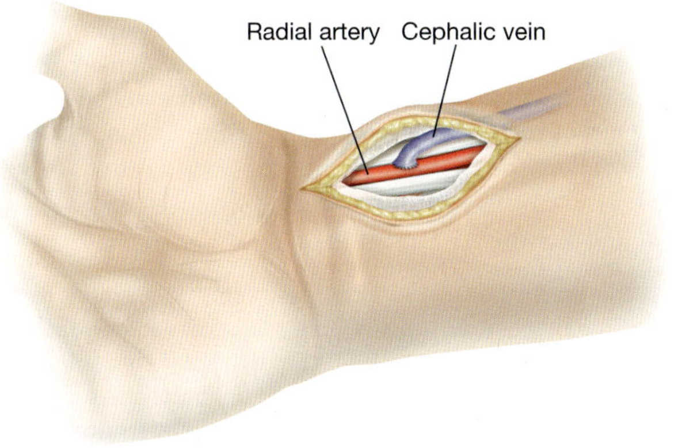

FIGURE 1 • A distal radial artery–cephalic vein AVF at the wrist. A longitudinal incision is made between the radial artery and cephalic vein at the wrist. The cephalic vein is mobilized and anastomosed to the radial artery in an end-to-side fashion.

- There should be a thrill in the proximal cephalic vein upon completion of the anastomosis, although this is not always detected intraoperatively due to the small caliber of the radial artery and any residual spasm resulting from the dissection and clamp placement. Regardless, a bruit should be detected using continuous wave Doppler.
- A pulsatile signal in the cephalic veins suggests an outflow stenosis that mandates further investigation, potentially a twist in the vein or stenosis resulting from inadequate mobilization.
- The patient's heparin effect is not usually reversed given the small caliber of the vessels. The skin is reapproximated with interrupted, absorbable sutures, and the skin is closed with a monofilament, absorbable suture.

Radial-Basilic AVF (FIGURE 2)

- A 3-cm longitudinal incision is made over the distal radial artery proximal to the wrist crease and the vessel is dissected free, similar to the approach for the radial-cephalic AVF.[5]
- An incision is made over the course of the basilic vein in the forearm from the antecubital fossa to the wrist. This vein is easily identifiable in thin patients, but its location can be facilitated by an intraoperative ultrasound if necessary.
- The basilic vein is completely dissected and the branches are ligated.
- The vein is transected at the wrist, gently distended with heparinized saline, and then passed across the volar aspect of the forearm immediately deep to the skin. This can be facilitated using an aortic clamp or a hollow tunneling device.

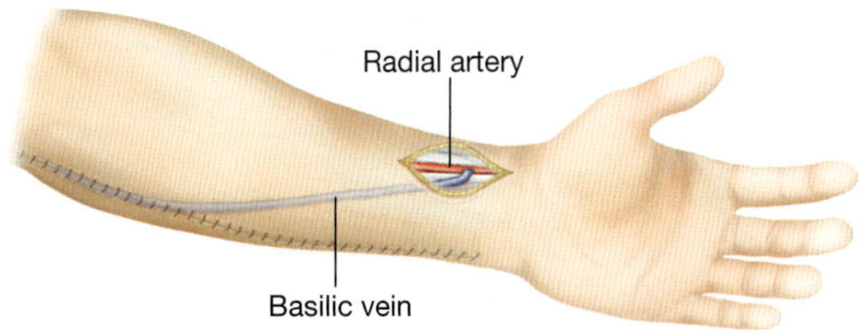

FIGURE 2 • A radial artery–basilic vein AVF. A longitudinal incision is made over the distal radial artery near the wrist. An incision is made over the basilic vein from the antecubital crease to the wrist, and the vein is dissected free. The vein is transposed over the volar aspect of the forearm in a subcutaneous plane, and an end-to-side anastomosis is performed.

Caution should be exercised to assure a gentle curve of the vein at the antecubital fossa to prevent compressing it on the adjacent soft tissue.

- The remaining components of the procedure including the anastomosis, completion assessment and closure are identical to the radial-cephalic AVF.

Alternatives

- The radial-cephalic AVF can be created distal to the wrist in the anatomic snuffbox located between the extensor pollicis brevis and the extensor pollicis longus tendons.[6] Although the radial artery and cephalic vein are somewhat smaller in this location, the reported outcomes are comparable with the more traditional configuration at the wrist.
- The distal radial artery at the wrist can be transected and anastomosed to the cephalic vein in an end artery–side vein configuration, termed the RADAR AVF (radial artery deviation and reimplantation).[7] This configuration may have better patency and a lower rate of anastomotic hyperplasia but concerns remain about the potential for hand edema resulting from the end artery–side vein configuration.
- The ulnar artery can be used for both cephalic- or basilic-based AVFs, although caution should be exercised given the fact that most individuals are ulnar dominant.

UPPER ARM AVF

Brachial-Cephalic AVF (FIGURE 3)

- A transverse incision is made across the antecubital crease and the cephalic vein (or median antecubital vein) is exposed. Care should be exercised when making the skin incision since the target vein runs very superficial and can be inadvertently injured.
- Alternatively, a sigmoidal incision over the distal cephalic vein in the upper arm extending across the antecubital crease and then longitudinally over the brachial artery can be used if additional mobilization of the cephalic vein is required (or if the proximal radial artery will be used for the anastomosis).
- The vein is dissected free and its branches are suture ligated. This may require mobilizing the vein more proximal on the upper arm by elevating the skin flap if the vein and brachial artery are somewhat far apart.
- We will occasionally use the median antecubital vein, preserving both the cephalic and basilic outflow, if the outflow veins are somewhat diminutive. This affords both the opportunity to dilate and mature, conceding that the basilic vein will need to be transposed in the future if it emerges as the dominant outflow and that the dual outflow configuration may be associated with a higher incidence of hand ischemia.

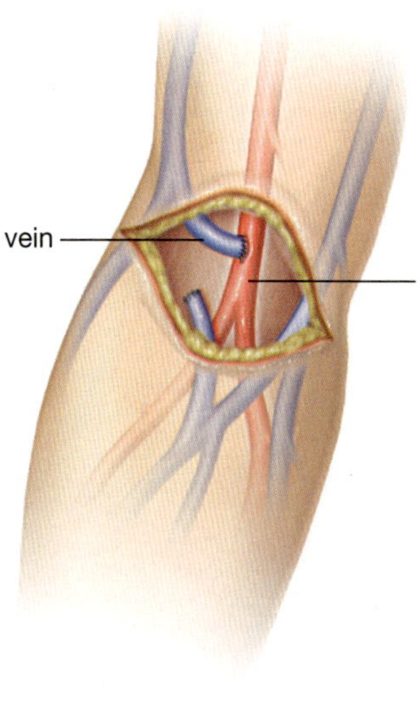

FIGURE 3 • A brachial artery–cephalic vein AVF. A transverse incision is made across the antecubital fossa, and the cephalic vein and brachial artery are dissected. The anastomosis is performed in an end-to-side fashion.

- The brachial artery is exposed by incising the overlying bicipital aponeurosis and a sufficient length is mobilized to facilitate applying the vascular clamps and creating the anastomosis.
- Approximately 20% of individuals will have an "early take-off" of the radial artery proximal to the antecubital fossa.[8] In this scenario, the radial artery courses superficial to the larger ulnar artery in the antecubital fossa and can be mistaken for the brachial artery. Concern for a high takeoff of the radial artery should be raised if the vessel seems smaller than anticipated.
- A 1-cm longitudinal arteriotomy is created after vascular control. The cephalic (or median antecubital) vein is spatulated and distended and the anastomosis performed using a 6-0 monofilament vascular suture. The deeper tributary branches of the cephalic vein may be partially preserved to create a more patulous anastomosis.
- A robust bruit and thrill should be detected upon completion of the anastomosis. The cephalic vein may occasionally be compressed by the adjacent soft tissue or tethered by one of its branches, which can be remediated by incising any concerning soft tissue and raising a larger skin flap or transecting the offending branch and further mobilizing the vein.
- The wound is reapproximated with interrupted, absorbable sutures, and the final layer of skin is closed using a subcutaneous monofilament suture. It is helpful to mark the skin using lines perpendicular to the planned transverse component of the skin incision to assure correct alignment of the skin flaps.

Brachial-Basilic AVF (FIGURE 4)

- The brachial-basilic AVF can be created as a single- or two-stage procedure. The available evidence is somewhat equivocal, but it suggests that the two-stage procedure may allow smaller veins to mature and ultimately be suitable for dialysis.[9] We prefer the two-stage procedure since it avoids a larger surgical procedure unless the vein has dilated sufficiently. Given the need to transpose the vein and elevate it from its deeper position compared with the skin, it is relatively contraindicated in obese patients.

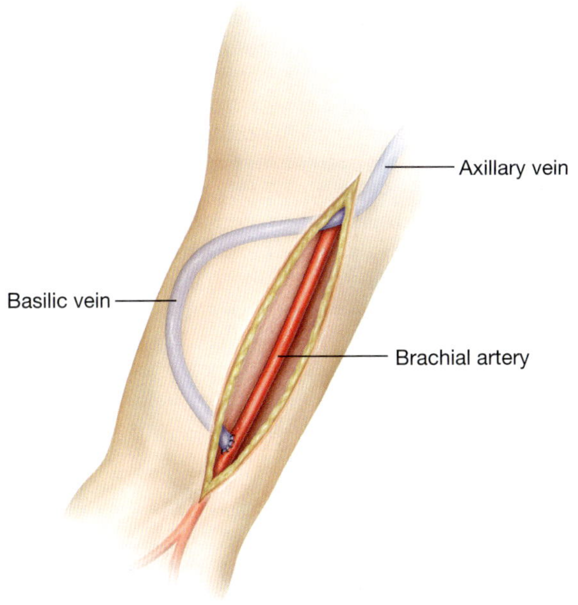

FIGURE 4 • A brachial artery–basilic vein AVF. Note that the image could represent a single- or the two-stage procedure. An incision is made from the antecubital fossa to the axilla, and the basilic vein is dissected free. The vein is transposed through a lateral, subcutaneous tunnel and anastomosed in an end-to-side fashion.

- A 3-cm incision is made halfway between the basilic vein and brachial artery in the distal upper arm, immediately proximal to the antecubital fossa, as the initial step of the two-stage procedure. The exposure of the basilic vein may be simplified by marking its course with duplex. The vein is identified, confirmed by the overlying median antecubital cutaneous nerve that bifurcates in the distal upper arm, and then circumferentially dissected. The adjacent brachial artery is dissected free by incising the brachial sheath and approximately 2 to 3 cm is exposed. The basilic vein is transected and its proximal portion (ie, distal extent) is suture ligated. The vein is spatulated and mobilized to create the end vein to side brachial artery anastomosis using a standard technique.
- The second stage procedure is performed when the outflow basilic vein has dilated sufficiently for cannulation, typically >5 mm in diameter. A longitudinal incision is made from the antecubital crease to the axilla, incorporating the incision from the first-stage operation. We will typically make a series of smaller, subtotal incisions (rather than one continuous initial incision) to make sure that the incision overlies the basilic vein, minimizing the extent of the skin flaps. The basilic vein is then circumferentially exposed from the anastomosis to the axilla and completely dissected free. The vein may elongate as well as dilate after the first stage thereby increasing the available length for transposition. The broader-based branches of the basilic vein should be suture ligated to reduce the likelihood of the tie inadvertently falling off. The dissection is continued to the anastomosis to optimize the available length despite the surrounding scar tissue, although we do not typically dissect out the brachial artery at the anastomosis.
- The vein can be elevated and/or transposed with several different techniques including simple mobilization and elevation, mobilization and elevation beneath a subcutaneous flap, or transection of the anastomosis and transposition through a new subcutaneous tunnel with re-siting the anastomosis more proximally. We prefer the later technique since it facilitates rerouting the vein more lateral on the upper arm, which is more anatomically favorable for cannulation, although it mandates redoing the anastomosis. Furthermore, this approach does not mandate transecting the cutaneous nerve.
- The initial anastomosis is dissembled by transecting the vein at the anastomosis and oversewing its hood. The vein is then distended and marked to prevent twisting. It is imperative to fully mobilize the vein in the axilla to avoid creating any tension at the swing segment (ie, "hinge point"), a common site of neointimal hyperplasia formation. The distended vein is then gently draped over the skin, and its proposed course is marked on the skin. A tunnel is created as lateral as possible, immediately deep to the skin, using a curved, hollow tunneller, and the vein is passed through the tunnel.
- The brachial artery adjacent to the exit site of the basilic vein tunnel is then exposed by incision of the overlying brachial sheath. The anastomosis is completed using standard technique.
- A #10 Jackson-Pratt drain is placed throughout the basilic vein harvest site, and the overlying soft tissue is closed, exercising care not to somehow crimp or narrow the AVF. The deep dermal and skin layers are closed using a continuous braided and monofilament absorbable suture, respectively.

Alternatives

- The distal radial artery can be used as an alternative to the brachial artery at the antecubital fossa as the inflow source for both the cephalic- and basilic-based upper extremity AVFs.[10] The potential advantage includes a lower access flow rate that can result in a lower incidence hand ischemia, venous hypertension, arm edema, and central vein stenoses.
- One of the deeper, perforating vessels off the antecubital vein can be used with the proximal radial or brachial radial arteries in a configuration traditionally referred to as the Gracz AVF.[11]
- The brachial vein may be used as an alternative to the basilic vein with either a single- or two-stage procedure as outlined above.[12] The brachial veins are paired structures that course along the brachial artery, and they tend to be fairly thin walled and friable. It is our preference to perform a two-stage procedure, selecting the largest of the two branches during the first stage.

TECHNIQUES

FOREARM AVG (FIGURE 5)

- A 3-cm incision is made across the antecubital crease, and the median antecubital vein and brachial artery are exposed. Alternatively, a horizontal incision can be made approximately 1 to 1.5 cm distal to the antecubital crease and skin flaps can be raised to expose the vessels. The cephalic, basilic, brachial, or median antecubital veins can be used as the venous outflow, and we traditionally just use the largest vein with the best outflow. Exposure of the brachial artery requires incising the overlying biceps aponeurosis. The course of the proposed prosthetic loop over the forearm is marked, extending approximately 2 to 3 cm from the wrist crease in a nice gentle curve. A separate longitudinal skin incision is made over this course near the wrist and a 6-mm nonringed graft, typically PTFE, is passed along the identified path using a hollow tunneller.
- The arterial and venous anastomoses are performed in sequence using a 6-0 monofilament vascular suture. We prefer to do the venous anastomosis first to minimize the amount of bleeding from the needle holes at the arterial anastomoses. A nice thrill should be detected at the venous anastomosis upon completion.
- The skin flaps are reapproximated with interrupted, absorbable sutures, and the final layer of the skin is closed with a monofilament, absorbable suture. The use of an early cannulation graft may avoid the use of a TDC in some settings.

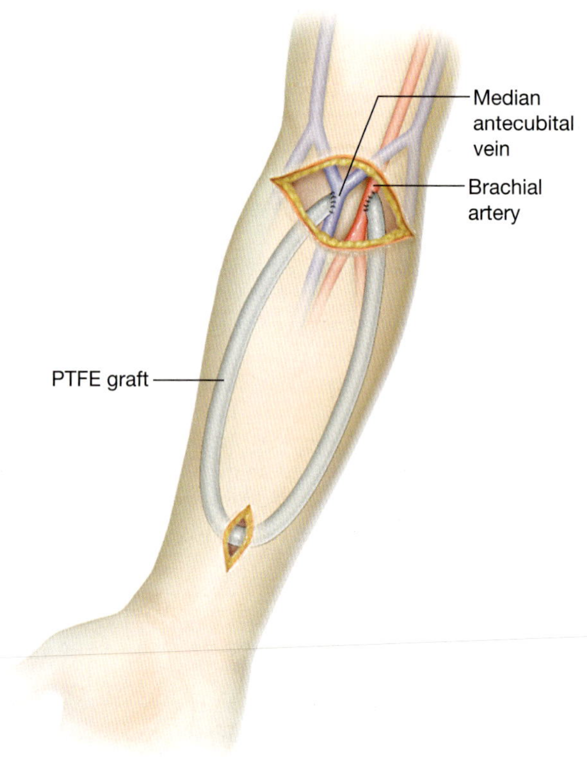

FIGURE 5 • A forearm brachial artery–median antecubital vein AVG. A transverse incision is made across the antecubital fossa, and the median antecubital vein and brachial artery are dissected free. A 6-mm polytetrafluoroethylene (PTFE) graft is tunneled in a looped configuration with the aid of a second counter incision. Both anastomoses are completed in an end-to-side fashion.

UPPER ARM AVG

- The upper arm AVG can be created in two configurations: a gentle, semicircle from the brachial artery immediately proximal to the antecubital fossa to the axillary vein in the axilla (**FIGURE 6A**) or a complete loop from the brachial artery in the axilla to the adjacent axillary vein (**FIGURE 6B**). Our preference is to use the brachial artery in the axilla for individuals at a higher risk of developing access-related hand ischemia given the higher incidence associated with the brachial artery near the antecubital fossa, typically women and older individuals. We favor using the more distal brachial artery for those at lower risk for ischemia (eg, younger men) because the tunnel is a bit easier to make, particularly for some of the early cannulation grafts that require removing an investing plastic sheath.
- The distal brachial artery is exposed through a 3-cm incision over its course proximal to the antecubital crease. This requires incising the overlying brachial sheath and dissecting 2 to 3 cm of the vessel. The axillary vein (and proximal brachial artery for the other looped configuration) is exposed using a 3- to 4-cm longitudinal incision over the course of the vessels that extends to the axillary skin fold. Adequate exposure may require proximal extension of the incision and retracting the pectoralis major muscle and adjacent soft tissue. Two deep Weitlander retractors oriented at about 60° from the longitudinal axis of the vessels provides adequate exposure.
- The venous anatomy in the axilla can be somewhat confusing. The paired brachial and basilic vein drain into the axillary vein, although these configurations are not universal and there can be paired outflow veins. Additional proximal dissection should be performed if the initially identified veins appear to be too small.
- The proximal brachial artery can be exposed by incising its overlying sheath, typically distal to the takeoff of the profunda brachial artery.
- The course of the graft is marked on the skin (ie, gentle curve for distal brachial artery and complete "tear drop" loop for proximal brachial artery). A separate incision sited at the mid portion of the tunnel in the distal, lateral upper arm is required to tunnel the complete loop for the proximal brachial artery configuration. The hollow tunneller is passed from the axillary incision to the separate arm incision in such a fashion that its course is relatively deep to the skin near the axilla but immediately below the dermis for the portion of the graft that will be used for cannulation, roughly all but the 3 to 4 cm length near the axilla.
- The anastomoses are completed using standard technique. We prefer to construct the venous anastomosis first since it is more challenging given its proximal location. The soft tissue of the axilla is closed in multiple layers using interrupted, absorbable sutures, and the final later of skin is closed in a subcuticular fashion.

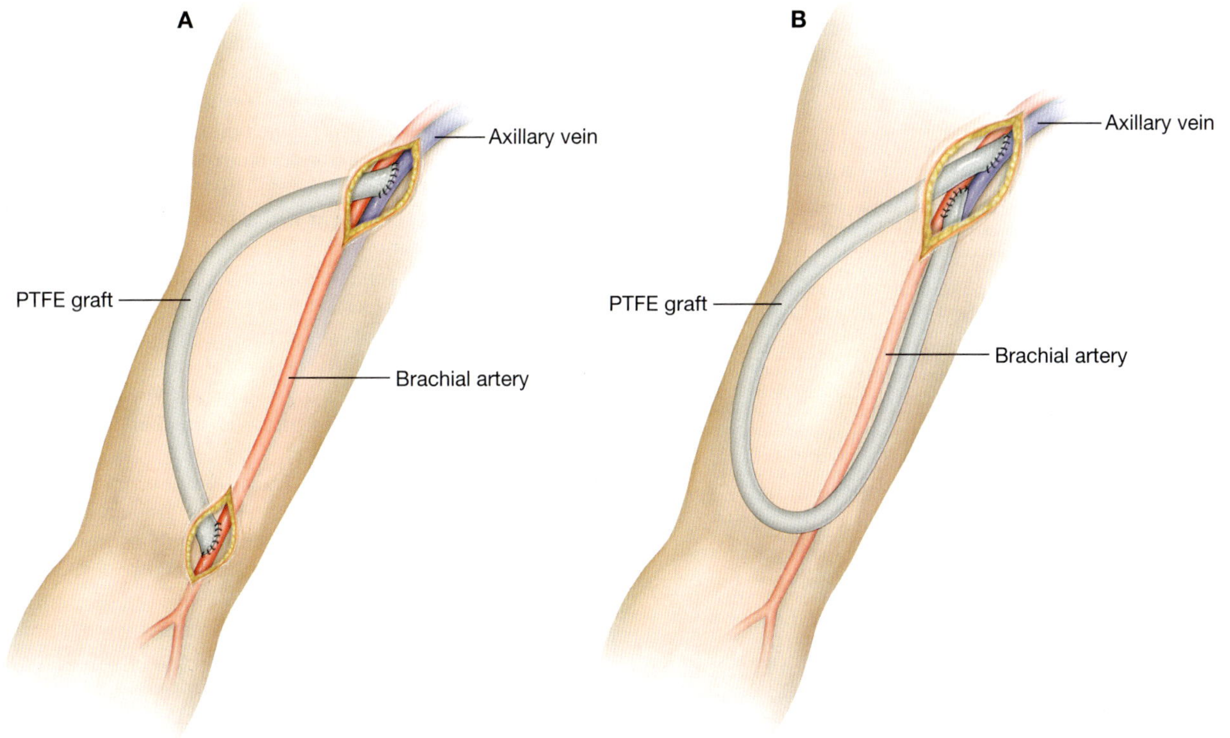

FIGURE 6 • **A,** An upper arm brachial artery–axillary vein AVG is shown with the brachial artery exposed near the antecubital fossa. The 6-mm PTFE graft is tunneled through a lateral, subcutaneous plane, and both anastomoses are completed in an end-to-side fashion. **B,** An upper arm brachial artery–axillary vein AVG is shown with both anastomoses located in the axilla. A separate counter incision is made to facilitate the tunnel.

PEARLS AND PITFALLS

Access choice	■ The choice of access procedure should be based upon anatomy, life expectancy, anticipated duration of dialysis, and patient preference within the context of the patient's ESKD Life Plan.
Access preservation	■ Strategies should be implemented to preserve all potential access configurations and salvage all failing or thrombosed accesses.
Anastomosis	■ The venous anastomosis should be constructed first when creating an AVG to minimize arterial bleeding from the needle holes.
Access Tunnel	■ The course of the tunnel should extend laterally over the upper arm when creating an AVG to facilitate a comfortable position for cannulation while the patient's arm rests on the table during dialysis. Flexing the elbow to 90° prior to marking the tunnel to ensure that the graft is tunneled sufficiently lateral is helpful.
Complication prevention	■ Strategies should be implemented preoperatively in patients deemed higher risk for ARHI including excluding any arterial inflow stenosis, avoiding the brachial artery at the antecubital fossa as the inflow source, and avoiding the use of large conduits (ie., transposed femoral vein). Furthermore, a potential remedial strategy should be generated *preoperatively* in the event that they develop ischemia. These higher-risk patients include the elderly, diabetic patients, those with peripheral vascular disease, and those with prior episodes of hand ischemia.

POSTOPERATIVE CARE

- A set of serum electrolytes should be obtained in the recovery room to determine the need for urgent hemodialysis. The new access and upper extremity pulses should be interrogated using a combination of physical examination and/or Doppler ultrasound. A brief neurological examination should be performed on the ipsilateral hand to assess both motor and sensory function.
- Patients undergoing second-stage brachial-basilic AVFs are routinely admitted overnight, and their drains are removed the following day at the time of discharge; all other patients are admitted selectively with the determinants being pain control, comorbidities, and urgent need for dialysis.
- Patients are seen in the outpatient clinic 2 weeks postoperatively and then monthly thereafter. The appearance of the wound and patency of the access are assessed along with the presence of any complications.
- Standard AVGs are cleared for use at 3 to 6 weeks postoperatively after the surgical incisions have healed, while early cannulation AVGs can be released almost immediately provided that the patient can tolerate graft cannulation through the surgical tunnel.
- An ultrasound of AVFs is obtained at 6 weeks to assess the outflow vein diameter and the access flow rates. AVFs are cleared for cannulation when the vein diameter exceeds 5 mm and the flow rates exceed 500 mL/min, typically in 3 to 4 months.[13]
- AVFs that fail to mature are evaluated further by AVF duplex. The etiology of this failure to mature includes inflow lesions, anastomotic stenosis, venous outflow stenosis, central vein lesions, accessory veins, excessive depth (ie, obesity), and diffuse narrowing.[4,14] Additional imaging with a catheter-based fistulagram or arteriogram is obtained with the choice dictated by the presumed problem and the need to image from the AVF anastomosis to the central veins or the whole access circuit including the arterial inflow. Remedial treatment with balloon angioplasty and/or an intraluminal stent can be performed as dictated by the findings. Unfortunately, up to one-third of AVFs require some type of remedial intervention to facilitate maturation.[4,14]

COMPLICATIONS

Access-Related Hand Ischemia

- The presence of any access-related hand ischemia (ARHI) or "steal" in the recovery room is particularly concerning. The symptoms of hand ischemia may range from mild (Grade 1—cool extremity, minimal symptoms) to moderate (Grade 2—pain during dialysis) to severe (Grade 3—rest pain, tissue loss).[15] Most of these complaints are more chronic, but the presence and any sensory or motor deficit in the immediate postoperative period merits further intervention. A small subset of patients, typically diabetic patients with peripheral arterial disease undergoing an AVG, can present with intense pain, paresthesia, and motor weakness in the early postoperative period despite normal wrist pulses. This condition, often termed ischemic monomelic neuropathy, is likely a variant of ARHI that primarily affects the nerves and is best treated with emergent access ligation, although some of the neurologic symptoms may not be reversible.[16,17]
- The management of ARHI or the steal syndrome remains an ongoing problem beyond the immediate postoperative period, and up to 20% of individuals receiving a brachial artery–based access at the antecubital fossa will develop some type of steal symptoms with roughly half of these requiring intervention.[18] The timing of the symptoms and ultimate need for intervention are somewhat variable with roughly one-third of the remedial interventions occurring within a week, one-third within a month, and the final one-third beyond a month.[18,19]
- The treatments for ARHI include correction of an arterial inflow stenosis, access flow restriction or "banding," proximalization of the arterial inflow (PAI), revision using distal inflow (RUDI), distal revascularization with interval ligation (DRIL), or ligation. The optimal choice is contingent access type (ie, AVF vs AVG), location (ie, brachial vs radial artery), comorbidities, patient life expectancy, available conduit, future access options, and anticipated dialysis access success. However, the practical choices for a brachial-axillary AVG with the anastomosis near the antecubital fossa include a PAI or ligation, while those for a brachial-based AVF include a RUDI, DRIL, or ligation.
- All patients with any motor compromise merit intervention to reduce the symptoms while, ideally, saving the access. The remedial treatment should include an arteriogram to exclude any inflow stenoses. Notably, the various treatment options (eg, DRIL, RUDI, banding) should be viewed as complementary rather than competitive strategies, with the DRIL and PAI potentially most beneficial for "low-flow" accesses (AVFs < 800 mL/min, AVG < 1200 mL/min) and the RUDI and banding techniques most beneficial for "high-flow" accesses.[20] We do not perform a DRIL or RUDI for steal symptoms associated with an AVG given their more limited patency but will correct the arterial inflow or perform a PAI.

Other Complications

- Patients undergoing permanent access procedures are prone to both systemic and access-specific complications. Owing to their comorbidities, these patients are prone to the typical cardiac and pulmonary complications.
- The access-specific complications commonly include ARHI, failing/thrombosed access, infection, arm edema, neuropathy, high-output congestive heart failure, and seroma. Although most of these complications are chronic, they can occur in the early postoperative period.
- Both AVFs and AVGs can thrombose in the early postoperative period with the incidence being around <10%.[21,22] Early access thromboses are typically attributed to technical issues or a hypercoagulable condition. We have taken an aggressive approach in this setting and have attempted access thrombectomy and surgical revision as dictated by the intraoperative findings and imaging.
- Surgical site infection can occur, and the spectrum of infection ranges from mild cellulitis to more extensive soft tissue infections. Minor wound infections can be treated with antibiotics targeted against the typical microorganisms. More extensive infections are less common and may mandate removal of all prosthetic material. These more extensive infections do not usually occur with autogenous AVFs.

- Postoperative edema is common. This usually resolves within the first couple of weeks. Persistent swelling merits further investigation with duplex ultrasound to exclude a hematoma or a venous outflow stenosis or occlusion. A catheter-based fistulagram may be necessary to evaluate for central venous stenosis. We typically wait 4 weeks after the access creation to obtain a fistulagram to allow the access to be incorporated in the surrounding soft tissue in an attempt to minimize cannulation complications at the time of the fistulagram.
- A seroma can develop in any of the surgical incisions from persistent lymph leak. These are usually self-limited and resolve with expectant management. Persistent leaks merit surgical exploration with ligation of all potential sources, although they can mandate access excision if they persist.

REFERENCES

1. NKF-DOQI clinical practice guidelines for vascular access. National Kidney Foundation-Dialysis Outcomes Quality Initiative. *Am J Kidney Dis*. 1997;30(4 suppl 3):S150-S191. http://www.ncbi.nlm.nih.gov/pubmed/9339150
2. Gold JA, Hoffman K. Fistula first: the National Vascular Access Improvement Initiative. *WMJ*. 2006;105(3):71-73.
3. Lok CE, Huber TS, Lee T, et al. KDOQI clinical practice guideline for vascular access: 2019 update. *Am J Kidney Dis*. 2020;75(4 suppl 2): S1-s164. (In Eng). doi:10.1053/j.ajkd.2019.12.001
4. Huber TS, Ozaki CK, Flynn TC, et al. Prospective validation of an algorithm to maximize native arteriovenous fistulae for chronic hemodialysis access. *J Vasc Surg*. 2002;36(3):452-459.
5. Silva MB, Jr., Hobson RW, Pappas PJ, et al. Vein transposition in the forearm for autogenous hemodialysis access. *J Vasc Surg*. 1997;26(6):981-986. http://www.ncbi.nlm.nih.gov/pubmed/9423713
6. Heindel P, Dieffenbach BV, Sharma G, Belkin M, Ozaki CK, Hentschel DM. Contemporary outcomes of a "snuffbox first" hemodialysis access approach in the United States. *J Vasc Surg* 2021;74(3):947-956. (In Eng). doi:10.1016/j.jvs.2021.01.069
7. Sadaghianloo N, Declemy S, Jean-Baptiste E, et al. Radial artery deviation and reimplantation inhibits venous juxta-anastomotic stenosis and increases primary patency of radial-cephalic fistulas for hemodialysis. *J Vasc Surg*. 2016;64(3):698-706.e1. (In Eng). doi:10.1016/j.jvs.2016.04.023
8. Kirksey L. Unrecognized high brachial artery bifurcation is associated with higher rate of dialysis access failure. *Semin Dial*. 2011;24(6):698-702.
9. Cooper J, Power AH, DeRose G, Forbes TL, Dubois L. Similar failure and patency rates when comparing one- and two-stage basilic vein transposition. *J Vasc Surg*. 2015;61(3):809-816.
10. Arnaoutakis DJ, Deroo EP, McGlynn P, et al. Improved outcomes with proximal radial-cephalic arteriovenous fistulas compared with brachial-cephalic arteriovenous fistulas. *J Vasc Surg*. 2017;66(5):1497-1503. (In Eng). doi:10.1016/j.jvs.2017.04.075
11. Gracz KC, Ing TS, Soung LS, Armbruster KF, Seim SK, Merkel FK. Proximal forearm fistula for maintenance hemodialysis. *Kidney Int*. 1977;11(1):71-75. http://www.ncbi.nlm.nih.gov/pubmed/839655
12. Jennings WC, Sideman MJ, Taubman KE, Broughan TA. Brachial vein transposition arteriovenous fistulas for hemodialysis access. *J Vasc Surg*. 2009;50(5):1121-1125.
13. Beathard GA, Lok CE, Glickman MH, et al. Definitions and end points for interventional studies for arteriovenous dialysis access. *Clin J Am Soc Nephrol*. 2018;13(3):501-512. (In Eng). doi:10.2215/cjn.11531116
14. Huber TS, Berceli SA, Scali ST, et al. Arteriovenous fistula maturation, functional patency, and intervention rates. *JAMA Surg*. 2021;156(12):1111-1118. (In Eng). doi:10.1001/jamasurg.2021.4527
15. Sidawy AN, Gray R, Besarab A, et al. Recommended standards for reports dealing with arteriovenous hemodialysis accesses. *J Vasc Surg*. 2002;35(3):603-610. http://www.ncbi.nlm.nih.gov/pubmed/11877717
16. Wilbourn AJ, Furlan AJ, Hulley W, Ruschhaupt W. Ischemic monomelic neuropathy. *Neurology*. 1983;33(4):447-451.
17. Thimmisetty RK, Pedavally S, Rossi NF, Fernandes JAM, Fixley J. Ischemic monomelic neuropathy: diagnosis, pathophysiology, and management. *Kidney Int Rep*. 2017;2(1):76-79. (In Eng). doi:10.1016/j.ekir.2016.08.013
18. Huber TS, Brown MP, Seeger JM, Lee WA. Midterm outcome after the distal revascularization and interval ligation (DRIL) procedure. *J Vasc Surg*. 2008;48(4):926-932.
19. Scali ST, Chang CK, Raghinaru D, et al. Prediction of graft patency and mortality after distal revascularization and interval ligation for hemodialysis access-related hand ischemia. *J Vasc Surg*. 2013;57(2):451-458.
20. Zanow J, Petzold K, Petzold M, Krueger U, Scholz H. Flow reduction in high-flow arteriovenous access using intraoperative flow monitoring. *J Vasc Surg*. 2006;44(6):1273-1278.
21. Farber A, Imrey PB, Huber TS, et al. Multiple preoperative and intraoperative factors predict early fistula thrombosis in the Hemodialysis Fistula Maturation Study. *J Vasc Surg*. 2016;63(1):163-170.e6. (In Eng). doi:10.1016/j.jvs.2015.07.086
22. Huber TS, Carter JW, Carter RL, Seeger JM. Patency of autogenous and PTFE upper extremity arteriovenous hemodialysis accesses: a systematic review. *J Vasc Surg*. 2003;38(5):1005-1011.

Chapter 42

Hemodialysis Catheter Placement and Maintenance

Nathan W. Kugler and Kellie R. Brown

DEFINITION

- Hemodialysis is defined as the direct mechanical alteration of both blood volume and composition through filtering of blood. This differs from other forms of dialysis, such as peritoneal dialysis, in which volume and composition are indirectly altered.
- Hemodialysis catheters are central venous catheters placed for the purpose of and to facilitate administration of hemodialysis, either in a continuous or intermittent fashion. Typically, these are large-bore (up to 16Fr) dual-lumen catheters designed to facilitate exchange of large volumes of blood at rates (up to 500 mL/min) required for dialysis. Based on the most recent KDOQI guidelines the recommended catheter blood flow rates should be >350 mL/min.[1]
- Catheters can be either tunneled or nontunneled. Tunneled catheters often have a cuffed portion positioned subcutaneously near the skin exit site designed to prevent catheter migration and to decrease the risk of infection.
- A multitude of different hemodialysis catheter tip configurations are on the market, all of which have their own benefits and drawbacks (**FIGURE 1**).
- Hemodialysis catheter placement is typically defined by the vessel of venous access:
  - Internal jugular vein
  - Subclavian vein
  - Femoral vein

PATIENT HISTORY AND PHYSICAL FINDINGS

- A detailed history and physical examination are crucial when evaluating patients in need of a hemodialysis catheter for access.
- History:
  - Special attention to previous central venous line (CVL), peripherally inserted central catheter (PICC), and pacemaker placement is key to understanding risk for central venous stenosis.
  - History of previous upper extremity or neck vein deep venous thrombosis (DVT) provides insight to potential access site difficulties. History of previous lower extremity DVT is important when planning femoral vein access.
- Physical examination:
  - Face and chest wall swelling, with or without chest wall collaterals, can indicate significant central venous stenosis, possibly within the superior vena cava.
  - Chest wall scars can be indicative of previous tunneled lines or implantable port. In addition, palpation of chest wall can aid with evaluation of an underlying pacemaker.
  - Evaluation of the bilateral upper and lower extremities should include investigation of scars consistent with previous hemodialysis access attempts.
  - Unilateral upper extremity swelling can be indicative of either deep venous thrombus or more central venous stenosis.
- Bedside ultrasound evaluation is an important adjunct available in many provider offices. Such technology is becoming more readily available and is now often taught in conjunction with physical examination skills.

IMAGING AND OTHER DIAGNOSTIC STUDIES

- Any available previous imaging should be reviewed in detail. Prior chest x-ray and computed tomography (CT) imaging may demonstrate the presence of a pacemaker, previous central venous lines, peripherally inserted central catheters, or venous stents.

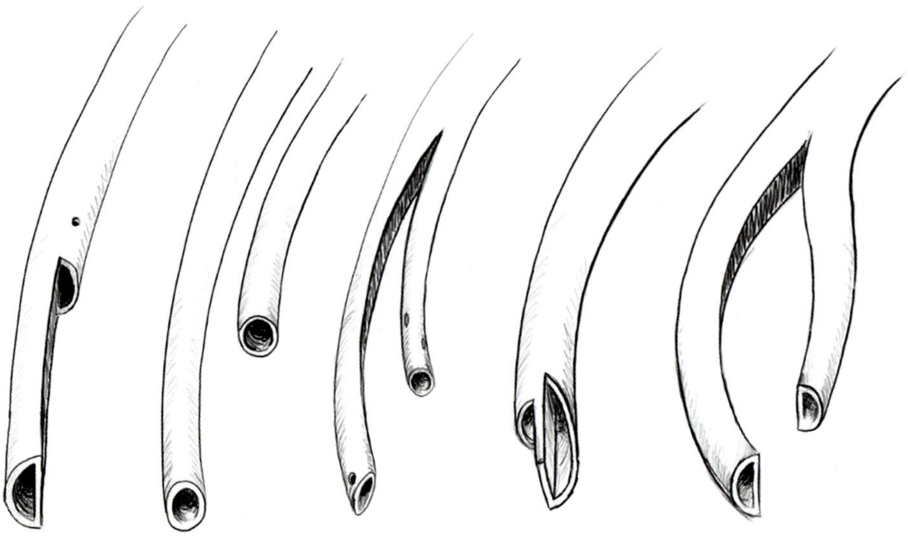

FIGURE 1 • Diagram outlining the different tip designs of tunneled hemodialysis catheters. (Courtesy of Jacob C. Wood, MD.)

- Imaging review can help clinicians understand anatomic challenges to central catheter placement. In addition, it may aid in the understanding of and predict potential issues that may result in catheter dysfunction following placement.
- Ultrasound evaluation of the venous system is helpful in establishing the presence of thrombus and evidence of central obstruction and determining technical feasibility.
- In the situation of numerous previous central venous lines and no previous imaging, a reasonable start to evaluation is a dedicated CT venogram of the chest. Such imaging will help assess central venous anatomy and patency.

SURGICAL MANAGEMENT

Preprocedural Planning

- Determining whether the hemodialysis catheter will be tunneled or temporary is key to procedural planning. Absolute contraindications to placement of tunneled dialysis catheters include ongoing bacteremia and uncorrected coagulopathy, and overlying skin infection or breakdown. Relative contraindications include severe metabolic abnormalities, chest wall neoplasms, anticipated site of radiation therapy, ongoing cellulitis, chest wall burns, and those requiring ongoing chest physiotherapy.
- Tunneled dialysis catheters are available in different calibers and appropriate lengths. Choice of the appropriate length is critical as the anticipated duration of these catheters is significantly longer.
- Temporary nontunneled catheters are preferred for short-term (less than 2 weeks) dialysis access, or in the case of ongoing bacteremia or when multiple line exchanges are anticipated. Nontunneled catheters are available in different calibers, configurations (straight vs curved), and lengths. Differences in configuration lend advantages and disadvantages based on the venous access location.
- Appropriate preprocedural laboratory studies should include a basic metabolic panel to assess potassium and uremia along with an international normalized ratio for all patients. Those receiving heparin products should have a recent activated partial thromboplastin time. Patients with a history of or risk factors for thrombocytopenia should have a recent platelet count.
- Preprocedural antibiotic administration should be used in accordance with your institutional policy.
- Venous access location
  - The preferred location for venous access is the right internal jugular vein.
  - Catheters should not be placed on the side of a maturing fistula or anticipated hemodialysis fistula or graft as ipsilateral placement puts the patient at risk for central stenosis and potential for failure to mature.

Patient Positioning

- Patient positioning for catheter placement is dependent upon planned location of venous access and whether tunneled or nontunneled catheter is being placed.
- When utilizing internal jugular or subclavian vein access, the head should be rotated to the contralateral side. This technique will open the jugular triangle facilitating the most direct venous access. Restrictions such as associated cervical spine injury or previous spinal fusion may preclude this maneuver and may play a role in choice of venous access location.
- Trendelenburg positioning is an important aspect of safe venous access when utilizing either an internal jugular or a subclavian venous approach.
- When placing a tunneled hemodialysis catheter, the operator must ensure patient positioning allows sufficient exposure of the venous access site, skin tunnel, and catheter exit site.
- Overall room setup is a consideration with the understanding that alternative venous access sites might be required. Patient and bed positioning if planned fluoroscopy with a C-arm ensures adequate working room with minimal movement. Planning of optimal room setup and patient position can minimize unnecessary movements that may compromise sterile technique.
- Supplies:
  - It is critical to ensure all needed supplies for catheter placement are gathered and present prior to beginning the procedure. This ensures the most efficient means of placement while lessening risk of breaks in your sterile field.
  - Typical setups include a central venous access kit including the necessary wires, dilators, and catheters. Local anesthetic, skin knife, and dressings are necessary for all line placements. When planning for tunneled line placement, a tunneler is essential along with suture and dressing to close with the counter incision at the venous access site.

GENERAL CONSIDERATIONS

- Ensuring adequate sterile technique is essential to reducing catheter-associated infections. Chlorhexidine and alcohol-based skin preparation products are best suited for prevention of infection,[2] and utilization of full body sterile draping minimizes potential exposure and equipment contamination.
- Utilization of a central line dressing kit, which typically includes an antimicrobial dressing such as BIOPATCH (Ethicon Inc., Cincinnati, OH) or Tegaderm CHG (3M Health Care, St. Paul, MN) dressing. There is some evidence that utilization of chlorhexidine dressings can reduce early catheter-associated blood stream infections.[3]
- Ultrasound should be utilized for both preprocedural assessment of the venous access site and for direct visualization of the needle and wire within the venous lumen. Use of ultrasound has been shown to improve first access attempt success while decreasing access site complications.[4]

GENERAL SELDINGER VENOUS ACCESS TECHNIQUE

- Step 1: Access site is chosen after ultrasound identification of the vessel. Local anesthesia is administered to the site. Ultrasound-guided needle access into the vein is performed with direct visualization of the needle tip within the lumen. This can be performed with an open needle technique or with negative aspiration utilizing a partially saline-filled syringe.
- Step 2: Evaluation of back bleeding can aid in confirmation of venous access. Back bleeding evaluation is often limited with micropuncture needle use. Back bleeding assessment can be confounded in severely hypotensive and/or hypoxic patients. If necessary, an arterial line transducer can be used to confirm that the access is within a vein, rather than an artery.
- Step 3: A wire is advanced through the needle to facilitate durable venous access. Ultrasound images of the wire within the venous lumen should be obtained and saved to the medical record. Wire position can then be manipulated under fluoroscopic guidance to ensure positioning within the inferior vena cava.

INTERNAL JUGULAR AND SUBCLAVIAN VEIN APPROACH

- Following Seldinger access of the appropriate vein the optimal position of the catheter must be determined with fluoroscopy. The wire can be positioned at the desired tip location and removed from the venous access sheath to measure the intravascular length for the catheter.
- Under fluoroscopy a 0.038-in wire is positioned within the inferior vena cava. In a subclavian vein approach or left internal jugular approach, directional catheters can be utilized to achieve proper wire position.
- A series of dilators are passed over the wire prior to introduction of the peel-away introducer sheath through which the dialysis catheter will be introduced and positioned under fluoroscopy. Trendelenburg positioning and a breath hold maneuver during removal of the dilator can minimize the risk of air embolism.
- The wire is removed from the peel-away introducer sheath prior to passing the hemodialysis catheter. Sheaths with a hemostatic valve will prevent significant back bleeding prior to advancing the catheter. If the peel-away sheath does not have a hemostatic valve, finger occlusion of the ostium can prevent significant back bleeding and minimize risk for air embolism.
- The hemodialysis catheter is advanced through the peel-away sheath into the venous system. Utilizing finger manipulation or small nontoothed forceps, the catheter is stabilized at the level of the venous access site as the peel-away sheath is removed.
- Following complete removal of the sheath the catheter should be evaluated with fluoroscopy to ensure no major kinks are identified and the appropriate tip position has been achieved (**FIGURE 2**).

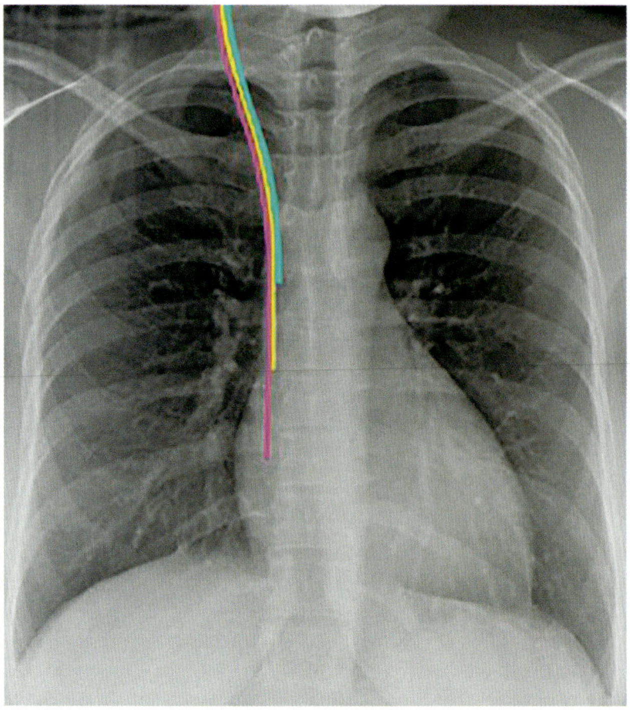

FIGURE 2 • Chest x-ray or fluoroscopy aids in determination of the hemodialysis catheter as too shallow (blue), appropriately positioned (yellow), or too deep (pink). (Courtesy of Jacob C Wood, MD.)

FEMORAL VEIN APPROACH

- The general Seldinger technique is utilized to achieve femoral vein access with confirmation of venous access as detailed above.
- Catheter length is typically less of a consideration as often the longest available catheter is chosen. If concern for central stenosis exists, a venogram can help identify any areas of stenosis. The appropriate position of a femoral catheter is within the inferior vena cava, central to any significant stenosis if one exists. Placement central to any stenosis minimizes the risk for recirculation during hemodialysis sessions.
- If tunneled catheter placement is performed, tunnels should be positioned to ensure changes in patient position do not result in kinks in the catheter.

TUNNELED DIALYSIS CATHETER PLACEMENT

- The traditional Seldinger technique is utilized to gain venous access with a small skin incision made at the venous access site. Compared with nontunneled line placement, a more lateral venous access approach is utilized to minimize the impact of the catheter course of the vein.
- Utilization of a small Kelly forceps can release the surrounding soft tissues. It is important to establish venous sheath access prior to removal of the wire, which will facilitate catheter measurement.
- The wire is positioned at the location of the desired catheter tip using fluoroscopic guidance. Removal of the wire facilitates measurement of the intravascular length of the catheter. The intravascular length of the catheter is subtracted from the overall catheter length to determine the external catheter length. This external catheter length determines the length of the tunnel and thus the position of the skin exit site on the chest wall.
- After determination of the skin exit site and tunnel course, local anesthesia is instilled along the tract to facilitate comfortable passage of the tunneler.
- All tunneled dialysis catheter kits include a tunneler that is attached to the catheter. This is utilized to pass the catheter in a subcutaneous fashion from the skin exit site to the venous access site. The cuff should be positioned approximately 1-2 cm from the skin exit site within the tunnel (**FIGURE 3**). After tunneling, all lumens of the catheter should be flushed and capped.
- After tunneling to the venous access site, a stiff 0.038-in guidewire is positioned through the venous sheath into the inferior vena cava with the aid of fluoroscopy.
- A series of dilators are advanced at the venous access site prior to placement of the peel-away introducer sheath. The tip of the dilators only needs to be advanced 2 to 3 cm into the vein as they aid primarily in subcutaneous tissue dilation. The peel-away introducer sheath should be advanced under fluoroscopy to ensure smooth placement without kinking or concern for a more central obstruction.
- The dilator is removed from the peel-away sheath after which the dialysis catheter is inserted. Expeditious placement of the catheter within the sheath after dilator removal minimizes the chances of an air entry. In addition, Trendelenburg positioning and breath holding techniques help minimize risk for air embolism.
- The dialysis catheter should be firmly held at the level of the venous access site while the split peel-away introducer sheath is carefully removed.

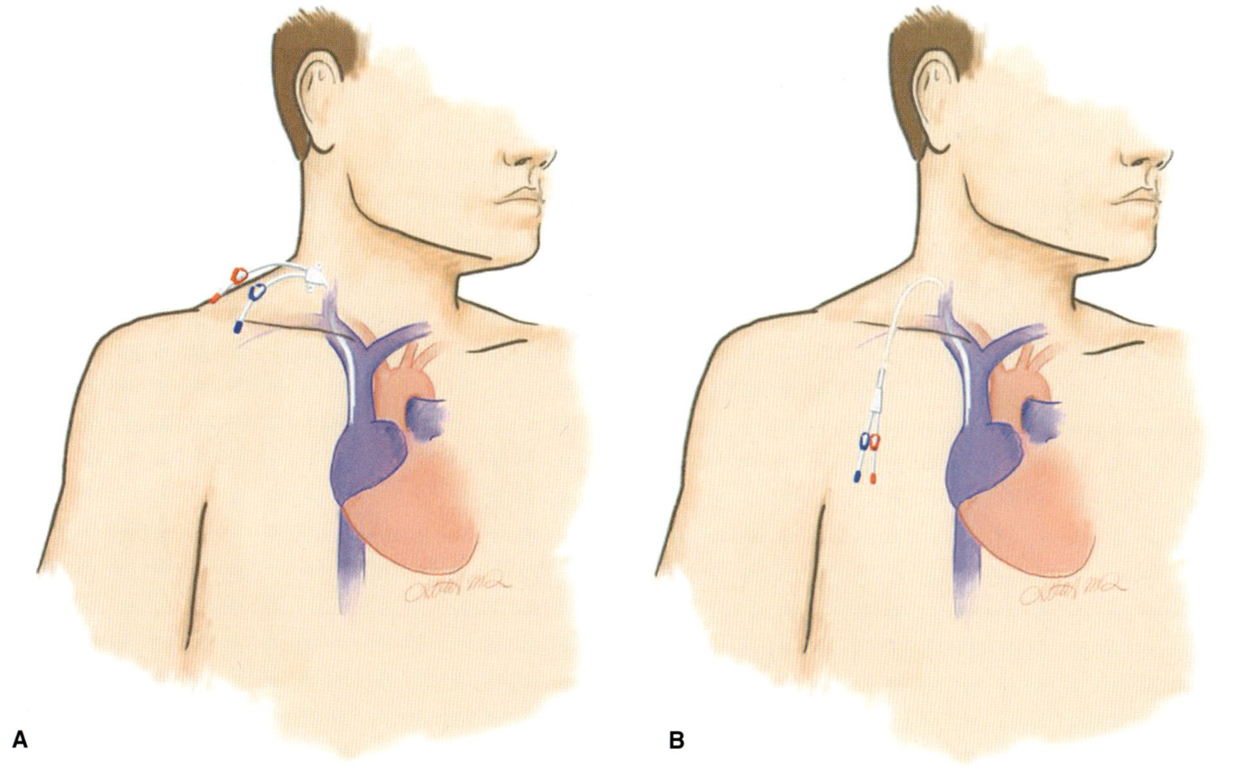

FIGURE 3 • Nontunneled **(A)** and tunneled lines **(B)** with appropriate subcutaneous cuff position. (Courtesy Jacob C. Wood, MD.)

TECHNIQUES

FINISHING CONSIDERATIONS

- All dialysis catheters, tunneled or not, should be flushed and aspirated prior to completion of the procedure to ensure appropriate line function.
- Prior to completion, all lines should be capped with the appropriate solution based on institutional protocols.
- For tunneled dialysis catheters the venous access site should be closed with both subcutaneous suture and a sterile dressing, often a sterile surgical adhesive.
- All catheters should be secured in place to ensure limited movement. Multiple different techniques and devices are available to proceduralists to accomplish this task.
- Sterile dressings in compliance with institution protocol should be placed prior to breaking down the sterile field. Antibiotic ointment can be applied at the catheter exit site during the initial healing period.[5]

HEMODIALYSIS CATHETER EXCHANGE

- Passage of a 0.035-in guidewire through the catheter port under fluoroscopy allows the operator to remove the dialysis catheter while maintaining venous access. The catheter should be inspected to ensure the tip is intact following removal.
- The guidewire should ideally be positioned into the inferior vena cava (IVC) prior to removal of the hemodialysis catheter. If having difficulty navigating to the IVC, use of an angled hydrophilic wire and torque device can facilitate IVC selection prior to catheter removal. A catheter can then be advanced over the hydrophilic wire to facilitate exchange for a stiffer 0.035-in wire. After removal of the catheter, pressure at the venous access site can help minimize bleeding.
- If bacteremia is present, wiping the wire with either Betadine or an alcohol-based solution can minimize risk of reinfection. When bacteremia exists and venous access options make it feasible, transition to a nontunneled catheter until bacteremia has completely resolved is best.
- When exchanging a nontunneled hemodialysis catheter, a new peel-away sheath can be advanced over the wire to facilitate placement of the new catheter.
- When exchanging a tunneled catheter, prior to passage of the guide wire, the catheter exit site is infiltrated with local anesthetic to allow adequate dissection of the subcutaneous cuff. Infiltration directly around the cuff can aid in dissection of the surrounding tissues. Adequate dissection of the cuff from the surrounding soft tissue is key to a smooth successful exchange.
- The guidewire is positioned within the IVC as noted above, and the replacement catheter is loaded onto the guidewire, and under fluoroscopic guidance the catheter is advanced to ensure passage without loss of wire position.

PEARLS AND PITFALLS

Patient selection	■ Thorough evaluation of all previous central venous lines and pacemakers is incredibly important when assessing for potential placement challenges.
Imaging evaluation	■ Optimal positioning of a nontunneled hemodialysis catheter is within the central superior vena cava. Nontunneled catheters are stiffer, and thus, atrium placement should be avoided. ■ Optimal positioning of the tunneled hemodialysis catheter tip is within the right atrium as catheters will retract several centimeters with upright positioning.[6] ■ Careful consideration of catheter length is crucial to the long-term function. Catheters terminating in the superior vena cava (SVC) risk dysfunction due to dislodging into the brachiocephalic or jugular veins. In addition, catheters terminating within the ventricle can be a source of ongoing arrhythmias.

Technique	■ In a tunneled dialysis catheter, the cuff of the catheter should not be placed more than 3 cm into the tract as it may complicate future removal. ■ For internal jugular venous access, entry into the jugular vein higher on the neck will create an unfavorable catheter course for tunneled lines leading to increased risk of kinking and dysfunction. ■ If unable to achieve stable wire access in the IVC, utilization of an angled catheter and glide wire under fluoroscopic guidance can facilitate IVC selection. ■ If positioning of the catheter is not ideal or if a kink exists within the catheter, placement of a stiff wire via one of the infusion ports can facilitate repositioning. ■ With tunneled dialysis catheter exchange, placement of an exchange length stiff glide wire in each catheter port facilitates a more stable platform over which to advance and position the replacement catheter (**FIGURE 4**).

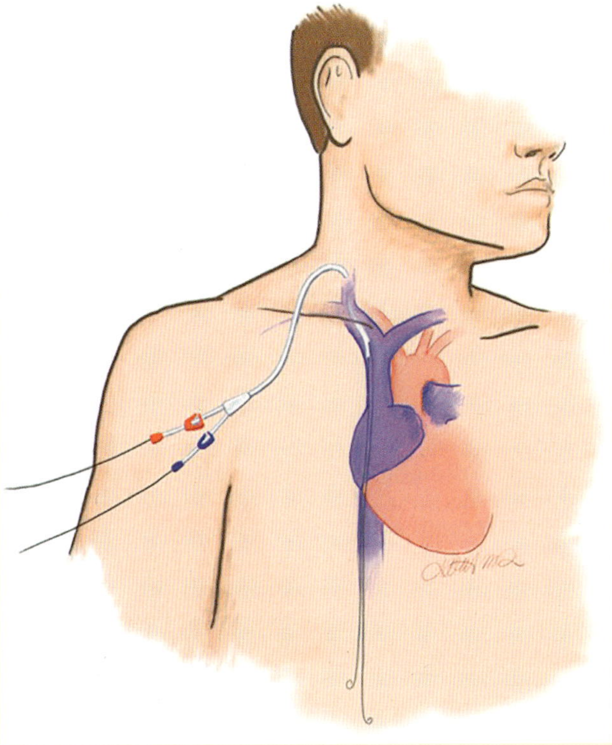

FIGURE 4 • Illustration showing stiff glide wire access through each port of the tunneled dialysis catheter and into the infrarenal aorta. (Courtesy of Jacob C. Wood, MD.)

POSTOPERATIVE CARE

- Hemodialysis catheter maintenance:
  - When initiating dialysis, the catheter hub should be sani-with a chlorhexidine-based solution. The locking solution should be withdrawn till blood is visualized prior to connecting to the dialysis circuit.
  - After hemodialysis is complete, the catheter should be flushed with a locking solution based on institutional policy. Flushing all blood from the catheter minimizes the risk of thrombus formation. The most common catheter locking solutions include saline or heparin-saline (variable concentrations). Alternative options include antibiotic locks, tissue plasminogen activator, sodium citrate, and sodium bicarbonate.
  - The catheter hubs and skin entry site should be cleaned with a chlorhexidine-based solution and new sterile dressings applied.
- Any catheter should be removed when no longer clinically necessary. Removal of a nontunneled temporary hemodialysis line is easily performed at the bedside. Appropriate positioning and adequate manual pressure reduce risks of air embolism and hematoma formation. Removal of a tunneled catheter is typically performed in a procedural suite due to need for dissection of the subcutaneous cuff, which requires local anesthesia along with a scalpel and a small hemostat to aid with the dissection.
- All nonfunctional catheters that fail conservative techniques aimed at restoring function will need to be exchanged. Preservation of the venous access site should be of the utmost importance unless it is thought this factor is the reason for dysfunction.
- In patients with bacteremia, based on the most recent guidelines, antibiotic treatment with delayed line exchange over a nonbraided wire is encouraged. In cases with persistent exit site infection, other venous access sites should be explored.[1]
- Trouble shooting
  - Most issues related to a malfunctioning hemodialysis catheter are related to positioning. Repositioning of the

catheter over a wire to preventing kinking, particularly in the situation of a recently place tunneled catheter, may resolve the issue.
- Power aspiration and flushing of hemodialysis catheters can aid with clearing potential thrombus debris in a line resulting in improved function. If such techniques are required frequently then line exchange should be considered.
- When pressure for urgent dialysis exists, maneuvers such as flipping the inflow and outflow ports may help improve flow rates if mechanical catheter issues exist. This is not a long-term solution but can alleviate the need for urgent line exchanges.

COMPLICATIONS

- Iatrogenic arterial injury is a well-documented complication of percutaneous venous access. While inadvertent arterial needle access has been estimated up to 10%, use of ultrasound guidance has significantly lessened this event.[7,8] The true incidence is hard to calculate as fortunately the majority are detected prior to cannulation. Intra-arterial catheter placement rates are reported in less than 1%.[8]
- Removal of an inadvertent central line placed in the arterial system utilizing manual pressure alone for hemostasis has high rates of bleeding complications.[9]
- Pneumothorax can occur after internal jugular or subclavian venous access. The incidence of pneumothorax varies greatly by location of access, failed previous attempts, underlying lung disease, and operator experience but remains highest with a subclavian approach in up to 2% of cases.[10] While the majority of these will require simple observation, routine postprocedural chest x-ray imaging should be obtained.
- Access site hematoma is a complication seen with both tunneled and nontunneled lines.
- SVC and/or myocardial perforation is a rare but potentially fatal complication of either hemodialysis catheter placement or delayed complication of inappropriate catheter length. Hemothorax can occur, and if discovered should prompt contrast-enhanced CT imaging to better define potential site of injury.
- Infection is a significant complication after catheter placement, which can be catheter related blood stream infections, catheter colonization, or exit site infections. Not all catheter-associated bloodstream infections require line removal or exchange, and based on the most recent guidelines there are very few instances where abandoning venous access for a line holiday is necessary.[1]
- Exit site infections are typically defined by hyperemia, induration, or tenderness less than 2 cm from the catheter exit site, and if associated with drainage this should be cultured. These infections can be treated with a 7- to 14-day course of appropriate antibiotic therapy. If unable to clear the associated infection, then line removal and/or exchange will be necessary.
- Catheter-associated thrombus is a common complication of any indwelling central catheter. Determination of ongoing need for the associated hemodialysis catheter is important when considering treatment options. Anticoagulation should be initiated per CHEST guidelines with line removal only if no longer clinically necessary.[11]
- Catheter-associated thrombus can affect catheter performance. Late catheter dysfunction is most commonly the result of thrombus formation either within or around the catheter. Anticoagulation remains the mainstay of external thrombus management with potential line removal if it is no longer necessary. Treatment should be continued based on the most recent CHEST guidelines. Internal thrombus can be managed with intraluminal lysis therapy or forceful saline flush techniques. Mixed results of the efficacy of these techniques have been reported. Ultimately, if unsuccessful in resolving the associated dysfunction, catheter exchange is necessary.
- Central venous stenosis is a well-documented complication of long-standing indwelling hemodialysis catheters and can affect longevity of future permanent dialysis access in that extremity.

OUTCOMES

- The general life expectancy of a hemodialysis catheter is highly variable, with tunneled catheters typically having a longer lifespan due to a decreased risk of infection.[12,13]
- Previous work has shown venous access location does significantly affect longevity of hemodialysis catheters, with right internal jugular (median 633 days) longer than either left internal jugular (430 days) or femoral (116 days).[14] Other studies have failed to replicate these results between right and left internal jugular approaches while femoral catheters universally have been shown to have the shortest life expectancy.
- Studies have demonstrated differences in longevity of hemodialysis catheters based upon distal tip design, with better catheter survival seen with split tips and/or split catheters.[14]
- While variability in institutional protocols for removal or exchange make long-term data difficult, no studies have shown that scheduled catheter exchanges improve long-term catheter-based hemodialysis success.
- Infection rates are often one of the greatest quality measures of catheter care following placement. The Centers for Disease Control and Prevention previously issued recommendations for interventions aimed at reducing catheter-associated infections including hand washing, full barrier precautions during insertion, chlorhexidine skin disinfection, avoidance of femoral cannulation, and removal when clinically indicated.[15] A study published in the *NEJM* evaluated the rate of catheter-related blood stream infections in ICU patients with indwelling central venous catheters following implementation of a safety bundle. They demonstrated a significant improvement in the mean number of infections per 1000 catheter days from 7.7 to 1.4 over an 18-month period.[16]

REFERENCES

1. Lok CE, Huber TS, Lee T, et al. KDOQI clinical practice guideline for vascular access: 2019 update. *Am J Kidney Dis*. 2020;75(4):S1-S164.
2. Yasuda H, Sanui M, Abe T, et al. Comparison of the efficacy of three topical antiseptic solutions for the prevention of catheter colonization: a multicenter randomized controlled study. *Crit Care*. 2017;21(1):320.
3. Puig-Asensio M, Marra AR, Childs CA, Kukla ME, Perencevich EN, Schweizer ML. Effectiveness of chlorhexidine dressings to prevent catheter-related bloodstream infections. Does one size fit all? A systematic literature review and meta-analysis. *Infect Control Hosp Epidemiol*. 2020;41(12):1388-1395.

4. Rabindranath KS, Kumar E, Shail R, Vaux EC. Ultrasound use for the placement of haemodialysis catheters. *Cochrane Database Syst Rev*. 2011(11):CD005279.
5. O'Grady NP, Alexander M, Burns LA, et al. Summary of recommendations: guidelines for the prevention of intravascular catheter-related infections. *Clin Infect Dis*. 2011;52(9):1087-1099.
6. Engstrom BI, Horvath JJ, Stewart JK, et al. Tunneled internal jugular hemodialysis catheters: impact of laterality and tip position on catheter dysfunction and infection rates. *J Vasc Intervent Radiol*. 2013;24(9):1295-1302.
7. Farrell J, Walshe J, Gellens M, Martin KJ. Complications associated with insertion of jugular venous catheters for hemodialysis: the value of postprocedural radiograph. *Am J Kidney Dis*. 1997;30(5):690-692.
8. Bowdle A. Vascular complications of central venous catheter placement: evidence-based methods for prevention and treatment. *J Cardiothorac Vasc Anesth*. 2014;28(2):358-368.
9. Dixon OGB, Smith GE, Carradice D, Chetter IC. A systematic review of management of inadvertent arterial injury during central venous catheterisation. *J Vasc Access*. 2017;18(2):97-102.
10. Vinson DR, Ballard DW, Hance LG, et al. Pneumothorax is a rare complication of thoracic central venous catheterization in community EDs. *Am J Emerg Med*. 2015;33(1):60-66.
11. Stevens SM, Woller SC, Kreuziger LB, et al. Antithrombotic therapy for VTE disease. *Chest*. 2021;160(6):e545-e608.
12. Dryden MS, Samson A, Ludlam HA, Wing AJ, Phillips I. Infective complications associated with the use of the Quinton "Permcath" for long-term central vascular access in haemodialysis. *J Hosp Infect*. 1991;19(4):257-262.
13. Mandolfo S, Acconcia P, Bucci R, et al. Hemodialysis tunneled central venous catheters: five-year outcome analysis. *J Vasc Access*. 2014;15(6):461-465.
14. Fry AC, Stratton J, Farrington K, et al. Factors affecting long-term survival of tunnelled haemodialysis catheters a prospective audit of 812 tunnelled catheters. *Nephrol Dial Transplant*. 2008;23(1):275-281.
15. O'Grady NP, Alexander M, Burns LA, et al. Guidelines for the prevention of intravascular catheter-related infections. *Clin Infect Dis*. 2011;52(9):e162-e93.
16. Pronovost P, Needham D, Berenholtz S, et al. An intervention to decrease catheter-related bloodstream infections in the ICU. *N Engl J Med*. 2006;355(26):2725-2732.

Chapter 43

Insertion of a Peritoneal Dialysis Catheter

An Alternative to Creating Vascular Access in the Treatment of Renal Failure

Ashley Nicole Krepline and Dean Edward Klinger

DEFINITION

- Peritoneal dialysis (PD) is a means of treating patients with end-stage renal disease. A catheter is placed within the peritoneal cavity to allow installation of a dextrose-based dialysate. PD uses the concept of diffusion gradients across a membrane. In PD, the membrane is all of the peritoneal surfaces within the abdomen.
- The diffusion gradient is created by the dialysate fluid instilled in the abdomen. Toxins, electrolytes, and water can diffuse across the membrane as dictated by the concentration gradients, the exposed surface area of peritoneum, and the length of time the dialysate is in the abdomen.

Alternatives to Peritoneal Dialysis

- The treatment options for patients with significant renal failure include kidney transplantation, hemodialysis, and PD. If possible, a kidney transplant is the preferred treatment. Renal replacement therapy with PD and hemodialysis offer comparable survival outcomes. PD, for the appropriate patient, offers several advantages to hemodialysis. Compared to hemodialysis, PD is associated with a slower decline in residual renal function. While hemodialysis is primarily performed in dialysis centers, PD is performed in the home allowing for more independence. Additionally, PD is associated with a lower cost per year as it does not require a dialysis center, requires fewer support staff, and patients require less erythropoietin stimulating agents when undergoing peritoneal dialysis.
- The rates of peritoneal dialysis vary widely across the world. Worldwide, approximately 11% of patients on dialysis undergo peritoneal dialysis; however, the rate of peritoneal dialysis is increasing at a faster rate than the utilization of hemodialysis (8% vs 6%-7%). Rates of peritoneal dialysis are highest in Hong Kong, Thailand, New Zealand, and Australia. Conversely, hemodialysis is utilized more frequently in Africa, North America, and Europe. In this chapter, we will focus on PD.

PATIENT HISTORY AND PHYSICAL FINDINGS

- A good history and physical exam will help ensure that you have a good candidate for PD. Hemodialysis is also an option for the treatment of renal failure and may be the better choice of dialysis for some patients.
- PD is a very good option for those patients that want to be independent as it is done at home. PD is less stressful on the heart and therefore is a good option in patients with heart failure. It is also a good option for patients with ascites from right sided heart failure and liver disease as PD provides treatment for both the renal failure and ascites.
- Patients with hernias should have them repaired at the time of insertion of the catheter unless the hernias are too large or complicated, in which case hemodialysis should be considered. Individuals that tell you of prior abdominal operations and having a lot of adhesions may not be able to have PD. Operations may leave the patient with too many adhesions such that a catheter cannot be inserted or there is insufficient surface area for adequate dialysis. Patients with ostomies and feeding tubes are also considered to be poor candidates for PD.

IMAGING AND OTHER DIAGNOSTIC STUDIES

- There is no preoperative imaging required prior to placement of a PD catheter. There is no imaging modality that quantifies the degree of adhesions that would prevent insertion of a catheter or predict adequate surface area and function of PD.

SURGICAL MANAGEMENT

Preoperative Planning

- Patients are required to meet with the home PD staff prior to insertion of the catheter. Assessments are made to ensure that the patient will be able to care for the catheter as well as do the dialysis. This requires adequate mental and physical abilities. An example of a patient where there could be problems might be in someone who has had a stroke. It is also advisable that the patient have a safe home environment that is clean and there is a live-in caregiver who can assist with the PD should the need arise. The PD staff make a home visit to assess the physical layout to assess the ability to store all the supplies and dispose of the waste.
- Care must be taken to keep in mind the patient's body habitus and disabilities when planning the location of the exit site of the PD catheter. The exit site should not be in a skin fold or at the beltline and when possible in a location that the patient can see.
- Chlorhexidine wipes or soap are given to the patient to use the day before and day of the operation. Prior to the operation, the patient is given preoperative antibiotics.

Positioning

- The patient is placed supine with arms out on the operating room table with appropriate padding of dependent areas. If the PD catheter is being inserted laparoscopically, a monitor is placed at the foot of the bed for visualization.

INSERTION OF A PD CATHETER

- The three means by which a PD catheter can be inserted are percutaneous, open, and laparoscopic. There are advantages and disadvantages to each (**TABLE 1**).
- The advantage of percutaneous and open insertion is that the procedure can be done under local anesthesia, with less cost as the procedure is shorter, and there is no requirement for use of the postanesthesia recovery unit. The advantage of laparoscopic insertion is that there is about 10% reduction in the patient having problems with the catheter being obstructed by the omentum.
- It is unknown if there is an increased risk of complications with insertion of the PD catheter using the laparoscopic technique compared to the open technique. This remains a controversy as some studies have demonstrated laparoscopic placement of PD catheters is associated with a higher rate of intraoperative complications; however, not all studies have demonstrated this.

Table 1: Advantages and Disadvantages of Each Method of PD Catheter Insertion

	Anesthesia	Cost	Catheter obstruction	Complications
Percutaneous	+	+	–	–
Open	+	+	–	+
Laparoscopic	–	–	+	+/–

PERCUTANEOUS PLACEMENT

- PD catheters can be placed using ultrasound and a percutaneous technique in a Seldigner fashion. Our practice does not utilize this technique and is beyond the scope of this chapter.

OPEN TECHNIQUE

- The operation begins with determining where to make the incision for insertion of the PD catheter. Markings are placed on the patient to indicate skin folds and where the patient's beltline is located. The surgeon's PD catheter of choice is used to help locate the position of the incision. The intra-abdominal portion of the catheter is positioned about 2 cm above the symphysis pubis. The first Dacron cuff on the catheter should be positioned in the rectus muscle through a paramedian incision. A mark is placed on the skin where the cuff will be positioned and marks can be placed on the skin to delineate the incision (**FIGURE 1**). At this time, assessment is made as to where the exit site will be located. The exit site of the catheter should not be in the skin folds or under the beltline. It is also preferred to have the exit site in a position where the patient is able to see it so as to make it easier to care for the catheter. The location of the incision can be shifted to accommodate the best position of the intra-abdominal portion of the catheter and exit site.
- The incision is carried through the skin and subcutaneous tissue down to the anterior rectus fascia (**FIGURE 2**). The fascia is incised in a craniocaudal direction to expose the rectus muscle. The rectus muscle is spread between its fibers to expose the posterior rectus fascia (**FIGURE 3**). A purse-string suture is placed in the posterior rectus fascia with care not to go too deep and catch underlying bowel (**FIGURE 4**). An opening is made in the posterior rectus and peritoneum. Care needs to be taken not to misinterpret bowel wall for the peritoneum.
- The PD catheter is thread onto a long stylet used to introduce the catheter. Initially, the catheter is thread on all

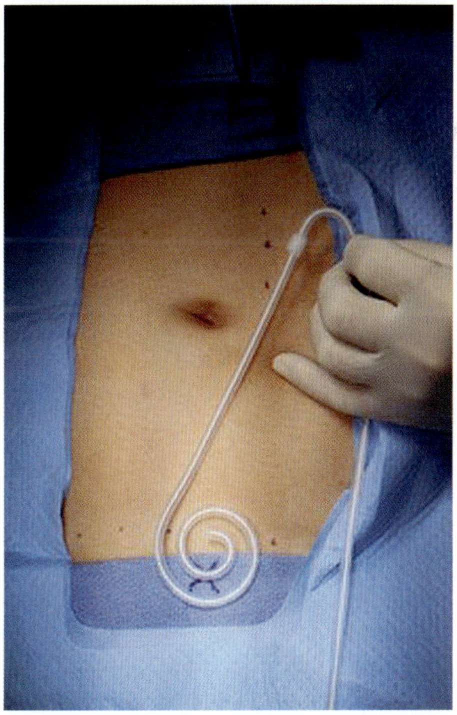

FIGURE 1 • Prior to making an incision, preoperative landmarks are identified. The pubic symphysis is marked and skin folds and the beltline are noted. The end of the PD catheter is placed 2 cm cranially to the pubic symphysis and the location of the paramedian incision is marked at the level where the deep cuff lands.

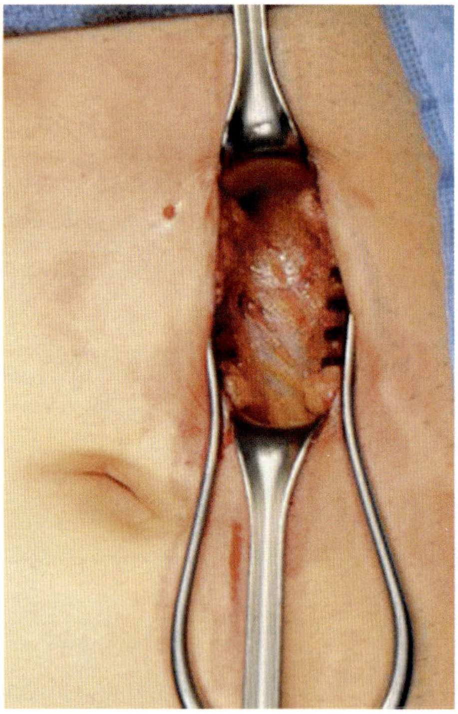

FIGURE 2 • The incision is made and dissection through the subcutaneous tissues is done to expose the anterior rectus fascia.

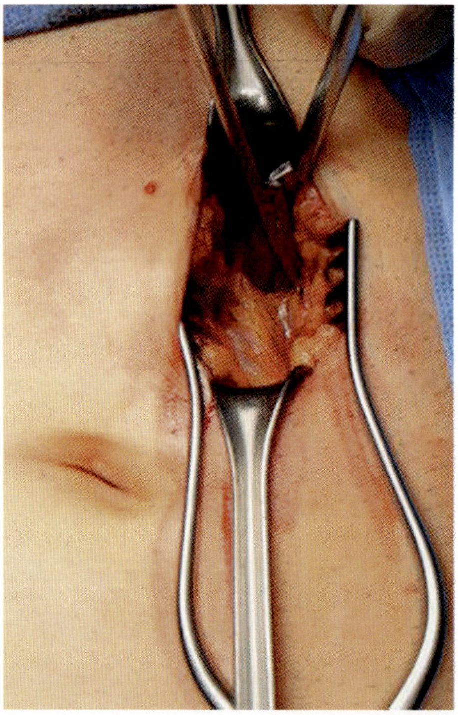

FIGURE 3 • The anterior rectus fascia is incised. A Metzenbaum scissors is placed between rectus muscle fibers and spread perpendicular to the muscle fibers to expose the posterior rectus sheath.

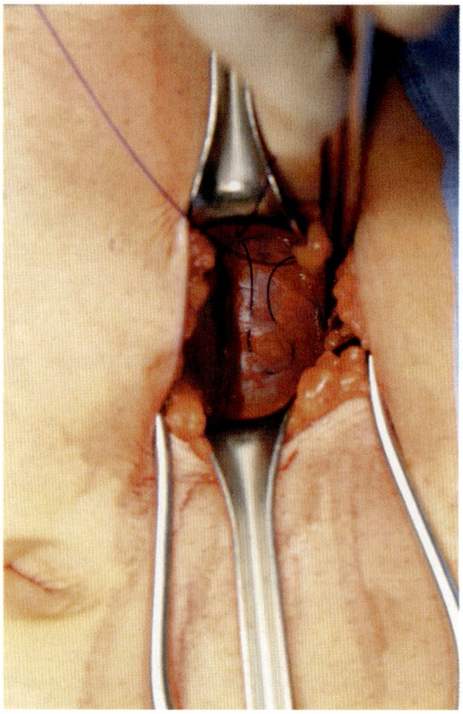

FIGURE 4 • A purse-string suture is placed in the posterior rectus sheath.

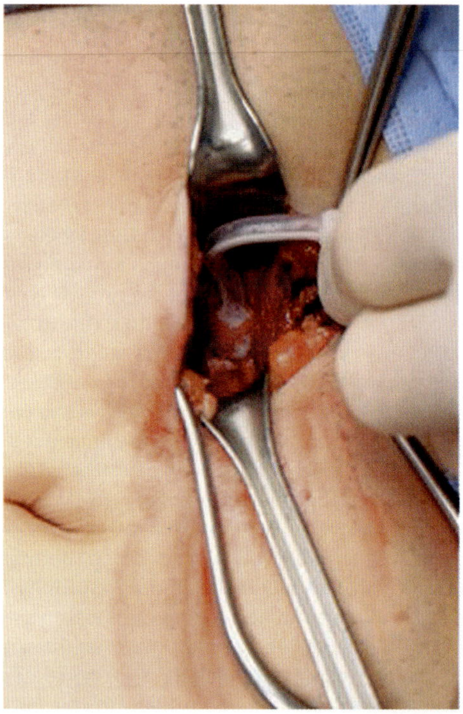

FIGURE 5 • Once the PD catheter is inserted, the purse-string suture is tied.

the way to the end of the stylet to aid in easier insertion, but once the catheter is in the abdomen, the catheter is advanced over the stylet by several centimeters so that the end is not rigid. The catheter is gently directed toward the symphysis pubis. Once the stylet is in the correct position, the remainder of the catheter is introduced into the pelvis. The first Dacron cuff should come to lie in the rectus muscle and the purse-string suture is tied down about the catheter (**FIGURE 5**).

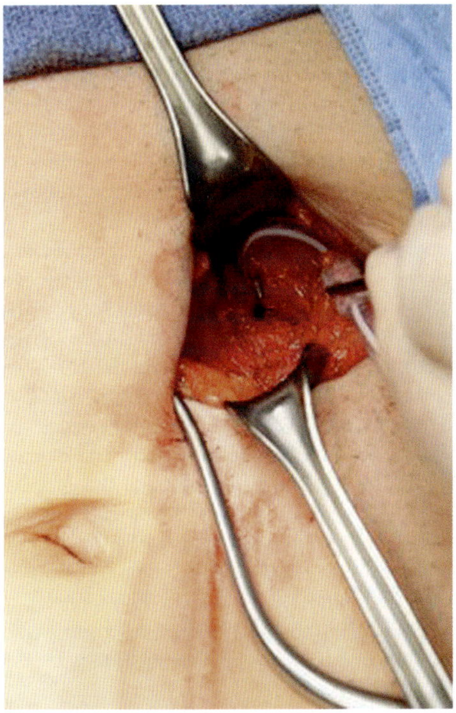

FIGURE 6 • The catheter is flushed with saline solution and fluctuations of the meniscus in the catheter is observed during respiration or changes in the intra-abdominal pressure indicating a patent catheter.

- The function of the catheter can now be tested. Approximately 20 to 30 mL of saline is instilled through the catheter. Ease of introduction is noted. Gentle aspiration can be attempted and the color of the fluid returned noted. It should be clear saline. A bit more saline is introduced and then the syringe is disconnected from the catheter. The meniscus of fluid in the catheter is observed. The meniscus should freely move up and down in the catheter, moving with changes of intra-abdominal pressure changes. Most often, variations can be seen just with respiration. If the meniscus freely fluctuates in the catheter, the catheter is in a good position (**FIGURE 6**).
- The anterior rectus fascia is closed from the caudal to cranial direction. The thought of closing it in this direction is to angle the catheter and get a bit of torque on the catheter to lever up the intra-abdominal end toward the anterior abdominal wall (**FIGURE 7**).
- The catheter is then tunneled to the exit site, avoiding skin folds and the beltline, and in a position where the second Dacron cuff is about 2 centimeters from the skin. The function of the catheter can be tested again and capped. The incision is closed and dressings applied (**FIGURE 8**, **Video 1**).

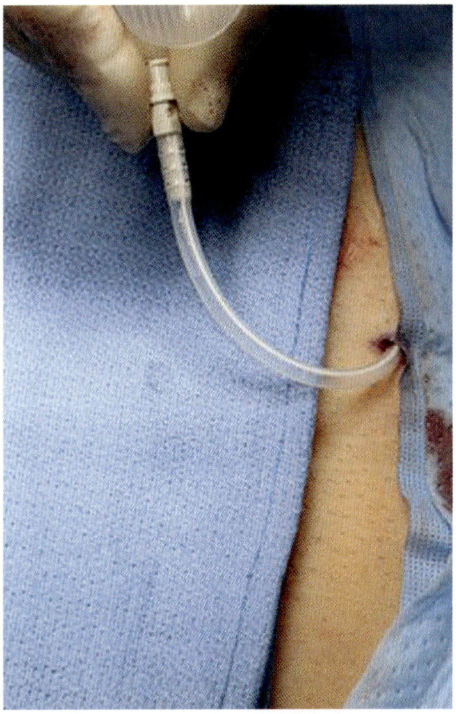

FIGURE 7 • After insertion of the PD catheter, suture is used to close the anterior rectus sheath in a running fashion. The anterior sheath is closed from caudal to cranial to allow for the creation of a tunnel.

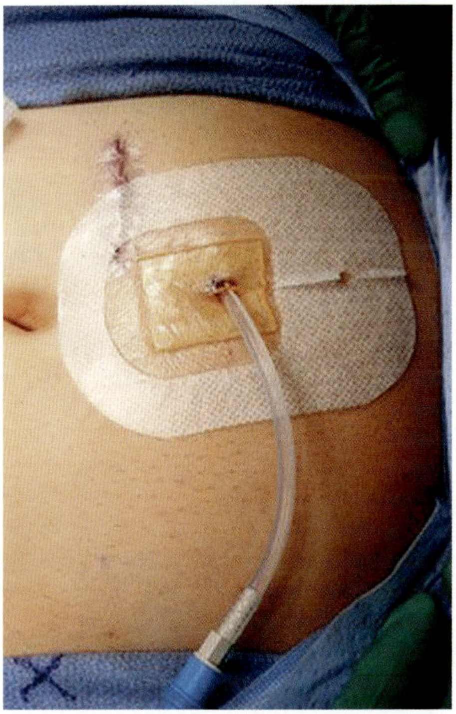

FIGURE 8 • The PD catheter exit site is dressed with a chlorhexidine-impregnated Tegaderm and the incisions are dressed with Dermabond.

LAPAROSCOPIC TECHNIQUE

- When inserting the PD catheter using the laparoscopic technique, considerations for the insertion site and exit site are the same as for the open technique. Pneumoperitoneum is obtained by placing a Veres needle at Palmer point in the left upper quadrant. A 5-mm radially dilating trocar is inserted in the left upper quadrant. A small incision is then made where the PD catheter is to be inserted and a second 5-mm trocar is inserted. A third 5-mm trocar is inserted in the opposite side of the abdomen from where the catheter is inserted.
- Using the three trocars, the omentum is pulled into the upper abdomen and sutured to the anterior abdominal wall in the right, middle, and left upper quadrants to prevent its migration back into the pelvis. A suture passing needle is used to place a stitch through the anterior abdominal wall. The suture is passed around a portion of the omentum, taking care to avoid vessels, and then taken back out the abdominal wall and secured. The purpose this maneuver is to prevent it from encasing and obstructing flow through the PD catheter.
- An alternative to suturing the omentum to the upper abdomen is to remove it. If this is to be done, we recommend placing a 12-mm Hasson cannula in the subxiphoid area. The insertion of the larger trocar is to help facilitate removal of the omentum from the abdomen. A harmonic scissors or LigaSure is used to remove the omentum following along the caudal border of the transverse colon.
- Attention is then directed toward inserting the PD catheter. The trocar at the PD catheter insertion site is removed. A peel away sheath and dilator is inserted at this site with the catheter going through the anterior rectus fascia, tunneling through the rectus muscle on an angle toward the pelvis, and exiting the posterior rectus fascia and peritoneum several inches caudal to the insertion site. The dilator is removed and the PD catheter is inserted through the sheath and directed toward the pelvis. The sheath is removed and the first Dacron cuff comes to lie in the rectus muscle. By tunneling the catheter at an angle through the rectus muscle, there is a torque on the catheter such that it will want to come to lie up against the anterior pelvic wall. The catheter is then tunneled to the exit site as described in the open technique, trocars removed, incisions closed, and dressings applied (**FIGURE 9**, **Video 2**).

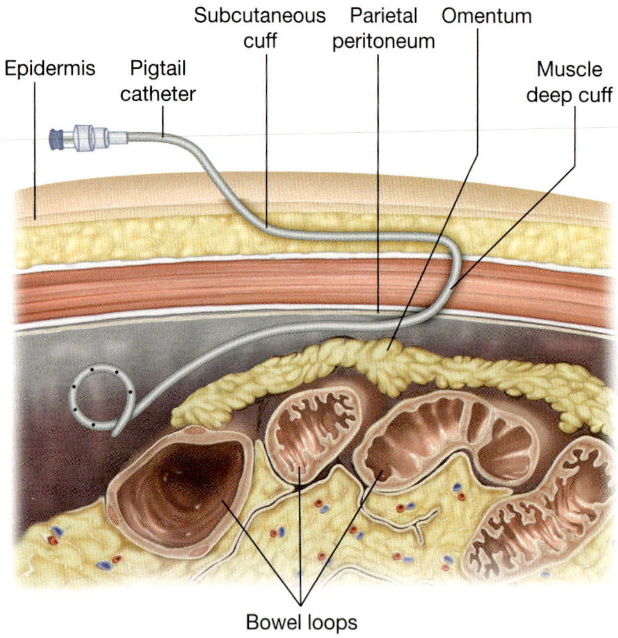

FIGURE 9 • A depiction of the tunnel created within the rectus muscle to allow the catheter to sit along the anterior abdominal wall.

PEARLS AND PITFALLS

Surgical management	■ When determining the position of the catheter in the pelvis, we aim to insert the catheter so the end of the catheter lays approximately 2 cm cephalad to the pubic symphysis so as to be just a bit further from the rectum and bladder. It has been our observation that patients may experience fewer symptoms of pressure in the pelvis during dialysis. ■ If the catheter is inserted laparoscopically, we recommend doing a concurrent omentectomy or pexy of the omentum to the upper abdomen. This is done to reduce the risk of the catheter being encased in the omentum, causing obstruction to drainage.

Technique	- Once the PD catheter is inserted, prior to leaving the operating room, it is important to flush the catheter to ensure patency. A syringe is used to inject approximately 20 to 30 mL of saline through the catheter. The saline should freely flow indicating the catheter is not kinked or obstructed. Once the saline is injected, the meniscus of the saline within the catheter tubing is observed and should vary with respiration or applying pressure to the abdominal wall. - When suturing about the catheter, care must be taken not to puncture the catheter with the needle as this would result in leakage from the catheter during use.

POSTOPERATIVE CARE

- Traditional teachings suggest application of a nonocclusive gauze dressing over the PD catheter exit site to prevent contamination and to secure the PD catheter to prevent tugging on the catheter. Our practice has been to apply a chlorhexidine-impregnated Tegaderm to the PD catheter exit site. Regardless of the type of dressing applied, it is suggested the dressing be changed by experienced PD nurses in the perioperative period to prevent contamination.
- PD catheter flushing is performed weekly to assess the functionality of the PD catheter and closely monitor the patient in the postoperative period. It is recommended to wait 3 weeks following insertion of the PD catheter prior to initiating PD. The risk of leakage about the catheter decreases from 28% at 1 week postoperatively to just 2.4% at 3 weeks.

COMPLICATIONS

- Complications occur in approximately 20% to 35% of peritoneal dialysis catheter placement.

Bladder and Rectal Discomfort

- Patients may experience bladder and rectal discomfort following placement of a PD catheter. This is thought to be associated with the PD catheter resting against the rectum or bladder. Anecdotally, patients less frequently experience this discomfort if the PD catheter is placed so the catheter terminates approximately 2 cm cephalad from the pubic symphysis.

Leakage

- Leakage of dialysate from around the exit site most commonly occurs within 30 days of placement of the PD catheter and is usually a result of initiating PD too early, a technical error when placing the PD catheter, or poor tissue integrity and healing leading to inadequate incorporation of the Dacron cuff. Cessation of PD and transition to hemodialysis for several weeks will allow the exit site to heal and will typically stop the leakage of dialysate from the exit site.

Hernia

- As with all abdominal operations, hernias may occur. The risk of developing a hernia following insertion of a PD catheter is approximately 8.3%. A hernia may develop at the PD catheter exit site, most commonly this will only contain dialysate and will manifest as a bulge under the skin at the tract site. Hernias may also develop at port sites when PD catheters are placed laparoscopically, as is the risk with all laparoscopic abdominal surgery.
- Additionally, the increased intra-abdominal pressure associated with installation of the dialysate may result in hernias that were not detected on preoperative physical exam apparent. If a hernia develops, the patient may undergo either open or laparoscopic repair and eventual resumption of PD.

Catheter Malfunction

- A catheter malfunction can occur as a result in obstruction of the catheter side holes or kinking of the catheter. If a catheter is obstructed by bowel or omentum, the catheter will flush; however, the omentum or bowel will cover the side holes when dialysate is being removed. If the PD catheter is kinked or if there is fibrinous debris or clot within the catheter, the catheter will not flush or allow for drainage of the dialysate.
- Approximately 10% of patients develop catheter dysfunction due to omentum wrapping around the catheter, whether the catheter was placed with an open or laparoscopic technique, unless omentectomy or pexy of the omentum was performed at the time of laparoscopic PD catheter insertion.
- If the catheter malfunctions, laparoscopic intervention should be entertained. There is a 97% success rate of catheter function with laparoscopic intervention when combined with omentectomy or pexy of the omentum.

Infection

- An exit site infection may be present if the exit site is erythematous, indurated, or purulent drainage is observed from the exit site. If the exit site symptoms do not improve with antibiotics or recur after cessation of antibiotics, it is likely the cuff is involved. If this is the case, antibiotics should be given to suppress the infection. A new PD catheter can be inserted on the opposite side of the abdomen and dressings are applied. Following this, the old catheter is removed.
- The PD catheter cuff can extrude through the skin if tunneled too superficially and will act as a reservoir for bacteria. If the PD catheter cuff is completely exteriorized, it can be excised with a scalpel or pulled off with a forceps. If the cuff is incompletely exteriorized, it should be removed from the PD catheter tract and removed from the catheter.
- If there is concern for peritonitis, a peritoneal fluid sample should be obtained. A peritoneal fluid white blood cell count greater than 100/μL or bacteria identified on culture are indicative of peritonitis. Peritonitis can frequently be treated with appropriate antibiotics instilled via the PD catheter. If the pathogen causing peritonitis is yeast or mycobacterium, if the patient does not improve with antibiotic therapy, or if the patient develops recurrent peritonitis, the catheter will

need to be removed and replaced after successful treatment of peritonitis with an interval transition to hemodialysis while undergoing treatment for peritonitis.

SUGGESTED READING

1. Crabtree JH, Shrestha BM, Chow KM, et al. Creating and maintaining optimal peritoneal dialysis access in the adult patient: 2019 update. *Perit Dial Int.* 2019;39(5):414-436. doi:10.3747/pdi.2018.00232
2. Hagen SM, Lafranca JA, IJzermans JN, Dor FJ. A systematic review and meta-analysis of the influence of peritoneal dialysis catheter type on complication rate and catheter survival. *Kidney Int.* 2014;85(4):920-932. doi:10.1038/ki.2013.365
3. Krezalek MA, Bonamici N, Lapin B, et al. Laparoscopic peritoneal dialysis catheter insertion using rectus sheath tunnel and selective omentopexy significantly reduces catheter dysfunction and increases peritoneal dialysis longevity. *Surgery.* 2016;160(4):924-935. doi:10.1016/j.surg.2016.06.005
4. Li PK, Chow KM, Van de Luijtgaarden MW, et al. Changes in the worldwide epidemiology of peritoneal dialysis. *Nat Rev Nephrol.* 2017;13(2):90-103. doi:10.1038/nrneph.2016.181
5. Mehrotra R, Devuyst O, Davies SJ, Johnson DW. The current state of peritoneal dialysis. *J Am Soc Nephrol.* 2016;27(11):3238-3252. doi:10.1681/ASN.2016010112
6. Sodo M, Bracale U, Argentino G, et al. Simultaneous abdominal wall defect repair and Tenckhoff catheter placement in candidates for peritoneal dialysis. *J Nephrol.* 2016;29(5):699-702. doi:10.1007/s40620-015-0251-8

Chapter 44 Toe and Foot Amputations: Ray/Transmetatarsal/Symes*

Jacob C. Wood and Stephen Heisler

DEFINITION

- In the pursuit of limb preservation, it unfortunately is frequent that a patient may need a foot amputation to avoid compromising the entire extremity or even the individual. The development of nonviable tissue in one's foot may be due to the rapid onset of disease, poor comorbidity management, or delay in seeking medical attention. Diabetic patients suffer from a unique propensity for developing foot wounds secondary to the presence of macro- and microvascular disease and neuropathy—foot wounds can develop and spiral out of control without the patient even being aware.
- In this chapter we will be discussing several levels of foot amputations. A toe amputation is transecting a digit at the level of the phalanges. A ray amputation is transecting a digit at the level of the metatarsal bone. A transmetatarsal amputation (TMA) is transecting all digits at the metatarsal level. A Symes amputation is amputation of the foot through the distal tibia and fibula above the level of the malleoli.

DIFFERENTIAL DIAGNOSIS

- Diabetes mellitus with ulceration or gangrene
- Osteomyelitis
- Pressure-induced wounds
- Frostbite
- Vasculitis
- Vasospasm
- Peripheral arterial disease
- Thromboembolism
- Venous insufficiency
- Trauma
- Malignancy

PATIENT HISTORY AND PHYSICAL FINDINGS

- There are many things to take into consideration when evaluating a patient presenting with a foot wound. A careful history and physical should be sufficient to discover the etiology, extent, and acuity of a foot wound.
- A patient presenting with tachycardia, hypotension, leukocytosis, or other signs concerning for onset of sepsis warrants more urgent intervention.
- Foot wounds, particularly in the diabetic patient, can be much more extensive than they externally appear. There should be a low threshold to further interrogate a wound with purulent drainage or if the patient has systemic symptoms.
- The chronicity of a wound may be difficult to determine for diabetic patients. Not infrequently, patients present who have been completely unaware of the wound of concern until discovered by another person.
- To ensure healing potential and to prevent wound recurrence one maximizes medical optimization of comorbid conditions. This often requires a multidisciplinary approach. At our institution we regularly refer diabetic patients with marginal blood glucose control who present with foot wounds to endocrinology for optimization.
- Healing a wound requires an adequate blood supply to the affected area. A full pulse examination should be undertaken to evaluate for concomitant arterial insufficiency.
- Ischemic wounds can occur for several reasons, including atherosclerotic disease and digital ischemia in the setting of vasopressor use. After a revascularization procedure or after resolution of the offending condition, it is prudent to allow the ischemic wound to equilibrate prior to performing an amputation. Often what appears to be ischemic may prove to be viable if given time to declare itself.
- The more proximal an amputation the more it will affect the mechanics of ambulation. This will not affect a younger patient with excellent rehabilitation potential as much as an elderly patient who already has difficulty ambulating.

IMAGING AND OTHER DIAGNOSTIC STUDIES

- General laboratory data can help glean a patient's physiologic status on presentation including a basic metabolic panel and a complete blood count.
- C-reactive protein and erythrocyte sedimentation rate are general markers for inflammation and can suggest presence of osteomyelitis.
- The status of a diabetic patient's blood glucose control should be assessed with a hemoglobin A1c. The blood glucose level alone should not be used for this purpose as hyperglycemia may be a reflection of inflammation rather than poor glycemic control.
- When concerned for presence of osteomyelitis, foot X-ray with multiple views is a good initial imaging modality given a relatively low cost and the speed at which it can be performed. If the X-ray is inconclusive, or if more information is required to determine the extent of disease, magnetic resonance imaging may be necessary.

*Illustrations by Jacob C. Wood.

- If tibial pulses are not palpable an ankle-brachial index (ABI) with toe pressure is obtained to assess the vascular status of the foot. Values that are favorable for healing include an ABI greater than 0.8 (between 0.5 and 0.8 are marginal values) and a toe pressure greater than 50 mm Hg.
- Additional information can be obtained with segmental blood pressures, transcutaneous oxygen measurement, arterial duplex, and arteriography.

SURGICAL MANAGEMENT

Preoperative Planning

- The operation performed is dictated by the extent of disease, the vascular supply, and the rehabilitation potential of the patient. Minimizing the extent of the foot that is taken will maximize postoperative function; however, enough tissue should be taken to allow enough healthy skin and soft tissue to create a tension-free flap coverage for the amputation.
- Proximal amputations may cause tendon and ligamentous alterations that will cause unopposed plantarflexion or other deformity. Additional operations may be necessary to help the remaining foot reside in a maximally functional position, such a calcaneal (Achilles) tendon lengthening procedure.
- Foot amputations are well suited for nerve block with sedation, which most patients should tolerate.

Positioning

- Supine position is ideal for most foot amputations.
- The foot and distal leg are prepped and draped in circumferential fashion.

TECHNIQUES

DIGIT AND RAY AMPUTATION

- When amputating a digit, the extent of the amputation dictates the incision that is made. A circumferential incision is sufficient for amputations at the phalangeal level or the distal aspect of a metatarsal bone. If the amputation must extend more proximally on the metatarsal bone a wedge-shaped incision or a racket-shaped incision is used. The incision should incorporate the ulcer if one is present with the goal of leaving behind only healthy and viable tissue. An incision should always be made with careful planning due to the unpredictable extent of underlying necrosis from infection. Making the incision about 1 cm or greater distal to the intended level of bone transection should allow for a tension-free closure (**FIGURES 1** and **2**).
- Electrocautery is used to divide the subcutaneous and soft tissues until the phalanx or metatarsal bone is encountered. Care is taken to not encroach on tissues in the territories of other digits so as to prevent unintentional devascularization of the adjoining digit. Electrocautery is usually sufficient to achieve hemostasis.
- If there is concern for vascular insufficiency, tissues should be handled as atraumatically as possible with sparing use of electrocautery, favoring suture ligation. Utilizing full-thickness flaps can lead to improved outcomes as these can protect vital vascular structures.
- Tendons are transected proximal to the incision. This is accomplished by grasping the tendons at the incision, putting tension on the tendons, and dividing them sharply at the incision. The remaining tendon should recoil within the foot proximal to the incision.
- The bone is isolated from the surrounding tissues using a periosteal elevator or other device. The bone should be transected along the diaphysis of the phalanx or metatarsal bone using bone shears or an oscillating saw. As mentioned above, the bone should be transected about 1 cm or greater proximal to the incision to allow a tension-free closure. Cartilage should not be left exposed at the wound surface. If any cartilage is exposed, it should be removed using a rongeur.
- If the amputation was done for osteomyelitis, a sample of the distal aspect of the remaining bone is sent for culture and pathology. This can be done using a rongeur. The specimen will guide further antibiotic needs and help dictate the length of antibiotic requirements.
- Any sesamoid bones within the affected area should be removed. This can be done using a combination of electrocautery and blunt dissection to divide the tissue surrounding the sesamoid bone(s). When enough of the bone is exposed

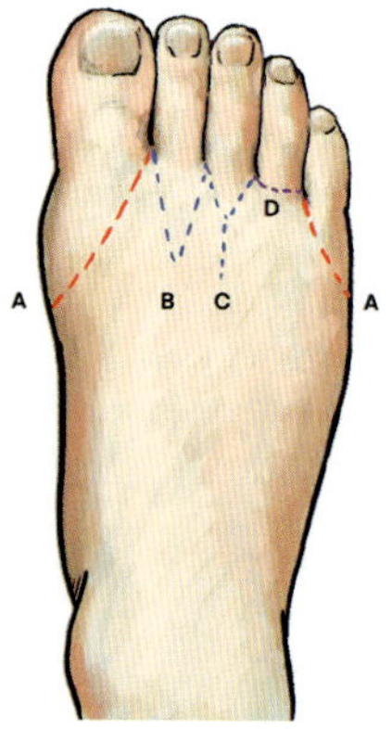

FIGURE 1 • Incisions for toe/ray amputation. **A,** Beveled incisions are made for digits 1 and 5. Incisions for digits 2 to 4 require a **(B)** wedge-shaped or **(C)** racket-shaped incision. **D,** A circumferential incision at the base of the digit can be performed on any digit if the pathology is confined to the digit. (Illustration by Jacob C. Wood.)

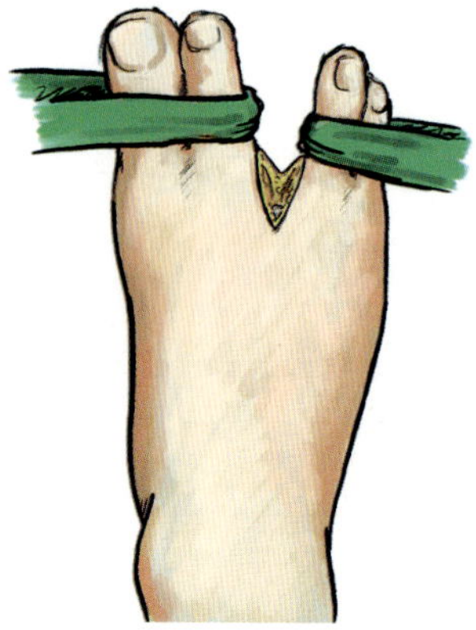

FIGURE 2 • A wedge-shaped incision is made to perform a 3rd digit ray amputation. Loops from a lap pad are used to retract the medial and lateral toes away from the operative field. (Illustration by Jacob C. Wood.)

as can be grasped by toothed forceps (such as Kocher forceps), tension can be applied to the bone, which will facilitate circumferential dissection and removal.

- After infected and/or devitalized tissue is removed and hemostasis is obtained, the wound is closed in two layers with deep absorbable sutures in buried fashion and the skin approximated with permanent, monofilament sutures, usually in vertical mattress fashion.
- One may choose to leave the incision open or partially open if there is concern for retained infected tissue, which may worsen if the wound is closed. The wound may then be closed in a staged fashion or by secondary intention (**FIGURE 3**).
- When the offending pathology is focal to the distal digit, leaving the proximal one-third of the proximal phalanx of the toe has been found to reduce toe deviation of adjacent toes leading to ulcerations after the patient recovers.

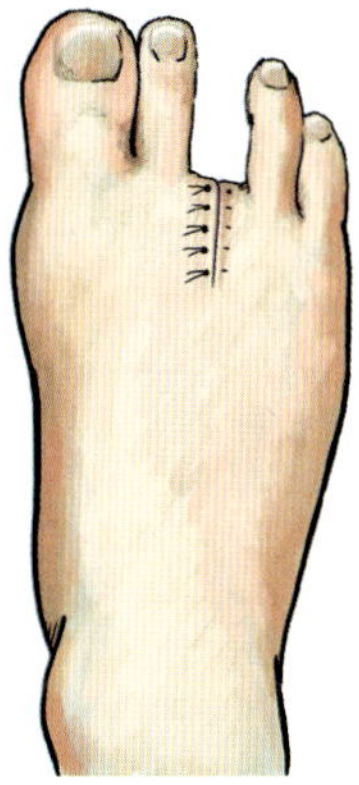

FIGURE 3 • A 3rd digit ray amputation is completed with a multilayered closure. (Illustration by Jacob C. Wood.)

TRANSMETATARSAL AMPUTATION

- TMA is performed when all digits of a foot must be removed. The level of amputation is dictated by how much viable tissue the surgeon has to work with. Ideally, the metatarsal bones are transected at the distal aspects of the diaphyses just proximal to the flaring of the metaphyses and the parabolic relationship of metatarsal bone lengths is maintained.
- A modified fish-mouth incision is made, with the plantar flap longer than the dorsal flap (**FIGURE 4**).
- The dorsal incision is made 1 to 2 cm distal to the intended location of the metatarsal bone resection. The incision is sharply carried to the level of the metatarsal bones in a plane perpendicular to the surface of the skin. The medial and lateral apices of the incisions are placed midway between the dorsal and plantar aspects of the foot. The dorsal flap is retracted from the metatarsal bones (**FIGURE 5**).
- Each bone is individually isolated from the periosteum and surrounding tissue at the intended location of transection, then divided using either oscillating saw or bone shears. A power saw is preferred over the bone shears due to fragility of the metatarsal bones that can occur with advanced age or infection leading to longitudinal fractures. The tissue between each metatarsal bone is preserved to maintain the intermetatarsal vessels.

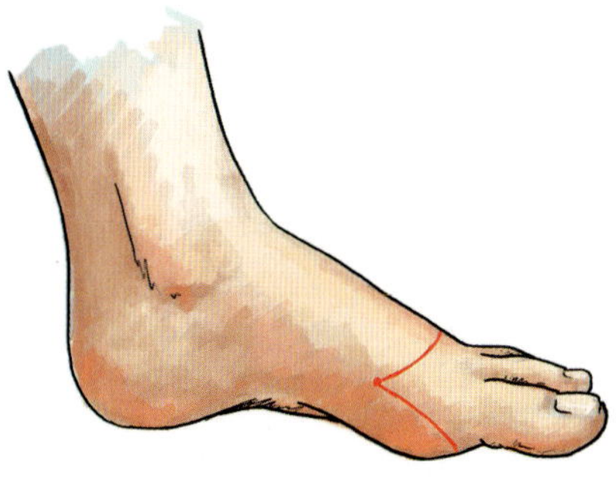

FIGURE 4 • A fish-mouthed incision for a TMA. The plantar flap is longer than the dorsal flap. (Illustration by Jacob C. Wood.)

- The first and second metatarsal bones are cut at approximately the same length. The subsequent metatarsal bones are divided in a gently tapered fashion, aiming to maintain the curvature of the native metatarsal configuration.
- The metatarsal bones are cut at a 45° angle in the dorsoplantar projection. Beveling the bones at this angle reduces prominences on the plantar surface, thereby lowering focal pressure during propulsion that can otherwise lead to additional ulcerations after resuming ambulation.
- Proximal bone fragments can be sent for culture and pathology to ensure complete resection of osteomyelitic bone or to help guide antibiotic therapy for retained osteomyelitis.
- The plantar incision is made distal to the level of the metatarsal heads. The metatarsal bones and the toes are detached as the unit from the plantar flap. Care is taken to retain the intermetatarsal tissue.

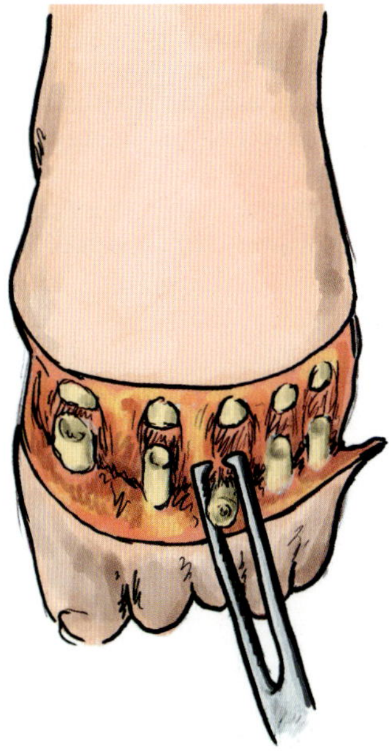

FIGURE 5 • During a TMA, the metatarsal bones are transected at lengths that maintain the parabolic shape of the forefoot. The intermetatarsal tissue is preserved as the plantar flap is created. (Illustration by Jacob C. Wood.)

TECHNIQUES

- Sesamoid bones and joint tissue are removed from the plantar flap to avoid development of heterotopic ossification and to decrease unnecessary bulk.
- After all compromised tissue has been removed and after hemostasis has been achieved, the flaps are brought together and closed. This is done using absorbable, braided suture in buried, interrupted fashion to approximate the deep tissues. The skin is brought together using either permanent, nonabsorbable suture in interrupted, vertical mattress fashion or with staples (**FIGURE 6**).
- When approximating tissue layers it is important to eliminate the amount of dead space as this can lead to wound dehiscence and reinfection of the amputation due to large flap remodeling and bone resection.
- If there is not enough tissue to accomplish complete closure or if there is concern for retained infected tissue that will not resolve with antibiotics, the surgeon may elect to perform partial closure or to leave the incision open.
- With good wound care, the wound may be able to be closed in delayed fashion if there is enough tissue, or closure can be obtained by secondary intention.

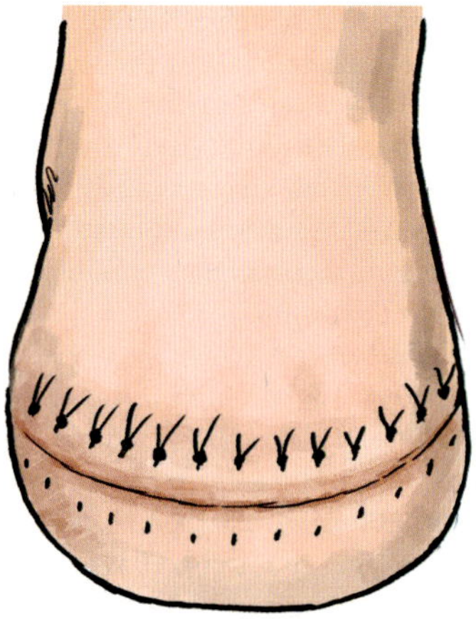

FIGURE 6 • A TMA is completed with a multilayered closure. (Illustration by Jacob C. Wood.)

- Negative pressure wound therapy can facilitate wound closure or can bridge the gap for and maximize the wound bed for skin graft attempts.

SYMES AMPUTATION

- A Syme level amputation is a tibiotalar disarticulation with division of the tibia and fibula at the level of the malleoli. The flap is based on the heel fat pad (**FIGURE 7**).
- This operation can be done in one or two stages. The two-stage method involves ankle disarticulation followed by transection of the tibia and fibula approximately 6 weeks later. This is done when there is concern for retained infection or nonviable tissue.
- A fish-mouth incision is made based on the anatomic landmarks of the malleoli. The apices of the incision are placed 1 cm inferior and 1 cm anterior to the lateral malleolus and 1 cm inferior and 1 cm anterior to the medial malleolus. These points are connected extending anteriorly across the dorsal aspect of the ankle and in a plantar-ward direction.
- Planning of the medial incision must take the location of the posterior tibial artery into consideration, which must be preserved.

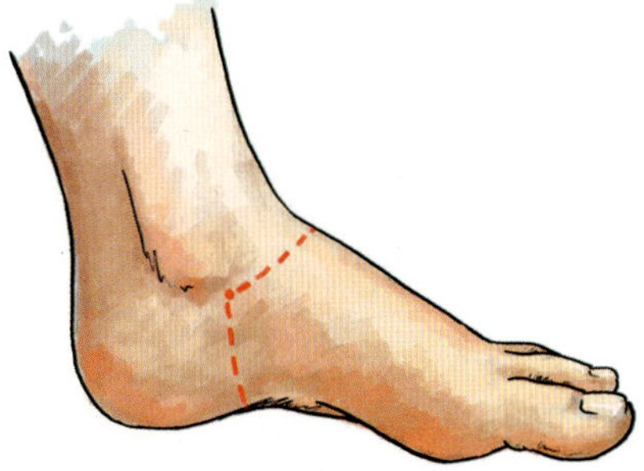

FIGURE 7 • Syme amputation is done with a fish-mouthed incision with the apices about 1 cm inferior and 1 cm anterior to the medial and lateral malleoli. (Illustration by Jacob C. Wood.)

- The anterior/dorsal incision is made and carried directly to bone in a plane perpendicular to the skin surface. The extensor tendons encountered are stretched and divided to allow them to retract into the remaining tissue. The anterior tibial artery is ligated and divided.
- The talus bone is encountered. The talus bone is retracted with a bone hook, allowing dissection to and through the tibiotalar joint capsule and disarticulation of the ankle joint. Care is taken to preserve the posterior tibial artery with its branches, which will be encountered posterior to the medial malleolus thereby maintaining perfusion to the myocutaneous flap (**FIGURE 8**).
- The calcaneus is dissected free in a subperiosteal plane moving posteriorly to the calcaneal tuberosity where the tendocalcaneus (Achilles tendon) is encountered and dissected free from its insertion.

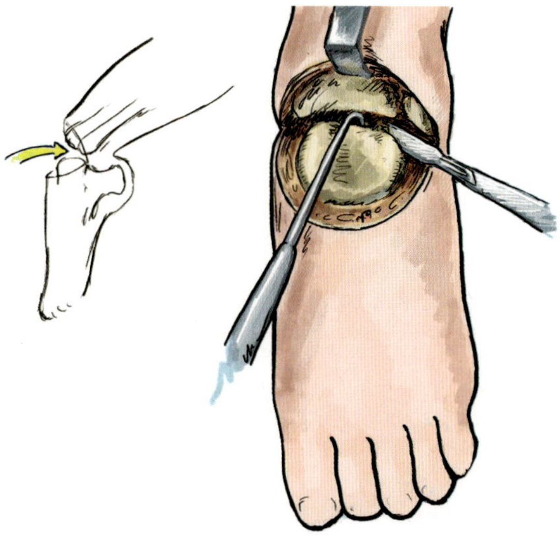

FIGURE 8 • The tibiotalar joint is separated. Dissection is carried posteriorly around the calcaneus in a subperiosteal plane. (Illustration by Jacob C. Wood.)

- The calcaneus is further dissected in a subperiosteal plan until encountering the inferiorly directed incision. The calcaneus and foot are removed in one piece.
- The periosteum will assist with the weight-bearing potential of the flap and tends to heal to the tibia and fibula quite well.
- The heel fat pad has a unique aptitude for weight bearing and should be preserved at all costs—if it cannot be preserved, a different amputation should be considered.
- The tibia and the fibula are divided using an oscillating bone saw at a level proximal to the articular cartilage segments and distal to the diaphyses. Retaining the flaring segments of the tibia and fibula will assist with prosthesis fitting. Also, transecting in a point with a large amount of cortical bone will maximize the weight-bearing potential of the limb (**FIGURE 9**).
- The medial and lateral aspects of the malleoli are beveled to minimize pressure points while still maintaining a bulbous distal aspect of the amputation for prosthetic fitting.
- All synovial tissue and articular cartilage should be removed.
- A misplaced heel flap is an important complication after this amputation. It can be avoided by careful placement of the plantar surface of the flap directly beneath the center of the tibia. Removal of dog-ears, which will resolve with time, is thought to be a cause of flap migration.
- The peroneal tendons are anchored to the anterior flap fascia and retinaculum.

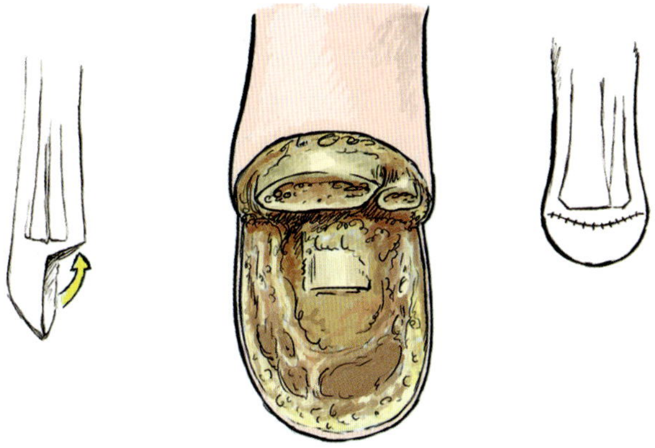

FIGURE 9 • The tibia and the fibula are transected. The medial and lateral aspects are beveled to avoid pressure points. The flap is made up of the Achilles tendon, the calcaneus periosteum, and the superficial tissues in this area including the plantar fat pad. The flap is rotated anteriorly to complete the amputation with a multilayered closure. Drains are often placed to eliminate the dead space under the flap—not pictured. (Illustration by Jacob C. Wood.)

- The wound is closed over drains to obliterate the dead space. Closure is performed in multiple layers using absorbable braided suture in deep interrupted fashion. The skin is closed using permanent monofilament suture in interrupted, vertical mattress fashion or with staples.

PEARLS AND PITFALLS

Closure	▪ Striving for a tension-free skin closure while minimizing the trauma to the myocutaneous flaps during the operation will maximize success of the amputation. ▪ Dog-ears from closure will resolve with time and healing.
Wound management and source control	▪ Removing all infected tissue may not be possible. Microscopic disease will likely resolve with antibiotics with the wound being able to be closed. A grossly infected wound should be left open as closure will likely result in wound breakdown or worsening of the infection, potentially requiring a more proximal amputation. Counter incisions may be necessary for source control in the setting of severe infections.
Tourniquet use	▪ Tourniquet can be used to minimize operative blood loss but should not be used in patients with severe ischemia or incompressible vessels. Tourniquet use is not only ineffective in patients with noncompressible arteries but is detrimental as it also causes venous hypertension resulting in more bleeding and bleeding that can be difficult to control.
Multidisciplinary approach	▪ Most amputation patients benefit from a multidisciplinary approach to their preoperative and postoperative care to optimize their comorbid conditions and their functional rehabilitation.

POSTOPERATIVE CARE

- The postoperative hospital stay is largely dedicated to coordinating the patient's rehabilitation needs, antibiotic needs, medical management needs, and preparing the patient for ultimately living at home.
- Weight bearing of distal individual toe amputations and metatarsal amputations is variable based on patient needs and functional status prior to amputation. The preferable option is to be non–weight-bearing or heel weight bearing. For transmetatarsal amputations it is preferable to maintain a non–weight-bearing status for 4 weeks in a 90° splint or a tall boot to prevent dehiscence.
- Foot amputations require pressure offloading, which can be accomplished using specialized orthotic shoes. Offloading measures should be continued until the amputation is healed.
- Rehabilitation: becoming accustomed to a new configuration to one's foot may be quite challenging. The rehabilitation needs of a patient depend on the level of amputation and the

degree of deconditioning prior to the amputation. Physical and occupational therapy are useful for assessing a patient's rehabilitation needs as well as teaching patients how to ambulate while offloading the affected segment of the foot.

- Infection is a common reason for needing an amputation. The antibiotic requirements after an operation may range from none if the operation completely eradicates the infection to requiring a lengthy course of intravenous antibiotics if treating ongoing osteomyelitis.
- If the bone culture is positive then there is osteomyelitis that should be treated. The antibiotic of choice can be dictated by the speciation and sensitivities. We routinely seek Infectious Disease consultation for these patients. A peripherally inserted central catheter or equivalent will often need to be placed.
- If the bone culture is negative but there is concern for residual infected tissue, a short course of oral antibiotics may be desired. The wound should be monitored closely for evidence of recurrence of infection.
- Postoperative care should be coordinated in a multidisciplinary fashion to optimize the patient's comorbid conditions.

COMPLICATIONS

- Wound infection
- Wound breakdown
- Neuroma
- Pressure wounds
- Phantom limb pain
- Foot malformation

SUGGESTED READING

1. Bibbo C. Modification of the Syme amputation to prevent postoperative heel pad migration. *J Foot Ankle Surg*. 2013;52(6):766-770. doi:10.1053/j.jfas.2013.07.006
2. Boffeli TJ, Waverly BJ. Transmetatarsal and Lisfranc amputation. In: Boffeli T, ed. *Osteomyelitis of the Foot and Ankle*. Springer; 2015. doi:10.1007/978-3-319-18926-0_19
3. Eliassen A, Coleman DM. Transmetatarsal amputation. In: Upchurch GR, Henke PK, eds. *Clinical Scenarios in Vascular Surgery*. 2nd ed. Wolters Kluwer; 2015:468-471.
4. Harris RI. Syme's amputation. *J Bone Joint Surg*. 1956:38 B(3):614-632. doi:10.1302/0301-620X.38B3.614
5. Jimenez JC. Lower extremity amputation. In: Moore WS, Lawrence PF, Oderich GS, eds. *Vascular and Endovascular Surgery: A Comprehensive Review*. 9th ed. Saunders Elsevier; 2019:956-992.
6. Lavery LA, Ahn J, Ryan EC, et al. What are the optimal cutoff values for ESR and CRP to diagnose osteomyelitis in patients with diabetes-related foot infections?. *Clin Orthop Relat Res*, 2019;477(7):1594-1602. doi:10.1097/CORR.0000000000000718
7. Rios AL, Eidt JF. Lower extremity amputation: operative techniques and results. In: Sidawy AN, Rutherford RB, Perler BA, eds. *Rutherford's Vascular Surgery and Endovascular Therapy*. 9th ed. Saunders Elsevier; 2019:1496-1513.

Chapter 45 Lower Extremity Amputation: BKA/AKA/Hip Disarticulation

Shernaz S. Dossabhoy and Shipra Arya

DEFINITION

- Lower extremity amputations are a necessary set of procedures for vascular, orthopedic, plastic, and general surgeons to employ in various situations, including trauma, infection, ischemia/atherosclerotic disease, diabetic complications, malignancy, congenital or acquired deformities, and intractable pain (neuropathic, ischemic).
- The goals of lower extremity amputation are to remove ischemic, infected, or devitalized tissue and allow for eventual wound closure and healing. Amputation can also treat pain and improve mobility and function with the aid of rehabilitation and prosthetic limbs.
- Major amputations are proximal to the tarsometatarsal joint (Chopart, Boyd, Syme, Below Knee, and Above Knee). Minor amputations are distal or through the tarsometatarsal joint (Forefoot, Transmetatarsal, and Lisfranc). This chapter will focus on three types of major amputation, including: below-the-knee amputation (BKA), above-the-knee amputation (AKA), and hip disarticulations.
- Key terms: below-the-knee amputation (BKA) is a transtibial amputation, above-the-knee amputation (AKA) is a transfemoral amputation, and hip disarticulation is dislocation at the hip joint to allow for removal of the lower limb.

DIFFERENTIAL DIAGNOSIS

- Most amputations can be categorized as traumatic or nontraumatic. In this section, we discuss the differential diagnoses that lead to amputation and how the decision is made to proceed with limb salvage (secondary amputation) vs primary amputation. Primary amputation is defined as amputation occurring without prior attempt at limb salvage (eg, revascularization, bone repair, soft tissue/muscle flap coverage). On the other hand, secondary amputation includes amputations occurring after a failed attempt at revascularization and tissue reconstruction. This section will primarily focus on nontraumatic amputations. The operative techniques for BKA, AKA, and hip disarticulation, however, remain the same for both traumatic and nontraumatic amputations.
- Indications for primary amputation include "wet gangrene" (**FIGURE 1A**), nonsalvageable limb with loss of sensorimotor function (traumatic mangled extremity or acute limb ischemia), end-stage peripheral arterial disease (PAD), or critical limb threatening ischemia (CLTI) that is unable to be revascularized, comorbidities that preclude revascularization (ie, endovascular or open-bypass surgery), severe tissue loss or infection that precludes attempts at limb-salvage, intractable pain of the lower limb, refractory to management by pain specialist (ischemic, traumatic, neuropathic, or mechanical instability), and malignant tumors.
- Wet gangrene is a limb- and life-threatening event, presenting with swelling, purulence, blistering, erythema, and drainage in the setting of ischemic/under-perfused tissue with superimposed infection. Immediate guillotine amputation followed by definitive closure is advised (**FIGURE 2**).
- If primary amputation is not immediately indicated, patients will likely fall into one of the following categories: diabetic or other foot ulcer, dry gangrene, osteomyelitis, traumatic injury, peripheral arterial disease, or malignant tumor. Each should be closely monitored for signs of worsening ischemia, infection, or pain, which may necessitate future amputation.
- Diabetic foot ulcer (DFU): Diabetes is a major risk factor for lower extremity amputations worldwide. Approximately 25% to 90% of amputations within studied populations are associated with diabetes mellitus.[1] In Medicare patients, the incidence of DFU was 6.0% and lower extremity amputation 0.5% with 11% and 22% associated annual mortality, respectively.[2] Complications from diabetes mellitus are responsible for 60% to 80% of amputations.[2] Of patients with DFU, nearly 50% have concomitant PAD, which increases the risk of overall complications and amputation.[3]
- Other foot ulcers (neuropathic, pressure, arterial, venous): Amputations may be recommended for nonhealing nondiabetic ulcers, including neuropathic, pressure-related, or arterial. It is rare for amputation to be necessary for venous ulcers unless there is an association with intractable osteomyelitis.
- "Dry gangrene" (**FIGURE 1B**): In contrast to "wet gangrene," "dry gangrene" occurs in an extremity where the tissue "mummifies" and becomes discolored and ischemic, appearing dark or black. If there is no evidence of overt infection, dry gangrene does not require immediate amputation. The affected extremity can be conservatively managed or undergo revascularization with debridement. Amputation may often be avoided as an ischemic extremity will not heal properly. Dry gangrene or mummified tissue does not pass macrobacteria into the circulation.[2]
- Osteomyelitis: Especially in patients with diabetes, osteomyelitis of the forefoot, foot, and ankle may necessitate amputation. Often these infections are comanaged with podiatry and specific foot amputations are beyond the scope of this chapter (Chapter 44). However, care must be taken to exclude osteomyelitis of the tibia or femur prior to transtibial or transfemoral amputation, respectively, to ensure adequate healing postoperatively.
- Traumatic injury: A mangled lower extremity in the setting of trauma may require amputation. Often, these injuries involve bone, muscle, and neurovascular structures, and it is helpful to involve specialists from orthopedic, vascular, and plastic surgery. Neurovascular structures should be assessed first as this will determine what portion of the limb may be salvageable as well as dictate level of amputation. Patient's age and functional status should be taken into consideration.
- PAD and nonsalvageable limb: Lower extremity ischemia is often due to chronic atherosclerotic disease, also known as PAD. Between 2000 and 2015, PAD was estimated to affect between 8.5 and 12 million Americans[4,5]—a 25% increase in prevalence over the prior decade. Risk factors for PAD

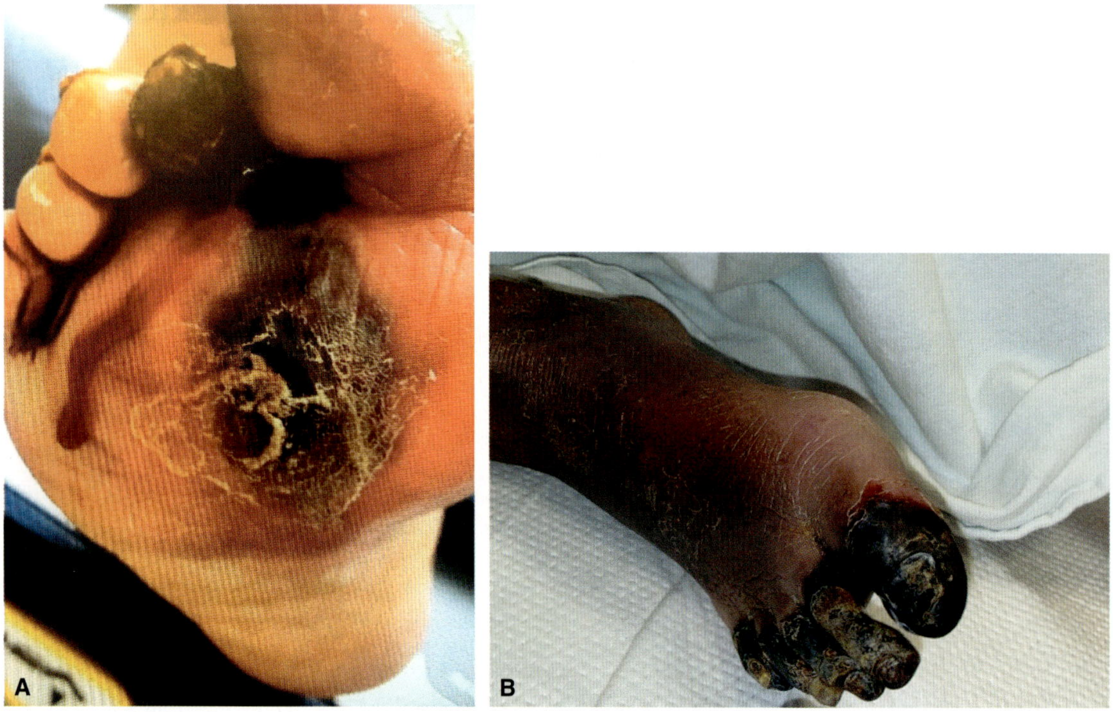

FIGURE 1 • Gangrenous changes of foot with **(A)** wet gangrene with presence of infection and purulence on top of ischemic gangrenous changes and **(B)** dry gangrene with ischemia and necrosis of entire forefoot.

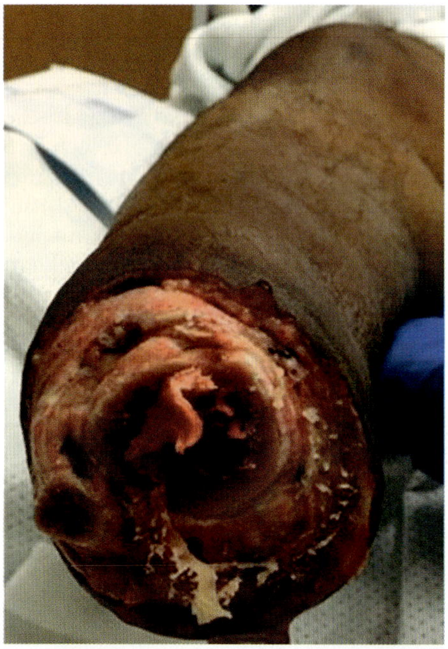

FIGURE 2 • Staged amputation of lower extremity, also called "guillotine" amputation.

include age, cigarette smoking, dyslipidemia, and diabetes mellitus.[6] Late-stage, severe PAD is referred to as chronic critical limb threatening ischemia (CLTI) in the vascular surgery literature. Approximately 11% of patients with PAD will go on to develop CLTI,[7] which carries an associated 1-year amputation rate of 15% to 20% and 1-year mortality of 15% to 40%.[8] Once a limb is deemed "nonsalvageable" either due to failed prior revascularizations or inability to further revascularize, the patient should be evaluated for amputation. Urgency of amputation depends on degree of pain, presence of wound and/or infection, and often patient's desire or willingness to proceed with amputation.

- Malignant tumors of the proximal lower extremity: Malignant bony or soft tissue tumors with extensive involvement of the femur and soft tissues, not amenable to lesser resections, are treated with hip disarticulation. Hip disarticulation is reserved "for tumors more distal than those requiring a hemipelvectomy and more proximal than those that can be treated with a high thigh amputation."[9]

PATIENT HISTORY AND PHYSICAL FINDINGS

- Evaluation and planning for lower extremity amputation includes a thorough history and physical exam to optimize patient risk factors and assess for appropriateness of amputation.
- History should include risk factor assessment, extent of wound, infection, and ischemia that would guide efforts at limb salvage and functional status assessment. Risk factor assessment and modification to decrease perioperative morbidity and mortality includes smoking cessation, optimization of diabetes, hypertension, and hyperlipidemia, and consideration of perioperative beta-blockers in certain patients.
- Severe infections may require a two-stage approach, that is, *"guillotine"* amputation (see in "Surgical Management" section) followed by amputation formalization.
- Perioperative DVT prophylaxis and blood glucose control is important to minimize postoperative complications.

- Overall rehabilitation potential is based on individual patient's ability to ambulate, functional status, mental state, and overall life expectancy.
- Physical exam should include full vascular exam, including bilateral lower extremity femoral, popliteal, dorsalis pedis, and posterior tibial pulses. Additionally, one should assess for signs of infection, wounds, tissue loss, and any anatomic variations.
- The extent of amputation is determined by degree of tissue loss, ischemia, and infection as determined by physical exam. Ideally, there should be a palpable pulse proximal to the level of planned amputation as this is highly associated with stump healing. However, a nonpalpable pulse does not preclude amputation or mean the planned amputation will not heal; in these cases, further imaging and diagnostic studies are required, as described below (see in "Imaging and Other Diagnostic Studies" section).
- The Society for Vascular Surgery (SVS) Wound, Ischemia, and Foot Infection (WIfI) classification system can be used to assess threatened lower extremities by assigning a grade from 0-3 for each component (**TABLE 1**).[10] Based on this grading, a WIfI class is assigned. For example, a patient who presents with ischemic rest pain with ankle brachial index (ABI) 0.3, no wound, and no signs or symptoms of infection would be classified as Wound-0, Ischemia-3, Foot Infection-0, thus WIfI 030. This clinical stage can then be used to estimate the (a) risk of 1-year amputation and (b) likely need for/benefit of revascularization (assumes infection is controlled) (**FIGURE 3**). It should be noted that these estimates have been prospectively validated by numerous studies in select patient groups.[11]

Table 1: SVS Wound, Ischemia, and Foot Infection (WIfI) Classification System

Grade	(W) wound	(I) ischemia	(fI) foot infection
0	No ulcer; no gangrene	ABI ≥0.80 Ankle SBP > 100 mm Hg TP/$TcPO_2$ ≥ 60 mm Hg	No s/sx of infection
1	Small, shallow ulcer; no exposed bone; no gangrene	ABI 0.6-0.79 Ankle SBP 70-100 mm Hg TP/$TcPO_2$ 40-59 mm Hg	Local infection with at least 2 s/sx: • Local swelling or induration • Erythema 0.5-2 cm around ulcer • Local tenderness or pain • Local warmth • Purulent drainage
2	Deeper ulcer with exposed bone; gangrene on digits	ABI 0.4-0.59 Ankle SBP 50-70 mm Hg TP/$TcPO_2$ 30-39 mm Hg	Local infection (as above) with • Erythema >2 cm, or • Involving deeper structures (eg, abscess, osteomyelitis, septic arthritis, fasciitis)
3	Extensive, deep ulcer; extensive gangrene	ABI ≤0.39 Ankle SBP <50 mm Hg TP/$TcPO_2$ <30 mm Hg	Local infection (as above) with s/sx of SIRS: • Temp >38 °C or <36 °C • HR >90 beats/min • RR >20 breaths/min or $PaCO_2$ <32 mm Hg • WBC >12,000 or <4000 cu/mm or 10% bands

ABI, Ankle-brachial index; s/sx, signs/symptoms; $TcPO_2$, transcutaneous oximetry; TP, toe pressure.

IMAGING AND OTHER DIAGNOSTIC STUDIES

- The initial evaluation of a patient who may undergo lower extremity amputation should include noninvasive evaluation of peripheral circulation with arterial waveforms, ABIs, toe pressures or toe-brachial indices (TBIs), segmental pressures with pulse volume recordings (PVRs), and transcutaneous oxygen tensions ($TcPO_2$).
- ABIs >0.5 are associated with 90% healing of BKAs, while ABIs <0.35 correlate with poor wound healing of toe amputations.
- TBIs (also called "toe pressures") are a more reliable indicator of peripheral vascular disease and limb perfusion in diabetic patients. TBIs > 0.3 and absolute toe pressures >30 mm Hg are acceptable for wound healing in nondiabetic patients. In patients with diabetes, toe pressures >45 to 55 mm Hg may be required for healing.
- Segmental pressures with plethysmography, or pulse volume recordings (PVRs), are obtained by measuring blood pressure at successive levels along the length of the extremity combined with Doppler, which allows the examiner to localize the specific level of arterial disease. PVRs measure volume changes within the limb and are most useful in identifying disease in calcified vessels, which tend to yield falsely elevated pressure measurements (and thus falsely elevated ABIs). Regarding amputation prognosis, a calf Doppler systolic pressure of 50 to 70 mm Hg and a Doppler systolic thigh pressure of 80 mm Hg predict high success rate for wound healing after BKA.
- Transcutaneous oxygen tensions ($TcPO_2$s) of the lower extremity are obtained through platinum oxygen electrodes with patients positioned supine and with elevation of the limb. A $TcPO_2$ >40 torr predicts healing in 98% of amputations while $TcPO_2$ <20 torr has been historically associated with failure. Moreover, Columbo et al found that patients with $TcPO_2$ <40 torr had a two-fold increase of conversion to AKA or death.[12] Thus, $TcPO_2$ is a strong predictor of wound healing and may be more reliable than skin perfusion or segmental pressures.
- Duplex ultrasound (DUS) has recently been suggested to predict the best level of lower extremity amputation in patients with CLTI, as examination of lower extremity pulses may be unreliable. For example, in one study, all patients with aortoiliac or deep femoral arterial occlusion who initially received a BKA required reoperation with AKA due to poor wound healing, suggesting that performing a primary AKA for these patients could significantly reduce reoperation rates.[13]
- Often, if there has been concern for infection or osteomyelitis, X-ray (XR) or magnetic resonance imaging (MRI) of the foot and lower leg has been obtained. Both XR and/or MRI should be reviewed to ensure the tibial and fibular bones are free from infection prior to proceeding with amputation.
- While dedicated lower extremity imaging with computed tomographic angiography (CTA) or magnetic resonance angiography (MRA) is typically not required before amputation, they can provide an overall assessment for the degree of atherosclerotic vascular disease if noninvasive imaging is

A Estimate risk of amputation at 1 year for each combination

	Ischemia – 0				Ischemia – 1				Ischemia – 2				Ischemia – 3			
W-0	VI	VI	L	M	VI	L	M	H	L	L	M	H	L	M	M	H
W-1	VI	VI	L	M	VI	L	M	H	L	M	H	H	M	M	H	H
W-2	L	L	M	H	M	M	H	H	M	H	H	H	H	H	H	H
W-3	M	M	H	H	H	H	H	H	H	H	H	H	H	H	H	H
	fI-0	fI-1	fI-2	fI-3	fI-0	fI-1	fI-2	fI-3	fI-0	fI-1	fI-2	fI-3	fI-0	fI-1	fI-2	fI-3

B Estimate likelihood of benefit of/requirement for revascularization (assuming infection can be controlled first)

	Ischemia – 0				Ischemia – 1				Ischemia – 2				Ischemia – 3			
W-0	VI	VI	VI	VI	VI	L	L	M	L	L	M	M	M	H	H	H
W-1	VI	VI	VI	M	L	M	M	M	M	H	H	H	H	H	H	H
W-2	VI	VI	VI	VI	M	M	H	H	H	H	H	H	H	H	H	H
W-3	VI	VI	VI	VI	M	M	M	H	H	H	H	H	H	H	H	H
	f-0	fI-1	fI-2	fI-3	fI-0	fI-1	fI-2	fI-3	fI-0	fI-1	fI-2	fI-3	fI-0	fI-1	fI-2	fI-3

fI. foot Infection; I, Ischemia; W, Wound.

Premises:

1. Increase in wound class increases risk of amputation (based on PEDIS, UT, and other wound classification systems)
2. PAD and infection are synergistic (Eurodiale): infected wound + PAD increases likelihood revascularization will be needed to heal wound
3. Infection 3 category (systemic/metabolic instability): moderate to high-risk of amputation regardless of other factors (validated IDSA guidelines)

Four classes: for each box, group combination into one of these four classes

Very low = VL = clinical stage 1
Low = L = clinical stage 2
Moderate = M = clinical stage 3
High = H = clinical stage 4

Clinical stage 5 would signify an unsalvageable foot

FIGURE 3 • Clinical staging of wound based on the SVS Wound, Ischemia, and Foot Infection (WIfI) classification system. (Reprinted from Mills JL Sr, Conte MS, Armstrong DG, et al. The Society for Vascular Surgery Lower Extremity Threatened Limb Classification System: Risk stratification based on Wound, Ischemia, and foot Infection (WIfI). *J Vasc Surg*. 2014;59(1):220-234.e2. Copyright © 2014 The Authors. With permission.)

inconclusive and demonstrate any anatomic variations not assessed by physical exam.

- An important note for DFU with infection: If there is tarsal and/or calcaneal bone involvement, then patient may require a BKA. If the infection is limited to only the forefoot, then can consider transmetatarsal amputation (TMA); however, further discussion is beyond the scope of this current chapter (Chapter 44).

SURGICAL MANAGEMENT

Algorithm for Approach to Amputation

- The approach to lower extremity amputation must first consider if the limb is salvageable or not, followed by consideration of the patient's clinical status (septic or not), and potential for postoperative ambulation (see **FIGURE 4**, Management Algorithm).
- Throughout this process, shared decision-making between the multidisciplinary care team (including vascular surgeons, plastic surgery, orthopedic surgery, podiatry, wound care, physical medicine and rehabilitation (PM&R), nutrition, and palliative care, etc.) and the patient is of highest importance.[14] Patients must consider what is important for their quality of life, as some would rather proceed with terminal wound care and defer amputation until their clinical status changes, while others prefer to undergo primary amputation with the goal of increased rehab potential and ambulation with a prosthetic. It is helpful to engage PM&R physicians, who can often provide a more realistic assessment to patients and surgeons regarding ambulatory potential.

Preoperative Planning

- For patient preoperative management, see in "Preoperative Preparation." In addition, standard preoperative workup including anesthesia preassessment, ECG, echo, and chest x-ray if indicated, should be considered.
- Determining the appropriate level of amputation is essential for successful would healing and rehabilitation potential. Various objective criteria have been described to determine the level of amputation according to the degree of vascular perfusion (see in "Imaging and Other Diagnostic Studies"). Surgeon clinical judgment and experience complement the use of these adjunctive measures.

Positioning

- For any lower extremity amputation, the patient should be positioned supine on standard operating room table. A tourniquet of appropriate size should be available but kept sterile and only placed on the patient after prep and draping. A "bump" can be fashioned out of folded blue towels on the back table and is helpful for elevation of the limb during the procedure.

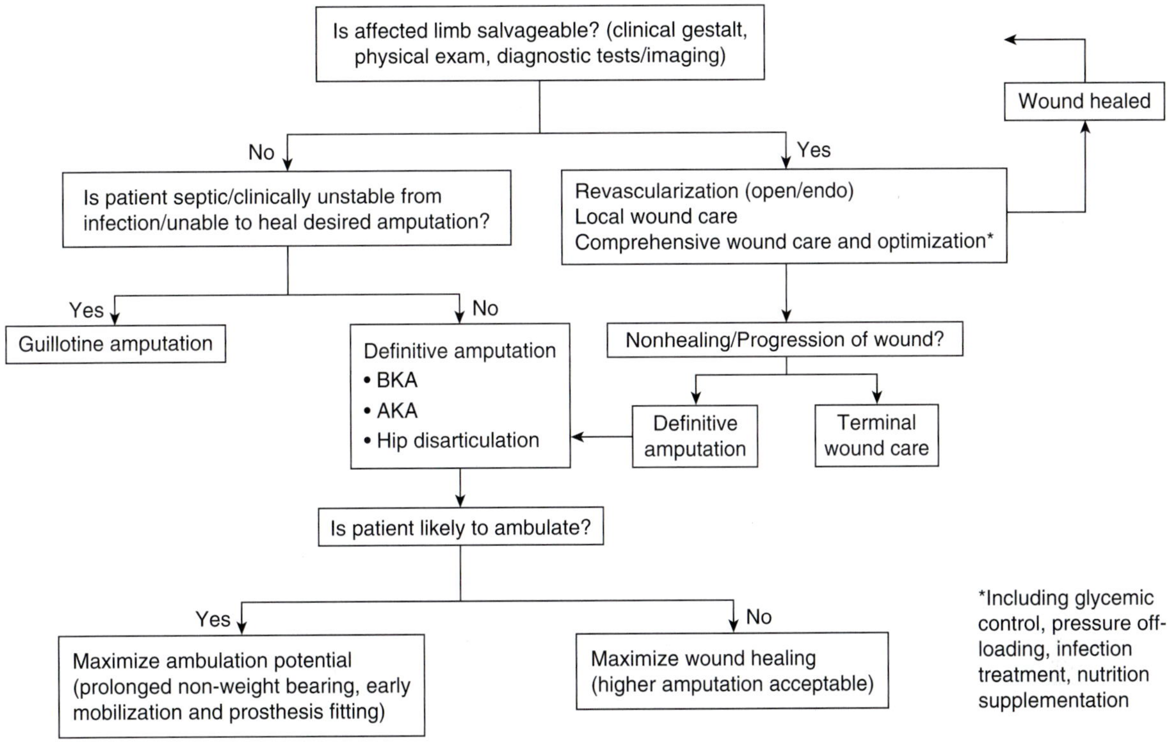

FIGURE 4 ● Algorithm for approach to limb salvage and amputation.

GENERAL PRINCIPLES

- Certain surgical principles can be applied to all amputation types. Selecting the appropriate amputation level is the first step and based on clinical and diagnostic factors (see in "Imaging and Other Diagnostic Studies") to assess vascular perfusion and structural bone integrity.
- Routine antibiotic and venous thromboembolism prophylaxis are administered. A tourniquet should be avoided in an ischemic limb unless the diseased arterial segment is located distally to the level of amputation only.
- Any dead or devitalized skin, muscle, and tissue is debrided and removed. Unnecessary trauma to healthy marginal tissue is minimized by careful dissection and avoiding excessive tissue handling with forceps or electrocautery.
- Skin and subcutaneous tissue should be kept intact with the fascia. Muscles are divided with electrocautery or sharply with scissors.
- Bone is divided with an electric or Gigli saw. Any bone dust is irrigated from the residual bone with saline. Bone edges are smoothed with a rasp. The anterior edge of larger bones (eg, femur or tibia) is beveled with an electric saw to minimize potential trauma with a future prosthesis.
- Large vessels are suture ligated.
- Nerves are tied off under stretch, divided sharply using scissors (not electrocautery), and allowed to retract into the residual limb. This prevents potential neuroma formation in the future. Injecting local anesthetic or neurolytic to the nerve stump prior to dividing has been proposed to ameliorate postoperative or phantom limb pain but is not in our routine practice.
- In patients who are at risk of having negative reactions to narcotic pain medications such as the elderly, the authors have had excellent results partnering with anesthesia to place preoperative nerve block catheters, which supply a continuous infusion of local anesthetic to the surgical limb and reduces postoperative opiate use.
- To keep the inferior muscle pad in place over the new residual limb in BKAs or AKAs, *myodesis* can be performed. The distal muscle is sutured to the bone through a predrilled hole, thereby securing the muscle to the bone. This prevents stump deformity and shifting of muscles during contraction, which can lead to progressive atrophy.
- In closing, the external fascia is reapproximated over the muscle and bone in a tension-free manner. Skin is approximated using staples, interrupted nonabsorbable sutures, or continuous suture (absorbable or nonabsorbable).
- No benefit has been shown to leaving drains in the wound and may increase the risk of infection. If drains are used, they should be removed by postoperative day 1 to 2 and placed away from the suture line.

TRANSTIBIAL OR BELOW KNEE AMPUTATION

- Transtibial amputation or BKA is the most common amputation used for lower extremity infection or ischemia (**FIGURE 5**). Typical BKA uses a long posterior flap that is well-vascularized, though other techniques have been described (eg, sagittal, skew, medial, or fish mouth flaps).
- An anterior skin incision is made 1 cm distal to the intended transection of the tibia, which is typically measured as one handbreadth (10-12 cm) below the tibial tuberosity. The incision is extended about one half to two thirds around the leg's circumference. The posterior flap includes the gastrocnemius and is 3 cm more than the transverse diameter of the calf to be eventually folded anteriorly and cover the tibia to cushion the bone for prosthesis.
- Muscles of the anterior and lateral compartments are divided with electrocautery.
- The tibia is divided 10 to 12 cm distal to the tibial tuberosity using a power saw perpendicular to the long axis of the bone. The anterior edge of the tibia is beveled to minimize prosthetic trauma. The fibula is next divided 1 to 2 cm proximal to the tibia, typically with Horsley bone cutters.
- Major vascular bundles are suture ligated. The tibial and peroneal nerves are divided sharply under stretch.
- The posterior flap is completed by dividing the residual posterior compartment musculature and soft tissue with a long amputation knife. To reduce bulk of the posterior flap, the soleus muscle can be excised at the level of the tibial osteotomy, preserving the gastrocnemius muscle and fascia.
- The deep fascia and skin are closed without tension.

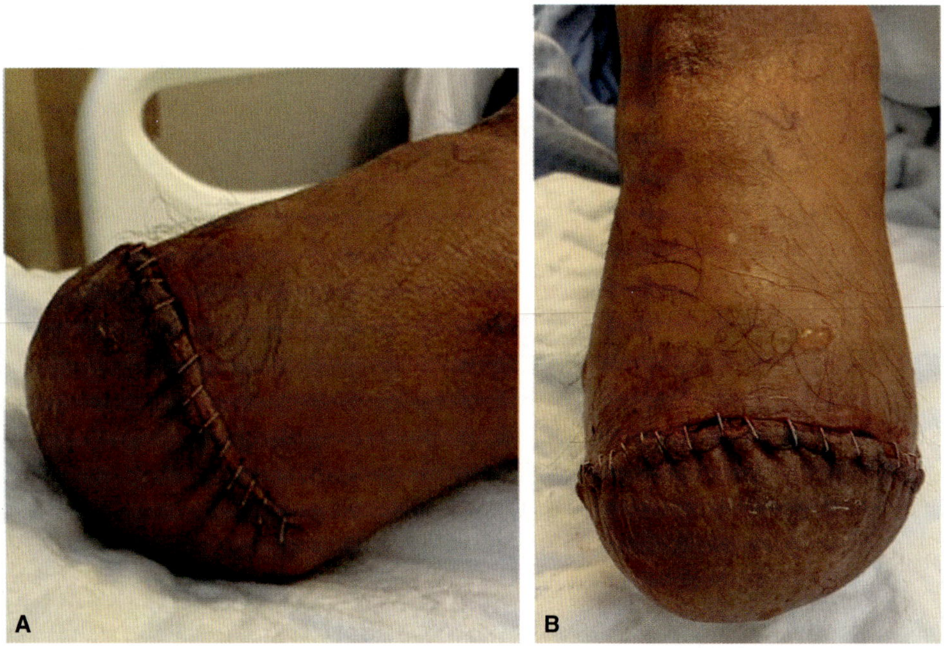

FIGURE 5 • Transtibial or below-knee-amputation (BKA).

TRANSFEMORAL OR ABOVE KNEE AMPUTATION

- Transfemoral amputations or AKA can be performed at one of three levels (high, mid, or low) depending on the patient's expected postoperative function status and/or the extent of ischemia or infection.
- A circular (fish mouth) or sagittal incision is made 2 to 3 cm below the expected level of dividing the femur, followed by carrying the dissection down through the skin, fascia, and muscles. The femoral artery and vein are suture ligated in Hunter's canal. The femur is divided using an electric saw, proximal to the level of the divided muscles. The sciatic nerve is divided under stretch as described in "General Principles."
- Myodesis can be performed, whereby distal tendons of muscles are attached directly to bone via predrilled holes in the bone to maintain function and provide distal padding (**FIGURE 6**). While more common in tumor surgery, myodesis can be performed during both below-knee or above-knee amputations. In BKA, myodesis of the major leg muscle groups to the distal tibia provides soft-tissue coverage to the stump.[15] In AKA, a two-layer myodesis can be performed over the end of the femur, which provides added muscle stabilization of the bone.[16] Typically, the quadriceps and hamstrings muscles are myodesed to one another covering the distal bony femur edge. These muscles and the adductors are then secured to the femur using drill holes. Both absorbable and nonabsorbable suture have been described for this use.
- Myodesis, if performed, is followed by fascial closure with interrupted sutures.
- Skin is closed using sutures or staples.

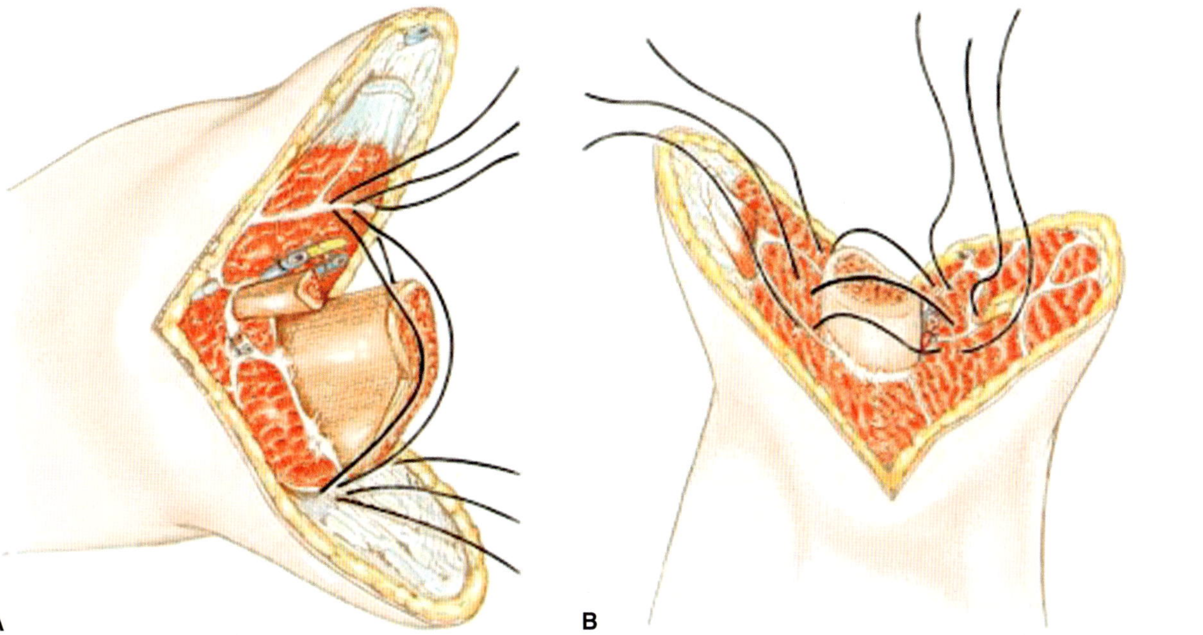

FIGURE 6 • **A,** Myodesis over the distal tibia in below-knee-amputation. **B,** Two-layer myodesis over the femur stump in above-knee-amputation. (Reprinted by permission from Springer: Sugarbaker P, Bickels J, Malawer M. Above-knee amputation. In: Malawer MM, Sugarbaker PH, eds. *Musculoskeletal Cancer Surgery. Springer*; Reprinted by permission from Springer: Malawer M, Bickels J, Sugarbaker P. Below-knee amputation. In: Malawer MM, Sugarbaker PH, eds. *Musculoskeletal Cancer Surgery*. Springer; 2004:366.)

HIP DISARTICULATION

- Disarticulation of the femur at the hip joint is a rare procedure, performed for nonhealing amputations at a lower level, life-threatening infection/gangrene, tumors, or trauma. Patients commonly have impaired arterial inflow at the level of the iliac arteries, and so are at high risk of decubitus pressure ulcers and nonhealing wounds. Wound complication (60%) and mortality (21%) rates are high, even more so in the context of ischemia or urgent/emergent surgery.
- The patient is positioned in the lateral decubitus position to facilitate both a posterolateral and anterior approach to the hip (**FIGURE 7**).[17] For the first stage, the surgeon stands in an anterior position to the patient to perform the neurovascular bundle exposure and ligation. After an anterior oblique skin incision is made along and below the level of the inguinal ligament, the femoral vessels and nerve are divided, and the muscles of the anterior thigh are transected off the pelvic bone from lateral to medial, beginning with the sartorius and ending with the adductor magnus.
- The iliopsoas and obturator externus muscles are divided at their insertion on the lesser trochanter of the femur; all other muscles are divided at their origin. The quadratus femoris muscle is identified and preserved. The hip flexor muscles are transected from the ischial tuberosity at their origin.
- In the next phase, the surgeon moves to the contralateral side in a posterior position to the patient to facilitate gluteal muscular dissection and joint disarticulation. The pelvis is rotated from posterolateral to anterolateral position. The posterior skin incision is made. The gluteal fascia, tensor fascia lata, and gluteus maximus muscles are divided at their posterior attachments to reveal the muscles inserting onto the greater trochanter (via a common tendon). These muscles are transected at their insertion on the bone. The posterior joint capsule is exposed and transected. The sciatic nerve is identified and divided and then retracts below the piriformis muscle.
- The wound is closed with preserved muscles reapproximated over the joint capsule. Suction drains are placed, and over these, the gluteal fascia is secured to the inguinal ligament. Skin is closed with interrupted sutures.

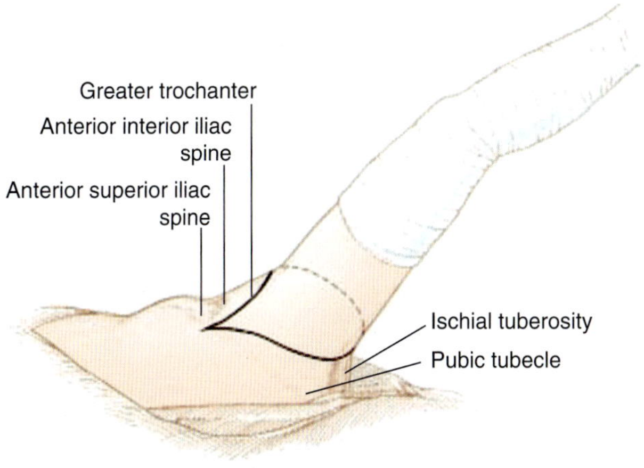

FIGURE 7 • Hip disarticulation patient positioning and surgical incision. (Reprinted by permission from Springer: Sugarbaker P, Malawer M. Hip disarticulation. In: Malawer MM, Sugarbaker PH, eds. *Musculoskeletal Cancer Surgery*. Springer; 2004:340.)

PEARLS AND PITFALLS

BKA	▪ For BKA, a long posterior flap is crucial to allow for successful padding and closure of the stump. The tibia should be resected 10-12 cm below the tuberosity with the fibula 1-2 cm above the level of the tibia. If the tibia is transected too proximally, the bony stump can erode through the anterior portion of the stump. If the fibula is left too long, then the patient will be unable to properly bear weight with a prosthesis.
AKA	▪ For AKA, the length of the femur should be considered for either high or low AKA. High AKA is recommended if there is occlusion of the external iliac artery or profunda femoris for healing of the surgical incision site or if the extent of infection is extensive (ie, infected prosthesis or bone).
Hip disarticulations	▪ For hip disarticulations, the lower extremity should be prepped and draped to allow for free manipulation of the hip joint, including hip flexion. Flexion at the knee joint is also important for developing the posterior amputation flap, which includes skin, subcutaneous tissue, fascia, and the gluteus maximus muscle maintaining its attachment at the deep surface to ensure adequate vascular supply for the flap. It is important to remember that the vascular supply to the posterior flap is dependent on leaving the gluteus maximus muscle attached to this flap.[9]

POSTOPERATIVE CARE

- Prior to leaving the operating room, the wound is commonly dressed in sterile fashion with vaseline gauze (Xeroform), layers of 4 × 4 cm gauze ("fluffs"), then wrapped with a Kerlix gauze bandage followed by an Ace compression bandage. This soft dressing with mild compression protects the wound and decreases edema. A knee immobilizer may be placed to keep the lower extremity extended at the knee joint to prevent contracture after BKA. The dressings are typically taken down on postoperative day 3 and further dressings with mild compression or shrinker stocking are continued until the wound is well healed (**FIGURE 8**). Compression over the patella should be avoided if possible as this can cause skin necrosis if placed too tightly.
- Instead, some surgeons have advocated for a rigid protective dressing. A rigid plaster of Paris stump dressing is applied immediately postoperatively and left on for 14 days. This dressing can be split longitudinally to allow for easy opening and closing (like a clamshell) for comfort and easier removal. This rigid dressing may reduce swelling and protect the stump from trauma and contracture. Disadvantages include its increased weight, inability to inspect the wound postoperatively, and possible compromise of blood flow to a stump with borderline perfusion.
- A recent Cochrane systematic review found no significant difference in benefits or harms when comparing rigid and soft dressings for patients undergoing transtibial amputations (BKAs).[18] Clinical judgment should be used after assessing the potential benefits and harms for each patient (ie, a high-fall risk patient may benefit more from a rigid protective dressing, while a patient with poor baseline skin integrity may benefit more from a soft dressing to decrease the risk of wound breakdown). While some studies favor rigid dressings immediately postoperatively for achieving faster stump healing[19] and reduction of stump volume, there is no apparent advantage in functional outcomes.
- Rigid removable dressings (RRDs) have also been utilized. These consist of sport tube socks to provide compression followed by a rigid plaster cast that is suspended by a stockinette to a supracondylar suspension cuff. Similar to a rigid

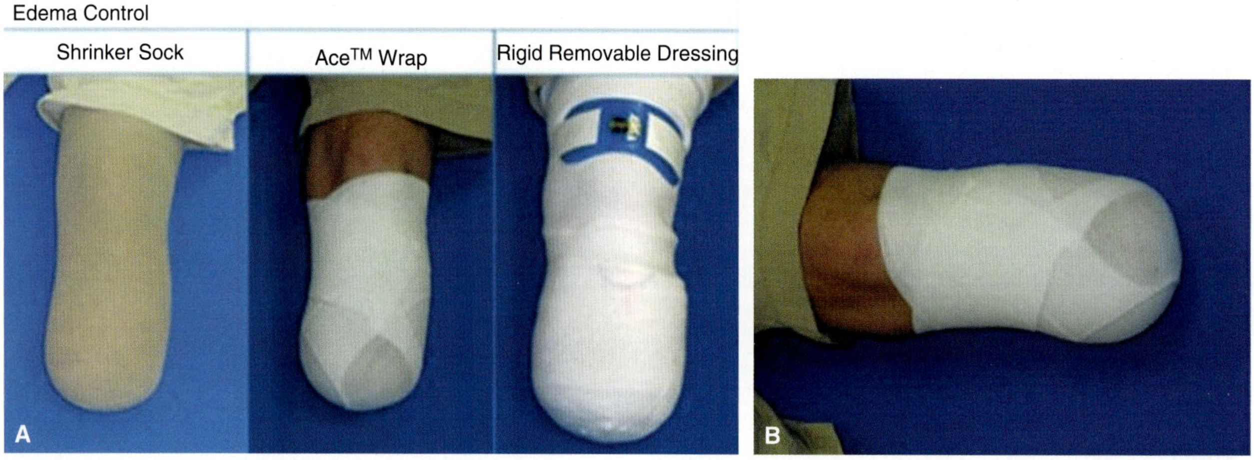

FIGURE 8 • **A,** Types of postoperative dressings for compression and controlling edema after amputation. **B,** Ace wrap in figure-of-8 pattern. (Republished with permission of Springer, from Spires M. Lower extremity amputation: postamputation and residual limb care. In: Spires MC, Kelly BM, Davis AJ, eds. *Prosthetic Restoration and Rehabilitation of the Upper and Lower Extremity*. Demos Medical Publishing; 2014:26, Chapter 3; permission conveyed through Copyright Clearance Center, Inc.)

dressing, these reduce edema formation, but unlike the rigid protective dressing described above, their removability allows for more frequent wound inspections. Compression of the limb can be carefully controlled by adding more tube socks under the rigid cast.

- Regardless of dressing used, patients are made non-weight-bearing on the affected limb until the wounds are healed. An accidental traumatic injury to a fresh amputation site is a common cause of wound breakdown and complications.
- Other postoperative management should include standard postsurgical management including advancement of diet, adequate pain control, bowel regimen, and management of other medical conditions.

Rehabilitation and Prosthesis Preparation

- When patients have the time and opportunity to prepare for life with an amputation, consultation with PM&R specialists should be arranged prior to the surgery.
- With an adequate postoperative pain control regimen, rehabilitation begins as early as postoperative day 1 with joint exercises, bed and transfer mobility, and strengthening exercises for the contralateral leg and upper body.
- Inpatient consultation with PM&R service is made early to guide physical and occupational therapy, educate the patient about prosthetics, assist with rehabilitation placement, and help patients regain independence. Physical and occupational therapy should be prescribed early to facilitate mobility and training for activities of daily living (ADLs).
- The residual limb is fitted with an elastic compression stocking or "shrinker sock" to decrease edema and help shape and mold the limb to fit into the socket of a prosthesis. The shrinker sock is worn 24 hours a day to maximize edema reduction and optimize the shape of the residual limb for prosthesis fitting. Once the wound has healed, usually after 1 to 2 months, slow progression of weight-bearing is allowed.
- Long-term rehabilitation begins once the surgical incision is healed, which can take up to several weeks or longer depending on if there are any wound healing complications. Once healed, the patient can be fitted with a temporary prosthesis for gait training. Later, usually a minimum of 6 months postoperatively, a definitive prosthesis is prescribed, once the residual limb has stabilized in size and the patient has shown adequate ambulatory skill and training.

COMPLICATIONS AND OUTCOMES

- Multiple postoperative complications may arise after lower extremity amputations (**TABLE 2**), often due in large part to underlying comorbidities. In a large, retrospective review from 1990 to 2001, Aulivola et al identified 959 major lower extremity amputations (704 BKA = 73%, 255 AKA = 27%) in 788 patients.[20] The most commonly occurring complications included cardiac (10.2%), wound infection (5.5%), and pneumonia (4.5%). Amputation stump wound breakdown and failure for the residual limb to heal occur more commonly after BKA (13%) as compared to AKA (4%) (**FIGURE 9**).
- Outcomes on healing and revisions after amputations have been well studied. Nehler et al reported outcomes of 154 patients undergoing 172 major lower extremity amputations (94 BKA, 78 AKA) from 1997 to 2002.[21] Healing rates were lower for BKA vs AKA (55% BKA vs 76% AKA at 100 days; 83% BKA vs 85% AKA at 200 days). Thirty-nine patients (25%) required revision (23 BKA, 16 AKA) with 18 BKAs (19%) converted to AKA. In a more recent single-institution review from Columbo et al, 130 limbs undergoing BKA in 120 patients were examined. Thirty-eight percent of all BKAs achieved healing and ultimately ambulation. One-quarter of BKAs required reintervention with 9 limbs (7%) requiring BKA revision and 24 limbs (18%) converted to AKA.[12] In the series from Aulivola et al, 5% of AKA and 18% of BKA limbs required additional operation with 10% of BKAs requiring conversion to AKA at average time of 77 days postoperatively.[20]
- Ability to ambulate or wear a prosthesis is dependent on patient characteristics and amputation extent. In one study, 83% of BKA patients were ambulatory as compared to 45% of AKA patients; at 6-month follow up, these declined to 58% and 25%, respectively.[22] Of the patients who were ambulatory preoperatively, 74% of BKA and 63% of AKA

Table 2: Complications Following Major Lower Extremity Amputation With Relative Incidence

Complication	Reported incidence (%)
Deep vein thrombosis (DVT)	50% (without prophylaxis, AKA 38% vs BKA 21%)
Stump bleeding or hematoma	3%-9%
Infection	13%-40%
Need for reamputation	10%-20%
Phantom limb pain	50%-85%
Flexion contracture	3%-5%

Adapted with permission of Springer, from Arya S, Escobar GA. Principles of Lower Extremity Amputation: Etiology, Goals, Limb Length Decisions and Impact on Prosthetic Management. In: Spires MC, Kelly BM, Davis AJ, eds. Prosthetic Restoration and Rehabilitation of the Upper and Lower Extremity. Demos Medical Publishing; 2014:9-20; permission conveyed through Copyright Clearance Center, Inc..

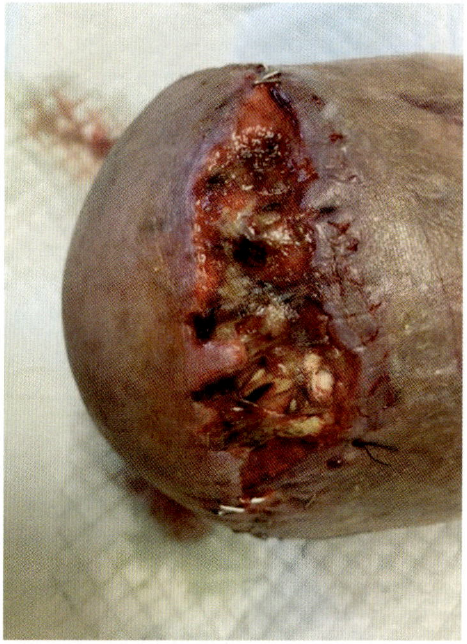

FIGURE 9 • Postoperative wound complication demonstrating below-knee-amputation (BKA) stump dehiscence.

remained so postamputation with similar rates observed at >1 year follow-up. Of all comorbidities studied (diabetes, renal insufficiency, PAD, or obesity), only age >70 years and female sex were independently associated with nonambulation postoperatively.

- Regarding mortality after amputation, in the large series from Aulivola et al, 30-day mortality was nearly 9% overall and significantly higher for AKA vs BKA (17% vs 6% $P < .001$) and for guillotine vs closed amputation (14% vs 8%, $P = .03$). Overall survival was 70% at 1 year and 35% at 5 years and significantly worse for AKA vs BKA (51% vs 75% at 1 year; 23% vs 38% at 5 years; $P < .001$). Gabel et al reviewed the Vascular Quality Initiative data registry for major lower extremity amputations (both BKA and AKA) from 2013 to 2015 and found an overall perioperative complication rate of 15% with 30-day mortality of 5%.[23] Patients undergoing AKA vs BKA were more likely to be female, >70 years old, underweight, nonambulatory, have ABI < 0.6, and have nonprivate insurance (all $P < .001$). AKA patients had a lower rate of 30-day postoperative complications (12% vs 18%) but a higher 30-day mortality (7% vs 3%) than BKA patients (all $P < .001$).
- Aspirin and statin therapy play an important role in risk prevention in PAD and nontraumatic amputations. In a population-based study from Arya et al, 155,647 patients with incident PAD were shown to have a significant reduction in both amputation and mortality with high-intensity statin therapy as compared to antiplatelet therapy only (HR 0.67; 95% CI 0.61-0.74 and HR 0.74; 95% CI 0.70-0.77, respectively).[24]

REFERENCES

1. Unwin N. Epidemiology of lower extremity amputation in centres in Europe, North America and East Asia. *Br J Surg*. 2000;87(3):328-337. doi:10.1046/j.1365-2168.2000.01344.x
2. Arya S, Escobar GA. Principles of lower extremity amputation: Etiology, goals, limb length decisions and Impact on prosthetic management. In: Spires MC, Kelly BM, Davis AJ, eds. *Prosthetic Restoration and Rehabilitation of the Upper and Lower Extremity*. Demos Medical Publishing; 2014:9-20.
3. Prompers L, Huijberts M, Apelqvist J, et al. High prevalence of ischaemia, infection and serious comorbidity in patients with diabetic foot disease in Europe. Baseline results from the Eurodiale study. *Diabetologia*. 2007;50(1):18-25. doi:10.1007/s00125-006-0491-1
4. Allison MA, Ho E, Denenberg JO, et al. Ethnic-specific prevalence of peripheral arterial disease in the United States. *Am J Prev Med*. 2007;32(4):328-333. doi:10.1016/j.amepre.2006.12.010
5. Thiruvoipati T, Kielhorn CE, Armstrong EJ. Peripheral artery disease in patients with diabetes: Epidemiology, mechanisms, and outcomes. *World J Diabetes*. 2015;6(7):961. doi:10.4239/wjd.v6.i7.961
6. Barnes JA, Eid MA, Creager MA, Goodney PP. Epidemiology and risk of amputation in patients with diabetes mellitus and peripheral artery disease. *Arterioscler Thromb Vasc Biol*. 2020;40(8):1808-1817. doi:10.1161/ATVBAHA.120.314595
7. Nehler MR, Duval S, Diao L, et al. Epidemiology of peripheral arterial disease and critical limb ischemia in an insured national population. *J Vasc Surg*. 2014;60(3):686-95.e2. doi:10.1016/j.jvs.2014.03.290
8. Duff S, Mafilios MS, Bhounsule P, Hasegawa JT. The burden of critical limb ischemia: a review of recent literature. *Vasc Health Risk Manag*. 2019;15:187-208. doi:10.2147/VHRM.S209241
9. Karakousis C. *Hip disarticulation*. In: *Operative Techniques in Orthopaedic Surgical Oncology*. Springer New York; 2014:217-222. doi:10.1177/0003134820923341
10. Mills JL, Conte MS, Armstrong DG, et al. The Society for vascular surgery lower extremity threatened limb classification system: risk stratification based on wound, ischemia, and foot infection (WIfI). *J Vasc Surg*. 2014;59(1):220-234.e2. doi:10.1016/J.JVS.2013.08.003
11. Darling JD, McCallum JC, Soden PA, et al. Predictive ability of the Society for Vascular Surgery Wound, Ischemia, and foot Infection (WIfI) classification system following infrapopliteal endovascular interventions for critical limb ischemia. *J Vasc Surg*. 2016;64:616-622. doi:10.1016/j.jvs.2016.03.417
12. Columbo JA, Nolan BW, Stucke RS, et al. Below-knee amputation failure and poor functional outcomes are higher than predicted in contemporary practice. *Vasc Endovasc Surg*. 2016;50(8):554-558. doi:10.1177/1538574416682159
13. Wagner WH, Keagy BA, Kotb MM, Burnham SJ, Johnson G. Noninvasive determination of healing of major lower extremity amputation: the continued role of clinical judgment. *J Vasc Surg*. 1988;8(6):703-710. doi:10.1016/0741-5214(88)90078-X
14. Gerhard-Herman MD, Gornik HL, Barrett C, et al. AHA/ACC guideline on the management of patients with lower extremity peripheral artery disease—Executive summary: a report of the American College of Cardiology/American Heart association task force on clinical practice guidelines. *J Am Coll Cardiol*. 2017;69(11):1465-1508. doi:10.1016/J.JACC.2016.11.008
15. Malawer M, Bickels J, Sugarbaker P. *Below-knee amputation*. In: *Musculoskeletal Cancer Surgery*. Springer; 2004:363-369. doi:10.1007/0-306-48407-2_23
16. Sugarbaker P, Bickels J, Malawer M. *Above-knee amputation*. In: *Musculoskeletal Cancer Surgery*. Springer; 2004:351-362. doi:10.1007/0-306-48407-2_22
17. Sugarbaker P, Malawer M. Hip disarticulation. In: *Musculoskeletal Cancer Surgery*. Springer; 2004:337-349. doi:10.1007/0-306-48407-2_21
18. Kwah LK, Webb MT, Goh L, Harvey LA. Rigid dressings versus soft dressings for transtibial amputations. *Cochrane Database Syst Rev*. 2019;6(6):CD012427. doi:10.1002/14651858.CD012427.pub2
19. Sumpio B, Shine SR, Mahler D, Sumpio BE. A comparison of immediate postoperative rigid and soft dressings for below-knee amputations. *Ann Vasc Surg*. 2013;27(6):774-780. doi:10.1016/j.avsg.2013.03.007
20. Aulivola B, Hile CN, Hamdan AD, et al. Major lower extremity amputation: outcome of a modern series. *Arch Surg*. 2004;139(4):395-399. doi:10.1001/archsurg.139.4.395
21. Nehler MR, Coll JR, Hiatt WR, et al. Functional outcome in a contemporary series of major lower extremity amputations. *J Vasc Surg*. 2003;38(1):7-14. doi:10.1016/S0741-5214(03)00092-2
22. MacCallum KP, Yau P, Phair J, Lipsitz EC, Scher LA, Garg K. Ambulatory status following major lower extremity amputation. *Ann Vasc Surg*. 2021;71:331-337. doi:10.1016/j.avsg.2020.07.038
23. Gabel J, Jabo B, Patel S, et al. Analysis of patients undergoing major lower extremity amputation in the Vascular Quality Initiative. *Ann Vasc Surg*. 2018;46:75-82. doi:10.1016/j.avsg.2017.07.034
24. Arya S, Khakharia A, Binney ZO, et al. Association of statin dose with amputation and survival in patients with peripheral artery disease. *Circulation*. 2018;137(14):1435-1446. doi:10.1161/CIRCULATIONAHA.117.032361

SECTION IX: Vascular Injury—Abdominal

Chapter 46 Zone I Injuries

Caroline Park and Joseph P. Minei

DEFINITION

- Zone I injuries carry a high mortality up to 60% due to the consequences of massive hemorrhage.[1]
- Injuries in the abdomen and pelvis can be classified by zone, including Zone I, Zone II, and Zone III (**FIGURE 1**). Zone I injuries are defined as an injury to the inferior vena cava or abdominal aorta within the retroperitoneum. The superior boundaries include the diaphragm, the inferior portion to the bifurcation of the iliac vessels, and the lateral borders, including the proximal renal vessels. Zone II injuries include the kidneys, spleen, adrenal glands, and may include ascending or descending colon. Zone III injuries encompass the inflow and outflow of the pelvis, including the common iliac vein and artery and internal and external iliac veins and arteries.
- Zone I injuries can be further divided into supra and inframesocolic, a border defined by the mesentery of the transverse colon. This is an important distinction that may influence the surgeon's operative approach.

DIFFERENTIAL DIAGNOSIS

- Patients presenting with blunt trauma carry a high probability of concurrent injuries given the severe mechanism of injury, including solid organ (liver, spleen, kidney) and hollow viscus injuries. Patients with penetrating trauma may also present with solid organ and hollow viscus injuries associated with the path of the missile or other object, and can include the duodenum, esophagus, stomach, pancreas, and colon (**FIGURE 2**).
- Hemorrhagic shock must be excluded first before investigating other types of shock, including spinal, neurogenic, or cardiogenic shock.

PATIENT HISTORY AND PHYSICAL FINDINGS

- Initial workup includes the primary survey to assess the airway, breathing, and circulation. Patients in hemorrhagic shock may be obtunded and require a definitive airway;

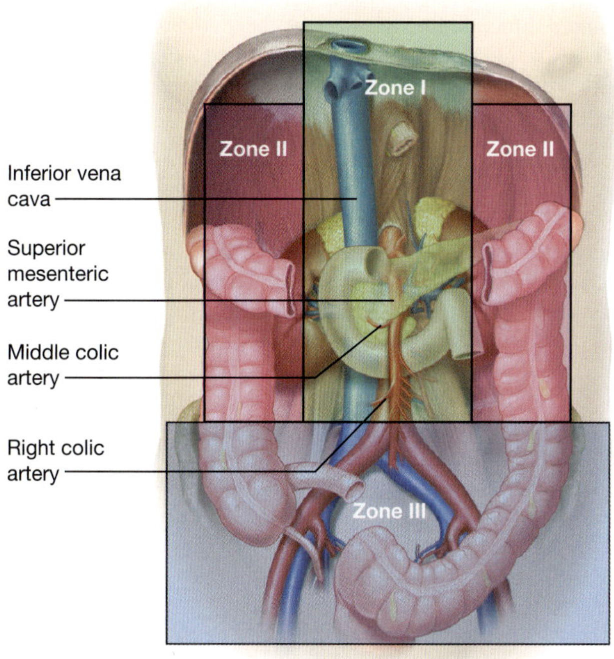

FIGURE 1 • Zone I, II, and III injuries. (Modified with permission from Fischer J. *Fischer's Mastery of Surgery*. 7th ed. Wolters Kluwer; 2019. Figure 231.1.)

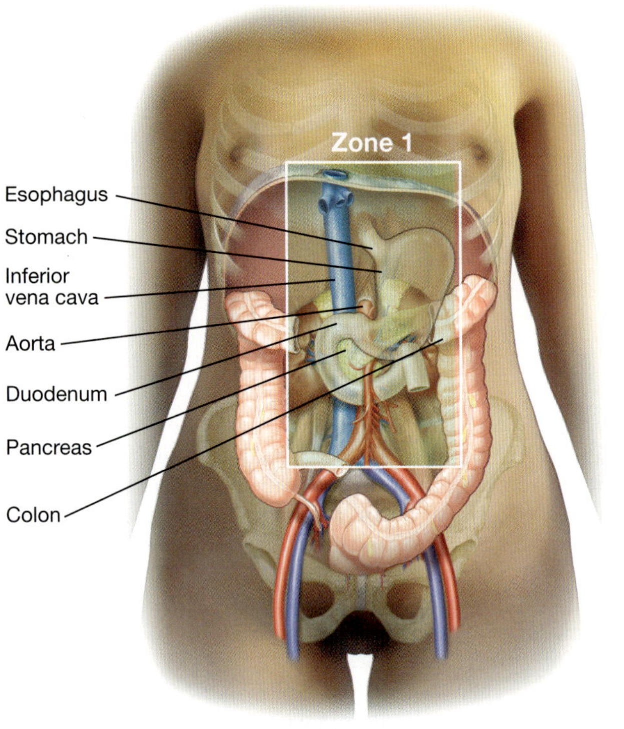

FIGURE 2 • Zone I and its relation to the abdominal organs and pelvis. Note the relation to the lesser curvature of the stomach and pancreas.

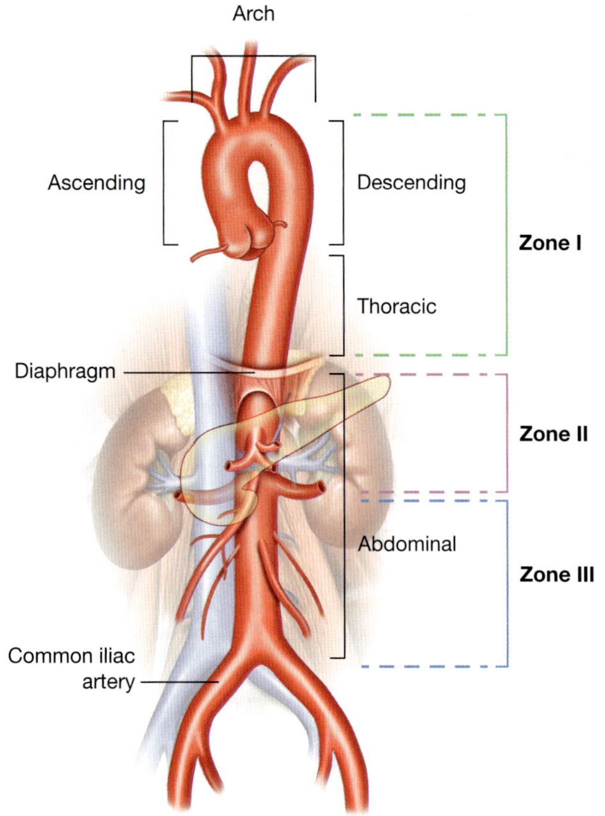

FIGURE 3 • Aorta, thoracic, and abdominal portions. Zone I = distal to the subclavian artery to the celiac trunk. Zone II = celiac trunk to the lowest renal artery. Zone III = just below the renal arteries to the bifurcation of the common iliac arteries. (Modified with permission from Kawamura D, Nolan T. *Abdomen and Superficial Structures*. 4th ed. Wolters Kluwer; 2018. Figure 4.1.)

however, if the patient is able to be bag-valve masked with satisfactory oxygenation, large-bore intravenous access should be obtained first with transfusion of blood prior to intubation.[2]

- Resuscitating the patient is critical prior to intubation to avoid precipitating cardiovascular collapse. If there is a suspicion for abdominal or pelvic hemorrhage, access should be secured above the heart (subclavian, internal jugular, or upper extremities).
- Injuries to the inferior vena cava and aorta often present with classic signs of hemorrhagic shock, including tachycardia, hypotension, and narrowed pulse pressure. Other signs or symptoms of shock may include diminished pulses, cool, clammy skin, confusion, or obtunded state in more severe cases. Patients with retroperitoneal hemorrhage may have bruising of the flank, "Grey Turner sign"; however, this is classically seen in more acute-on-chronic presentations and is not a reliable sign in the patient presenting acutely with hemorrhagic shock.

IMAGING AND OTHER DIAGNOSTIC STUDIES

- Injuries to the retroperitoneum are difficult to diagnose on primary and secondary survey and plain films, including chest X-ray, abdominal X-ray, or pelvis X-ray. Plain films should be utilized for blunt torso trauma for cavitary triage, to rule out hemothorax, pneumothorax, or pelvis fracture. Focused Assessment with Sonography in Trauma exam may be helpful to triage the abdomen for intraperitoneal fluid, but is not sensitive in detecting retroperitoneal injuries.[3]
- Computed tomography is reserved for patients who are otherwise stable and should be performed with contrast in both arterial and delayed phases to evaluate for active extravasation.

SURGICAL MANAGEMENT

Preoperative Planning and Equipment

- Patients with zone I injuries requiring operative intervention will often present with hemodynamic instability and may transiently respond to blood transfusions. Two large bore IVs in the bilateral arms are sufficient for rapid administration of blood and medications. If a multiple-access catheter or percutaneous sheath introducer is required, consider placing a subclavian or internal jugular venous catheter as femoral venous catheters may directly drain through an inferior vena cava (IVC) injury. However, these injuries are often recognized in the operating room, in which case a femoral line should be discontinued and switched to venous drainage above the heart.
- Resuscitative Endovascular Balloon Occlusion of the Aorta (REBOA)[4] is a minimally invasive technique to occlude the inflow of blood into the chest, abdomen, and pelvis based on zone of deployment (**FIGURE 3**—aorta and its zones). It has

been compared to the traditional resuscitative thoracotomy in occluding inflow to areas of hemorrhage and diverting blood to the heart and brain during a traumatic arrest with disputed outcomes.[5]

- This endovascular technique is minimally invasive and less painful and morbid than a thoracotomy incision, which is not without its own occupational hazards. The catheter can be delivered through a 7-Fr sheath in the common femoral artery and the balloon inflated to obtain partial or full occlusion to decrease blood loss (reference). For intra-abdominal bleeding, the catheter should be inflated at zone I.
- These catheters however are not without their own risks, including access problems (dissection, thrombosis), rupture of the iliac artery, aorta, or common femoral artery, and are generally not recommended for use in a patient with suspected thoracic aorta or cardiac injury, as this can potentially propagate the injury.

SURGICAL APPROACH

Positioning

- Patients should be prepped widely from chin to knees for maximum exposure and placed supine with the arms out for the anesthesiologists to access and administer anesthesia, products, and medications. Patients in extremis should be prepped awake and transfusions continued from the trauma bay. Excellent and timely communication with the anesthesiology team is paramount during intubation, as entering the abdomen and releasing any tamponade effect of a retroperitoneal hematoma could precipitate a traumatic arrest.

EXPLORATION

- A generous midline laparotomy incision from xyphoid to pubis is made and all hematoma evacuated, and all four quadrants packed with laparotomy pads. A quick survey and palpation of the spleen and liver can rule out injury that requires compression and packing. Any enteric violation should be quickly stopped with sutures or Babcock clamps. Next the zones of the abdomen should be explored.

ZONE I—ABDOMINAL AORTA AND INTRA-ABDOMINAL CONTROL

- Abdominal aortic injuries can be classified by region, including diaphragmatic, suprarenal, and infrarenal.
- Zone I injuries are most easily identified by mobilizing the left hepatic ligament, retracting on the body of the stomach, entering pars flaccida medial to the lesser curvature, and examining the hiatus where the esophagus and aorta exit the thoracic cavity (**FIGURE 4**).
- Once pars flaccida is opened, the left and right crura are identified and spread away from the aorta (**FIGURE 5**).
- Zone I injuries can also be grossly evaluated by lifting the transverse colon out of the abdomen and onto the chest—the middle colic vein and artery drain down through the transverse mesocolon and join the superior mesenteric artery and vein. However, massive injuries to zone I may result in large hematomas that track to zone II; thus, it is imperative to explore these injuries in the setting of hemorrhage shock.
- If the surgeon suspects an injury to the inferior vena cava, obtaining proximal aortic control may still be required to mitigate ongoing bleeding while determining which—or if both—has been injured.

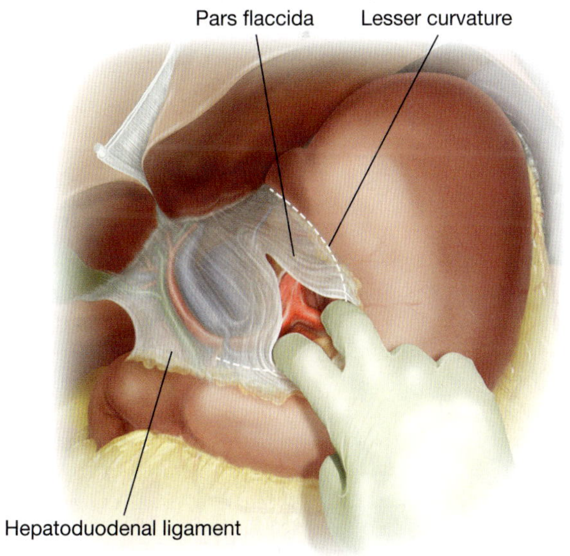

FIGURE 4 • Surgeon dissecting the pars flaccida along the lesser curvature of the stomach. (Modified with permission from Britt LD, Peitzman AB, Barie PS, et al. *Acute Care Surgery*. 2nd ed. Wolters Kluwer; 2019. Figure 11.12A.)

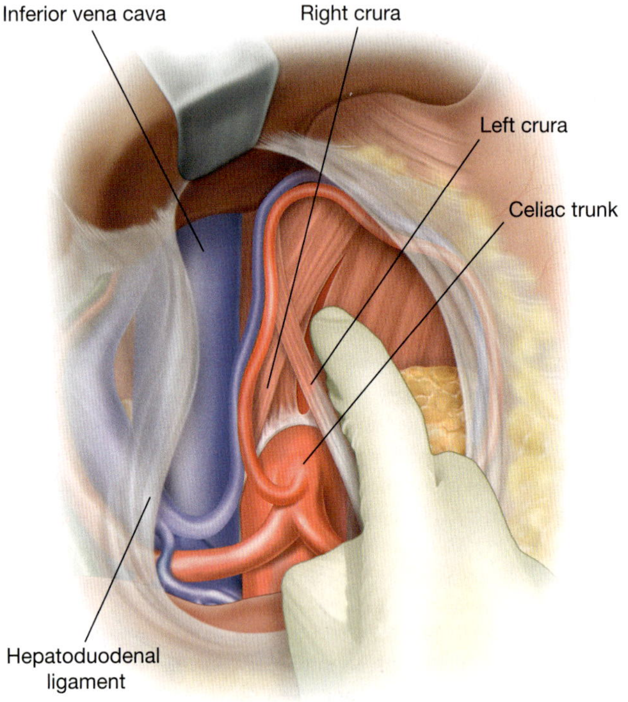

FIGURE 5 • Left and right crura of the diaphragm are identified above the celiac trunk. (Modified with permission from Britt LD, Peitzman AB, Barie PS, et al. *Acute Care Surgery*. 2nd ed. Wolters Kluwer; 2019. Figure 11.12B.)

MANUAL COMPRESSION AND OCCLUSION

- A sponge stick can also be placed in this area and pressed along the spine to obtain immediate proximal control while waiting for an aortic clamp. The celiac trunk is also accessible in this space (**FIGURES 6** and **7**).

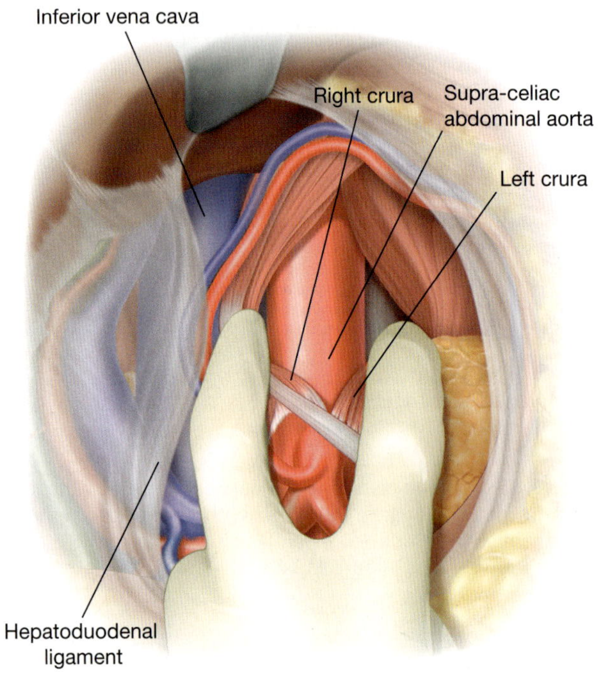

FIGURE 6 • The crura are spread away from the abdominal aorta, freeing up space for a clamp or sponge stick. (Modified with permission from Britt LD, Peitzman AB, Barie PS, et al. *Acute Care Surgery*. 2nd ed. Wolters Kluwer; 2019. Figure 11.12C.)

- If aortic bleeding is identified below the celiac trunk, a sponge stick or an aortic clamp should be applied and ischemic time noted. The surgeon should take care to place this clamp cephalad to maximize space for exploration in the abdomen. Oftentimes the patient in extremis and in hemorrhagic shock or arrest may have a weakly palpable pulse. Defining the aorta from the esophagus may be challenging in this situation. An orogastric tube should be placed to palpate the esophagus, encircle it with a Penrose drain, and retract it aside to accurately identify and place a clamp on the aorta (**FIGURE 8**).

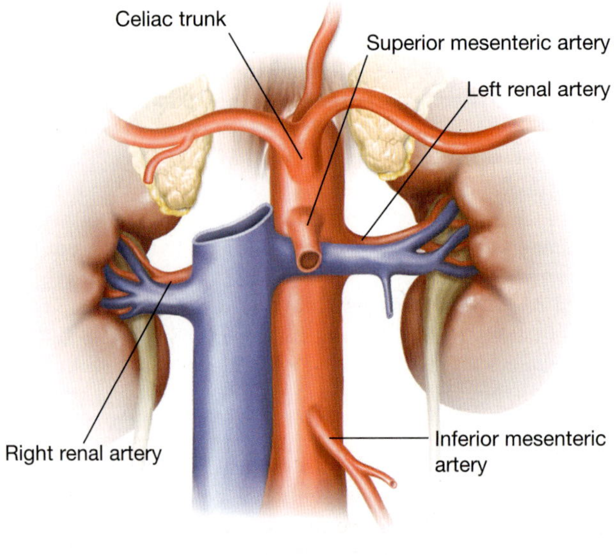

FIGURE 7 • Relation of the celiac trunk and its proximity to the diaphragm, superior mesenteric artery, left and renal arteries.

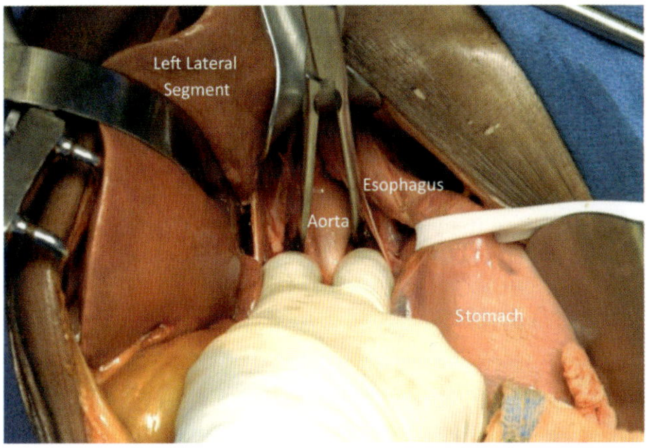

FIGURE 8 • Spreading the crura away from the abdominal aorta and placement of a clamp for aortic occlusion. Penrose encircles the distal esophagus/gastroesophageal junction laterally. (Used with permission by Cambridge University Press, from Teixeira P, Magee G, Rowe V. Abdominal aorta and splachnic vessels. In: Demetriades D, Inaba K, Velmahos G, eds. *Atlas of Surgical Techniques in Trauma*. Cambridge University Press; 2020:268-285.)

PROXIMAL ABDOMINAL AORTIC INJURIES—APPROACH FROM THE LEFT CHEST

- If the abdominal aortic injury is at or above the celiac trunk, then a left anterolateral thoracotomy should be performed to access the thoracic aorta. The inferior pulmonary ligament tethers the left lower lobe to the diaphragm and is taken down. The lower lobe can then be retracted cephalad to expose the posterior mediastinum. The pleura over the aorta is incised above the diaphragm, taking care to avoid the left inferior pulmonary vein.
- An orogastric tube within the esophagus can help guide delineation between the thin plane between the esophagus and aorta. The thoracic aorta should be cross-clamped as low as possible to avoid injury to the hilar structures.

ZONE I—INTRA-ABDOMINAL AORTA, INJURIES, AND EXPOSURES

- The abdominal aorta is best exposed by a left medial visceral rotation, or a Mattox maneuver, although a retroperitoneal approach can also provide an unparalleled view of the abdominal aorta (**FIGURE 9**).
- In a trauma laparotomy, however, a left medial visceral rotation is most practical and efficient given the risk of concomitant intraperitoneal injury.

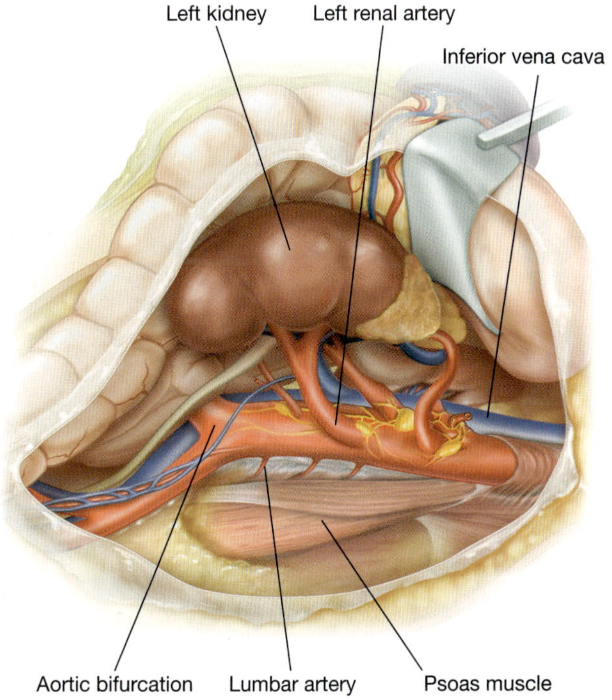

FIGURE 9 • Exposure of the abdominal aorta through a retroperitoneal approach. Note the spleen, pancreas, and left kidney are all mobilized medially, exposing the abdominal aorta and psoas muscle.

LEFT MEDIAL VISCERAL ROTATION

- In this exposure, the descending colon is taken down at the peritoneal reflection, and cephalad toward the splenic flexure. The splenic flexure is taken down, taking care to avoid injury to the spleen. The spleen and all of its attachments, including the gastrosplenic, splenocolic, phrenocolic, and splenorenal ligaments, are taken down. In a complete left medial visceral rotation, the left kidney, including the hilum and ureter, is mobilized off the peritoneum and rotated medially.

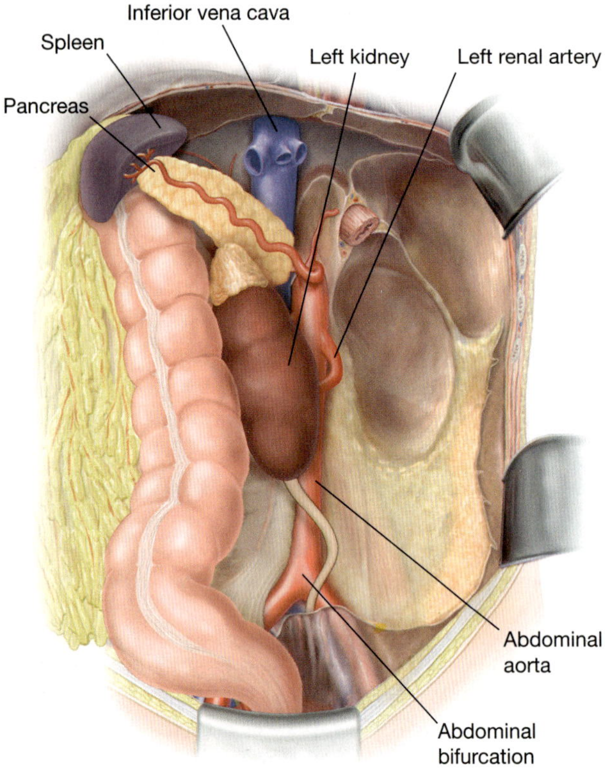

- This exposure will provide access to the abdominal aorta and bifurcation of the common iliac arteries. The left common iliac artery and vein can also be accessed through this exposure (**FIGURE 10**).
- In a modified Mattox maneuver, the left kidney remains in the retroperitoneum and Gerota fascia left intact. The surgeon should take care to avoid traction injuries when mobilizing the viscera to avoid avulsing the left renal vein (**FIGURE 11**).

FIGURE 10 • Left medial visceral rotation. Full rotation of the spleen, pancreas, left kidney, and colon. (Modified with permission from Fischer J. *Fischer's Mastery of Surgery*. 6th ed. Wolters Kluwer; 2012. Figure 254.2.)

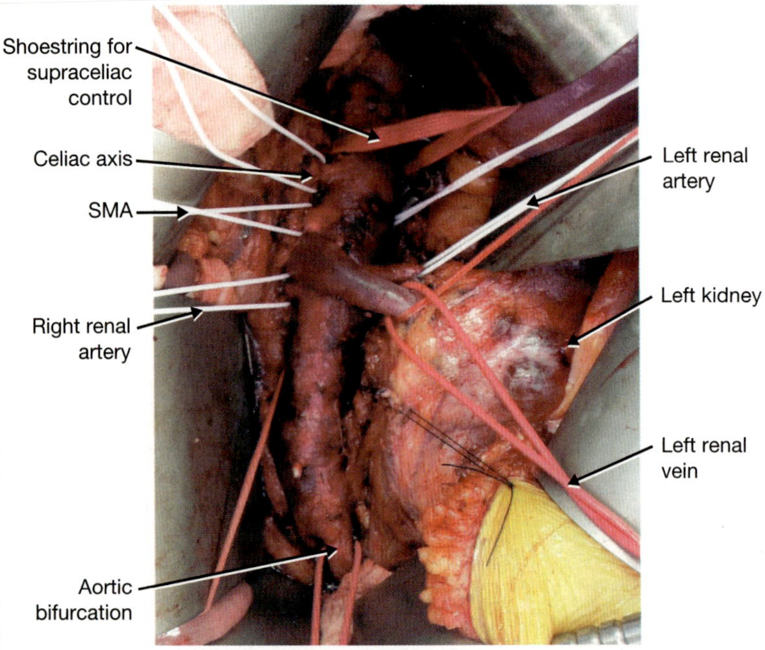

FIGURE 11 • Modified Mattox maneuver with left kidney and renal vein/artery down. Abdominal aorta from above the celiac access to the bifurcation is exposed. Note the length of the left renal vein as it crosses over the aorta and its relation to the renal artery. (Reprinted with permission from Dalman R. *Operative Techniques in Vascular Surgery*. Wolters Kluwer; 2016. Figure 22.10.)

ZONE I—ISOLATED INJURIES TO ABDOMINAL AORTA

- Injuries to the infrarenal aorta can be better localized by mobilizing the fourth portion of the duodenum medially and incising the peritoneum over the aorta and IVC. This exposure allows to maintain the integrity of Gerota fascia of the left kidney and examine the left renal vein, inferior mesenteric artery, aorta, and some parts of the IVC. This maneuver may be helpful when encountering and controlling aortoduodenal fistulae (**FIGURE 12**).
- Penetrating injuries to the infrarenal aorta are in several ways easier to manage than venous injuries as the location is noted by pulsatile bleeding and can be controlled

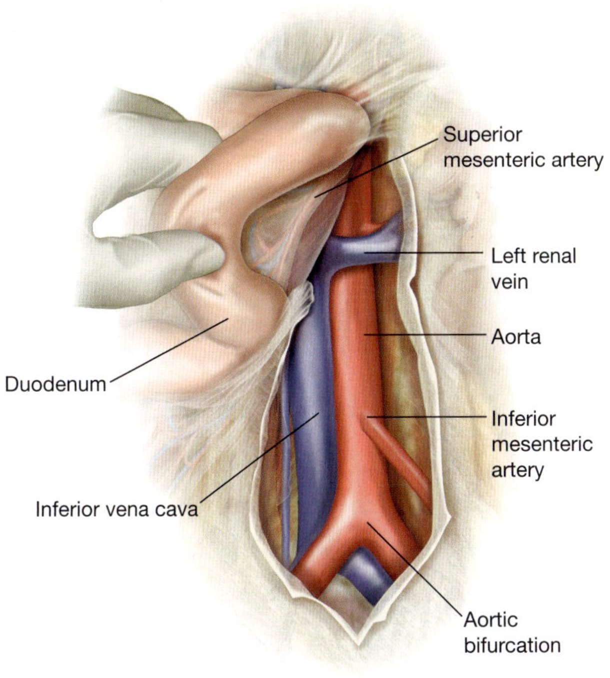

immediately with the surgeon's finger. If the patient's condition allows, systemic heparinization should be administered prior to clamping for proximal and distal control, either with vessels loops, Rummel tourniquets, or vascular clamps (**FIGURE 13**).

- The most expeditious way to approach an infrarenal aorta injury includes a left medial visceral rotation and clamps proximal and distal to the injury. In penetrating injuries, it is critical to evaluate the posterior wall of the aorta for a concomitant injury. In **FIGURE 13**, the infrarenal aorta is controlled with vascular clamps. For a small injury that can be repaired primarily, a patch repair with bovine pericardium or primary repair may be sufficient. One must ensure there is brisk inflow and back-bleeding prior to definitive repair.

FIGURE 12 • Alternative approach to injuries to the infrarenal aorta. (Modified with permission from Upchurch, GR Jr. *Clinical Scenarios in Vascular Surgery*. 2nd ed. Wolters Kluwer; 2016. Figure 36.3.)

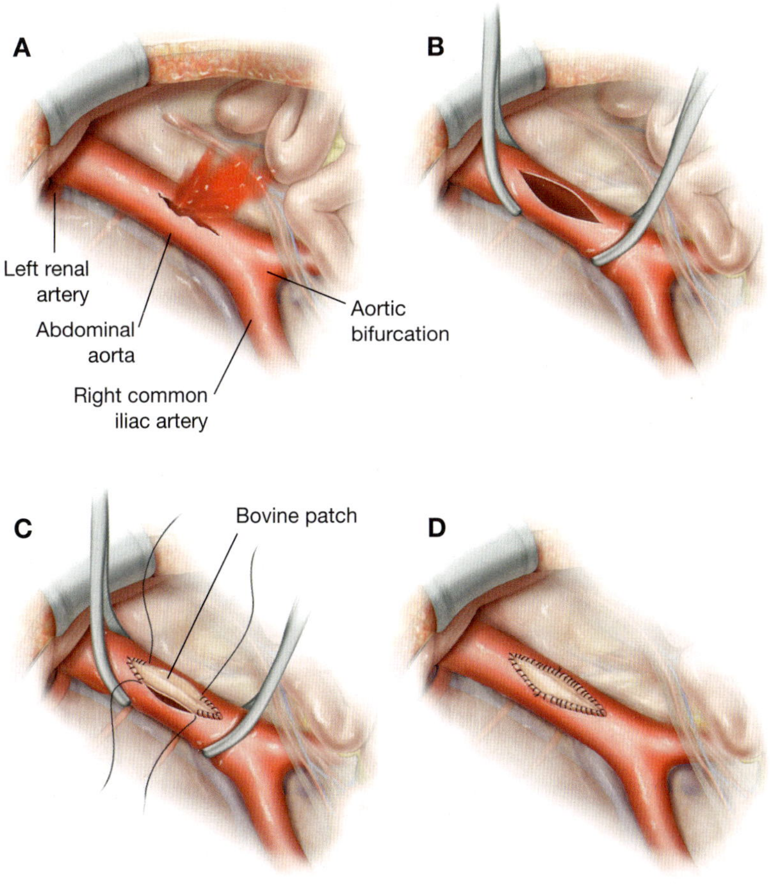

FIGURE 13 • Contained rupture of aortic aneurysm. Proximal and distal control of an aortic repair with vascular clamps, followed by bovine patch placement. **A-D**, Obtaining proximal and distal control of an infrarenal aortic injury using vascular clamps, followed by bovine patch placement.

ZONE I—INTRA-ABDOMINAL AORTA AND JUNCTIONAL INJURIES

- Junctional injuries involving the iliac artery and vein can also be approached by a left medial visceral rotation. It is important to note that the right common iliac artery crosses over left common iliac vein. Careful use of dissection is warranted when encircling the common iliac artery to avoid injury to the iliac vein, which can precipitate massive bleeding. The ureter crosses over the common iliac artery before the bifurcation of the external and internal iliac arteries and is a reliable landmark if one needs to identify and ligate the internal iliac arteries for massive pelvic bleeding (**FIGURE 14**).
- Synthetic grafts or autologous conduits can be used, favoring the latter for contaminated cases (**FIGURES 15** and **16**).

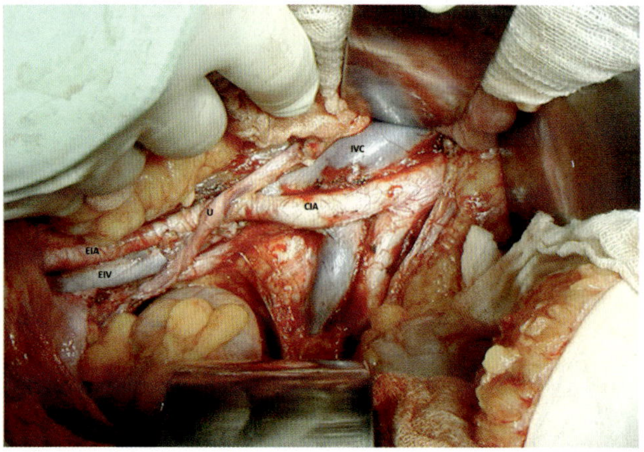

FIGURE 14 • Intraoperative photo of IVC and aortic bifurcations and relation to ureter. CIA, common iliac artery; EIA, external iliac artery; EIV, external iliac vein; IVC, inferior vena cava; U, ureter. (Reprinted with permission from Dimick JB, Upchurch, GR Jr, Sonnenday CJ, Kao LS. *Clinical Scenarios in Surgery*. 2nd ed. Wolters Kluwer; 2019. Figure 21.3.)

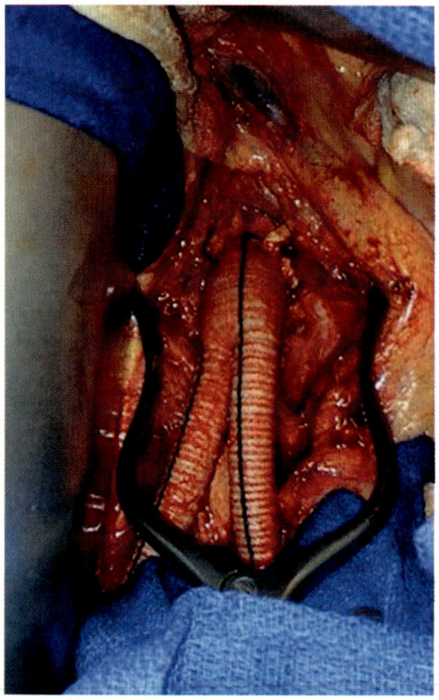

FIGURE 15 • Infrarenal aortic synthetic graft. (Courtesy of Michael Siah, MD, University of Texas Southwestern Medical Center, Division of Vascular Surgery.)

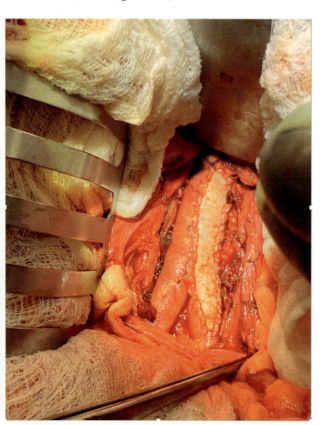

FIGURE 16 • Bovine pericardium patch of aortoiliac vessels. (Courtesy of Michael Siah, MD, University of Texas Southwestern Medical Center, Division of Vascular Surgery.)

ZONE I—INFERIOR VENA CAVA AND INITIAL HEMORRHAGE CONTROL

- The inferior vena cava drains the common iliac veins, lumbar veins, renal, adrenal, hepatic veins, and phrenic veins before it drains into the suprahepatic IVC and right atrium (**FIGURE 17**). The retrohepatic vena cava, though it spans a short distance behind the liver, is the most difficult portion to access if injured (**FIGURE 18**).
- Massive IVC injuries often present with an expanding zone I hematoma, and in penetrating injuries can be devastating if the tamponade effect within the retroperitoneum is lost. Securing IV access, notably access above the heart (internal jugular vein, subclavian vein), is critical to prevent ongoing losses within the abdomen.
- Aortic occlusion should be obtained by the steps outlined previously in this chapter OR by endovascular occlusion with a REBOA catheter, keeping in mind the inherent risks of catheter placement with an existing aortic injury.

Injuries to the Inferior Vena Cava—Exposure

Right Medial Visceral Rotation

- A complete right medial visceral rotation offers the best approach to the infrahepatic IVC. The ascending colon is taken down along the peritoneal reflection, including the hepatic flexure. The avascular fusion plane between the small bowel mesentery and posterior peritoneum is scored to lengthen this plane. The duodenum is reflected medially via Kocher maneuver to include the head of the pancreas. This complete maneuver should allow for small bowel evisceration onto the patient's chest (**FIGURE 19**). Be wary of the inferior mesenteric vein, which can be avulsed in this maneuver.
- Once this is complete, the infrahepatic inferior vena cava and hepatoduodenal ligament are readily exposed.

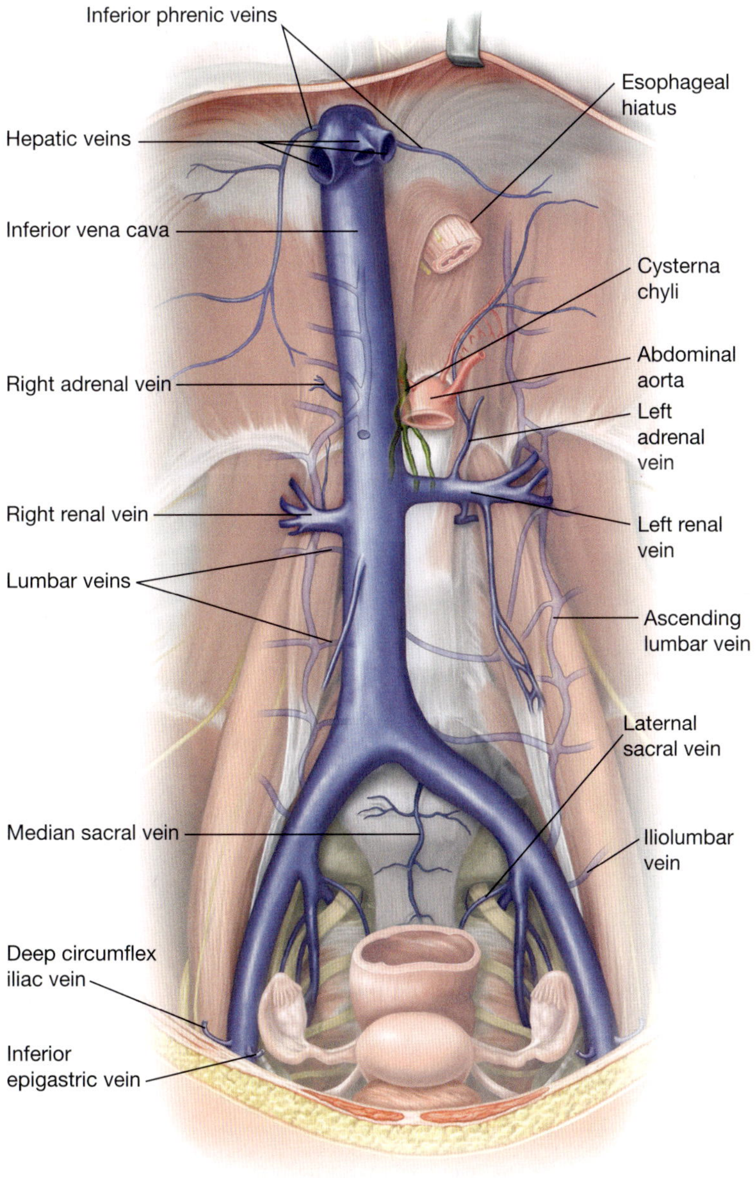

FIGURE 17 • Inferior vena cava and its drainage.

- The right renal vein can be seen anteriorly draining the kidney, but the left renal vein, which typically drains into the inferior vena cava slightly more superior, should also be exposed and visualized (**FIGURE 20**). This is important to identify if an inferior vena cava injury is so destructive that it requires ligation.

Control of Hemorrhage

- Venous injuries are typically more difficult to control given the large volume but low pressure system. Oftentimes there is significant hemorrhage with poor visualization. Sponge sticks should be readily available and applied with direct compression above and below the injury. Vascular clamps can also be applied (**FIGURE 21**).
- Expanding Zone I injuries necessitate exploration. Both the posterior and anterior walls of the inferior vena cava should be explored.

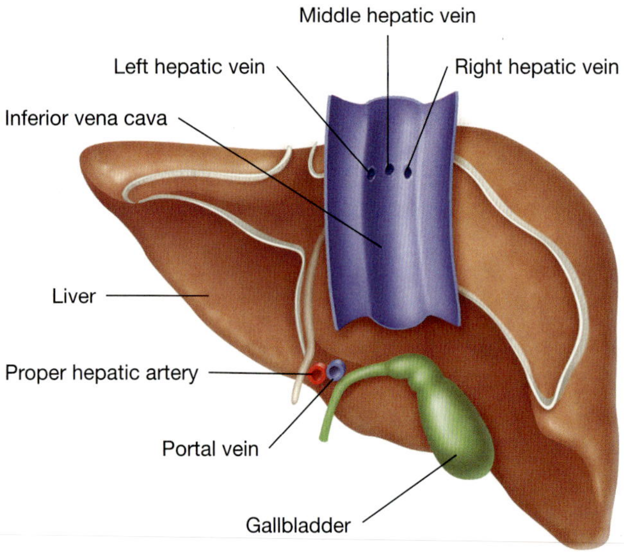

FIGURE 18 • Retrohepatic inferior vena cava and its relation to the hepatic veins (posterior view). (Reprinted with permission from Olinger AB. *Human Gross Anatomy*. Wolters Kluwer; 2016. Figure 2.86c.)

Anterior, Posterior Injuries

- The back wall or posterior aspect of the inferior vena cava should be repaired primarily first prior to repairing the anterior wall using prolene suture (**FIGURE 21**). Be wary of severe stenosis or narrowing of the inferior vena cava. (If the inferior vena cava is so significantly narrowed with "waisting" (>40% narrowing), the incidence of deep venous thrombosis is predictably greater in patients after ligation. The risk of pulmonary embolus is unclear between patients who undergo ligation vs repair.[6])

Complete Laceration

- If the inferior vena cava is completely disrupted, it is unlikely to be approximated without significant tension. The tissue is usually tenuous and will not allow for a primary repair. An interposition graft is a suitable conduit in a stable patient without massive contamination (**FIGURE 22**). Otherwise, the infrarenal inferior vena cava can be ligated if the patient is in hemorrhagic shock and repair cannot be attempted. These patients are at high for massive swelling of the lower extremities and compartment syndrome. Prophylactic bilateral four-compartment fasciotomies may be necessary to mitigate the risk of ischemia.

Suprarenal and Retrohepatic Inferior Vena Cava Injuries—Approach

- Suprarenal inferior vena cava injuries can still be accessed by a right medial visceral rotation. Injuries in this area carry a high

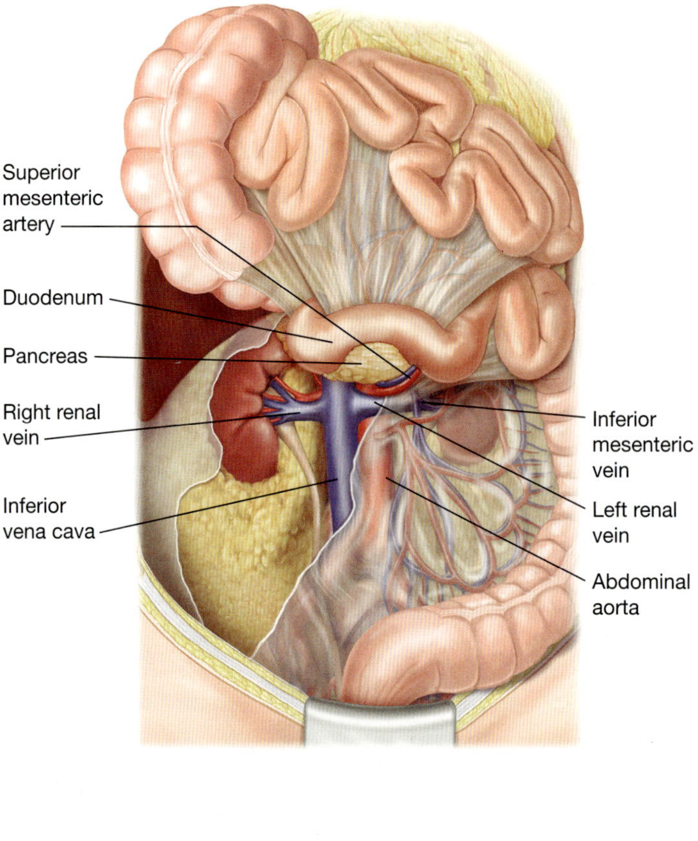

FIGURE 19 • Right medial visceral rotation, or Cattell-Braasch maneuver to access the inferior vena cava.

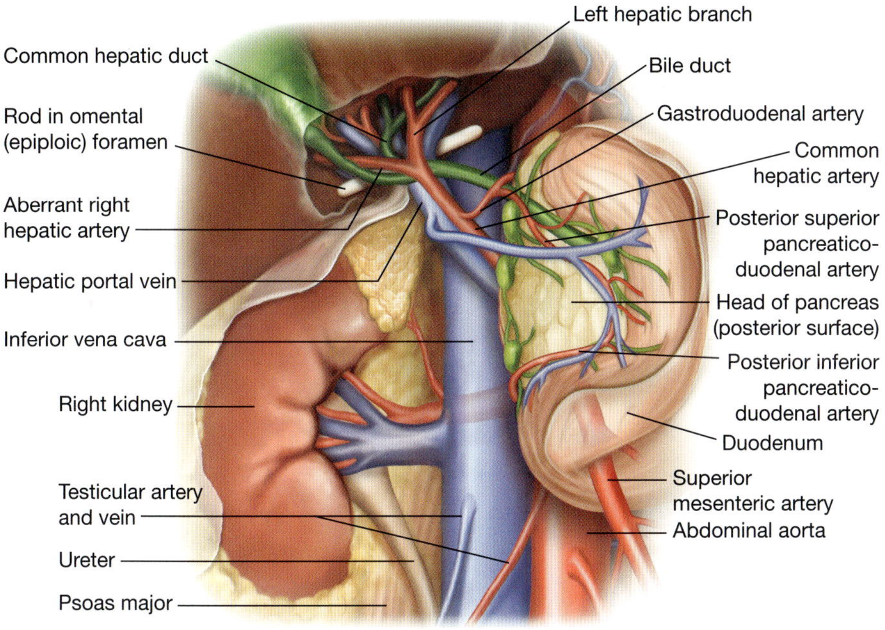

FIGURE 20 • Exposure of the infrahepatic inferior vena cava after right medial visceral rotation. Note the hepatoduodenal ligament and relation to the head of the pancreas and inferior vena cava.

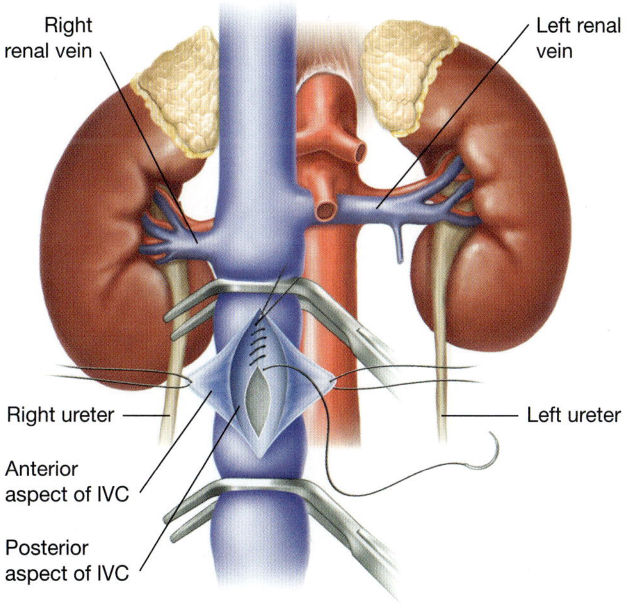

FIGURE 21 • Occlusion of the infrahepatic inferior vena cava and suture repair of a posterior inferior vena cava injury.

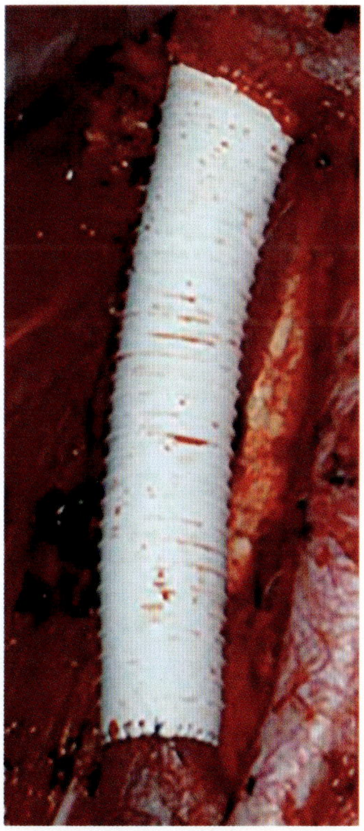

FIGURE 22 • Inferior vena reconstruction with synthetic graft. (Courtesy of Michael Siah, MD, University of Texas Southwestern Medical Center, Division of Vascular Surgery.)

risk of injury to the renal hilum, adrenal glands, aorta, duodenum, pancreas, and portal triad. Surgeons should take note of the anterior position of the renal veins and the length of the left renal vein as it crosses over the aorta (**FIGURES 23** and **24**).

Retrohepatic Inferior Vena Cava Injuries—Approach

- Retrohepatic caval injuries are the perhaps the most dreaded vascular injuries given their inaccessibility and associated

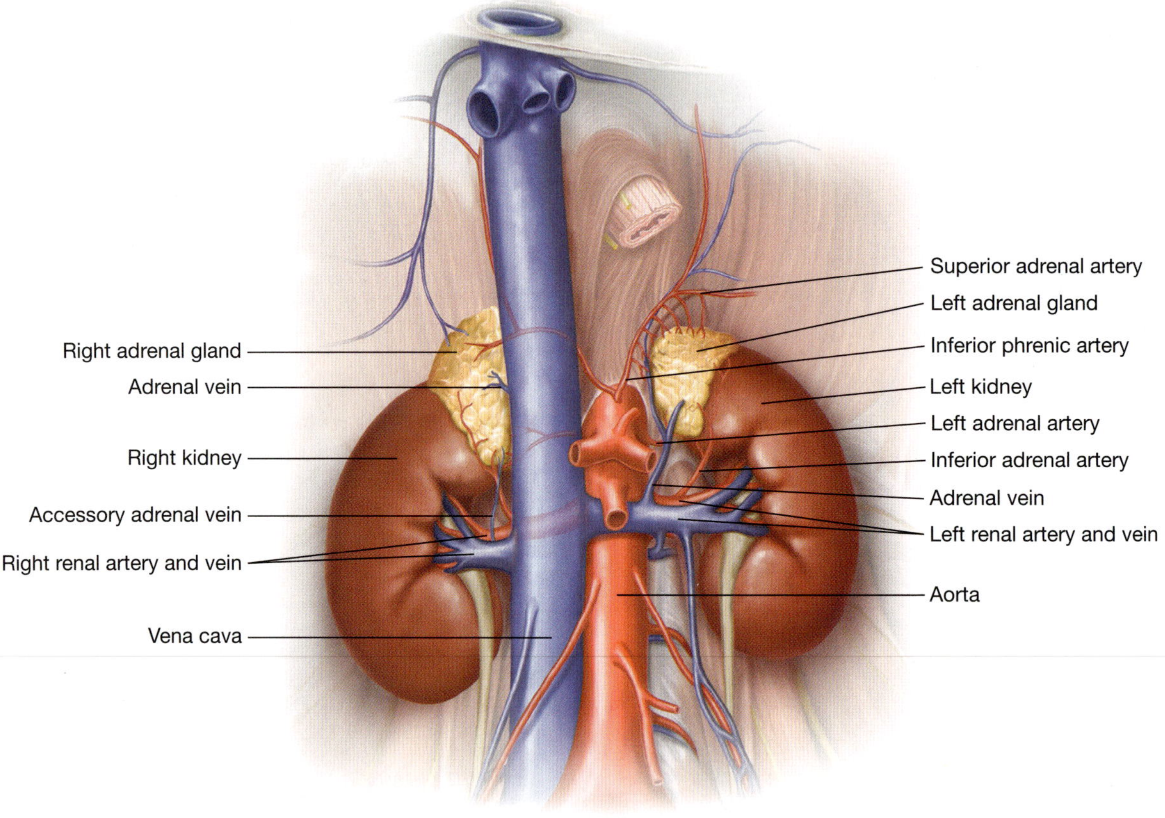

FIGURE 23 • Inferior vena cava and relation to the renal hilum, aorta, and adrenal glands.

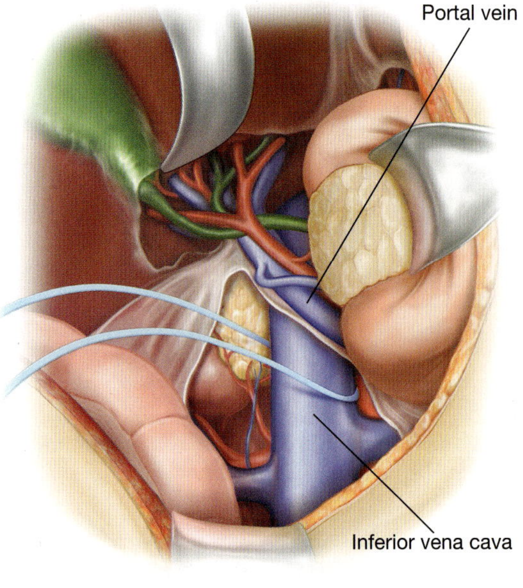

FIGURE 24 • Suprarenal inferior vena cava and relation to renal veins and portal veins. (Modified with permission from Fischer J. *Fischer's Mastery of Surgery*. 7th ed. Wolters Kluwer; 2019. Figure 130.7.)

mortality. The dictum has classically been to "pack and not look." Mobilizing the ligaments, including the right triangular ligament, can release any tamponade effect and precipitate torrential bleeding.

- Measures to exclude other types of bleeding, including hepatic veins and arteries should be excluded by packing and compression above and below the liver, and a Pringle maneuver by encircling the hepatoduodenal ligament with a Rummel tourniquet.
- Total hepatic vascular isolation is the second to last alternative to an atriocaval shunt and entails clamping of the suprahepatic inferior vena cava, followed by the infrahepatic inferior vena cava, and a Pringle maneuver.
- If these measures are exhausted, and if the injury is suprahepatic, the last consideration should be toward mobilization of the liver and preparation for an atriocaval shunt.
- Prior to mobilizing the liver, it is critical to communicate with the anesthesiologist on the anticipated blood loss and to secure the following equipment prior to shunting the retrohepatic inferior vena cava:
  - Sternal saw or Lebsche knife
  - 28-Fr chest tube with created perforations
  - Rummel tourniquets or umbilical tape
  - Kelly Clamp

Obtaining Proximal Control

- The right triangular ligament is taken down and the right liver medialized. Multiple short veins to the inferior vena cava should be clipped and divided (**FIGURE 25**). Sponge sticks should be placed directly above and below the injury to temporize massive bleeding.

Securing Distal Control

- The intrapericardial inferior vena cava can be accessed above the liver and through the diaphragm, through the right chest or via median sternotomy.
- The central tendon is divided to access the intrapericardial inferior vena cava, taking care to avoid any injury to either one.
- The intrapericardial inferior vena cava can also be accessed through a right anterolateral thoracotomy; however, the most efficient way to approach the intrapericardial inferior vena cava is through a sternotomy, opening up the pericardium and clamping the inferior vena cava before it drains into the right atrium. Occluding the inferior vena cava can precipitate cardiovascular collapse; thus, the abovementioned equipment is critical to have stand-by.
- The thoracostomy tube should be prepared in advance by creating separate side holes that can drain into the right atrium and cut to length. The right atrial appendage should be elevated with an Allis clamp and a pursestring placed with prolene. The appendage should be opened readily clamped down to avoid ongoing blood loss.
- This extremely rare procedure requires the coordination of at least two surgeons placing the thoracostomy tube in through the injury of the inferior vena cava and the other anticipating its exit through the right atrial appendage. Once the thoracostomy tube stents open the right atrium and inferior vena cava, the pursestring suture should be tied down around the right atrial appendage and Rummel tourniquets tied down below the level of the injury and at the level of the atrial appendage. The thoracostomy tube will now act as stent to divert most of the blood from the abdomen to the heart to allow for next steps (**FIGURE 26**).

Superior Mesenteric Artery and Vein, Hepatic Artery and Portal Vein Injuries—Approach

- Injuries to the mesenteric vessels, notably the superior mesenteric vein and artery and portal vein, are commonly associated with injuries to the small and large bowel and pancreas.

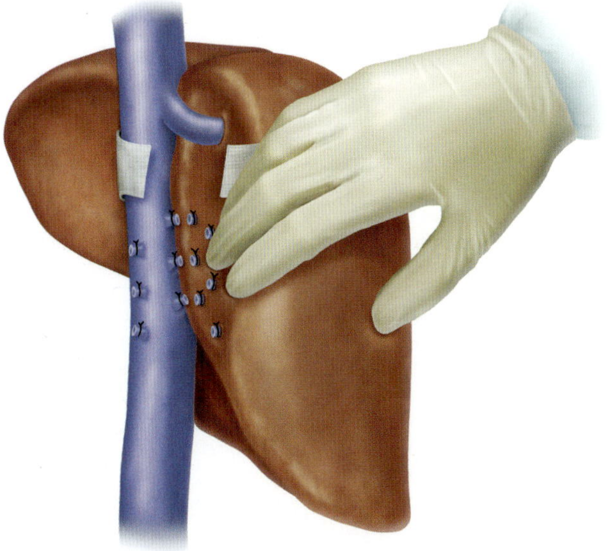

FIGURE 25 • Medializing the right liver lobe to visualize and ligate short veins of the retrohepatic vena cava. (Reprinted with permission from Dimick JB. *Mulholland & Greenfield's Surgery*. 7th ed. Wolters Kluwer; 2022. Figure 37.9.)

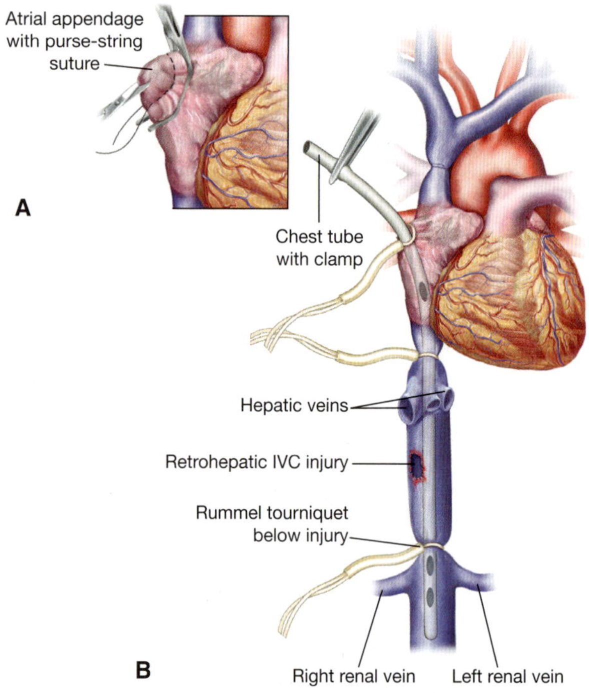

FIGURE 26 • Atriocaval shunt for retrohepatic inferior vena cava injuries.

- The hepatic flexure is taken down and the duodenum medialized. A Pringle maneuver and clamping with a Rummel tourniquet can temporize bleeding from injuries toward the liver.
- Depending on whether the injury is on the left or right, a medial visceral rotation can improve visualization of the superior mesenteric artery and vein. Destructive injuries to either can cause massive small bowel ischemia with overall increased morbidity and mortality. Restoration of flow should be attempted, either with primary repair, patch angioplasty, or interposition graft.

PEARLS AND PITFALLS

Zone I—Abdominal	■ The aorta can be occluded by a clamp or by endovascular approach. Take note of the ischemic time, particularly if above the mesenteric or renal vessels. ■ Consider using a shunt (large Argyle or thoracostomy tube) in damage control situations. ■ Avoid the use of synthetic grafts in cases with massive contamination due to the risk of graft infection and pseudoaneurysm. If a graft is used, consider rifampin-soaked grafts after a thorough wash-out and cover with peritoneum to exclude from the abdomen.
Zone I—Inferior vena cava and initial hemorrhage control	■ In cases with massive contamination, and injuries requiring resection that cannot be brought together without tension, a synthetic graft is usually discouraged due to the risk of seeding and infection. Autologous graft (internal jugular vein, saphenous vein) and bovine pericardium may be used. ■ Infrarenal inferior vena cava injuries: The infrarenal vena cava can be ligated but may cause massive swelling of the extremities, warranting prophylactic bilateral lower extremity fasciotomies. Avoid narrowing the inferior vena cava >40% due to the risk of venous thromboembolism. ■ Suprarenal inferior vena cava injuries: One may consider using a large shunt (thoracostomy tube) in a damage control situation and returning for definitive repair with synthetic graft.

POSTOPERATIVE CARE

Zone I—Abdominal

- Patients after aortic repair should be followed with serial abdominal, neurovascular examinations, and laboratory studies as CBC, chemistry, and lactate. Patients with prolonged ischemic time, massive transfusion, and hypotension are at risk for mesenteric ischemia and renal failure.
- Systematic heparinization is typically not necessary given the large diameter and high-pressure state.
- Damage control surgery and resuscitation should be considered in patients in hemorrhagic shock requiring massive transfusion with subsequent acidosis, hypothermia, and coagulopathy. A second look within 24 hours is warranted to evaluate for ischemic bowel.

Zone I—Inferior Vena Cava and Initial Hemorrhage Control

- All patients are at risk for venous thromboembolism and should be on chemoprophylaxis. Patients who undergo repair with narrowing are also at risk for pulmonary embolus. Both lower extremities should be wrapped and elevated to decrease swelling.
- Patients are at risk for mesenteric ischemia from prolonged clamp time, hypotension, and possible venous congestion and should be followed with serial exams, complete blood county (including WBC), and lactate.

COMPLICATIONS

Zone I—Abdominal

- Graft infection: Patients presenting with concomitant bowel injury and vascular injuries requiring bypass are at risk for graft infection. Synthetic grafts typically carry a higher risk of infection compared to autologous tissue. Any signs of infection, flank pain, change in neurovascular status, or change in hemoglobin should prompt a computed tomography angiography (CTA) to evaluate for graft infection.
- Thrombosis: thrombosis of an arterial graft is rare but may be related to kinking, compression, dissection, infection, or hematologic disorders. CTA should be performed to evaluate for these complications and systemic anticoagulation initiated while planning next steps for revision, endovascular approach for thrombectomy, etc.
- Mesenteric ischemia: Patients may develop ischemia in watershed areas, develop lower gastrointestinal bleeds, or pain from ischemia. Early endoscopy is critical to diagnosis and treatment.
- Pseudoaneurysm: Be suspicious for pseudoaneurysm in the setting of back pain, bleeding, or change in vascular exam and image with CTA. Treatment will likely require endovascular treatment with stenting and coil embolization.

Zone I—Inferior Vena Cava and Initial Hemorrhage Control

- Complications of inferior vena cava injuries relate to drainage of the venous system, including thromboembolism and compartment syndrome.
- Surgeons should maintain a low threshold to perform fasciotomies in the presence of pain out of proportion and swelling. Loss of pulses and neurologic changes are very late signs of ischemia.
- Patients with suprarenal inferior vena cava injuries are at risk for acute renal injury and failure from hypotension and possible thrombus secondary to occluded inflow; thus, it is important to monitor urine output and creatinine.

REFERENCES

1. Kobayashi LM, Costantini TW, Hamel MG, Dierksheide JE, Coimbra R. Abdominal vascular trauma. *Trauma Surg Acute Care Open*. 2016;1(1):e000015.
2. Ferrada P, Callcut RA, Skarupa DJ, et al. Circulation first – the time has come to question the sequencing of care in the ABCs of trauma; an American Association for the Surgery of Trauma multicenter trial. *World J Emerg Surg*. 2018;13:8.
3. Rozycki GS, Ochsner MG, Feliciano DV, et al. Early detection of hemoperitoneum by ultrasound examination of the right upper quadrant: a multicenter study. *J Trauma*. 1998;45(5):878-883.
4. Stannard A, Eliason JL, Rasmussen TE. Resuscitative endovascular balloon occlusion of the aorta (REBOA) as an adjunct for hemorrhagic shock. *J Trauma*. 2011;71(6):1869-1872.
5. DuBose JJ, Scalea TM, Brenner M, et al. The AAST prospective Aortic Occlusion for Resuscitation in Trauma and Acute Care Surgery (AORTA) registry: data on contemporary utilization and outcomes of aortic occlusion and resuscitative balloon occlusion of the aorta (REBOA). *J Trauma Acute Care Surg*. 2016;81(3):409-419.
6. Byerly S, Cheng V, Plotkin A, Matsushima K, Inaba K, Magee GA. Impact of inferior vena cava ligation on mortality in trauma patients. *J Vasc Surg Venous Lymphat Disord*. 2019;7(6):793-800.

Chapter 47 Abdominal Vascular Injury Zone II

Melike N. Harfouche and David T. Efron

DEFINITION

- An abdominal vascular injury is defined as any injury to abdominal vascular structures located primarily in the retroperitoneal space. They are traditionally separated into three zones—I, II, and III. Zone I refers to the midline retroperitoneal vessels—the aorta and the inferior vena cava (IVC). Zone II refers to the lateral, upper retroperitoneal vessels, namely, the renal hilar vessels, and zone III refers to the pelvic vessels—the iliac artery and vein and their branches.

DIFFERENTIAL DIAGNOSIS

- Patients with abdominal vascular injury can have several concomitant injuries, depending on the mechanism. Abdominal vascular injuries from a blunt mechanism are very rare and can present more insidiously if the vascular injury is limited to the intima or contained by surrounding structures. In these cases, associated solid organ injuries affecting the liver, spleen, and/or kidney can also result in significant hemorrhage and may be the primary indication for operative intervention. Penetrating trauma more commonly results in abdominal vascular injury, with an acutely bleeding patient in hemorrhagic shock. In these cases, associated hollow viscus injuries are common, but the primary aim of operative intervention is expedient hemorrhage control.

PATIENT HISTORY AND PHYSICAL FINDINGS

- Patients with abdominal vascular injuries often present with hypotension and tachycardia, although this may not be present if the injury is incomplete, a clot has formed overlying the injury, or tamponade has been provided by surrounding structures; the absence of abnormal vital signs does not rule out abdominal vascular injury.
- A distended abdomen can also indicate retroperitoneal vascular injury, although this finding has a wide differential diagnosis in the setting of penetrating abdominal trauma.
- Injuries to the renal hilar structures often involve the collecting duct and/or the renal parenchyma, which can be seen as hematuria upon Foley insertion.

IMAGING AND OTHER DIAGNOSTIC STUDIES

- A foreign body series should be obtained in the trauma bay for all patients with penetrating injuries. The portable x-rays should include skin and soft tissue borders to ensure that all ballistic fragments are identified, and usually extend from the chest down to the pelvis. Defining the trajectory of penetrating wounds early in the trauma assessment is key to identifying potential injuries.
- A Focused Assessment with Sonography in Trauma (FAST) examination should be performed in all patients with blunt mechanism of injury and hemodynamic instability; it can be performed selectively in other groups (penetrating trauma, normal vital signs).
- A positive abdominal FAST is usually absent in isolated zone II injuries but may be seen if intraperitoneal structures are bleeding or the retroperitoneal hematoma is no longer contained within the retroperitoneum.
- Patients with stable vital signs without other indications for laparotomy (peritonitis, evisceration, clear intraperitoneal trajectory) should proceed to computed tomography (CT) of the abdomen and pelvis with intravenous contrast. Rectal contrast can be administered to increase detection of retroperitoneal colon injuries. Images should include both an arterial and venous phase to allow for identification of venous injuries and to distinguish the presence of pseudoaneurysms from active arterial extravasation. A 5-minute delayed phase can also be obtained to identify collecting duct and ureteral injuries.

SURGICAL MANAGEMENT

- In general, all patients with penetrating zone II abdominal vascular injury should undergo operative exploration. However, patients with stable vital signs who undergo CT scan demonstrating grades I to IV renal parenchymal injury can undergo selective nonoperative management (SNOM) based on clinician discretion.[1]
- Patients with blunt zone II abdominal vascular injuries identified on CT scan can be observed if they are hemodynamically stable. If a zone II injury is identified at the time of laparotomy, operative exploration of the retroperitoneum is indicated in the setting of hemodynamic instability and/or an expanding perinephric hematoma.
- Hemodynamically stable individuals with renal injury who undergo SNOM can be managed with angioembolization in cases where active bleeding is identified, and long-term complications of urinoma and/or urine leak can be managed with percutaneous drainage and/or ureteral stent placement.[2]

Preoperative Planning

- It is imperative to communicate with the OR staff regarding the planned procedure to ensure all necessary equipment is available.
- Patients presenting with signs of shock should have a massive transfusion protocol initiated, with blood product available in the operating room. Cell saver should be requested in settings where significant blood loss is anticipated.

Positioning

- Patients should be positioned supine, with both arms extended away from the body at 90°. This allows access to the chest cavity if necessary.

SETUP

- Skin preparation should extend from the chin to the knees, and down toward the operating table laterally. This ensures that additional procedures, if required, can be performed without breaking sterility.

INCISION

- The skin incision for all emergent trauma laparotomies should be generous, extending from below the xyphoid to the pubis.

EXPOSURE OF ZONE II

- Once the decision has been made to explore a zone II abdominal vascular injury, the first step consists of medial mobilization of the colon.
- On the right, medial mobilization of the colon should be initiated by identifying the avascular plane tethering the cecum to the retroperitoneum known as the white line of Toldt (**FIGURE 1**). Once this plane is entered, it can be extended cephalad along the right retroperitoneum toward the hepatic flexure of the colon. It is important to remain close to the colon during this dissection to prevent inadvertent injury to the ureter (**FIGURE 2**). As one extends toward the hepatic flexure, the retroperitoneal portions of the duodenum course very closely to the ascending colon and should be protected by ensuring the surgeons fingers dissect immediately posterior to the border of the colon (**FIGURE 3**).
- Immediately posterior to the duodenum lies the infrahepatic portion of the IVC and further cephalad the right renal vein can be identified (**FIGURE 4**). The kidney lies within Gerota fascia and can be challenging to fully expose due to its retrohepatic location (**FIGURE 5**).
- On the left, medial mobilization of the colon is similarly initiated at the left paracolic gutter by entering the avascular plane along the line of Toldt and extended cephalad, taking care to protect the ureter. The left kidney lies considerably lower than on the right, making it easier to expose (**FIGURE 6**).

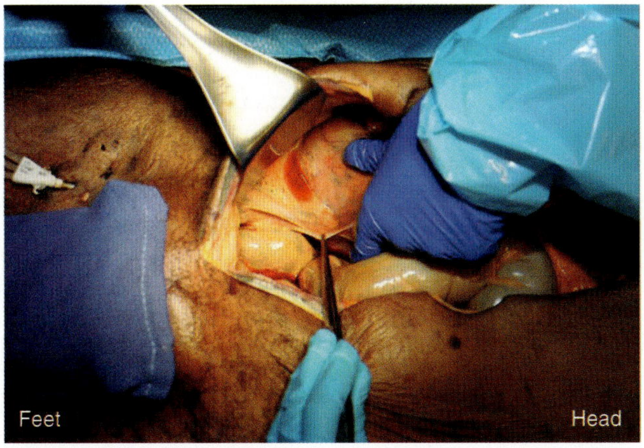

FIGURE 1 • Line of Toldt to begin colon mobilization for access to the kidney in the retroperitoneum.

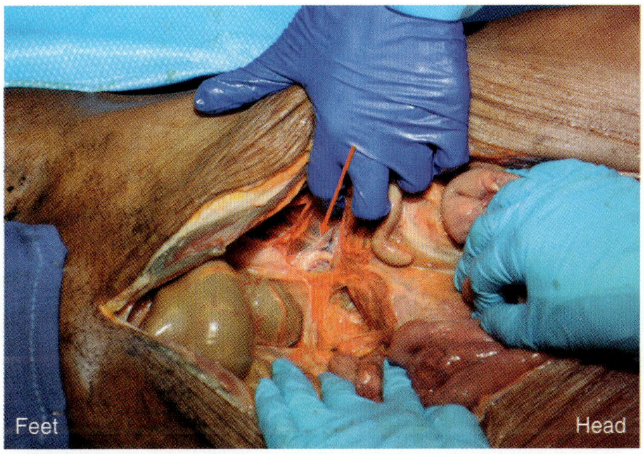

FIGURE 2 • With the cecum retracted superiorly the ureter is identified in the retroperitoneum as it crosses the iliac vessels. *Red arrow* = ureter.

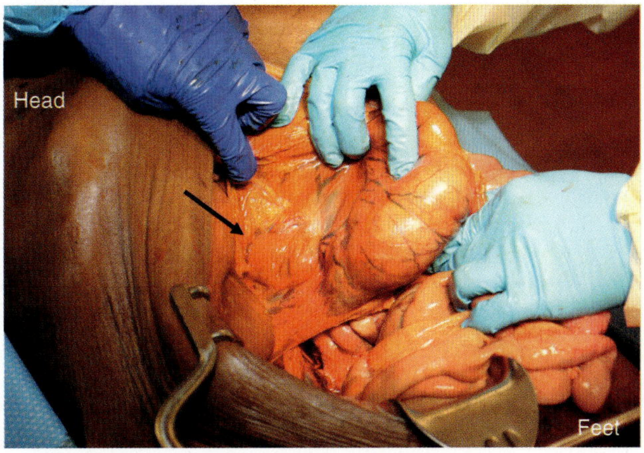

FIGURE 3 • The retroperitoneal portions of the duodenum course very closely to the posterior border of the colon and should be protected. *Black arrow* = duodenum.

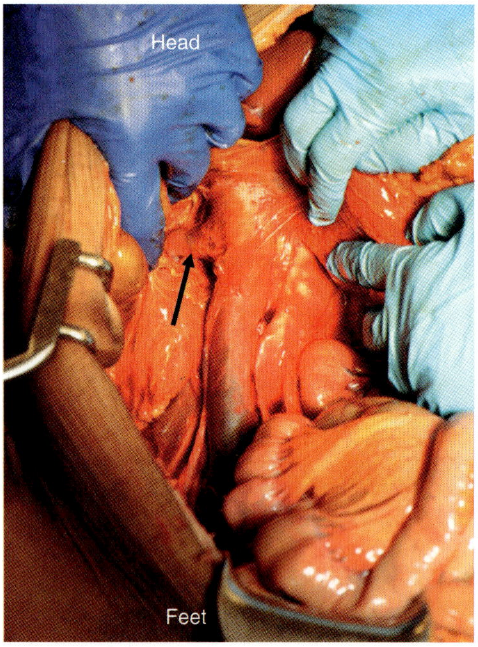

FIGURE 4 • Further cephalad dissection along the inferior vena cava will reveal the right renal vein (*black arrow*). The kidney itself is obscured by the right lobe of the liver.

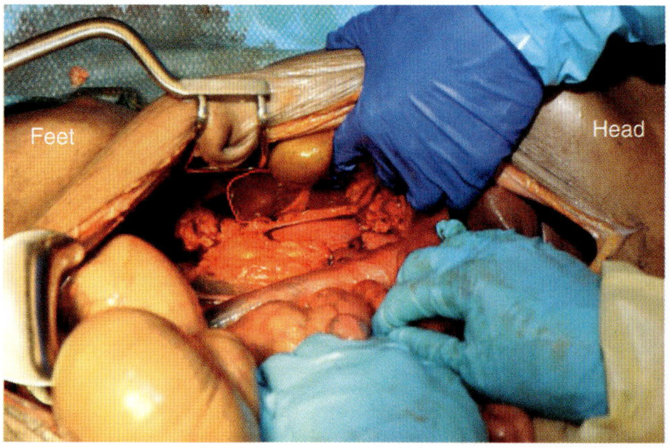

FIGURE 5 • Right kidney visible within Gerota fascia rests underneath the right lobe of the liver (*red outline*).

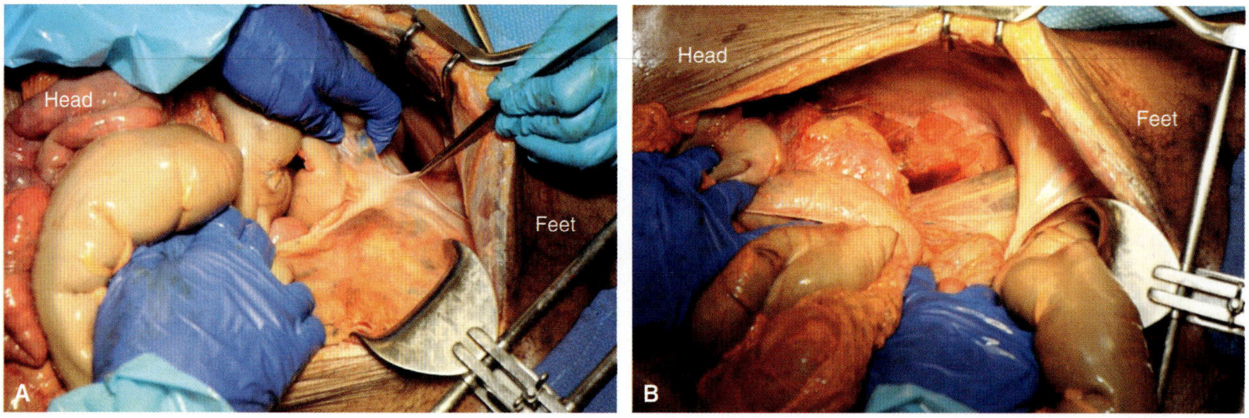

FIGURE 6 • Mobilization of the line of Toldt **(A)** along the left paracolic gutter reveals the left kidney **(B)**, which sits considerably lower than the right kidney.

MANAGEMENT OF RENAL HILAR INJURY

- Exploration of zone II injuries often results in nephrectomy, which is most expediently performed by medial mobilization of the kidney to the midline, followed by hilar control. Experienced surgeons may prefer to obtain hilar control first prior to mobilization of the kidney at the risk of prolonging operative time.[3]
- Once the kidney is elevated and mobilized to the midline, the renal artery and vein can be identified and individually ligated. In a damage control setting, they can be ligated en bloc, with a low risk of long-term development of arteriovenous fistulae. As shown in **FIGURE 7**, several variants of renal hilar vasculature can exist with paired veins and/or paired arteries. The ureter can be traced to the pelvic brim and ligated to reduce the likelihood of development of urothelial cancer, although this is not necessary.

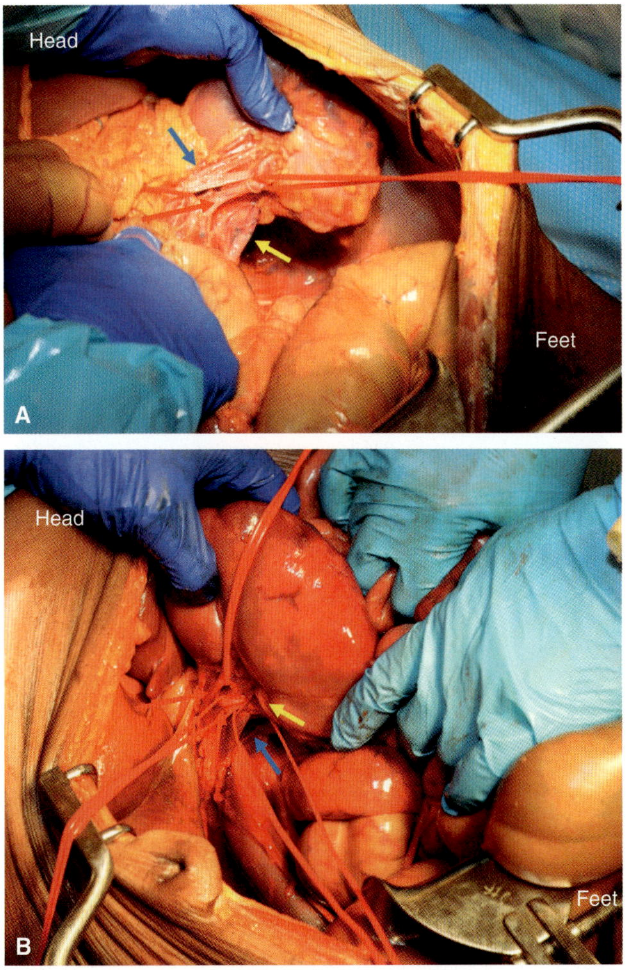

FIGURE 7 • Hilar control of renal vessels of the left kidney from an anterior view **(A)** and right kidney from a posterior view **(B)**. *Red arrows* point to the renal arteries, blue arrows point to the renal veins, and yellow arrows point to the ureters.

PEARLS AND PITFALLS

Partial nephrectomy	▪ Partial nephrectomy should only be performed in the hemodynamically stable patient with an isolated injury to upper or lower pole of the kidney; most zone II injuries mandating operative intervention will result in nephrectomy.
Contralateral kidney	▪ Palpation of the contralateral kidney prior to proceeding with nephrectomy can be performed to determine if renal salvage should be attempted; in cases of damage control surgery (DCS), the absence of a contralateral kidney should not preclude life-saving procedures such as nephrectomy.
Endovascular approach	▪ In hemodynamically stable patients with blunt renal trauma, an endovascular approach can be utilized for repair of intimal injuries to the renal artery to prevent development of renal ischemia and infarction.

POSTOPERATIVE CARE

- Patients should be monitored closely for evidence of ongoing bleeding or missed injuries, as right renal hilar injuries are also associated with pancreatic and duodenal injuries. Missed injuries often present in the first 24 hours with worsening hypotension, fever, and signs of peritonitis.
- DCS can be performed if patients have had massive blood loss, with evidence of coagulopathy (INR > 2), acidosis (pH < 7.2), or hypothermia (T < 34 °C). During DCS, an abbreviated surgery aims to control bleeding and hollow viscus injury, followed by temporary abdominal closure and planned return to the operating room in 48 to 72 hours.

COMPLICATIONS

- Urine leaks/urinomas can be managed effectively with percutaneous drainage.
- Endovascular coil embolization or deployment of a covered stent can be performed to treat the development of arteriovenous fistulae between the renal artery and vein.
- The risk of delayed bleeding and/or abscess formation increases with the presence of hollow viscus or pancreatic injury. In these cases, pancreatic injuries should be well drained and bowel anastomoses should be isolated from renal hilar vascular structures.

REFERENCES

1. Schellenberg M, Benjamin E, Piccinini A, Inaba K, Demetriades D. Selective nonoperative management of renal gunshot wounds. *J Trauma Acute Care Surg*. 2019;87(6):1301-1307.
2. Keihani S, Xu Y, Presson AP, et al. Contemporary management of high-grade renal trauma: results from the American association for the surgery of trauma genitourinary trauma study. *J Trauma Acute Care Surg*. 2018;84(3):418-425.
3. Gonzalez RP, Falimirski M, Holevar MR, Evankovich C. Surgical management of renal trauma: is vascular control necessary? *J Trauma*. 1999;47(6):1039-1042; discussion 1042-1044.

Chapter 48 Abdominal Vascular Injury Zone III

Elizabeth Dauer and Abhijit S. Pathak

DEFINITIONS

- Zone III of the retroperitoneum extends from the bifurcation of the aorta and confluence of the inferior vena cava to the level of the inguinal ligament and pelvic floor.
- The vascular structures in zone III are (**FIGURE 1**):
  - Common iliac artery and vein
  - External iliac artery and vein
  - Internal iliac artery and vein and its branches
  - Sacral venous plexus
  - Distal portions of the gonadal vessels

DIFFERENTIAL DIAGNOSIS

- Injuries to the vascular structures in zone III that require surgical management are most often associated with penetrating injuries, with missile injuries being the most common and outnumbering stab wounds. Blunt mechanisms and crush injuries of the pelvis are less common. These injuries are usually identified during exploration of the abdomen and present as retroperitoneal hematomas in zone III, which may or may not be contained. They are commonly associated with other visceral injuries including the ureter, bladder,

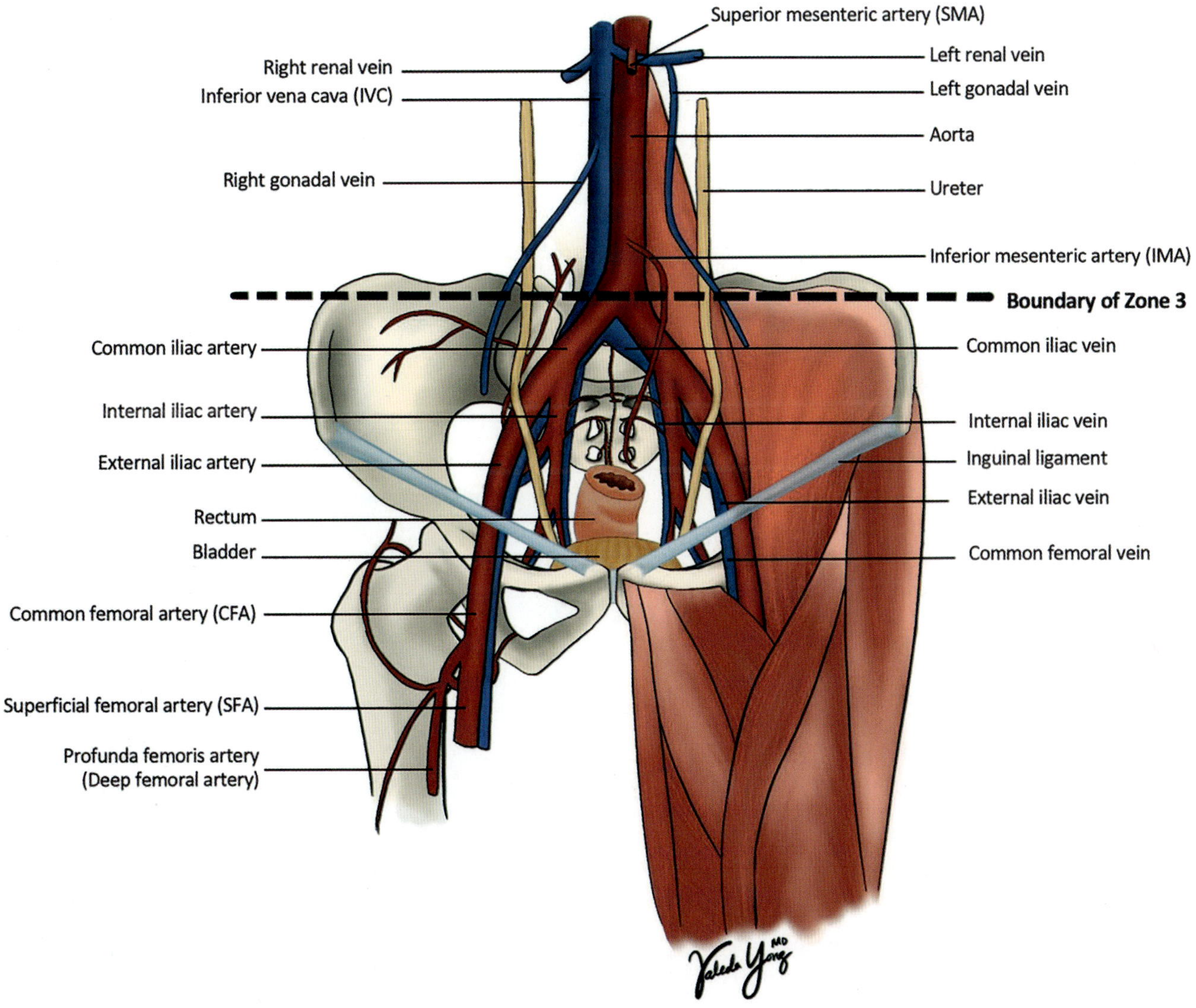

FIGURE 1 • Vascular structures of zone III. (Courtesy of Valeda Yong, MD.)

rectum, small bowel, and colon. Furthermore, a diagnosis of zone III vascular injuries preoperatively requires a high index of suspicion based on the evaluation of the patient and the mechanism of injury. For instance, a gunshot wound to the abdomen or pelvic region with transpelvic trajectory as determined by clinical examination and plain radiographs along with hypotension may signify an iliac vascular injury.

PATIENT HISTORY AND PHYSICAL FINDINGS

- The patient history and physical examination may be limited depending on the severity of injury, the mechanism, and other associated injuries. The history should be focused on the mechanism of injury, forces that may have been applied due to that mechanism, and areas of perceived pain. Blunt mechanisms that should raise concern for bleeding from structures in zone III are those that are associated with high-energy forces and the development of pelvic fractures. These include fall from a significant height, pedestrian struck, high-speed motor vehicle collisions, and significant crush injury to the pelvic region. In penetrating trauma, zone III vascular injuries are considered when the estimated trajectory takes a course through the lower abdomen and pelvic region.
- Physical examination findings include:
  - Evidence of hemorrhagic shock: tachycardia, hypotension, poor distal perfusion, widened pulse pressure, altered mental status
  - Pulse discrepancy on palpation of the femoral pulses
  - Lack of dorsalis pedis or posterior tibial pulse or Doppler signals with concern for intracavitary injury
  - Abdominal tenderness or peritoneal signs on abdominal examination
  - Concerning penetrating injury trajectory
  - Significant bleeding from a penetrating wound
  - Pelvic instability or pelvic fracture on imaging
  - Scrotal/perineal hematoma

IMAGING AND OTHER DIAGNOSTIC STUDIES

- The focused assessment with sonography in trauma (FAST) examination may provide evidence of intra-abdominal or pelvic hemorrhage that can occur with zone III vascular injuries. The patients may have a positive FAST examination in the pelvis, right upper quadrant, or left upper quadrant views with zone III injuries; however, a negative FAST does not preclude injury. In a systemic review of randomized controlled trials from 1965 through 2009, Quinn et al found that FAST examination had a high specificity (94%-100%) and low sensitivity (28%-100%) in determining intra-abdominal hemorrhage after penetrating torso trauma. They concluded that a positive FAST examination should prompt exploratory laparotomy but a negative FAST examination should prompt further investigation through available diagnostic modalities.[1]
- The presence of a pelvic fracture on pelvic radiograph may suggest bleeding in the area of zone III, particularly if an open book pelvic fracture exists. Also, pelvic radiographs may give insight to missile trajectory in penetrating trauma, and if both a lateral and anteroposterior view of the pelvis is obtained, cavitary violation may be able to be excluded based on the location of the wounds and any retained foreign bodies.
- Computed tomography (CT) scan can be used to assess for zone III injury in patients who are hemodynamically acceptable to undergo CT scan imaging. CT scan can provide valuable diagnostic information with regards to vessel injury, areas of active hemorrhage, penetrating trajectory, and associated injuries. Active contrast extravasation on CT scan has been shown to be the most reliable indicator of significant arterial bleeding identified on subsequent angiography and can provide a roadmap for interventional radiologist to more accurately and expeditiously localize the site of bleeding.[2]
- Angiography can serve as both a diagnostic and therapeutic imaging modality. It can assess for ongoing arterial bleeding, pseudoaneurysm formation, or abrupt vessel cutoff, which is indicative of potential vessel injury. Angiographic embolization is a safe and effective tool for control of hemorrhage in surgically difficult areas such as deep in the pelvis (**FIGURES 2-4**).[3]

SURGICAL MANAGEMENT

- In patients with blunt trauma and potential pelvic bleeding, the decision for operative intervention may not always be clear. The patient's hemodynamics and other associated injuries must be taken into consideration when deciding how to proceed after the initial trauma assessment. In addition, simultaneous management of associated injuries, such as pelvic fractures, may be indicated in order to stabilize the patient.
- In the case of complex pelvic ring injuries with widening of the pubic symphysis, placement of a pelvic binder to decrease the volume of the pelvis may assist in creating tamponade for pelvic bleeding. It is imperative that these devices be placed correctly, in order to approximate the pubic symphysis without causing widening of the posterior elements of the pelvis. A sheet or a commercially available pelvic binder

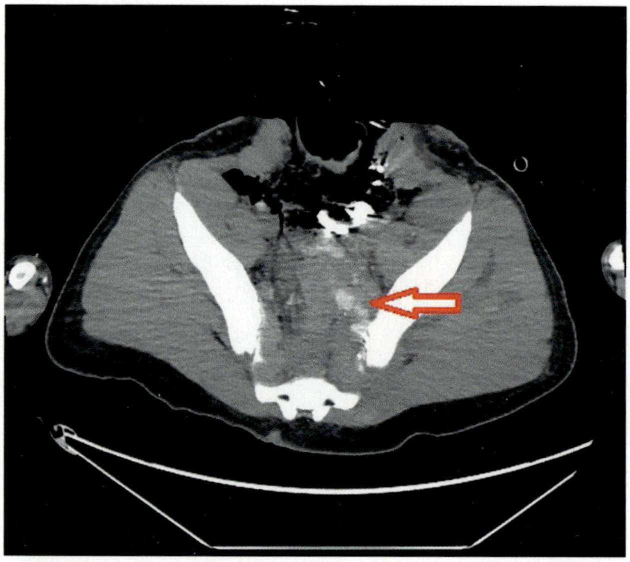

FIGURE 2 • Postoperative computed tomography angiography demonstrates contrast blush from distal left internal iliac artery branches (*arrow*).

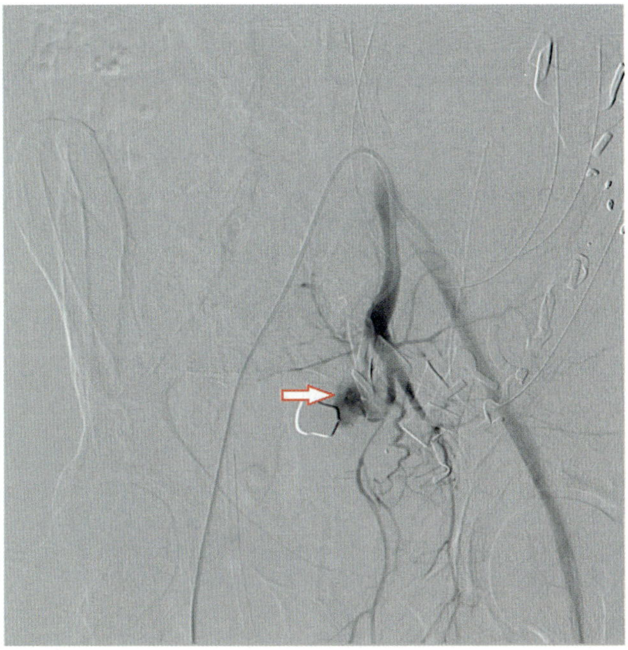

FIGURE 3 • Angiogram demonstrates injury with blush/pseudoaneurysm from distal left internal iliac artery branches (*arrow*).

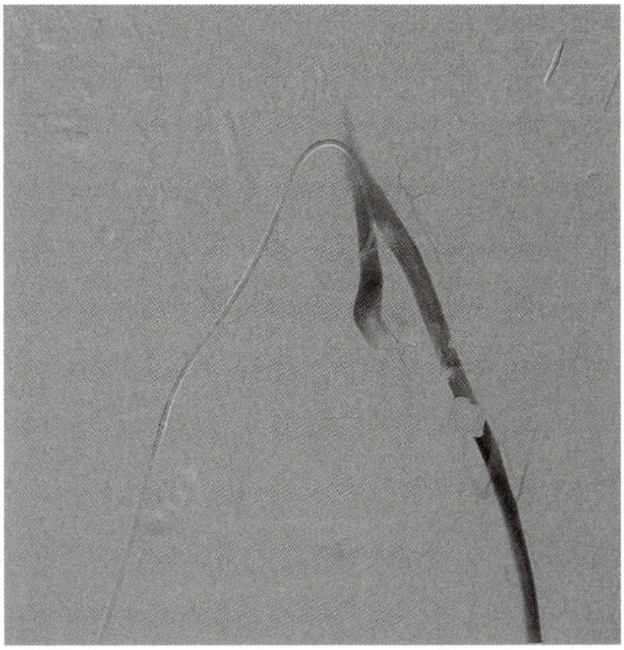

FIGURE 4 • Gelfoam embolization of the distal left internal iliac artery performed with cessation of flow into the distal injured branch.

may be used to accomplish this task and should be placed at the level of the greater trochanters of the femurs to allow for proper reapproximation of the pubic symphysis. Blunt iliac artery injuries associated with pelvic fractures are rare; however, when they do occur they have a high complication and mortality rate.[4]

TECHNIQUES

- In blunt trauma, injury to the large pelvic vessels, including the common iliac artery and external iliac artery are rare but can range from small intimal irregularities to complete transection. These injuries are associated with severe pelvic fractures, hypotension, genitourinary injury, and bowel injury and have a high overall risk of morbidity and mortality.[4]
- When proceeding to the operating room for suspected zone III vascular injury, the patient should be placed supine on the operating room table in order to allow access to both the abdomen and thighs in the event it is necessary to gain vascular control at the level of the femoral vessels or if greater saphenous vein needs to be harvested to use as a conduit in the management of a vascular injury.
- A generous midline laparotomy incision should be used and taken caudally to the level of the pubic symphysis in order to provide the widest exposure of the pelvic structures as possible. The abdomen is packed tightly to allow for tamponade of bleeding, for placement of the self-retaining retractor for exposure, and for the anesthesiologists to properly resuscitate the patient prior to opening any retroperitoneal hematomas that may result in copious hemorrhage.
- In penetrating trauma, injury to the vascular structures of zone III must be in the differential diagnosis for every patient with a trajectory that enters the lower abdomen and pelvis. All zone III hematomas from penetrating injury obligate exploration for a source of hemorrhage, whereas, in blunt trauma, the presence of a zone III hematoma does not mandate exploration, as up to 85% of pelvic bleeding is venous.[5] Exploration of a zone III hematoma in blunt trauma risks release of tamponade and exsanguinating hemorrhage from the pelvic venous plexus. In the absence of significant ongoing major arterial injury, these injuries are better treated with a combination of preperitoneal packing, angiographic embolization, and pelvic stabilization. When major vascular injury is suspected, the basic tenets of vascular surgery with obtaining proximal and distal control should be followed to limit hemorrhage and to provide appropriate exposure of the injury.
- Based on trajectory and location of the zone III hematoma, the approximate level of the injury should be able to be estimated to help the surgeon determine where to gain control of the vasculature. If bleeding is significant and precluding identification of the structures, sponge sticks placed both proximally and distally or direct manual compression can be used to control bleeding and improve visibility in order to gain proximal and distal control of the vessels.
- To gain proximal control, a right medial visceral rotation (see **FIGURE 5**) is performed to expose the aorta and inferior vena cava at the level of the aortic bifurcation. This maneuver ensures the ability to isolate the arterial and venous structures at their most cranial extent, if necessary. If there is significant ongoing bleeding, the aorta can then be compressed or a vascular clamp applied at this level to greatly diminish inflow to the area. Also, the right medial visceral rotation

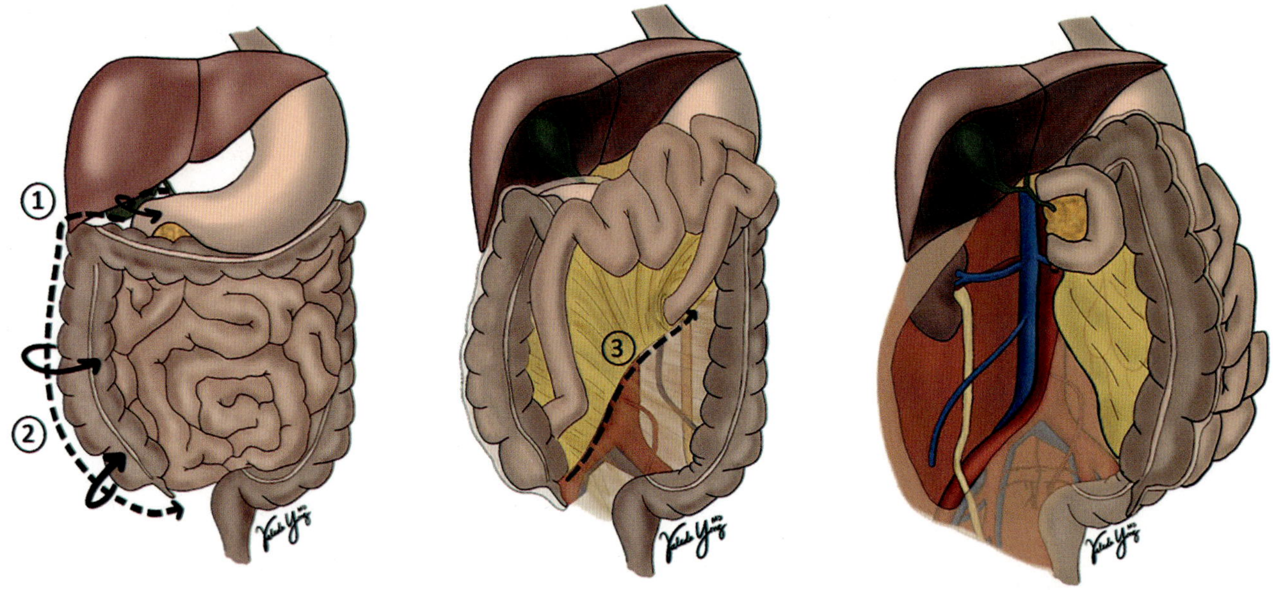

FIGURE 5 • Right-sided medial visceral rotation (Cattell-Braasch-Kocher maneuvers). This maneuver involves mobilization of the right colon including the hepatic flexure (Cattell)[2] and mobilization of the small bowel (Braasch)[3] along the avascular plane between the small bowel mesentery and the posterior peritoneum. This will allow access to the subhepatic inferior vena cava and aorta, to the entirety of the right iliac vessels and the proximal left iliac vessels. (Courtesy of Valeda Yong, MD.)

provides optimal exposure for the right-sided iliac vessels. The most proximal portion of the left-sided iliac vessels can be accomplished in this way; however, the bifurcation of the left common iliac vessels is covered by the sigmoid and descending colon mesentery. To expose this area, the left colon and sigmoid colon should be released from its lateral attachments to the abdominal wall and be reflected medially to expose the left iliac vessels all the way to the level of the inguinal ligament. Depending on the assumed level of the injury, a vessel loop can be placed to encircle both the artery and vein or, alternatively, a vascular clamp applied on the side of injury at this time. Gaining control of the common iliac vein can prove to be challenging as it sits posterior to the common iliac artery on the right and posterior and medial to the common iliac artery on the left. It may be necessary to transect the right common iliac artery in order to gain access to a right common iliac vein injury, although this is rarely needed and, if performed, will necessitate reconstruction or placement of a temporary vascular shunt in order to ensure distal flow. In addition, it may be necessary to gain control of the internal iliac artery and internal iliac vein. The takeoff of the internal iliac artery and vein usually occurs at the level of the fourth lumbar vertebra, and the vessels course posteromedial and inferior to supply the pelvic structures. the internal iliac artery and vein can be ligated to control hemorrhage or to facilitate repair of the common or external iliac vessels if the injury spans the bifurcation of the common iliac artery and the confluence of the internal and external iliac veins. If this is done, the patient should be carefully monitored for the development of gluteal compartment syndrome on the effected side. If bilateral internal iliac vessels are ligated, the patient can develop ischemia or necrosis to the pelvic structures.

- To gain distal control, the external iliac artery and vein can be encircled below the suspected level of injury. For injuries occurring just before or at the level of the inguinal ligament, a counter incision can be made in the groin to isolate the common femoral artery and vein to gain distal control. The inguinal ligament can be divided to expose injuries at the level of the inguinal ligament. The most distal extent of the external iliac artery and vein and the most cranial extent of the common femoral artery and vein give rise to the circumflex vessels, which may need to be ligated to limit ongoing back bleeding into the surgical field.
- Once vascular control has been obtained, the injury can be exposed in its entirety. The vessels should be inspected circumferentially to ensure identification of all injuries as well as the extent of the injury as blast effect can lead to a larger area of injury than first appreciated (**FIGURE 6**).
- Management of arterial injuries to the common iliac artery and external iliac artery is determined based on the extent of the injury, available conduits, and clinical stability of the patient. Injuries that involve less than 50% circumference of the vessel can be considered for primary repair if no evidence of intimal injury or blast injury exists. The wound edges should be debrided and closed transversely to avoid narrowing of the vessel, which may impede distal flow. For larger injuries, the vessels should be debrided back to healthy tissue with excision of the edges and can be repaired primarily in an end-to-end fashion provided there is not a significant defect in length (usually <1 cm) or tension. If there is a significant resultant segmental defect then using a graft to span the vessel defect will be necessary. An interposition graft using autologous vein using polypropylene suture is ideal; however, a polytetrafluoroethylene prosthetic conduit may be necessary if no suitable autologous vein using polypropylene suture is available. If able, the retroperitoneum should be closed over the graft to isolate it from the intra-abdominal contents. The placement of either autologous or

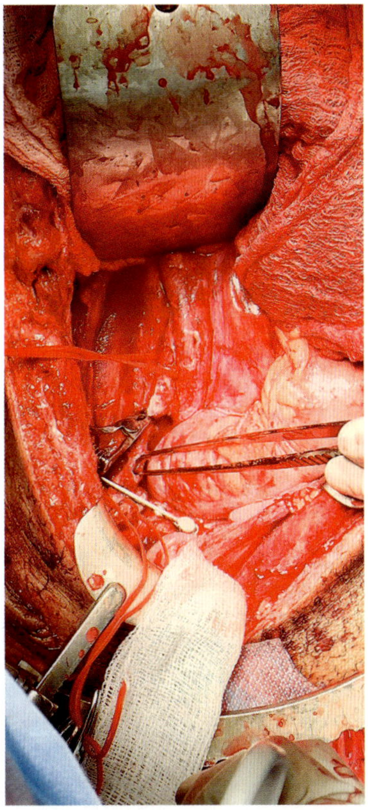

FIGURE 6 • Injury to the right external iliac artery with proximal control at the right common iliac artery and distal control at the right external iliac artery with vessel loops and vascular clamps used immediately proximal and distal to the injury.

prosthetic graft in a grossly infected field from spillage of bowel contents remains a serious problem due to concern for graft infection. Development of graft infection can lead to anastomotic pseudoaneurysm formation, recurrent bacteremia and sepsis, and even graft blowout, which can lead to life-threatening bleeding. Owing to these potential complications, some have advocated the use of iliac artery ligation with reconstruction using extra-anatomic bypass to restore flow to the lower extremity in extreme circumstances,[6] but this has not gained widespread acceptance.

- In damage control situations, the use of a temporary intravascular shunt (TIVS) can be used to restore flow and abbreviate operating room time to allow for resuscitation and rewarming in the intensive care unit. There are a large number of commercially available vascular shunts that can be used in this situation. The shunt chosen should be an appropriate size match for the vessel and should be adequately secured to prevent dislodgement. The use of TIVS in damage control situations is not related to increased shunt-related complications in comparison with nondamage control use, and there is no attributable mortality to the shunt procedure itself in reported series.[7,8]
- The use of systemic anticoagulation during these procedures remains controversial. In a multicenter retrospective review of 323 patients, Maher et al found that the use of systemic anticoagulation during the repair of major arterial injuries was associated with better arterial patency without an increase in bleeding complications.[9] The surgeon must weigh the risks of arterial clot formation with the risk of ongoing bleeding to determine the utility of intraoperative systemic anticoagulation in each clinical situation.
- Venous injuries to the iliac vessels can be managed via ligation or repair. When comparing ligation vs repair in patients with isolated iliac vein injuries, Magee et al. found that patients who underwent ligation had increased mortality in comparison with those who had repair; however, rates of venous thromboembolism, fasciotomy, amputation, and acute kidney injury were comparable.[10] Venous repair is a viable option in injuries that are small or easily approximated; however, it may not be feasible in destructive venous injuries or if the patient is in extremis and the injury needs to be managed expeditiously. Also, the surgeon must have the experience and surgical expertise in order to perform the repair. Different repair strategies have been used including simple lateral venorrhaphy, vein patch, and interposition grafts. When looking at venous repair patency, early patency rates are approximately 60% to 70% with less early extremity edema, but long-term extremity morbidity is similar.[11,12] Hence, complex venous repairs or reconstruction should be avoided.
- Once hemorrhage control has been achieved and the vascular injuries managed with either definitive repair or damage control techniques, the abdomen should be thoroughly inspected for other associated injuries. Care should be taken to identify the trajectory of penetrating injuries to allow for meticulous assessment of the structures within that path. Specific attention should be paid to evaluation of the ureters as they cross the external iliac vessels below the level of the iliac bifurcation.
- After the intra-abdominal injuries and other major associated injuries are managed, the need for adjunctive procedures should be determined. The risk of ischemia and reperfusion to the lower extremity after injury to the iliac vessels, particularly in the setting of hemodynamic instability and massive resuscitation, is of great concern. Performance of four-compartment lower extremity prophylactic fasciotomy in this setting should be considered, and the decision to proceed should be based on the injury complex, the patient's clinical status, existing evidence of compartment syndrome in the operating room, and ability to effectively monitor the patient in the postoperative setting for the development of compartment syndrome. Prophylactic thigh fasciotomy is rarely performed and should be considered on a case-to-case basis. Early fasciotomy and the judicious use of crystalloid resuscitation has been associated with a decrease in amputation rates after vascular injuries effecting the lower extremity.[13,14]
- Patients who require ligation of the internal iliac vasculature, especially if needed bilaterally, can develop gluteal compartment syndrome over time. Routine prophylactic gluteal fasciotomy is unwarranted, but serial gluteal compartment checks should be performed to assess the need for compartment release.

PEARLS AND PITFALLS

Patient presentation	■ Any patient presents with a penetrating mechanism to the abdomen and pelvic region with associated abdominal tenderness and hypotension should go to the operating room. Diagnostic imaging studies should only be undertaken in those patients who are hemodynamically acceptable without concern for intracavitary injury that would require operative intervention.
Preoperative planning	■ The patient should be prepped from the chin to both knees and from table to table on either side in order to access the chest, abdomen, and both proximal extremities. A midline incision extending from the xiphoid to the pubis is the most versatile in an unstable trauma patient in order to access all regions of the peritoneal cavity and retroperitoneum. An inadequate incision will lead to difficulty in exposure of the injuries and may prolong time to hemorrhage control.
Operative pearls	■ Once the peritoneal cavity is entered, remove clots and free blood and then pack the abdomen. Inspect all retroperitoneal zones. Properly identifying the presence of and location of a retroperitoneal hematoma will dictate the next steps in the conduct of the exploration. All zone III hematomas from a penetrating injury should be explored. Proximal control to the iliac vessels is obtained via a right medial visceral rotation. The sigmoid and left colon will need to be mobilized medially to access the left iliac vessels. If necessary, a groin incision or splitting of the inguinal ligament can be undertaken to obtain distal control. Use sponge sticks or manual pressure to control any hemorrhage until proximal and distal vascular control is achieved.
Hemodynamic stability	■ The patient's identified injuries and hemodynamic stability should dictate the management strategy at the time of the initial operative intervention. Injuries to the common or external iliac arteries should be repaired or managed via temporary intravascular shunt in damage control situations. Ligation of these vessels leads to ischemia distally and the need for above-knee amputation or hip disarticulation. Iliac vein injuries can be ligated to shorten operative time in damage control scenarios. Avoid complex venous repairs in these circumstances. Consider lower extremity fasciotomies, especially in patients with both arterial and venous injuries.

POSTOPERATIVE CARE

- The general postoperative care is similar to that of any trauma patient who has undergone an exploratory laparotomy or damage control laparotomy. They should be monitored for any signs of bleeding, as well as frequent vascular examinations of the lower extremities should be done to monitor for any change. If the patient has undergone damage control laparotomy and has a temporary shunt in place, it is crucial to monitor the lower extremity by vascular examination for any signs that the shunt may have thrombosed. In addition, patients should be monitored for the development of compartment syndrome of the gluteal region, thigh, and lower leg. Patients should return to the operating room (OR) for pack removal and definitive management of their injuries as well as abdominal closure once their metabolic failure has been corrected.

COMPLICATIONS

- Postoperative bleeding is a true concern with these injuries since it is not only the main iliac vessels that may be injured but also other smaller distal branches in the pelvis as well as the presacral venous plexus. These patients can continue to bleed even after definitive control and may mandate damage control with packing and temporary abdominal closure. Even with packing, these patients may continue to bleed especially in the setting of metabolic failure, which should be aggressively corrected. Despite this, these patients may require a return to the OR for hemorrhage control. Delayed hemorrhage with significant bleeding can occur and is usually associated with pelvic sepsis, many times when there is a concomitant bowel injury with a leak from a repair or anastomosis. This can result in an anastomotic failure of a vascular repair/graft with pseudoaneurysm formation or graft blow out. Many times, the first indication of this complication is a herald bleed with new blood present in intra-abdominal drains placed for intra-abdominal infection or from an unexplained drop in hemoglobin or hematocrit levels. Depending on the time period from the index operation, the subsequent management of the abdomen, and perceived risk for reoperation in a "hostile" pelvis, this can be managed with endovascular techniques or a combination of endovascular techniques and extra-anatomic bypass on a case-by-case basis (**FIGURES 7-9**).

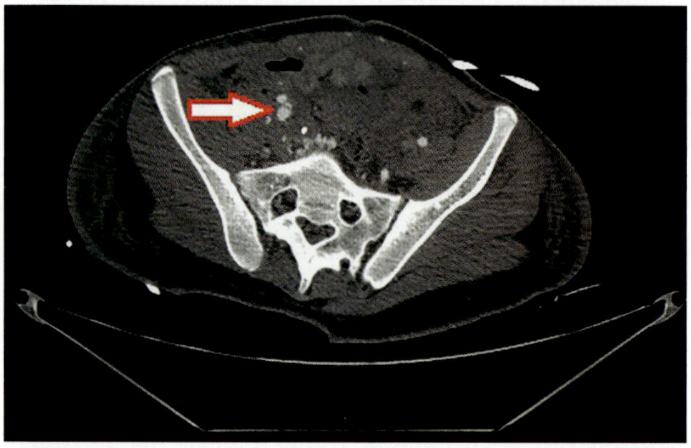

FIGURE 7 • Computed tomography angiography demonstrates pseudoaneurysm from the proximal right iliofemoral bypass graft (*arrow*).

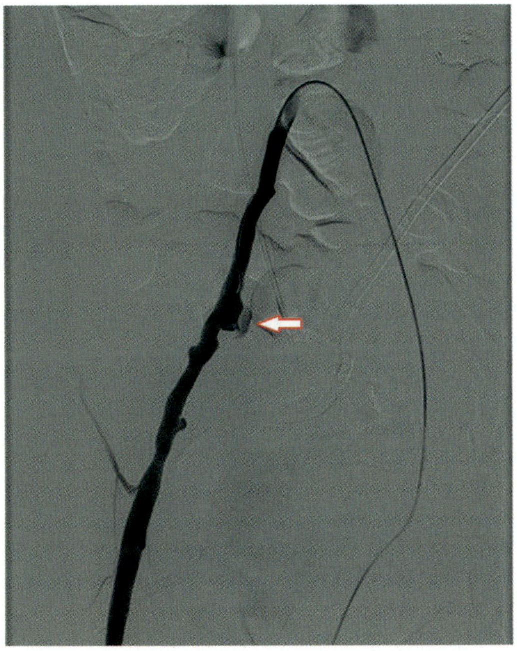

FIGURE 8 ● Angiogram demonstrates pseudoaneurysm from the proximal right iliofemoral bypass graft (*arrow*).

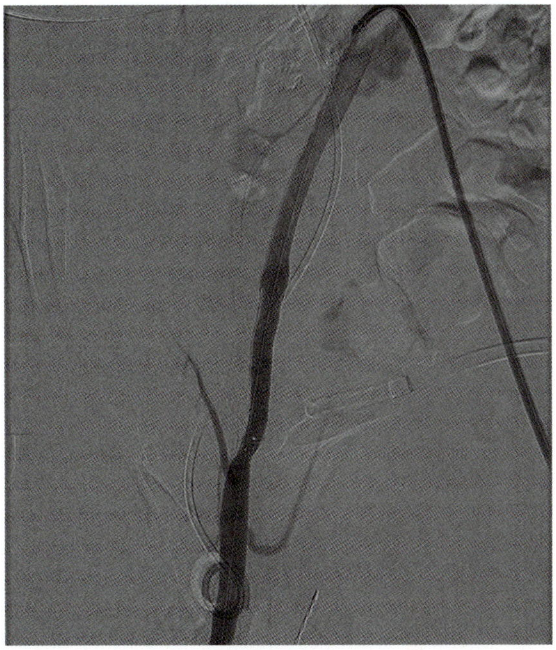

FIGURE 9 ● A covered endovascular stent was placed from the right common iliac artery to the right common femoral artery with resolution of the pseudoaneurysm.

- Patients may develop gluteal, thigh, or lower leg compartment syndrome, which is related to the ischemia and reperfusion injury to the affected extremity depending on the level of the vascular injury. If prophylactic fasciotomies had not been performed, one must be vigilant to monitor for its occurrence and proceed with early fasciotomy as indicated.
- Abdominal compartment syndrome can develop even in association with damage control surgery especially in the setting of intra-abdominal packing. There can be an accumulation of ascites, retroperitoneal edema, and/or blood and bowel edema, which can lead to increased intra-abdominal pressures. Patients should be monitored for intra-abdominal hypertension and development of abdominal compartment syndrome even in the setting of an "open" abdomen.
- Serial vascular examinations of the lower extremities after any repair or shunt are paramount. Any change in the examination may signify a concern for thrombosis. If there is any concern then prompt reexploration in the early operative period is the best chance for limb salvage. Delayed thrombosis can also occur and is usually associated with pelvic sepsis, many times due to a concomitant bowel injury with a leak from a repair or anastomosis. Depending on the time period from the index operation, the subsequent management of the abdomen, and perceived risk for reoperation in a "hostile" pelvis, this can be managed with endovascular techniques or a combination of endovascular techniques and extra-anatomic bypass on a case-by-case basis.

REFERENCES

1. Quinn AC, Sinert R. What is the utility of the Focused Assessment with Sonography in Trauma (FAST) exam in penetrating torso trauma? *Injury*. 2011;42(5):482-487.
2. Yoon W, Kim JK, Jeong YY, et al. Pelvic arterial hemorrhage in patients with pelvic fractures: detection with contrast-enhanced CT. *Radiographics*. 2004;24:1591-1605.
3. Velmahos G, Toutouzas K, Vassiliu P, et al. A prospective study on the safety and efficacy of angiographic embolization for pelvic and visceral injuries. *J Trauma*. 2002;53(2):303-308.
4. Cestero R, Plurad D, Green D, et al. Iliac artery injuries and pelvic fractures: a national trauma database analysis of associated injuries and outcomes. *J Trauma*. 2009;67(4):715-718.
5. Huittinen VM, Slatis P. Postmortem angiography and dissection of the hypogastric artery in pelvic fracatures. *Surgery*. 1973;73:454-462.
6. Feliciano D. Approach to major abdominal vascular injury. *J Vasc Surg*. 1988;7(5):730-736.
7. Tung L, Leonard J, Lawless R, et al. Temporary intravascular shunts after civilian arterial injury: a prospective multicenter Eastern Association for the Surgery of Trauma study. *Injury*. 2021;52(5):1204-1209.
8. Inaba K, Aksoy H, Seamon M, et al. Multicenter evaluation of temporary intravascular shunt use in vascular trauma. *J Trauma Acute Care Surg*. 2016;80(3):359-364.
9. Maher Z, Frank B, Salliant N, et al. Systemic intraoperative anticoagulation during arterial injury repair. *J Trauma Acute Care Surg*. 2017;82(4):680-686.
10. Magee G, Cho J, Matsushima K, et al. Isolated iliac vascular injuries and outcome of repair versus ligation of isolated iliac vein injury. *J Vasc Surg*. 2018;67(1):254-261.
11. Meyer J, Walsh J, Schuler J, et al. The early fate of venous repair after civilian vascular trauma. A clinical, hemodynamic, and venographic assessment. *Ann Surg*. 1987;206(4):458-464.
12. Agarwal N, Shah P, Clauss R, et al. Experience with 115 civilian venous injuries. *J Trauma*. 1982;22(10):827-832.
13. Farber A, Tan T, Hamburg N, et al. Early fasciotomy in patients with extremity vascular injury is associated with decreased risk of adverse limb outcomes: a review of the National Trauma Data Bank. *Injury*. 2012;43(9):1486-1491.
14. Dauer E, Yamaguchi S, Yu D, et al. Major venous injury and large volume crystalloid resuscitation: a limb threatening combination. *Am J Surg*. 202;219(1):38-42. doi:10.1016/j.injury.2011.06.006.

SECTION X: Vascular Injury: Extremities

Chapter 49 Lower Extremity Vascular Trauma—Femoral and Popliteal With Infrapopliteal Fasciotomy

Kelly M. Sutter and Christine T. Trankiem

DEFINITION

- Lower extremity trauma is defined as trauma to an extremity below the inguinal ligament. Specifically, this includes trauma to all vessels distal to the iliofemoral junction, including the common femoral artery, superficial femoral artery, femoral vein, greater saphenous vein, and tibial artery.

DIFFERENTIAL DIAGNOSIS

- When a patient presents with hemorrhage from the lower extremity or with a tourniquet in place, named blood vessels are frequently not the culprit of bleeding.
- Venous bleeding can be exacerbated secondary to tourniquet placement and resultant venous congestion.
- Muscular bleeding, particularly hematomas resulting from muscular injury, can raise concern for serious vascular trauma.
- Motor deficits and sensory changes, harbingers for acute limb ischemia or compartment syndrome, may result from direct traumatic injury to the nerve.
- Vasospasm can mimic arterial injury, especially on imaging.

PATIENT HISTORY AND PHYSICAL FINDINGS

Presentation

- Lower extremity vascular trauma can result from both blunt and penetrating trauma.
  - Penetrating trauma to a blood vessel can be more easily identifiable than blunt injury because of the penetration defect. However, given the sometimes unpredictable ballistic or stab trajectory, it is important to examine the patient completely.
    - Overall, penetrating lower extremity trauma is more common in military settings. The majority of proximal lower extremity vascular injuries are penetrating, whereas distal lower extremity trauma is equally associated with penetrating and blunt mechanisms.[1]
    - Blunt vascular injury may be more challenging to diagnose as a patient may present with a constellation of injuries in multiple anatomic regions.
    - A commonly missed musculoskeletal injury is posterior knee dislocation. This can be seen in patients whose knees strike the dashboard during a motor vehicle collision or who fall on their knee; this injury is often associated with popliteal artery injury.
    - Additional orthopedic injuries associated with lower extremity vascular injury are tibial plateau fracture (popliteal artery injury) and femoral shaft fracture (superficial femoral artery injury).

Exam Findings

- Vascular injuries are typically assessed with respect to HARD and SOFT signs.
  - Hard signs in penetrating trauma usually require emergent intervention, while soft signs can provide time for diagnostic tests.
    - Hard signs: Pulsatile bleeding, expanding hematoma, thrill at injury site, pulseless limb
    - The "6 Ps" seen in advanced acute limb ischemia or compartment syndrome also fall into this category—Pain, Pallor, Paresthesia, Paralysis, Pulseless, and Poikilothermia
  - Soft signs: bleeding in transit, unexplained hypotension, injury near a major vessel, nonexpanding hematoma, or nonpulsatile bleeding.
- Patients who are in shock should be taken to the operating room for exploration, irrespective of hard or soft signs of vascular injury.

IMAGING AND OTHER DIAGNOSTIC STUDIES

- In any patient with lower extremity trauma, whether it is penetrating or blunt (dislocation, fracture, or contusion), it is important to complete a thorough neurovascular exam of the affected extremity. Commonly, palpable pulses on exam are thought to obviate the need for further workup, but this can be misleading, especially in a healthy, hemodynamically normal patient.
- In vascular trauma, the management algorithms are often geared toward whether to proceed directly to operation or whether to image first. Imaging has been linked to delay in management, which in the case of limb ischemia can lead to tissue loss, compartment syndrome, or even limb loss. When appropriate, the following image modalities are recommended.

Ankle-Brachial Index

- Historically, the ankle-brachial index (ABI) was used to determine the necessity of angiography in occult vascular injuries; that is, vascular trauma without hard signs.
  - Current guidelines recommend that patients who meet this demographic should undergo computed tomography (CT) angiography if ABI <0.9. ABIs of <0.9 are 95% sensitive and 97% specific in diagnosing clinically significant vascular trauma.[2] There is increasing literature that supports lowering the ABI threshold to avoid unnecessary radiation in both blunt and penetrating trauma.[3]
  - In cases of unilateral extremity trauma, some institutions advocate the use of the ankle-ankle index (also known as the Injury Extremity Index), comparing the systolic blood pressure of the normal extremity to that of the affected limb; if the ankle-ankle ratio is <0.9, the patient is sent for CT angiography.

CT Angiography

- In its 2020 guidelines for evaluation of lower extremity trauma, the American Association for the Surgery of Trauma recommends CT angiography as the preferred modality in evaluating lower extremity vascular trauma as compared with conventional angiography.[4]
- CT scan is convenient in most large centers and is much less invasive than traditional angiography. CT angiography can be used to evaluate both the arterial and venous injuries. The former is used to identify active arterial bleeding by demonstrating active extravasation, disruption of arterial flow, and intimal dissection and flaps, and the latter to identify injury to large veins, hematomas, or other less brisk sources of bleeding.
- When a patient cannot tolerate obtaining an ABI due to pain, has a mangled extremity, or when there are multiple possible sources of vascular injury, we recommend forgoing the ABI and sending the patient straight to CT for angiography.
- CT can also help guide operative management of concomitant injuries.

Mangled Extremity Severity Score

- In 1990, Johansen et al introduced a scoring system to assist in the decision to amputate in patients with severe lower extremity injuries.[5] A mangled extremity is, by definition, an extremity with injury to a combination bone, soft tissue, nerves, or blood vessels.[6]
- High-energy trauma, shock, increased age, and advanced signs of limb ischemia have been associated with higher rates of amputation (see **TABLE 1**). Given the advances in vascular and orthopedic surgery and in imaging since 1990, there is new literature to support utilizing mangled extremity severity score (MESS) with caution. Importantly, Loja et al in the AAST PROOVIT study showed that in their patient population, a MESS of 8 predicted in-hospital amputation in only 43.2% of patients,[7] compared with 100% of patients in Johansen's 1990 study.
- In mass casualty or limited resource settings, MESS can be considered for use as a triage tool. However, in advanced trauma centers, functionality, quality of life, and limb salvage options should be discussed in a multidisciplinary setting with input from the trauma, vascular, plastic, and orthopedic surgery teams prior to proceeding to amputation, regardless of MESS.

Table 1: MESS Scoring System

Skeletal/Soft-Tissue Injury	
Very high energy (high energy + contamination)	4
High energy (military GSW/close range GSW)	3
Medium energy (open fracture)	2
Low energy (stab, simple fx, civilian GSW)	1
*Limb Ischemia**	
Cool, paralyzed, numb, insensate	3
Pulseless, paresthesia, slow capillary refill	2
Diminished pulse, normal perfusion	1
*Double score if ischemia time > 6 h	
Shock	
Persistent hypotension	3
Transiently hypotensive	2
Systolic > 90 mm Hg	1
Age	
>50	3
30-50	2
<30	1

SURGICAL MANAGEMENT

Preoperative Management

- The management of the patient prehospital and preoperatively will play a large part in determining the appropriate operation.
- Use of tourniquets is widely advocated at most major trauma centers, prehospital (**FIGURE 1**), in the trauma bay, and intraoperatively (**FIGURE 2**). Historically, there had been concerns that tourniquet use could propagate limb ischemia and cause nerve injury. However, in recent years, tourniquet use has become more prevalent. Studies have shown that use of tourniquets in lower extremity trauma has both a mortality benefit[8] and a reduction in shock and blood product use in the hospital.[9]
- The life-saving yet basic principles of hemorrhage control in the prehospital setting have propelled an initiative by the American College of Surgeons Committee on Trauma through the **Stop the Bleed®** program. This program encourages both clinicians and nonhealth care workers to become trained in **Stop the Bleed®** so that the community can be armed in putting a stop to preventable death by hemorrhage.
- In addition to hemorrhage control, ischemia time is a factor that is integral to outcomes following lower extremity trauma, regardless of operative technique. For several decades, 6 hours has been used as the threshold for irreversible ischemia in lower extremity vascular trauma.
  - Alarhayem et al performed a retrospective review of 4406 patients who sustained lower extremity trauma between the years 2012 and 2015. The amputation rate overall was 11.3% but decreased to 6% when revascularization was done within 1 hour of injury. Increased amputation risk was associated with blunt trauma, nerve injury, corresponding lower extremity fractures, popliteal injury, age, and Injury Severity Score.[10] It is therefore imperative that revascularization be performed as soon as it is safe and reasonable to do so.

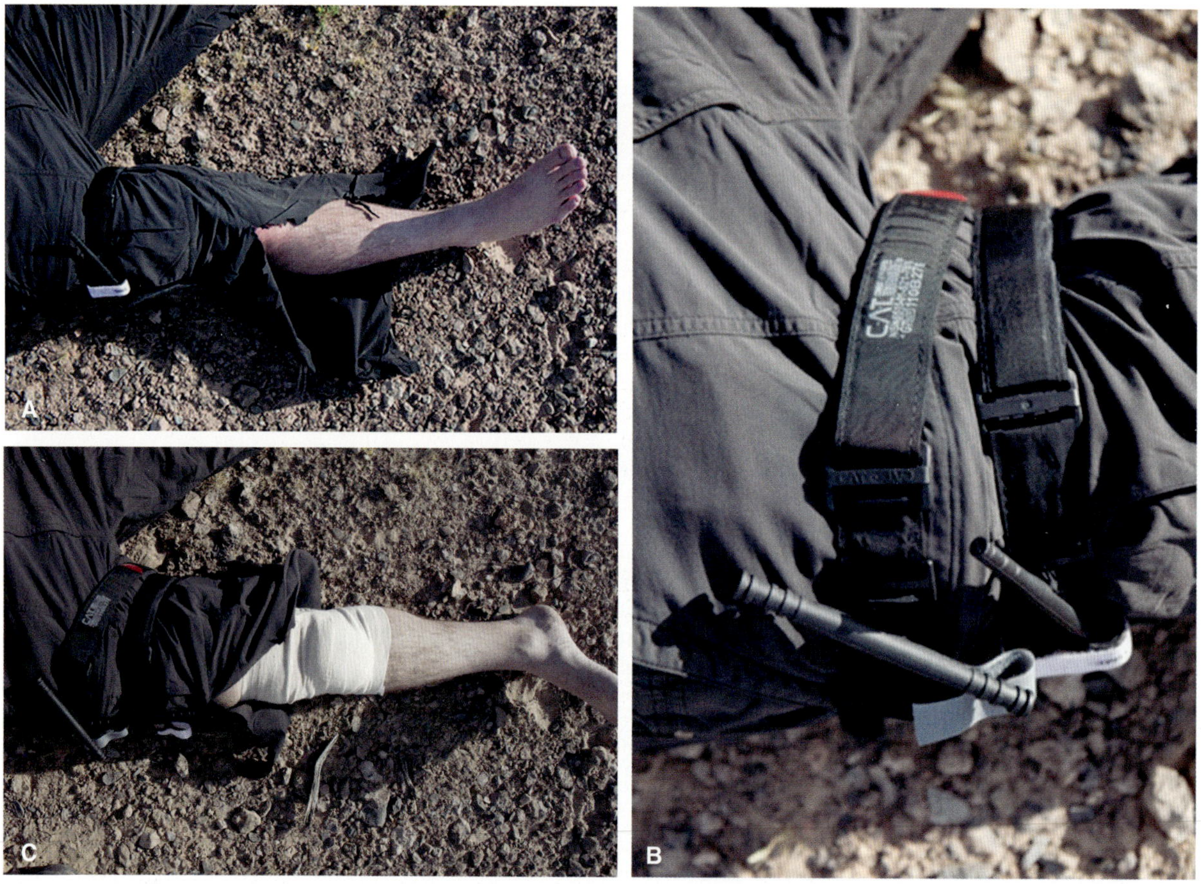

FIGURE 1 • Tourniquet conversion. **A,** The original tourniquet in place proximal to the site of injury. **B,** First, place a second tourniquet in addition to the original, but do not tighten. This is in case bleeding cannot be controlled and the first tourniquet breaks as it is being retightened. **C,** Slowly release the tourniquet while evaluating the wound for bleeding, attempt to control with direct pressure or pressure dressing if needed. If hemorrhage is controlled, leave tourniquets in place in the event that severe bleeding resumes. If hemorrhage is not controlled, tighten tourniquet and reassess at a later time, if possible. (Courtesy of Matthew Horbal. Reprinted with permission from: Hawkins SC. Wilderness EMS. Wolters Kluwer; 2018. Figure 21.1C.)

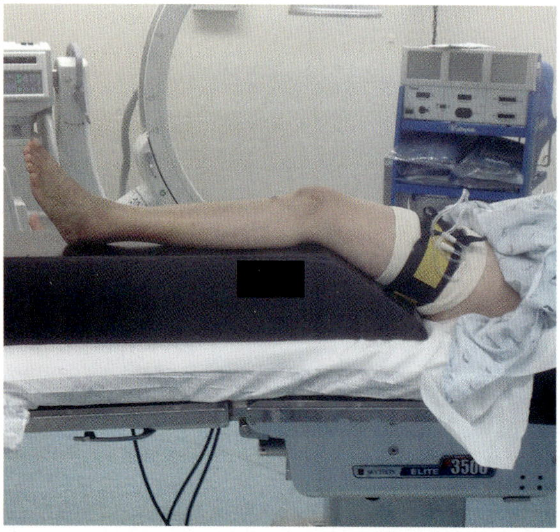

FIGURE 2 • Supine positioning of the injured ankle. A thigh tourniquet is applied, a rolled sheet bump is placed under the hip to internally rotate the leg so the patella is pointed directly anterior, and the ankle is elevated on an inclined bump (foam bump or sheets) to allow for lateral fluoroscopic images without moving the ankle. (Used with permission from Wiesel SW, Albert T. *Operative Techniques in Orthopaedic Surgery*. 3rd ed. Wolters Kluwer; 2022. Part 2 Figure 24.4.)

OPERATIVE TECHNIQUES

- We will discuss operative techniques in lower extremity trauma, organized from proximal to distal

COMMON FEMORAL/SUPERFICIAL FEMORAL ARTERY

Prepping and Draping

- As with all lower extremity traumas, we recommend prepping and draping the patient from at least the chin to the knees including the groins and genitalia, with Foley catheter placement. It is important to prep in the contralateral groin and extremity for consideration of saphenous vein harvest (**FIGURE 3A-C**). The contralateral vein is preferable so that venous outflow in the affected (injured) extremity is not compromised, especially in the setting of undiagnosed deep venous injury.

Incision—Proximal and Distal Control of Hemorrhage

- One of the principal tenets of vascular trauma is obtaining control of hemorrhage proximal and distal to the injury. Preoperatively and intraoperatively, tourniquet use may be helpful in obtaining proximal control while the surgeon continues exploration of the involved vascular structures. Trauma involving the iliofemoral junction can be challenging to obtain proximal control of hemorrhage.
  - External control of hemorrhage using a tourniquet or direct pressure may not be possible in this region so expedient management is key.
  - Resuscitative endovascular balloon occlusion of the aorta (REBOA) use may be considered for proximal control in select patients.[11]
- We recommend first creating an incision spanning from the anterior posterior iliac spine to the inguinal canal and caudally (distal to the injury). If it is possible to obtain proximal control below the inguinal ligament, the artery can be controlled with an iliac clamp or a bulldog clamp. If control is required proximal to the inguinal ligament, the surgeon can perform a low midline incision in the abdomen, and isolation

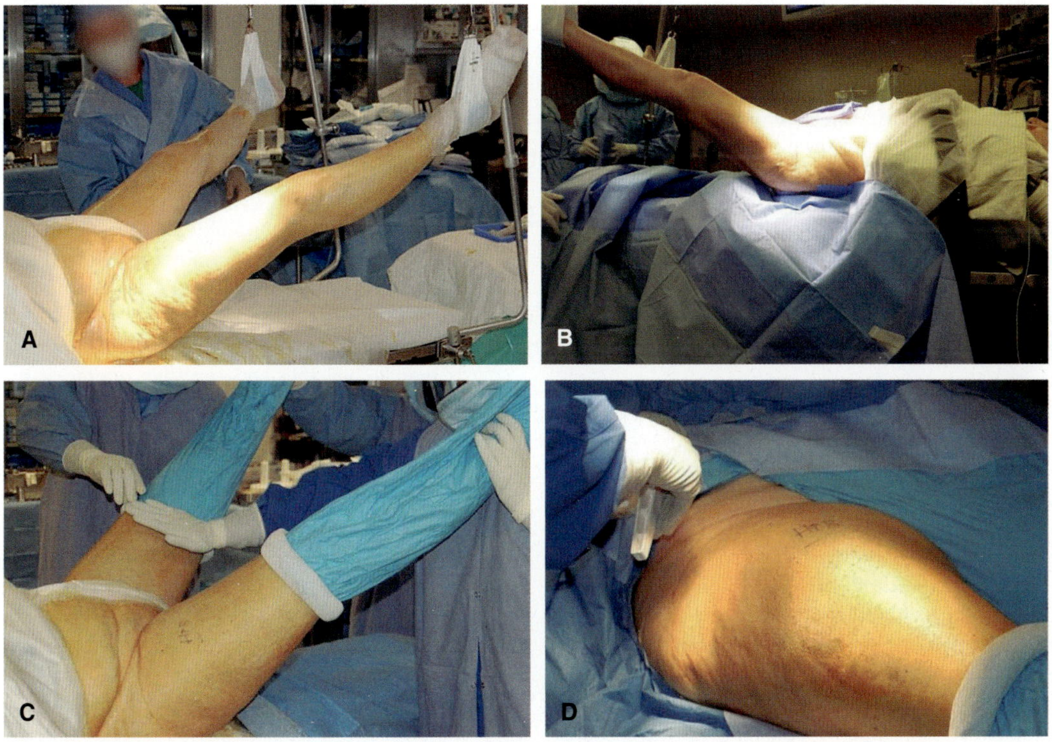

FIGURE 3 • **A,** Both legs prepped. **B,** First sterile U-drape. **C,** Bilateral stockinettes. **D,** Operative side isolated. (Used with permission from Wiesel SW, Albert T. *Operative Techniques in Orthopaedic Surgery*. 3rd ed. Wolters Kluwer; 2022. Part 3 Tech Figure 18.1.)

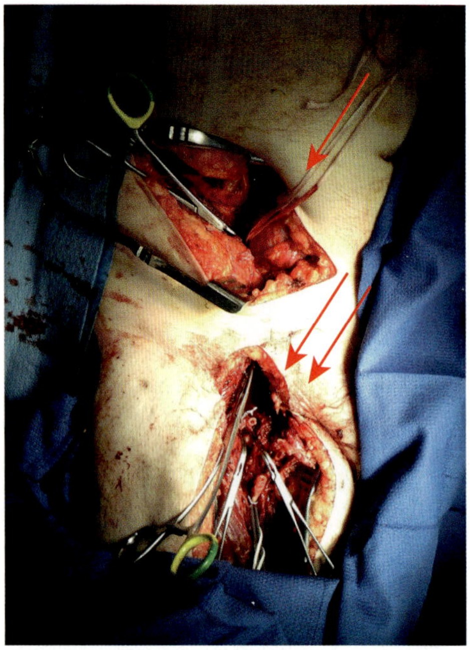

FIGURE 4 • Retroperitoneal exposure for proximal control (*arrow*). Standard femoral exposure for the distal control (*double arrow*). (Reprinted with permission from Upchurch GR, Henke PK. *Clinical Scenarios in Vascular Surgery.* 2nd ed. Wolters Kluwer; 2016. Figure 124.1.)

of the external iliac vessels either via a peritoneal or retroperitoneal approach (**FIGURE 4**).

- We recommend whichever approach facilitates the safest and quickest control; this is often achieved with laparotomy. Takedown of the inguinal ligament may be required for adequate exposure; we recommend overcoming any hesitation in dividing this structure in the face of life- or limb-threatening bleeding.

- In the instance where injury prohibits ready access to the proximal aspect of the injured artery, a Fogarty balloon can be inserted and the balloon inflated to control hemorrhage. Distal control is usually more easily achieved via the superficial femoral artery with a vascular clamp (**FIGURE 5**). It is acceptable to make an initial or additional incision(s) away from the site of injury (in "virgin" territory) if this will facilitate or expedite control of hemorrhage.

Shunting

- In extremity trauma, it is particularly important to balance control of hemorrhage with ischemia time. Hemorrhage control is always the priority; however, once control is obtained, a focus on establishing distal perfusion should be the next step. In the setting of multiple injuries such as orthopedic trauma or severe hemorrhage shock, a shunt can be placed in the area of injury as a damage control measure.
- Shunts temporarily restore blood flow, allowing the patient to undergo additional resuscitation or other prioritized procedures prior to definitive vascular repair, such as reduction or external fixation of fractures. There are many commercial shunts available in the civilian setting; 14F chest tubes can also be used as a shunt in resource-limited situations. A shunt is used in **FIGURE 6**, for a patient who sustained a popliteal artery injury.

Primary Repair

- Once the patient is in an acceptable physiologic condition, the options for definitive repair must be addressed. Partially injured femoral arteries (<50%) can be debrided and repaired primarily or with a patch. Patch is favored to avoid narrowing of the vessel unless the injury is punctate, in which case a primary repair can be performed. Patch repair can be used with vein, biologic, or synthetic material and is usually not appropriate in smaller vessels.
- In patients with a transected common femoral or superficial femoral artery, end-to-end anastomosis is an option provided there is enough length after debridement of the vessel. Typically, a 2-cm defect can be resected with enough mobilization to perform a tension-free anastomosis. Primary anastomosis typically requires mobilization of both the distal and proximal ends of the artery.
- While all efforts are made to preserve arterial branches, however, a tension-free repair takes priority. Bridging veins may also need to be ligated; however, care should be taken to avoid ligating named veins if possible.

Interposition Graft

- It is when there is an injury prohibiting primary anastomosis that the surgeon will need to decide on the appropriate conduit for the patient (**FIGURE 7**). There is a paucity of current literature which discusses outcomes in civilians with synthetic grafts vs autologous vein grafts in the proximal lower extremity. In the military setting, synthetic graft infections are prevalent and vein graft is highly recommended if it meets size criteria. Feliciano et al found that in noncontaminated wounds, the infection rate and patency of synthetic grafts are comparable to vein grafts, especially when the conduit is >6 mm in diameter (which is usually the case with proximal lower extremity arteries) and in a noncontaminated setting.[12]
- In the civilian setting, ringed polytetrafluoroethylene (PTFE) is readily available and can save operative time compared to harvesting the saphenous vein. This is a major consideration in the polytrauma patient who may require multicavity surgery.

Extraanatomic Bypass

- Bypass, particularly in the thigh, is less frequently used in trauma. There is no particular size defect which mandates bypass. The main reason for bypass in most cases is inadequate, necrotic, or infected soft tissue over the area of defect. If there is no adjacent muscle or soft tissue to cover the vessels, then bypass must be considered to mitigate infection risk of the repaired vessel.

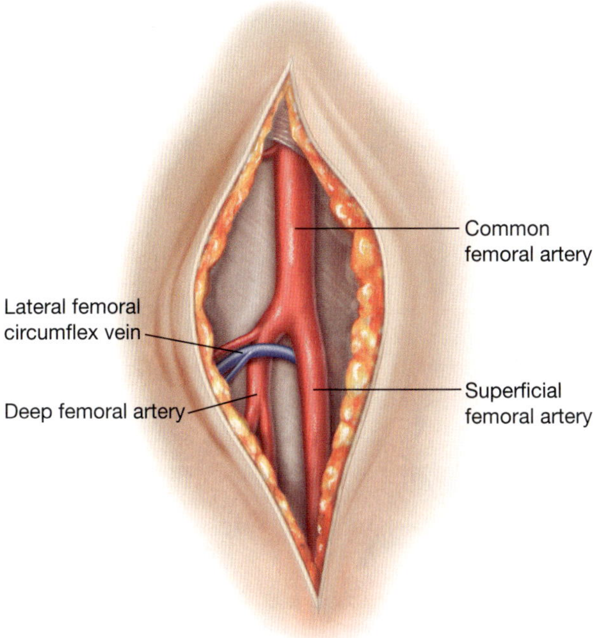

FIGURE 5 • The deep femoral artery normally arises laterally off the common femoral trunk about 3.5 cm distal to the inguinal ligament. Its origin is crossed by the lateral femoral circumflex vein. (Reprinted with permission from Wind GG, Valentine RJ. *Anatomic Exposures in Vascular Surgery*. 3rd ed. Wolters Kluwer; 2014. Figure 15.21.)

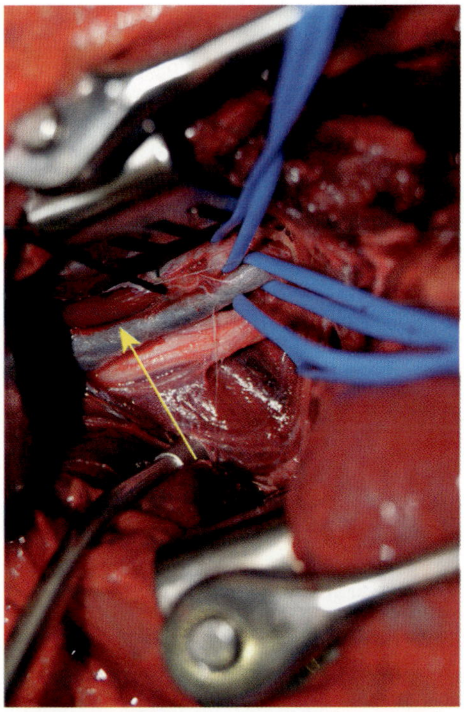

FIGURE 6 • A close view of the structures of the below-knee popliteal space including the popliteal artery with a patent vascular shunt in place, the popliteal vein, and the tibial nerve. In this case, the popliteal vein was uninjured and has been dissected free from the medial portion of the artery and encircled with a blue vessel loop to allow retraction away from the artery. (Yellow arrow points to the popliteal arterial shunt and its securement by a silk suture.) (Reprinted with permission from Upchurch GR, Henke PK. *Clinical Scenarios in Vascular Surgery*. 2nd ed. Wolters Kluwer; 2016. Figure 122.4.)

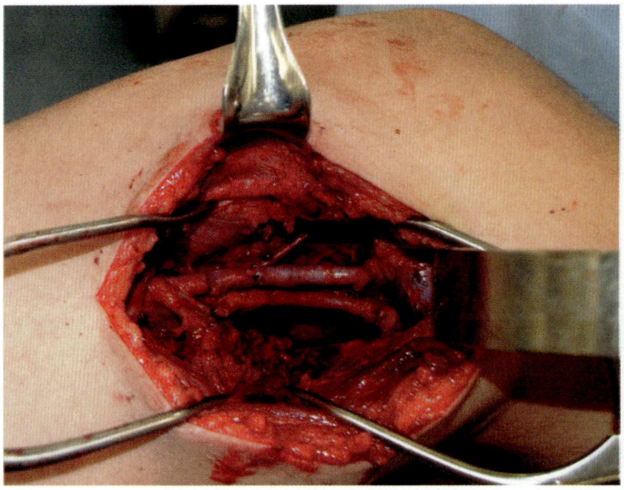

FIGURE 7 • Operative photograph showing an interposition vein graft repair of the left proximal popliteal artery and vein. The interposition greater saphenous vein grafts were harvested from the right (contralateral) leg and performed following removal of the temporary vascular shunts. (Reprinted with permission from Dimick JB. *Mulholland & Greenfield's Surgery*. 7th ed. Wolters Kluwer; 2022. Figure 27.7.)

Technique

- From a technical standpoint, vascular anastomoses follow similar steps once exposure has been obtained:
  - Proximal and distal control of the injured vessel should be obtained using vessel loops or vascular clamps/bulldog clamps.
  - The ends of the artery should be debrided to expose healthy intima. Regardless of conduit, the ends should be spatulated to allow for expansion of the graft since

many vessels will be in significant vasospasm from injury.

- A Fogarty catheter should be passed at least twice distally and proximally to ensure no clot or occlusion of the injured vessel.
- Systemic heparinization or regional heparinized saline can be administered; the latter is typically favored in trauma due to the high bleeding risk.
- Using a 5-0 or 6-0 nonabsorbable monofilament suture, bites should be taken from internal to external on the artery in order to secure the intima using a double-armed needle. The suture is then run at 3 o'clock or 9 o'clock posteriorly and then anteriorly. It is often preferred to start posteriorly as this is the more technically challenging angle.
- Prior to securing the suture, the vessel will be flushed with additional heparinized saline while unclamping the vessels in each respective direction to ensure patency and remove debris.
- With the proximal clamp or loop reapplied, the distal clamp is left open to evaluate for backflow. This is universally used as a sign of distal patency. Distal pulses should be obtained before closure of the repaired vessel. If angiography is available, on-table angiogram is the best method to confirm distal patency. The suture can then be tied.

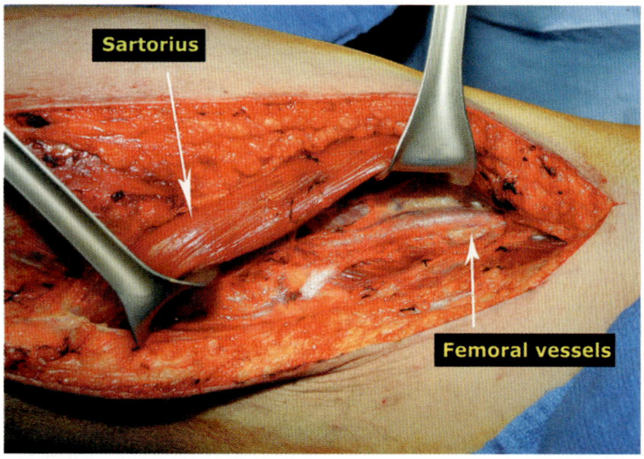

FIGURE 8 • In the proximal thigh, retracting the sartorius anterior and lateral allows exposure of the femoral vessels, all the way to the inguinal ligament if necessary. (Used with permission from Wiesel SW, Albert T. *Operative Techniques in Orthopaedic Surgery*. 3rd ed. Wolters Kluwer; 2022. Tech Figure 25.1E.)

- If possible, a muscle flap should be placed over the vessel to protect the vessel from contamination (**FIGURE 8**).
- Evaluate need for fasciotomy (discussed later in this chapter).

POPLITEAL ARTERY

Prepping and Draping

- The posterior location along the knee joint of the popliteal artery makes this arterial injury more challenging to manage than the femoral vessels. The patient should be prepped in the same manner as described above and positioned with the hip abducted and externally rotated in the "frog-leg" position.
- A blanket or sterile towels (a "bump") can be used under the thigh to improve exposure. If a tourniquet is in place, this can be prepped in the field and can be useful as a method of proximal control during dissection.

Incision—Proximal and Distal Control of Hemorrhage

- A medial approach is typically taken (see **FIGURE 9**). Incision is made posterior to the distal femur, spanning the knee joint down to the tibia. The distal femoral artery and proximal popliteal artery are in Hunter canal within the adductor magnus. An incision over the sartorius is made. In order to best expose the popliteal vessels, take down of the sartorius, semimembranosus, and semitendinosus muscles is often necessary; this transection can be achieved most efficiently with cautery. A clean transection of these muscles (as time allows) will allow a sounder reconstruction which will play a role in the recovery and function of the limb.
  - Care must be taken to avoid injury to the greater saphenous vein which often underlies the sartorius. Depending on the level of the injury, the two heads of the gastrocnemius may need to be taken down as well with the soleus muscle to obtain distal control.
- Once the popliteal fossa has been exposed, the tibial nerve will be the most superficial structure. Care should be taken to identify and carefully retract this nerve out of the field of view, typically with a vessel loop. The popliteal vein will be superficial and slightly lateral to the artery. This should be skeletonized and controlled with vessel loops proximally and distally to obtain better exposure of the artery. Once the artery is in view, the tourniquet may be relaxed to identify the area of injury and then reinflated as needed. Proximal and distal control should then be obtained with vessel loops.
  - The geniculate vessels should not be ligated unless they are contributing to hemorrhage; collateralization from these vessels is important in perfusing the leg, especially in the setting of injury to the popliteal artery.

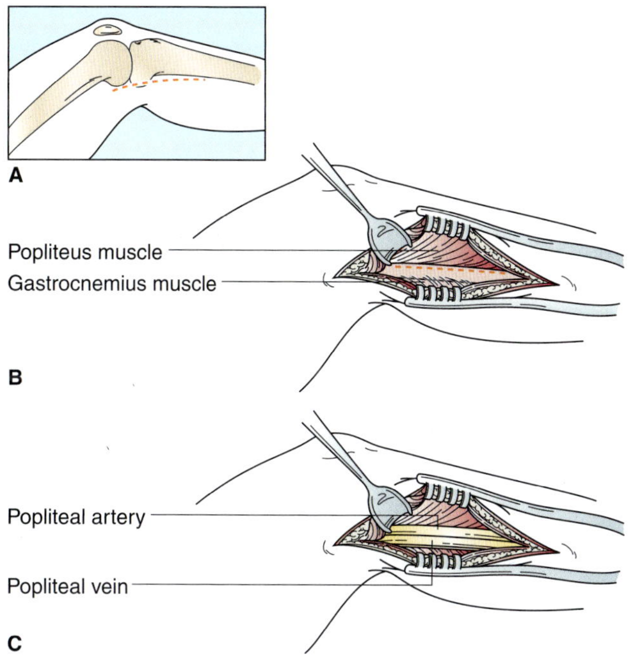

FIGURE 9 • Exposure of the popliteal artery below the knee. The medial incision is made directly overlying the course of the greater saphenous vein **(A)**, with posterior retraction of the gastrocnemius muscle **(B)**, to reveal the popliteal vessels in the popliteal fossa **(C)**. (Reprinted with permission from Dimick JB. *Mulholland & Greenfield's Surgery*. 7th ed. Wolters Kluwer; 2022. Figure 91.8.)

Primary Repair

- As described in the above section, repair will depend on the nature of the injury. Popliteal artery injuries have a higher incidence of amputation than femoral vessel injuries; this is due to its association with blunt polytrauma and undiagnosed arterial injury.[13]
- For injuries <30% circumference of the vessel, primary repair can be considered. However, primary repairs are more prone to failure as the caliber of the vessel is smaller than that of the femoral vessels. To mitigate risk of stenosis, an alternative to primary repair is to excise the lesion and perform an end-to-end anastomosis or perform a patch repair.

Interposition Graft

- A tension-free end-to-end anastomosis becomes more challenging to achieve beyond 2 cm, and therefore, interposition graft (bypass) is typically the next best step in management. As with all vascular surgeries, the choice of conduit and technical approach will be integral in determining patency of the repair. Interposition graft is usually recommended in popliteal artery trauma with exceptions outlined below.
- Autologous vein graft is the preferred conduit at or below the knee. Historically, synthetic grafts were avoided overall due to findings that PTFE in popliteal artery injury has worse outcomes and inferior patency to autologous vein.[14] However, synthetic graft is often necessary in patients in whom suitable vein is not available (small caliber, diseased or injured vein). In fact, there is emerging literature that supports use of PTFE as a below the knee conduit, showing no difference in secondary amputation rate, wound infection, or graft infection.[15]
- We recommend using the largest caliber ringed PTFE graft available for interposition popliteal grafts to the extent that a size mismatch does not undermine the integrity of the repair. As described above, spatulation of the graft is important to accommodate the change in caliber of the vessel after reperfusion.

Alternative Revascularization Methods

- As with femoral artery injuries, extraanatomic bypass of the injury is typically reserved in patients whose native artery site is destroyed or at risk of severe contamination (eg, severe soft tissue or orthopedic injury resulting in an inability to cover the vessel with viable tissue postoperatively).
- In patients with small popliteal artery injuries or pseudoaneurysms, endovascular stenting has been suggested as a bridge to definitive repair, especially in patients with significant soft tissue and bone trauma. Specifically, endovascular therapy has been shown to be the safe alternative to open repair in patients with greater injury severity scores and blunt polytrauma.[16]

TECHNIQUES

VENOUS INJURIES

- In patients with venous extremity trauma, the general trend in these patients is to ligate veins. In concomitant arterial injury or soft tissue injury, it is important to consider the importance of venous drainage. In the event of an isolated venous injury, however, repair may not prove as beneficial as ligation. Military literature has shown that repair of venous injury is associated with a lower amputation rate than ligation.[17] Therefore, if the patient's clinical status allows time for repair, it may be worth pursuing venous repair in instances of multivessel trauma or significant soft tissue damage.
- When a vein is ligated, it is important to remember that while collateralization may allow the patient to compensate for its lost drainage, in the immediate postoperative period, impaired venous drainage can result in DVT and/or significant edema. It is for this reason that in the acute setting, ligation of named veins is usually best accompanied by fasciotomy. Additionally, the lower extremity should be wrapped ankle to thigh and elevated above the heart to aid in adequate venous drainage.

BELOW KNEE FASCIOTOMY

- It is important to have a low threshold to perform fasciotomy in the trauma setting, especially when risk of compartment syndrome is high, such as with mangled extremities, venous injury, crush injury, reperfusion, etc.

Prepping and Draping

- The authors favor the standard approach to four-compartment fasciotomy, using two longitudinal incisions at the medial and lateral aspects of the calf. The patient's lower extremity from above the knee and including the foot should be prepped and draped.

Incision

- The medial incision is used to release the superficial and deep posterior compartments. An incision is made one fingerbreadth posterior to the palpable tibia and should be carried along the gastrocnemius muscles to 2 fingerbreadths/3 cm superior to the medial malleolus (**FIGURE 10A**).
  - Once the skin is incised, care should be taken to avoid the saphenous vein. Skin flaps can be raised several centimeters anteriorly and posteriorly, exposing the fascia. An incision should be created in the fascia and continued longitudinally overlying the gastrocnemius muscles for the entire length of the incision. This will open the superficial posterior compartment.
  - To ensure entry into the posterior compartment which contains the popliteal vessels and nerve, the soleus muscle should be taken down from its tibial attachments and the neurovascular bundle visualized (**FIGURE 10E**).
- The lateral incision is used to release the anterior and lateral compartments. The incision will start proximally two fingerbreadths below the fibular head and carried distally to 2 fingerbreadths/3 cm superior to the lateral malleolus. Once the skin is incised, care should be taken to avoid the superficial peroneal nerve. Skin flaps can be raised several centimeters anteriorly and posteriorly, exposing the fascia.
  - In order to eliminate the risk of missing a compartment, a transverse incision should be created in the fascia; once this is done, visualization reveals the following from anterior to posterior: anterior compartment, fascial septum separating anterior and lateral compartments, lateral compartment, fascial septum separating lateral and superficial compartments, and superficial posterior compartment.
  - Two incisions should be created in the fascia and continued longitudinally for the entire length of the incision, one releasing the anterior compartment and one releasing the lateral compartment.
  - Lateral fascial incisions create the risk of transecting superficial vasculature and the superficial peroneal nerve, so care must be taken to evaluate the anatomy prior to incision (**FIGURE 11**).
- Once fasciotomy is complete, the wounds can be covered with saline moistened gauge (**FIGURE 12A**) or petrolatum dressing covered with a dry gauze dressing and evaluated on a twice or once daily basis. Once the initial edema appears to have stabilized, return to OR should be planned for closure. A staged closure with a Jacob ladder technique (**FIGURE 12C**), negative pressure wound therapy (**FIGURE 12B**), or a combination (**FIGURE 12D**) of the two may be required. In the case of loss of domain, skin grafting may be considered. If only one incision can be closed under minimal to no tension, we advise that the lateral incision closure be prioritized for cosmetic reasons.

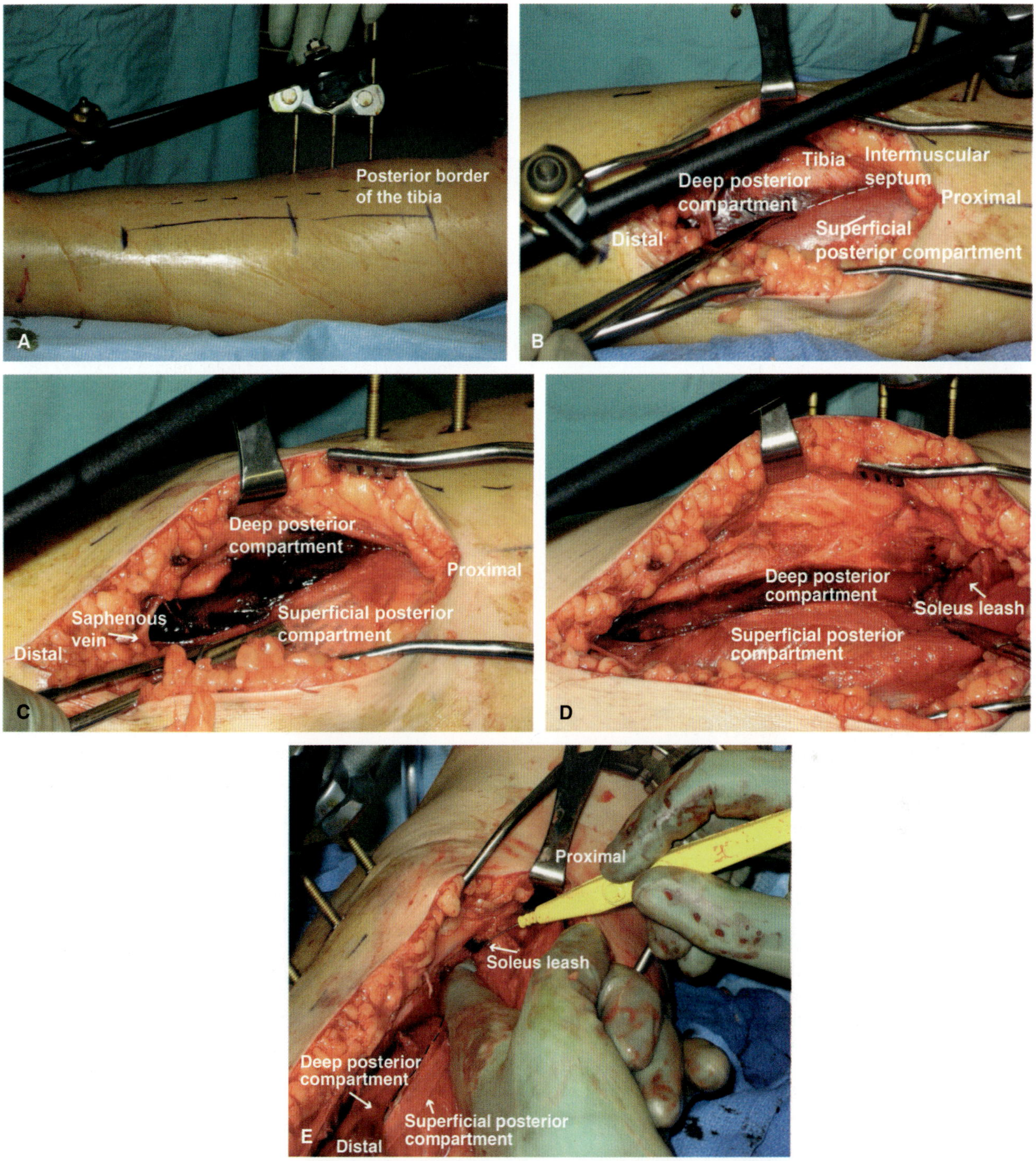

FIGURE 10 • Medial incision of the two-incision technique. **A,** The medial incision lies approximately 2 cm posterior to the posterior tibial margin. **B,** Care is taken to avoid injury to the saphenous vein. The picture shows the posterior border of the tibia exposed along with the deep and superficial posterior compartments. The tips of the dissecting scissors lie on the deep posterior compartment. **C,** A small transverse incision is made to identify the intermuscular septum between the deep and superficial posterior compartments. Dissecting scissors are used to release the fascia over the deep posterior compartment proximally and distally. Proximally, the fascia is released under the soleus bridge. Scissors are shown under the fascia of the superficial posterior compartment. **D,** The deep and superficial compartments are released. The superficial posterior compartment looks healthy, whereas the deep posterior compartment is dusky. The tips of the clamp lie under the soleus bridge, which also needs to be released from its origin on the tibia. **E,** The surgeon releases the soleus bridge using electrocautery, taking care to protect the deep structures. (Used with permission from Wiesel SW, Albert T. *Operative Techniques in Orthopaedic Surgery*. 3rd ed. Wolters Kluwer; 2022. Part 2 Tech Figure 22.2.)

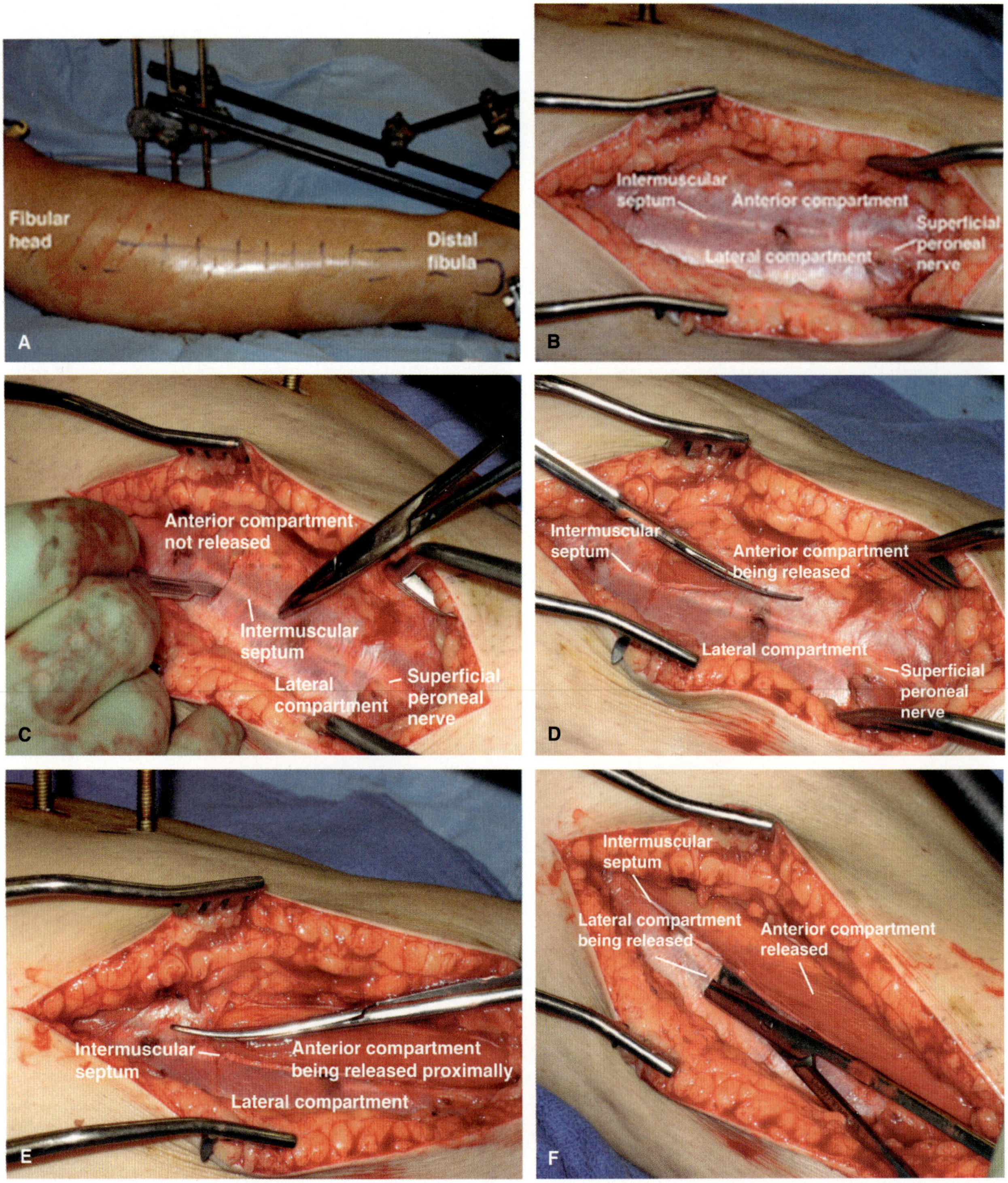

FIGURE 11 • Lateral incision of the two-incision technique. **A,** The anterolateral incision is made halfway between the fibula and the tibial crest overlying the intermuscular septum dividing the anterior and lateral compartments. **B,** Close-up picture of the fasciotomy site after skin incision before the fascia is open, showing the intermuscular septum between the lateral and anterior compartments and the course of the superficial peroneal nerve. **C,** With a knife, a small transverse incision is made over the intermuscular septum. Care is taken to avoid injury to the superficial peroneal nerve. **D,** The surgeon inserts the tips of the scissors into the small rent in the fascia, and keeping the tips of the scissors up and away from the superficial peroneal nerve, the surgeon incises the fascia over the anterior compartment distally. **E,** The scissors are turned with the tips proximally, and the fascia of the anterior compartment is released proximally. **F,** The tips of the scissors are then inserted into the rent created in the fascia of the lateral compartment. Keeping the tips of the scissors up and away from the superficial peroneal nerve, the surgeon releases the fascia over the lateral compartment proximally and distally. (Used with permission from Wiesel SW, Albert T. *Operative Techniques in Orthopaedic Surgery*. 3rd ed. Wolters Kluwer; 2022. Part 2 Tech Figure 22.1.)

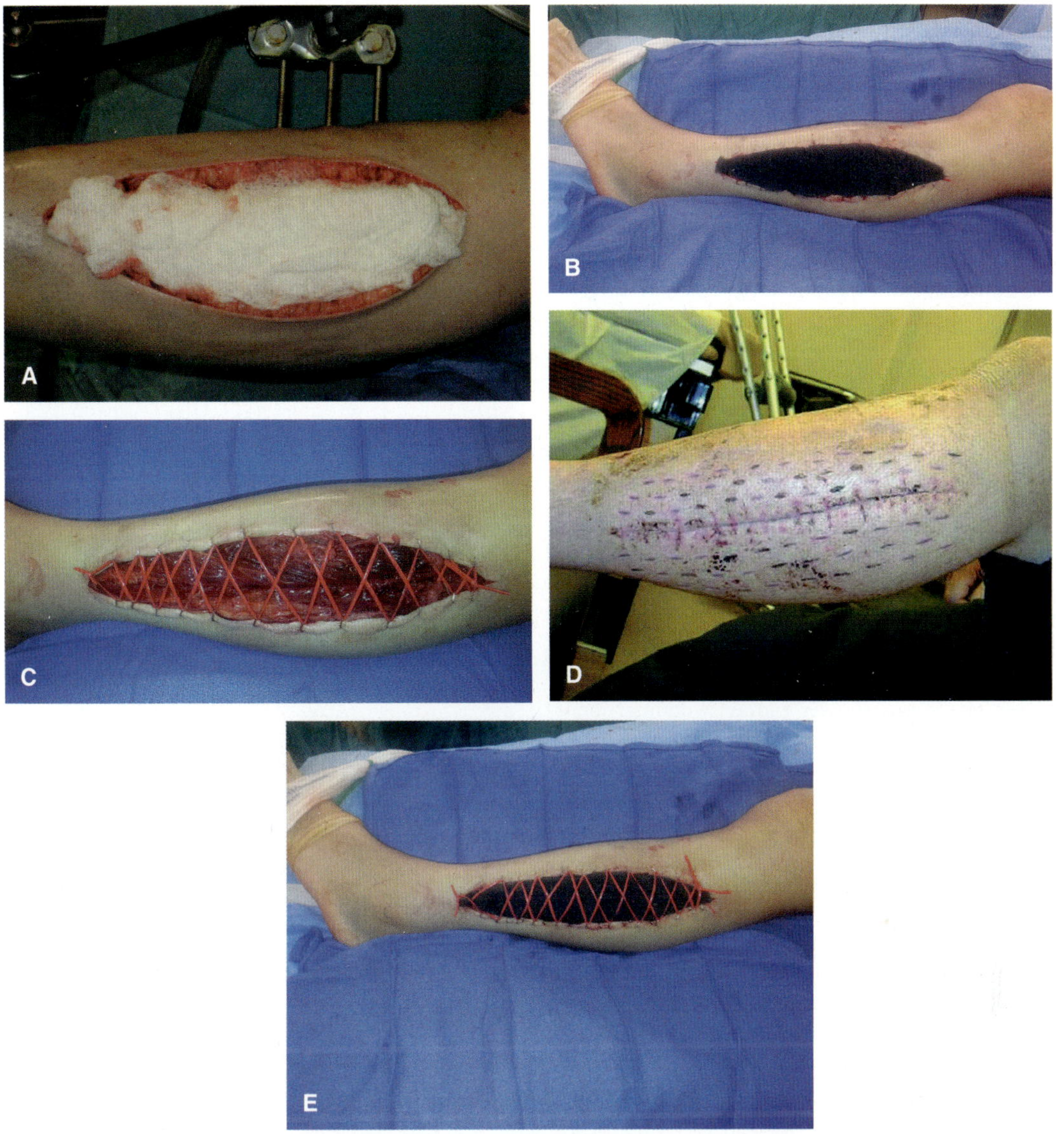

FIGURE 12 • Closure of fasciotomies. **A,** Moist dressings covering the fasciotomy wound. **B,** Sterile vacuum system applied to the fasciotomy site. **C,** Bootlace technique for approximating the edges of a fasciotomy wound. **D,** Small relaxing incisions made around the fasciotomy site to release tension and allow easier closure. **E,** Bootlace technique combined with sterile vacuum system. (Used with permission from Wiesel SW, Albert T. *Operative Techniques in Orthopaedic Surgery*. 3rd ed. Wolters Kluwer; 2022. Part 2 Tech Figure 22.4.)

PEARLS AND PITFALLS

Prepping and draping	■ Prepare contralateral groin and lower extremity for potential vein harvest.
Leg fasciotomy	■ Be sure to take down the soleus muscle fibers from the tibia and visualize the neurovascular bundle to ensure the deep compartment is entered and decompressed.
Timely diagnosis	■ Have a high index of suspicion for vascular injury in all patients with extremity trauma. ABIs remain useful.
Exposure in junctional vasculature injuries	■ Do not be afraid to divide the inguinal ligament or perform laparotomy in order to obtain proximal control.
Document vascular exam	■ Be sure to document vascular exam immediately following revascularization ("index exam"). Communicate this clearly to the care team. Should the exam change, consider imaging vs return to OR.

POSTOPERATIVE CARE

- Following vascular surgery, it is most important that the patient undergoes frequent (hourly) neurovascular checks.
- Postoperative anticoagulation or antiplatelet therapy may not be indicated following vascular surgery for trauma and may be contraindicated in the setting of polytrauma and hemorrhagic shock.
  - In many cases, traumatized vessels will not have baseline disease and therefore do not require additional treatment. This contrasts with more elective vascular surgery in patients with atherosclerotic disease whose pathology originates from plaque build-up and embolic disease.
  - Recent evidence from the AAST's PROOVIT registry demonstrated that there was no difference in outcomes in anticoagulated patients compared with nonanticoagulated patients following traumatic vascular surgery; other than that the anticoagulated patients required more blood products than the latter group.[18]

COMPLICATIONS

- Complications from traumatic vascular surgery have primarily been highlighted in each of the sections above but the following are the most devastating:
  - **Compartment syndrome**—Lower extremity compartment syndrome can occur as a result of reperfusion after a period of ischemia, swelling from injury alone, or edema secondary to venous injury. There should be a low threshold to perform preemptive fasciotomy in patients who have sustained vascular trauma.
  - **Graft failure**—In the immediate postoperative period, graft failure is a technical complication. This can be avoided by shunt placement to reduce ischemia time. Some may consider intraoperative vascular surgery consultation; new data demonstrates noninferiority for extremity vascular repairs by trauma surgeons compared to vascular surgeons.[19]

REFERENCES

1. Kauvar DS, Sarfati MR, Kraiss LW. National trauma databank analysis of mortality and limb loss in isolated lower extremity vascular trauma. *J Vasc Surg*. 2011;53(6):1598-1603.
2. Fox N, Rajani RR, Bokhari F, et al. Evaluation and management of penetrating lower extremity arterial trauma. *J. Trauma and Acute Care Surgery*. 2012;73(5):315-320.
3. Hemingway J, Adjei E, Desikan S, et al. Re-evaluating the safety and effectiveness of the 0.9 ankle-brachial index threshold in penetrating lower extremity trauma. *J Vasc Surg*. 2020;72(4):1305-1311.
4. Kobayashi L, Coimbra R, Goes AMO, et al. American association for the surgery of trauma—World Society of emergency surgery guidelines on diagnosis and management of peripheral vascular injuries. *J Trauma Acute Care Surg*. 2020;89(6):1183-1196.
5. Johansen K, Daines M, Howey T. Helfet D, Hansen S. Objective criteria accurately predict amputation following lower extremity trauma. *J Trauma Inj Infect Crit Care*. 1990;30(5):568-572.
6. Prasarn ML, Helfet DL, Kloen P. Management of the mangled extremity. *Strategies Trauma Limb Reconstr*. 2012;7(2):57-66.
7. Sriussadaporn S, Pak-art R. Temporary intravascular shunt in complex extremity vascular injuries. *J Trauma Inj Infect Crit Care*. 2002;52(6):1129-1133.
8. Texiera P, Brown CVR, Emigh B, et al. Civilian prehospital tourniquet use is associated with improved Survival in patients with peripheral vascular injury. *J Am Coll Surg*. 2018;226(5):769-776.
9. Smith A, Ochoa JE, Wong S, et al.. Prehospital tourniquet use in penetrating extremity trauma: decreased blood transfusions and limb complications. *J Trauma Acute Care Surg*. 2019;86(1):43-51.
10. Alarhayem AQ, Cohn SM, Cantu-Nunez O, Eastridge BJ, Rasmussen TE. Impact of time to repair on outcomes in patients with lower extremity arterial injuries. *J Vasc Surg*. 2019;69(5):1519-1523.
11. Bulger EM, Perina DG, Qasim Z, et al. Clinical use of resuscitative endovascular balloon occlusion of the aorta (REBOA) in civilian trauma systems in the USA, 2019: a joint statement from the American College of surgeons committee on trauma, the American College of emergency physicians, the national association of emergency medical Services physicians and the national association of emergency medical technicians. *Trauma Surg Acute Care Open*. 2019;4(1):e000376.
12. Feliciano D. For the patient—evolution in the management of vascular trauma. *J Trauma Acute Care Surg*. 2017;83(6):1205-1212.
13. Mullenix P, Steel S, Anderson C, Starnes B, Salim A, Martin MJ. Limb salvage and outcomes among patients with traumatic popliteal vascular injury: an analysis of the National Trauma Data Bank. *J Vasc Surg*. 2006;44(1):94-100.
14. Feliciano DV, Mattox KL, Graham JM, Bitondo CG. Five-year experience with PTFE grafts in vascular wounds. *J Trauma*. 1985;25(1):71-82.
15. Rehman Z. Outcomes of popliteal artery injuries repair: autologous vein versus prosthetic interposition grafts. *Ann Vasc Surg*. 2020;69:141-145.
16. Worni M, Scarborough JE, Gandhi M, Pietrobon R, Shortell CK. Use of endovascular therapy for peripheral arterial lesions: an analysis of the National Trauma Data Bank from 2007 to 2009. *Ann Vasc Surg*. 2013;27(3):299-305.
17. Rich NM, Hobson RW, Collins GJ Jr., Andersen CA. The effect of acute popliteal venous interruption. *Ann Surg*. 1976;183(4):365-368.
18. Loja MN, Galante JM, Humphries M, et al. Systemic anticoagulation in the setting of vascular extremity trauma. *Injury*. 2017;48(9):1911-1916.
19. Parihar S, Benarroch-Gampel J, Teodorescu V, Ramos C, Minton K, Rajani RR. Vascular surgeons carry an increasing responsibility in the management of lower extremity vascular trauma. *Ann Vasc Surg*. 2021;70:87-94.

Chapter 50

Upper Extremity: Axillary, Brachial, Radial/Ulnar Fasciotomy

Brian K. Yorkgitis, Jeanette Zhang, and Matthew P. Kochuba

DEFINITION

- The content discussed in the following text assumes the reader has familiarity with standard upper extremity arterial anatomy and its most common variations along with the general principals of trauma evaluation and management. Management of traumatic vascular injury includes restoration of the distal circulation, and should be prioritized based on other injuries the patient may have sustained.
  - Upper extremity traumatic vascular injury accounts for close to 30% of all traumatic vascular injuries, with the majority being from a penetrating mechanism. Fractures and/or dislocation can injure neighboring vessels by direct laceration or stretch on the vessel.[1]
  - Vascular injury can be divided into five different types[2]
    - Intimal injuries
    - Vessel wall defect with bleeding, hematoma, or pseudoaneurysm
    - Transection with bleeding and/or occlusion
    - Arteriovenous fistula
    - Spasm
  - Concomitant injury to nerves that accompany arteries is common[3]

DIFFERENTIAL DIAGNOSIS

- Arterial injuries as described previously
- Compartment syndrome
- Venous injuries
- Fracture(s)
- Thrombosis/embolus from other conditions or injuries

PATIENT HISTORY AND PHYSICAL FINDINGS

- Assessment of extremity injury should take place within the context of overall Advanced Trauma Life Support (ATLS) resuscitation. Consideration should be given to the mechanism of injury, whether blunt, penetration, hyperextension, crush, or avulsion, as it can inform on the likely nature of the resulting arterial pathology.[4]
- Hemorrhage from upper extremity vascular injury can affect circulation that needs to be addressed in the "C" section of the Primary Survey. Strategies for hemorrhage control, in order of preference, include direct pressure, application of a commercial tourniquet, or direct clamping of a visible vessel. Blind clamping is discouraged as it is more likely to cause additional injury than control bleeding.[5]
- In the absence of ongoing bleeding, assessment of the extremity takes place during the Secondary Survey. Thorough vascular, sensory, and motor exams should be completed. Specifically, pulses palpated or signals achieved via Doppler, capillary refill, color, and temperature of the extremity should be checked and compared to the contralateral uninjured limb. If there are obvious fractures or dislocations, exams should be documented both before and after reduction or realignment.[6]
- Physical exam findings concerning for arterial injury have traditionally been categorized into "hard signs" or "soft signs" of injury. Hard signs include active hemorrhage, a large, expanding or pulsatile hematoma, any of the 6 "Ps" classically associated with arterial occlusion (pulselessness, pallor, paresthesias, pain out of proportion, paralysis, and poikilothermia), and a palpable thrill or audible bruit. Patients presenting with these findings are typically managed with immediate operation. Soft signs include a history of arterial bleeding at the scene or in transit, proximity of a penetrating wound or blunt injury to an artery, small nonpulsatile hematoma over an artery, and neurologic deficit in a nerve adjacent to a named artery. Further diagnostic studies may be necessary in these patients to evaluate for vascular injury.[2]
- Recent literature has questioned the focus on hard vs soft signs of injury, arguing that the defined hard signs are limited in their ability to characterize injuries. They argue that categorizing exam findings into hemorrhagic or ischemic signs provides a more clinically relevant paradigm.[7] For instance, those presenting with hemorrhagic signs were more likely to have arterial transection, while those with ischemic signs were more likely to be due to occlusive injury. This can have implications for the mode of diagnosis and subsequent management options, especially considering advances in and increased utilization of endovascular or hybrid approaches.
- Evaluation for compartment syndrome is needed as this can lead to a pulseless extremity or could result from ischemic insult. The forearm is comprised of four compartments: superficial and deep volar, dorsal, and the mobile wad of Henry. The interosseous membrane of the radius and ulna divides the dorsal and volar compartments. Compartment syndrome is largely a clinical diagnosis. The etiology of forearm compartment syndrome includes fractures (18%), soft tissue trauma without fracture (23%), along with vascular injuries, ischemia with reperfusion injury, rhabdomyolysis, burn/electrical injury, bleeding/hematoma, IV extravasation, insect bites, constricting bandage/splint, and infection. Timely diagnosis and treatment are needed to avoid sequelae.[8,9]
- Fractures and dislocations can be associated with vascular injury. For shoulder dislocation the rate of axillary artery injury is close to 1% and for elbow dislocations injury to the brachial artery is close to 0.5%.[10]

IMAGING AND OTHER DIAGNOSTIC STUDIES

- Adhering to principles of ATLS when obtaining imaging is important to not miss life-threatening conditions. Chest radiograph can assist in identifying pneumothorax, hemothorax, or signs suggesting injury to great vessels.[4]

- Radiographs of the injured extremity can identify fractures and/or dislocations that can be the etiology of vascular compromise. After any reduction maneuvers, repeat imaging should be obtained.[4]
- In patients presenting with soft signs of vascular injury, an Ankle or Brachial/Brachial Index (ABI or BBI = systolic blood pressure in extremity distal to the area of injury/systolic blood pressure in brachial artery of uninjured upper extremity) or Arterial Pressure Index (API = Doppler arterial pressure distal to injury/Doppler arterial pressure in uninvolved upper extremity) can be performed. A value of ≤0.9 or a difference between the extremities of >0.1 is considered abnormal, and is diagnostic or suspicious of an arterial injury and warrants further investigation.[4] However, normal ABI may be present in a subclavian or axillary injury due to its rich collaterals.
- Computed tomography angiography (CTA) in the hemodynamically stable patient can assist in the identification of vascular injury or abnormality. This is a readily available test that can assist with diagnosis of vascular injuries along with any associated injuries. In upper extremity and lower extremity vascular injuries, CTA has a sensitivity and specificity of 95% to 100% and 87%, respectively.[11] A single-institution prospective study found CTA to have 100% sensitivity and specificity in detecting clinically relevant vascular injury and was associated with favorable cost profile compared to conventional angiography.[12] Limitations include proximity of shrapnel and difficulty differentiating spasm from occlusion.
- Emergent diagnostic angiogram can be performed in select situations if the CTA was nondiagnostic (ex. secondary to artifact from shrapnel). It may also be used as a primary modality in the operating room (OR) in localizing an injury in a patient who is unable to undergo CTA.[1,2]
- Duplex ultrasonography can be used to identify arterial injury. The major limitation is having experienced staff to obtain and interpret the study. The specificity has been reported as high as 95%, but the sensitivity ranges from 50% to 100%.[1,2]

SURGICAL MANAGEMENT

Preoperative Planning

- Assuring adequate volume resuscitation with evidence-based strategies and availability of blood products is crucial to the patient's outcome. This requires good communication with the anesthesia team and blood bank.
- It is important to identify all life-threating injuries the patient may have sustained to assist the surgical team in the conduct of operative procedures. Often hemorrhage from extremities can be controlled by methods listed previously. Torso hemorrhage, on the other hand, is difficult to control without operative intervention and should be addressed expeditiously. Concomitant suspected or confirmed neurotrauma presents a challenge and spinal motion restriction should be maintained as able, and discussion with neurotrauma colleagues about any neurologic monitoring needed is crucial.[4]
- Perioperative antibiotics should be given. In the event of an open fracture, antibiotic selection and duration should be guided by the Gustilo-Anderson classification.
- Surgical management of the arterial injury will depend on patient acuity, mechanism of injury, and other traumatic injuries. Early discussion with orthopedic surgery should address any skeletal fixation that is needed for fractures of the upper extremity.[2,5,13] Restoration of arterial flow should be prioritized over skeletal fixation to minimize ischemic time. Temporary shunting allows for stabilization of unstable fractures or dislocations when not easily reduced prior to definitive repair, whereas immediate definitive repair can be performed when the skeletal injury is not significantly displaced. Fasciotomies should be performed early in combined vascular-skeletal injuries. Inspection of the vascular repair should be performed at the conclusion of skeletal fixation.
- Axillary artery exposure is dependent on the area of the injury along the course of the artery. The proximal artery is typically exposed via a transverse infraclavicular incision. Exposure of the second portion is approached through a deltopectoral incision and the third portion through axillary approach. In traumatic axillary artery injuries, exposure of the entire artery may be needed for injury identification and proximal and distal control.[14]
- The brachial artery is relatively superficial at the antecubital fossa, making it vulnerable to injury. Most injuries to the brachial artery are from penetrating trauma. Posterior elbow dislocations and supracondylar fractures may cause injury requiring inspection of the injured segment for intimal disruption or thrombosis.[15]
- The ulnar artery at the wrist is the dominant hand artery in the majority of patients. Achieving or maintaining sufficient arterial outflow at the wrist is essential to the hemodynamic and clinical success of the management of arterial injury to the radial and/or ulnar arteries. The status of both the radial and ulnar arteries at the wrist should be confirmed in the course of evaluating all patients for upper extremity revascularization options. An Allen test utilizing a Doppler on the palmar arch can assist in identification of flow into the hand.[16]
- Systemic intraoperative anticoagulation (SIAC) during traumatic vascular repair should be used with caution if the patient has trauma-induced coagulopathy, suspected, or confirmed additional sources of hemorrhage including the torso or central nervous system. There is varying literature on its efficacy. In a recent study examining mostly gunshot wounds, SIAC utilization experienced better arterial patency without additional bleeding complications.[17] In another study, SIAC was not associated with a difference in repair thrombosis or limb loss but increased blood product utilization and hospital length of stay.[18] The decision to use SIAC should be driven by the surgical team's risk–benefit analysis. Local heparin flushing (50units/mL), 20 to 25 mL into the injured artery proximal and distal to repair, is commonly used.[19]
- Temporary vascular shunts are used to establish arterial flow in a damage control setting. Plastic commercially available intraluminal shunts are available in a variety of sizes and configurations. Scenarios for consideration of a temporary shunt include patient hemodynamic instability, coagulopathy, acidosis, hypothermia, unstable skeleton, major wound contamination/infection, defects in soft tissue impeding wound coverage, need to address other life-threatening injuries, and austere environment with limited resources.[5]

Operating Room Setup

- Trauma patients may have multiple injuries and the ability to address the burden of injuries should guide the OR setup.

Ideally, a hybrid room or an OR equipped with radiolucent operating table, arm/hand table, and fluoroscopic equipment, preferably with digital subtraction angiography and last-image hold capabilities, is necessary.

- In trauma patients, general anesthesia is usually preferred, as regional anesthesia hampers neurologic examination of the upper extremity.
- For the majority of upper extremity vascular procedures, the affected limb is typically abducted 90°. To avoid stretch on the brachial plexus, care should be taken to avoid hyperabduction and extension of the limb. The operative field should take into account other injuries the patient may have sustained to the torso. In isolated upper extremity injuries, the operative field should include the ipsilateral axilla, chest, and neck.[14] The head should be rotated and extended to the contralateral side if no spinal trauma is suspected. A shoulder roll may be used under the ipsilateral shoulder to assist with neck and shoulder extension if able (**FIGURE 1**). For access to the deltopectoral region of the axillary artery, the arm can be externally rotated and abducted 30° relative to the lateral chest.
- In situation where a venous conduit may be needed, a lower extremity should be appropriately prepared into the surgical field to allow access for vein harvesting. The vein, if needed, should be harvested from the least affected lower extremity.

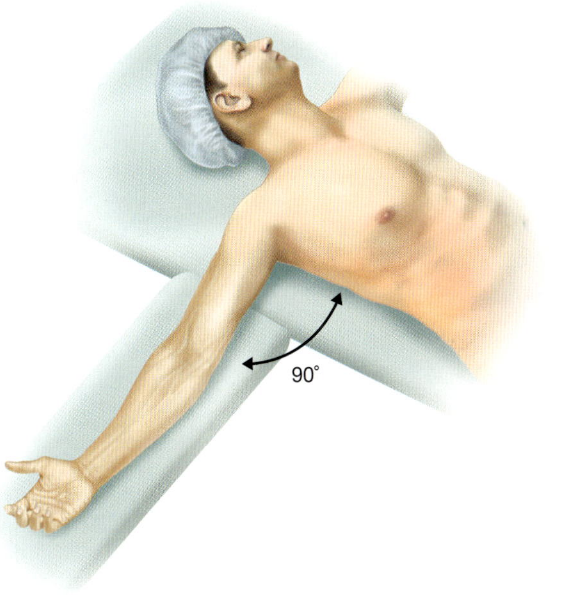

FIGURE 1 • With the patient supine, the arm of interest is pronated and extended at 90° relative to the chest. The head is externally rotated to the contralateral side to expose the ipsilateral neck segment.

PROXIMAL AXILLARY ARTERY

First Step

- An approach to the proximal (first) portion of the axillary artery can be performed through an infraclavicular incision one fingerbreadth below the middle third of the clavicle and can extend to the deltopectoral groove when needed (**FIGURE 2A**). This may be needed to assist with delineation of tissue planes in an injured field.
- The pectoral fascia is opened longitudinally. The pectoralis major muscle is divided with a muscle-splitting incision if able. Otherwise the muscle should be divided approximately 2 cm from its attachment to the humerus to better access the vessel in traumatic injuries with significant hematoma or hemorrhage. The clavipectoral fascia is then divided to expose the proximal axillary sheath. Lateral retraction or division of the pectoralis muscle near its insertion on the coracoid process may be needed to aid in exposure.
- The arm may need to be repositioned to reduce position-related anatomic alteration.

Second Step

- Delicate dissection is performed to expose and control the axillary artery deep to the clavipectoral fascia. Care must be taken with dissection and retraction to minimize injury to the cords of the brachial plexus that surround the artery. The lateral pectoral nerve and proximal cephalic vein must be identified to avoid injury during dissection or traction from retraction (**FIGURE 2B**).

Third Step

- The axillary vein lies anteromedial to the artery and partially overlaps the artery. Retraction of the vein in a caudal direction with a vessel loop or small retractor is often needed to access the artery. Ligation of venous tributaries and the thoracoacromial artery and vein may be required. Again, care is needed to prevent injury to the lateral pectoral nerve.

Fourth Step

- Proximal and distal control of the injured segment of the axillary artery is achieved with vessel loops once circumferential dissection and exposure is obtained. If vascular clamps are used, assure nerve structures are not included when applying the clamp to the artery. Examination of the injured artery should be performed to identify the extent of the injury. If the patient is unstable or other injuries need to be addressed, consider temporary vascular shunt placement.

Fifth Step

- If the injury is small without significant vessel destruction, simple repair or debridement back to healthy intima and end-to-end anastomosis can be performed using nonabsorbable permanent monofilament, such as polypropylene (Prolene, Johnson & Johnson, New Brunswick, NJ, USA), suture.
- Gunshot wounds usually require a more extensive debridement and interposition. When performing interposition grafting, the damaged artery is transected and removed. The proximal and distal arterial segments should be examined for trauma, dissection, or thrombus formation. Repair of traumatic injuries should follow basic principles

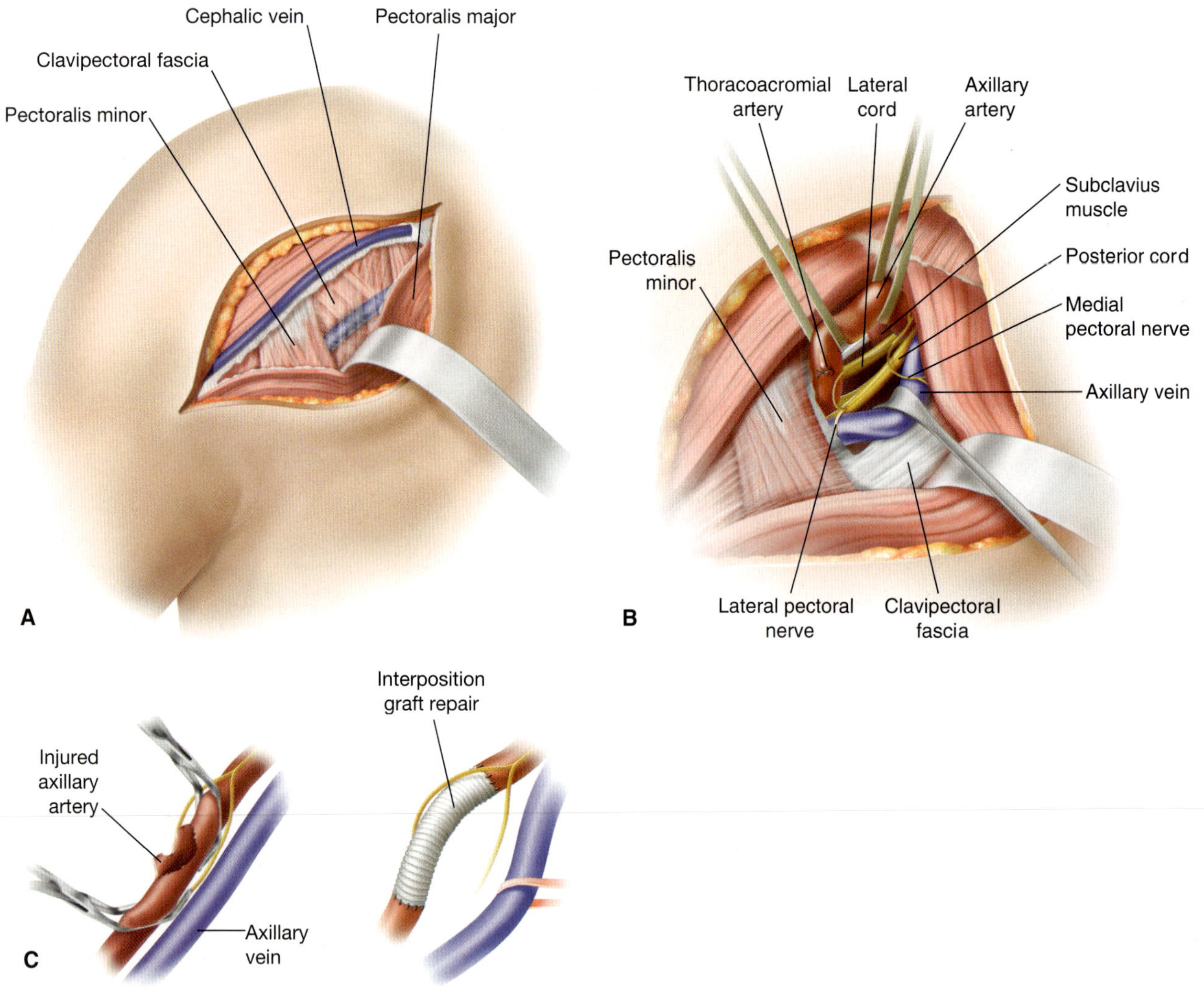

FIGURE 2 • **A,** Infraclavicular exposure of the proximal axillary artery. **B,** Components of the infraclavicular axillary sheath. **C,** Interposition graft repair of a proximal axillary artery traumatic partial transection.

of vascular repairs, beginning with minimal debridement back to healthy intima. The vessel can be flushed with heparinized saline.

- Autologous vein is the preferred conduit if bypass is required and is harvested from the least injured extremity, typically the saphenous veins. Prosthetic material for the conduit may be needed. The use of stretch polytetrafluoroethylene can prevent excessive traction on the anastomosis with arm movement (**FIGURE 2C**). Appropriate length of the conduit should be confirmed to prevent kinking with arm motion.
- Proximal and distal anastomoses are performed in an end-to-end or end-to-side fashion depending on respective diameters of the inflow and outflow segments.
- Catheter embolectomy should be employed as needed if concern for thrombus exists. Imaging guidance can be used to assist in the decision and performance of this step.
- Performance of a completion angiogram may be performed to evaluate the graft and its flow.
- Venous injury repair should be attempted if quick and feasible. Otherwise, ligation results in limited long-term morbidity.

MID-DISTAL AXILLARY ARTERY

First Step

- Exposure of the mid-distal axillary artery can be performed through an axillary incision or deltopectoral incision. An incision through the posterolateral border of the pectoralis major muscles allows for partial mobilization and medial retraction to access the artery (**FIGURE 3A**).
- In a deltopectoral exposure, dissection is carried along the anterior border of the deltoid muscle extending through the subcutaneous tissue in the deltopectoral groove. Medial retraction of the pectoralis major muscle exposes the clavipectoral fascia, under which the neurovascular bundle lies.

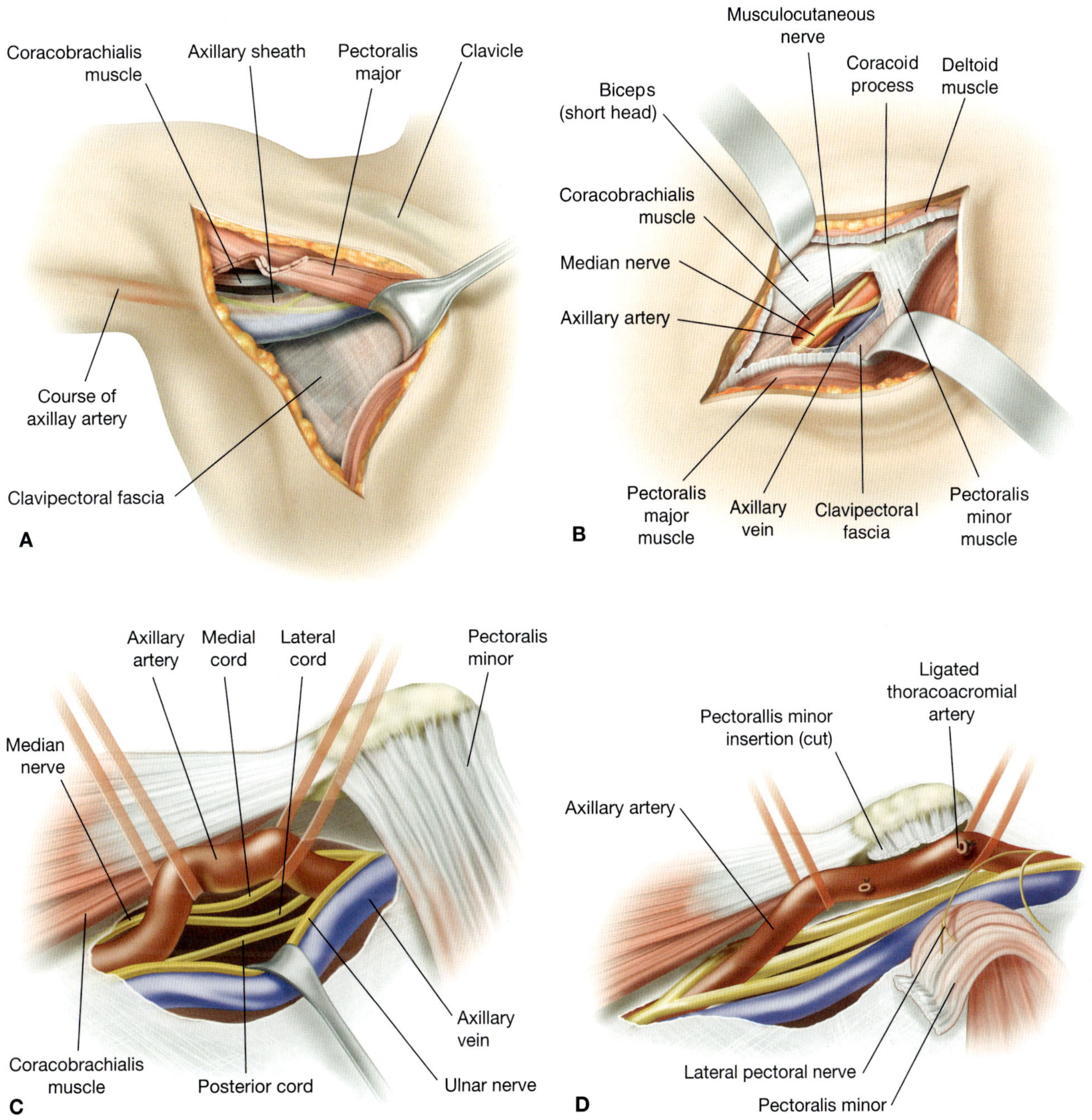

FIGURE 3 • **A,** Axillary exposure of the mid-distal axillary artery. **B,** Deltopectoral exposure of a long segment of axillary artery. **C,** Exposure of the distal axillary artery and associated axillary sheath structures. **D,** Exposure of the midaxillary artery via reflection of the pectoralis minor muscle.

Second Step

- Inside the axillary sheath, the artery is under the median nerve (**FIGURE 3B**). The medial and lateral cords form the median nerve lateral to the border of the pectoralis major muscle. The ulnar nerve lies inferoposterior to the border of the axillary artery in this area. Identification of these surrounding structures is important to minimize risk of damage.
- Vessel loops can be applied proximal and distal to the injury. If vascular clamps are used, assure nerve structures are not included when applying the clamp to the artery. Caudal traction can be applied to the vessel loops to augment exposure and reduce the risk of injuring adjacent nerves (**FIGURE 3C**).

Third Step

- The pectoralis minor muscle can be divided with care to prevent injury to the lateral pectoral nerve when further exposure is needed.
- The second portion of the axillary artery is surrounded by brachial plexus nerves on all sides but the anterior surface. To allow circumferential exposure, the thoracoacromial artery can be ligated and divided at its origin (**FIGURE 3D**).

Fourth Step

- Addressing the injured artery follows the steps previously described through careful inspection and reconstruction.

BRACHIAL ARTERY

First Step

- Exposure of the brachial artery is best accomplished by making a longitudinal incision over the bicipital sulcus between the biceps and triceps muscles (**FIGURE 4A**).
- As dissection is carried out through the subcutaneous tissue, care should be taken to visualize the basilic vein. The vein can be retracted. Branches of the vein can be ligated and divided to facilitate artery exposure or if they are damaged from the trauma. If the vein is heavily damaged, it may require ligation and resection.

Second Step

- The deep fascia is incised at the medial border of the biceps. The neurovascular bundle is then encountered. The median nerve will be the first structure encountered in the brachial sheath. To allow gentle retraction of the nerve, wide mobilization should be performed to access the artery (**FIGURE 4B**).
- Branches of the brachial artery may require control during exposure. The deep brachial artery arises from the posteromedial surface of the brachial artery just distal to the lateral border of the teres major muscle. The superior and inferior ulnar collateral arteries are found in the distal upper arm arising from the brachial artery.
- To access the artery in the distal upper arm, the bicipital aponeurosis may need to be divided to obtain maximal exposure of the artery. At the level of the antecubital fossa, the incision should make a laterally oriented S curve to allow access to the bifurcation and to prevent joint contracture (**FIGURE 5A**). The median nerve is found posteromedial to the brachial artery in this location and care should be taken to avoid injury (**FIGURE 5B**).

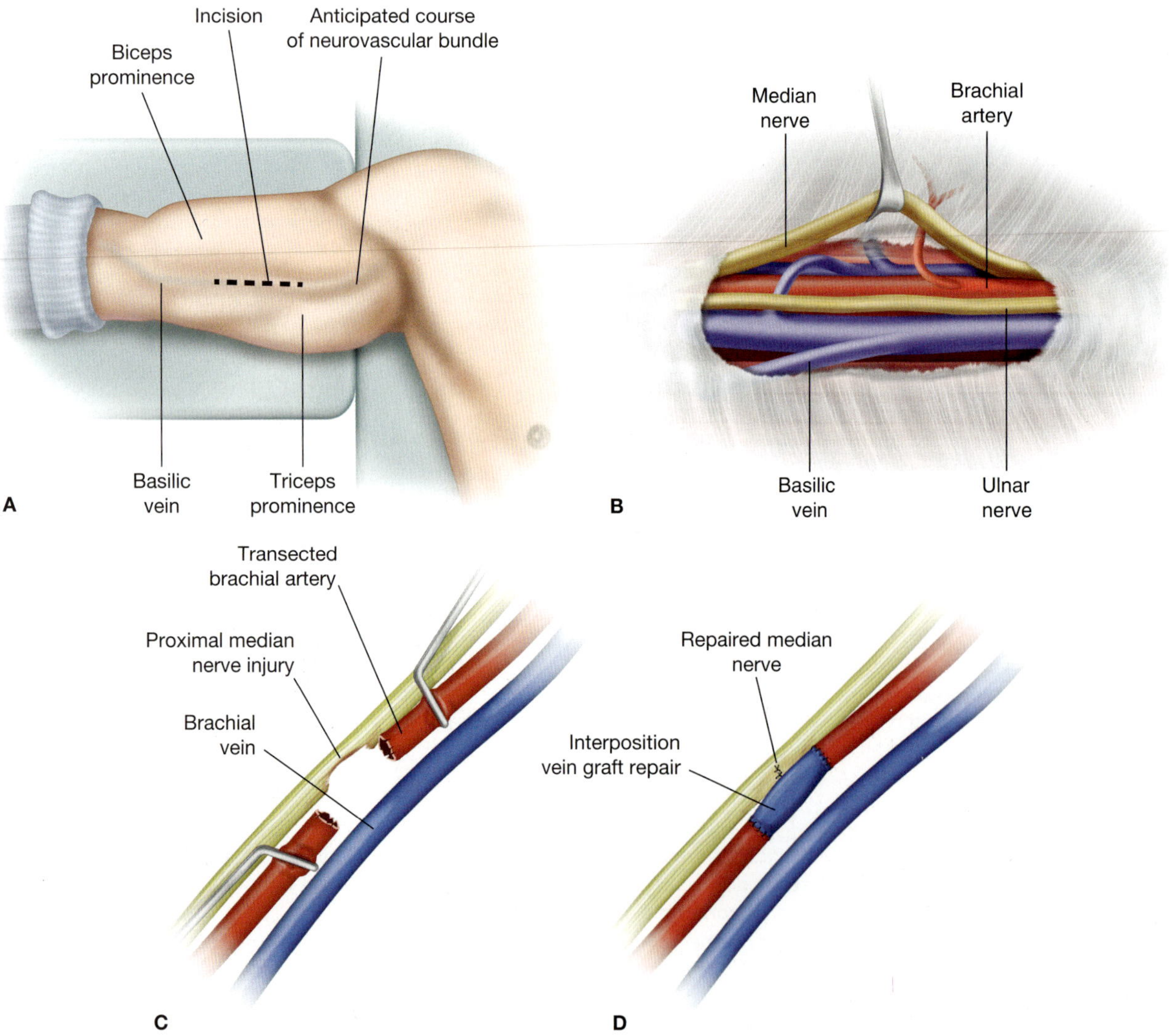

FIGURE 4 • **A,** Incision created for exposure of the proximal brachial artery in the upper arm. **B,** The brachial artery in the upper arm is adjacent to the median and ulnar nerves. **C,** Traumatic transection of the brachial artery with associated intimal damage, along with partial injury to the median nerve. Subsequent repair is performed with a brachial artery interposition graft using a vein conduit and median nerve repair **(D)**.

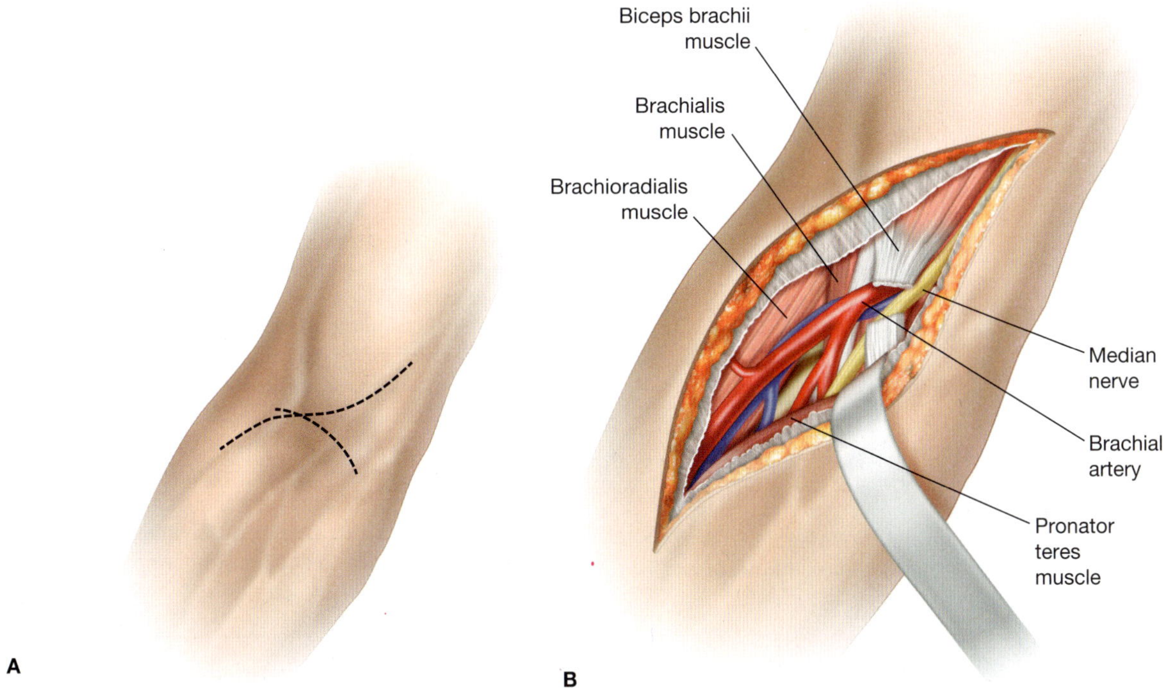

FIGURE 5 • **A,** Typical incisions used for exposure of the distal brachial artery and proximal radial and ulnar arteries at the antecubital fossa. **B,** Relative anatomy of the brachial, radial, and ulnar arteries and adjacent median nerve.

Third Step

- Proximal and distal control must be obtained with vessel loops or vascular clamps. Examine the injured vessel to identify the extent of trauma (**FIGURE 4C**).
- Repair of traumatic arterial injuries should follow basic principles of vascular repairs, beginning with minimal debridement back to healthy intima. Small wounds of the artery may be repaired primarily or with debridement and reapproximation. Larger injury to the vessel and partial transections may be amenable to patch angioplasty. For destructive wounds often seen with gunshots, interposition grafting is recommended. Autologous vein is the preferred conduit harvested from the least injured extremity, typically the saphenous veins (**FIGURE 4D**). If the patient is unstable or other injuries need to be addressed, consider temporary vascular shunt placement.
- Ensure appropriate length to allow elbow motion without traction on the anastomosis. Kinking is reduced by reconstructing other injured structures in the area to limit graft motion during elbow flexion.
- Proximal and distal anastomoses are performed in an end-to-end or end-to-side fashion depending on respective diameters of the inflow and outflow segments.
- Catheter embolectomy should be employed as needed if concern for thrombus exists. Imaging guidance can be used to assist in the decision and performance of this step. This should be carried out in an antegrade fashion and may require a proximal incision if concerns about the proximal artery exist to avoid emboli into the systematic circulation.
- Performance of a completion angiogram may be done to evaluate the graft and its flow.

RADIAL ARTERY

First Step

- Direct exposure of the radial artery can be performed along the length of the forearm. Exposure needs to be adequate to achieve control proximal and distal to the injury.
- The brachial artery bifurcates into the radial and ulnar arteries at the level of the radial tuberosity (**FIGURE 5B**). Some patients may have high bifurcation, and in these cases, the radial artery originates proximal to the antecubital fossa.
- The proximal radial artery can be exposed via a transverse incision approximately two fingerbreadths distal to the antecubital crease. If distal brachial artery exposure is needed or the antecubital fossa is crossed, an alternate approach is a "lazy-S" incision beginning at the medial aspect of the biceps tendon, crossing the midpoint of the antecubital fossa, and extending toward the lateral aspect of the volar forearm.
- The mid- and distal radial artery is exposed via longitudinal incision over the course of the vessel. After emerging from the brachioradialis muscle, the radial artery travels between the brachioradialis and flexor carpi radialis muscles. Distally,

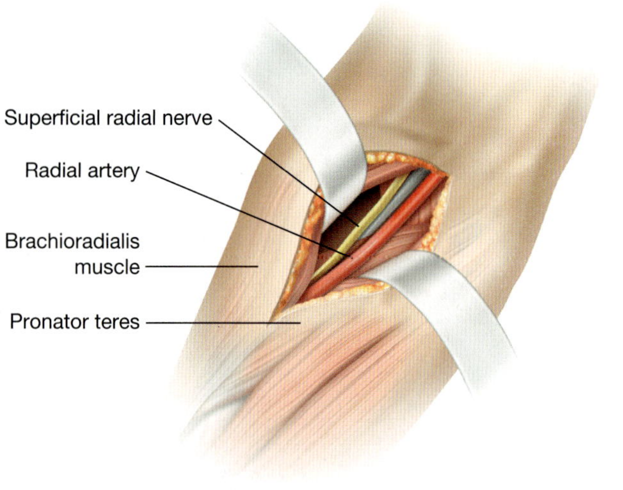

FIGURE 6 • Exposure of the radial artery in the proximal forearm.

it is found between the flexor pollicis longus and lateral border of the radius until it passes behind the flexor retinaculum into the hand.

Second Step

- The radial artery is covered by antebrachial fascia, and therefore, this must be incised along the length of the incision. The brachioradialis muscle can then be retracted laterally to expose the radial artery (**FIGURE 6**).
- Paired radial veins travel with the radial artery along its course in the forearm. The superficial branch of the radial nerve can also be found laterally in closeness, proximity to the mid- and distal radial artery. Care should be taken not to injure these associated structures.

Third Step

- Isolated injury to the radial artery, in the presence of intact ulnar artery flow and complete palmar arch, is unlikely to result in ischemia to the forearm or hand. Repair is not mandatory and ligation is a reasonable approach.
- Repair of traumatic transections should follow basic principles of vascular repairs, beginning with minimal debridement back to healthy intima. Stab wounds are more likely to have minimal surrounding damage, whereas ballistic wounds with associated blast injury are more likely to result in more extensive tissue loss. Depending on the degree of tissue loss, an end-to-end anastomosis or interposition graft can be completed.

ULNAR ARTERY

First Step

- Similar to the radial artery, the ulnar artery can be exposed via an S-shaped incision at the antecubital fossa or via longitudinal incision over its course along the forearm.
- Proximally, the ulnar artery lies on the brachialis muscle, then the flexor digitorum profundus distally. It is deep to the pronator teres, flexor carpi radialis, and flexor digitorum superficialis. The distal ulnar artery emerges between the flexor digitorum superficialis and the flexor carpi ulnaris (FCU).
- The ulnar nerve lies just medial to the artery distally, and care should be taken not to injure this (**FIGURE 7**).

Second Step

- As with radial artery injuries, isolated ulnar artery injury is also unlikely to result in distal ischemia. The ulnar artery is more often the dominant inflow to the hand, and therefore in instances where both forearm vessels are injured, ulnar artery repair is preferred.
- Repair of injuries once again begins with debridement to healthy intima, followed by end-to-end anastomosis or interposition graft.

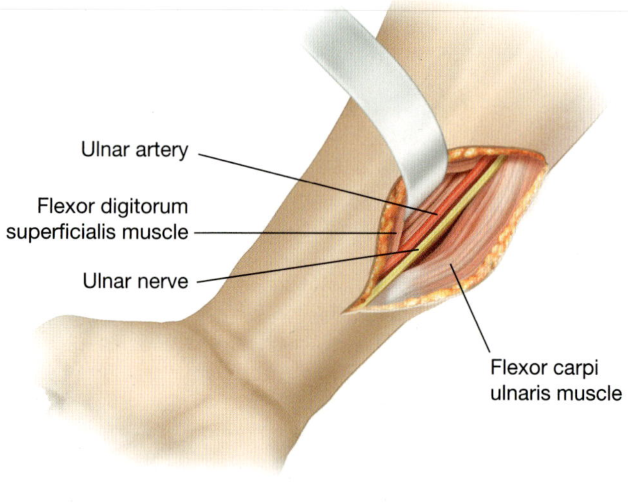

FIGURE 7 • Exposure of the proximal midulnar artery in the forearm.

TEMPORARY VASCULAR SHUNT

First Step

- Expose the proximal portion of the injured artery. Then, locate the distal end of the injured artery. Control the ends of the vessel with a vessel loop using a double pass around the vessel tagged with a hemostat that is used to provide tension to occlude the vessel or a Rummel tourniquet.

Second Step

- Inspect the ends of the injured vessel and locate the true lumen. Debridement may be needed in heavily damaged vessels to locate the lumen.

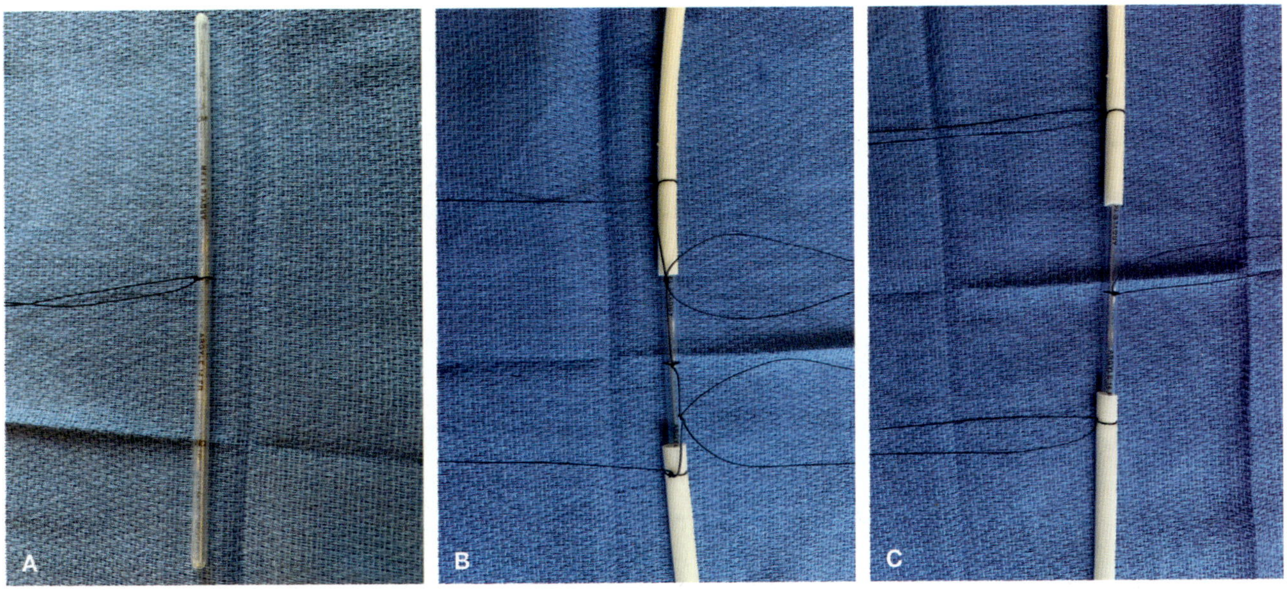

FIGURE 8 • **A,** Commercial intraluminal shunt. **B,** Shunt in proximal and distal artery. **C,** Shunt and artery secured with suture.

Third Step

- Commercially available plastic intraluminal shunts are selected of appropriate size that closely mirrors the size of the injured vessel (**FIGURE 8A**). Flush the selected shunt with heparinized saline.

Fourth Step

- Place the shunt into the lumen of the proximal and distal segments of the injured vessel. Care is needed to avoid any further injury to the arterial lumen when inserting the shunt. Assure adequate shunt length of several centimeters inside each end of the injured vessel to prevent dislodgement. Secure the shunt by placing silk suture tied around the vessel over the shunt (**FIGURE 8B**). These sutures can then be tied together and around the mid-portion of the shunt to protect against dislodgement (**FIGURE 8C**).

Fifth Step

- A Doppler device can be used to assess the shunt through evaluation of signal presence. Assure patency of the shunt through palpation of distal artery pulsation or the use of a Doppler device to detect distal signals. If flow is not detected, thrombectomy with an embolectomy balloon catheter may be needed for the injured vessel and/or the shunt itself. If not contraindicated, systemic heparin can be administered to facilitate shunt flow. Assure flow periodically by palpation or Doppler device. If skeletal stabilization is needed after perfusion is restored, monitor the flow and shunt position (if able) prior to, during, and after stabilization maneuvers.

FOREARM FASCIOTOMIES

First Step

- The volar compartment is usually addressed first as it is most susceptible to ischemic and compressive injury due to fascial boundaries that limit expansion of the muscle bellies' swelling. An incision is planned over the volar forearm proximally, medial to the antecubital fossa and ends distally on the ulnar side of the wrist in a curvilinear fashion (**FIGURE 9A**). Several other incisions have been used including a zig-zag incision, ulnar- or radial-based single incision that extends proximally and distally, or separate radial- and ulnar-sided incisions (**FIGURE 9B**). No matter the incision selected, avoiding orthogonal incisions over the elbow and wrist joint is suggested. Adequate skin flap should allow coverage of the median nerve- and radial-sided neurovascular structures. The incision can be extended to perform a carpal tunnel release if needed.
- A skin incision is made over the planned path. A small fascial incision is made. If able, blunt dissection is performed below the fascia to protect underlying structures as the fasciotomy is performed. The fascia is released distally to the wrist and proximally to the lacertus fibrosis covering the FCU.

Second Step

- After decompression of the superficial compartment, the deep volar compartment should be assessed and decompressed if needed. Retraction of the FCU ulnarly and the flexor digitorum superficialis medially allows access to the deep compartment. Incise and open the deep fascia for its entire length with caution to avoid injury to underlying structures. Epimysiotomy of individual muscle bellies is done if muscles look pale and tense after fasciotomy. Particular attention is needed for the pronator quadratus as controversy remains over whether it is contained in its own compartment.
- If needed, the carpal tunnel and Guyon canal can be released through the volar approach by extending the distal incision over the transverse carpal ligament. Careful planning of the incision to be no further radially than the mid-axis of the ring finger or ulnar side of the palmaris longis is essential to

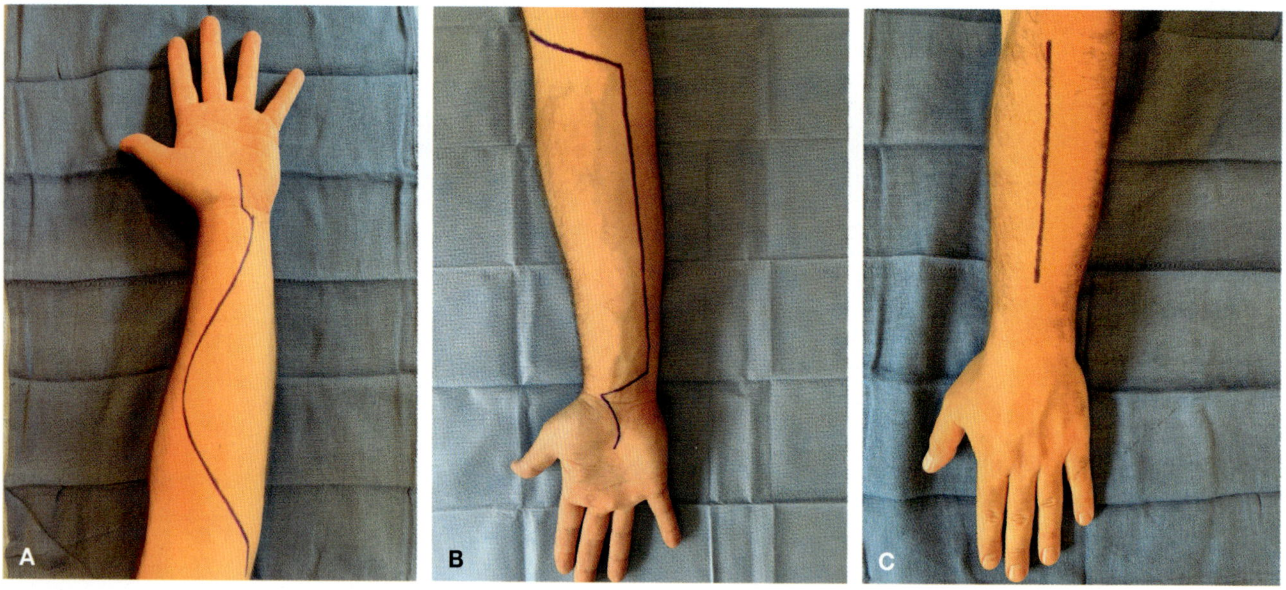

FIGURE 9 ● **A,** Volar forearm curvilinear fasciotomy incision. **B,** Volar forearm ulnar based fasciotomy incision. **C,** Dorsal forearm fasciotomy incision.

avoid injury to the recurrent motor and superficial palmar branches of the median nerve.

- After all volar compartments have been released adequately, inspection for necrotic muscle and debridement if present is performed. Inspection of the anatomy including nerves, blood vessels, and musculoskeletal structures should be performed to identify any injuries.

Third Step

- Assessment of the dorsal compartment is undertaken. Decompression of the volar compartment may provide adequate relief of the dorsal compartment. If dorsal compartment fasciotomy is needed, it is accomplished through a single midline incision (**FIGURE 9C**).

Fourth Step

- The incision is planned several centimeters distal to the lateral epicondyle extending to several centimeters proximal to the midline of the wrist.
- The skin incision is carried out over the planned path. A small fascial incision is made. If able, blunt dissection is performed below the fascia to protect underlying structures as the fasciotomy is performed. Divide the dorsal fascia. The dorsal muscles often are contained in separate fascial septae that will need to be decompressed individually.
- After the dorsal compartment has been released adequately, inspection for necrotic muscle and debridement if present is performed. Inspection of the anatomy should be performed to identify any injuries.

Fifth Step

- After adequate decompression of the compartments, inspection of anatomic structures and debridement of necrotic tissue within the wound is done.
- The wounds are often left open. Some surgeons advocate the use of retention sutures to assist with closure. The wound can be dressed with sterile wet-to-dry dressing or negative pressure wound therapy (NPWT). The dressing should be applied carefully to allow for further swelling as this is common in the first 24 to 48 hours.

Sixth Step

- The arm should be inspected regularly to assess swelling and neurovascular status. The patient typically returns to the OR every 48 to 72 hours to examine the wound and debride any further necrotic tissue. The wound can be closed once the swelling subsides. NPWT can assist with decreasing edema and facilitating wound closure. If wound closure cannot be achieved, the use of skin grafting can be employed.

PEARLS AND PITFALLS

Identification of injuries	Following standard evaluation of the trauma patient using ATLS principles assists in identifying injuries rather than focusing on the upper extremity injury.
Upper extremity nerve injuries	Upper extremity arterial injuries often are associated with concomitant nerve injuries. Early recognition and diagnosis of nerve injuries is important to long-term functional outcome. Consultation at the time of identification or suspected nerve injury with specialist trained in management of these injuries is prudent.
Iatrogenic nerve injury during axillary artery exposure	Whenever possible, axillary exposure proximal to the axilla should be obtained as proximal as possible, to limit the risk of nerve injury as the cords of the brachial plexus become more intimately related to the axillary artery as it proceeds laterally from the clavicle. Far proximal anastomotic positioning of the axillary artery minimizes artery displacement and traction with arm movement. The preferred choices for axillary artery exposure are proximal or distal to the second portion of the axillary artery unless repair requires deltopectoral exposure.
Arterial repair following segmental resection	The extent of injury to the artery should be delineated prior to attempts at reconstruction. Failure to identify the extent of injury will lead to complications of the repair.
Inflow assessment	Prior to completion of an arterial repair, the surgeon must ensure adequate inflow. A preoperative CTA can be reviewed if available or intraoperative angiogram can be performed.
Outflow assessment	Adequate arterial outflow is paramount to maintain patency of proximal repairs to reduce potential extremity ischemic symptoms. Intraoperative outflow assessment should be performed in circumstances where the distal vascular examination is abnormal following revascularization.
Compartment syndrome	Injury to the arm induces tissue edema, bleeding, and possibly ischemia. These factors can lead to compartment syndrome particularly if there is prolonged ischemic times (>4-6 hours). Early consideration for fasciotomy of the extremity is warranted. The carpal tunnel may need to be released if median nerve dysfunction is suspected or confirmed. Consultation with a specialist versed in compartment syndrome of the hand may be warranted if decompression of the hand is being considered.
Spasm	Spasm often occurs after injury. Restoration of normal hemodynamics, correction of hypothermia, and topical warming of the injured extremity may reverse spasm. In patients with limb-threatening arterial spasm intra-arterial injection with papaverine with or without infusion. Additionally, other vasodilators can be administered to attenuate spasm if the patient is stable to tolerate.

POSTOPERATIVE CARE

- Motor, sensory, and pulse status (including a Doppler and pulse examination) should be performed immediately postoperatively to determine the new baseline for subsequent serial examinations and to document improvement.
- Observation should be performed for bleeding, hematomas, or change in serial neurovascular status, as well as development of compartment syndrome.
- Antithrombotic medications should be considered for arterial repair or reconstruction. In a meta-analysis, the use of anticoagulation following vascular trauma reduced the risk of amputations and reoperative events.[20] Often aspirin 81 mg or 162 mg orally daily is recommended with reconstruction or concerns about distal runoff when concern for other etiologies of bleeding is tempered.[19]
- Patients with combined vascular injury with musculoskeletal injuries, nerve injuries, or large wound burdens may require a multidisciplinary discussion on further reconstructive procedures as well as the possibility of amputation.[1,5,19]

COMPLICATIONS

- Intraoperative arterial vasospasm or occlusion
- Missed concomitant venous or nerve injuries
- Iatrogenic brachial plexus, median, or ulnar nerve injuries from intraoperative electrocautery, traction, or accidental transection
- Arterial repair or bypass graft stenosis or thrombosis
- Bleeding
- Wound or graft site infection
- Compartment syndrome

REFERENCES

1. Huber GH, Manna B. Vascular extremity trauma. *STATPearls*. 2021. Available at: https://www.ncbi.nlm.nih.gov/books/NBK536925/
2. Feliciano DV, Moore FA, Moore EE, et al. Western Trauma Association/critical decisions in trauma evaluation and management of peripheral vascular injury. Part 1. *J Trauma*. 2011;70(6):1551-1556.
3. Shaw AD, Milne AA, Christie J, et al. Vascular Trauma of the upper limb and associated nerve injuries. *Injury*. 1995;26:515-518.
4. American College of Surgeons Committee on Trauma. *Advanced Trauma Life Support: Student Course Manual*. 10th ed. American College of Surgeons; 2018.
5. American College of Surgeons Committee on Trauma. *Management of Complex Extremity Trauma*. 2005. Available at: https://imsva91-ctp.trendmicro.com:443/wis/clicktime/v1/query?url=http%3a%2f%2fjasoncartermd.com%2fems%2fmedia%2fpdf%2facs%2fmancompexttrauma.pdf&umid=01BE9A7D-E350-8A05-A962-F45AD0ED0D29&auth=f717728ea12e7e4b3bc261b22673ae2801b01ac9-068020fc621ee86617f9a8de50a828c791ed6729

6. Mavrogenis AF, Panagopoulos GN, Kokkalis ZT, et al. Vascular injury in orthopedic trauma. *Orthopedics*. 2016;39(4):249-259.
7. Romagnoli AN, DuBose J, Dua A, et al. Hard signs gone soft: a critical evaluation of presenting signs of extremity vascular injury. *J Trauma Acute Care Surg*. 2020;90(1):1-10.
8. Prasan ML, Ouellette EA. Acute compartment syndrome of the upper extremity. *J Am Acad Orthop Surg*. 2011;19:49-58.
9. Kistler JM, Ilyas AM, Thoder JJ. Forearm compartment syndrome evaluation and management. *Hand Clin*. 2018;34:53-60.
10. Pillai L, Luchette FA, Romano KS, Ricotta JJ. Upper-extremity arterial injury. *Am Surg*. 1997;63:224-227.
11. Miller-Thomas MM, West OC, Cohen AM. Diagnosing traumatic arterial injury in the extremities with CT angiography: pearls and pitfalls. *Radiographics*. 2005;Suppl 1:S133-S142.
12. Seamon MJ, Smoger D, Torres DM, et al. A prospective validation of a current practice: the detection of extremity vascular injury with CT angiography. *J Trauma*. 2009;67:238-244.
13. Wahlgren CM, Riddez L. Penetrating vascular trauma of the upper and lower limbs. *Curr Trauma Rep*. 2016;2:11-20.
14. Demetriades D, Asensio JA. Subclavian and axillary vascular injuries. *Surg Clin North Am*. 2001;81(6):1357-1373.
15. Degiannis E, Levy RD, Silwa K, et al. Penetrating injuries of the brachial artery. *Injury*. 1995;26(4):249-252.
16. Thai JN, Pacheco JA, Margolis DS, et al. Evidence-based comprehensive approach to forearm arterial laceration. *West J Emerg Med*. 2015;165(7):1127-1134.
17. Maher Z, Frank B, Saillant N, et al. Systemic intraoperative anticoagulation during arterial injury repair: implications for patency and bleeding. *J Trauma Acute Care Surg*. 2017;82(4):680-686.
18. Loja MN, Galante JM, Humphries M, et al. Systemic anticoagulation in the setting of vascular extremity trauma. *Injury*. 2017;48(9):1911-1916.
19. Feliciano DV, Moore FA, Moore EE, et al. Western Trauma Association/critical decisions in trauma evaluation and management of peripheral vascular injury. Part II. *J Trauma*. 2013;75(3):391-397.
20. Khan S, Elghazally H, Mian A, Khan M. A meta-analysis on anticoagulation after vascular trauma. *Eur J Trauma Emerg Surg*. 2020;46(6):1291-1299.

Index

Note: Page numbers followed by *f* indicate figures and *t* indicate tables.